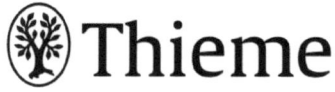

Body Imaging: Thorax and Abdomen

Anatomical Landmarks, Image Findings, Diagnosis

Gabriele A. Krombach, MD
Professor and Director of the Clinic for Diagnostic and Interventional Radiology
Justus Liebig University Giessen
Giessen University Hospital
Giessen, Germany

Andreas H. Mahnken, MD, MBA, MME
Professor
Diagnostic and Interventional Radiology
Philipps University
Marburg University Hospital
Marburg, Germany

1509 illustrations

Thieme
Stuttgart • New York • Delhi • Rio de Janeiro

Library of Congress Cataloging-in-Publication Data is available from the publisher.

This book is an authorized translation of the 1st German edition published and copyrighted 2015 by Georg Thieme Verlag, Stuttgart. Title of the German edition: Radiologische Diagnostik Abdomen und Thorax. Bildinterpretation unter Berücksichtigung anatomischer Landmarken und klinischer Symptome.

Translator: Terry Telger, Fort Worth, TX, USA
Illustrator: Christine Lackner, Ittlingen, Germany. Selected anatomical images by M. Voll and K. Wesker taken from Schünke M, Schulte E, Schumacher U. Prometheus:
LernAtlas der Anatomie: Innere Organe. 2nd ed. Stuttgart, Thieme 2009; LernAtlas der Anatomie: Allgemeine Anatomie und Bewegungssystem. 3rd ed. Stuttgart, Thieme 2011; LernAtlas der Anatomie: Kopf, Hals und Neuroanatomie. 2nd ed. Stuttgart, Thieme 2009.

Important note: Medicine is an ever-changing science undergoing continual development. Research and clinical experience are continually expanding our knowledge, in particular our knowledge of proper treatment and drug therapy. Insofar as this book mentions any dosage or application, readers may rest assured that the authors, editors, and publishers have made every effort to ensure that such references are in accordance with **the state of knowledge at the time of production of the book.**

Nevertheless, this does not involve, imply, or express any guarantee or responsibility on the part of the publishers in respect to any dosage instructions and forms of applications stated in the book. **Every user is requested to examine carefully** the manufacturers' leaflets accompanying each drug and to check, if necessary in consultation with a physician or specialist, whether the dosage schedules mentioned therein or the contraindications stated by the manufacturers differ from the statements made in the present book. Such examination is particularly important with drugs that are either rarely used or have been newly released on the market. Every dosage schedule or every form of application used is entirely at the user's own risk and responsibility. The authors and publishers request every user to report to the publishers any discrepancies or inaccuracies noticed. If errors in this work are found after publication, errata will be posted at www.thieme.com on the product description page.

Some of the product names, patents, and registered designs referred to in this book are in fact registered trademarks or proprietary names even though specific reference to this fact is not always made in the text. Therefore, the appearance of a name without designation as proprietary is not to be construed as a representation by the publisher that it is in the public domain.

© 2018 Georg Thieme Verlag KG

Thieme Publishers Stuttgart
Rüdigerstrasse 14, 70469 Stuttgart, Germany
+49 [0]711 8931 421, customerservice@thieme.de

Thieme Publishers New York
333 Seventh Avenue, New York, NY 10001, USA
+1-800-782-3488, customerservice@thieme.com

Thieme Publishers Delhi
A-12, Second Floor, Sector-2, Noida-201301
Uttar Pradesh, India
+91 120 45 566 00, customerservice@thieme.in

Thieme Publishers Rio, Thieme Publicações Ltda.
Edifício Rodolpho de Paoli, 25º andar
Av. Nilo Peçanha, 50 – Sala 2508
Rio de Janeiro 20020-906 Brasil
+55 21 3172 2297 / +55 21 3172 1896

Cover design: Thieme Publishing Group
Typesetting by DiTech Process Solutions Pvt. Ltd., India

Printed in Germany by CPI Books GmbH   5 4 3 2 1

ISBN 978-3-13-205411-0

Also available as an e-book:
eISBN 978-3-13-205421-9

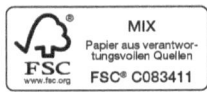

This book, including all parts thereof, is legally protected by copyright. Any use, exploitation, or commercialization outside the narrow limits set by copyright legislation without the publisher's consent is illegal and liable to prosecution. This applies in particular to photostat reproduction, copying, mimeographing, preparation of microfilms, and electronic data processing and storage.

To our teachers

Contents

Foreword xiii
Preface xiv
Acknowledgments xv
Contributors xvi
Abbreviations xvii

Part 1: Chest

1. Mediastinum 2
Gabriele A. Krombach

1.1	**Anatomy** 2		Extragonadal Germ Cell Tumors 13	
			Liposarcoma 15	
1.2	**Evaluation of the Mediastinum on Conventional Radiographs** 4		Sarcomas 15	
			Cystic Masses 17	
1.2.1	Silhouette Sign 4		Lymphangioma and Cystic Hygroma 19	
1.2.2	Edge-on Effect 4	1.4.2	**Middle Mediastinum** 19	
			Sarcoidosis 20	
1.3	**Diffuse Mediastinal Diseases** 6		Lymphoma 20	
			Castleman's Disease (Angiofollicular Hyperplasia) ... 22	
1.3.1	Acute Mediastinitis 6	1.4.3	**Posterior Mediastinum** 24	
1.3.2	Chronic Mediastinitis and Multifocal Fibrosclerosis ... 8		Neurogenic Tumors 24	
			Extramedullary Hematopoiesis 26	
1.4	**Mediastinal Masses** 9		Bochdalek, Morgagni, and Larrey Hernias ... 27	
1.4.1	Anterior Mediastinum 9	1.5	**Trauma with Mediastinal Injury: Pneumomediastinum** 28	
	Intrathoracic Goiter 9			
	Thymic Hyperplasia 11			
	Thymoma and Thymic Carcinoma .. 11			
	Thymic Cysts 12		**Bibliography** 29	
	Neuroendocrine Tumors of the Thymus; Thymic and Mediastinal Carcinoids ... 13			

2. Heart and Pericardium 30
Gabriele A. Krombach

2.1	**Heart** 30	2.2	**Pericardium** 65
2.1.1	Anatomy 30	2.2.1	Anatomy 65
	Cardiac Borders 30	2.2.2	Diseases 66
	Cardiac Chambers 30		Pericarditis 66
2.1.2	Diseases 32		Constrictive Pericarditis 68
	Heart Failure 32		Pericardial Masses 69
	Coronary Heart Disease and Myocardial Infarction ... 34		Pericardial Aplasia 70
	Cardiomyopathies 42		
	Cardiac Tumors 49		**Bibliography** 70
	Acquired Valvular Disease 60		

3. Large Vessels 72
Andreas H. Mahnken

3.1	**Aorta** 72		Aberrant Right Subclavian Artery and Kommerell Diverticulum ... 74
3.1.1	Anatomy 72		Patent Ductus Arteriosus 74
3.1.2	Development 73		Coarctation of the Aorta 76
3.1.3	Congenital Anomalies 73		Double Aortic Arch 77
	Variants in the Origins of Supra-aortic Vessels 74		Right Aortic Arch 78
			Congenital Abdominal Aortic Stenosis 79

3.1.4	Diseases	79	3.2.4	Diseases	104	

3.1.4 Diseases 79
- Aortic Aneurysms 79
- Acute Aortic Syndrome 84
- Aortic Dissection 85
- Intramural Hematoma 87
- Penetrating Aortic Ulcer 89
- Aortic Rupture 90
- Leriche Syndrome 92
- Coral Reef Aorta 92
- Aortitis 94
- Vasculitis 96
- Malignant Vascular Tumors 97
- Aortic Fistulas 98
- Subclavian Steal Syndrome 99
- Thoracic Outlet and Thoracic Inlet Syndrome 101

3.2 Vena Cava and Large Veins 102
- 3.2.1 Anatomy 102
- 3.2.2 Development 102
- 3.2.3 Congenital Anomalies 103
  - Persistent Left Superior Vena Cava 103
  - Left-Sided and Duplicated Inferior Vena Cava 103
  - Azygos or Hemiazygos Continuation 104
- 3.2.4 Diseases 104
  - Nutcracker Syndrome 104
  - May–Thurner Syndrome 106
  - Superior Vena Cava Syndrome 107
  - Vena Cava Thrombosis 108
  - Tumor Thrombi in the Vena Cava 108

3.3 Pulmonary Vessels 109
- 3.3.1 Anatomy 109
- 3.3.2 Development 111
- 3.3.3 Congenital Anomalies 111
  - Pulmonary Artery Agenesis 111
  - Pulmonary Artery Sling 111
  - Anomalous Pulmonary Venous Return 112
- 3.3.4 Diseases 112
  - Pulmonary Artery Aneurysm 112
  - Pulmonary Embolism 113
  - Pulmonary Hypertension 116
  - Arteriovenous Malformations 118

Bibliography 121

4. Lung and Pleura 122
Gabriele A. Krombach

4.1 Anatomy 122
- 4.1.1 Pleura and Interlobar Fissures 122
- 4.1.2 Trachea and Pulmonary Segments 122
- 4.1.3 Vessels 123
- 4.1.4 Pulmonary Veins 125
- 4.1.5 Lung Parenchyma 127

4.2 Tracheobronchial System 128
- 4.2.1 Normal Variant: Tracheal Bronchus 128
- 4.2.2 Tracheal Stenosis and Tracheopathia Osteochondroplastica 129
- 4.2.3 Bronchiectasis 129
- 4.2.4 Bronchiolitis 129
- 4.2.5 Constrictive Bronchiolitis 131
- 4.2.6 Emphysema, Alpha$_1$-Antitrypsin Deficiency, and Chronic Obstructive Pulmonary Disease 131
- 4.2.7 Atelectasis 133

4.3 Lung 135
- 4.3.1 Congenital Malformations 135
  - Malformations of the Lung 135
- 4.3.2 Infections 139
  - Pneumonia 139
  - Septic Emboli 141
  - Tuberculosis 142
  - Aspergillosis 144
  - Swyer–James–MacLeod Syndrome 147
- 4.3.3 Neoplasms 147
  - Pulmonary Nodules 147
  - Lung Cancer 149
  - Hamartoma 150
- 4.3.4 Diffuse Lung Diseases 151
  - Interstitial Lung Diseases: Idiopathic Interstitial Pneumonias ... 151
  - Sarcoidosis 158
  - Langerhans Cell Histiocytosis, Histiocytosis X 159
  - Lymphangioleiomyomatosis and Pulmonary Involvement by Tuberous Sclerosis 159
  - Cystic Fibrosis 161
- 4.3.5 Pneumoconioses 162
  - Silicosis 162
  - Asbestosis 163
  - Other Pneumoconioses 164
  - Summary 165
- 4.3.6 Extrinsic Allergic Alveolitis 165
- 4.3.7 Pulmonary Trauma 165
  - Trauma Due to Smoke Inhalation, Fire, or Toxic Gases 165
  - Mixed Aspiration Events 166
- 4.3.8 Vasculitides 166
  - Wegener's Granulomatosis 166
  - Churg–Strauss Syndrome 167
- 4.3.9 Connective Tissue Diseases 168
- 4.3.10 Amyloidosis 169
- 4.3.11 Goodpasture's Syndrome, Intrapulmonary Hemorrhage 170
- 4.3.12 Alveolar Microlithiasis 170
- 4.3.13 Alveolar Proteinosis 171
- 4.3.14 Pulmonary Infarction 172
- 4.3.15 Respiratory Distress Syndrome 172
  - Adult Respiratory Distress Syndrome 172
  - Infant Respiratory Distress Syndrome 174

4.4 Pleura 175
- 4.4.1 Pneumothorax 175
- 4.4.2 Pleural Effusion 176
- 4.4.3 Pleural Empyema 176
  - Pleural Mesothelioma 176

Bibliography 178

Part 2: Abdomen

5. Liver 182
Guenther Schneider and Gabriele A. Krombach

5.1	**Anatomy**	182		Mesenchymal Lesions	193
				Primary Hepatocellular Lesions	206
5.2	**Anatomical Variants**	182	**5.5.2**	Secondary Hepatic Lesions	218
				Hepatic Metastases	218
5.3	**Imaging**	182		Inflammatory Changes: Hepatic Abscess ...	221
5.3.1	Landmarks...	182		Parasitic Lesions	221
5.3.2	Imaging Techniques	182	**5.5.3**	Pseudolesions of the Liver Parenchyma ...	227
	Ultrasonography	182		Focal Fatty Infiltration and Fatty Sparing ...	227
	Computed Tomography..........................	183			
	Magnetic Resonance Imaging	184	**5.6**	**Diffuse Liver Diseases**	227
	Unenhanced Imaging Techniques	185	5.6.1	Cirrhosis	227
	Contrast-Enhanced Imaging Techniques ...	185	5.6.2	Iron Storage Diseases	230
				Hemochromatosis	230
5.4	**Vascular Diseases**	186		Hemosiderosis	231
5.4.1	Portal Vein Thrombosis	186		Hepatic Steatosis	232
5.4.2	Budd–Chiari Syndrome	190	**5.7**	**Liver Injuries**	235
5.4.3	Rendu–Osler–Weber Disease	192			
5.5	**Focal Hepatic Lesions**	193		**Bibliography**	239
5.5.1	Primary Hepatic Lesions	193			

6. Gallbladder and Biliary Tract 242
Horst D. Litzlbauer

6.1	**Anatomy**	242	**6.5**	**Acquired Diseases**	256
6.1.1	Biliary Fluid..	242	6.5.1	Gallstones and Their Sequelae	256
6.1.2	Biliary Capillaries and Bile Ducts	242		Silent Cholelithiasis	258
6.1.3	Gallbladder	242		Symptomatic Cholecystolithiasis	261
6.1.4	Blood Vessels, Lymphatics, and Nerves	243		Gallbladder Hydrops and Empyema	264
				Chronic Cholecystitis and Porcelain Gallbladder	266
6.2	**Physiology and Pathophysiology**	243		Mirizzi's Syndrome	268
6.2.1	Cholestasis (Obstructive Jaundice)	243	6.5.2	Inflammatory and Infectious Biliary Tract Diseases .	270
				Ascending Cholangitis	270
6.3	**Imaging**	245		Primary Sclerosing Cholangitis	272
6.3.1	Conventional Radiography	245	6.5.3	Benign Tumors and Hyperplastic Changes	273
6.3.2	Ultrasonography	245		Gallbladder Polyps	273
	Initial Ultrasound Examination	245		Benign Hyperplasia of the Gallbladder Wall (Adenomyomatosis and Cholesterolosis).........	275
	Ultrasound Evaluation of Gallbladder Function	246		Intraductal Papillary Mucinous Neoplasm ..	277
6.3.3	Computed Tomography..........................	246	6.5.4	Malignant Tumors	277
6.3.4	Magnetic Resonance Imaging and Magnetic Resonance Cholangiopancreatography	246		Gallbladder Carcinoma...........................	277
				Biliary Cystadenocarcinoma	280
6.3.5	Percutaneous Transhepatic Cholangiodrainage	247		Cholangiocarcinoma	281
6.4	**Normal Variants, Developmental Anomalies, and Congenital Disorders**..............	248	6.5.5	Injuries and Posttherapeutic Changes	283
				Injuries of the Gallbladder and Biliary Tree ...	283
6.4.1	Anatomical Variants	249		Changes after Cholecystectomy...............	287
	Variants of the Gallbladder.....................	249		Changes after Endoscopic Retrograde Cholangiopancreatography and Percutaneous Transhepatic Cholangiodrainage	289
	Variants of the Bile Ducts and Biliary Vessels	249		Chemotherapy-induced Cholangitis and Cholecystitis.........	291
6.4.2	Biliary Atresia	250			
6.4.3	Choledochal Cysts	253		**Bibliography**......................................	293
6.4.4	Caroli's Disease and Caroli's Syndrome	254			

7. Pancreas 295
Lars Grenacher and Franziska Fritz

7.1	**Anatomy**	295	7.1.1	Position	295
				Histology..	295

7.1.2	Blood Supply	295	7.3.3	Cystic Lesions		308
7.1.3	Development	295		Unilocular Cysts: Pseudocysts		308
7.1.4	Imaging Landmarks	295		Microcystic Lesions: Serous Cystadenoma		309
7.1.5	Normal Variants and Congenital Anomalies	297		Macrocystic Lesions		311
	Pancreas divisum	297		Cysts with Solid Components: Solid Pseudopapillary Tumor		313
	Annular Pancreas	297		Differential Diagnosis of Cystic Tumors		313
				Summary		313
7.2	**Nonneoplastic Diseases**	297	**7.4**	**Generalized Pancreatic Changes**		313
7.2.1	Acute Pancreatitis	297	7.4.1	Pancreatic Lipoma		313
7.2.2	Chronic Pancreatitis	300	7.4.2	Cystic Fibrosis		314
	Subtype: Autoimmune Pancreatitis	303	7.4.3	Primary Hemochromatosis		317
7.3	**Neoplastic Diseases**	303		**Bibliography**		319
7.3.1	Ductal Adenocarcinoma	303				
7.3.2	Neuroendocrine Tumors	306				

8. Gastrointestinal Tract ... 322
Thomas C. Lauenstein and Lale Umutlu

8.1	**Anatomy**	322	8.4.7	Gastric Carcinoma	337
8.1.1	Position and Divisions	322	**8.5**	**Diseases of the Jejunum and Ileum**	338
8.1.2	Imaging Landmarks	323	8.5.1	Meckel's Diverticulum	338
8.2	**Imaging**	325	8.5.2	Intestinal Obstruction	338
8.2.1	Radiography	325	8.5.3	Intussusception	339
8.2.2	Computed tomography and Magnetic Resonance Imaging	326	8.5.4	Mesenteric Ischemia	340
			8.5.5	Hemorrhage	342
8.2.3	Contrast Media	326	8.5.6	Crohn's Disease	342
8.3	**Diseases of the Esophagus**	326	8.5.7	Adenocarcinoma	345
			8.5.8	Carcinoid Tumors	346
8.3.1	Achalasia	326	**8.6**	**Diseases of the Colon and Rectum**	347
8.3.2	Esophageal Diverticula	327	8.6.1	Volvulus	347
8.3.3	Esophageal Varices	328	8.6.2	Appendicitis	348
8.3.4	Esophageal Atresia and Tracheoesophageal Fistula	329	8.6.3	Epiploic Appendagitis	349
8.3.5	Hiatal Hernia	330	8.6.4	Pseudomembranous Colitis	349
8.3.6	Esophageal Carcinoma	330	8.6.5	Ulcerative Colitis	349
8.4	**Diseases of the Gastroduodenum**	331	8.6.6	Imaging signs	350
			8.6.7	Clinical features	350
8.4.1	Hypertrophic Pyloric Stenosis	332	8.6.8	Diverticulosis and Diverticulitis	351
8.4.2	Diverticula	333	8.6.9	Colorectal Carcinoma	351
8.4.3	Peptic Ulcer Disease	333	8.6.10	Ogilvie's Syndrome	353
8.4.4	Zollinger–Ellison Syndrome	335		**Bibliography**	354
8.4.5	Gastrointestinal Stromal Tumors	336			
8.4.6	Lymphoma	336			

9. Spleen and Lymphatic System ... 355
Christoph Thomas

9.1	**Introduction**	355		Splenic Infarction	359
				Splenic Cysts	360
9.2	**Spleen**	355		Splenic Abscess	361
				Neoplastic Diseases	362
9.2.1	Anatomy	355		Splenic Metastases	362
9.2.2	Imaging	355		Splenic Rupture	364
	Radiography	355		Splenic Artery Aneurysm	364
	Ultrasound	356	**9.3**	**Lymph Nodes**	365
	Computed Tomography	356			
	Magnetic Resonance Imaging	357	9.3.1	Anatomy	365
9.2.3	Anomalies and Normal Variants	357	9.3.2	Imaging	365
	Accessory Spleen	357		Ultrasound	366
	Asplenia and Polysplenia	357		Chest Radiography	366
9.2.4	Diseases	358		Computed Tomography	366
	Differential Diagnosis of Splenomegaly	358		Magnetic Resonance Imaging	366

	Positron Emission Tomography–Computed Tomography	366		Sarcoidosis	370
9.3.3	Diseases	366		Multiple Myeloma	370
	Differential Diagnosis of Lymph Node Enlargement	366		**Bibliography**	373
	Malignant Lymphoma	367			
	Castleman's Disease	370			

10. Adrenal Glands 374
Andreas Saleh

10.1	**Anatomy**	374		Hypercortisolism	381
				Hyperaldosteronism	381
10.2	**Imaging**	374		Pheochromocytoma	382
10.2.1	Ultrasound	374		Virilization	384
	Adults	374		Adrenocortical Insufficiency	385
	Children	374	10.3.3	Tumors	385
10.2.2	Computed Tomography	376		Adrenal Cysts	385
10.2.3	Positron Emission Tomography–Computed Tomography	377		Adrenal Myelolipoma	385
10.2.4	Magnetic Resonance Imaging	377		Adrenal Adenomas	387
10.2.5	Adrenal Vein Sampling	379		Adrenal Metastases	387
				Neuroblastoma	388
10.3	**Diseases**	379		Adrenal Hematoma	388
10.3.1	Incidentalomas	379		Adrenocortical Carcinoma	390
10.3.2	Functional Disorders	381		**Bibliography**	391

11. Kidney and Urinary Tract 393
Ulrike Attenberger, Johanna Nissen, and Metin Sertdemir

11.1	**Kidney**	393	11.1.4	Renal Transplantation	420
11.1.1	Imaging	393		Preoperative Evaluation	420
	Ultrasound	393		Postoperative Period	420
	Radiography	393	**11.2**	**Urinary Tract**	420
	Voiding Cystourethrography	393	11.2.1	Retroperitoneal Masses	420
	Computed Tomography	393	11.2.2	Congenital Variants	421
	Magnetic Resonance Imaging	394	11.2.3	Bladder Masses	422
11.1.2	Anatomy and Congenital Variants	394	11.2.4	Urothelial Carcinoma of the Upper Urinary Tract	425
	Anatomy	394	11.2.5	Ureteral Stones	427
	Congenital Variants	395	11.2.6	Urachal Cysts	429
11.1.3	Diseases	396		**Bibliography**	429
	Masses	396			
	Inflammatory Changes	413			
	Vascular Changes	417			

12. Female Pelvis 430
Céline D. Alt

12.1	**Anatomy**	430	12.3.1	Bicornuate Uterus, Uterus Didelphys, and (Sub)Septate Uterus	435
12.1.1	External and Internal Genitalia	430	12.3.2	Hymenal Atresia	435
12.1.2	Suspensory Apparatus	432	12.3.3	Uterovaginal Agenesis	436
12.1.3	Pelvic Floor	432			
12.1.4	Blood Supply	432	**12.4**	**Diseases**	436
12.1.5	Lymphatic Drainage	432	12.4.1	Inflammatory Changes	436
12.2	**Imaging**	432		Tuberculosis of the Genital Tract	437
12.2.1	Transabdominal Ultrasound	433		Vaginal Fistulas	438
12.2.2	Magnetic Resonance Imaging	433	12.4.2	Benign Lesions and Pseudotumors	438
12.2.3	Computed Tomography	434		Cysts of the Uterus, Vulva, and Vagina	438
12.2.4	Differential Diagnosis	434		Ovarian and Tubal Torsion	440
12.3	**Congenital Anomalies**	435		Polyps	440
				Leiomyomas	441
				Endometriosis	442

12.4.3	Malignant Lesions	447	Sarcomas of the Pelvic Organs	455
	Endometrial Carcinoma	447	Pelvic Lymphoma	457
	Cervical Carcinoma	449	Ovarian Tumors	458
	Vaginal Carcinoma	451	Fallopian Tube Carcinoma	461
	Vulvar Carcinoma	453	**Bibliography**	464
	Recurrent Tumors	455		

13. Male Pelvis 467
Tobias Franiel

13.1 Testis and Epididymis 467

- 13.1.1 Imaging 467
- 13.1.2 Anatomy 467
- 13.1.3 Congenital Disorders: Cryptorchidism (Undescended Testis) 469
- 13.1.4 Vascular Diseases 469
  - Varicocele 469
  - Testicular Torsion 470
- 13.1.5 Inflammatory Diseases: Epididymitis and Epididymo-orchitis 471
- 13.1.6 Traumatic Disorders: Testicular Trauma 471
- 13.1.7 Benign Intrascrotal Masses 471
  - Hydrocele 471
  - Spermatocele 472
  - Testicular Microlithiasis 473
- 13.1.8 Malignant Neoplasms 474
  - Testicular Tumors 474
  - Epididymal Tumors 477

13.2 Penis 477

- 13.2.1 Imaging 477
- 13.2.2 Anatomy 477
- 13.2.3 Vascular Disorders 478
  - Priapism 478
  - Cavernosal Thrombosis 479
- 13.2.4 Inflammatory Disorders: Peyronie's Disease 479
- 13.2.5 Traumatic Disorders: Penile Fracture 479
- 13.2.6 Penile Carcinoma 482

13.3 Prostate and Seminal Vesicles 483

- 13.3.1 Imaging 483
- 13.3.2 Anatomy 483
- 13.3.3 Prostatitis 484
- 13.3.4 Benign Prostatic Hyperplasia 486
- 13.3.5 Prostate Cancer 487

Bibliography 489

Index 491

Foreword

Anyone who has seen the lively public interest in the printed media sold at conferences and book fairs might easily conclude that the "electronic media revolution" does not exist.

On the other hand, it is clear that growing numbers of younger people are no longer reading printed media, especially newspapers and periodicals. Fortunately, this trend has not yet reached the world of science and professional education, which still values the classic printed text and still thirsts for technical information drawn from the print medium. This climate has helped to motivate the authors of this book.

Diagnostic imaging of the chest and abdomen accounts for much of the routine daily work in radiology. Anyone who has written a book knows how much work and effort are needed to convey facts and knowledge in a didactically appealing way. That challenge has been met here with outstanding success. A book of this kind can expect a wide readership, especially in the setting of specialist training and also as a reference work for practicing radiologists and interested physicians in other disciplines.

The editors of this book are from the radiology department at Aachen University Hospital, Germany, which I directed for many years, and I am pleased that they have worked together from their academic offices in Giessen and Marburg to complete this challenging project.

I hope, therefore, that *Body Imaging: Thorax and Abdomen* will be well received, will gain a wide readership, and will resonate strongly with the medical community.

Professor Rolf W. Guenther, MD
Department of Radiology
Charité Hospital
Berlin, Germany

Preface

Radiology plays a central role in the diagnostic algorithm for most patients. Selecting a modality that is best for a particular case represents the first challenge on the path to a correct diagnosis. Guidelines or evidence-based recommendations have already been established for most indications and inquiries, helping physicians to make the correct decision for any given case. Once the appropriate modalities have been selected and the images have been obtained, the results must be interpreted within the context of the clinical presentation. This process requires an awareness of possible causative disorders, a directed look at specific body regions, and a systematic image analysis that includes the critical evaluation of all available findings. For an experienced radiologist, anatomical landmarks provide an indispensable aid for image analysis. Radiologists have honed their skills over many years and apply them on an intuitive basis. But this option is not available to beginners, who must painstakingly learn and learn to recognize anatomical landmarks and the typical signs of pathologic changes.

The authors contributing to this book are all experts in their respective fields. Their goal was to introduce less experienced readers to diagnostic imaging of the chest and abdomen, placing special emphasis upon linical signs and symptoms and relevant anatomical landmarks.

The modalities of plain radiography, ultrasonography, CT, and MRI are all covered in this textbook. The scope of the book reflects the application of these modalities in routine clinical use. Every author has made a special effort to take note of current guidelines and recommendations. The images have been selected for their value as teaching aids and are supplemented by diagrams and drawings.

The text in each section is arranged by subheads—Brief Definition, Clinical Features, Imaging Signs, Differential Diagnosis, and Key Points (and occasionally others)—so that readers can quickly and easily locate specific areas of interest relating to radiological interpretation. Important teaching points have been condensed and highlighted in color boxes.

In presenting the triad of clinical symptoms, anatomical landmarks, and radiological findings, this book seeks to familiarize current and future generations of radiologists and allied specialties with this systematic approach to image interpretation.

We hope that our readers will derive the greatest possible benefit from this approach and will gain a lasting understanding of radiological interpretation in the chest and abdomen.

Gabriele A. Krombach, MD
Andreas H. Mahnken, MD, MBA, MME

Acknowledgments

We thank all our authors for their contributions, which they managed so capably while meeting the demands of their clinical practice. We also thank all of our colleagues at radiology centers and departments, whose excellent work has brought forth the illustrations used in this book.

We express special thanks to the team at Georg Thieme Verlag, especially Dr. Siegfried Steindl, who was instrumental in conceiving the idea for this book; Ms. Susanne Huiss, MA, who made the concept a reality with unparalleled warmth and dependability; and Dr. Christian Urbanowicz and Mr. Florian Toniutti—all of whom pooled their talents to create a highly professional and efficient team.

We also thank our referring colleagues for the close, ongoing dialogue that is essential for the substantive practice of radiology.

Gabriele A. Krombach, MD
Andreas H. Mahnken, MD, MBA, MME

Contributors

Editors

Gabriele A. Krombach, MD
Professor
Department of Diagnostic and Interventional Radiology
Justus Liebig University Giessen
Giessen University Hospital
Giessen, Germany

Andreas H. Mahnken, MD, MBA, MME
Professor
Diagnostic and Interventional Radiology
Philipps University
Marburg University Hospital
Marburg, Germany

Contributing Authors

Céline D. Alt, MD
Department of Diagnostic and Interventional Radiology
Düsseldorf University Hospital
Düsseldorf, Germany

Ulrike I. Attenberger, MD
Professor
Department of Clinical Radiology and Nuclear Medicine
Mannheim University Hospital
Specialty: Oncologic and Preventive Medicine
Mannheim, Germany

Tobias Franiel, MD
Associate Professor
Department of Diagnostic and Interventional Radiology
Jena University Hospital
Jena, Germany

Franziska L. Fritz, MD
Department of Diagnostic and Interventional Radiology
Heidelberg University Hospital
Heidelberg, Germany

Lars Grenacher, MD
Professor
Department of Diagnostic and Interventional Radiology
Heidelberg University Hospital
Heidelberg, Germany

Thomas C. Lauenstein, MD
Professor
Department of Diagnostic and Interventional Radiology and Neuroradiology
Essen University Hospital
Essen, Germany

Horst D. Litzlbauer, MD
Center for Radiology
Giessen University Hospital
Giessen, Germany

Johanna Nissen, MD
Department of Clinical Radiology and Nuclear Medicine
Mannheim University Medical Center
Mannheim, Germany

Andreas Saleh, MD
Professor
Department of Diagnostic and Interventional Radiology and Pediatric Radiology
Schwabing Hospital
Munich, Germany

Guenther Schneider, MD
Professor
Department of Diagnostic and Interventional Radiology
Saarland University Hospital
Homburg, Germany

Metin Sertdemir, MD
Diagnostic Group Practice
Karlsruhe, Germany

Christoph Thomas, MD
Associate Professor
Department of Diagnostic and Interventional Radiology
Düsseldorf University Hospital
Düsseldorf, Germany

Lale Umutlu, MD
Associate Professor
Department of Diagnostic and Interventional Radiology and Neuroradiology
Essen University Hospital
Essen, Germany

Abbreviations

AAST	American Association for the Surgery of Trauma	HU	Hounsfield unit
ACE	angiotensin-converting enzyme	IASLC	International Association for the Study of Lung Cancer
ACTH	adrenocorticotropic hormone	ICU	intensive care unit
ADC	apparent diffusion coefficient	IgA	immunoglobulin A
ADPKD	autosomal dominant polycystic kidney disease	IGCCCG	International Germ Cell Cancer Collaborative Group
AECC	American–European Consensus Conference	IIP	idiopathic interstitial pneumonia
AFP	alpha-fetoprotein	ILO	International Labor Organization
AHA	American Heart Association	INSS	International Neuroblastoma Staging System
AIP	acute interstitial pneumonia	IPAS	intrapancreatic accessory spleen
AJCC	American Joint Committee on Cancer	IPF	idiopathic pulmonary fibrosis
ANCA	antineutrophil cytoplasmic antibody	IPMN	intraductal papillary mucinous neoplasm
ANP	atrial natriuretic peptide	IRDS	infant respiratory distress syndrome
AP	anteroposterior	IV	intravenous
APACHE	acute physiology and chronic health evaluation	LAVA	liver acquisition with volume acceleration
ARDS	acute respiratory distress syndrome	LIP	lymphoid interstitial pneumonia
ARPKD	autosomal recessive polycystic kidney disease	LLD	left lateral decubitus
ATP	adenosine triphosphate	μm	micrometer
ATS	American Thoracic Society	MALT	mucosa-associated lymphoid tissue
AWMF	(German) Association of Scientific Medical Societies	MEN	multiple endocrine neoplasia
BALT	bronchus-associated lymphoid tissue	MIBG	metaiodobenzylguanidine
BPH	benign prostatic hyperplasia	MP RAGE	magnetization-prepared rapid-acquisition gradient echo
BW	body weight	MRA	magnetic resonance angiography
cANCA	cytoplasmic antineutrophil cytoplasmic antibodies	MRCP	magnetic resonance cholangiopancreatography
CNS	central nervous system	mRECIST	modified response evaluation criteria in solid tumors
COP	cryptogenic organizing pneumonia	MRI	magnetic resonance imaging
COPD	chronic obstructive pulmonary disease	MRS	magnetic resonance spectroscopy
CPAP	continuous positive airway pressure	ms	millisecond
CREST	calcinosis, Raynaud phenomenon, esophageal dysmotility, sclerodactyly, and telangiectasia	M_z	longitudinal magnetization
CRP	C-reactive protein	NASH	nonalcoholic steatohepatitis
CSF	cerebrospinal fluid	NSAIDs	nonsteroidal anti-inflammatory drugs
CT	computed tomography	NSIP	nonspecific interstitial pneumonia
CTA	CT angiography	NSTEMI	non–ST segment elevation myocardial infarction
DIP	desquamative interstitial pneumonia	*PA*	*posteroanterior; pulmonary artery*
DSA	digital subtraction angiography	PACS	picture archiving and communication system
DWI	diffusion-weighted imaging	pANCA	perinuclear antineutrophil cytoplasmic antibodies
ECG	electrocardiogram, electrocardiography	PaO_2	arterial oxygen partial pressure
EPI	echo planar imaging	PCR	polymerase chain reaction
ER	emergency room	PEEP	positive end-expiratory pressure
ERCP	endoscopic retrograde cholangiopancreaticography	PET	positron emission tomography
ERS	European Respiratory Society	PPFE	pleuroparenchymal fibroelastosis
ESR	erythrocyte sedimentation rate	PSA	prostate-specific antigen
ESUR	European Society of Urogenital Radiology	PTC	percutaneous transhepatic cholangiography
FDG	fluorodeoxyglucose	PTCD	percutaneous transhepatic cholangiodrainage
FIGO	International Federation of Gynecology and Obstetrics	PUD	peptic ulcer disease
FiO_2	fraction of oxygen concentration in the inspired air	RB-ILD	respiratory bronchiolitis associated interstitial lung disease
GBM	glomerular basement membrane	RECIST	response evaluation criteria in solid tumors
Gd-DTPA	gadolinium diethylenetriamine pentaacetic acid	ROI	region of interest
GIST	gastrointestinal stromal tumor	SALT	skin-associated lymphoid tissue
gRE	global relative enhancement	SE	spin echo
GRE	gradient echo (sequence)	SI	signal intensity
HASTE	half-Fourier acquisition single-shot turbo spin-echo	SIOPEL	International Childhood Liver Tumor Strategy Group
HCG	human chorionic gonadotropin	SE	spin echo
HHT	hereditary hemorrhagic telangiectasia	SIOP	International Society of Pediatric Oncology
HIDA	hepatobiliary iminodiacetic acid	SIRT	selective internal radiation therapy
HIV	human immunodeficiency virus	SOFA	sequential organ failure assessment
HNPCC	hereditary nonpolyposis colorectal cancer	SPECT	single-photon emission computed tomography
HRCT	high-resolution computed tomography		

Abbreviations

SPIO	supraparamagnetic iron oxide	TSE	turbo spin echo
STEMI	ST segment elevation myocardial infarction	TWIST	time-resolved angiography with interleaved stochastic trajectories
STIR	short tau inversion recovery		
T1W	T1-weighted	UICC	Union for International Cancer Control (*Union Internationale contre le Cancer*)
T2W	T2-weighted		
TACE	transarterial chemoembolization	UIP	usual interstitial pneumonia
TASC	Transatlantic Inter-Society Consensus	VIBE	volume-interpolated breath-hold examination
TAVI	transcatheter aortic valve implantation	VIN	vulvar intraepithelial neoplasia
Tc	technetium	WHO	world health organization
TIPS	transjugular intrahepatic portosystemic shunt	XDR	extremely drug-resistant
TrueFISP	true fast imaging with steady precession		

Part 1
Chest

1	**Mediastinum**	*2*
2	**Heart and Pericardium**	*30*
3	**Large Vessels**	*72*
4	**Lung and Pleura**	*122*

1 Mediastinum

Gabriele A. Krombach

1.1 Anatomy

▶ **Location and divisions.** The mediastinum extends from the thoracic inlet to the diaphragm and is bounded laterally by mediastinal pleura. The mediastinum constitutes a single, coherent space that has no natural (fascial) barriers to the spread of tumors or inflammation. Nevertheless, it is useful conceptually to divide the mediastinum into parts because various diseases tend to occur at specific sites within the mediastinum, and the location of a pathologic process can be helpful in narrowing the diagnosis. The mediastinum is divided into anterior, middle, and posterior parts (▶ Fig. 1.1). The cervical fasciae communicate freely with the mediastinum, allowing inflammatory processes to spread contiguously from the neck into the mediastinum.

The mediastinum is further subdivided into the superior mediastinum and inferior mediastinum. The superior mediastinum extends downward from the thoracic inlet to the pericardium.

▶ **Radiographic landmarks.** ▶ Fig. 1.2 shows the mediastinal landmarks that appear on a standard chest radiograph.

Note

- The *anterior mediastinum* contains the thymus, lymph nodes, and fat. Its upper portion extends from the chest wall to the ascending aorta and superior vena cava, its lower portion from the retrosternal surface to the pericardium.
- The largest of the three compartments, the *middle mediastinum*, contains the heart, trachea, and large vessels arising from the aortic arch.
- The *posterior mediastinum* contains the esophagus, descending aorta, azygos and hemiazygos veins, and thoracic duct.

Caution

The pericardial reflection extends far in a cranial direction anteriorly and encloses almost the entire ascending aorta as far as the horizontal segment of the aortic arch.

▶ **CT landmarks** (▶ Fig. 1.3)
- The sternum and ascending aorta provide landmarks for the *thymic bed*, which is located between those structures.

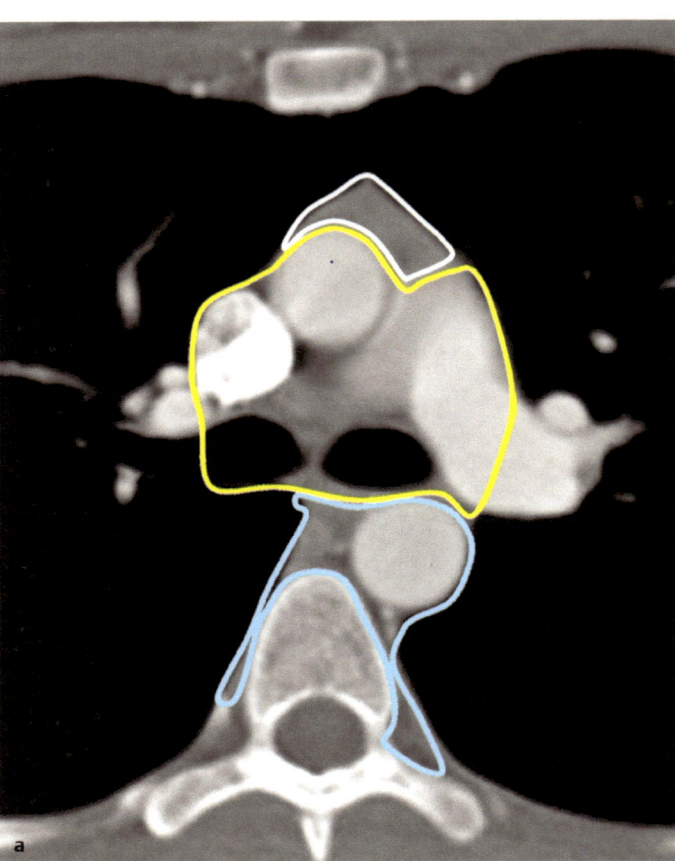
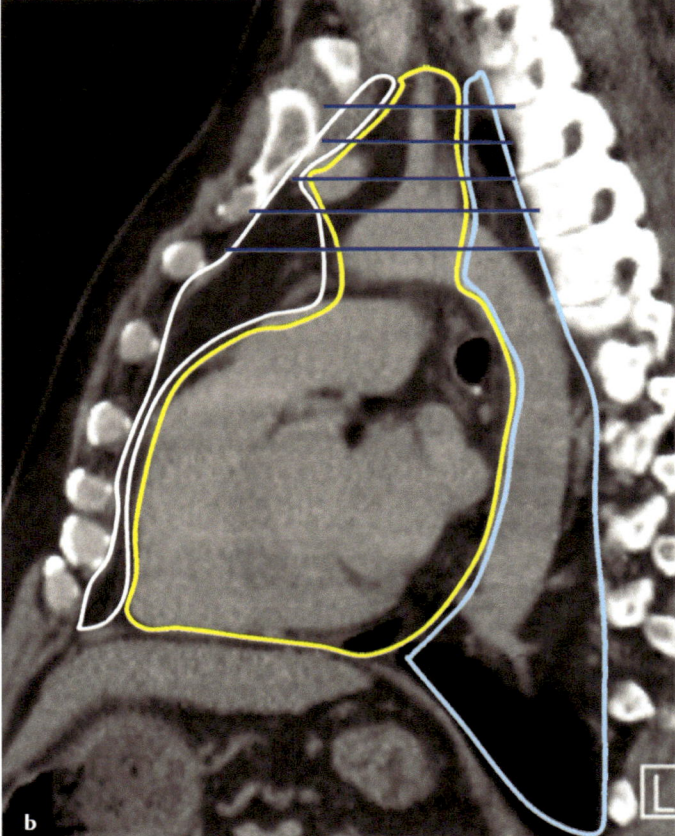

Fig. 1.1 Divisions of the mediastinum. (a) The divisions outlined in an axial CT scan. (b) The divisions outlined in a sagittal reformatted CT image. White indicates the anterior mediastinum (thymus, lymph nodes, and fatty tissue); yellow indicates the middle mediastinum (heart, aortic arch, pulmonary artery trunks, vena cava, trachea); light blue indicates the posterior mediastinum (descending aorta, esophagus, azygos and hemiazygos veins, thoracic duct); horizontal darker blue lines indicate the superior mediastinum (space above the pericardial reflection).

1.1 Anatomy

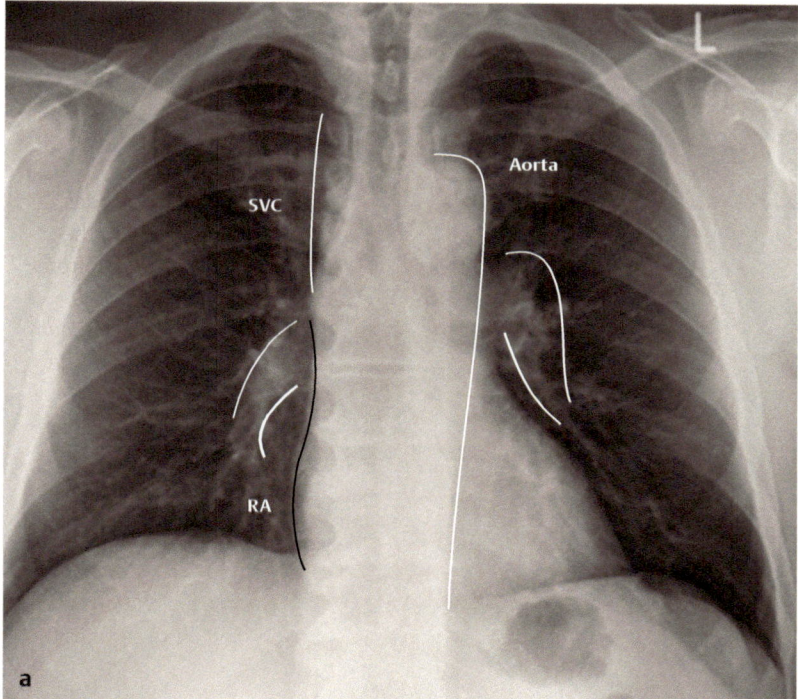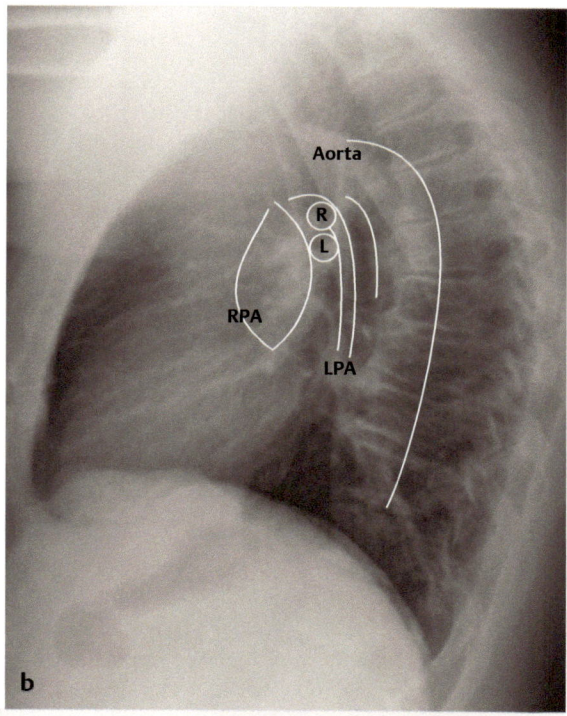

Fig. 1.2 Landmarks for mediastinal structures on chest radiographs. (a) PA view: the right mediastinal borders are formed by the superior vena cava (SVC), the pulmonary arteries in the hilum, and the right atrium (RA). The aortic contour is prominent on the left side. The left atrial appendage and left ventricle form the cardiac borders. The paravertebral line (black) is an edge-on projection of the pleura and immediate paravertebral soft tissues. (b) Lateral view: the left pulmonary artery (LPA) forms a cane-shaped figure that arches over the left main bronchus (L). The right pulmonary artery (RPA) runs for some distance across the mediastinum and appears end-on in the lateral view, creating an elliptical figure. The right main bronchus (R) runs just above it. The left main bronchus is projected below the right main bronchus. The aortopulmonary window is the gap between the left pulmonary artery and the aorta visible in the lateral projection.

- The most important landmarks in the superior mediastinum are the *supra-aortic branch vessels*. From right to left they are the brachiocephalic trunk, which branches into the right subclavian artery and common carotid artery; the left carotid artery; and the left subclavian artery (see ▶ Fig. 1.3a). The next vessel to the right is the superior vena cava. The trachea is located behind those vessels and is just anterior to the esophagus.
- The *thoracic duct* ascends to the right of the aorta and opens into the junction of the left subclavian vein and left jugular vein. It collects lymphatic fluid from the lower extremities and abdominal organs in the upper left half of the body except for the left lower lobe of the lung. Its maximum diameter in the mediastinum is approximately 5 mm. The remaining areas on the right side are drained by the smaller right lymphatic duct.
- The *vagus nerve* descends with the major vessels in the neck, entering the chest through the thoracic inlet. Below the level of the aortic arch it accompanies the esophagus in its descent through the mediastinum.
- The right *recurrent laryngeal nerve* leaves the vagus nerve at the level of the subclavian artery, winds around that vessel, and ascends to the neck in the groove between the trachea and esophagus. The left recurrent laryngeal nerve is longer; it leaves the vagus nerve at the level of the aortic arch, passes behind the ductus arteriosus and around the aorta, and runs cephalad between the trachea and esophagus (▶ Fig. 1.4). Compression or infiltration of the nerve by a tumor leads to hoarseness.
- The *phrenic nerve* arises from the C3–C5 nerve roots, leaves the brachial plexus, and accompanies the subclavian artery and vein through the thoracic inlet. It descends in the middle mediastinum along the pericardium to the diaphragm. Infiltration of the phrenic nerve by a mass leads to unilateral elevation of the diaphragm (▶ Fig. 1.5).

▶ **Selection of modalities.** The most common mediastinal diseases are masses. These present clinically with nonspecific complaints caused by the compression of surrounding structures. Typical presenting complaints are dyspnea, foreign-body sensation, and dysphagia. Chest radiographs in two planes are the imaging study of first choice in these cases; they can further narrow the diagnosis and may indicate a need for sectional imaging by CT or MRI. When mediastinal imaging is required in patients with a known disease entity or in cases where the history and symptoms are suspicious for a particular disease, CT is the modality of choice for defining the location and extent of the changes and for tumor staging. MRI should be added in selected cases where CT alone cannot detect or exclude conditions such as tumor infiltration of the pericardium or invasion of the spinal canal through the neural foramina. Ultrasound imaging has a minor role and may have limited applications in the anterior superior mediastinum. Transesophageal ultrasonography is needed to access the posterior mediastinum with ultrasound.

Mediastinum

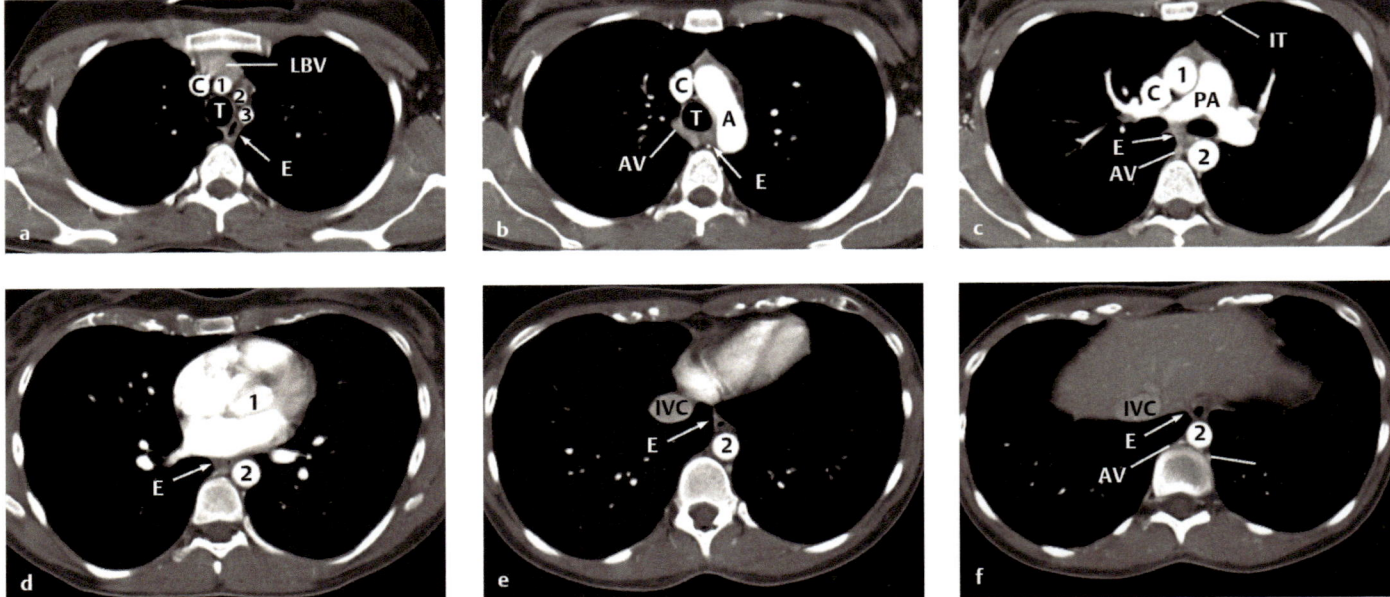

Fig. 1.3 Landmarks for mediastinal structures on axial CT. (a) Superior mediastinum, supra-aortic branches. Just posterior to the sternum is the left brachiocephalic vein (LBV). Just to the left of it are the vessels arising from the aortic arch, the brachiocephalic trunk (1), left common carotid artery (2), and left subclavian artery (3), which run anterior to the trachea (T). Just posterior to the trachea is the esophagus (E), whose small lumen can be traced through all the slices down to its passage through the diaphragm at the esophageal hiatus. The superior vena cava (C) can be traced through all slices from the union of both brachiocephalic veins to the right atrium. It occupies a right anterolateral position relative to the trachea and borders the brachiocephalic trunk on the right side. (b) At the level of the aortic arch (A), the azygos vein (AV) curves around the right main bronchus and opens into the superior vena cava (C). Additional landmarks for identifying the vessel are the spinal column and trachea (T). The azygos vein follows a right prevertebral path. (c) Below the aortic arch are the main trunk of the pulmonary artery and its division into the right and left pulmonary arteries, which forms a typical Y-shaped structure (PA). The left and right internal thoracic artery and vein, which arise from the subclavian artery and drain into the subclavian vein, respectively, follow a parasternal path on the inner chest wall. 1, ascending aorta; 2, descending aorta; C, superior vena cava; E, esophagus; IT, internal thoracic artery; AV, azygos vein. (d) The ascending aorta (1) arises from the middle of the heart. The descending aorta (2) occupies a left anterolateral position relative to the spinal column. E, esophagus. (e) The inferior vena cava (IVC) is identified at this level. 2, descending aorta; E, esophagus. (f) The hemiazygos vein ascends in a left prevertebral path to approximately the level of the T7 vertebral body, where it empties into the azygos vein (AV). 2, descending aorta; E, esophagus; IVC, inferior vena cava.

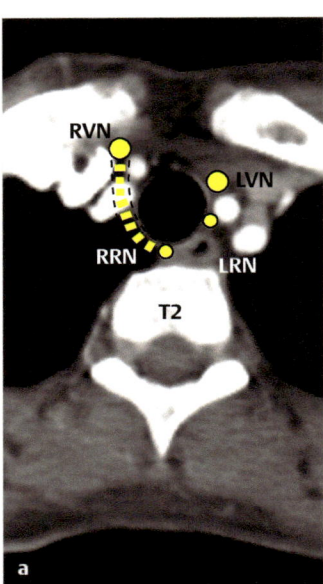
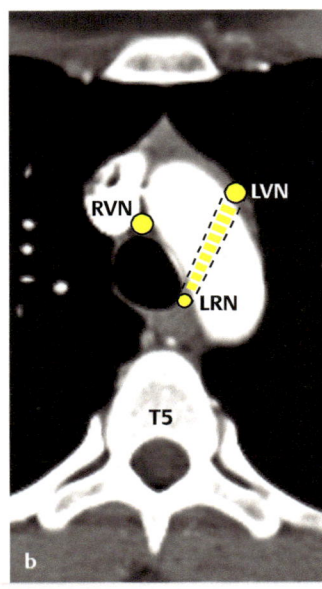

Fig. 1.4 The course of the vagus nerve and the recurrent laryngeal nerve. Axial scans demonstrate the course of the right vagus nerve (RVN) and left vagus nerve (LVN) and the right and left recurrent laryngeal nerve (RRN, LRN). The vagus nerve emerges from the skull base through the jugular foramen and runs behind the carotid artery in the carotid sheath. (a) The right recurrent laryngeal nerve leaves the vagus nerve at the level of the subclavian artery origin, loops around the vessel, and ascends to the larynx between the trachea and esophagus. (b) The left recurrent laryngeal nerve leaves the vagus nerve at the level of the aortic arch and runs below the aortic arch between the trachea and esophagus, where it ascends toward the head.

1.2 Evaluation of the Mediastinum on Conventional Radiographs

1.2.1 Silhouette Sign

When seen on conventional radiographs, soft tissues such as muscles, organs, and fluid are indistinguishable from one another in terms of their radiographic density. The radiographic phenomenon termed the silhouette sign may be helpful in determining the location of a mass.

- When organs of equal density border directly on one another, they form a composite silhouette of uniform density when viewed on a projection radiograph. This image resembles a paper cutout (the original "silhouette") with one continuous outline and no internal gradations of shading or color (▶ Fig. 1.6).
- When two structures of equal density are located at different depths in the chest and are separated by a third structure of lower density, the two structures will appear sharply outlined relative to each other (▶ Fig. 1.7). They do not exhibit the silhouette sign.

1.2.2 Edge-on Effect

In conventional radiography, the edge-on effect describes the visualization of a very thin structure, such as the pleura, when

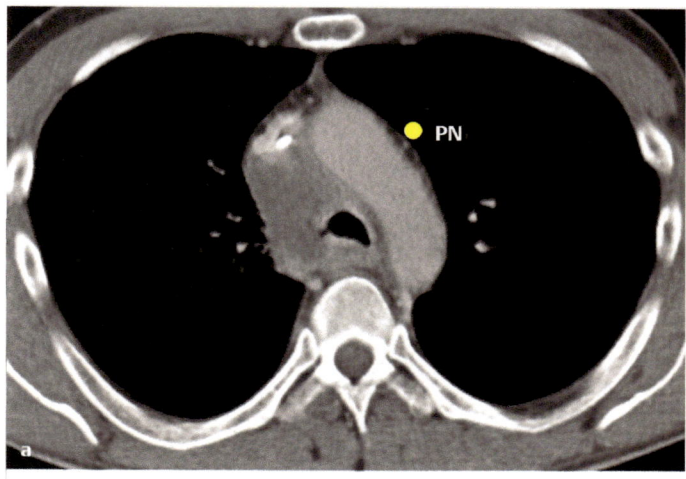
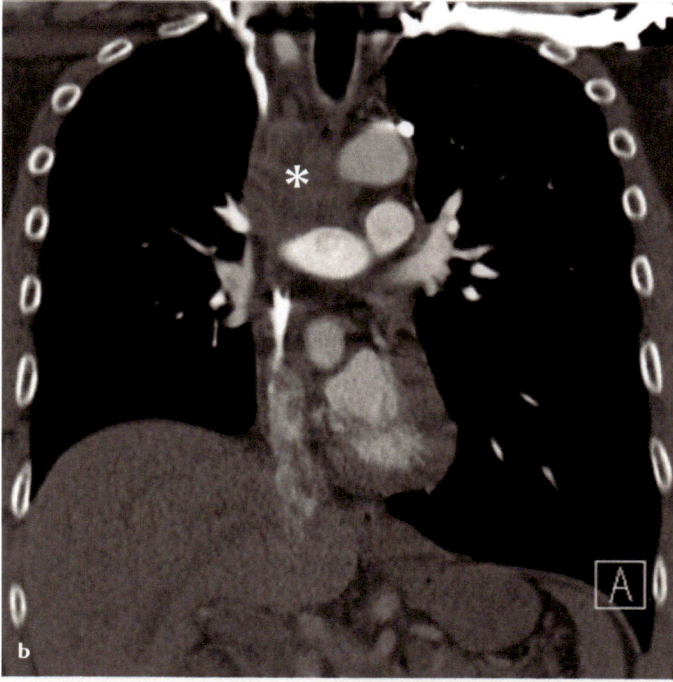

Fig. 1.5 **Infiltration of the right phrenic nerve by a mediastinal metastasis** (asterisk in [b]) has led to elevation of the diaphragm on the affected side. The location of the phrenic nerve (PN) is indicated in image (a). (a) Axial CT after IV injection of contrast medium. (b) Coronal reformatted image.

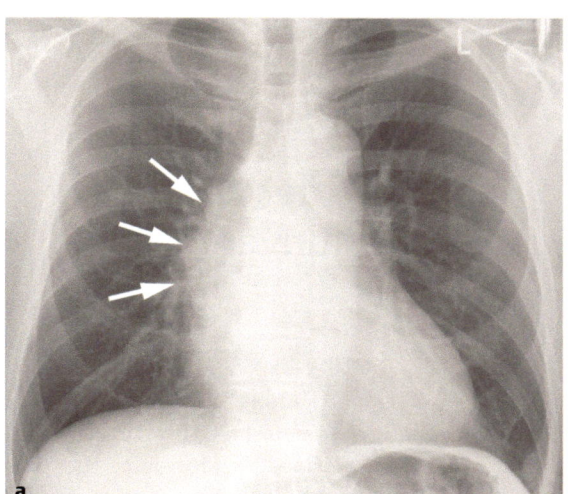
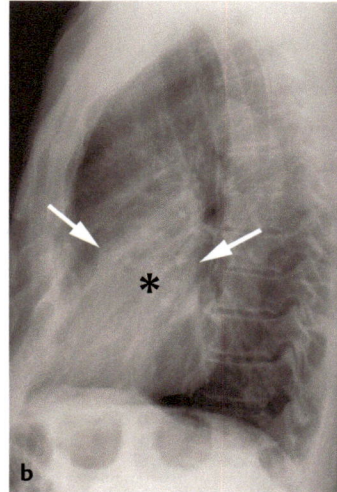

Fig. 1.6 **Positive silhouette sign of a thymoma.** (a) AP chest radiograph: the right mediastinal border is widened by a mass (arrows) abutting the heart and hilum. The mass and heart appear to have the same density in this frontal projection, so the boundary between them is indistinct (negative silhouette sign). (b) The lateral view confirms the anterior location of the tumor (asterisk; arrows indicate the tumor margins). (c) Axial CT demonstrates the enhancing mass (asterisk) in the anterior and middle mediastinum.

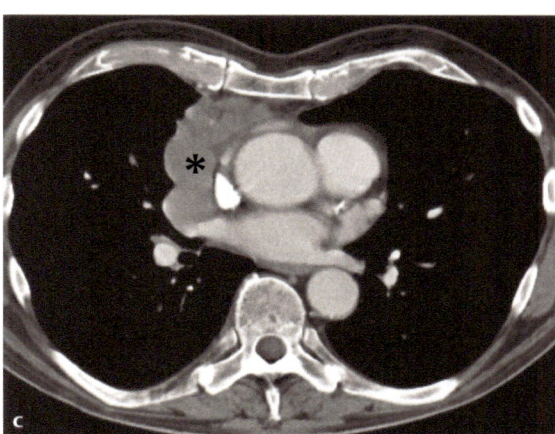

Mediastinum

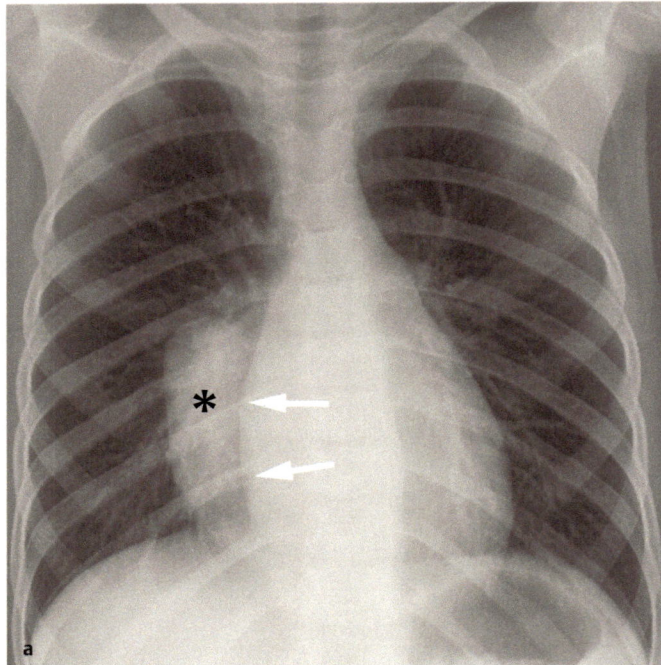
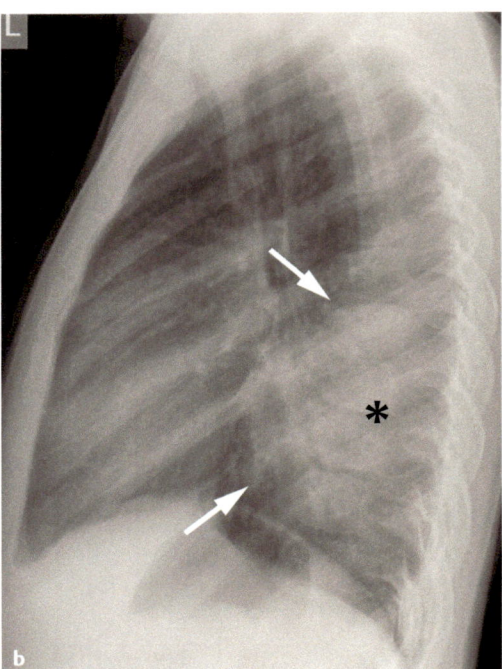
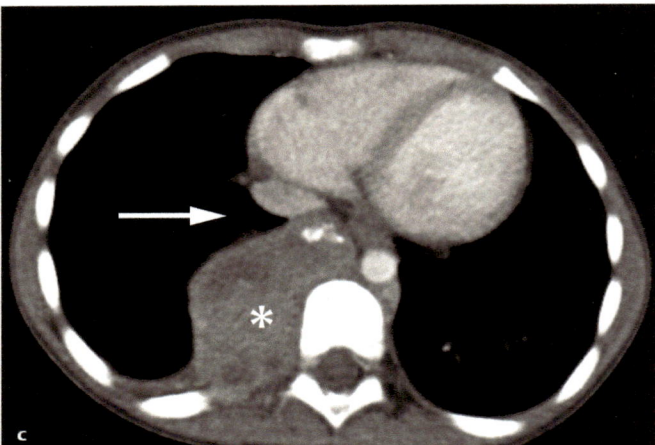

Fig. 1.7 Negative silhouette sign of neuroblastoma. (a) In the PA chest radiograph, a sharp line separates the cardiac border (arrows) from the mass (asterisk). This sign proves that a structure of different density—in this case aerated lung—is located between the cardiac border and mass and that both are in different planes. This radiographic sign is called a "negative silhouette sign". (b) Lateral view: the tumor (asterisk; arrows indicate the tumor margins) is posterior to the heart and is not in direct contact with it. (c) Axial CT confirms the location of the mass (asterisk) in the posterior mediastinum. The arrow indicates lung tissue that is interposed between the heart and mass and is responsible for the positive silhouette sign.

several centimeters of that structure occupy a plane that is oriented "edge-on" relative to the detector. Another common example of this effect is the visualization of the pulmonary interlobar fissures in a lateral chest radiograph.

When the mediastinum is viewed in a PA chest radiograph, multiple lines can be seen due to the edge-on effect as well as the density difference between the soft tissues and lung. Lines visible in the anterior and middle mediastinum include the right paraesophageal line, the anterior pleural interface line, and the paracaval line (▶ Fig. 1.8). Lines visible in the posterior mediastinum include the paravertebral and para-aortic lines. The close proximity of masses or inflammatory processes may disrupt these lines (e.g., obliteration of the right paravertebral line [see ▶ Fig. 1.7]).

Note

It is important to realize that lines produced by an edge-on projection are visible in healthy subjects only if the structures in question are aligned in the plane of the detector. It is very rare for all the lines to be visualized in a healthy individual.

1.3 Diffuse Mediastinal Diseases

1.3.1 Acute Mediastinitis

▶ **Brief definition.** Acute mediastinitis is a bacterial infection of the mediastinal fat and connective tissue that may be a mixed

1.3 Diffuse Mediastinal Diseases

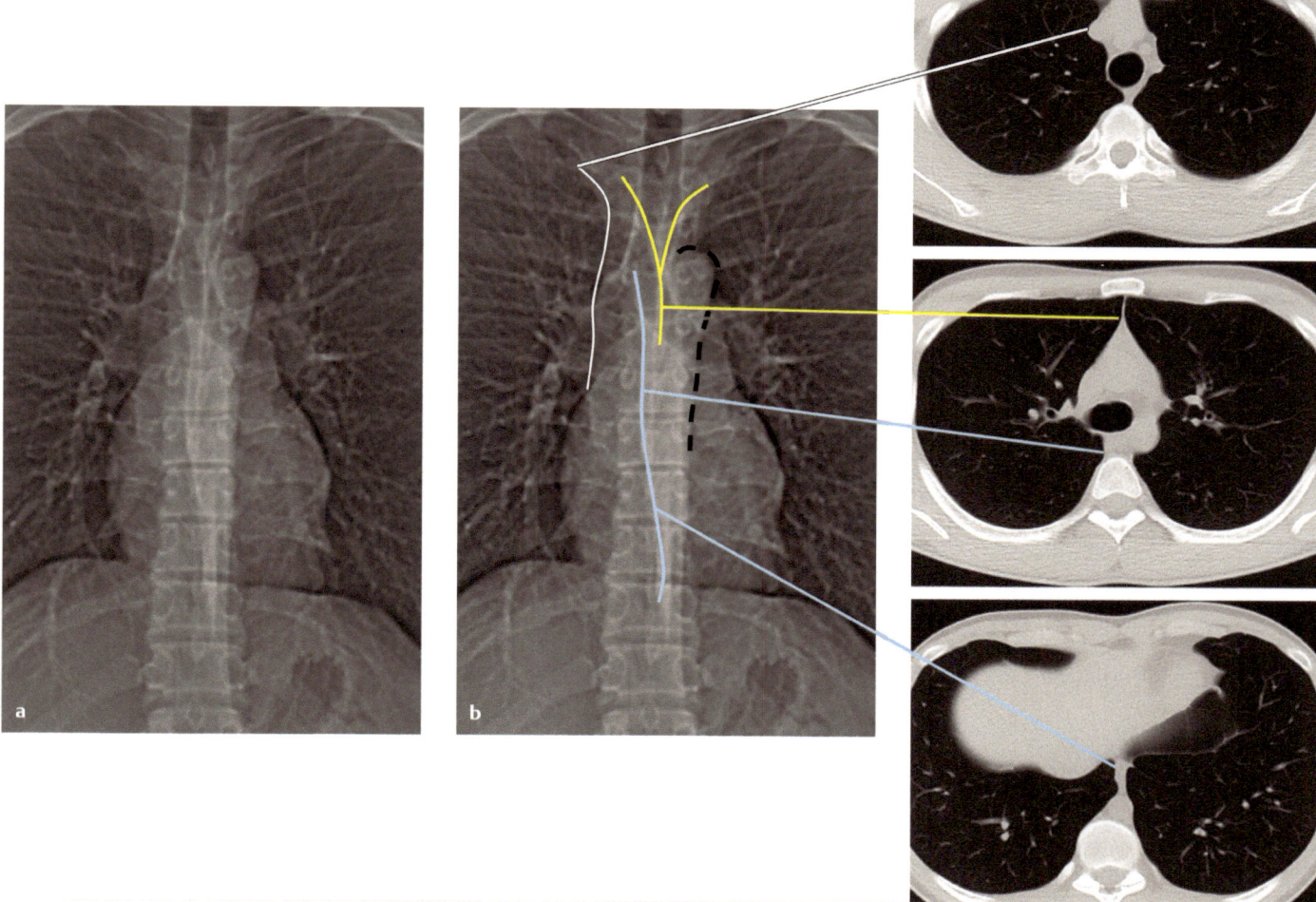

Fig. 1.8 Boundary lines in the anterior and middle mediastinum that are visible in the chest radiograph, with corresponding CT scans.

infection (type I) or may be caused by group A beta-hemolytic streptococci (type II). It may develop as a postoperative complication, after trauma including esophageal perforation, or in the form of descending necrotizing mediastinitis secondary to a deep soft tissue infection in the neck.[1] The majority of cases result from an esophageal perforation. The negative intrathoracic pressure generated by each inspiration promotes the contiguous spread of infectious organisms from the cervical soft tissues to the mediastinal connective tissue. This leads to a high tissue concentration of bacterial toxins, resulting in tissue necrosis. Predisposing factors are diabetes mellitus, obesity, and alcohol and nicotine abuse. If untreated, the necrotizing mediastinitis will lead to generalized sepsis and death. In recent decades the mortality rate of this disease has declined from 49% in the early 1900s to the current level of 11 to 15% as a result of prompt imaging evaluation combined with aggressive surgical and interventional therapy (excision of the necrotic tissue and drain insertion).[2]

▶ **Imaging signs**
- The chest radiograph shows widening of the mediastinum as a nonspecific sign. CT after IV administration of contrast medium is the modality of choice for confirming the diagnosis and planning treatment.

- Mediastinitis may present as a diffuse, suppurative inflammation of the mediastinal fat and connective tissue, or may lead to the formation of necrotic tracks and abscesses in the mediastinum. In diffuse mediastinitis, the mediastinal fat initially shows streaky infiltration followed later by homogeneous, diffusely increased density with positive attenuation values (▶ Fig. 1.9). Reactive lymphadenopathy is often present.
- If the mediastinitis results from an esophageal perforation, imaging may reveal small air inclusions or larger collections including mediastinal emphysema.
- Fluid collections are found in mediastinitis with abscess formation. Like abscesses elsewhere in the body, a mediastinal abscess may display an enhancing rim formed by inflammatory cells. This rim is not always initially defined in early acute cases, however, so the absence of enhancement in the tissue surrounding a fluid collection does not exclude mediastinitis.
- In very pronounced cases, mediastinitis may spread into the lung through the hila. This creates a streaky pattern of perihilar density.
- Mediastinal abscess may be complicated by perforation of the abscess into the esophagus or trachea.

▶ **Clinical features.** Acute mediastinitis presents as a highly acute, severe illness of sudden onset with rapid debilitation,

Mediastinum

fever, chills, elevated ESR, left shift, and elevated C-reactive protein. The history may suggest the correct diagnosis, for example:
- Previous esophageal perforation (either iatrogenic or due to vomiting as in Boerhaave syndrome).
- Previous endoscopy.
- Esophageal carcinoma (perforation).
- Sinusitis.
- Tonsillitis.
- Dental root infection.
- Retropharyngeal abscess.

▶ **Differential diagnosis.** Postoperative air inclusions, postoperative hematomas, and chronic mediastinitis with increased mediastinal density and pruning of vessels should be considered in the differential diagnosis.

▶ **Pitfalls.** Mediastinitis is difficult to diagnose in the early postoperative period. Mediastinal air inclusions may persist for up to 3 weeks after surgery. Postoperative hematomas may lead to increased density of mediastinal fat and persist for up to 2 months after surgery. They are difficult to distinguish from mediastinitis by their imaging appearance, as the changes are similar. The clinical presentation is the decisive factor.

▶ **Key points.** Acute mediastinitis has a high mortality rate without treatment. Cardinal CT features are increased density of the mediastinal fat, fluid collections, and air inclusions. In patients who have just undergone surgery, these features require differentiation from postoperative changes that may display the same imaging characteristics. Laboratory values and clinical symptoms aid differentiation.

1.3.2 Chronic Mediastinitis and Multifocal Fibrosclerosis

▶ **Brief definition**
- *Chronic mediastinitis* is a fibrosing inflammation that may have a variety of causes such as infection (e.g., *Actinomyces israelii* or *Aspergillus* species), prior radiotherapy, or autoimmune processes.
- *Multifocal fibrosclerosis* is a disorder characterized by the occurrence of fibrous lesions at various sites. The fibrosis may be retroperitoneal (Ormond's disease), intraorbital, or may occur in the form of a Riedel goiter.[3] To date, fewer than 50 cases of multifocal fibrosclerosis with mediastinal involvement have been described in the literature. The disease is characterized histologically by the presence of lymphocytes and plasma cells. Leukocytes are absent, so the disease is interpreted as an autoimmune inflammation. The extracellular collagen proliferation and fibrosis are attributed to cell mediators from eosinophilic granulocytes.[4] No causative organism has been isolated in any case of multifocal fibrosclerosis described to date. The current treatment of choice is anti-inflammatory steroid therapy.

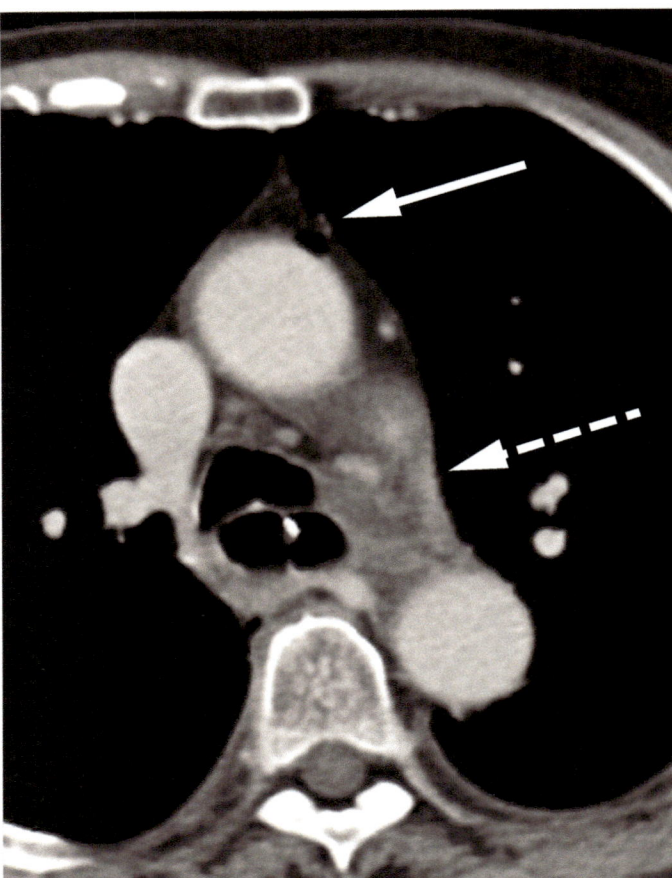

Fig. 1.9 Mediastinitis. The mediastinal fat (dashed arrow) shows increased density and contains air inclusions (solid arrow).

▶ **Imaging signs.** Increased density is noted in the mediastinal fat (▶ Fig. 1.10). CT and MRI frequently show narrowing of the mediastinal vessels.

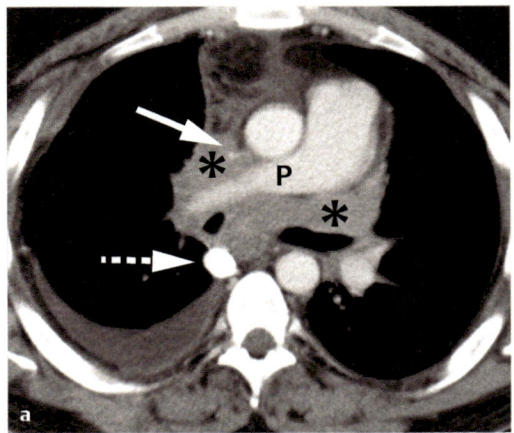
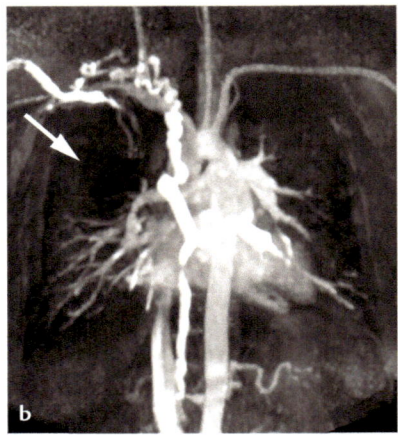

Fig. 1.10 Mediastinal fibrosis. (a) CT shows increased density in the mediastinum with connective tissue proliferation (asterisks). The superior vena cava is occluded (arrow), giving rise to collateral flow through the azygos vein (dashed arrow) and hemiazygos vein into the inferior vena cava. The right pulmonary artery (P) is narrowed. The mediastinal fat and perivascular areas provide useful landmarks for image interpretation. (b) MR angiography shows the decreased perfusion of the right upper lobe (arrow) due to stenosis of the anterior trunk (upper lobar artery).

▶ **Clinical features.** Symptom onset is insidious, occurring gradually over a period of time. Inflammatory markers are only slightly elevated. The most common signs and symptoms relate to compression of the superior vena cava with "superior vena cava syndrome" (swelling of the neck and face, bluish discoloration of the face, distended veins in the face and neck, headache, vision problems). Other common findings are narrowing of the trachea (stridor) and stenosis of the pulmonary arteries with decreased lung perfusion and dyspnea. The stenosing processes are responsible for the mortality in chronic mediastinitis, and the stenoses should be treated surgically or by interventional radiology in accordance with the symptoms.

▶ **Differential diagnosis.** Unlike acute mediastinitis, chronic mediastinitis is not associated with the presence of fluid collections.

▶ **Key points.** Chronic mediastinitis is a rare disorder. Dominant clinical findings relate to the stenosis of blood vessels or the trachea. Inflammatory markers are not elevated. On imaging, increased density is noted on CT and fibrotic tissue is found on MRI. Fluid collections do not occur.

1.4 Mediastinal Masses

Mediastinal masses caused by malignant tumors may manifest clinically through B symptoms or symptoms relating to the compression or invasion of neighboring structures:
- Narrowing of the *trachea* leads to dyspnea, while obstruction of the *superior vena cava* by the mass leads to superior vena cava syndrome. Sudden onset of clinical complaints requiring emergency diagnosis may result from a fast-growing tumor or from decompensated stenosis due to a slower-growing tumor. When vascular narrowing occurs gradually, circulation can be maintained by the development of collaterals, and superior vena cava syndrome does not occur.
- If the recurrent laryngeal nerve is damaged by compression or infiltrated by a mass, the result is unilateral vocal cord paralysis with hoarseness. Persistent hoarseness may be the only symptom of a small tumor impinging on the recurrent laryngeal nerve.

Note
In patients with longstanding hoarseness and no associated cold symptoms, exclusion of a tumor involving the recurrent laryngeal nerve is necessary.

▶ **Selection of modalities.** The initial imaging study is often a plain chest radiograph, which can demonstrate the location and extent of a mediastinal tumor. The radiographic signs described earlier are helpful in determining the location of a mass. Sectional imaging can then accurately define the extent of the lesion while also revealing the compression or possible infiltration of adjacent organs. CT is most commonly used for this purpose, as it can display structures in high resolution while scanning the entire chest for any metastases that may already be present. MRI, on the other hand, is more time-consuming and usually does not add new information. It should be reserved for specific questions that could not be answered by CT.

Important considerations:
- The *location* of mediastinal tumors will often suggest the correct diagnosis.
- Morphological imaging criteria such as the *distribution of enhancement* within a mass and the *morphological appearance* of the tissue (homogeneity, necrosis, calcifications, fat content, relationship to neighboring structures with possible displacement, invasion, or cystic components) can further narrow the diagnosis. Cystic masses can be differentiated from solid tumors.

The correlation of imaging findings with the clinical presentation, including patient age and gender, is sufficient for making a differential diagnosis and may even allow characterization of the lesion in many cases. The presumptive diagnosis is then confirmed histologically by CT-guided percutaneous biopsy or excision.

Note
In the reporting of mediastinal masses, it is important to describe the exact size, location, and relationship of the mass to neighboring structures.

1.4.1 Anterior Mediastinum

The most common masses in the anterior mediastinum are goiters with intrathoracic extension, thymoma and thymic carcinoma, extragonadal germ cell tumors (usually the benign variant of teratoma but occasionally malignant teratomas, seminomas, embryonic cell carcinomas, and other germ cell tumors).

Intrathoracic Goiter

▶ **Brief definition.** Iodine deficiency leads to enlargement of the thyroid gland in patients with a euthyroid or hypothyroid metabolic state. Approximately 15 to 30% of all adults, depending on eating habits, have an enlarged thyroid gland. If more than 50% of the enlarged gland extends into the chest, the patient is said to have an intrathoracic (or retrosternal) goiter. Intrathoracic goiter is a common incidental finding on chest radiographs, CT, and MRI in iodine-deficient geographic regions.

▶ **Imaging signs.** When viewed on chest radiographs, an intrathoracic goiter appears as a sharply circumscribed density in the superior mediastinum that displaces the trachea laterally at the level of the thoracic inlet in the PA view (▶ Fig. 1.11) and displaces it anteriorly in the lateral view. This feature is useful in distinguishing goiters from other diseases in the superior mediastinum, since other tumors as well as mediastinal widening due to other causes will rarely cause tracheal displacement. If tracheomalacia (pressure injury to the cartilage leading to tracheal instability during respiration) is suspected on clinical grounds, a standard tracheal radiograph should be obtained during a Valsalva maneuver (bearing down against a closed glottis to raise the intrathoracic pressure) and a Müller maneuver (inspiring against a closed glottis with the nostrils held shut to increase the negative intrathoracic pressure). If the luminal width changes by more than 50% during these maneuvers, tracheomalacia is present (▶ Fig. 1.12). A sectional imaging diagnosis of intrathoracic goiter relies on two main criteria:
- The mediastinal mass is in continuity with the thyroid gland.
- The tissue has the same density (CT) or signal intensity (MRI) as the thyroid gland.

Mediastinum

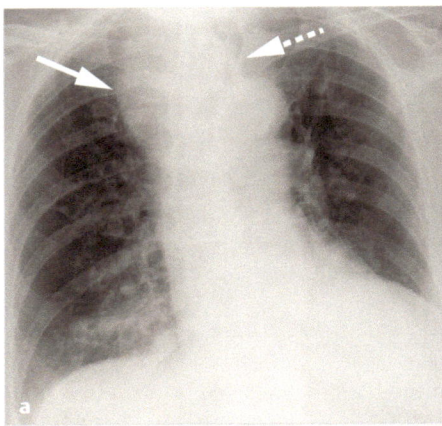 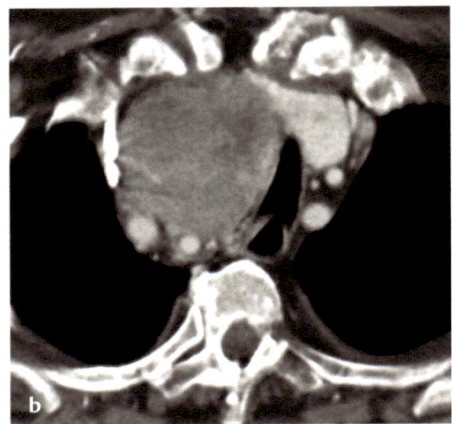 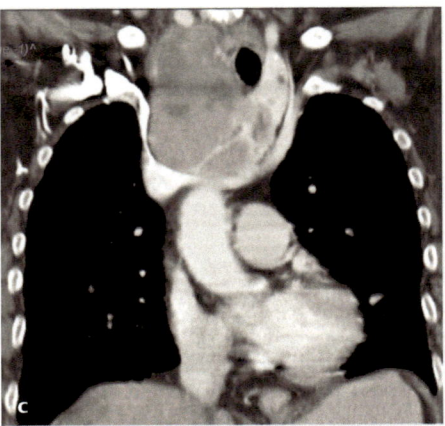

Fig. 1.11 **Multinodular goiter.** (a) Chest radiograph demonstrates mediastinal widening (arrow). The trachea is markedly displaced to the left (dashed arrow). (b) Axial CT: the thyroid parenchyma appears inhomogeneous after IV injection of contrast medium. (c) Coronal reformatted image shows continuity of the goiter from the cervical to intrathoracic level.

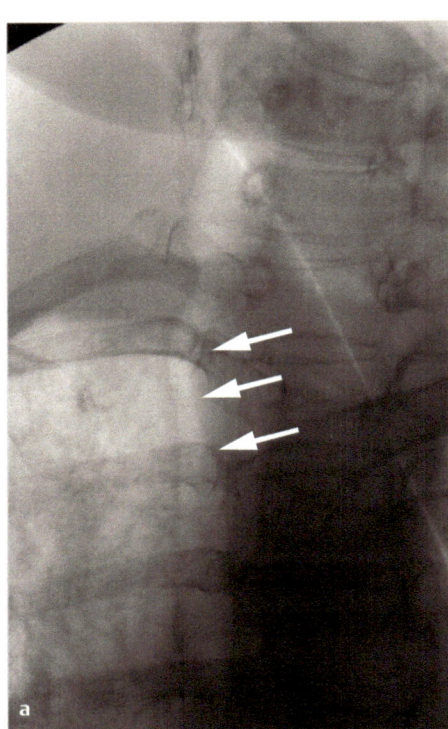 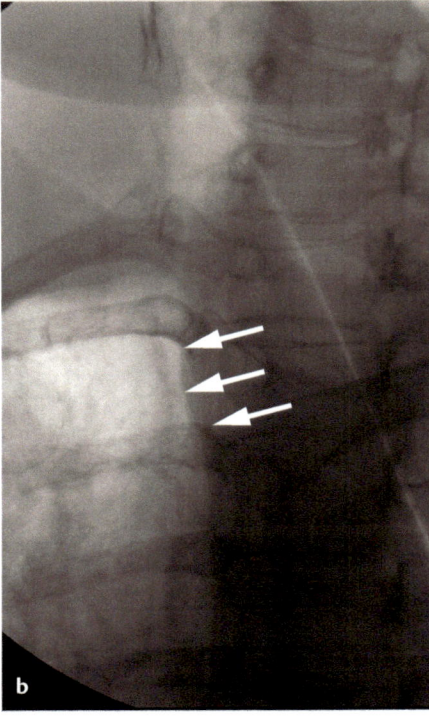

Fig. 1.12 **Tracheomalacia due to extrinsic compression by a goiter.** In tracheal spot views, the luminal width of the trachea changes by more than 50% (arrows) in response to Valsalva maneuver (a) and a Müller maneuver (b).

Both the thyroid gland and ectopic thyroid tissue are markedly hyperdense to muscle on plain CT scans due to their high iodine content. Their unenhanced attenuation values are in the range of 65 to 120 HU. Thyroid tissue shows intense contrast enhancement owing to its rich blood supply. Large goiters generally contain calcifications. Most extend into the anterior mediastinum, and some may even extend as far as the middle or posterior mediastinum. Because most goiters are multinodular and contain colloid cysts, intrathoracic goiters often have a heterogeneous CT appearance and include areas that enhance less than the surrounding thyroid tissue.

▶ **Clinical features.** Patients usually present clinically with visible enlargement of the thyroid gland, typically located at a supraclavicular level in the midline. The goiter may become symptomatic due to tracheal displacement, and large goiters may cause tracheomalacia with cough, dyspnea, and inspiratory stridor.

▶ **Differential diagnosis**
- Enlargement of the thyroid gland may be a result of *thyroiditis* or *thyroid carcinoma*. CT scans of thyroid carcinoma may show only indirect signs such as extraglandular growth or the invasion of adjacent structures. Small carcinomas in the thyroid gland are indistinguishable from regressive nodules or thyroid adenomas by ultrasound or CT. Thyroid carcinoma may also contain calcifications, so the presence of calcifications is not a useful criterion for benign/malignant differentiation. Iodine 123 (^{123}I) (or iodine 131 [^{131}I]) thyroid scintigraphy can detect nodules that do not concentrate iodine. Suspicious nodules are then evaluated by ultrasound-guided fine needle aspiration biopsy to exclude thyroid carcinoma.

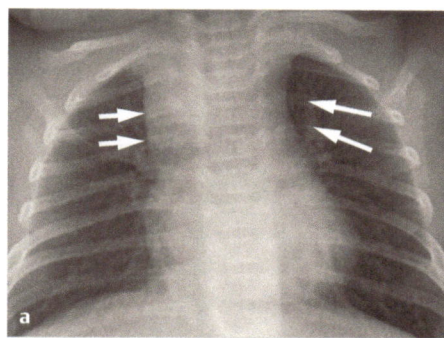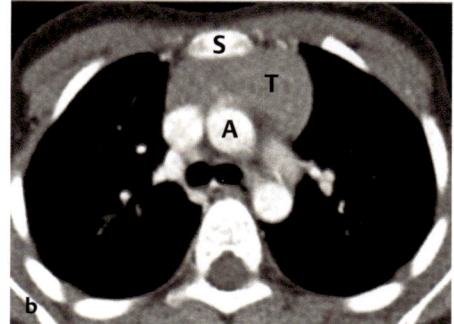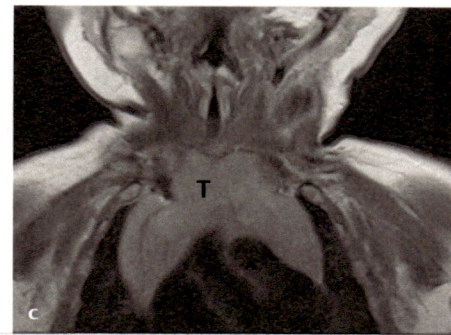

Fig. 1.13 Normal thymus in three patients. (a) Chest radiograph of an 8-week-old infant. The superior mediastinum is markedly widened by the thymus (arrows). (b) CT scan in a 6-year-old girl. The thymus (T) shows homogeneous contrast enhancement. The sternum (S) and aorta (A) serve as landmarks, as the thymus is located between them. (c) Coronal T2 W MR image in a 6-week-old infant. The thymus (T) extends well beyond the heart.

- *Ectopic thyroid tissue* in the mediastinum is rare. It has smooth margins and its enhancement characteristics are identical to those of thyroid tissue. With an ectopic thyroid gland in the mediastinum, the compartment normally occupied by the thyroid gland will be empty.

▶ **Key points.** Intrathoracic goiter is a common incidental radiological finding in iodine-deficient geographic regions. In imaging, the intrathoracic tissue is continuous with the thyroid gland and has the same attenuation values on CT and same signal intensity on MRI.

Thymic Hyperplasia

▶ **Brief definition.** The thymus originates from the third pharyngeal pouch, and during embryogenesis it ascends from the level of the pharynx into the anterior mediastinum in front of the aortic arch. Thymic cysts may form anywhere along this path. The imaging appearance of the thymus varies with age. In newborns, the thymus may be larger than the heart (▶ Fig. 1.13). It begins to atrophy at puberty, continues to regress with aging, and by age 40 years is visible on CT scans in only about 5 to 17% of the population. Reactive thymic hyperplasia, known also as rebound hyperplasia, may occur as a result of chemotherapy, chemoradiotherapy, or severe illness and characterizes recovery of the immune system. During this period the thymus may grow up to 50% larger than its original size. On average, reactive thymic hyperplasia occurs 6 months after the cessation of chemotherapy in children and 9 months after in adults, but intervals from 2 months to 5 years have been reported in the literature.[5] Rebound hyperplasia may occur in just 2 to 3 weeks in children who discontinue steroid therapy, taking somewhat longer in adults. Thymic hyperplasia also occurs in response to thyrotoxicosis, lupus erythematosus, Behçet's syndrome, Addison's disease, and Hashimoto's thyroiditis.

▶ **Imaging signs.** Viewed in axial images, the thymus in adults usually presents a triangular shape with the apex pointing toward the sternum. Severe diseases, chemotherapy, and steroid therapy elicits rapid atrophy of the thymus, which later recovers to a state of reactive hyperplasia. The hyperplastic thymus may abut blood vessels but never displaces them, whereas actual tumors of the thymus will cause vascular displacement. Another criterion for the diagnosis of reactive hyperplasia is the arrowhead shape that is typical of the thymus.

▶ **Clinical features.** Thymic hyperplasia has no clinical manifestations.

▶ **Differential diagnosis.** An important differential diagnosis is a thymoma, which usually has an oval shape unlike that of a normal or hyperplastic thymus. Recurrent lymphoma also requires differentiation from reactive hyperplasia, especially if there has been previous thymic involvement by lymphoma. It may be difficult in any given case to distinguish a recurrence from reactive thymic hyperplasia after the cessation of chemotherapy.

▶ **Key points.** The thymus slowly atrophies after puberty. This atrophy may occur rapidly after severe illness or chemotherapy, followed by rebound enlargement of the gland after recovery from the disease or the withdrawal of chemotherapy. This reactive hyperplasia requires differentiation from recurrent lymphoma, especially if there was primary involvement of the thymus.

Thymoma and Thymic Carcinoma

▶ **Brief definition.** Thymoma is a tumor originating from the epithelial cells of the thymus that are responsible for the maturation of T lymphocytes. Often the thymus is also found to contain collections of abnormal T cells that have been influenced by the excessive proliferation of altered epithelial cells. These cells form autoantibodies that may cause myasthenia gravis by blocking acetylcholine receptors at the motor end plates of striated muscle. Approximately 15% of patients with myasthenia gravis have a thymoma. By the same token, the thymus is not always enlarged in patients with a clinical diagnosis of myasthenia gravis. Histology in these patients shows a lymphoid reaction with an increased number of T lymphocytes in the thymus, which does not correlate with imaging abnormalities. Thymoma is most commonly diagnosed in the fourth to sixth decades and accounts for approximately 20% of all masses in the anterior mediastinum. As a general rule, thymomas have a smooth round or oval shape and enhance markedly after administration of contrast medium. Thymomas are typically located in the anterior superior mediastinum (▶ Fig. 1.14, see also ▶ Fig. 1.6), but 10% are found in the posterior mediastinum. Thymomas may contain cysts or calcifications. Numerous classifications were used for thymoma until 1999, when the WHO proposed a uniform classification that is often used today in its 2004 modification. This histological classification is based on the presence and number of cellular atypias. Types A,

Mediastinum

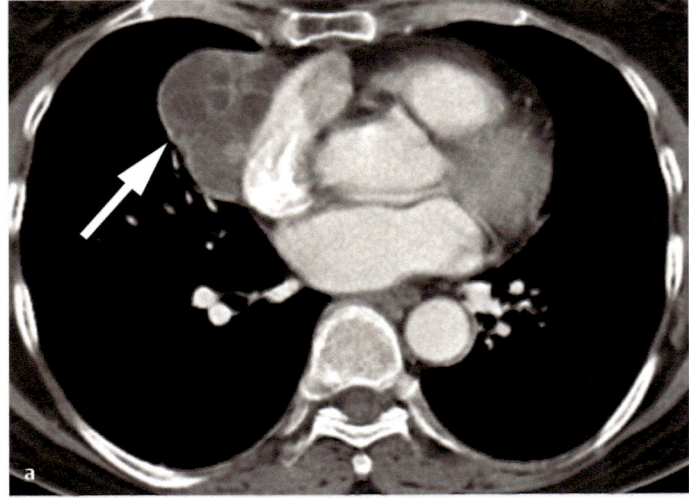
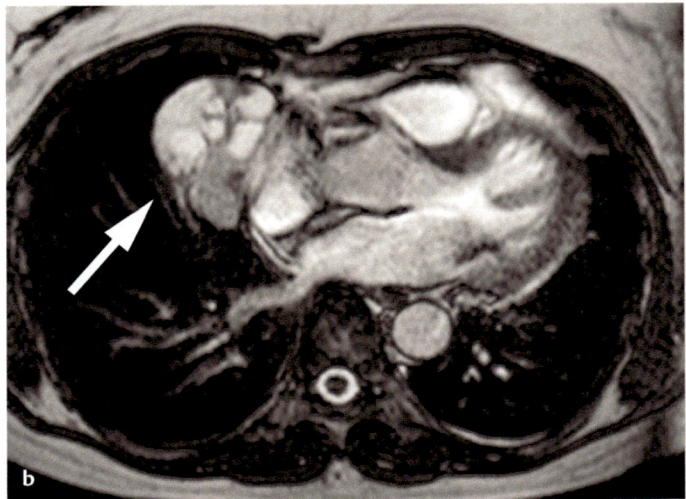

Fig. 1.14 **Thymoma.** (a) On axial CT the tumor (arrow) displays cystic and solid components. Its solid portions enhance faintly after administration of contrast medium. (b) T2 W/T1 W TrueFISP MRI sequence demonstrates the multiple cysts (arrow). (TrueFISP, true fast imaging with steady precession.)

AB, and B1 are low-risk thymomas, types B2 and B3 are high-risk thymomas; and type C is thymic carcinoma.[6] All thymomas, even type A, may be locally invasive and may give rise to distant metastases, leading many authors to question the validity of the WHO classification. The incidence of thymoma and thymic carcinoma in the United States and Europe is 1 per 1 million population.

▶ **Imaging signs.** Thymomas have soft tissue attenuation on CT and enhance markedly with administration of intravenous contrast medium. They may contain cysts. Thymic carcinoma frequently invades blood vessels, with associated intravascular extension into the heart (▶ Fig. 1.15). If the tumor does not transgress the boundaries of the thymus, only histology can distinguish between thymoma and thymic carcinoma and provide an accurate classification. Recent studies suggest that thymic carcinoma has a higher standardized flurodeoxyglucose (FDG) uptake value on PET/CT than low- and high-risk thymomas.[7] On MRI, thymomas are hyperintense in T2 W images, are isointense to muscle on unenhanced T1 W images, and enhance intensely after administration of contrast medium. If thymoma is suspected, the entire chest and upper abdomen should be evaluated by CT, as 15% of patients will be found to have drop metastases along the pleura, and intra-abdominal metastasis may occur through the physiologic apertures in the diaphragm.

▶ **Clinical features.** One-third of all thymomas lead to myasthenia gravis, with presenting symptoms of muscle weakness, fatigue, and ptosis. Another one-third of thymomas present with signs and symptoms attributable to local tumor growth. These include chest pain, superior vena cava syndrome, and a visible and palpable cervical mass with tumors that have grown up through the thoracic inlet. Another one-third of thymomas are detected incidentally by imaging done for a different indication. Given the difficulty of distinguishing benign thymoma from thymic carcinoma, all lesions should be resected.

▶ **Differential diagnosis.** Enlargement of the thymus in adults may also result from its involvement by Hodgkin's disease, non-Hodgkin's lymphoma, or acute lymphocytic leukemia. It is important to be aware of the presence or otherwise of these diseases in making a differential diagnosis.

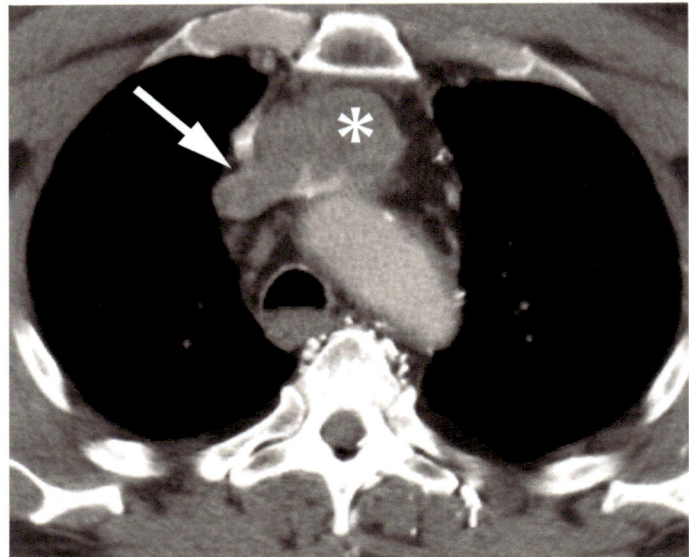

Fig. 1.15 **Thymic carcinoma** (asterisk). The tumor has invaded the left brachiocephalic vein (arrow).

▶ **Key points.** Thymoma and thymic carcinoma are distinguishable by imaging only if the invasion of surrounding structures can be demonstrated.

Thymic Cysts

▶ **Brief definition.** Cysts of the thymus may be congenital or acquired. The thymus originates from the third pharyngeal pouch, and cysts may develop along the path by which it descends from the level of the pharynx to the anterior mediastinum at the level of the aortic arch. The peak incidence is from 3 to 15 years of age.

▶ **Imaging signs.** Thymic cysts display CT features that are characteristic of cysts: an enhancing wall with contents that are

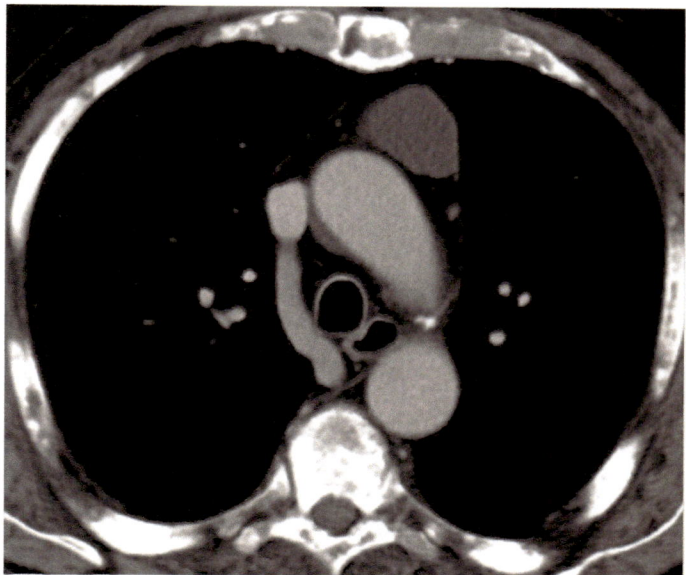

Fig. 1.16 **Thymic cyst.** CT scan demonstrates the thin-walled cyst anterior to the aortic arch.

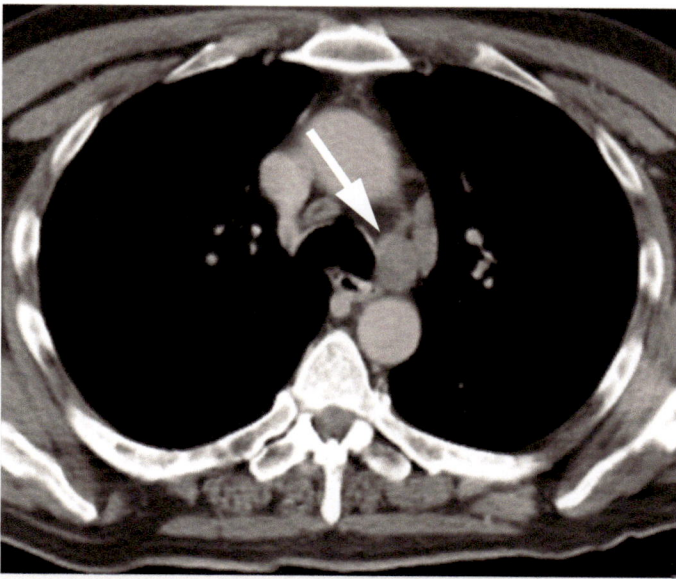

Fig. 1.17 **Carcinoid** (arrow) **and adjacent lymph node metastases.**

isodense to water, or hyperdense if intracystic hemorrhage has occurred (▶ Fig. 1.16). MRI shows the high T2 W signal intensity and low T1 W signal intensity that are typical of cysts. Thymic cysts may form outside or inside the thymus.

▶ **Clinical features.** Thymic cysts are usually an asymptomatic incidental finding on chest radiographs or sectional images.

▶ **Differential diagnosis.** Cysts located within the thymus require differentiation from seminomas, which may also develop large cysts. Equivocal cases should be resolved by percutaneous biopsy. Thymic cysts may also be associated with carcinomas of variable size.

▶ **Key points.** Thymic cysts may develop within the thymus or outside the thymus along its path of descent during embryogenesis. They have typical attenuation values on CT (0 HU) and typical cystic signal intensity on MRI (high T2 W signal, low T1 W signal, with a reversal of signal intensities in cysts with a high protein content). Most thymic cysts are incidental imaging findings.

Neuroendocrine Tumors of the Thymus; Thymic and Mediastinal Carcinoids

▶ **Brief definition.** Carcinoids are tumors of neuroendocrine origin that arise from primitive stem cells. Carcinoids are usually slow-growing and may metastasize. They are most common in middle age, and men are affected more frequently than women.

▶ **Imaging signs.** Carcinoids of the thymus are often indistinguishable from thymoma or thymic carcinoma by their imaging appearance. They may occur in the mediastinum and other sites and may not be localized to a particular organ (▶ Fig. 1.17), appearing on CT as an enhancing mass of soft tissue density. Carcinoids have high T2 W signal intensity on MRI. They are isointense to muscle on T1 W images and show marked contrast enhancement.

▶ **Clinical features.** Symptoms result from hormones produced in the tumor. Approximately one-third of carcinoids form adrenocorticotropic hormone leading to Cushing's syndrome. Hypertension, diarrhea, and paroxysmal flushing due to capillary vasodilation may also occur.

▶ **Differential diagnosis.** The differential diagnosis should include thymoma, thymic carcinoma, and sarcoma.

▶ **Pitfalls.** Carcinoids cannot be diagnosed from imaging findings alone. Diagnosis requires the correlation of imaging findings with clinical symptoms relating to hormone production or with histology.

▶ **Key points.** Carcinoids may occur within the thymus or separately in the mediastinum. They do not have typical imaging features that permit a definite diagnosis. This requires clinical and laboratory correlation.

Extragonadal Germ Cell Tumors

"Extragonadal germ cell tumors" is a collective term for all tumors that originate from embryonic germ cells and are histologically indistinguishable from tumors of the gonads. They include teratomas (benign and malignant forms), seminomas, dermoid cysts, embryonic cell carcinomas, and chorionic carcinomas. Extragonadal germ cell tumors occur predominantly in the mediastinum and comprise 15% of all mediastinal tumors. Approximately 80% are benign teratomas. Seminomas follow teratomas in absolute numbers and account for most malignant forms (ca. 40% of malignant germ cell tumors in the mediastinum).

Teratomas; Dermoid and Epidermoid Cysts

▶ **Brief definition**
- *Teratomas* may contain tissue elements derived from all three germ layers (mesoderm, endoderm, and ectoderm). Ectodermal cells may give rise to cutaneous appendages such as hair and

sebaceous glands as well as teeth. Muscle, cartilage, and bone may develop from mesodermal cells, while epithelium and pancreatic glands may arise from endodermal cells. Mature teratomas are benign, with a peak age of incidence in young adulthood (20 to 40 years).

- *Dermoid cysts* are composed of ectodermal and mesodermal elements and are not distinguishable from cystic teratomas by their imaging morphology. In 5% of cases, squamous cell carcinoma develops in dermoid cysts.
- *Epidermoid cysts* are composed entirely of ectodermal elements. They contain squamous epithelium and may gradually enlarge through desquamation.

The great majority of teratomas, dermoid cysts, and epidermoid cysts occur in the anterior superior mediastinum. Only about 8% of all cases occur in the posterior mediastinum.

▶ **Imaging signs.** Imaging of teratomas often reveals cystic components (88% of teratomas) and fatty components (76% of teratomas) that contrast with areas of soft tissue density found in almost every teratoma. Calcified areas are found in 53% of teratomas (▶ Fig. 1.18). Teratomas or dermoid cysts that form teeth or bone are easily diagnosed by CT. Teratomas and dermoid cysts present a heterogeneous tissue structure on both CT and MRI. Diffusion imaging of dermoid and epidermoid cysts shows severe diffusion abnormalities: imaging at high b values ($b = 1000$) shows an intense signal with a marked decrease in the apparent diffusion coefficient. Fat–fluid levels in cystic areas have repeatedly been described as pathognomonic in individual case reports but are very rarely found. Epidermoid cysts are purely cystic in almost all cases. All three tumor entities are smoothly marginated. Malignant teratoma has indistinct margins and an inhomogeneous matrix; it is also composed of elements of all three germ layers and may therefore contain fatty tissue and calcifications. Their other imaging features coincide with those of teratomas.

▶ **Clinical features.** Teratomas and dermoid and epidermoid cysts are generally asymptomatic. Large teratomas or dermoid cysts may compress adjacent structures, resulting in symptoms that may include chest pain. Intralesional hemorrhage in a teratoma or dermoid cyst may cause sudden enlargement of the mass, leading to sudden compression of mediastinal structures with associated symptoms. The treatment of a mature teratoma or mature dermoid or epidermoid cyst is complete resection of the mass. If this is accomplished, the tumor will not recur.

▶ **Differential diagnosis.** Differential diagnosis of teratomas requires mainly differentiation from sarcomas. With malignant teratomas, differential diagnosis cannot always rely on imaging findings. Lymphomas are another possibility but are more homogeneous. Dermoid and epidermoid cysts can be classified more accurately by diffusion-weighted MRI.

▶ **Key points.** Teratomas have components derived from all three germ layers and a heterogeneous imaging appearance. Dermoids are composed of ectodermal and mesodermal elements, while epidermoids are purely ectodermal. Dermoids and epidermoids can be differentiated from other cysts by diffusion-weighted MRI.

Primary Seminomas

▶ **Brief definition.** Primary extragonadal seminomas are rare malignant masses. The most common site of occurrence is the anterior mediastinum, followed by the pineal gland and retroperitoneum. Approximately 10% of all malignant mediastinal tumors are primary seminomas. Over 90% of all primary seminomas in the mediastinum occur in males, with a peak age of incidence at 20 to 40 years. It is now believed that primary extragonadal seminomas arise from pluripotent primitive germ cells that become trapped in the mediastinum as they migrate across the midline into the gonads during early embryogenesis. These heterotopic cells may differentiate into both ectodermal and endodermal tissues; they are believed to be responsible for the development of chorionic carcinoma, embryonic cell carcinoma, and other germ cell tumors in the mediastinum.

▶ **Imaging signs.** Primary seminomas of the mediastinum are usually quite large by the time they are diagnosed. They have smooth, lobulated margins. Seminomas may contain stippled calcifications and cysts along with other areas showing slight, homogeneous enhancement. They have homogeneous signal intensity on MRI, appearing hyperintense in T2W images and showing intense contrast enhancement.

▶ **Clinical features.** The symptoms of primary mediastinal seminoma are nonspecific and result from the compression of structures in the superior mediastinum. Compression of a recurrent laryngeal nerve may cause cough and hoarseness. Other possible symptoms are dyspnea, dysphagia, and chest pain; obstruction of the superior vena cava is rare. Approximately one-third of patients are asymptomatic. Tumor markers such as alpha-fetoprotein (AFP) and human chorionic gonadotropin (β-HCG) (see ▶ Table 1.1) are not elevated. Primary seminomas of the mediastinum are treated by excision, followed if necessary by adjuvant radiation. Recent reports describe the addition of cisplatin chemotherapy and indicate very high survival rates with this combination.

▶ **Differential diagnosis.** Seminomas resemble lymphomas in their imaging appearance. Unlike lymphomas, however, seminomas compress surrounding structures, most notably vessels, and

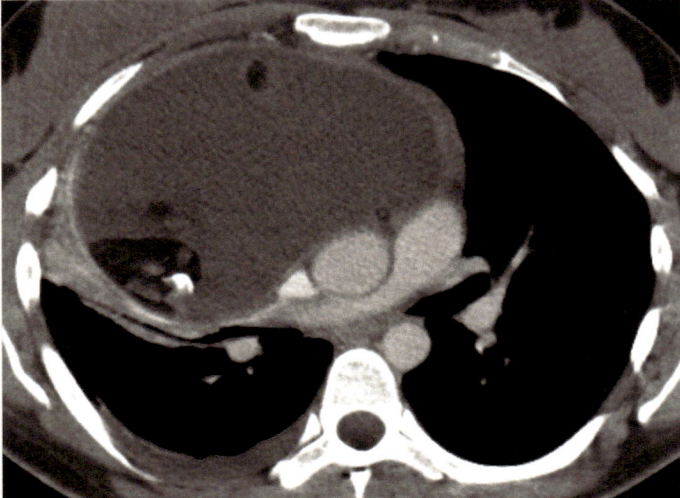

Fig. 1.18 Teratoma. CT scan shows the well-circumscribed mass with mixed attenuation values

Table 1.1 Markers for various extragonadal germ cell tumors

Tumor entity	Typical tumor markers
Seminoma	None
Embryonic cell carcinoma	AFP
Chorionic carcinoma	β-HCG
Malignant teratoma	AFP, β-HCG
Yolk sac tumor	AFP

Abbreviations: AFP, alpha-fetoprotein; HCG, human chorionic gonadotropin.

may also show vascular invasion. Differentiation is mainly required from sarcomas and thymomas, which may also contain cysts and calcifications.

Note
Primary seminomas are not distinguishable from other mediastinal tumors by their imaging appearance; their diagnosis requires biopsy.

▶ **Pitfalls.** Following the histological diagnosis of a mediastinal seminoma or other mediastinal germ cell tumor, a primary gonadal tumor should be definitively excluded before a mediastinal extragonadal germ cell tumor is diagnosed.

▶ **Key points.** Extragonadal seminomas of the mediastinum arise from pluripotent primitive germ cells that become trapped in the mediastinum as they migrate across the midline to the gonads during early embryogenesis. The peak age of incidence is 20 to 40 years with a male predilection. The tumors show prominent enhancement at imaging and may contain cysts and calcifications. Given the lack of pathognomonic imaging features, the diagnosis of extragonadal seminoma should be confirmed histologically.

Chorionic Epithelioma, Embryonic Cell Carcinoma, and Mixed Germ Cell Tumors

▶ **Brief definition.** Malignant germ cell tumors that are histologically distinct from primary mediastinal seminoma are associated with a poorer prognosis. Like seminomas, these tumors arise from pluripotent primitive germ cells that become trapped in the mediastinum. These cells may differentiate in various ways:
- *Embryonic cell carcinoma* is composed of various poorly differentiated cell types.
- *Chorionic carcinoma* contains syncytiotrophoblasts and cytotrophoblasts. Hematogenous metastasis is common. This property is analogous to the ability of the placenta to invade blood vessels.
- As noted earlier, *malignant teratoma* is composed of cells derived from all three germ layers.

Germ cell tumors may be considered "caricatures" of embryogenesis. The various tumor types differentiate from pluripotent germ cells along different lines and reflect the varying cellular components of embryogenesis.[8] These tumors, unlike seminomas, form tumor markers (▶ Table 1.1) that are useful in monitoring treatment response and detecting recurrence. Like other tumors, they occur predominantly in the anterior mediastinum.

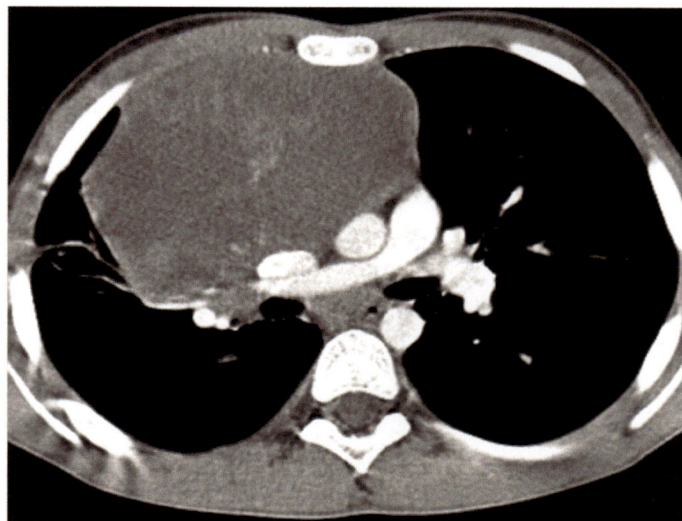

Fig. 1.19 **Germ cell tumor in the anterior mediastinum.** On CT the mass shows low attenuation and inhomogeneous enhancement. It has compressed the superior vena cava and right pulmonary artery.

▶ **Imaging signs.** Extragonadal germ cell tumors of the mediastinum have a heterogeneous appearance on CT and MRI with areas of varying density or signal intensity. They show a nonhomogeneous pattern of enhancement (▶ Fig. 1.19). Because of their rapid growth, malignant germ cell tumors other than seminoma are prone to intratumoral hemorrhage and often exhibit necrotic areas. They may also contain cysts. The various tumor types may not be clearly distinguishable from one another by their imaging features and require a histological diagnosis.

▶ **Clinical features.** Clinical features are the same as for seminoma. These germ cell tumors typically produce tumor markers (see ▶ Table 1.1). Treatment consists of surgical resection followed by radiation and chemotherapy.

▶ **Differential diagnosis.** Sarcoma, lymphoma, thymoma, and thymic carcinoma should be included in the differential diagnosis. Extragonadal germ cell tumors that are histologically distinct from seminoma also require a histological diagnosis.

▶ **Key points.** Extragonadal germ cell tumors have a heterogeneous appearance on CT and MRI, with areas of varying density or signal intensity, and show inhomogeneous contrast enhancement. They are diagnosed histologically.

Liposarcoma

▶ **Brief definition.** Primary liposarcomas of the mediastinum are very rare malignant masses of adipose tissue with a peak incidence in the fifth decade. Different types are distinguished by their grade of differentiation.

Sarcomas

▶ **Brief definition.** Sarcomas are mesenchymal malignancies that may occur in all mediastinal compartments. Primary sarcomas of the mediastinum are very rare. Types other than liposarcoma include fibrosarcoma, chondrosarcoma, osteosarcoma, and

Mediastinum

rhabdomyosarcoma. The overall incidence of soft tissue sarcomas (including gastrointestinal stromal tumor) in all body regions in adults is 2 per 100,000 population.

▶ **Imaging signs.** Well-differentiated liposarcoma is composed mainly of fatty tissue, has negative CT attenuation values, and is isointense to fat on MRI. The presence of septa thicker than 2 mm or of enhancing areas within the tumor are signs of well-differentiated liposarcoma on sectional imaging. Mixed tumors additionally contain other cell types such as fibrocytes. Poorly differentiated liposarcomas contain large areas of denser tissue that shows intense enhancement (▶ Fig. 1.20). The treatment of choice is surgical excision. Sarcomas appear on radiographs as well-circumscribed masses that may have lobulated margins. The tumors are usually inhomogeneous on CT and MRI (▶ Fig. 1.21). Osteosarcomas may contain calcifications and bone matrix, which are more clearly depicted by CT than MRI.

▶ **Clinical features.** Symptoms result from the compression of adjacent structures such as the heart, trachea, or esophagus. If compression is absent, B symptoms may be predominant. The treatment of choice is excision followed by radiation.

▶ **Differential diagnosis.** Lymphomas encase vessels but do not compress them. Seminomas and other extragonadal germ cell tumors cannot be distinguished from sarcomas. Thymomas are located in the thymic compartment and may contain cysts but otherwise show the same characteristics on CT and MRI. Lipomatosis mediastinalis (▶ Fig. 1.22) usually occurs in obese patients.

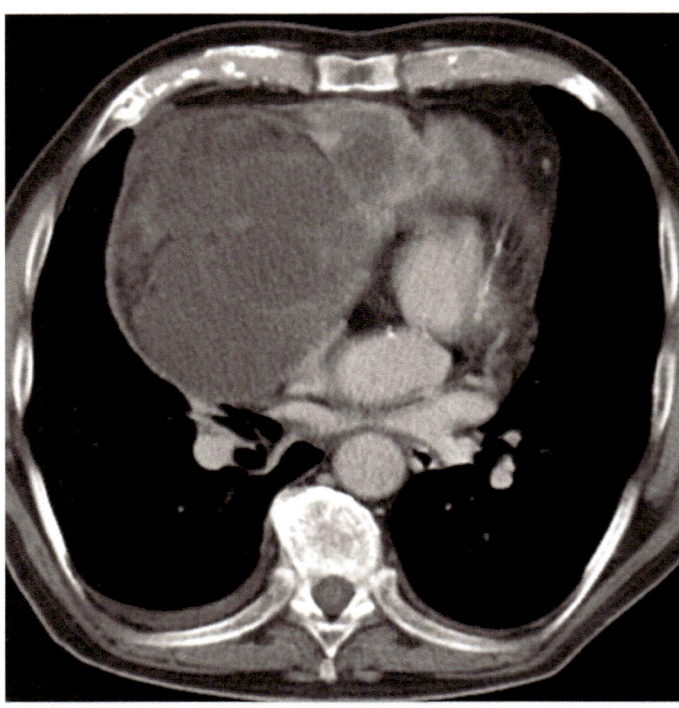

Fig. 1.20 Liposarcoma. CT after IV injection of contrast medium. The mass contains areas of variable density and shows inhomogeneous enhancement.

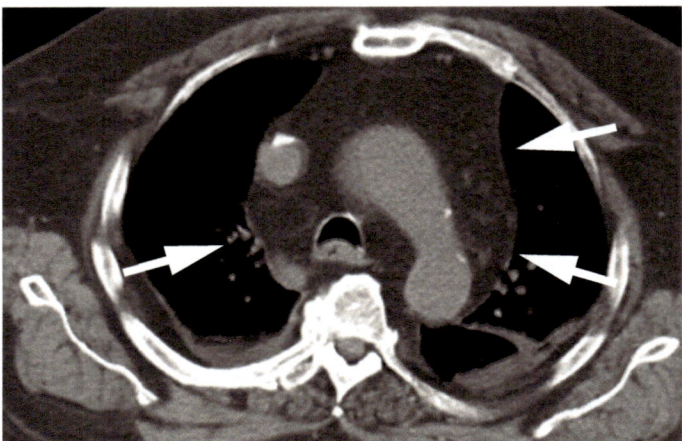

Fig. 1.22 Mediastinal lipomatosis. An increased volume of mediastinal fat is noted in this obese patient. The mediastinal structures are uniformly surrounded by fat (arrows). The thymic compartment is a useful landmark in older patients. The perivascular tissue in the superior mediastinum provides a landmark in patients of all age groups.

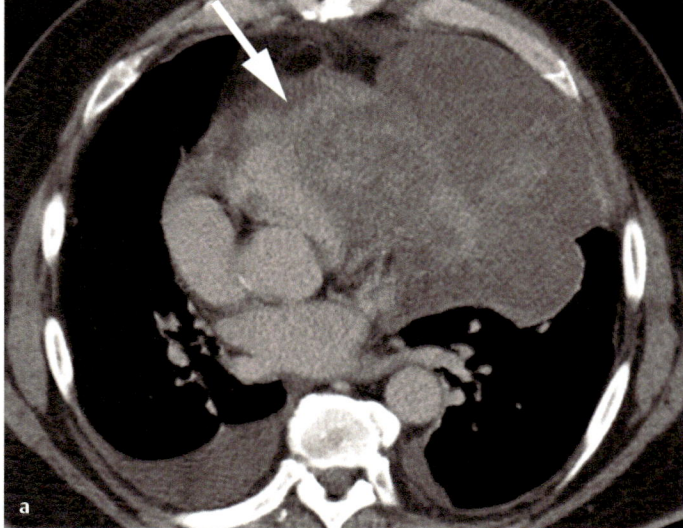
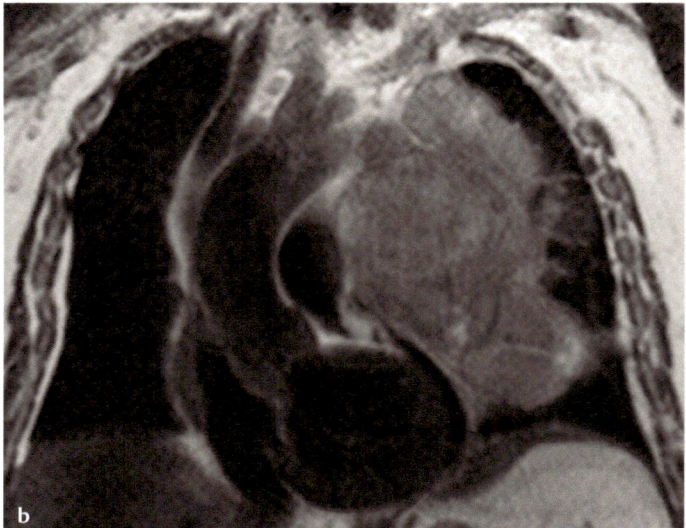

Fig. 1.21 Rhabdomyosarcoma. (a) On CT the tumor shows inhomogeneous density with areas of varying enhancement. Its boundary with the pericardium and heart is indistinct (arrow), suggesting possible invasion. (b) Coronal T2 W MRI shows that the tumor has reached the pericardium but has not yet penetrated it.

1.4 Mediastinal Masses

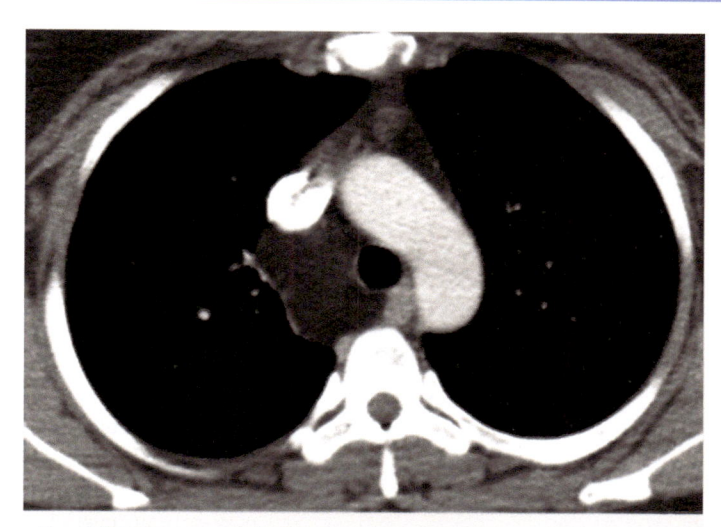

Fig. 1.23 Lipoma. Axial CT demonstrates a circumscribed mass of fat density.

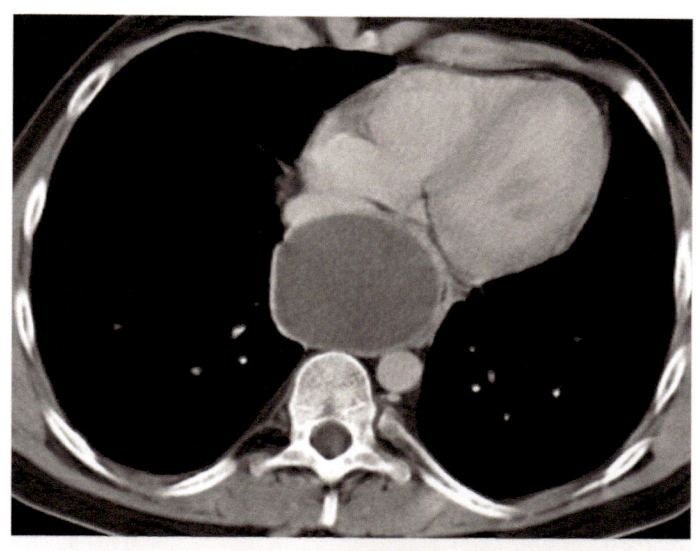

Fig. 1.24 Bronchogenic cyst. CT demonstrates a thin-walled cyst with contents of water attenuation. The esophagus is displaced. There is no apparent relationship to the trachea or large bronchi. After resection, the cyst was found to be lined by respiratory epithelium. By its imaging appearance the cyst is indistinguishable from a duplication of the esophageal wall (see ▶ Fig. 1.27).

As with lipomas (▶ Fig. 1.23), density is similar to that of fat in other locations.

▶ **Key points.** Sarcomas enhance in all modalities. They present a heterogeneous pattern, depending on the parent tissue, and are diagnosed histologically. The role of imaging is to accurately describe the size, location, and surrounding structures. A specific diagnosis requires histology.

▶ **Differential diagnosis.** Bronchogenic cysts are often indistinguishable from esophageal duplication in terms of their imaging appearance, and a specific diagnosis requires cyst resection and histological identification of respiratory epithelium lining the cyst.

Cystic Masses

Cystic masses of the mediastinum are very rare. Bronchogenic cysts and cysts of the esophagus fall in the category of foregut duplication cysts.

Note
As a general rule, morphological imaging studies will not demonstrate the relationship of bronchogenic cysts to the trachea or segmental bronchi.

Bronchogenic Cysts

▶ **Brief definition.** Bronchogenic cysts are congenital changes that result from abnormal budding of the trachea between the fourth and sixth gestational weeks. They are lined by respiratory epithelium and may contain cartilage. Up to 85% of bronchogenic cysts are located in the mediastinum, usually at the infracarinal level; the rest occur in the lung parenchyma. These cysts develop somewhat later in embryogenesis and are more likely to communicate with the tracheobronchial tree than mediastinal bronchogenic cysts.

▶ **Imaging signs.** Bronchogenic cysts appear as homogeneous, well-circumscribed densities on chest radiographs. CT and MRI identify them as fluid-filled structures with thin walls (▶ Fig. 1.24). Only the walls enhance after administration of contrast medium. CT attenuation and MRI signal intensity depend on the protein content of the cyst fluid. Bronchogenic cysts may be air-filled if they communicate with the tracheobronchial tree.

▶ **Clinical features.** Bronchogenic cysts may cause dyspnea and stridor, depending on their location. If they are located close to the main bronchi, they may lead to areas of compression atelectasis even in infants. Smaller cysts may remain asymptomatic for some time. If the cyst becomes infected, symptoms develop as a result of associated inflammatory signs and rapid enlargement of the cyst with compression of surrounding structures.

▶ **Key points.** Bronchogenic cysts are developmental anomalies of the tracheobronchial tree. They are lined by respiratory epithelium and may become symptomatic due to compression of surrounding structures or superinfection. Often they are indistinguishable from esophageal duplication cysts by their imaging appearance.

Pericardial Cysts and Diverticula

▶ **Brief definition.** Pericardial cysts are rare masses that account for approximately 7% of all mediastinal tumors. They are located predominantly in the left (70%) or right (30%) cardiophrenic angle (▶ Fig. 1.25). They are of mesothelial origin and represent outpouchings of the parietal pericardium (persistence of a pericardial recess during embryogenesis) that do not communicate with the rest of the pericardium. By contrast, pericardial diverticula communicate directly with the pericardial cavity. They may also be acquired and may occur postoperatively. Rapid enlargement over time suggests a pericardial diverticulum rather than a true pericardial cyst (▶ Fig. 1.26).

▶ **Imaging signs.** Pericardial cysts and diverticula have smooth, well-defined margins on chest radiographs and abut the cardiac silhouette. CT and MRI show their direct relationship to the heart. Pericardial cysts and diverticula have an extremely thin cyst wall, and internal septa are rarely present. CT attenuation and MRI

Mediastinum

signal intensity depend on the protein content of the cyst. Because pericardial cysts usually contain a clear, serous fluid, they have also been termed "spring water cysts." This results in high T2W signal intensity and low T1W signal intensity. CT attenuation is approximately 10 HU. Asymptomatic patients do not require treatment. The treatment of choice for symptomatic cases is surgical removal; resected cysts do not recur. The cysts can be decompressed by percutaneous aspiration but will refill over time unless obliterated by the injection of alcohol or tissue adhesive.

▶ **Clinical features.** Most pericardial cysts and diverticula are detected incidentally at imaging. In very rare cases where other structures, such as lung, are compressed by a mass effect, pericardial cysts may lead to dyspnea or even symptoms of heart failure (e.g., by hemodynamically significant compression of the right ventricle). Persistent cough and atypical chest pain have also been described in a few instances. Intracystic hemorrhage may cause significant cyst enlargement with acute onset of symptoms due to compression of adjacent organs. Cyst infection and rupture are extremely rare.

▶ **Differential diagnosis.** The differential diagnosis of well-circumscribed masses on the chest radiograph should include large epicardial fat pads as well as mediastinal tumors. CT or MRI is useful for the differentiation of solid tumors and fat.

Note
The cardiophrenic angle is the principal landmark for pericardial cysts and diverticula.

▶ **Pitfalls.** The pericardial reflections at the level of the ascending aorta show small amounts of fluid, even in healthy individuals, and should not be taken to indicate small pericardial cysts.

▶ **Key points.** Pericardial cysts communicate with the pericardium, while pericardial diverticula communicate with the pericardial cavity. Both entities show the typical characteristics of cysts in sectional imaging studies.

Esophageal Duplication Cysts

▶ **Brief definition.** Duplication cysts of the esophagus are rare congenital malformations that result from abnormal budding of the foregut in the third to fourth gestational week. The wall of the cyst may contain smooth or striated muscle. The cysts are lined by esophageal epithelium, which rarely may include areas of ectopic gastric epithelium. Secretions from this tissue may erode through the cyst wall, leading to intracystic hemorrhage or perforation of the cyst.[9]

▶ **Imaging signs.** Esophageal duplication cysts are often detected incidentally on chest radiographs of asymptomatic patients, appearing as well-circumscribed, oblong densities projected over the posterior inferior mediastinum. The contents are

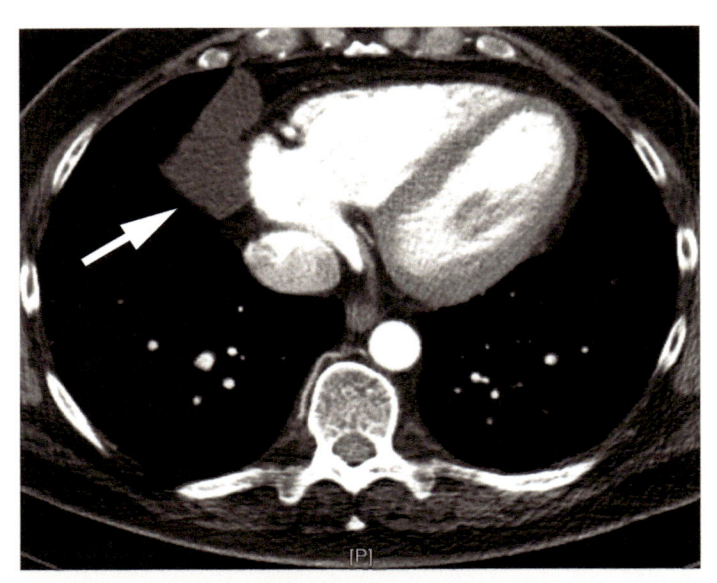

Fig. 1.25 Pericardial cyst. CT demonstrates a thin-walled cyst (arrow) of water attenuation that abuts the pericardium.

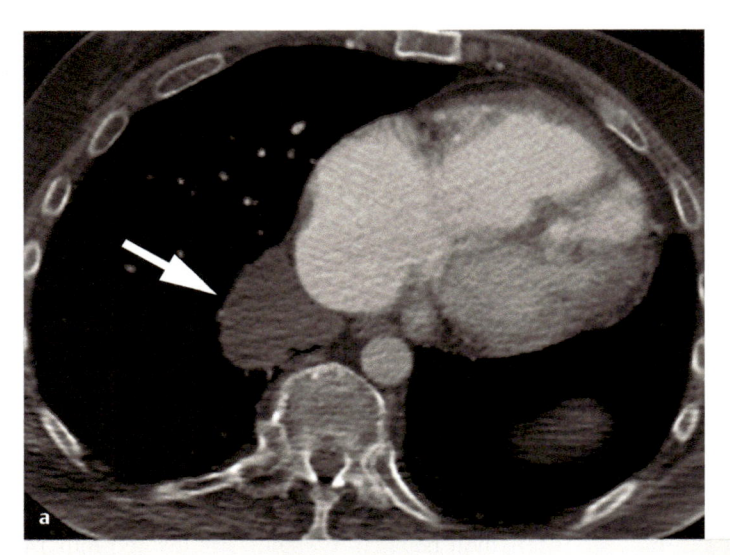

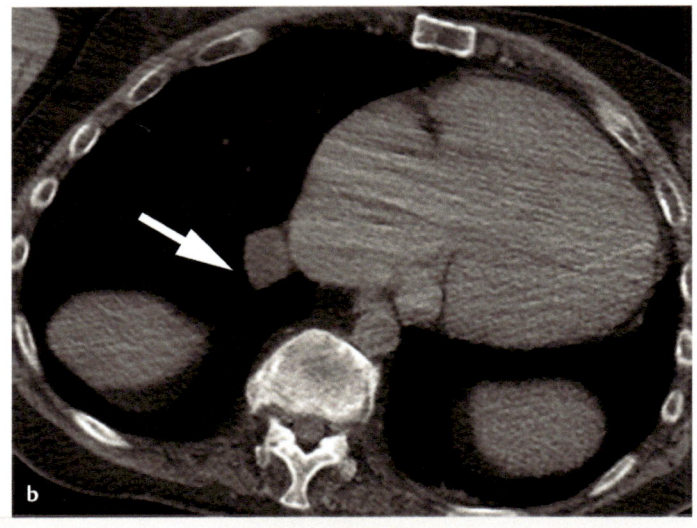

Fig. 1.26 Pericardial diverticulum detected incidentally in a patient with cor pulmonale. (a) CT shows a thin-walled paracardial mass of fluid attenuation (arrow). (b) A later scan documents spontaneous reduction in the size of the mass (arrow). This distinguishes it from a pericardial cyst and confirms the diagnosis of pericardial diverticulum.

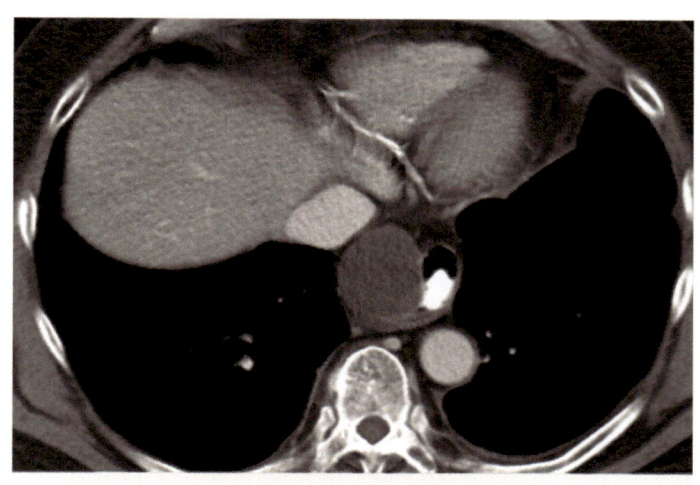

Fig. 1.27 Duplication of the esophagus. CT shows an immediate paraesophageal cyst that does not communicate with the esophageal lumen.

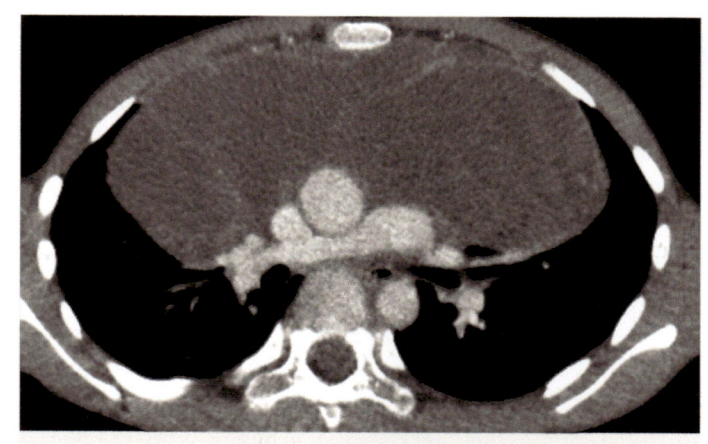

Fig. 1.28 Lymphangioma in the anterior mediastinum. Axial CT demonstrates the septated cystic mass.

isodense to water on CT and may show soft tissue density due to intracystic hemorrhage. Postcontrast enhancement is limited to the cyst wall. As with other types of cyst, T2 W MRI shows high signal intensity (or low intensity after intracystic hemorrhage), while T1 W images show absent or moderate signal depending on the protein content of the cyst fluid. Esophageal duplication cysts occur in the distal part of the esophagus in the posterior mediastinum. Most are entirely extramural, but some may be located within the esophageal wall (▶ Fig. 1.27). They often have an elliptical shape with a longitudinal orientation.

▶ **Clinical features.** Esophageal duplication cysts may lead to esophageal compression and dysphagia, but most are asymptomatic and are detected incidentally on chest imaging.

▶ **Differential diagnosis.** Differentiation from bronchogenic cysts is not always possible on the basis of imaging appearance alone.

▶ **Key points.** Esophageal duplication cysts are usually an incidental imaging finding. They are in contact with the esophagus and display the typical characteristics of cysts on sectional images, depending on the protein content of the cyst and possible intracystic hemorrhage.

Lymphangioma and Cystic Hygroma

▶ **Brief definition.** Lymphangioma and cystic hygroma are congenital malformations of the lymphatic system formed by heterotopic tissue from one of the five embryonic lymph sacs. This sequestration most commonly arises from the jugular lymph sac, with the result that 75% of these cystic masses are located in the neck. Lymphangiomas may already be present at birth or may present clinically during the second year of life, when the greatest growth of the lymphatic system takes place. A lymphangioma may be of the capillary or the cavernous type, depending on the size of its internal spaces. Cystic hygroma is a special form that consists of multiple large cysts.

▶ **Imaging signs.** Lymphangioma and cystic hygroma may contain solid components interspersed among the cysts. Ultrasonography can demonstrate the cystic nature of the mass. Hygromas are hypodense on CT scans, and only their solid portions enhance (▶ Fig. 1.28). The cysts are hyperintense on T2 W MRI. Their signal intensity on T1 W images depends on their protein content and on possible intracystic hemorrhage, which produces visible fluid levels within the cyst. Only the solid components enhance.

▶ **Clinical features.** Lymphangioma and cystic hygroma are usually apparent at birth, appearing as a tense swelling in the neck or upper chest. Infection may lead to acute enlargement and compression of the trachea, esophagus, or vessels. Dysphagia and dyspnea may occur acutely or develop over time.

> **Note**
> An accurate description of the tumor's extent and surrounding structures is important if surgical excision of the lymphangioma or cystic hygroma is intended.

▶ **Differential diagnosis.** Lymphangioma and cystic hygroma may occur in all areas of the mediastinum. They are composed almost entirely of cysts, so generally their diagnosis should present no difficulties. The lack of enhancement of the contents of the cyst serves to distinguish them from vascular malformations and cavernomas.

▶ **Key points.** Lymphangioma and cystic hygroma are congenital malformations of the lymphatic system. They may contain solid elements in addition to typical cystic components. Intracystic hemorrhage with fluid levels is a typical imaging finding.

1.4.2 Middle Mediastinum

Conditions in the middle mediastinum predominantly involve the lymph nodes.

▶ **Anatomy.** The lymph nodes in the chest are divided into 14 stations described by the American Joint Committee on Cancer (AJCC) and the Union for International Cancer Control (UICC; or

Table 1.2 Lymph node stations of the mediastinum based on the 1997 classification of the AJCC and UICC[17]

Station	Location
Mediastinal	
1 R/L	Superior mediastinum (cranial to brachiocephalic vein)
2 R/L	Upper paratracheal
3	• Retrotracheal (designated as 3P) • Prevascular (designated as 3A)
4 R/L	Lower paratracheal (R: includes the azygos nodes)
5	Aortic window, pulmonary trunk
6	Para-aortic to the level of the aortic arch
7	Subcarinal
8	Paraesophageal, subcarinal
9	Pulmonary ligament
Pulmonary (within the visceral pleura)	
10 R/L	Hilar
11 R/L	Interlobar
12 R/L	Lobar
13 R/L	Segmental
14 R/L	Subsegmental

Note: R/L designates the right or left side. Lymph node stations without an R/L designation are located in the midline.

Union Internationale Contre le Cancer), as shown in ▶ Table 1.2. Nine of the lymph node stations are located in the mediastinum (▶ Fig. 1.29).

Sarcoidosis

▶ **Brief definition.** Sarcoidosis is a multisystem disease of unknown etiology in which an abnormal immune response provokes the formation of noncaseating granulomas that contain epithelioid cells, multinucleated giant cells, and lymphocytes. These granulomas may form almost anywhere in the body but occur predominantly in the lung and mediastinal lymph nodes. The peak incidence of the disease is at 40 years of age, with a slight female predilection. The number of new cases per year is approximately 10 to 12 per 100,000 population. Pulmonary and mediastinal sarcoidosis is classified into four radiographic stages (▶ Table 1.3). Bilateral lymphadenopathy develops in 80% of sarcoidosis patients. The treatment of sarcoidosis is geared toward clinical complaints; acute cases are managed with oral steroids. Up to 95% of acute sarcoidosis cases resolve spontaneously over a period of several months. Chronic sarcoidosis is associated with permanent impairment of lung function in 20 to 30% of patients, with progression to pulmonary fibrosis occurring in 10%.

▶ **Imaging signs.** The chest radiograph shows symmetrical enlargement of the hilar lymph nodes. Enlargement of the mediastinal lymph nodes causes widening of the mediastinum. The mediastinal lymphadenopathy in sarcoidosis has a markedly symmetrical appearance on axial CT (▶ Fig. 1.30). Symmetrical involvement of the hila is also seen in most cases. Over time, approximately 40% of patients develop an eggshell pattern of lymph node calcification. Stage 2 disease is marked by the appearance of reticulonodular changes with nodules up to 5 mm in diameter; they are usually bilateral. The granulomas show a typical subpleural distribution along lymphatic vessels, along interlobar fissures, accompanying the bronchovascular bundles, and along interlobular septa. This pattern of involvement on CT is diagnostic of sarcoidosis.

▶ **Clinical features.** The clinical presentation includes B symptoms that may be associated with dry cough, dyspnea, arthritis, erythema nodosum, and facial nerve palsy depending on the pattern of involvement. Clinical and radiological suspicion is confirmed by bronchoalveolar lavage, which indicates a greater than 2:1 ratio of $CD4^+$ to $CD8^+$ T cells (T-helper cells and T-suppressor cells).

▶ **Key points.** Symmetrical enlargement of the hilar lymph nodes (station 10) and mediastinal nodes is characteristic of sarcoidosis. The nodules in stage 2 disease show a typical distribution on CT: peribronchial along the lymphatics, subpleural, and along the interlobar fissures.

Lymphoma

▶ **Brief definition.** Lymphomas are neoplasms of the lymphatic system. They are divided into two main groups: Hodgkin's lymphoma (lymphogranulomatosis) and non-Hodgkin's lymphoma. The incidence of all lymphomas is approximately 12 new cases per 100,000 population per year.

- *Hodgkin's lymphoma* has a bimodal age distribution with peaks in young adults (15 to 35 years) and after age 50 years. Generally the disease starts in a localized nodal region and then spreads to adjacent lymph node stations. Affected lymph nodes are enlarged and painless. The lymph nodes of the anterior mediastinum are affected in 60% of patients (▶ Fig. 1.31, ▶ Fig. 1.32). Over time the disease spreads from the initial site to adjacent nodal stations and then to extranodal tissues. Untreated, it leads to death. Treatment depends on histological subtype in the Rye classification (lymphocyte-predominant, nodular sclerosis, mixed cellularity, lymphocyte depletion). One histological characteristic of Hodgkin lymphoma is the presence of (multinucleated) Sternberg–Reed giant cells and large blasts (Hodgkin cells).
- *Non-Hodgkin's lymphomas* are a heterogeneous group of lymphomas composed of various cell types, include T-cell and B-cell lymphomas, and have a peak incidence in older adults. The incidence is greatly increased in immunosuppressed patients (organ recipients, AIDS sufferers). Besides the dysregulation of immune homeostasis, chromosomal translocations play an important role in the pathogenesis of non-Hodgkin's lymphoma. The majority of cases present with painless lymph node swelling, similar to lymphogranulomatosis. The abdominal lymph nodes are more commonly affected than the mediastinal nodes. Non-Hodgkin's lymphoma tends to affect lymph node stations not typically involved by Hodgkin's lymphoma (▶ Fig. 1.33) such as the posterior mediastinal nodes. Low- and high-grade non-Hodgkin's lymphomas are distinguishable by their clinical course and histology. The Kiel classification identifies subtypes based on the predominance of "cytes" or "blasts." As with Hodgkin's lymphoma, treatment is based on tumor histology.

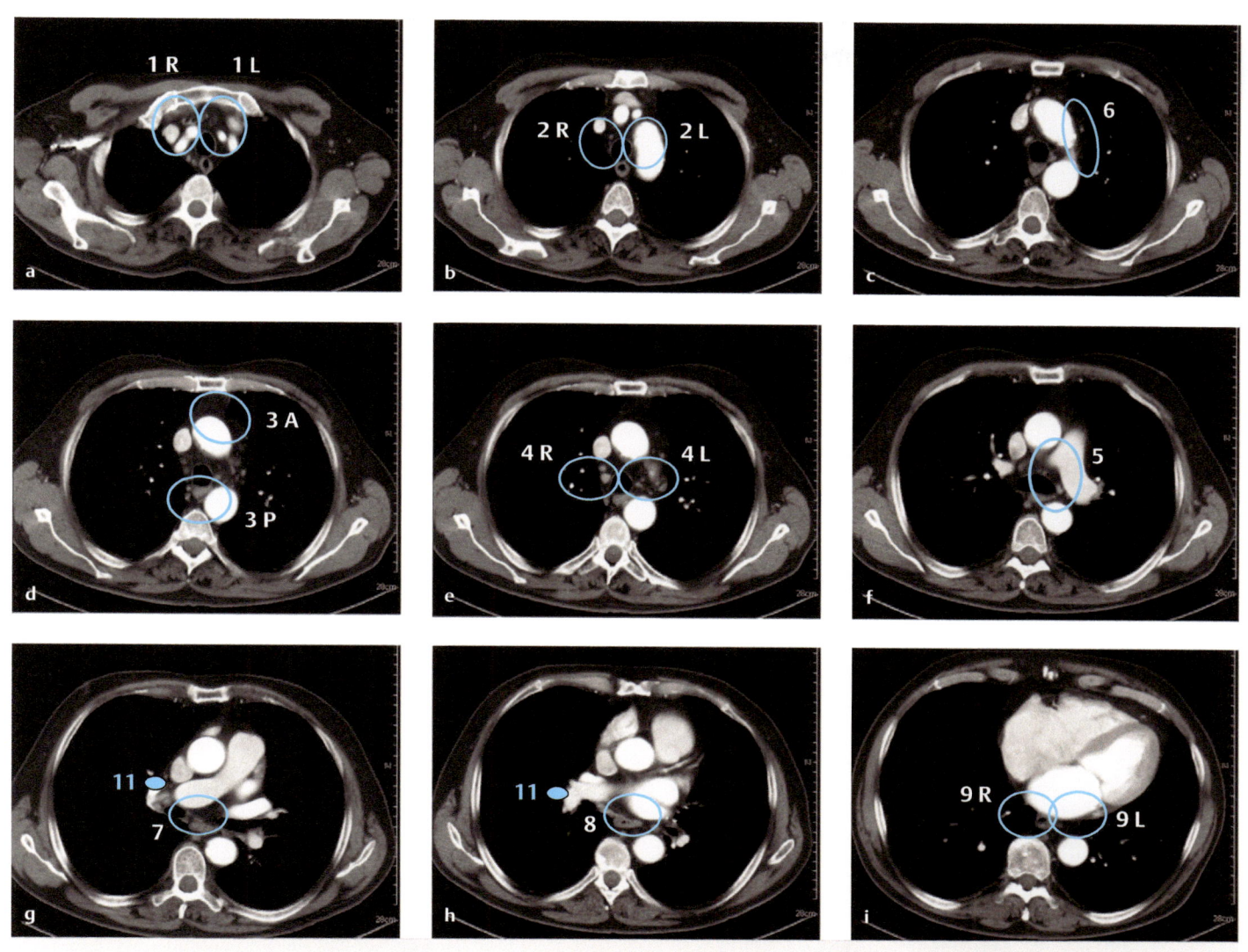

Fig. 1.29 Lymph node stations (light blue outlines) **in the mediastinum based on the 1997 classification of the AJCC and UICC.**[17] R/L designates the side (right/left). Lymph node stations without a R/L designation (5 to 8) refer to unpaired sites. Other, unmarked lymph node stations are station 12 (lobar), station 13 (segmental), and station 14 (segmental). Stations 11 to 14 are parabronchial. **(a)** Station 1 (high mediastinal). **(b)** Station 2 (high paratracheal). **(c)** Station 6 (para-aortic). **(d)** Station 3 (prevascular, retrotracheal). **(e)** Station 4 (low paratracheal, tracheobronchial). **(f)** Station 5 (subaortic [aortopulmonary window]). **(g)** Station 7 (subcarinal) and station 10 (hilar). **(h)** Station 8 (paraesophageal) and station 11 (interlobar). **(i)** Station 9 (pulmonary ligament).

Table 1.3 Staging of sarcoidosis

Stage	Description
0	Normal chest radiograph
1	Thoracic lymphadenopathy
2	Thoracic lymphadenopathy and lung changes
3	Nodular lung changes without thoracic lymphadenopathy
4	Pulmonary fibrosis

▶ **Imaging signs.** The chest radiograph shows enlargement of the hilar lymph nodes and opacity of the aortopulmonary window due to lymphadenopathy, or a large well-circumscribed mass usually located in the anterior mediastinum or at other sites in the case of non-Hodgkin's lymphoma. Large lymphomas generally encase vessels without occluding them (see ▶ Fig. 1.32). Vascular compression occurs only with very large tumors and then is limited chiefly to veins.

▶ **Clinical features.** Lymphomas typically present with B symptoms, consisting of fever, night sweats, and weight loss. Affected lymph nodes are enlarged and painless.

Caution

In the work-up of lymphoma, do not use a fine needle for the percutaneous biopsy of lymph nodes. Use an 18G or 16G core needle to ensure that the pathologist will have enough tissue with which to determine the histological type.

▶ **Differential diagnosis.** The differential diagnosis of large lymphomas should include sarcoma. The enhancement characteristics of the two entities may be identical. Sarcomas are distinguished by their tendency to compress and occlude blood vessels.

▶ **Key points.** Lymphomas are divided into *Hodgkin's lymphoma*, characterized histologically by Sternberg–Reed giant cells with

Mediastinum

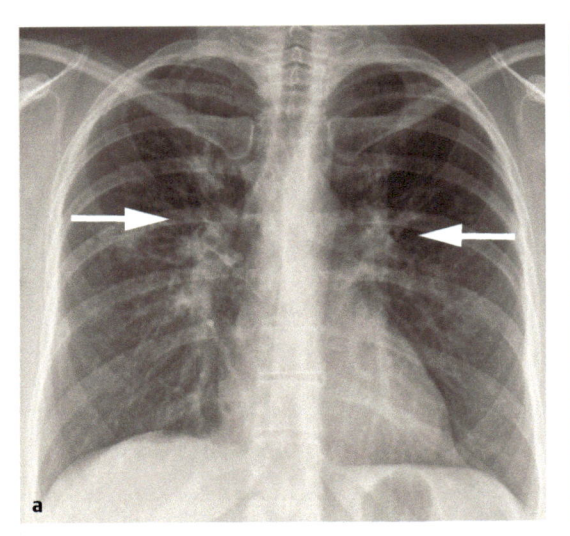

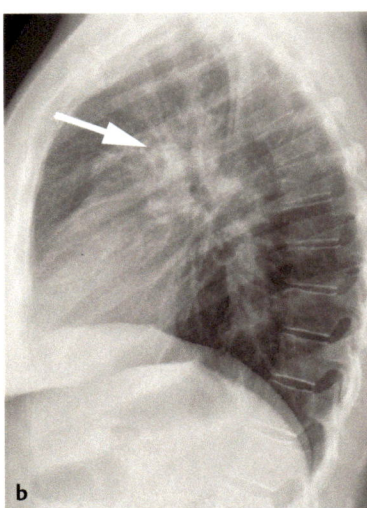

Fig. 1.30 Sarcoidosis. (a) Stage 1 and 2 disease is marked by symmetrical, bihilar lymphadenopathy (arrows). **(b)** Opacity of the aortopulmonary window due to lymphadenopathy (arrow; for landmarks see ▶ Fig. 1.2). **(c)** Axial CT shows symmetrical enlargement of the lymph nodes at stations 7, 8, and 10 R and L.

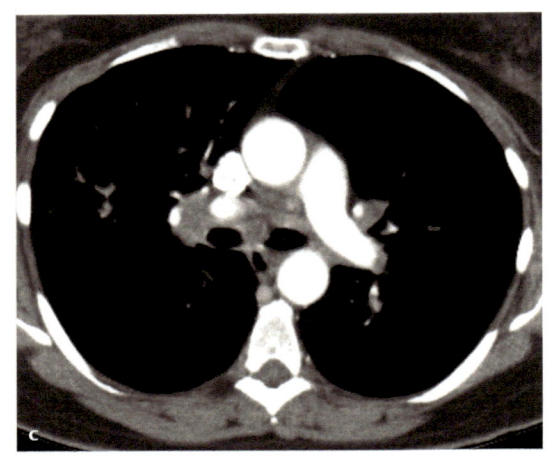

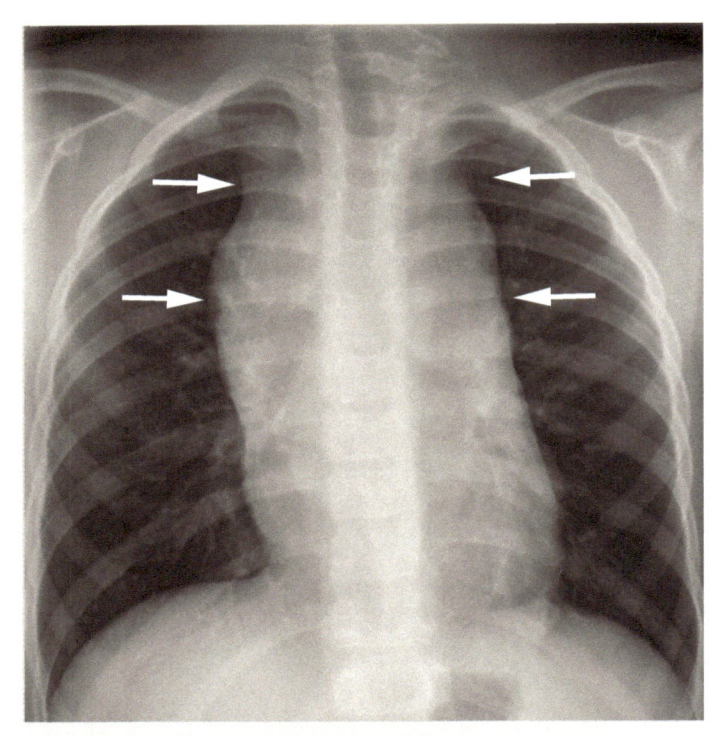

Fig. 1.31 Hodgkin's lymphoma. The lymphoma has caused a typical "chimney" appearance of mediastinal widening (arrows). The lateral radiograph showed opacity of the retrosternal space and superior mediastinum.

multiple cell nuclei and Hodgkin cells (large blasts), and *non-Hodgkin's lymphomas*, a histologically diverse group of B-cell and T-cell tumors. Lymph node enlargement is a characteristic feature. Lymphomas are diagnosed histologically. Percutaneous CT-guided biopsy requires a core needle, as fine-needle aspiration is inadequate for classification. The role of CT is to provide an accurate description of all affected lymph node stations and sites of extranodal involvement.

Castleman's Disease (Angiofollicular Hyperplasia)

▶ **Brief definition.** The pathologist Benjamin Castleman's first described this rare disease in the 1950s.[10] Its prevalence is estimated at 1 per 1 million population. Today the disease is attributed to infection with human herpesvirus 8, which is also responsible for Kaposi sarcomas in AIDS. The cytokine interleukin-6 leads to immune dysregulation with the proliferation of lymphocytes. In the more common hyaline vascular type of Castleman's disease, the lymph node follicles are characterized by regressive changes in the germinal centers and thickening of the mantle zone, which contains many very small lymphocytes. In the plasma cell type of Castleman's disease, the germinal centers are hypertrophic due to the accumulation of polyclonal plasma cells. In addition, a localized form of Castleman's disease is distinguished from a multicentric form with multiple sites of occurrence. The localized form

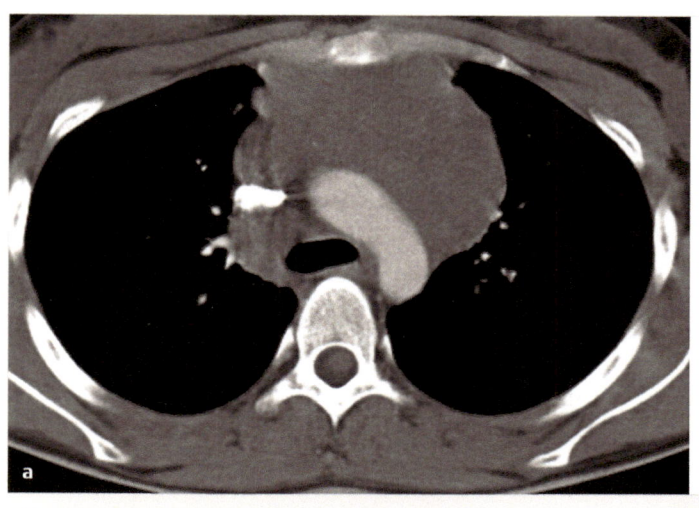

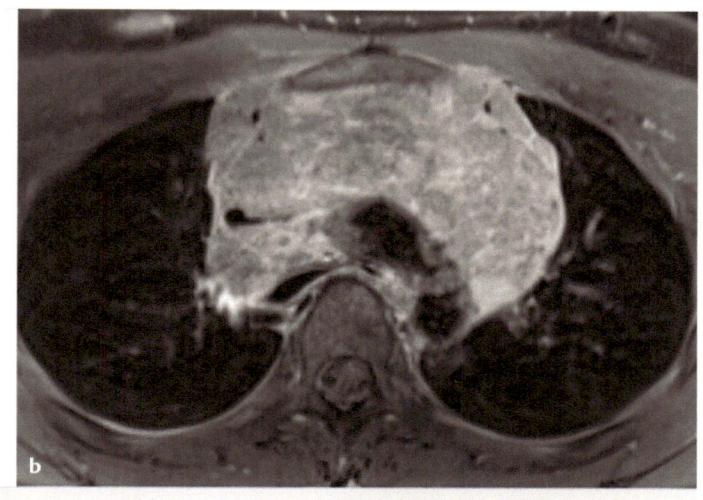

Fig. 1.32 Hodgkin's lymphoma. (a) The mass shows slight contrast enhancement on CT. There is no evidence of vascular compression. **(b)** T1 W MRI with fat suppression after IV injection of contrast medium.

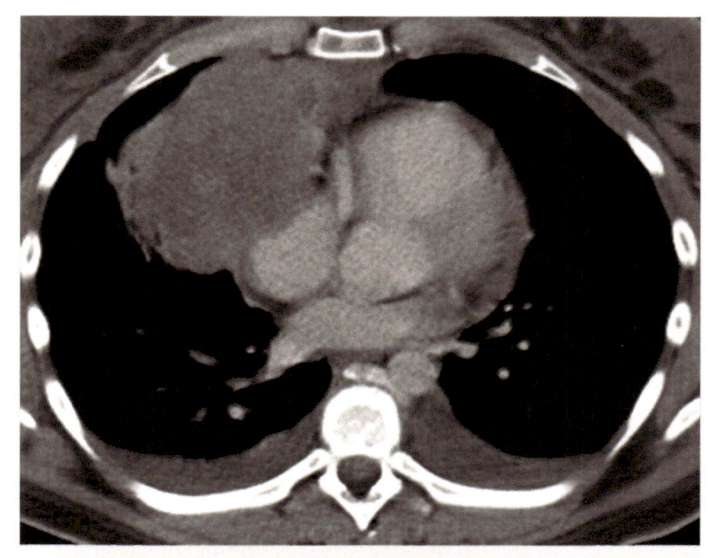

Fig. 1.33 B-cell lymphoma. The tumor shows slight, inhomogeneous enhancement on CT. The differential diagnosis would include sarcoma.

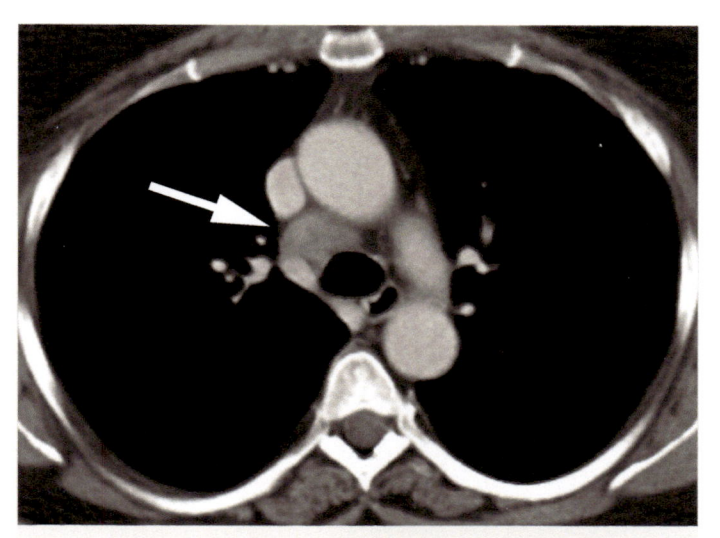

Fig. 1.34 Castleman's disease. CT demonstrates markedly enlarged station 4R lymph nodes (arrow) that show intense, homogeneous enhancement.

has an excellent prognosis, and excision of the isolated focus is generally curative. The multicentric form is associated with a much poorer prognosis.

▶ **Imaging signs.** The chest radiograph shows a mediastinal mass or lymphadenopathy that is indistinguishable from the changes characteristic of lymphoma. Both types of Castleman's disease are associated with the proliferation of blood vessels among the affected enlarged and confluent lymph nodes, resulting in intense enhancement on CT and MRI (▶ Fig. 1.34). Three distinct CT patterns have been described[11]:
- Approximately 50% of all patients have a solitary, noninvasive mass.
- In 40% of patients the mass is invasive and accompanied by lymphadenopathy.
- The remaining 10% of patients show lymph node enlargement at a single nodal station in the mediastinum.

Calcifications are found within the masses in up to 10% of cases.

▶ **Clinical features.** The more common hyaline vascular type of Castleman's disease is usually asymptomatic. The less common plasma cell type is associated with B symptoms, most notably fever and anemia. The unifocal form has a very good prognosis, and surgical resection of the tissue is curative in most cases. The multifocal form is associated with a poorer prognosis. It is treatable with chemotherapy and radiation, but often the disease will still progress to lymphoma. One study in patients with the plasma cell type reported a 20% incidence of non-Hodgkin's lymphoma over an approximately 2-year period.[12]

▶ **Differential diagnosis.** The main differentiation required is that from lymphoma and this is aided by the intense, homogeneous lesion enhancement that occurs in Castleman's disease.

▶ **Key points.** The localized form limited to a single site is distinguished from the multifocal form and is curable by local excision. The hyaline vascular type of Castleman's disease is distinguished from the plasma cell type. Both are characterized by enlarged lymph nodes that show intense, homogeneous enhancement.

1.4.3 Posterior Mediastinum

The most common masses in the posterior mediastinum are neurogenic tumors. Extramedullary hematopoiesis and hernias may also manifest in that region.

Neurogenic Tumors

Schwannoma (Neurinoma)

▶ **Brief definition.** Schwannomas (synonym: neurinomas) are common benign tumors that arise from the Schwann sheath cells of peripheral nerves and have a true fibrous capsule. Schwannomas may occur at any age but are most prevalent in young adults (the fourth to sixth decades). Histologically, areas with compact cells in a "shoal-of-fish" arrangement, palisading nuclei, and high vascular density (Antoni type A) are distinguished from hypocellular areas with a myxoid stroma (Antoni type B).

▶ **Imaging signs.** Schwannomas appear on chest radiographs as well-circumscribed tumors in the posterior mediastinum. Schwannomas show intense contrast enhancement on CT and MR images. On MRI, schwannomas are hypointense on unenhanced T1 W images and hyperintense on T2 W images. Regressive changes (cystic areas, calcifications, fat deposits) are common and are independent of tumor size. Generally speaking, the nerve from which the tumor arises can be visualized (▶ Fig. 1.35).

> **Note**
>
> It is typical for schwannomas to protrude from neural foramina, forming a dumbbell-shaped mass that enlarges the foramen. It is also common for schwannomas to grow along a nerve in the posterior mediastinum below the ribs.

▶ **Clinical features.** Most benign neurogenic tumors (schwannoma/neurinoma, neurofibroma) are asymptomatic and are detected incidentally at chest radiography, CT, or MRI. Some lesions may cause dysesthesia if sensory nerve branches are involved. The treatment of choice is complete surgical excision.

▶ **Key points.** Schwannomas are benign tumors of Schwann cells that develop on peripheral nerves. Spinal schwannomas tend to widen the neural exit foramina. They appear on sectional imaging as well-circumscribed, intensely enhancing lesions.

Neurofibroma

▶ **Brief definition.** Neurofibromas are benign tumors that arise from peripheral nerve sheaths. They are distinguished histologically from schwannomas by the involvement of mesenchymal cells of the peri- and epineurium (endo- and perineural fibroblasts) and the absence of a capsule. Neurofibromas may show a localized or diffuse growth pattern, and the lesions may be solitary (negative family history) or multiple in neurofibromatosis type 1 (von Recklinghausen's disease). Neurofibromatosis type 1 is a phacomatosis with neurocutaneous manifestations and the involvement of multiple organ systems. The disease has an autosomal dominant mode of inheritance and an incidence of 1 in 3,000 births. Approximately 50% of all new cases are spontaneous mutations. A defect on the long arm of chromosome 17 is responsible for neurofibroma formation. Neurofibromatosis type 1 is characterized by the development of multiple neurofibromas on peripheral nerves, café au lait spots on the skin, sphenoid dysplasia, pigmented iris nodules, and optic nerve glioma. Plexiform neurofibromas are pathognomonic for neurofibromatosis type 1. They occur in very early childhood, preceding the appearance of cutaneous neurofibromas, and involve a long nerve segment including its branches. The neurofibromas in neurofibromatosis type 1 have a 4% likelihood of malignant transformation. One clinical feature of neurofibromas is their rapidly progressive growth. Only about 10% of patients with a solitary neurofibroma are diagnosed with neurofibromatosis.

▶ **Imaging signs.** Neurofibroma appears on CT as a well-circumscribed mass that is isodense or hypodense to muscle on unenhanced images and usually shows predominantly central enhancement. On MRI, neurofibromas are hyperintense in T2 W images due to their myxoid stroma (▶ Fig. 1.36) and enhance intensely on T1 W images after IV administration of contrast medium.

▶ **Clinical features.** Neurofibromas may be asymptomatic or may cause symptoms due to the compression of surrounding structures. Rapid growth of a neurofibroma suggests malignant transformation.

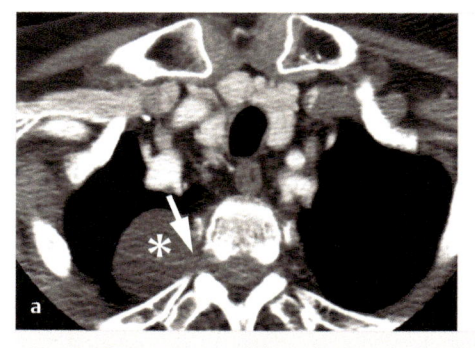

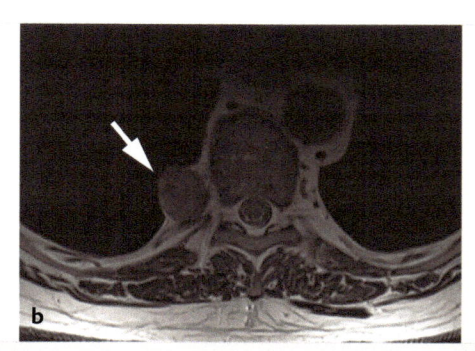

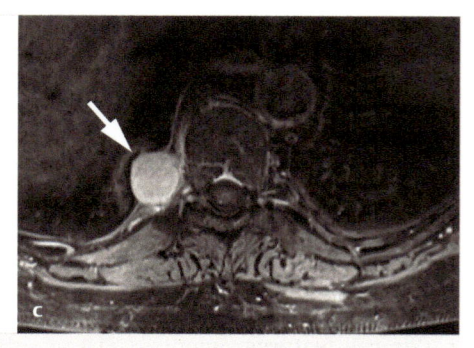

Fig. 1.35 Neurinoma. (a) CT displays the tumor (asterisk) as a dumbbell-shaped mass growing through the neural foramen and enlarging it (arrow). (b) T2 W MRI in a different patient demonstrates the location of the tumor (arrow) in relation to surrounding structures. (c) T1 W image in the same patient after IV administration of contrast medium shows marked enhancement of the neurinoma (arrow).

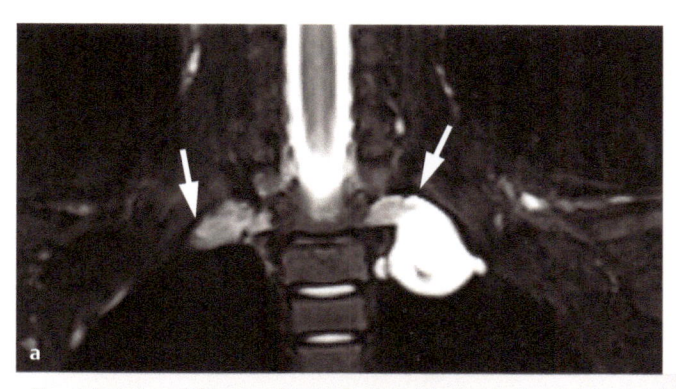

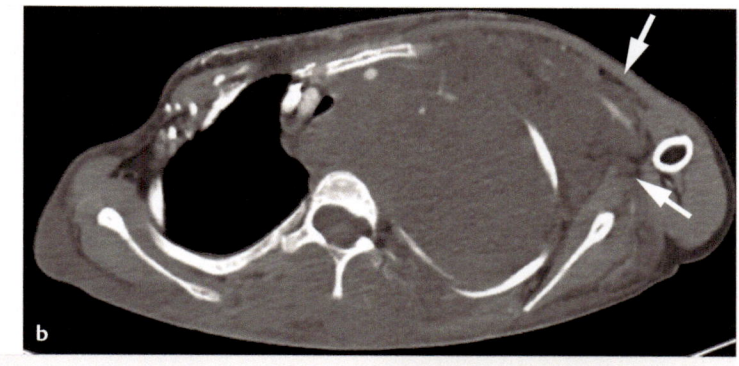

Fig. 1.36 Neurofibroma. (a) The tumors (arrows) show high signal intensity on T2 W MRI. **(b)** CT scan in a different patient with a large neurofibroma involving peripheral nerves (arrows). The tumor shows only slight enhancement.

▶ **Differential diagnosis.** Neurofibromas and malignant nerve sheath tumors cannot always be positively differentiated from one another at imaging. Nevertheless, a well-circumscribed tumor with predominantly central enhancement and a target pattern on T2 W MRI is typical of neurofibroma, whereas irregular, predominantly peripheral enhancement of a tumor with indistinct margins is suggestive of malignant transformation.

▶ **Key points.** Neurofibromas are benign tumors that arise from peripheral nerve sheaths. They are distinguished histologically from schwannoma by the involvement of mesenchymal cells of the perineurium and epineurium. Neurofibromatosis type 1 is characterized by the formation of multiple tumors along peripheral nerves. At imaging, neurofibromas have smooth margins and show intense, predominantly central enhancement after IV administration of contrast medium. Neurofibromas are hyperintense on T2 W MRI due to their myxoid stroma.

Neuroblastoma

▶ **Brief definition.** Neuroblastoma is an embryonic cell tumor derived from neural-crest progenitor cells of the autonomic nervous system. The peak incidence of this tumor occurs in infancy; the average age at diagnosis is 17 months. The incidence is 1 in 5,000 births. After Wilms's tumor, neuroblastoma is the second most common malignancy in children under 3 years of age.[13] Only 15% of all neuroblastomas occur in the mediastinum. Mediastinal neuroblastomas arise from the sympathetic trunk.

▶ **Imaging signs.** Chest radiographs show a posterior mass that disrupts the paraspinal line on the affected side (see ▶ Fig. 1.37). On CT, calcifications are found in the tumor matrix of thoracic neuroblastomas in up to 80% of cases. The masses are inhomogeneous and contain areas of relatively low density. Only moderate enhancement is seen on CT and MRI. The T1 and T2 times are prolonged on MRI, resulting in low signal intensity on unenhanced T1 W images and high signal intensity on T2 W images. A characteristic feature is tumor ingrowth into the spinal canal through the neural foramina. In some cases this is defined more clearly by MRI than by CT (▶ Fig. 1.37).

▶ **Clinical features.** Symptoms in most children result from catecholamine production by the primary tumor or from metastasis. Elevated urinary vanillylmandelic acid, a catecholamine breakdown product, is found in 78% of patients. Elevated catecholamine levels in the blood may induce episodes of flushing and hypertension. Neuroblastomas of the sympathetic trunk may extend into the spinal canal and cause symptoms due to cord compression (paraparesis, pain, dysesthesia).

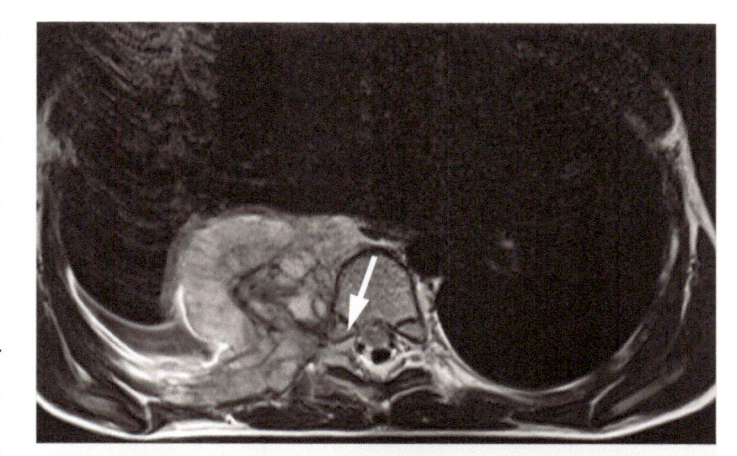

Fig. 1.37 Neuroblastoma. Same patient as in ▶ Fig. 1.3. Tumor ingrowth into the neural foramina (arrow) is clearly depicted in this T2 W MR image (but not on CT).

Note
Neuroblastomas occur at immediate paravertebral sites along the sympathetic trunk.

▶ **Differential diagnosis.** Neuroblastoma is virtually the only differential diagnosis for posterior mediastinal masses in very small children.

▶ **Key points.** Neuroblastoma is the first differential diagnosis for posterior mediastinal masses in small children. Laboratory findings and sectional imaging narrow the diagnosis. Ingrowth into the spinal canal through the neural foramina is typical and is clearly visualized by MRI.

Paraganglioma

▶ **Brief definition.** Paragangliomas are derived from the chromaffin cells of the paraganglia. Paragangliomas in the mediastinum arise from the vagus nerve and para-aortic ganglia. They may occur sporadically or may be inherited as an autosomal dominant trait. Although the tumor shows no histological signs of malignancy, it still metastasizes in 5% of cases. It has a reported growth rate of approximately 5 mm per year, with a peak age of incidence in the fourth and fifth decades. The incidence of paraganglioma is 1 per 1 million population per year. Paragangliomas are composed of chief cells and surrounded by a fibrous pseudocapsule. The tumor matrix is richly vascularized. Paragangliomas may show locally invasive growth.

▶ **Imaging signs.** Paragangliomas may occur in the course of the vagus nerve in the anterior mediastinum, at para-aortic sites, and at cardiac sites in the roof of the right atrium, in the posterior wall of the left ventricle, and in the atrial septum. Due to their rich blood supply, paragangliomas show prominent enhancement in all modalities. Paragangliomas appear as well-circumscribed tumors on CT (▶ Fig. 1.38). They are hyperintense in T2 W MR images and isointense to muscle in unenhanced T1 W images. A specific diagnosis requires clinical correlation with attention to potentially elevated catecholamine breakdown products in the urine. Hormonally inactive tumors require a histological diagnosis.

▶ **Clinical features.** Hormonally inactive tumors (50% of paragangliomas) mainly cause symptoms by compressing adjacent organs. Hormonally active (catecholamine-secreting) tumors lead to hypertension, hyperhydrosis, and flushing. The treatment of choice is complete surgical removal. Irradiation can be used for paragangliomas located at unfavorable sites or in inoperable patients, but radiotherapy is palliative.

▶ **Differential diagnosis.** The differential diagnosis should include neurinomas and metastases from hypervascular tumors such as renal cell carcinoma or neuroendocrine tumors.

▶ **Key points.** Paragangliomas may be locally invasive and metastasize in 5% of cases. They are richly vascularized and show correspondingly intense enhancement. Laboratory values (vanillylmandelic acid, a catecholamine breakdown product) should be considered in making the diagnosis.

Extramedullary Hematopoiesis

▶ **Brief definition.** Extramedullary hematopoiesis is a compensatory mechanism for severe anemia, usually occurring in the organs of the reticuloendothelial system (spleen, liver, and lymph nodes) and very rarely in other organs such as the kidneys, adrenal glands, or even the brain. It is attributed to the presence of ectopic pluripotent stem cells in parenchymal organs and lymph nodes. Intrathoracic extramedullary hematopoiesis may occur at paravertebral sites in the posterior inferior mediastinum. Based on current information, this results from the contiguous spread of hematopoietic marrow from the medullary cavities of the vertebral bodies and ribs. The recent literature consists mainly of individual case reports. In a small series of 29 patients with thalassemia, 65% of the patients were found to have paravertebral sites of extramedullary hematopoiesis in the chest.[14]

▶ **Imaging signs.** Imaging reveals lobulated paravertebral masses with smooth margins (▶ Fig. 1.39). CT shows masses of soft tissue density that are isoattenuating to spleen and have the same enhancement characteristics as the spleen. The hematopoietic tissue is isointense to spleen on MRI.

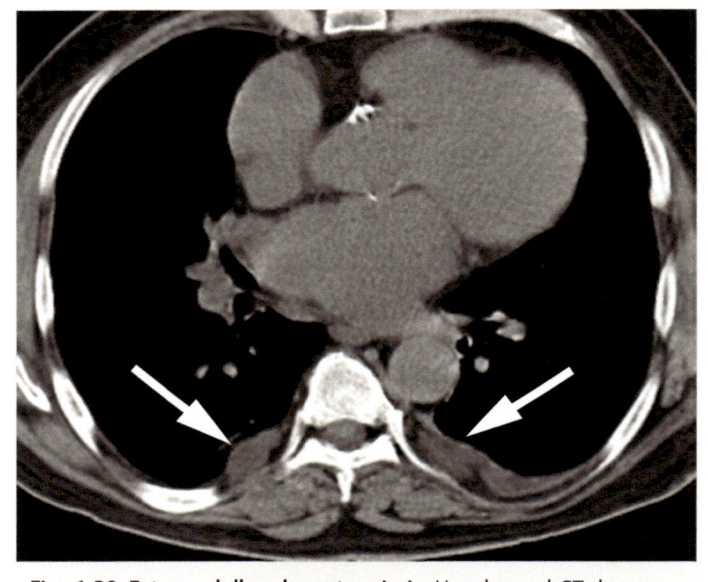

Fig. 1.39 Extramedullary hematopoiesis. Unenhanced CT shows multiple bilateral, paravertebral masses of soft tissue density (arrows).

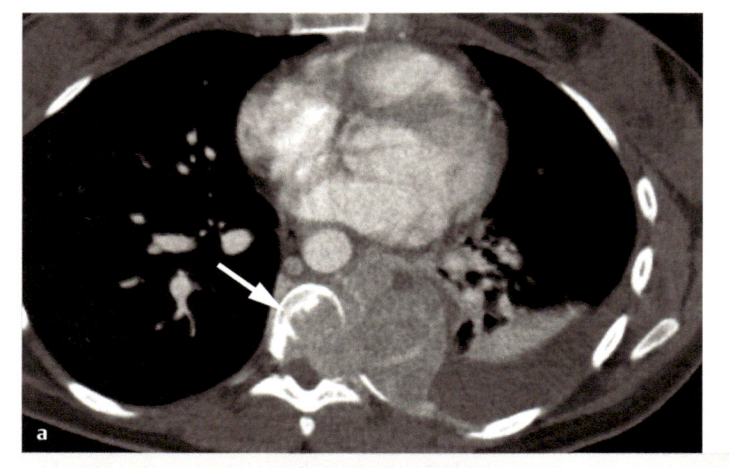

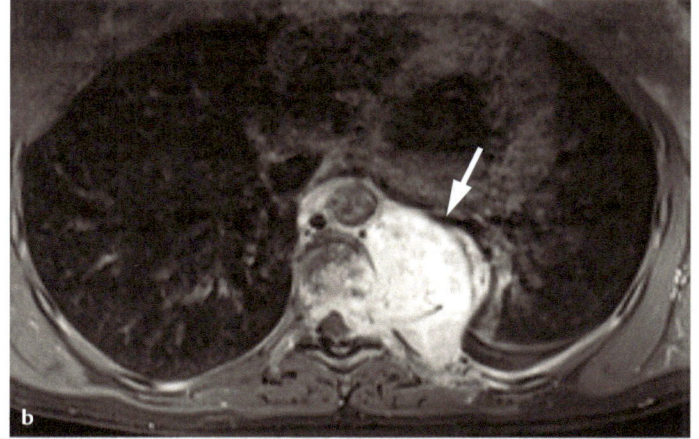

Fig. 1.38 Paraganglioma arising from a para-aortic ganglion. (a) CT demonstrates a paravertebral mass that is infiltrating the vertebral body (arrow) and shows homogeneous enhancement. (b) On T1 W MRI after IV administration of contrast medium, the tumor shows intense homogeneous enhancement (arrow).

1.4 Mediastinal Masses

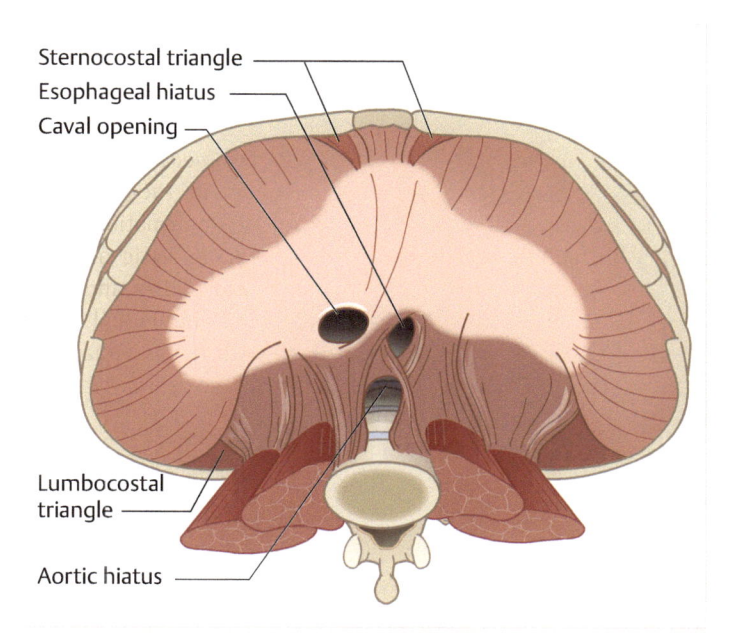

Fig. 1.40 Schematic representation of the diaphragm and its weak spots. Anterior: sternocostal triangle; posterolateral: Bochdalek triangle (lumbocostal triangle).

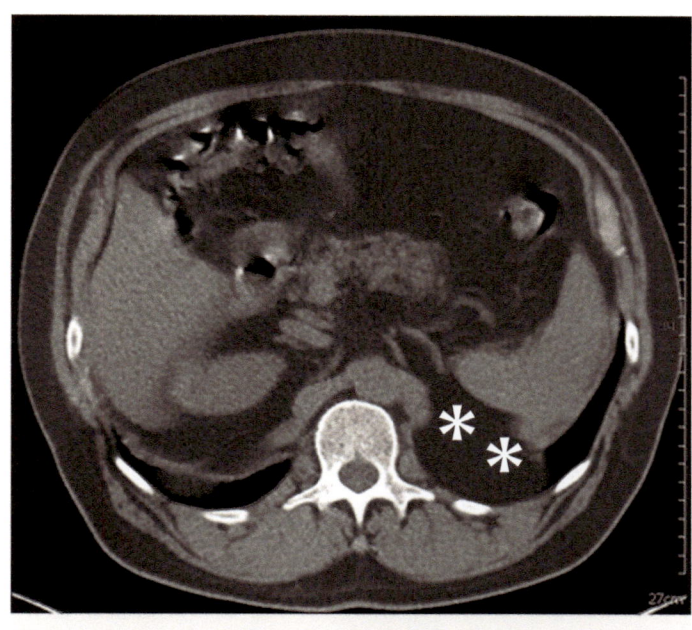

Fig. 1.41 Bochdalek hernia on the left side. CT demonstrates the hernia opening (asterisks), which is located posterolaterally at approximately the level of the renal upper pole.

▶ **Clinical features.** The dominant clinical features are those of the known disease underlying extramedullary hematopoiesis (myelofibrosis and hereditary anemias: thalassemia, sickle cell anemia, hereditary spherocytosis), while the extramedullary hematopoiesis itself is generally asymptomatic. Intraspinal extension with neurologic symptoms relating to cord compression has been described in a few cases.

> **Note**
>
> In equivocal cases where an underlying disease has not yet been identified, the diagnosis of extramedullary hematopoiesis can be established by fine needle aspiration biopsy.

▶ **Key points.** Sites of extramedullary hematopoiesis in the mediastinum appear as prevertebral and paravertebral masses that have the same characteristics as splenic tissue on sectional imaging.

Bochdalek, Morgagni, and Larrey Hernias

▶ **Brief definition.** The diaphragm has two anterior and two posterior regions that are devoid of muscle, are covered only by connective tissue, and form sites of predilection for diaphragmatic hernias (▶ Fig. 1.40):
- The *Bochdalek triangle* is a posterior region on each side of the diaphragm, located between the costal and lumbar muscle bundles, where a Bochdalek hernia may occur (▶ Fig. 1.41).
- The *sternocostal triangle* is an anterior parasternal region located at the sternocostal junction on each side. Abdominal contents, usually consisting of fat, greater omentum, or loops of small or large bowel, may herniate into the anterior inferior mediastinum through the right sternocostal triangle to form a Morgagni hernia (▶ Fig. 1.42) or through the left sternocostal triangle to form a Larrey hernia. Hiatal hernias are described in the chapter on the gastrointestinal tract.

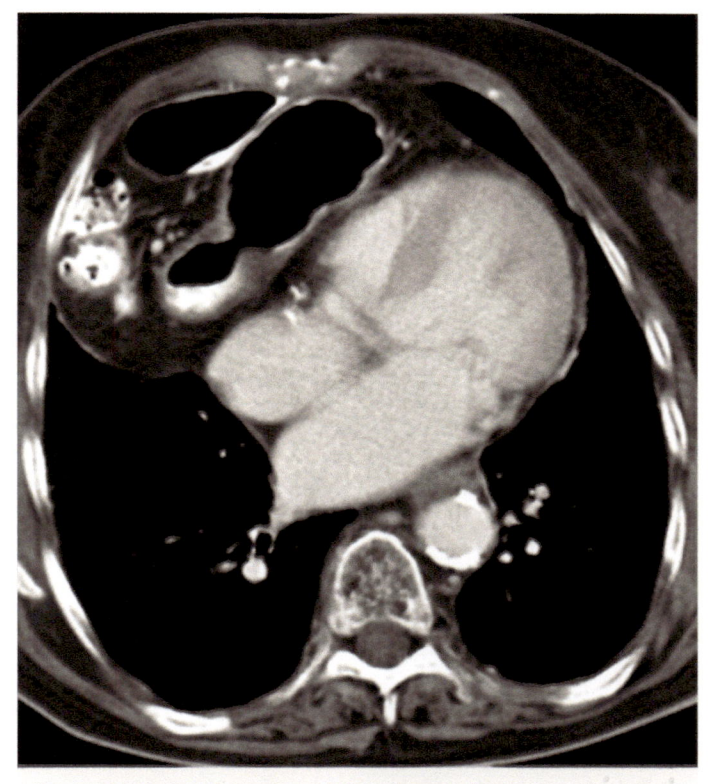

Fig. 1.42 Morgagni hernia with intrathoracic herniation of mesenteric fat and bowel loops.

▶ **Imaging signs**
- A *Bochdalek hernia* is usually detected incidentally on the lateral chest radiograph, appearing as a well-circumscribed opacity in the posterior inferior mediastinum. It is differentiated from a solid tumor (e.g., neurinoma) by CT, which demonstrates the herniation of fat or the upper renal pole through the lumbosacral triangle on the left side. A Bochdalek hernia on the right side is very rare because the liver covers the lumbosacral triangle on that side.

Mediastinum

- A *Morgagni hernia* or a *Larrey hernia* appears on the PA chest radiograph as a well-circumscribed paracardiac mass. The lateral radiograph localizes it to the anterior mediastinum. The Morgagni hernia (right-sided) is more common than the Larrey hernia (left-sided).[15] The defect in the diaphragm can be directly visualized by sectional imaging and the herniated fat, omentum, or bowel can be visually traced from the chest into the abdomen.

▶ **Clinical features**
- *Bochdalek hernias* are usually asymptomatic. With a small hernia, there may be pain due to incarceration of the herniated tissue. With a large hernia, displacement of the mediastinum and lung may lead to dyspnea and, less commonly, tachycardia. The defect should be surgically repaired in symptomatic patients.
- The majority of *Morgagni* and *Larrey hernias* are also asymptomatic and detected incidentally on the chest radiograph, CT, or MRI. Symptomatic patients may complain of retrosternal pressure, upper abdominal pain, or sudden and severe retrosternal pain in extremely rare cases of incarceration. As a general rule, Morgagni and Larrey hernias do not require treatment. Symptomatic patients can be treated by laparoscopic repair of the defect in the sternocostal triangle.

▶ **Pitfalls.** The lumbosacral triangle is located far laterally and posteriorly, well away from the esophageal hiatus. Axial and para-axial hernias should not be confused with a Bochdalek hernia. The upper pole of the kidney is located below the lumbosacral triangle and can provide a differentiating landmark.

▶ **Differential diagnosis.** If only the chest radiograph is available, the main differentiation required is from solid masses, depending on the nature of the herniated tissue.

▶ **Key points.** The sternocostal triangle, an anterior region located at the sternocostal junction on each side, is the site where a Morgagni hernia may occur on the right side or a Larrey hernia on the left side. The Bochdalek triangle is located posterolaterally between the costal and lumbar muscle bundles on each side and is the site where the eponymous hernia may form. These hernias appear on chest radiographs as masses of soft tissue density unless they include air-filled bowel loops. They are easily diagnosed on sectional images, which can define the hernial opening and herniated tissue.

1.5 Trauma with Mediastinal Injury: Pneumomediastinum

▶ **Brief definition.** Pneumomediastinum (mediastinal emphysema) refers to air in the mediastinum. It occurs in approximately 10% of patients who have sustained blunt trauma to the chest. It may also occur spontaneously due to a rise of intra-alveolar pressure in response to weight lifting, a Valsalva maneuver, vigorous coughing or vomiting, or barotrauma in divers or stunt pilots, for example. The pathogenic mechanism has been well understood since animal studies conducted in the 1930s: small tears in the alveoli permit air to escape into the interstitium. Because the pressure in the mediastinum is lower than in the peripheral lung, the air migrates centrally along the bronchovascular bundles. From there the air spreads along the anatomical structures of the mediastinum in the interstitium and may continue to spread into the neck and into the subcutaneous tissues of the limbs.[16] This mechanism also underlies the pneumothorax that occurs with blunt thoracic trauma. Generally these cases will resolve spontaneously, although this process will take several days due to the high nitrogen content of approximately 78% in room air (nitrogen has low solubility in blood). CT cannot demonstrate the small tears in the alveoli and therefore is not indicated in patients with a small pneumomediastinum whose cause cannot be determined from the history. CT is appropriate only in patients with a suspected severe tracheal injury following difficult intubation, for example. In contrast to pneumopericardium, in which the air collection is confined to the pericardium, the air crescent associated with a pneumomediastinum may extend far into the superior mediastinum (▶ Fig. 1.43).

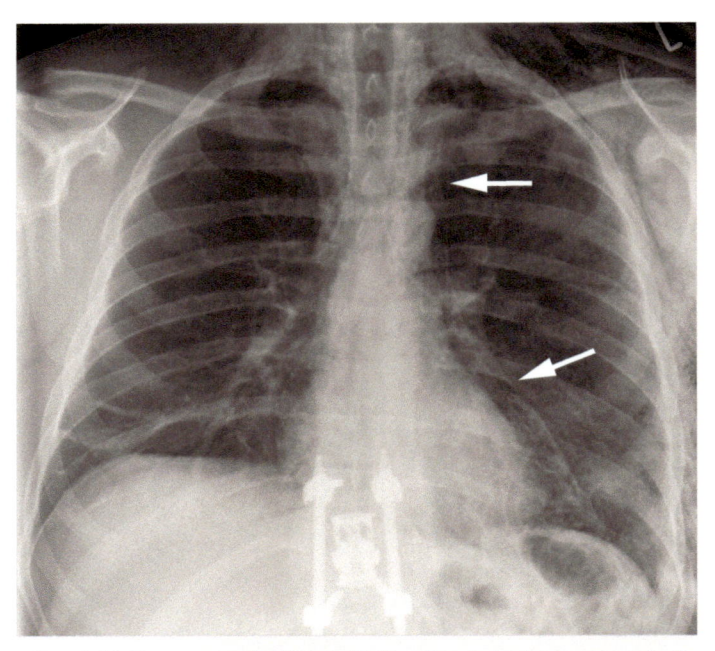

Fig. 1.43 Pneumomediastinum. Air has elevated a long segment of pleura away from the mediastinum (arrows).

▶ **Imaging signs.** Pneumomediastinum can usually be diagnosed on standard chest radiographs and a number of typical signs have been identified:
- The *continuous diaphragm sign* occurs when air is trapped between the pericardium and the diaphragm, and the diaphragm can be traced continuously across the midline from both sides of the chest in the AP or PA radiograph. The continuous diaphragm sign should not be mistaken for free air in the abdominal cavity.
- The *V sign* describes a V-shaped air collection in the left hemithorax between the diaphragm and paravertebral line.
- Air might be detectable as areas of hypertransparency around large vessels such as the aortic arch, superior vena cava, or azygos vein.
- Air in the interstitium around the bronchial wall creates high contrast between the bronchial wall and surrounding structures, causing the bronchus to form a visible ring when viewed in an end-on projection (the *bronchial ring sign*).

- Air around the thymus in young adults, adolescents, and children accentuates its typical bilobar structure. The *thymus sign* results from the silhouette phenomenon, in which structures of equal density are delineated by intervening material of a different density, in this case air.

▶ **Clinical features.** Pneumomediastinum leads to crepitus as a result of soft tissue emphysema in the neck. Patients with mild to moderate pneumomediastinum are usually asymptomatic. Some patients complain of pain radiating to the back of the neck. A large pneumomediastinum may cause dyspnea in rare cases.

▶ **Key points.** Pneumomediastinum (mediastinal emphysema) denotes the presence of air in the mediastinum, which occurs in approximately 10% of patients who have sustained blunt thoracic trauma but may also occur spontaneously due to a rise of intra-alveolar pressure (from weight lifting, vigorous coughing or vomiting, or barotrauma in divers or stunt pilots). It is caused by minute tears in the alveoli. CT is indicated only in patients with a suspected severe tracheal injury (usually iatrogenic after difficult intubation or bronchoscopy).

Bibliography

[1] Sandner A, Börgermann J. Update on necrotizing mediastinitis: causes, approaches to management, and outcomes. Curr Infect Dis Rep. 2011; 13 (3):278–286

[2] Ridder GJ, Maier W, Kinzer S, Teszler CB, Boedeker CC, Pfeiffer J. Descending necrotizing mediastinitis: contemporary trends in etiology, diagnosis, management, and outcome. Ann Surg. 2010; 251(3):528–534

[3] Jain D, Fishman EK, Argani P, Shah AS, Halushka MK. Unexpected sclerosing mediastinitis involving the ascending aorta in the setting of a multifocal fibrosclerotic disorder. Pathol Res Pract. 2011; 207(1):60–62

[4] Romagnoli M, Poletti V. Multifocal fibrosclerosis with lung, mediastinal, pancreatic and retroperitoneal involvement in a 58-year-old man. Sarcoidosis Vasc Diffuse Lung Dis. 2009; 26(1):73–75

[5] Nasseri F, Eftekhari F. Clinical and radiologic review of the normal and abnormal thymus: pearls and pitfalls. Radiographics. 2010; 30 (2):413–428

[6] Ströbel P, Marx A, Zettl A, Müller-Hermelink HK. Thymoma and thymic carcinoma: an update of the WHO Classification 2004. Surg Today. 2005; 35 (10):805–811

[7] Otsuka H. The utility of FDG-PET in the diagnosis of thymic epithelial tumors. J Med Invest. 2012; 59(3–4):225–234

[8] Sperger JM, Chen X, Draper JS, et al. Gene expression patterns in human embryonic stem cells and human pluripotent germ cell tumors. Proc Natl Acad Sci U S A. 2003; 100(23):13350–13355

[9] Mourra N, Lewin M, Parc Y. Clinical challenges and images in GI. Esophageal tubular duplication. Gastroenterology. 2008; 134(3):669–899

[10] Castleman B, Iverson L, Menendez VP. Localized mediastinal lymphnode hyperplasia resembling thymoma. Cancer. 1956; 9(4):822–830

[11] McAdams HP, Rosado-de-Christenson M, Fishback NF, Templeton PA. Castleman disease of the thorax: radiologic features with clinical and histopathologic correlation. Radiology. 1998; 209(1):221–228

[12] Oksenhendler E, Boulanger E, Galicier L, et al. High incidence of Kaposi sarcoma-associated herpesvirus-related non-Hodgkin lymphoma in patients with HIV infection and multicentric Castleman disease. Blood. 2002; 99 (7):2331–2336

[13] Papaioannou G, McHugh K. Neuroblastoma in childhood: review and radiological findings. Cancer Imaging. 2005; 5:116–127

[14] Dore F, Cianciulli P, Rovasio S, et al. Incidence and clinical study of ectopic erythropoiesis in adult patients with thalassemia intermedia. Ann Ital Med Int. 1992; 7(3):137–140

[15] Schubert H, Haage P. Images in clinical medicine. Morgagni's hernia. N Engl J Med. 2004; 351(13):e12

[16] Macklin CC. Histological indications of the sites of air leakage from the lung alveoli into the vascular sheaths during local overinflation of the living cat's lung. Can Med Assoc J. 1938; 38(4):401–402

[17] Mountain CF, Dresler CM. Regional lymph node classification for lung cancer staging. Chest. 1997; 111(6):1718–1723

2 Heart and Pericardium

Gabriele A. Krombach

2.1 Heart

2.1.1 Anatomy

Cardiac Borders

During embryogenesis, the heart initially forms as a symmetrical midline organ in the chest and subsequently undergoes a rotation in which the cardiac apex is slightly raised and rotated to the left. This process moves the right ventricle to a position directly behind the sternum. Approximately two-thirds of the heart is to the left of the midline and one-third is to the right. The left atrium rotates posteriorly; a blind pouch in its wall, the left atrial appendage, contains stretch receptors and forms atrial natriuretic peptide (ANP) in response to atrial wall distension.

▶ **Selection of modalities.** Chest radiography is the imaging modality of first choice for examining patients with unexplained cardiac disease. It is also useful in the follow-up of patients with known heart disease. CT is used for risk stratification and for imaging the coronary arteries in patients with an intermediate pretest probability. In evaluation of transcatheter aortic valve implantation (TAVI), CT is used to measure the dimensions of the aortic annulus and the distance between the origins of the coronary arteries. MRI is the gold standard for the quantification of regional and global cardiac function. For this the ventricles are covered with contiguous slices and their volumes are measured. This differs from echocardiography, in which the chamber volumes are not measured directly but derived from geometric assumptions based on short-axis and long-axis scans. As a result, the determination of functional parameters by echocardiography is imprecise, especially in diseased hearts with changes in ventricular shape. When it comes to perfusion imaging, MRI is superior to single-photon emission computed tomography (SPECT) in its sensitivity and specificity, and its use for detecting perfusion defects is already recommended in professional guidelines.[1] MRI is used for the assessment of myocardial viability after heart attacks. Additionally, MRI has become well established for the characterization of cardiomyopathies, the examination of patients with cardiac tumors, and the examination of patients with congenital heart disease based on its ability to measure flow and also to quantify cardiac function.

▶ **Radiographic landmarks**
- *PA radiograph* (standard projection for radiographs in the standing position):
  - The right atrium forms the right border of the cardiac silhouette. It forms a convex bulge toward the lung and is continuous superiorly with the superior vena cava (▶ Fig. 2.1).
  - The left ventricle forms the left border of the cardiac silhouette. Just above it is a small portion of the left atrial appendage and the left pulmonary trunk, followed by the aorta (see ▶ Fig. 2.1).
- Lateral radiograph:
  - The right ventricle forms the retrosternal border of the cardiac silhouette. It is continuous superiorly with its outflow tract, the pulmonary trunk.
  - The left atrium forms the posterior border (see ▶ Fig. 2.1). The inferior vena cava is visible inferiorly as a small triangle.

Cardiac Chambers (▶ Fig. 2.2)

The left ventricle is conical in shape. In a healthy heart, imaging of the left ventricle in slices directed at 90° to its long axis yields a series of circular cross sections of the chamber (▶ Fig. 2.3). Called "short-axis views" of the left ventricle, they represent the standard slice orientation for cardiac imaging by MRI, echocardiography, and CT. Volume measurements are easily performed in this slice orientation by scanning the left ventricle from the apex to the base (valvular plane) in contiguous slices and then summing the areas of the slices. The maximum wall thickness measured in the septum during diastole should not exceed 12 mm (▶ Fig. 2.4). The left ventricle contains the two papillary muscles (anterior and posterior papillary muscles). The muscles are connected to the mitral valve by fine tendons called the chordae tendineae. The left ventricle is less trabeculated than the right ventricle. This difference is grounded in embryogenesis: The myocardium of both ventricles initially has a spongy structure and is composed of very heavily trabeculated muscle tissue. The outer portions of each ventricle subsequently fuse to form a compact wall. This process is more pronounced on the left side than on the right, with the result that the left ventricle is less trabeculated but has a thicker wall.

> **Note**
>
> The maximum wall thickness of the left ventricle should not exceed 12 mm (measured in the septum during diastole). The maximum wall thickness of the right ventricle in a healthy individual is generally less than 6 mm, measured in the free wall of the right ventricle (see ▶ Fig. 2.4). Measurements that exceed those values indicate hypertrophy of the chamber in question. This hypertrophy may result from a chronic pressure increase due, for example, to pulmonary or aortic valve stenosis, arterial hypertension, or pulmonary hypertension. It may also result from a chronic (obstructive) hypertrophic cardiomyopathy due to a genetic cause.

▶ **Imaging landmarks.** A uniform slice orientation must be used in comparing different imaging modalities such as echocardiography or SPECT with MRI. The slice orientations in MRI are referred to the axes of the left ventricle, as in echocardiography, so as to obtain reproducible imaging planes (see ▶ Fig. 2.3). The position of the diaphragm, which is influenced by the volume of intraabdominal fat, contributes to positional variants such as a heart that is broadly apposed to the diaphragm or one that is narrower and more upright. The orientation of the slices must accordingly

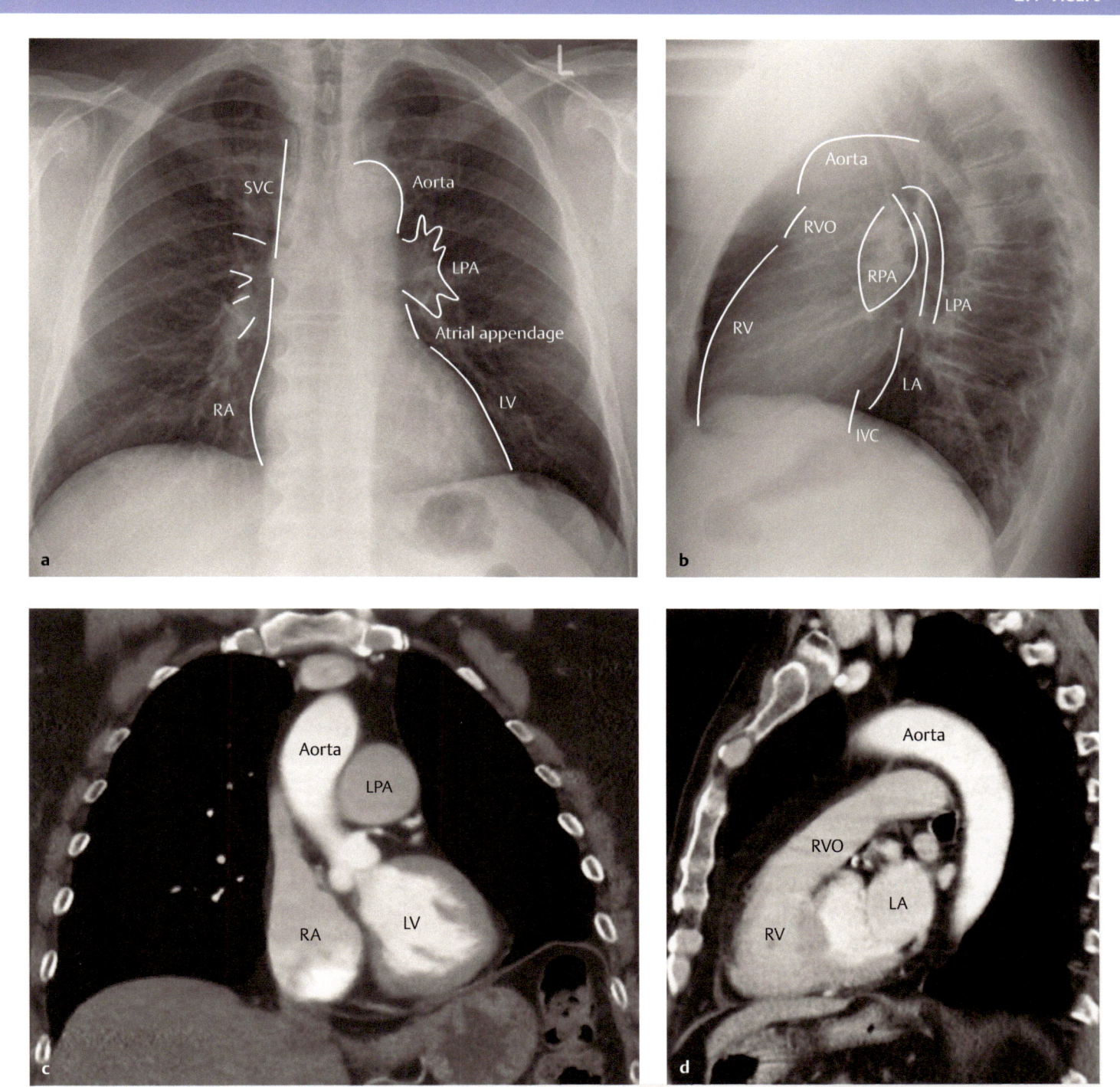

Fig. 2.1 Radiographic borders of the heart and great vessels. (a) PA chest radiograph. (b) Lateral radiograph. (c) Coronal image reformatted from a CT data set. (d) Sagittal image reformatted from a CT data set. LA, left atrium, LPA, left pulmonary artery, LV, left ventricle, RA, right atrium, RPA, right pulmonary artery, RV, right ventricle, RVO, right ventricular outflow tract, IVC, inferior vena cava, SVC, superior vena cava.

be individually adapted. To aid location description for the pathologist, the left ventricle is divided into a basal portion (valvular third), a midventricular portion (middle third), and an apical portion (apical third; ▶ Fig. 2.5). It is also customary to further subdivide the left ventricle into 17 segments based on a system first adopted for echocardiography in the late 1980s and later applied to MRI. Each third is systematically divided into segments that are designated with the appropriate descriptors. The anterior wall has one segment at each of at the basal, midventricular, and apical levels, and each segment is designated by its level and the word "anterior"—thus, basal anterior, midventricular anterior, and apical anterior. The same is done with the posterior wall, using the designation "inferior" (basal inferior, and so on). The septum and lateral wall are each divided into a basal and midventricular segment (inferoseptal and inferolateral, anteroseptal and anterolateral). This segmentation scheme is illustrated in ▶ Fig. 2.6. The anterior and inferior attachments of the right ventricle serve as landmarks for determining the position of the septal segments. The segments in the lateral wall are designated accordingly (basal inferolateral, and so on).

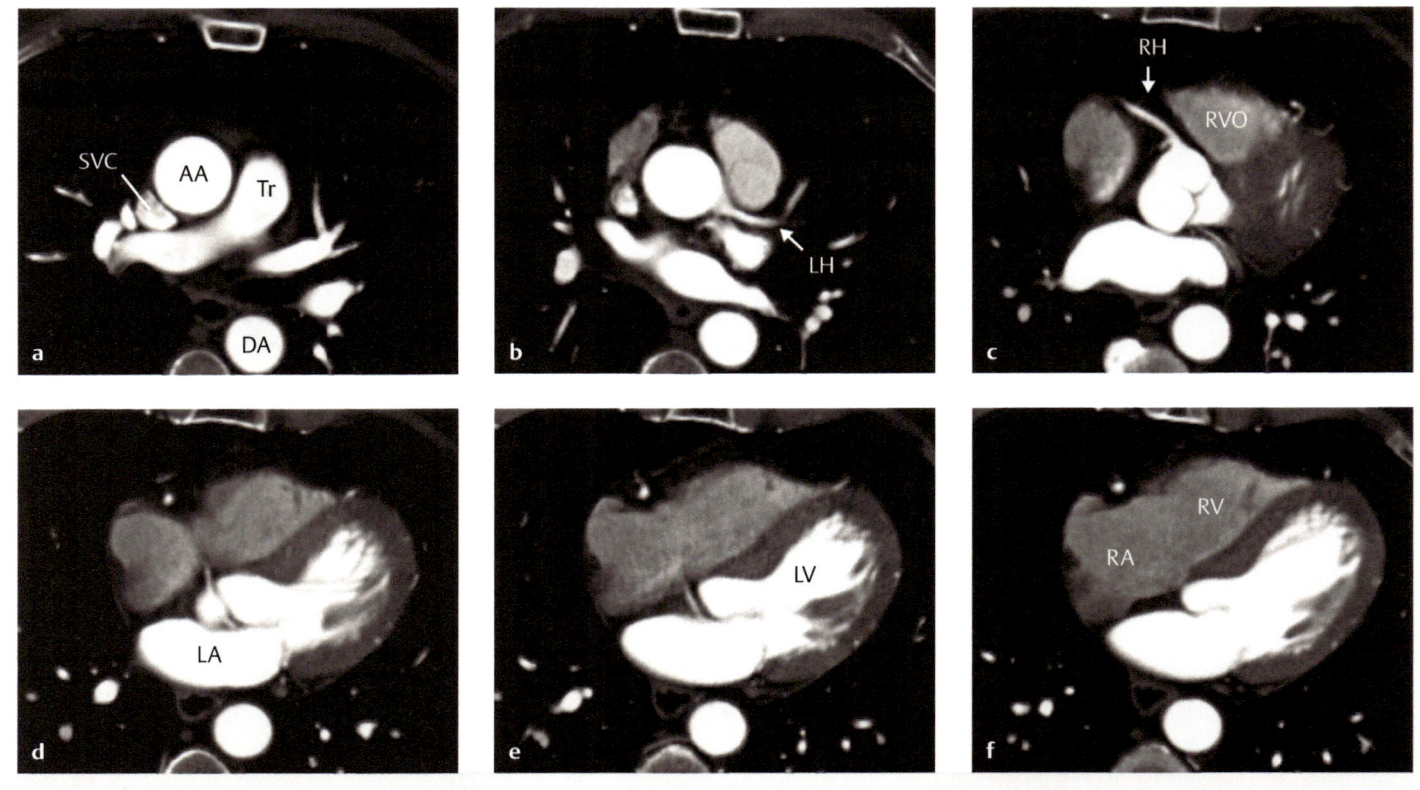

Fig. 2.2 **Cardiac chambers and great vessels** on axial CT scans. **(a)** Pulmonary trunk (Tr), ascending aorta (AA), descending aorta (DA), and superior vena cava (SVC). **(b)** Left coronary artery (LH). **(c)** Right coronary artery (RH) and right ventricular outflow tract (RVO). **(d)** Left atrium (LA). **(e)** Left ventricle (LV). **(f)** Right ventricle (RV) and right atrium (RA).

Note

In patients with ischemic heart disease, the location of the ischemic region helps to identify the affected coronary vessel. If the coronary circulation is "balanced," the anterior and anterolateral segments are supplied by the anterior interventricular branch of the left coronary artery, the inferolateral and anterolateral segments by the circumflex branch of the left coronary artery, and the inferoseptal and inferior segments by the right coronary artery. The segmental distribution pattern is different in hearts with a right-dominant or left-dominant coronary circulation.

The PA chest radiograph is taken with the patient standing upright and the X-ray source placed 2 meters from the detector (▶ Fig. 2.7a). Because the heart occupies a retrosternal position and is close to the detector, it is projected in approximately its true size. For the same reason, the lateral radiograph is taken with the patient lying on his or her left side. The situation is different with an AP radiograph taken in a supine position. In this case the X-ray tube is positioned closer to the cassette, while the heart is farther away. This causes the heart to be projected larger than its actual size (▶ Fig. 2.7b).

Note

In an upright chest radiograph taken at full inspiration, the transverse cardiac diameter should not exceed 50% of the transverse thoracic diameter (▶ Fig. 2.8). In a supine radiograph, it should not exceed 60% of the transverse thoracic diameter.

When the heart decompensates in response to a chronic pressure load or volume load, the result is cardiac enlargement.

2.1.2 Diseases

Heart Failure

▶ **Brief definition.** Heart failure develops as a result of myocardial damage, which can have many potential causes. With heart failure due to coronary disease, an acute infarction and, in certain cases of myocarditis, pulmonary congestion develop as a result of backward failure. This congestion can be recognized from typical radiographic signs. In patients with right ventricular failure, on the other hand, the principal effect is a damming back of blood in the systemic circulation, with associated lower leg edema and nocturia. Frequently both chambers are affected, resulting in mixed symptoms. In these cases, however, minimal changes may be noted in the chest radiograph if the inability of the left ventricle to deliver adequate blood to the systemic circulation is balanced by an absence of congestion in the pulmonary circulation due to right ventricular failure.

Caution

An acute pressure load on the heart, due for example to acute fulminant pulmonary embolism, leads to cardiac dilatation in the acute stage. In contrast, a chronic pressure load on the heart due to aortic or pulmonary valve stenosis, arterial hypertension, or pulmonary arterial hypertension leads to cardiac hypertrophy. This hypertrophy leads to wall thickening with no increase in outer diameter (concentric hypertrophy) and is not detectable on chest radiographs (▶ Fig. 2.9).

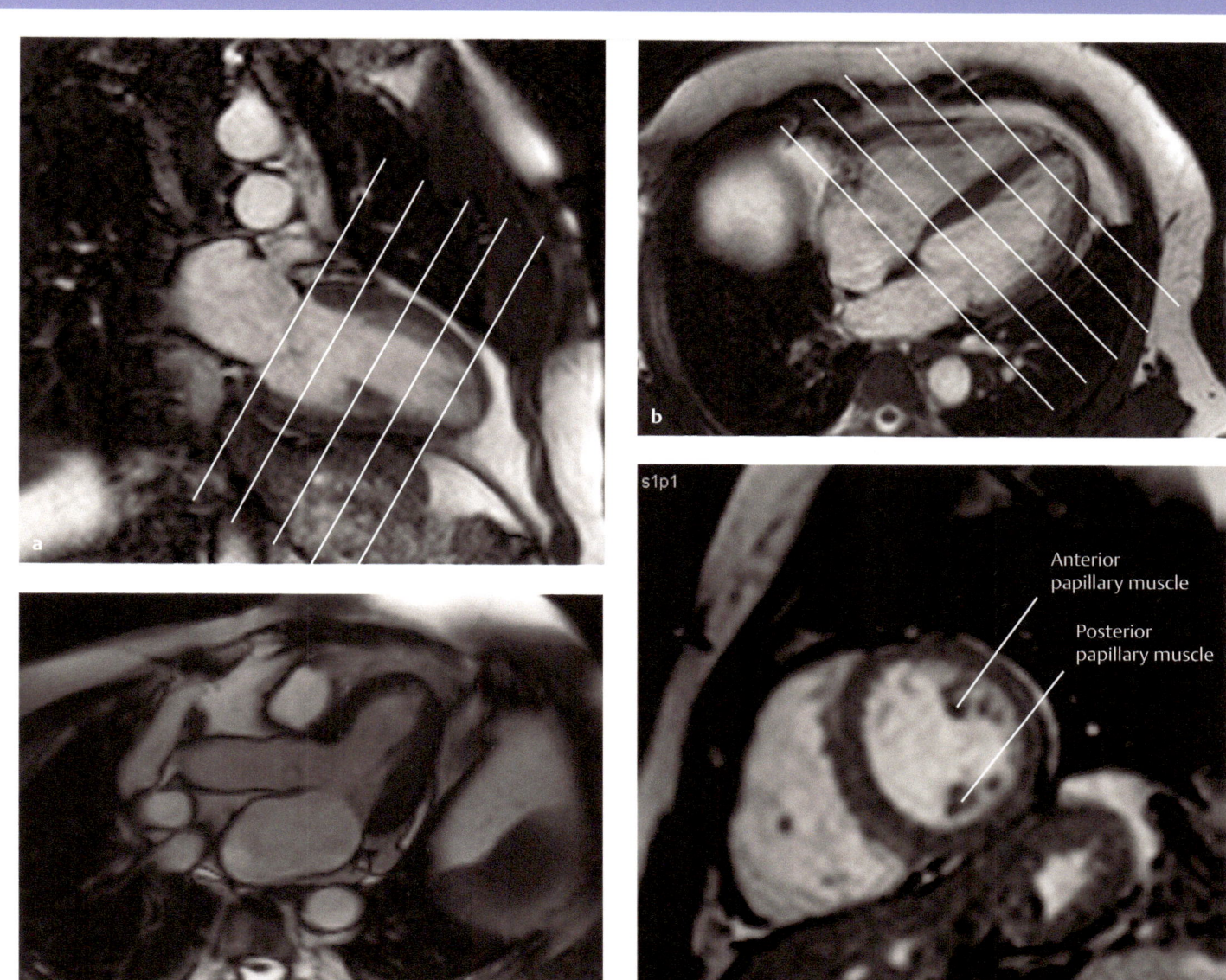

Fig. 2.3 Standard slice orientations for cardiac imaging. **(a)** The two-chamber view displays the left atrium and left ventricle. **(b)** The four-chamber view displays both atria and ventricles. **(c)** The three-chamber view shows the left atrium, left ventricle, and left outflow tract. **(d)** The image plane can be angled, as indicated in **(a)** and **(b)**, to obtain short-axis slices of the left ventricle. A series of these slices can provide complete coverage of the left ventricle.

▶ **Imaging signs.** Standard chest radiographs will usually provide an acceptable initial imaging work-up. If the cause of heart failure is still unknown and must be established, MRI is the modality of choice in patients with suspected myocarditis or cardiomyopathy. The imaging signs of pulmonary congestion due to acute left ventricular failure are:

- *Upper lobe diversion*: The first and most sensitive sign is the redistribution of blood to the upper lobes in the standing patient. In a normal chest radiograph, the vessels in the lower lung zones are more prominent than the vessels in the upper zones due to the hydrostatic pressure gradient. In patients with left heart failure, the upper lobe vessels are prominent (passively dilated) due to the increased blood volume in the pulmonary circulation (▶ Fig. 2.10).
- *Fluid accumulation in bronchial walls and vessels*: As the intravascular pressure in the pulmonary veins continues to rise, fluid leaks into the interstitium. The interstitial fluid accumulates around bronchi and causes thickening of the bronchial walls. Vessels become indistinct due to edema in the perivascular connective tissue.
- *Thickening of interlobular septa*: The edema also causes thickening of the fibrous interlobular septa (▶ Fig. 2.11), which appear as lines at sites where they are orthogonal to the X-ray beam. These septal lines are called Kerley lines (after Sir Peter Kerley, who first described them). On the PA radiograph, Kerley lines most commonly appear at the lung base close to the cardiophrenic angle. Lines at that location are called Kerley B lines (▶ Fig. 2.12). Kerley A lines extend radially from the hila to the periphery. Kerley C lines are short lines distributed in a reticular pattern over the lung parenchyma. Kerley A and C lines are rarely visible.
- *Alveolar edema*: A further pressure rise in the pulmonary veins causes fluid leakage into the alveoli. Auscultation at this time

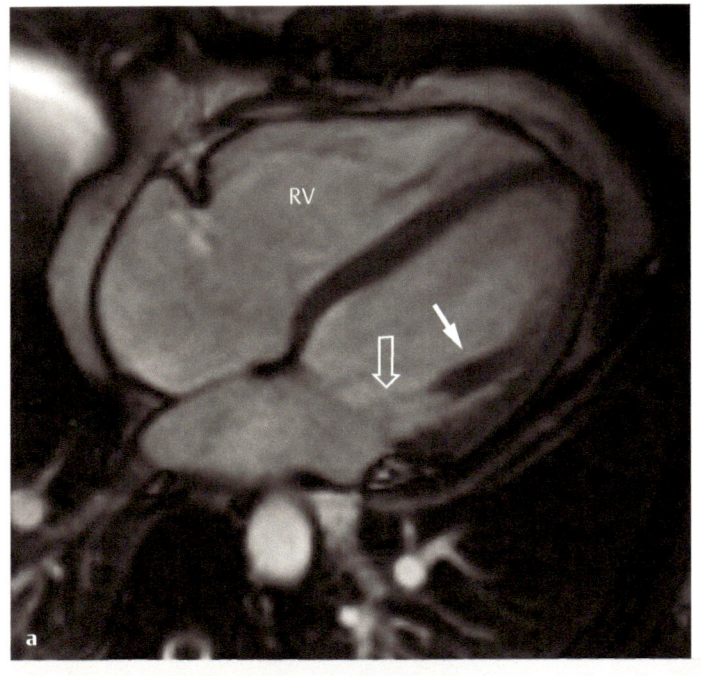

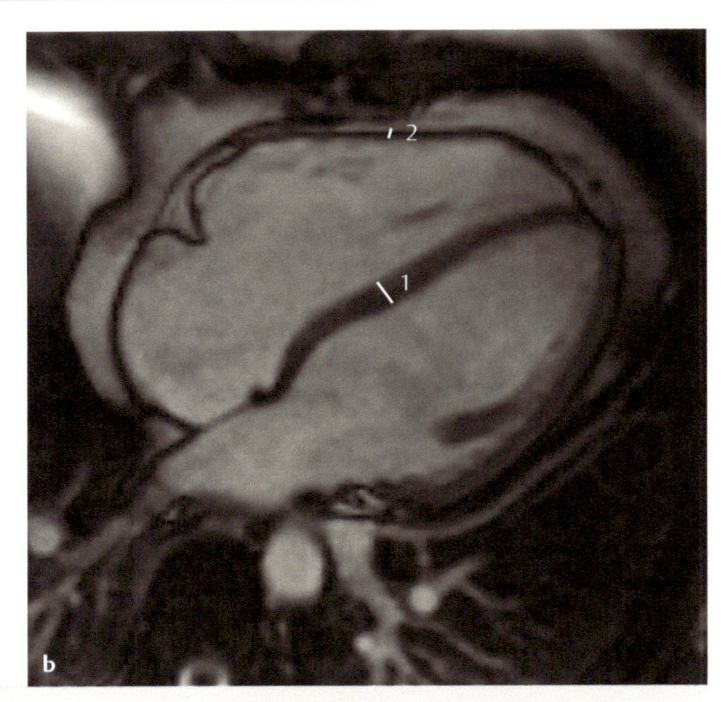

Fig. 2.4 Four-chamber view. (a) Solid arrow: anterior papillary muscle; open arrow: chordae tendineae. The right ventricle (RV) is more trabeculated than the left ventricle. (b) To check for myocardial hypertrophy in the left ventricle, the septum is measured as shown (line 1) in an end-diastolic view. The diameter should not exceed 12 mm. To check for right ventricular hypertrophy, the diameter of the free wall (line 2) is measured. It should not exceed the normal value of 4.5 mm. With a value of 6 mm or more, hypertrophy is present.

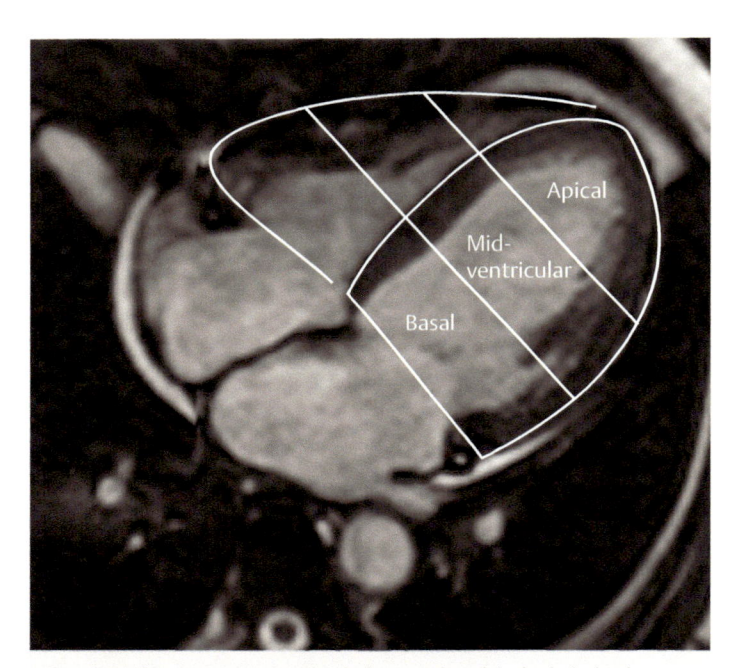

Fig. 2.5 The ventricles are divided into a basal (valvular) third, midcavity third, and apical third.

may detect audible rales. The chest radiograph shows pulmonary edema and congestive infiltrates (see ▶ Fig. 2.12). The lung opacities may show a butterfly pattern that initially spares the periphery.

- *Pleural effusion*: The additional development of right heart failure leads to dilatation of the superior vena cava and azygos vein and to pleural effusion. The pleural effusion may be limited to one side.

Caution

Congestive infiltrates are sometimes difficult to distinguish from pneumonic infiltrates. In doubtful cases the radiographic findings should be correlated with clinical symptoms. Pulmonary edema and congestive infiltrates, unlike pneumonic infiltrates, will improve within a few hours when the patient is treated for heart failure.

▶ **Differential diagnosis.** With a unilateral pleural effusion and no other abnormalities (no infiltrates, normal cardiac size, no other signs of pulmonary congestion), tuberculosis should be considered in the differential diagnosis. A malignant pleural effusion due to pleural carcinomatosis may also be limited to one side. In this case the history is usually helpful in narrowing the diagnosis.

▶ **Pitfalls.** Overhydration, which may result from rapid IV volume infusion or a positive fluid balance in renal failure, has to be differentiated from heart failure.

▶ **Key points.** Acute heart failure may have diverse causes. The initial imaging study is the chest radiograph. CT and MRI are available for further evaluation, depending on the cause.

Coronary Heart Disease and Myocardial Infarction

▶ **Brief definition.** Coronary heart disease refers to myocardial ischemia resulting from atherosclerosis of the coronary arteries that has led to coronary stenosis or occlusion. An acute occlusion may cause myocardial infarction. With its predominantly aerobic

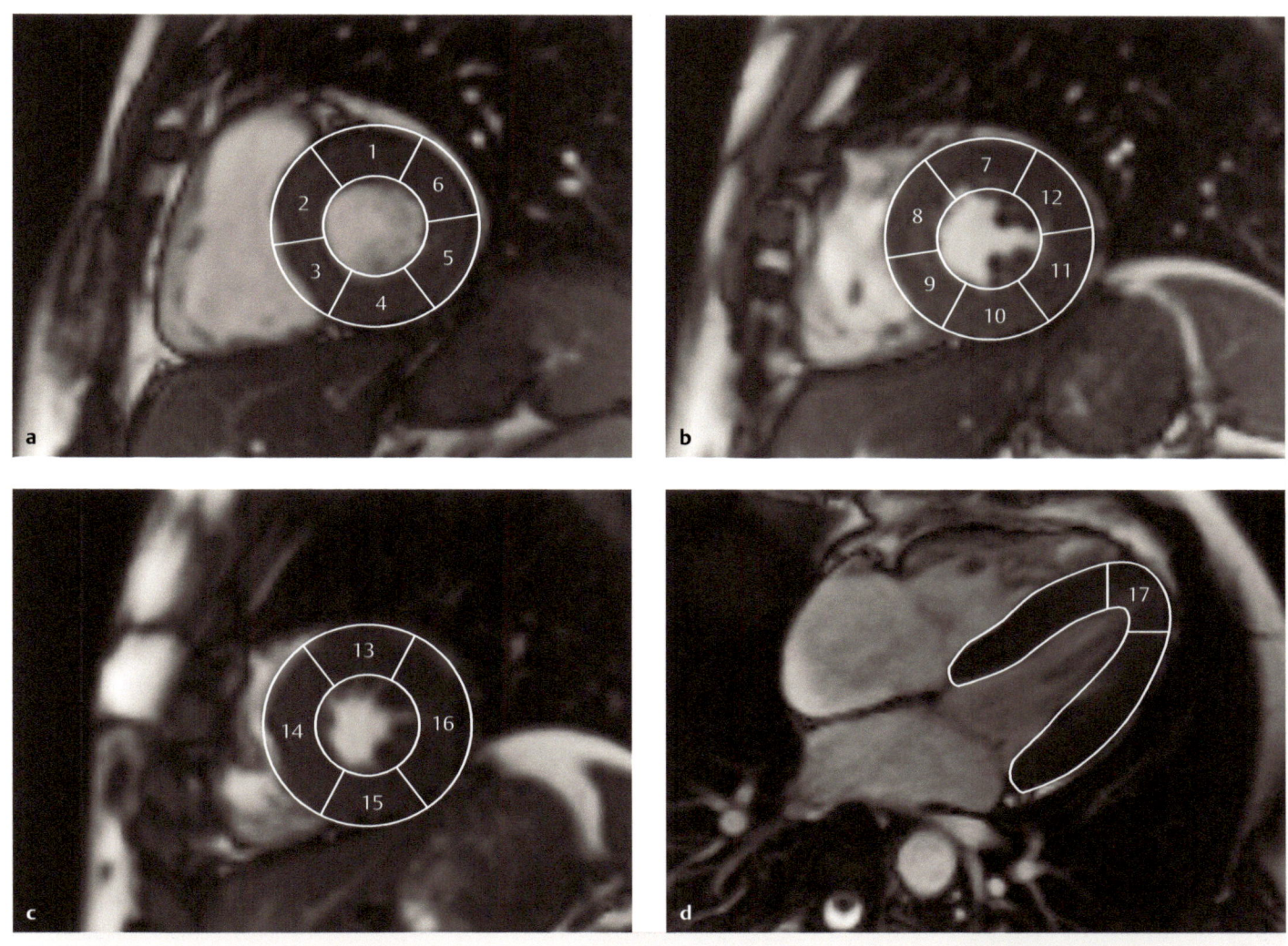

Fig. 2.6 Segmentation of the left ventricle. (a) Basal third. 1, basal anterior; 2, basal anteroseptal; 3, basal inferoseptal; 4, basal inferior; 5, basal inferolateral; 6, basal anterolateral. **(b)** Midventricular third. 7, midanterior; 8, midanteroseptal; 9, midinferoseptal; 10, midinferior; 11, midinferolateral; 12, midanterolateral. **(c)** Apical third. 13, apical anterior; 14, apical septal; 15, apical inferior; 16, apical lateral. **(d)** Apex (17).

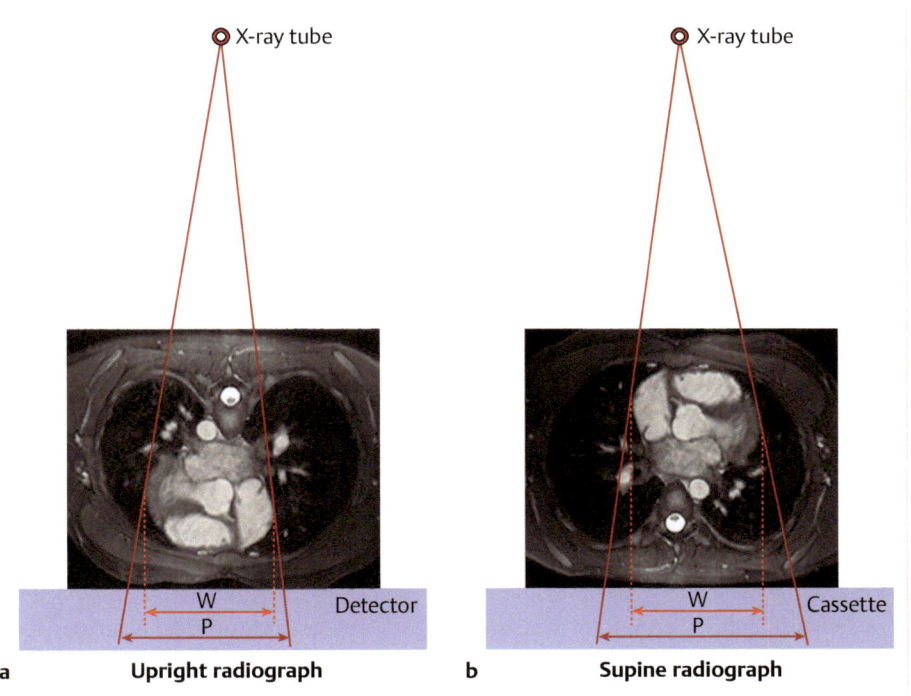

Fig. 2.7 Magnification effect of cardiac projections on chest radiographs. Diagrammatic representation. W, actual heart size, P, projected heart size. **(a)** The magnification effect is minimal in the upright PA radiograph owing to the proximity of the heart to the detector. **(b)** With a supine AP radiograph, the heart is projected considerably larger than its true size.

Heart and Pericardium

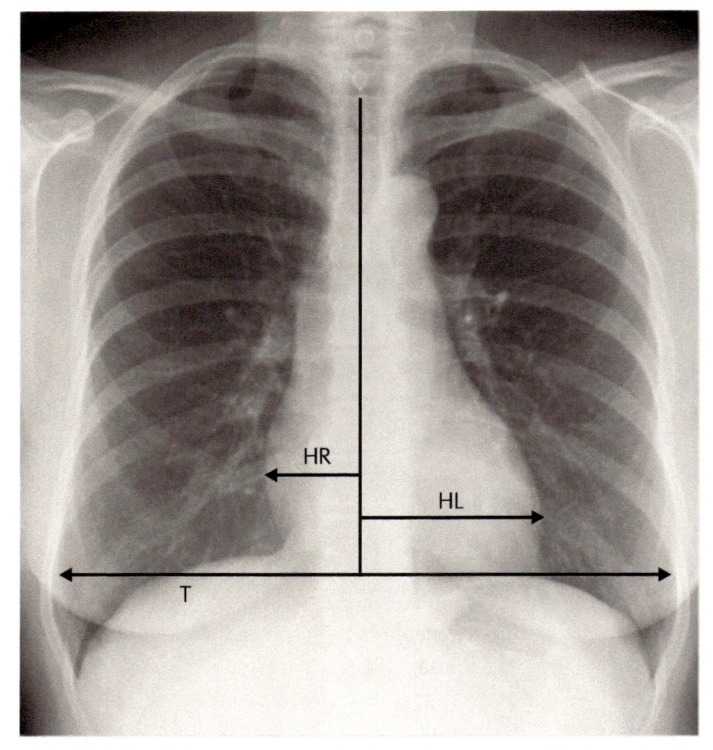

Fig. 2.8 Cardiothoracic ratio. The thoracic diameter T is determined between the inner rib margins at the level of the left hemidiaphragm. The transverse diameter on each side is measured at right angles from the midline to the outermost point of the cardiac silhouette (HL and HR) and the values are summed. The normal cardiothoracic ratio is less than 0.5 when measured in the upright radiograph and less than 0.6 in the supine radiograph.

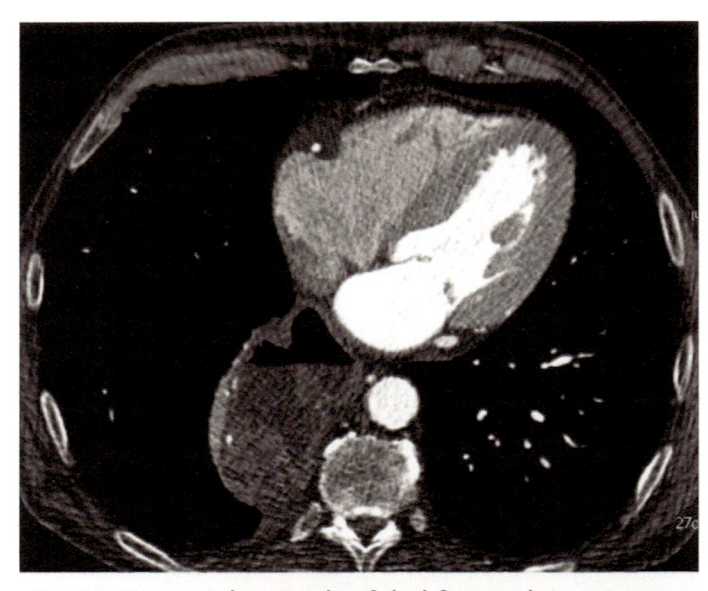

Fig. 2.9 Concentric hypertrophy of the left ventricle in a patient with aortic stenosis. The septum has a wall thickness of 18 mm at end diastole. The heart is not enlarged.

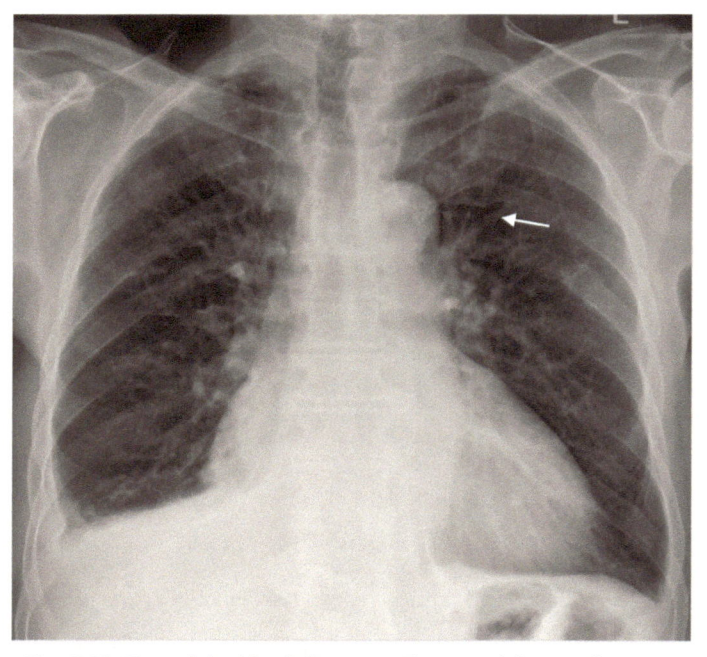

Fig. 2.10 Upper lobe blood diversion. The upper lobe vessels are markedly dilated (arrow) compared with the vessels in the lower zones. The heart is enlarged, and a right-sided pleural effusion is present.

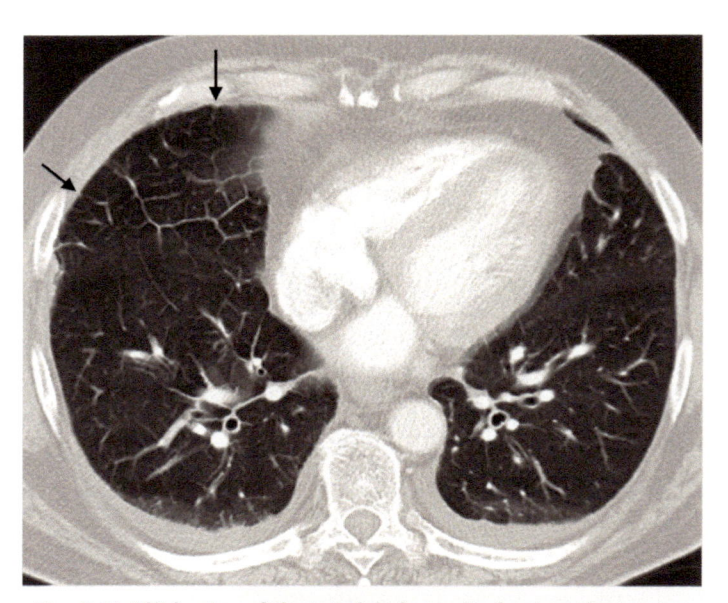

Fig. 2.11 Thickening of the interlobular septa due to pulmonary venous congestion. The arrows point to the interlobular septa. The bronchial walls are thickened.

metabolism, the myocardium has a high oxygen demand even at rest. Oxygen saturation is depleted to approximately 20% by the time the blood has passed through the myocardium and reached the venous vessels. With stress or exercise, the myocardial oxygen demand may increase 4- to 6-fold. The increased demand is met by dilation of the coronary arteries; this mechanism increases blood flow without changing the blood volume in the tissue. Blood flow increases from approximately 1.2 mL/min/g to approximately 4.0 to 6.7 mL/min/g during exercise. The pathophysiology of coronary stenosis and occlusion is as follows:

- *Stenosis*: The oxygen demand of myocardium supplied by a stenotic vessel is met by dilation of that vessel. As a result, luminal narrowing by up to 85% will not cause a reduction of myocardial perfusion at rest. With stress or exercise, however, adequate blood flow cannot be maintained because the vessel has already exhausted its potential for dilation. Stenoses of approximately 50% or more become hemodynamically significant during exercise. Moreover, a "steal effect" occurs as exercise induces dilatation of the nonstenotic vessels, thereby increasing blood flow to regions supplied by those vessels at the expense of the area supplied by the stenosed vessel. The pressure falls in the area beyond the stenosis, and blood flow declines significantly compared with myocardium supplied by nonstenotic vessels and also with the affected area at rest. The tissue becomes hypoperfused, and an ischemic cascade begins (▶ Fig. 2.13). The earliest manifestation of this process is a perfusion defect that is detectable by MRI. The decreased oxygen supply in the area supplied by the stenosed coronary artery initially leads to a reduction in the activity of the respiratory chain as an aerobic metabolic pathway. The synthesis of creatine phosphate and adenosine triphosphate (ATP) is diminished. Initially this leads only to diastolic dysfunction, but this is followed later by systolic dysfunction. As the duration and severity of the ischemia increase, changes begin to appear in the electrocardiogram (ECG). Further progression of the ischemic changes is manifested by anginal symptoms. The maintenance metabolism of the cells is still intact, however, so that even a high-grade stenosis, unlike occlusion, will usually not precipitate an infarction.

- *Occlusion*: After the acute occlusion of a coronary artery the respiratory chain is almost completely disrupted within 10 seconds. The intracellular levels of creatine phosphate and ATP show a steady decline. Meanwhile, the myocytes redirect their metabolism to anaerobic pathways, leading to lactic acidosis and the formation of free radicals. After an ischemic period of 20 to 30 minutes, the membrane potential of the myocytes can no longer be maintained. Calcium and potassium ions flow into the cell, and this electrolyte shift leads to cellular edema. Eventually the cellular edema and free radicals cause a loss of cell membrane integrity, resulting in cellular necrosis. The necrosis and interstitial edema in an acute infarction increase the distribution volume for extracellular contrast media that are routinely used in clinical imaging. When an acute myocardial infarction occurs, the myocytes in the area supplied by the occluded vessel do not all die simultaneously. Necrosis begins at the subendocardial level. As the duration of the ischemia increases, the necrosis spreads like a wavefront from the subendocardial zone across the central wall layers to the epicardial wall layers.[2] The lateral boundaries of the necrosis depend on the size of the area supplied by the occluded vascular branch. The transmural extent of necrosis depends on the duration of ischemia. If the infarcted area is large, acute heart failure with pulmonary venous congestion may develop. If the vessel remains occluded for more than 2 hours, percutaneous vascular recanalization will not consistently restore blood flow to the capillaries because the swelling of endothelial cells, capillary microthrombi, and arteriolar spasms lead to microvascular obstruction, with a failure of reperfusion at the tissue level. Microvascular obstruction is defined as an absence of

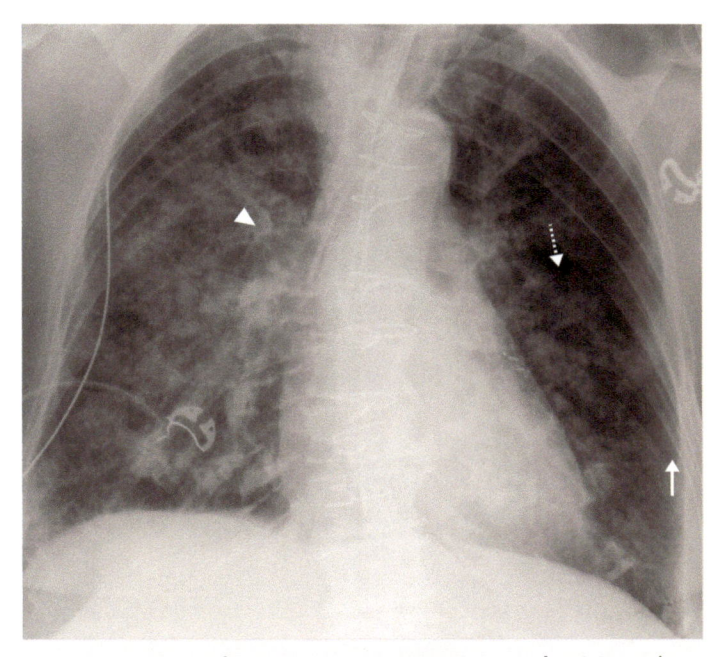

Fig. 2.12 Acute pulmonary venous congestion, grade IV. Note the Kerley A lines (dotted arrow), Kerley B lines (arrow), bronchial wall thickening (arrowhead), and alveolar edema.

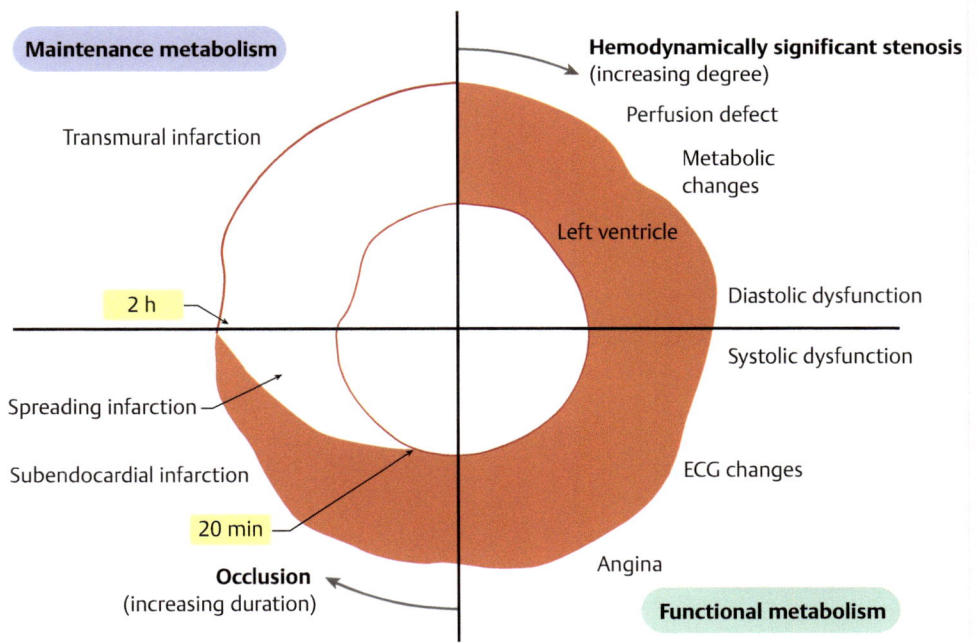

Fig. 2.13 Ischemic cascade. Diagrammatic representation of the pathophysiologic events associated with increasing stenosis of a coronary vessel (right half of diagram) and an occlusion of increasing duration (left half of diagram). MRI can detect a perfusion defect before any other changes appear. As a result, diastolic dysfunction is present even before ECG changes are visible or the patient develops anginal complaints. With the occlusion of a coronary vessel, infarction spreads from the subendocardial to subepicardial level over a period of approximately 20 minutes. By approximately 2 hours the infarction is transmural.

Heart and Pericardium

myocardial perfusion following successful recanalization of the coronary supply artery. Morbidity and mortality are increased in patients with microvascular obstruction. During the first 72 hours after an infarction, depending on the extent of the infarcted myocardium and on the preload and afterload, thinning of the necrotic tissue occurs due to the decreased strength of the affected tissue and its lack of stabilization by scarring, which has yet to occur. The thinning causes an apparent enlargement of the infarcted area. In extreme cases these changes may lead to ventricular rupture. Over a period of approximately 6 weeks, the necrotic myocardium is replaced by scar tissue. Its wall is markedly thinner compared with noninfarcted tissue. The remodeling processes are not limited to the infarcted area, however, but involve the entire heart. The increased wall tension leads to hypertrophy of the myocytes and enlargement of the left ventricular cavity.

▶ **Clinical features.** Coronary heart disease with hemodynamically significant coronary stenosis presents clinically with stable angina pectoris, which is characterized by exertional dyspnea and chest pain or discomfort in response to stress or exercise. The complaints are relieved within minutes by rest. Patients with an acute infarction experience crushing chest pain radiating to the left arm and neck as well as dyspnea.

▶ **Selection of modalities.** The appropriate imaging modality depends on the clinical question and is selected as follows:
- *Asymptomatic patients*: These patients first undergo a risk assessment based on the risk factors identified in the Framingham Study.[3] In patients with an intermediate risk of 10 to 20% of experiencing a cardiovascular event within the next 10 years, risk assessment can be improved by CT quantification of coronary artery calcium to obtain an Agatston score. This test uses unenhanced, ECG-gated/triggered cardiac CT to determine the calcium volume in the coronary vessels.

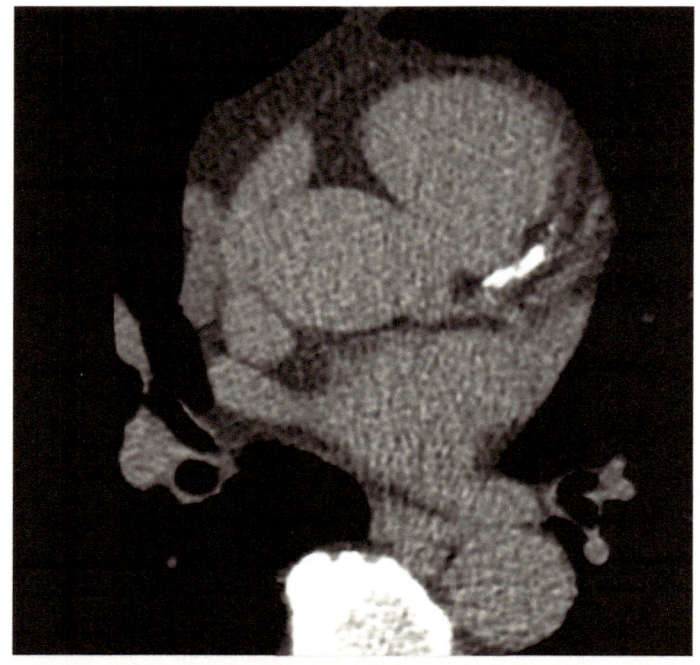

Fig. 2.14 Calcification in the right coronary artery. Single frame from an unenhanced ECG-gated CT data set.

- *Symptomatic patients with stable angina pectoris and intermediate pretest probability*: Initial evaluation of these patients consists of an MRI perfusion study and CT angiography (CTA) of the coronary arteries to avoid invasive testing.
- *Patients with unstable angina pectoris and no ECG or laboratory changes*: When clinically stabilized, these patients can undergo an MRI perfusion study to exclude hemodynamically significant stenoses.
- *Patients with non–ST segment elevation myocardial infarction (NSTEMI)*: CTA is performed in these patients to exclude coronary stenoses. MRI can be performed to rule out suspected myocarditis or takotsubo cardiomyopathy.
- *Patients with ST segment elevation myocardial infarction (STEMI)*: In this case MRI can define the infarcted area and detect the presence of microvascular obstruction as a basis for making a prognosis and planning further treatment.

▶ **Imaging signs**
- *CT*: An unenhanced, ECG-gated data set (▶ Fig. 2.14) is acquired and computer-analyzed to determine the calcium load of the coronary arteries and obtain an Agatston score (named for Arthur Agatston, who developed this technique in the mid-1980s). First, the maximum plaque density is determined in 3-mm-thick image slices. Based on this value, a weighting factor is assigned (130–199 HU, weighting factor = 1; 200–299 HU, weighting factor = 2; 300–399 HU, weighting factor = 3; 400 HU or more, weighting factor = 4). Next, the area of all calcified plaques in the entire data set is determined. The measured area in square millimeters is multiplied by the weighting factor to give the Agatston score (▶ Table 2.1). This score, when correlated with age and gender, supplies information on the probability of an infarction. Stenoses in the coronary vessels can be visualized by ECG-gated CT after IV injection of contrast medium. Landmarks on CT are the left and right coronary arteries, which arise respectively from the right and left aortic sinuses (see ▶ Fig. 2.2). The left coronary artery branches almost at once into the anterior interventricular branch and the circumflex branch. The anterior interventricular branch runs on the anterior surface of the heart in the sulcus between the ventricles. The circumflex branch runs on the posterior surface of the heart. The coronary arteries can be visualized by multiplanar reformatting of CT data (▶ Fig. 2.15), which can differentiate soft plaques from calcified plaques (▶ Fig. 2.16). The degree of stenosis is quantified by comparing the vascular diameters proximal and distal to the stenosis with the vascular diameter at the stenosis.
- *MRI*: For assessment of viability, regional and global myocardial function are quantified and the scarred area is visualized with IV contrast medium for direction of treatment planning or

Table 2.1 The Agatston score for evaluating the calcium load in coronary arteries

Agatston score	Interpretation
0	No calcification
1–10	Minimal coronary calcification
11–100	Mild coronary calcification
101–400	Moderate coronary calcification
401 or more	Severe coronary calcification

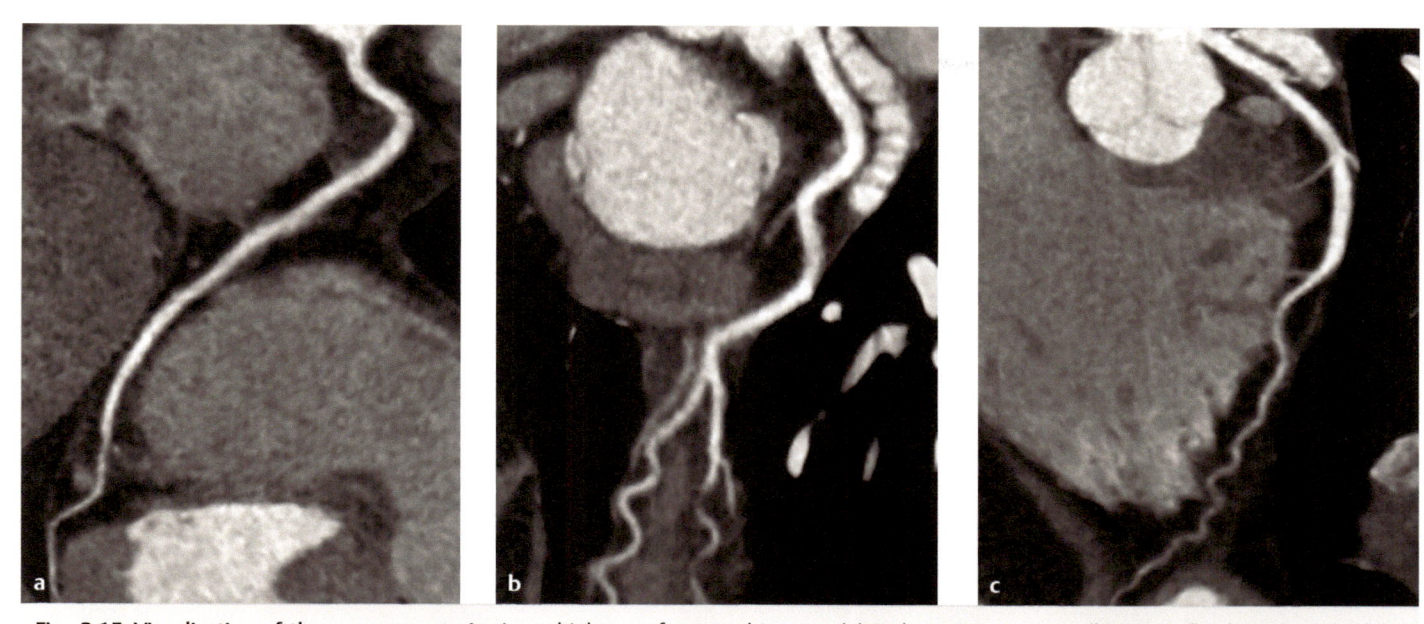

Fig. 2.15 Visualization of the coronary arteries in multiplanar reformatted images. **(a)** Right coronary artery. **(b)** Circumflex branch of the left coronary artery. **(c)** Anterior interventricular branch of the left coronary artery.

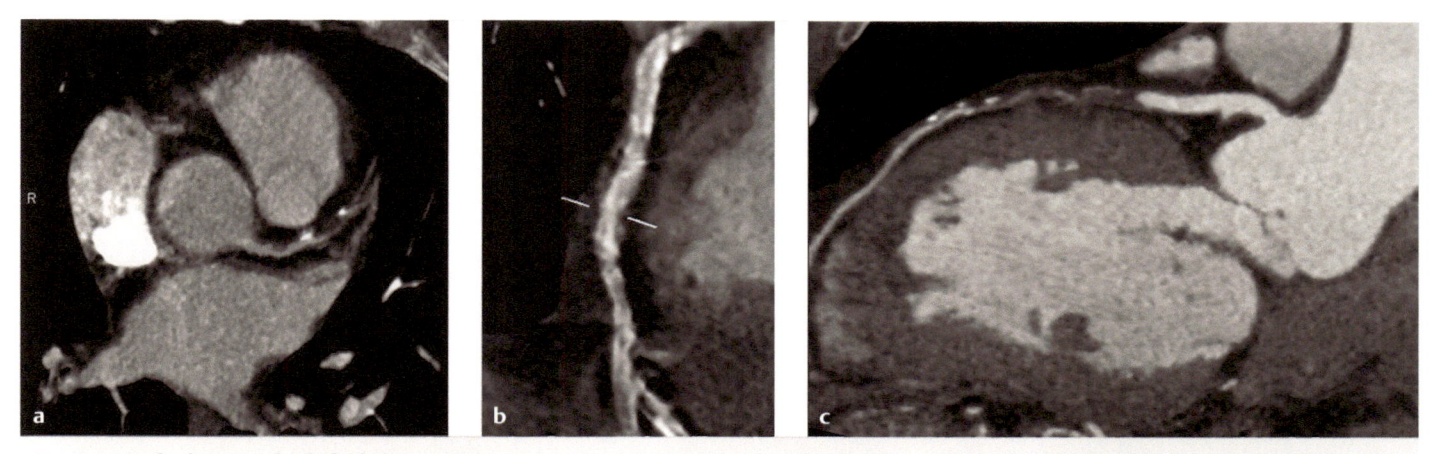

Fig. 2.16 Soft plaque and calcified plaques in coronary arteries. CT, axial scan and multiplanar reformatted images. **(a)** Soft plaque causing a high-grade stenosis in the right coronary artery. **(b)** Chronic complete occlusion of the left coronary artery. **(c)** Short segmental occlusion of the anterior interventricular branch.

forming a prognosis. Perfusion imaging can be added to the protocol to determine the presence or significance of coronary artery stenoses.
- *Assessment of regional function*: Regional function is evaluated with an ECG-gated TrueFISP (true fast imaging with steady precession) sequence (▶ Fig. 2.14) or, less commonly, with a GRE sequence. At least 30 image frames are acquired to document the cardiac cycle. Data acquisition is done sequentially so that the k-space lines of a single frame are acquired during several consecutive heartbeats (▶ Fig. 2.17), and the cine sequence for a given slice is acquired over several R–R cycles. This leads to poor image quality in patients with an arrhythmia. For functional analysis, individual slices are acquired in the two-, three-, and four-chamber views, producing a stack of slices that cover the left ventricle from base to apex. In this way each segment is imaged in two planes. Areas of regional dysfunction in the left ventricle are described with regard to their location and extent. Regional function is defined as follows:
  – Normokinesis: normal contractile function.
  – Hypokinesis: reduced contractile function.
  – Akinesis: contractile function is absent, or at most the affected areas move passively with the motion of adjacent unaffected regions.
  – Dyskinesis: paradoxical outward motion of the affected wall segments during systole.
- *Assessment of global function*: Global cardiac function is evaluated by the Simpson disk method. At a workstation, end systole and end diastole are first determined in short-axis slices, then the endocardial and epicardial myocardial borders are outlined in the slices. The area is multiplied by the slice thickness, including the interslice gap, and these values are added together to give the end-diastolic and end-systolic volumes. The stroke volume is the difference between the end-diastolic and end-systolic volumes. The ejection fraction is calculated by dividing the stroke volume by the end-diastolic volume. Multiplying the stroke

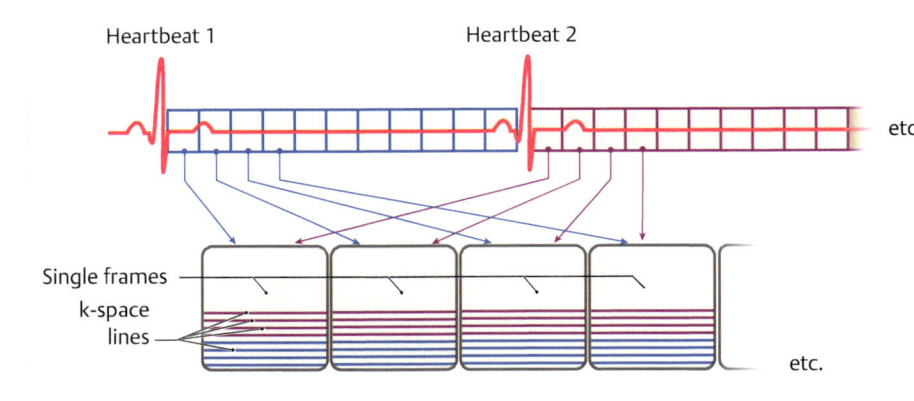

Fig. 2.17 The cardiac cycle imaged in cine mode with segmented data acquisition. Several phases of the cardiac cycle are imaged in single frames, which are composited to form a video sequence. Acquisition is continued for several heartbeats (R–R intervals). Multiple k-space cells are acquired in each frame per cardiac cycle until the k-space for a single image is filled with data from multiple heartbeats.

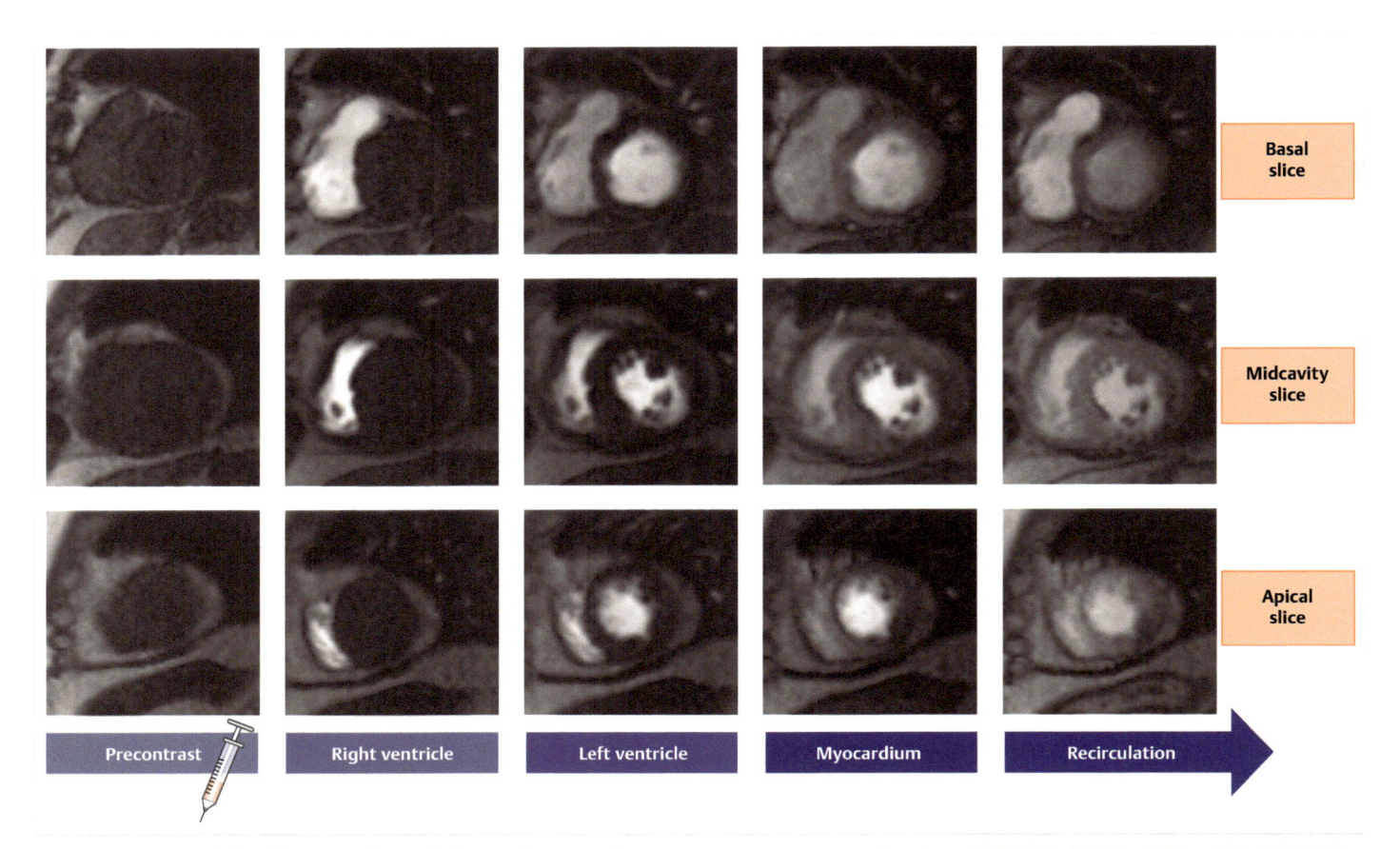

Fig. 2.18 Myocardial perfusion study. Single frames from a perfusion sequence. Image acquisition is started before injection of contrast medium to image the first pass of the contrast bolus through the heart. Generally at least three slices can be acquired within the allotted timeframe.

volume by the heart rate gives the cardiac output. Myocardial mass can be determined by also outlining the epicardial boundary of the ventricle so that the specific weight (1.05 g/mL) can be multiplied by that volume. Myocardial mass is an independent predictor of cardiac mortality. The myocardial mass can be normalized to body surface area to improve the comparability of the data. The Dubois method can be used to determine body surface area.

- Assessment of perfusion: Perfusion imaging may employ a fast GRE sequence, TrueFISP sequence, or hybrid GRE-EPI sequence. Stress perfusion imaging should precede imaging at rest. The left ventricle is scanned with a minimum of three slices. These slices are acquired in short-axis planes and are individually positioned for each patient by spacing the slices so that the apical, midventricular, and basal portions of the ventricle are each imaged with one slice. Unlike the cine sequences, each slice is acquired during one R–R interval to image the passage of the contrast bolus with acceptable temporal resolution (▶ Fig. 2.18).
- Delayed enhancement: In most protocols, perfusion imaging is followed by a heavily T1-weighted GRE sequence to evaluate delayed enhancement (▶ Fig. 2.19). In patients with an old myocardial infarction, capillary density is decreased in the scarred myocardium, resulting in a perfusion defect at rest and stress that coincides with the infarcted area. This is called a "fixed perfusion defect" (▶ Fig. 2.20). If imaging shows a perfusion defect without a myocardial infarction on delayed enhancement imaging, this indicates a stenosis in the vessel

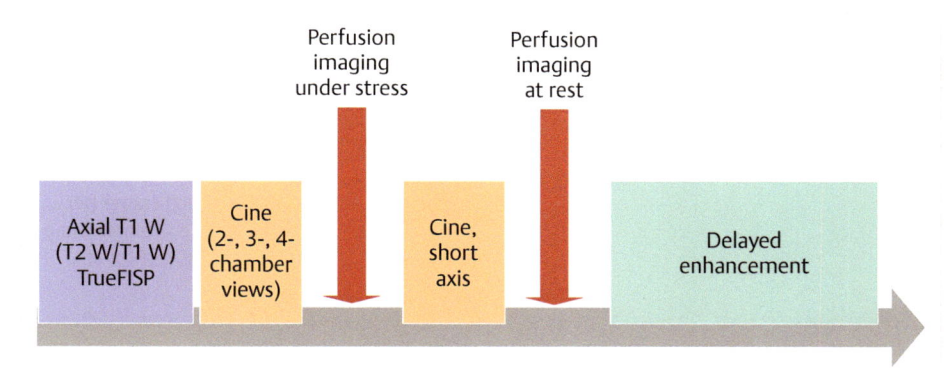

Fig. 2.19 Schematic representation of a typical protocol for a myocardial viability study that includes perfusion imaging.

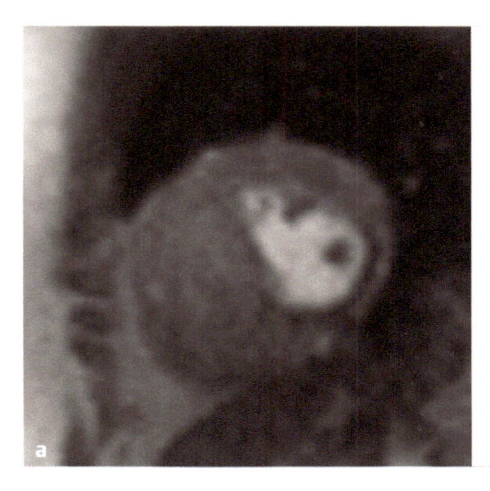

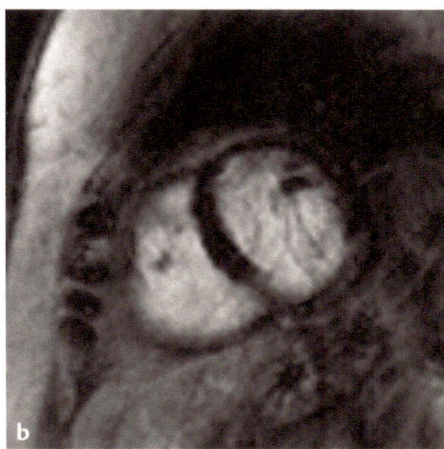

Fig. 2.20 Fixed perfusion defect. (a) Midinferior perfusion defect. (b) T1 W inversion recovery GRE sequence to show delayed enhancement. Transmural infarction corresponds to the perfusion defect in (a).

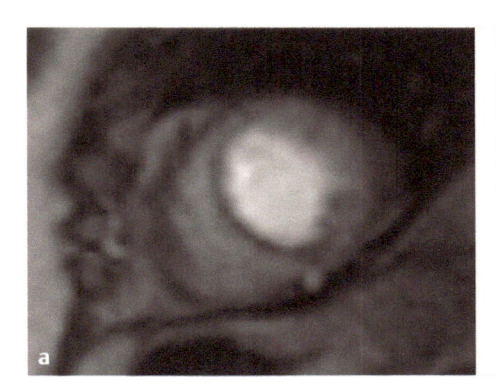

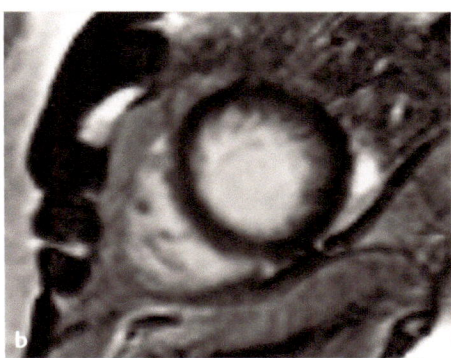

Fig. 2.21 Perfusion defect without myocardial infarction. (a) Septal perfusion defect. (b) T1 W inversion recovery GRE sequence to show delayed enhancement. Absence of a visible infarction confirms viability of the myocardium supplied by the stenotic artery.

supplying the affected area (▶ Fig. 2.21). The distribution volume for extracellular contrast medium is increased in acutely infarcted myocardium due to edema and cellular necrosis because contrast medium can also enter the necrotic cells as a result of loss of cell membrane integrity. With an old infarction, the enlarged extracellular matrix again provides a greater distribution volume for extracellular contrast medium (▶ Fig. 2.22). The location and transmural extent of delayed enhancement is a very useful indicator for prognosis and treatment planning (▶ Fig. 2.23, ▶ Fig. 2.24). When the myocardium in the area supplied by a stenosed vessel is viable, revascularization offers a significantly better prognosis for morbidity and mortality than that with conservative drug therapy. Conversely, the risk of arrhythmia after revascularization is increased in patients found to have nonviable tissue.

Note

- Viable myocardium—including "hibernating" myocardium (hypoperfused tissue that is functionally suppressed due to coronary stenosis but is not necrotic) and "stunned" myocardium (tissue that is functionally suppressed following an ischemic insult)—does not show delayed enhancement.
- With regard to prognosis, regional function may recover if the infarction involves less than 50% of the wall thickness. If more than 75% of the wall thickness is affected, functional recovery can no longer occur.
- Wall thickness in the peri-infarct zone—noninfarcted myocardium bordering the infarction—can be used to evaluate ventricular remodeling. If it is more than 4.5 mm in diastole, it is reasonable to predict a recovery of contractile function.

Healthy myocardium　**Acute infarction**　**Chronic infarction** (scar)

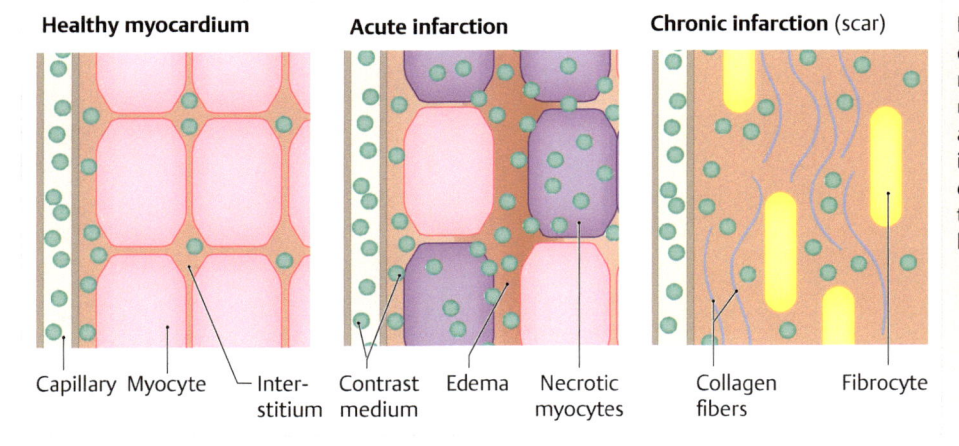

Capillary　Myocyte　Inter-　Contrast　Edema　Necrotic　Collagen　Fibrocyte
　　　　　　　　stitium　medium　　　　myocytes　fibers

Fig. 2.22 **Diagrammatic representation of the distribution volume of extracellular contrast medium in the myocardium.** Distribution volume in healthy myocardium (intravascular space and interstitium, total of 18 to 22%), in acutely infarcted myocardium (up to 100%), and chronically infarcted myocardium (variable due to varying cellularity of the scar, but markedly higher than in healthy myocardium).

Cardiomyopathies

In 2006 the American Heart Association (AHA) published a classification of cardiomyopathies that defines "primary cardiomyopathies" as those that are confined to the heart muscle.[3] They are further classified by etiology as genetic, acquired, or mixed genetic and nongenetic. "Secondary cardiomyopathies" are those that occur in the setting of systemic diseases.

Myocarditis

▶ **Brief definition.** Myocarditis is an inflammatory disease of the myocardium due to various causes. On the basis of the 1995 WHO classification, which is the most up-to-date classification at the time of writing (2017), myocarditis is classified as a "specific (inflammatory) cardiomyopathy."[4] The 2006 definition of the AHA classifies it as a "primary cardiomyopathy" in the acquired subgroup.[3] The gold standard for diagnosis is myocardial biopsy. Histological evaluation is based on the Dallas criteria for myocarditis, which require the presence of inflammatory infiltrate and associated myocyte necrosis. Most cases of myocarditis have a viral etiology. The most common viral pathogens are enteroviruses, parvoviruses, Coxsackie B virus, HIV, and hepatitis C virus. If the inflammatory process involves the pericardium, the condition is called "perimyocarditis." The incidence is estimated at 10 per 100,000 population per year but is not precisely known due to the large number of asymptomatic cases.

▶ **Clinical features.** Acute myocarditis is clinically silent in a great many cases or is associated with flulike symptoms such as fatigue, aching limbs, and dyspnea. Arrhythmias are sometimes present at rest or during exercise, however, and may even lead to sudden cardiac death. Additionally, acute myocarditis may produce ischemic complaints with chest pain. Sepsis may develop in some cases, especially those with a bacterial etiology. Acute myocarditis usually resolves without sequelae, but 10% of patients will develop dilated cardiomyopathy.

▶ **Imaging signs.** The diagnostic algorithm includes clinical examination, blood work, ECG (which may show extrasystoles and ST elevation), and echocardiography (for heart size, function, possible pericardial effusion). The chest radiograph may be normal, given the variable presentation of myocarditis, but patients with left ventricular dysfunction may show signs of pulmonary

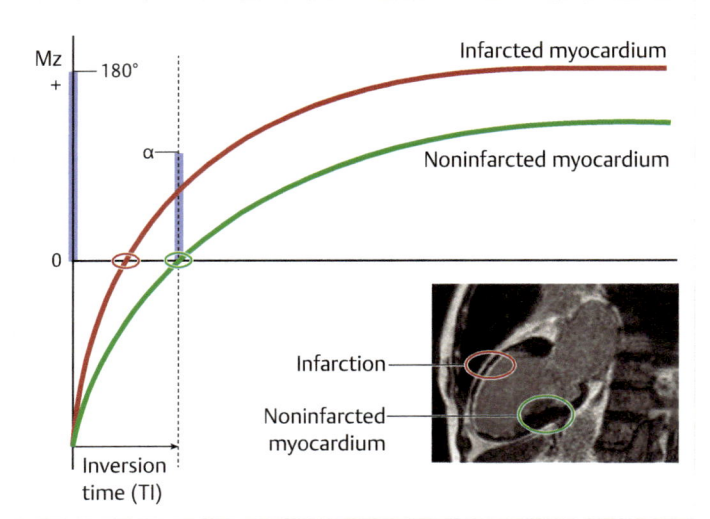

Fig. 2.23 **Diagram of delayed enhancement in the myocardium.** T1 W inversion recovery GRE sequence. The initial 180° pulse inverts all the spins, which then return to their original position in accordance with their T1 time. The excitation pulse (α) is applied at the null point of healthy myocardium in order to null the signal from that tissue. Mz = magnetization.

venous congestion or ventricular dilatation (▶ Fig. 2.25). The modality of choice is MRI, which is particularly useful in differentiating myocarditis from myocardial infarction in patients with ischemic symptoms. A comprehensive protocol should be followed in patients with suspected myocarditis.[5] Cine sequences are acquired in standard planes to evaluate regional and global function. Guidelines recommend fat-suppressed T2 W imaging of the left ventricle in short-axis and long-axis planes. This will reveal circumscribed edema in many patients with acute myocarditis (▶ Fig. 2.26). Diffuse involvement or persistent viral replication may lead to generalized myocardial edema with increased signal intensity throughout the myocardium.[6] Generalized edema is not apparent on visual assessment. Instead, the signal intensity of the myocardium should be measured and divided by the signal intensity of the skeletal muscle. The resulting value, called the edema ratio, is less than 1.9 in healthy subjects. A higher value is predictive of myocarditis with a sensitivity of 76% and a specificity of 95.5%.[5] Next, T1 W (T)SE images are acquired before IV injection of contrast medium and in the equilibrium phase 9 to

2.1 Heart

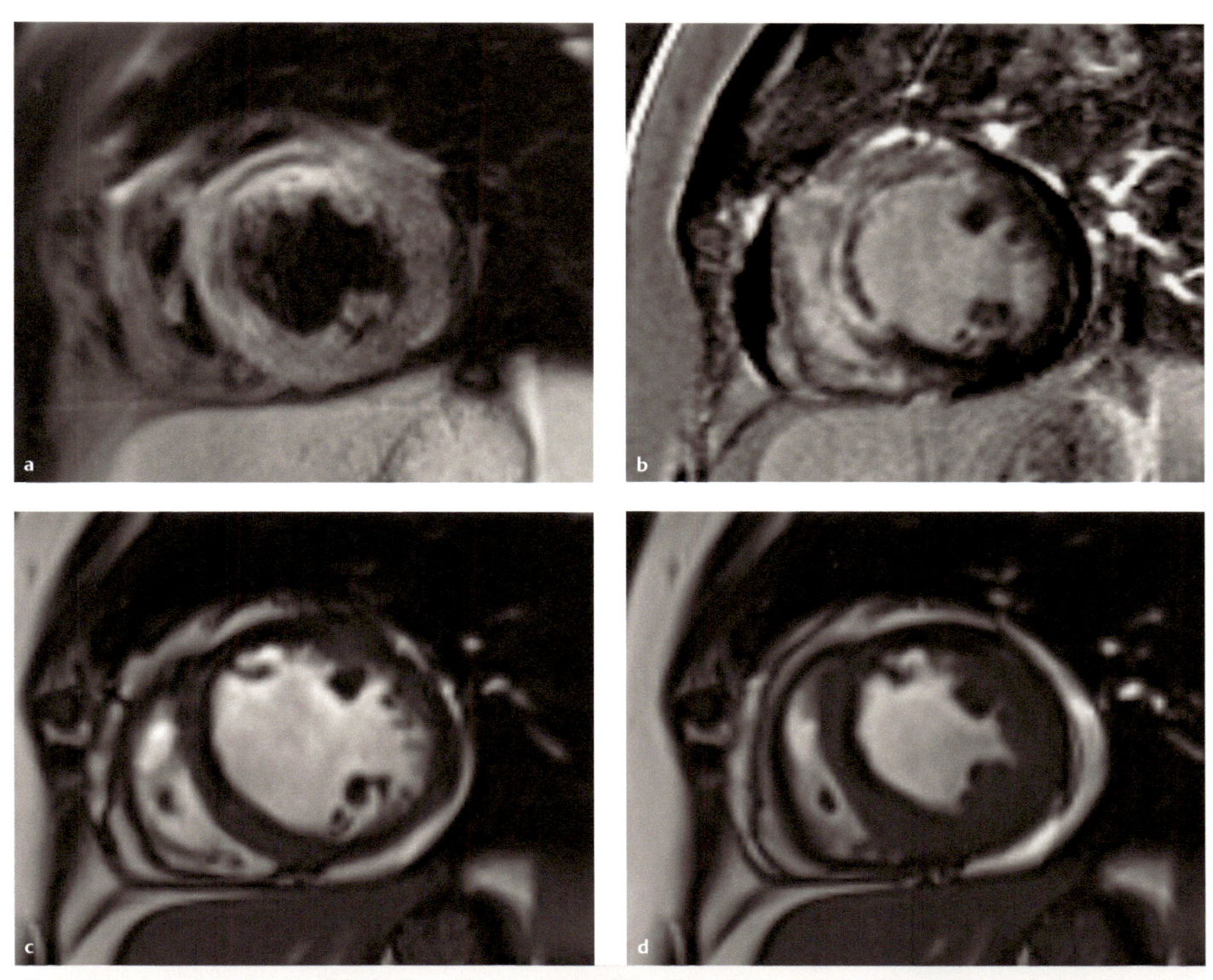

Fig. 2.24 Acute transmural myocardial infarction with microvascular obstruction in the septum. (a) T2 W image shows edema in the septum. (b) T1 W inversion recovery GRE sequence shows delayed enhancement consistent with transmural infarction. The absence of subendocardial enhancement indicates microvascular obstruction. (c) Cine image at end diastole. (d) Cine image at end systole. The infarcted area is akinetic.

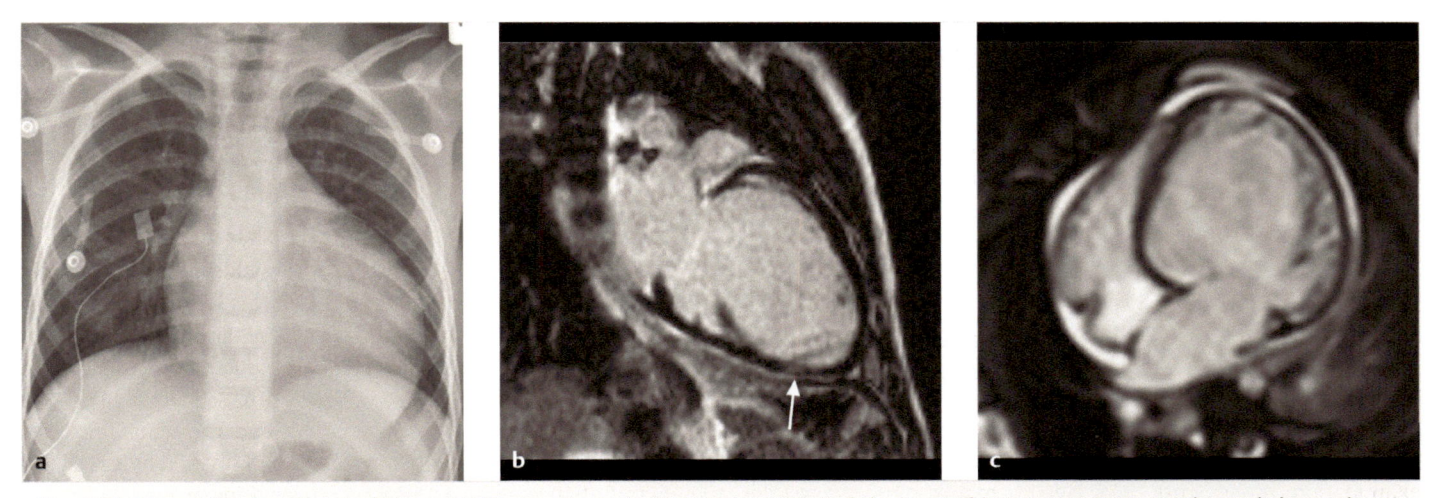

Fig. 2.25 Myocarditis in a 6-year-old boy. (a) Chest radiograph shows enlargement of the heart. (b) Postcontrast image shows slight patchy enhancement (arrow). (c) Four-chamber view, TrueFISP sequence. The left ventricle is markedly dilated.

12 min after injection of contrast medium (0.2 mmol/kg BW of a gadolinium-based extracellular contrast medium). This sequence is obtained to determine early enhancement. As in the determination of edema ratio, global relative enhancement is calculated from the signal intensity of the myocardium and skeletal muscle using the following formula:

$$gRE = \frac{SI_{myocardium\ postc} - SI_{myocardium\ prec}}{SI_{myocardium\ prec}} : \frac{SI_{muscle\ postc} - SI_{muscle\ prec}}{SI_{muscle\ prec}}$$

where

gRE = global relative enhancement.

$SI_{myocardium\ postc}$ = signal intensity of myocardium after administration of contrast medium.

$SI_{myocardium\ prec}$ = signal intensity of myocardium before administration of contrast medium.

$SI_{muscle\ postc}$ = signal intensity of skeletal muscle after administration of contrast medium.

$SI_{muscle\ prec}$ = signal intensity of skeletal muscle before administration of contrast medium.

The cutoff value for healthy myocardium is < 4. The early-enhancement phase of the examination is followed by the delayed-enhancement protocol. This may show patchy enhancement, which differs from the enhancement seen in ischemic disease in that it does not follow a subendocardial pattern (see ▶ Fig. 2.26). Depending on the extent of necrosis and edema, this enhancement pattern may regress with healing or may persist if confluent necrotic areas are present and scars have formed.

> **Caution**
>
> Contrary to former belief, the distribution of edema and delayed enhancement in the myocardium is not helpful in identifying the causative agent of myocarditis. Different causative agents do not have specific sites of predilection in the myocardium.

▶ **Key points.** MRI is the imaging modality of choice for myocarditis. It can detect myocardial edema and can quantify edema and early enhancement.

Dilated Cardiomyopathy

▶ **Brief definition.** Dilated cardiomyopathy is characterized by dilatation of the cardiac chambers accompanied by severe systolic and diastolic dysfunction. It is usually secondary to an underlying systemic cause. Causative agents may include toxins (chemotherapy drugs), alcohol, prior myocarditis that triggered an autoimmune response, or hemochromatosis. No cause can be identified in one-half of patients. In 30% of patients the disease is familial with an autosomal dominant mode of inheritance. Dilated cardiomyopathy is the second most common cause of heart failure and the most frequent reason for heart transplantation, as the disease is progressive regardless of its cause and is associated with an annual mortality rate as high as 14%.

▶ **Clinical features.** The severity of heart failure determines the clinical presentation.

▶ **Imaging signs.** The chest radiograph shows global cardiac enlargement. Echocardiography, MRI, and CT show a dilated ventricular chamber with normal wall thickness but decreased stroke volume. On MRI, 30% of patients show midmural delayed enhancement (▶ Fig. 2.27).[7]

▶ **Differential diagnosis.** The differentiation required is mainly that from cardiac dilatation due to ischemic heart disease. Thus,

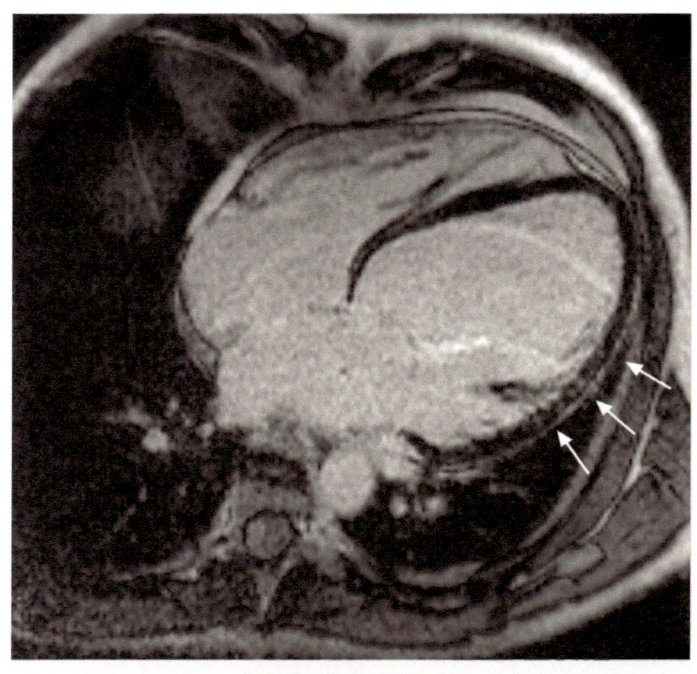

Fig. 2.27 **Dilated cardiomyopathy.** Delayed enhancement. Global cardiac enlargement is present. Slight midmural enhancement is noted in the lateral wall (arrows).

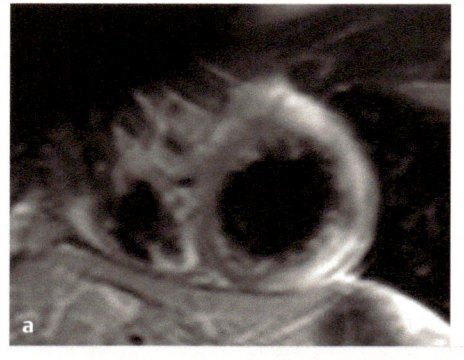

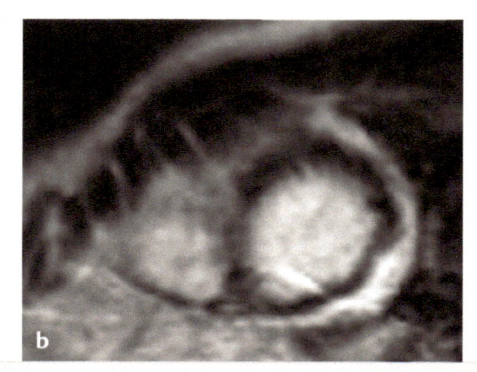

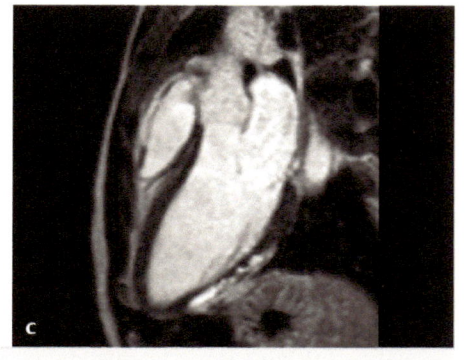

Fig. 2.26 **Myocarditis.** (a) T2 W short-axis view shows patchy subendocardial edema. (b) Area of delayed enhancement (short axis) corresponds to the edema. (c) Delayed enhancement (three-chamber view).

the work-up of dilated cardiomyopathy should always include the exclusion of significant coronary stenosis. The coronary arteries can be evaluated by CT coronary angiography or MR perfusion imaging. MRI can exclude prior myocardial infarction by excluding an infarction-type enhancement pattern (involving a coronary artery territory and showing a subendocardial-to-epicardial pattern of spread).

▶ **Key points.** Dilated cardiomyopathy develops as a result of myocardial damage and can have numerous causes. Global dilation is the common endpoint of this damage and appears as generalized cardiac enlargement on chest radiographs. MRI can quantify cardiac function and is useful for follow-up.

Hemochromatosis and Hemosiderosis

▶ **Brief definition.** (Primary) Hemochromatosis is a genetically mediated disease in which there is too high absorption of iron in the small intestine. In hemosiderosis, the iron overload in the body is an iatrogenic result of repeated blood transfusions. Both conditions are treated with chelating agents that can effectively lower the tissue iron concentration.

> **Note**
>
> In evaluating the heart, it is important to know that the iron overload in the liver can be reduced faster than that in the heart and that serum ferritin levels also respond more quickly. Consequently, these two parameters are not reliable indicators of the iron overload in the myocardium. For patients who are already in heart failure, it is very difficult to provide effective treatment to achieve myocardial iron reduction.

▶ **Clinical features.** The myocardial iron overload is initially asymptomatic. Eventually the patient develops dilated cardiomyopathy with signs and symptoms of heart failure. This stage is associated with a high mortality rate.

▶ **Imaging signs.** Due to the superparamagnetic properties of iron, an iron overload in the myocardium shortens the T2 time. For many years, measurement of the T2* time of the myocardium has been performed as a routine clinical test because of its technical simplicity. A normal value is 40 milliseconds. Values less than 20 milliseconds indicate an iron overload, and values of approximately 10 milliseconds have a high association with dilated cardiomyopathy and heart failure.

▶ **Differential diagnosis.** Since a low T2* value indicates iron overload, no other conditions need be considered in the differential diagnosis.

▶ **Key points.** The iron overload in hemosiderosis and hemochromatosis can be quantified with MRI.

Arrhythmogenic Right Ventricular Cardiomyopathy

▶ **Brief definition.** Arrhythmogenic right ventricular cardiomyopathy is characterized by a loss of myocytes and tissue replacement by fat and connective tissue. The left ventricle is also affected in 75% of cases. The disease is familial in approximately 30% of cases, with an autosomal dominant mode of inheritance. The apoptosis of myocytes initially leads to regional dysfunction of the right ventricle, followed by global dysfunction of the right ventricle and functional impairment of the left ventricle.

▶ **Clinical features.** The cardinal symptom is stress-induced arrhythmia with a risk of sudden cardiac death. Right-sided heart failure develops over the course of the disease.

▶ **Imaging signs.** MRI has become the gold standard for the diagnosis of arrhythmogenic right ventricular cardiomyopathy as it is superior to echocardiography for right ventricular imaging. Because the necrotic myocardium in arrhythmogenic right ventricular cardiomyopathy is replaced mainly by scar tissue and to a much lesser degree by fat, and fat deposits are also found in the right ventricle of healthy individuals, delayed enhancement on MRI has assumed a major diagnostic role.[8] MRI has a sensitivity of 96% and a specificity of 78%.[9] In 1994 an international task force proposed major and minor criteria for the diagnosis of arrhythmogenic right ventricular cardiomyopathy,[10] which were updated in 2010.[11] A diagnosis requires either two major criteria or one major criterion plus two minor criteria:

- Major criteria:
  - Severe dilatation of the right ventricle or outflow tract, or localized aneurysms of the right ventricle or outflow tract (▶ Fig. 2.28).
  - Fibrofatty replacement of right ventricular myocardium on endocardial biopsy.
  - Localized prolongation of the QRS complex to more than 110 milliseconds or epsilon waves in leads V1–V3 on ECG.
  - Positive family history with histological confirmation.
- Minor criteria:
  - Mild dilatation of the right ventricle or outflow tract.
  - Regional hypokinesis.
  - Inverted T waves in patients over 12 years of age.
  - Late potentials.
  - Ventricular tachycardia with left bundle branch block.
  - More than 1000 ventricular extrasystoles per 24 hours.

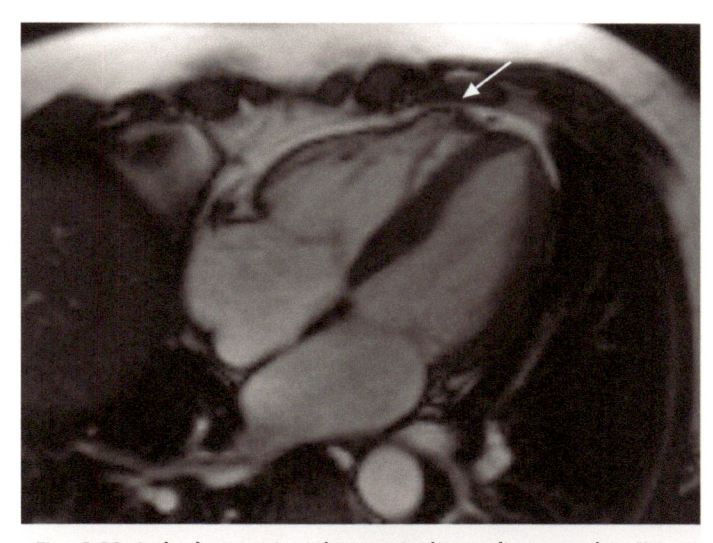

Fig. 2.28 Arrhythmogenic right ventricular cardiomyopathy. Cine image in the four-chamber view demonstrates a right ventricular aneurysm (arrow), which is a major diagnostic criterion for arrhythmogenic right ventricular cardiomyopathy.

- Sudden cardiac death in a first-degree relative under 35 years of age.
- Suspected family history of arrhythmogenic right ventricular dysplasia not confirmed histologically.

▶ **Key points.** MRI is the gold standard for the diagnosis of arrhythmogenic right ventricular cardiomyopathy. Major and minor criteria are considered in making the diagnosis.

Restrictive Cardiomyopathies

Restrictive cardiomyopathies are a group of diseases characterized by restricted diastolic function due to stiffening of the myocardium. Various pathogenic mechanisms have been identified:
- Infiltration of the myocardium.
- Various kind of deposits in storage diseases (extracellular amyloid deposits in amyloidosis, granulomas in sarcoidosis, glucocerebrosides in Gaucher's disease, mucopolysaccharides in Hurler's disease, Fabry's disease [lysosomal storage disease], glycogen storage diseases).
- Endomyocardial fibrosis (e.g., in hypereosinophilia syndrome, after radiotherapy, or drug-induced).

Amyloidosis

▶ **Brief definition.** Amyloidosis is characterized by the deposition of abnormally folded glycoproteins in the form of insoluble fibrils in the extracellular space. This leads to thickening of the myocardium and later of the valve leaflets and atria. In primary amyloidosis, these changes occur in the absence of other precipitating disease. Plasmacytoma is often associated with amyloid deposition. "Reactive" amyloidosis may develop in chronic inflammatory diseases such as osteomyelitis, Crohn's disease, or rheumatoid arthritis. Amyloidosis may affect almost any organ. Cardiac involvement has major prognostic significance in patients with primary amyloidosis, in whom heart and renal failure are the principal causes of death.

▶ **Imaging signs.** Imaging shows myocardial thickening of both cardiac chambers without dilatation. This is the same appearance seen in concentric hypertrophy (▶ Fig. 2.29). Valves and atrial walls become thickened later in the course of the disease. Cine MRI shows a restrictive pattern with decreased diastolic filling of the ventricles. T2 W imaging shows decreased signal intensity in the myocardium due to amyloid deposition. Diffuse myocardial involvement makes this change difficult to detect, however, since healthy myocardium is not available for comparison. Given the restrictive filling mechanism, T2 W black-blood imaging often shows an absence of signal suppression in the atria because insufficient unsaturated blood flows into the slice between the inversion pulses. T1 W mapping before injection of contrast medium shows a prolonged T1 time. The interstitial deposition of glycoproteins leads to expansion of the extracellular space. This increases the distribution volume for extracellular MRI contrast medium, causing increased signal intensity on T1 W images after injection of contrast medium. Because the amyloid deposition is diffuse and begins at the subendocardial level, delayed enhancement imaging shows a diffuse enhancement pattern that is most prominent at the subendocardial level (see ▶ Fig. 2.29). Rapid contrast washout from the blood occurs in patients with a large total amount of glycoprotein deposition, because the contrast medium accumulates rapidly in the large interstitial space (see ▶ Fig. 2.29).[12] For this reason, and because of the diffuse myocardial enhancement, it is difficult to select an appropriate inversion time for delayed enhancement and it is extremely difficult to null the myocardium.

▶ **Differential diagnosis.** Differentiation is mainly required from hypertrophic cardiomyopathy, as approximately one-half of patients with amyloidosis show asymmetrical thickening of the interventricular septum.[13]

▶ **Key points.** Cardiac involvement in patients with amyloidosis can be evaluated with MRI.

Sarcoidosis

▶ **Brief definition.** Sarcoidosis involves (p. 158) the heart in up to 30% of cases.[14] Cardiac involvement has a multifactorial pathophysiology and pathogenesis. At 58%, the frequency of cardiac involvement with sarcoidosis in Japan is significantly higher than in other countries and is responsible for 85% of all sarcoidosis deaths (compared with ca. 25% in Europe and the United States).[9] The pathophysiologic correlate of sarcoidosis is a noncaseating granuloma composed of macrophages and lymphocytes.[15] These cells secrete cytokines, which subsequently promote scar formation at the site of the healing granuloma. Diagnosis is extremely difficult

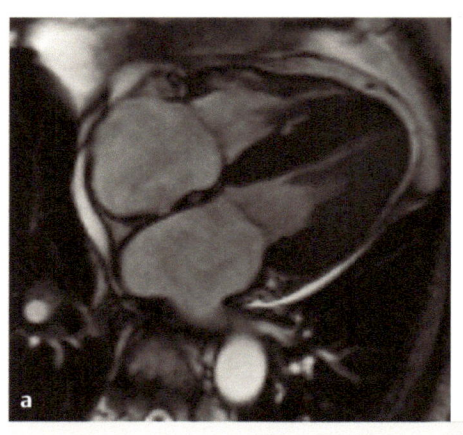

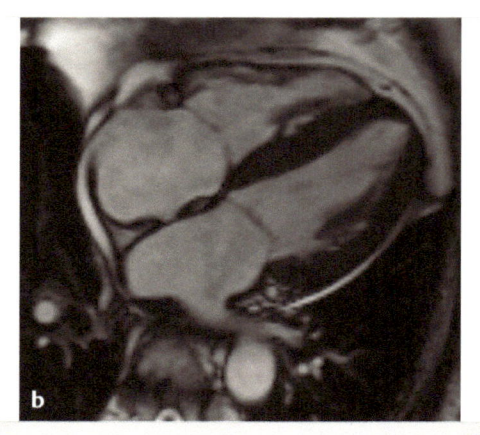

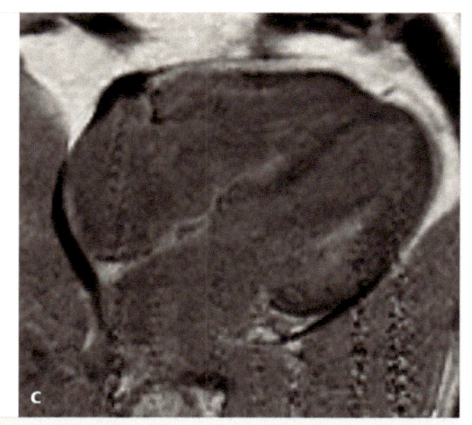

Fig. 2.29 Amyloidosis. (a) TrueFISP sequence, end systole. (b) TrueFISP sequence at end diastole shows myocardial thickening in both ventricles and restrictive dysfunction. (c) T1 W inversion recovery GRE sequence. Delayed enhancement image shows a global increase in myocardial signal intensity. Blood signal intensity is markedly decreased just 10 minutes after injection of contrast medium.

if only the heart is affected because no specific tests are available and it is difficult to obtain a representative biopsy due to sampling error (i.e., sampling of tissue from an unaffected site). The sensitivity of myocardial biopsy in sarcoidosis is only about 20%.[9]

▶ **Clinical features.** The dominant symptoms of systemic sarcoidosis relate to pulmonary involvement. Only 5% of patients develop cardiac symptoms. Most of these cases involve conduction disorders or tachyarrhythmias with risk of sudden cardiac death.

▶ **Imaging signs.** T2W MRI often shows circumscribed edema in areas of granuloma formation. The myocardium is thickened at these sites (▶ Fig. 2.30). The granulomas enhance after IV injection of contrast medium. "Burned out" granulomas leave behind scars that are clearly visualized by delayed enhancement but no longer show edema in T2W sequences. Circumscribed myocardial thickening has usually resolved by that time. The basal portions of the left ventricle are sites of predilection for granuloma formation.

▶ **Differential diagnosis.** Because of the patchy enhancement, myocarditis is an important differential diagnosis.

▶ **Key points.** MRI can detect cardiac involvement by sarcoidosis, which implies a poorer prognosis.

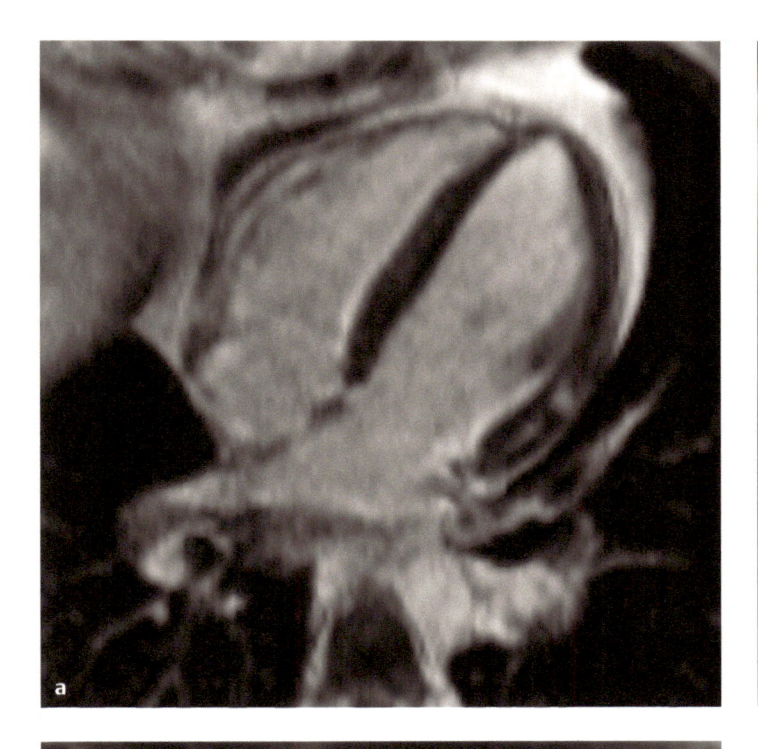

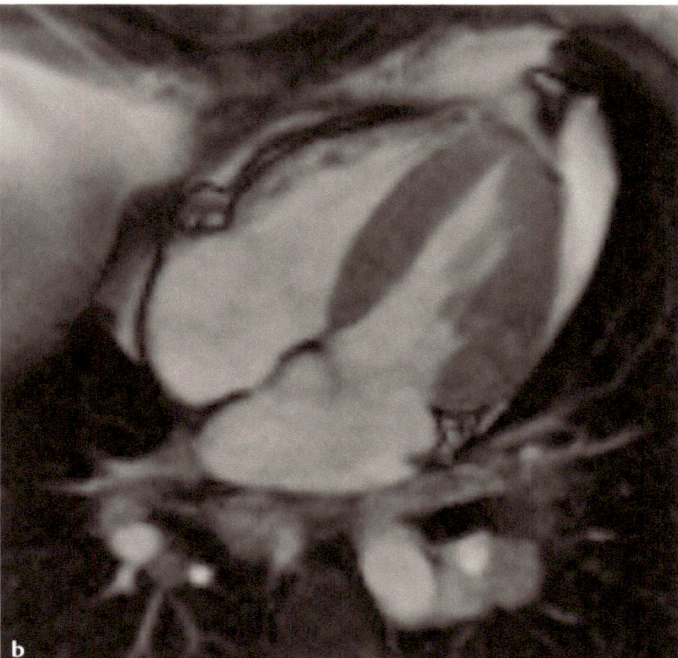

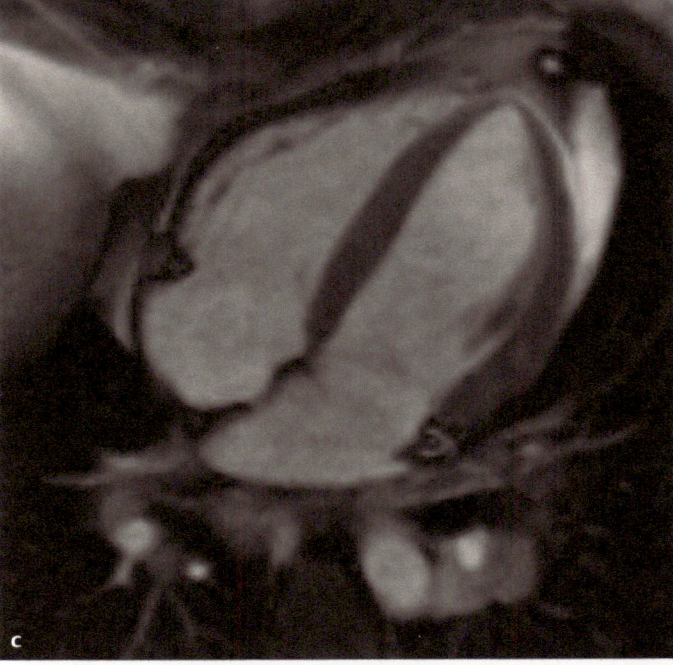

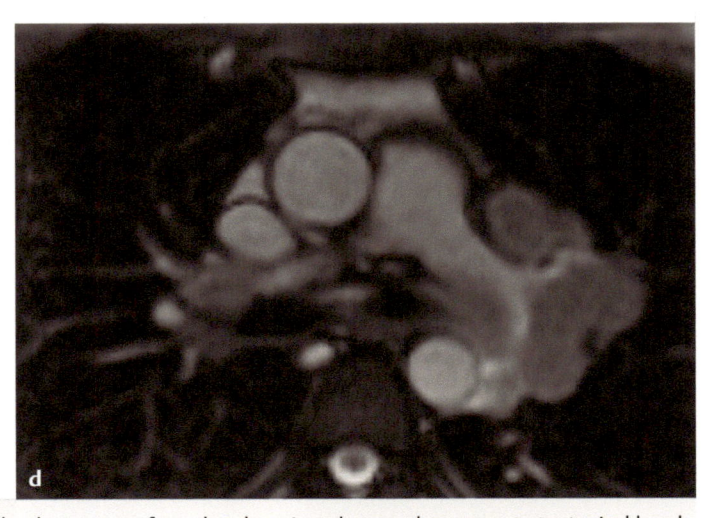

Fig. 2.30 Sarcoidosis. (a) T1W inversion recovery GRE sequence. Delayed-enhancement four-chamber view shows enhancement at a typical basal site in the lateral wall of the left ventricle. **(b)** TrueFISP sequence, end diastole. **(c)** TrueFISP sequence at end systole shows wall thickening in the affected area. **(d)** Axial TrueFISP image demonstrates bilateral lymphadenopathy.

Heart and Pericardium

Takotsubo Cardiomyopathy

▶ **Brief definition.** Takotsubo cardiomyopathy, also called "broken heart syndrome," is caused by an excess of catecholamine or a sudden sharp rise of epinephrine in the blood. It is usually precipitated by a highly stressful event such as the death of a spouse, a serious accident, or a failed suicide attempt. The midcavity and apical wall segments exhibit severe hypokinesis or akinesis with no associated coronary stenosis or occlusion. The two-chamber view shows ballooning of those wall segments during systole. The disease was first described by Japanese scientists, who noticed the similarity of the affected heart to the clay pots used as octopus traps (▶ Fig. 2.31a). The pathogenic mechanism of takotsubo cardiomyopathy is not fully understood but presumably relates to a catecholamine-induced vasospasm that particularly affects the smaller vessels. However, myocardial biopsies have also shown that the catecholamines have a direct injurious effect on cardiomyocytes and activate "stress genes" that eventually lead to apoptosis. Takotsubo cardiomyopathy occurs predominantly in postmenopausal women; this group has been found to have increased numbers of adrenergic receptors in the apical region of the heart. In younger patients, by contrast, these receptors are more numerous in the basal region; this group is subject to "reverse" takotsubo cardiomyopathy, which affects the basal wall segments while sparing the apical myocardium. This form of the disease is much rarer, however.

▶ **Clinical features.** Two-thirds of patients have chest pain and dyspnea that mimic the symptoms of a heart attack. If left ventricular dysfunction is severe, it may lead to cardiogenic shock. ECG changes are not seen in 66% of patients. The troponin level is slightly elevated in most cases. Potentially fatal arrhythmias may occur, so treatment with beta blockers is advised. These agents also have a beneficial effect on basal hyperkinesis. Angiotensin-converting enzyme (ACE) inhibitors are also used for treatment of acute heart failure. Ventricular thrombus formation in akinetic wall regions has been described, so treatment with coumarins is also recommended. Mortality is approximately 8%.

▶ **Imaging signs.** The diagnosis is suggested by apical or midcavity hypokinesis or dyskinesis in the ECG and by absence of coronary artery stenosis on MRI, CT, or angiography (▶ Fig. 2.31b–e). Delayed enhancement is not found in most patients. Left ventricular dysfunction will resolve spontaneously in 3 to 4 weeks.

▶ **Key points.** Takotsubo cardiomyopathy is precipitated by a catecholamine excess in response to a stressful event. Impaired left ventricular function shows an almost pathognomonic pattern of dysfunction that persists for several weeks. Fatal arrhythmias may occur during this time. MRI shows the typical functional abnormality with no evidence of myocardial infarction or an ischemic perfusion defect. The condition resolves spontaneously within a few weeks.

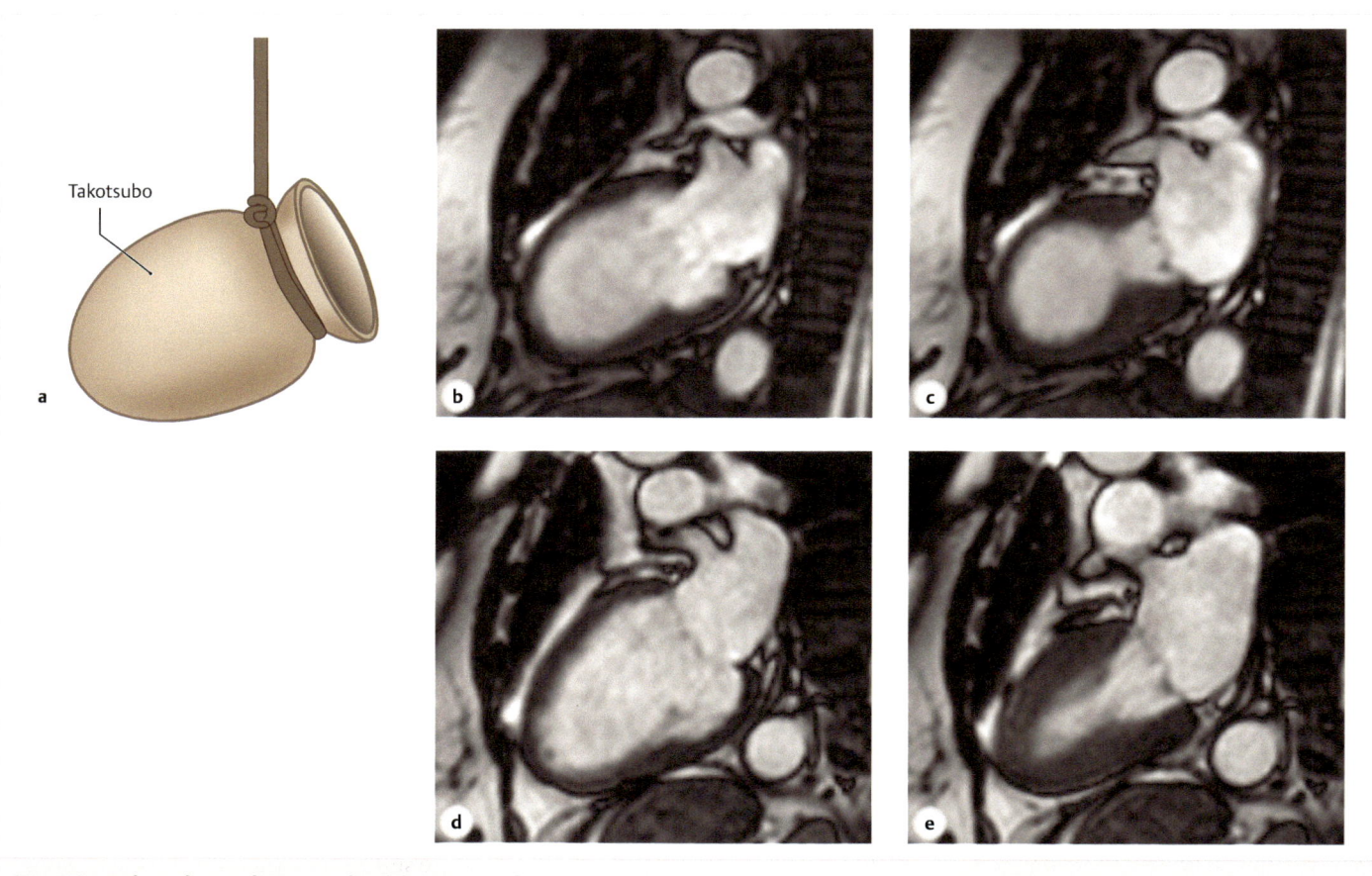

Fig. 2.31 Takotsubo cardiomyopathy. (a) Drawing of the "octopus pot" for which the disease is named. (b) End-diastolic TrueFISP image. (c) End-systolic TrueFISP image. The left ventricle shows apical and midventricular hypokinesis. (d) End-diastolic TrueFISP image 3 weeks later. (e) Corresponding end-systolic image documents complete resolution of hypokinesis.

Hypertrophic Cardiomyopathy

▶ **Brief definition.** Hypertrophic cardiomyopathy may be inherited as an autosomal dominant trait or may result from a spontaneous mutation. It is characterized by a usually asymmetrical thickening of the myocardium. The genetic defect involves sarcomere proteins. Hypertrophic obstructive cardiomyopathy is distinguished from the nonobstructive form. In patients with obstructive cardiomyopathy, the left ventricular outflow tract is narrowed at rest or during exercise. This occurs in slightly more than half of patients with nonobstructive hypertrophic cardiomyopathy. The first major pathophysiologic event is diastolic dysfunction. Later a disproportion arises between oxygen demand and microperfusion (capillary density).

▶ **Clinical features.** Hypertrophic cardiomyopathy is extremely variable in its severity and symptomatology. The phenotype usually presents in young adulthood. Genetic tests are available for establishing an early diagnosis. Young, asymptomatic family members of affected individuals are advised to have a screening examination every 5 years, as the disease may have a late onset. The dominant pathophysiologic feature is diastolic dysfunction. Patients with hypertrophic cardiomyopathy may remain asymptomatic for life; others may develop heart failure necessitating a heart transplant; fatal arrhythmias may also occur. Chest pain and exertional dyspnea are a common result of the diastolic dysfunction. Obstruction of the left ventricular outflow tract, usually associated with anterior motion of the anterior mitral valve leaflet, that is refractory to drug therapy should be managed by an invasive reduction of septal thickness.

▶ **Imaging signs.** Echocardiography and MRI show wall thickening to more than 12 mm in diastole. Cine MRI can demonstrate regional and global function, including obstruction of the left ventricular outflow tract. In a cine TrueFISP sequence, the obstruction appears as a flow jet in the outflow tract and at the level of the anterior mitral valve leaflet. Another feature of nonobstructive hypertrophic cardiomyopathy is hypercontraction, which appears on MRI as a very small ventricular cavity in systole (▶ Fig. 2.32). Perfusion imaging can identify hypoperfused myocardium. With symmetrical involvement of the left ventricle, a circumferential pattern of hypoperfusion will be seen. Delayed enhancement shows a patchy (tiger-stripe) pattern of uptake of contrast medium (▶ Fig. 2.33). The extent of enhancement correlates with the risk of arrhythmia.

▶ **Differential diagnosis.** Differentiation is required from hypertrophy due to hypertension and from hypertrophy in competitive athletes. Both can be identified when the history is taken. Myocardial storage diseases can usually be differentiated from nonobstructive hypertrophic cardiomyopathy on the basis of their systemic manifestations and associated symptoms.

▶ **Key points.** MRI can be used to evaluate the obstruction in hypertrophic obstructive cardiomyopathy and can demonstrate the pattern of spread of myocardial hypertrophy. Several studies have shown that the extent of delayed enhancement can predict the likelihood of developing an arrhythmia.

Noncompaction Cardiomyopathy

▶ **Brief definition.** Noncompaction cardiomyopathy is based on an arrest during embryogenesis of normal compaction of the heavily trabeculated left ventricular myocardium, resulting in failure to form a compact wall.

▶ **Clinical features.** Noncompaction cardiomyopathy may be an asymptomatic incidental finding. In other cases, thrombus formation may occur in the heavily trabeculated myocardium. Rare cases present with congestive heart failure.

▶ **Imaging signs.** The ratio of trabeculated myocardium to compact myocardium is greater than 2:1 (▶ Fig. 2.34). The changes are typically located at an apical to midcavitary level. Delayed enhancement does not occur.

▶ **Key points.** MRI can establish the diagnosis of noncompaction cardiomyopathy.

Cardiac Tumors

Primary cardiac tumors, or masses that originate from the heart, are very rare and have a prevalence of only 0.001 to 0.05% in autopsy series. Approximately 80% of all primary cardiac tumors are benign but may cause heart failure by obstructing the cardiac chambers or inciting arrhythmia. Malignant secondary cardiac tumors, consisting of metastases and mediastinal or pulmonary masses that invade the heart by contiguous spread, have a 40 times higher prevalence.[16] But the most common "cardiac masses" in the broadest sense are intracardiac thrombi, which have a tendency to form in akinetic areas.

▶ **Selection of modalities.** Echocardiography is the most common initial study, as it is for most cardiac diseases. MRI is used for the accurate determination of extent, invasion of adjacent structures, and resectability. CT may be used if MRI is contraindicated. In accordance with established guidelines, MRI should define the location and extent of the mass and any infiltrated structures, determine whether the lesion is benign or malignant whenever possible, and also determine vascularity by perfusion imaging at rest.[17] CT, on the other hand, is used mainly for the evaluation of paracardiac and mediastinal masses with intracardiac extension. Details of protocol based on current recommendations are outlined below[17]:

- Tumors that do not transcend the pericardium:
  1. Axial T1 W sequence (jugular fossa to below the diaphragm).
  2. Cine TrueFISP sequence in the two, three-, and four-chamber views and along the short axis of the left ventricle.
  3. T2 W sequence focused on the tumor in the best standard plane (sagittal, coronal or axial).
  4. T1 W sequence focused on the tumor in the best standard plane.
  5. Resting perfusion imaging of the tumor in the best standard plane.
  6. Repeat sequence no. 4.
  7. Delayed enhancement in the two, three- and four-chamber views and along the short axis of the left ventricle.
- Tumors that transcend the pericardium:
  1. Axial T1 W sequence (jugular fossa to below the diaphragm).
  2. Coronal T1 W sequence (whole chest).

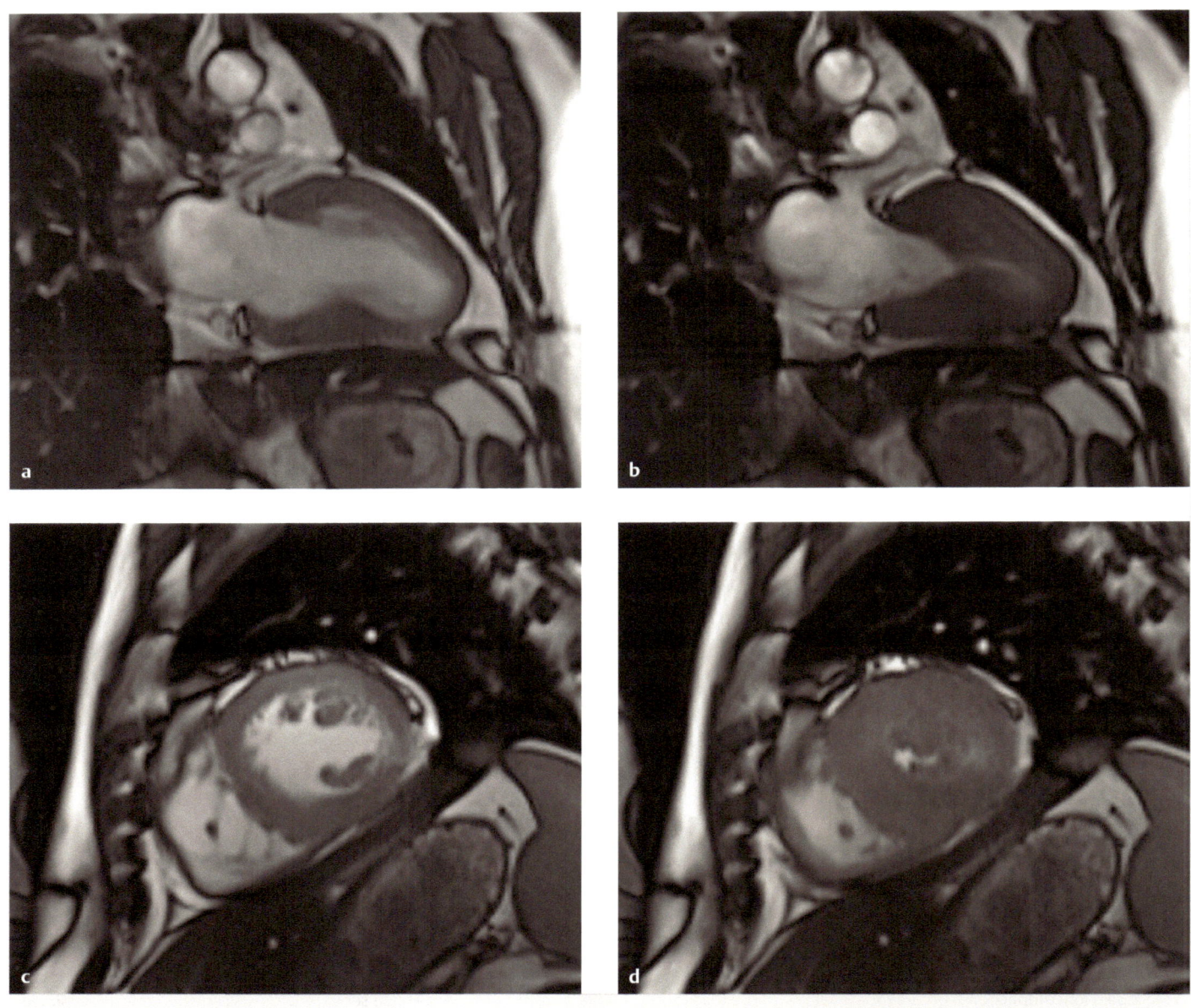

Fig. 2.32 **Hypertrophic cardiomyopathy.** The very small cavity size at end systole is a typical feature of hypertrophic cardiomyopathy. **(a)** End-diastolic TrueFISP image, four-chamber view. **(b)** End-systolic TrueFISP image, four-chamber view. **(c)** End-diastolic short-axis view. **(d)** End-systolic short-axis view.

3. Sagittal T1 W sequence (whole chest).
4. Cine TrueFISP sequence in the two, three-, and four-chamber views; add the short axis if the tumor reaches the ventricles.
5. T2 W sequence focused on the tumor in the best standard plane.
6. Rest perfusion imaging of the tumor in the best standard plane.
7. T1 W sequence focused on the tumor in the best standard plane.
8. Delayed enhancement in the two, three- and four-chamber views and along the short axis of the left ventricle.
9. If the great vessels are encased, follow perfusion imaging with MR angiography of the pulmonary artery and aorta and the central venous system.

First the location and extent of the cardiac mass should be described. The tumor may have an intracavitary, intramural, intrapericardial, or paracardial (extrapericardial) location (▶ Fig. 2.35). Then it should be determined whether the mass is benign or malignant.

Note

Malignancy criteria for cardiac tumors:
- Extension into more than one cardiac chamber.
- Extension into central vessels (vena cava, aorta, pulmonary arteries or veins).
- Broad attachment to the heart wall.
- Combined intramural and intracavitary growth.
- Presence of large necrotic areas in the tumor.
- Invasion of the mediastinum.
- Hemorrhagic pericardial effusion.
- Blood supply derived from the coronary arteries.

Malignant cardiac tumors are supplied by the coronary arteries. This can be determined by rest perfusion imaging. If the tumor is perfused by the coronary arteries, its nonnecrotic portions will show prominent first-pass enhancement.

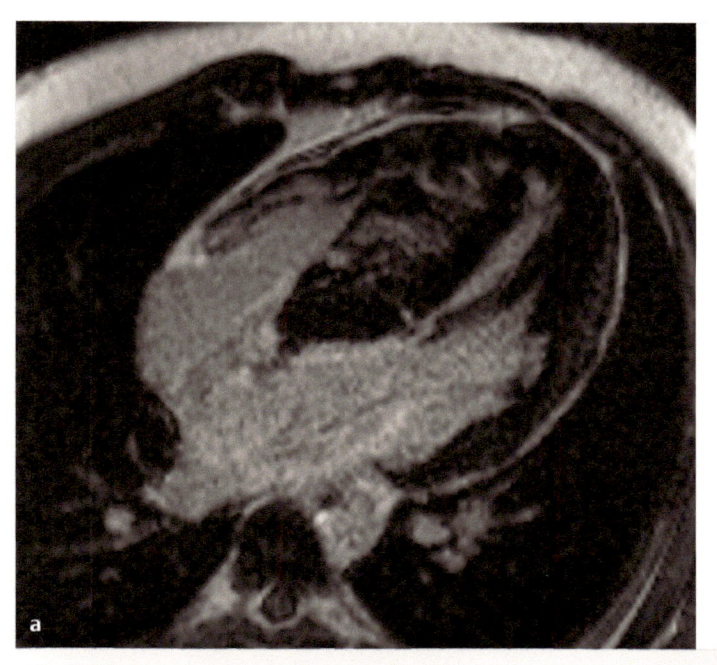

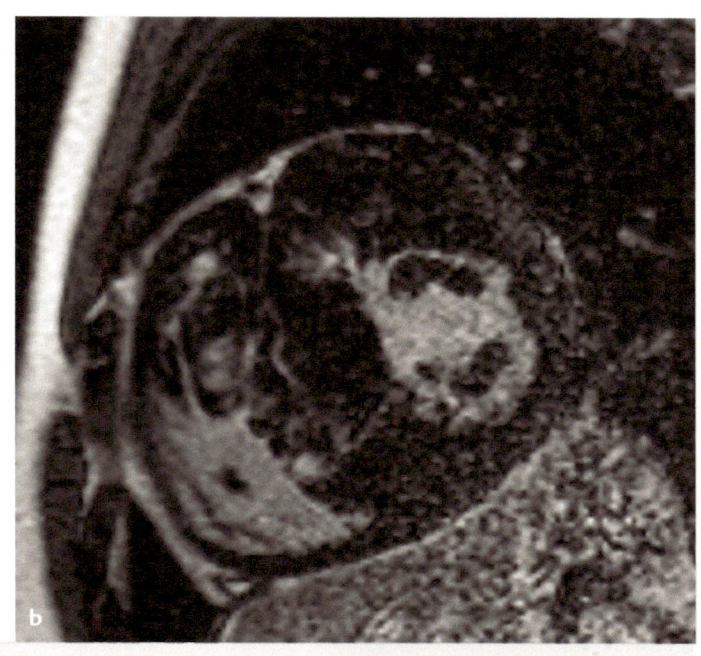

Fig. 2.33 **Hypertrophic cardiomyopathy.** (a) T1 W inversion recovery GRE sequence. Four-chamber view shows patchy delayed enhancement in the septum. (b) T1 W inversion recovery GRE sequence. Short-axis view also shows patchy delayed enhancement in the free wall of the true ventricle.

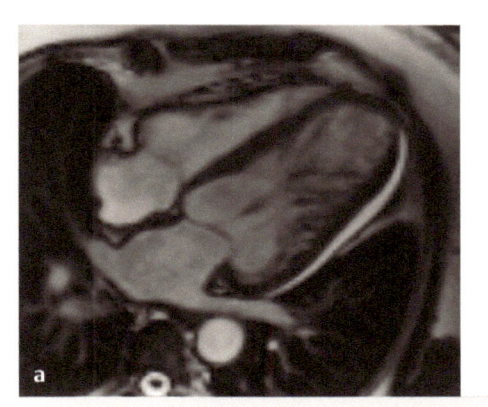

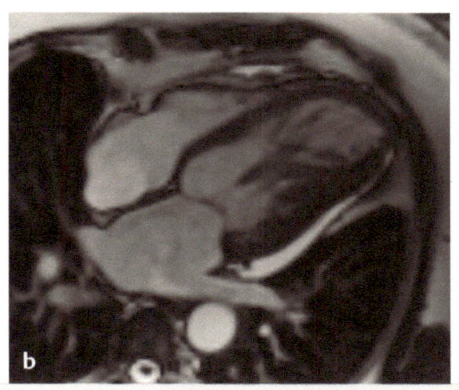

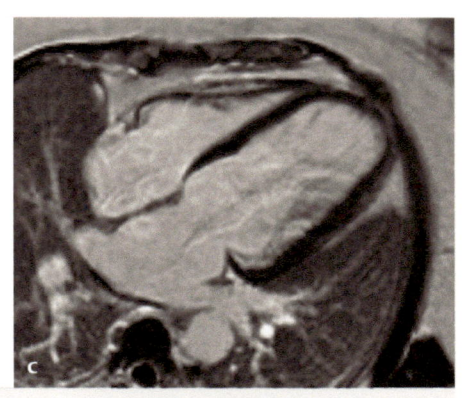

Fig. 2.34 **Noncompaction cardiomyopathy.** (a) End-diastolic four-chamber view from a TrueFISP cine sequence. The thickness of the trabeculated myocardium is more than twice the wall thickness of the left ventricle. (b) End-systolic image from a TrueFISP cine sequence. Left ventricular function is markedly impaired. (c) T1 W inversion recovery GRE sequence in the four-chamber view shows absence of delayed enhancement.

Benign Primary Cardiac Tumors

Myxoma

▶ **Brief definition.** Myxoma is the most common benign cardiac tumor and the most common of all primary cardiac tumors. Myxomas are located in the left atrium in 75% of cases and in the right atrium in 20% of cases. Females are predominantly affected by an approximately 3:1 ratio.[10] The peak age of incidence is broad, ranging from 30 to 60 years. Myxomas usually occur sporadically. The recurrence rate after surgical excision is only 1 to 3%. Up to 7% of all myxomas have a genetic etiology, however, and the may occur in syndromic conditions such as Carney's syndrome. Myxomas originate from mesenchymal cardiomyocyte progenitor cells,[18] which explains their predilection for the left atrium and their attachment to the atrial septum.

▶ **Imaging signs.** Two different types of myxoma are distinguished by their imaging morphologies: a rounded type and a polypoid villous type. Polypoid myxoma has a friable consistency and may shed peripheral arterial emboli.[19] Because they are composed of tumor fragments, these emboli are unresponsive to thrombolytic therapy, and anticoagulation has no prophylactic benefit. Myxomas of the left atrium are usually attached to the fossa ovalis by a pedicle (▶ Fig. 2.36, ▶ Fig. 2.37). With very large tumors that occupy the atrium almost completely, the attachment site may be difficult to identify and can mimic a sessile attachment to the atrial septum. Cine MRI shows the motion of the tumor during the cardiac cycle, making it easier to locate the point of attachment. When applied to larger tumors, this technique has documented tumor sliding from the atrium into the ventricle during diastole. Due to their soft consistency, atrial myxomas may grow into the right atrium through a patent foramen ovale, and even extra-atrial extension has been found in very rare cases. Myxomas often contain calcifications, which are well defined by CT. Myxomas are isointense to myocardium on T1 W SE images. They are generally hyperintense to myocardium

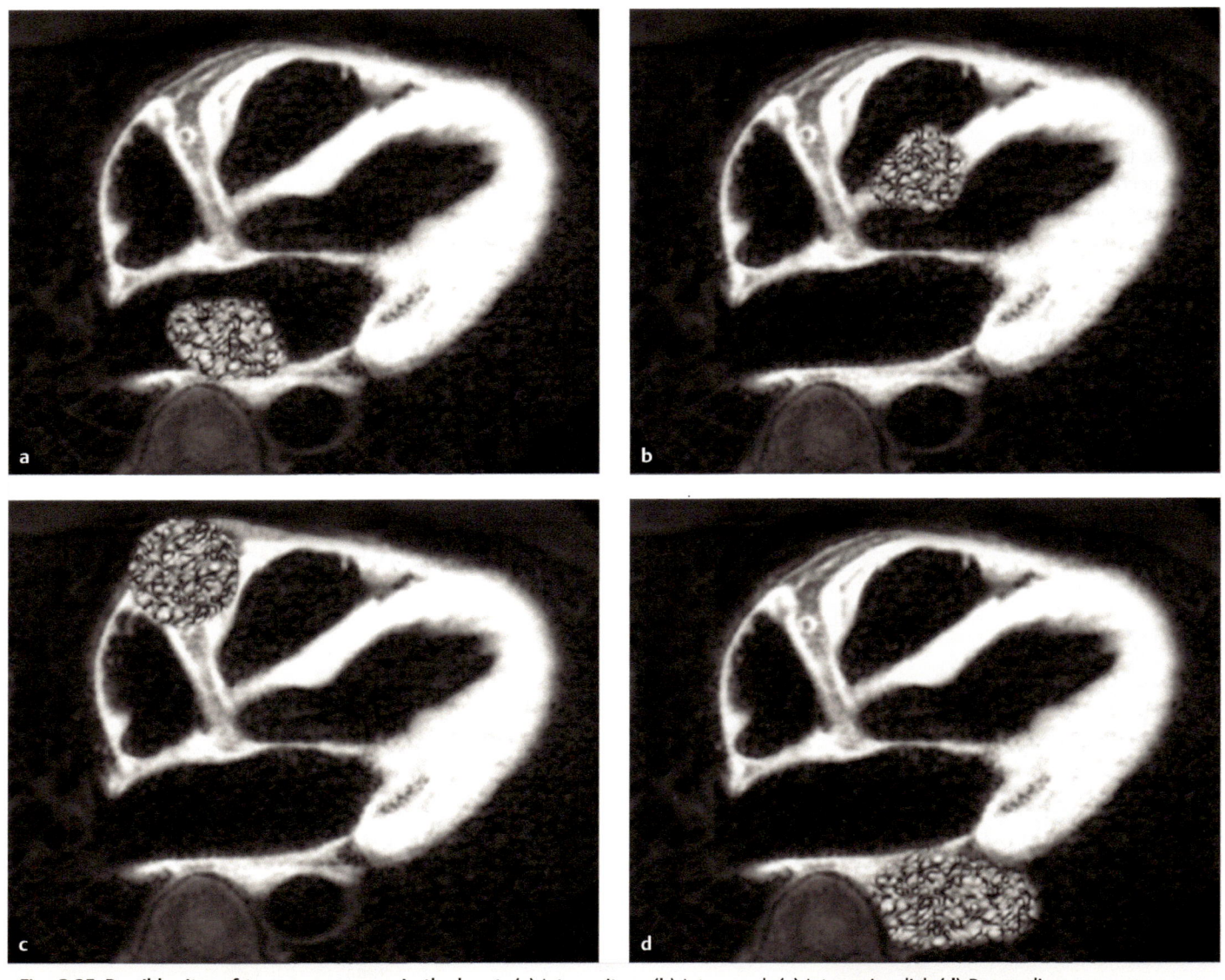

Fig. 2.35 Possible sites of tumor occurrence in the heart. (a) Intracavitary. (b) Intramural. (c) Intrapericardial. (d) Paracardiac.

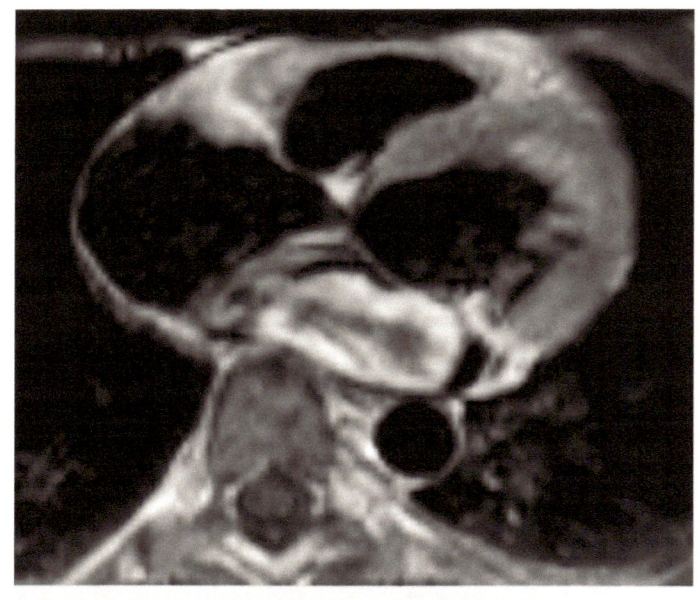

Fig. 2.36 Atrial myxoma. T1 W GRE sequence. The myxoma is located in the left atrium and shows peripheral enhancement.

on T2 W SE images due to their myxoid stroma, although there are myxomas that are hypointense to myocardium. Their variable signal intensity relates to a variable proportion of myxomatous stroma with a high water content and varying amounts of T2-shortening components, mostly interstitial calcifications, fibrotic areas, and deposits of paramagnetic hemoglobin breakdown products after interstitial hemorrhage.[20] Myxomas usually show increased signal intensity on T1 W images. On CT, myxomas are hypodense and show a moderate delayed contrast enhancement after IV administration of contrast medium. This signal increase is attributable to the enlarged interstitial space and greater distribution volume compared with myocardium.

▶ **Clinical features.** The initial symptoms may be transient ischemic attacks or an ischemic insult. Generally speaking, myxoma tissue may be a source of arterial emboli to all body regions, especially the coronary arteries. Symptoms caused either by mechanical obstruction of the cardiac chambers or by the release of cytokines are also commonly reported. Myxomas in the left atrium may lead to mitral valve obstruction with enlargement of the left atrium and right ventricle. Pedunculated myxomas may prolapse into the left ventricle in diastole, causing acute mitral valve obstruction with consequent heart failure. Mitral valve obstruction presents clinically with dyspnea and cyanosis, acute pulmonary edema, syncopal attacks, and possible cardiogenic shock. The diagnosis is suggested by symptom improvement in response to position change. The formation of interleukin-6 and tumor necrosis factor-α can lead to weight loss or cachexia, Raynaud's phenomenon, and an elevated ESR.

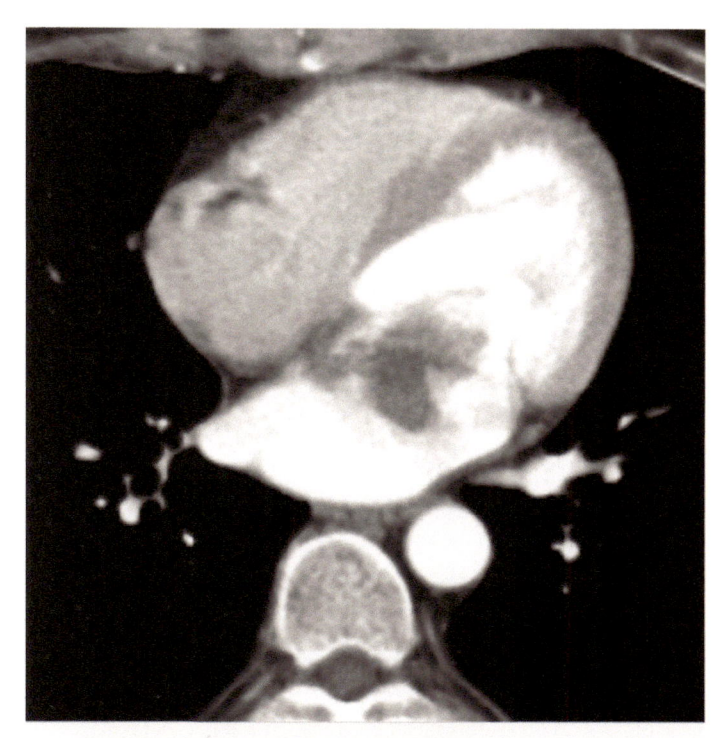

Fig. 2.37 **Atrial myxoma.** CT scan in a patient different from the one shown in ▶ Fig. 2.36 shows a myxoma attached to the atrial septum by a pedicle.

▶ **Key points.** Myxoma is the most common primary cardiac tumor. Its site of predilection is the left atrium.

Lipoma and Lipomatous Hypertrophy of the Atrial Septum

▶ **Brief definition**
- *Lipoma*: Lipomas are the second most commonly diagnosed primary cardiac tumors in adults. They may even be the most common adult cardiac tumors in general, as only large lipomas are symptomatic while many small tumors are undiagnosed. The peak age at diagnosis is 50 to 70 years. Lipomas are composed of mature and embryonic fat cells and are usually surrounded by a true capsule. Most cardiac lipomas are intracavitary, being located in the right atrium or atrial septum.
- *Lipomatous hypertrophy of the atrial septum*: This is defined as fatty infiltration of the interatrial septum that is more than 2 cm in thickness and spares the fossa ovalis. Lipomatous hypertrophy of the atrial septum is morphologically and histologically distinct from lipoma and, unlike lipoma, contains brown fat. Lacking a capsule, it has indistinct margins and may infiltrate the myocardium.

▶ **Clinical features**
- *Lipoma*: Large or intramural lipomas may cause atrial or ventricular arrhythmias. Small tumors are asymptomatic.
- *Lipomatous hypertrophy of the atrial septum*: This condition is an asymptomatic incidental finding in the great majority of patients. Given its intramural location, it may cause an impulse conduction disorder and arrhythmias in very rare cases.

▶ **Imaging signs**
- *Lipoma*: Lipoma forms close to the endocardial surface and has a broad area of attachment. Lipomas have fat attenuation on CT with negative HU values (▶ Fig. 2.38). On MRI they have the same signal intensity as subcutaneous or

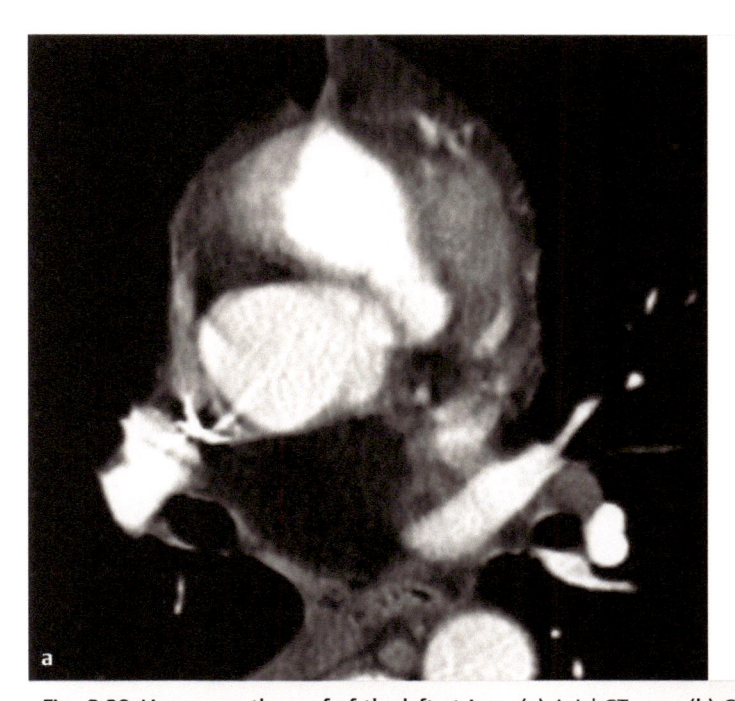

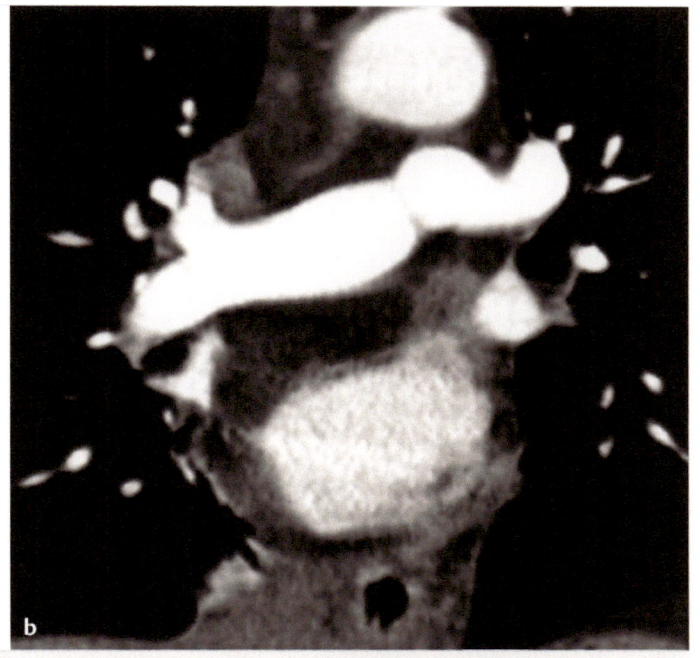

Fig. 2.38 **Lipoma on the roof of the left atrium.** (a) Axial CT scan. (b) Coronal reformatted image. The mass shows fat attenuation and smooth margins.

Heart and Pericardium

epicardial fat in all sequences. The signal can be completely suppressed with a fat-saturation pulse (▶ Fig. 2.39). Lipomas, like fatty tissue, have scant perfusion and a small interstitial space. For these reasons they generally do not enhance after IV injection of contrast medium. On cine images lipomas have a dark margin caused by the extinction effect of fat and blood spins in the same voxel. Unlike liposarcomas, which are extremely rare in the heart, lipomas are soft and change their shape during the cardiac cycle.

- *Lipomatous hypertrophy of the atrial septum*: Lipomatous hypertrophy and lipomas have the same signal characteristics and CT appearance (▶ Fig. 2.40). Lipomatous hypertrophy is distinguished by its location in the atrial septum and sparing of the fossa ovalis.

▶ **Differential diagnosis.** Unlike liposarcomas, which are extremely rare in the heart, lipomas are soft and undergo deformation during the cardiac cycle. This is clearly appreciated in cine MRI. Fat-saturated sequences can completely suppress the lipoma signal.

▶ **Key points**
- *Lipoma*: Cardiac lipomas have the same attenuation or signal intensity as subcutaneous fat on CT and MRI. Their signal on MRI can be suppressed with a fat-saturation pulse.

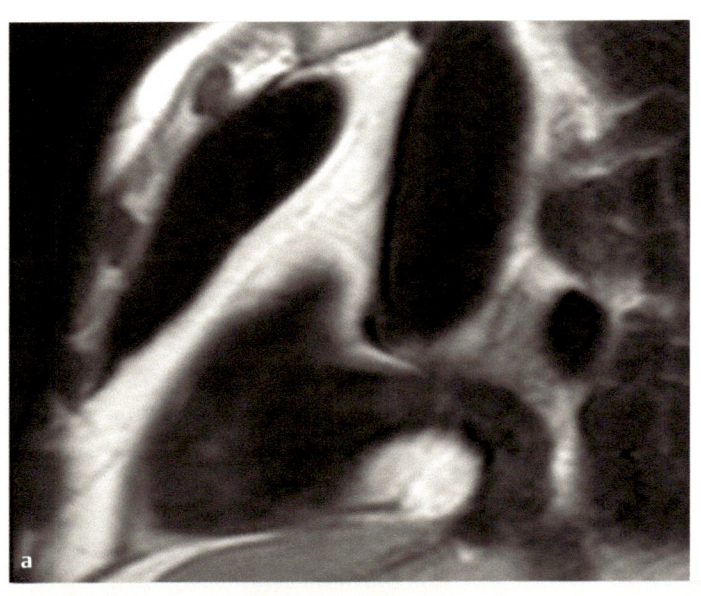

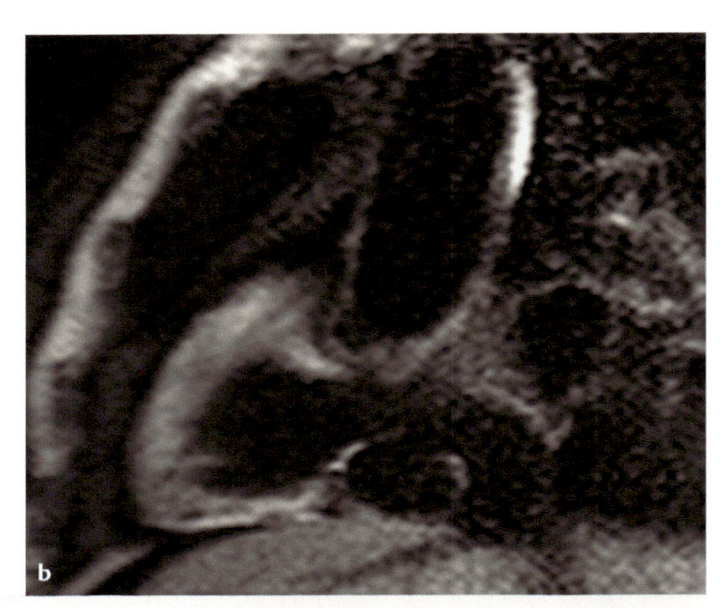

Fig. 2.39 Lipoma in the right atrium. (a) T1 W TSE sequence. The tumor is hyperintense. (b) The signal from the tumor has been completely suppressed with a fat-saturation pulse.

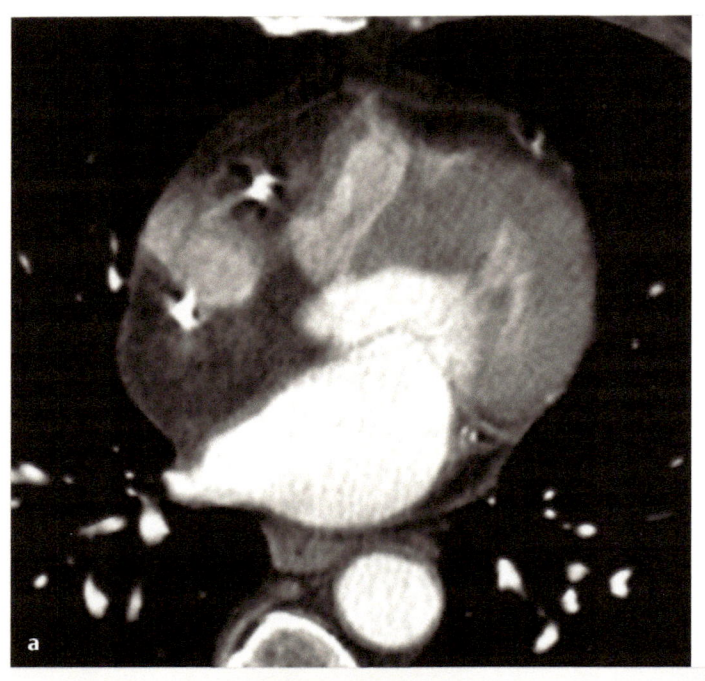

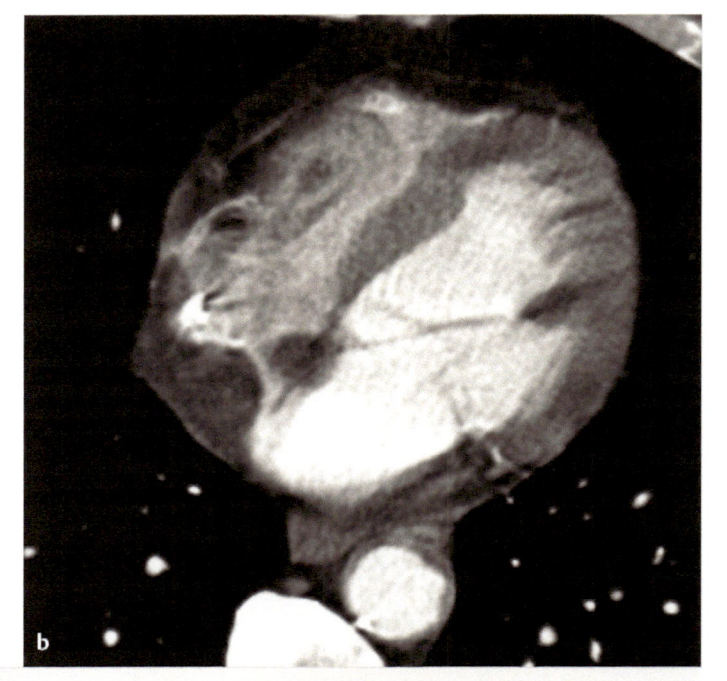

Fig. 2.40 Lipomatous hypertrophy of the atrial septum. (a) The atrial septum is thickened by fatty tissue. Due to the absence of a capsule, its margins appear irregular. (b) Sparing of the fossa ovalis is pathognomonic.

- *Lipomatous hypertrophy of the atrial septum*: This entity has a pathognomonic shape and spares the fossa ovalis.

Papillary Fibroelastoma

▶ **Brief definition.** Papillary fibroelastomas comprise only 10% of all primary cardiac tumors but 70% of all primary tumors of cardiac valves. The peak age of incidence is 60 to 70 years. Fibroelastomas are composed of avascular fibrous strands covered with endothelium. As a general rule, fibroelastomas are less than 1 cm in diameter. In approximately 90% of cases the tumor is attached to the valves by a short pedicle. The aortic valve is involved in 29% of cases, the mitral valve in 25%, the tricuspid valve in 17%, and the pulmonary valve in 13%.[21]

▶ **Clinical features.** Fibroelastomas of the aortic or mitral valve may become symptomatic when thrombi form on their surface and embolize into the arterial circulation.

▶ **Imaging signs.** Owing to their tissue composition, fibroelastomas are hypointense in unenhanced T1 W sequences and hyperintense on T2 W SE images (▶ Fig. 2.41). They enhance markedly after IV administration of contrast medium. The enhancement may be difficult to detect, however, due to their small size. On CT, fibroelastomas appear as filling defects in the arterial phase (▶ Fig. 2.42).

▶ **Differential diagnosis.** Differentiation is required from valvular myxoma and endocardial vegetations due to valvular endocarditis.

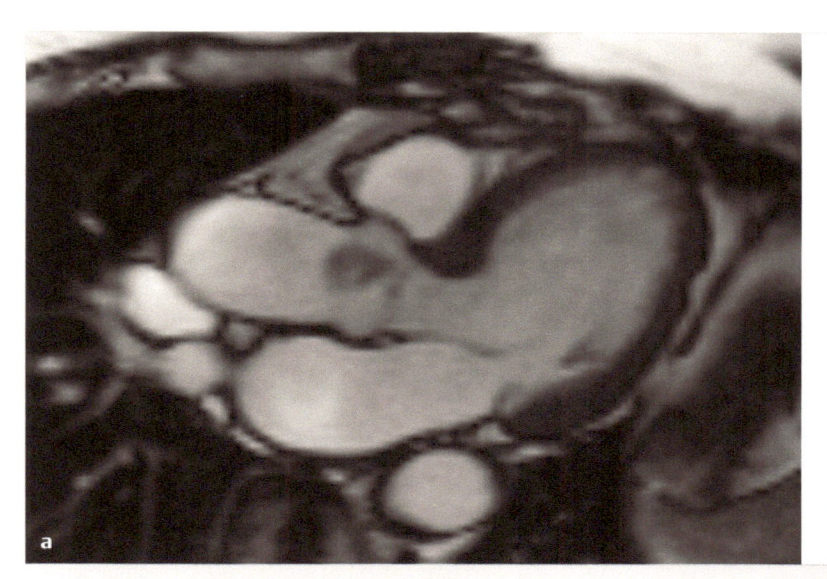

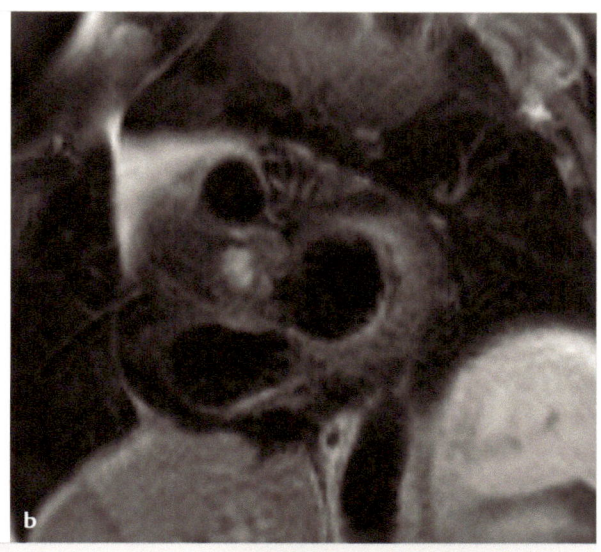

Fig. 2.41 Fibroelastoma. (a) Frame from a cine TrueFISP sequence in the three-chamber view. A small tumor is attached to the aortic valve by a pedicle. (b) T2 W TSE sequence with fat suppression. The fibroelastoma has high signal intensity.

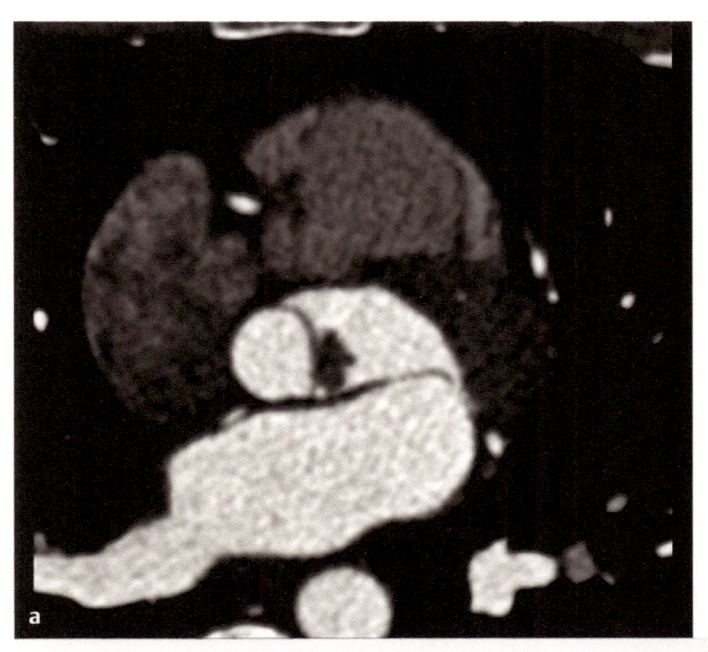

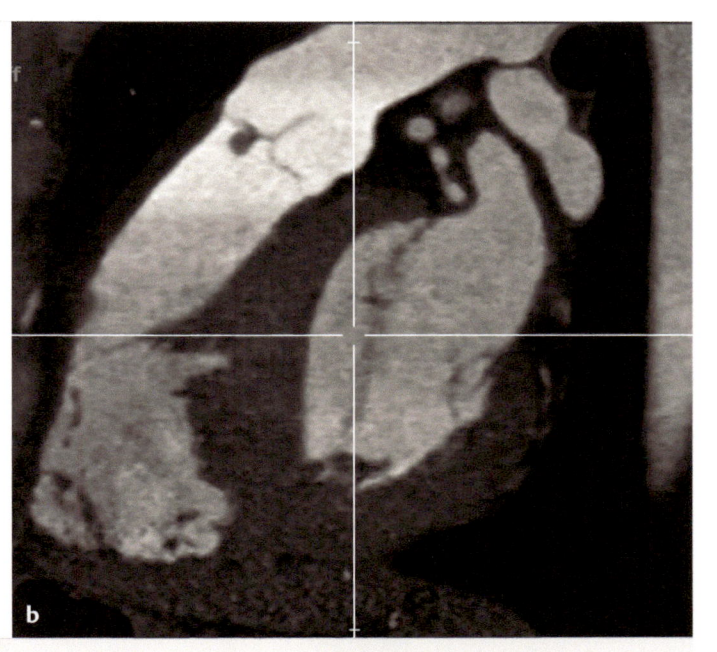

Fig. 2.42 Fibroelastomas. (a) Axial scan of a fibroelastoma on the aortic valve. (b) Sagittal reformatted image of a fibroelastoma on the pulmonary valve.

▶ **Key points.** A papillary fibroelastoma is typically attached to cardiac valves and is usually less than 1 cm in diameter.

Hemangioma

▶ **Brief definition.** Hemangiomas are composed of vascular cavities lined by endothelial cells. As in other organs, the following types are distinguished:
- Cavernous hemangioma: endothelium-lined cavities with large spaces and thin walls.
- Capillary hemangioma: small-caliber capillaries.
- Arteriovenous hemangioma: a tangled mass of thick-walled, dysplastic vessels.

Cardiac hemangiomas may have an intracavitary, intramural, intrapericardial, or paracardiac location. They do not show a predilection for specific chambers.

▶ **Imaging signs.** Intratumoral calcifications are a common finding. Hemangiomas are hyperintense on T2 W images. They are usually isointense to myocardium on T1 W images but may show heterogeneous signal intensity due to the presence of calcifications and signal voids from flowing blood. With their rich vascularity, they enhance intensely on MRI and CT after IV administration of contrast medium.

▶ **Key points.** Hemangiomas occur rarely in the heart and show intense enhancement on CT and MRI.

Benign Primary Cardiac Tumors in Children

▶ **Brief definition.** Primary cardiac tumors are even rarer in children than in adults. Benign primary cardiac tumors in the pediatric age group occur most commonly in the fetal period. Their overall incidence is 0.14%.[22]
- *Rhabdomyoma*: Rhabdomyoma accounts for 90% of all primary cardiac tumors in infancy and the prenatal period and is the most common cardiac tumor in this age group. Between 30 and 50% of rhabdomyomas occur in patients with tuberous sclerosis. The tumors range in size from microscopic cell clusters to masses several centimeters in diameter. Most are diagnosed by prenatal ultrasound. Rhabdomyomas are hamartomas and tend to regress spontaneously during the first few months of life, suggesting a possible dependency on maternal hormones.[23] Thus, resection is indicated only in cases where life-threatening symptoms arise. Rhabdomyomas usually have an intramural location and occur at multiple sites. Both ventricles are affected with equal frequency.
- *Fibroma*: Fibroma is a congenital neoplasm and the second most common cardiac tumor in children. A 2011 meta-analysis of all published cases found a mean age of 11.4 years and a median age of 2.8 years at diagnosis. The mean tumor size was 5.3 cm. By correlating age with tumor size, the authors hypothesized that fibromas stop growing when cardiac growth ceases at approximately 17 to 20 years of age.[24] Fibromas are composed of fibroblasts embedded in firm connective tissue fibers (collagen and elastic fibers). Individual myocytes have an intramural location, usually in the septum or in the anterior wall of the left or right ventricle. Interstitial calcifications are often found.

▶ **Imaging signs**
- *Rhabdomyoma*: Rhabdomyomas appear on echocardiography as an expansion of the myocardium. They are isointense to surrounding myocardium on T1 W images and hyperintense on T2 W images. Rhabdomyomas enhance intensely after IV administration of contrast medium. Administration of contrast medium is often required for the detection of small tumors.
- *Fibroma*: Most fibromas are several centimeters in diameter. Consistent with their composition of fibroblasts and collagen fibers, fibromas are hypointense to surrounding myocardium on T2 W SE images. They are isointense to myocardium on T1 W images. They usually do not show contrast enhancement.

▶ **Clinical features.** Rhabdomyomas are usually asymptomatic and therefore do not require treatment. Rarely they may cause arrhythmia or obstruction of cardiac chambers. Excision is indicated only for tumors that have caused refractory arrhythmia or hemodynamically significant effects on cardiac function.

▶ **Clinical features.** Due to their intramural location, fibromas may lead to conduction abnormalities and arrhythmias with a potential for sudden cardiac death. Intraseptal fibromas are associated with the highest risk of arrhythmias.[24]

▶ **Differential diagnosis.** The differential diagnosis of intramural cardiac tumors in children should include fibroma and rhabdomyoma. With a solitary tumor that is hypointense on T2 W images, fibroma is the most likely diagnosis. Multifocal tumors with high T2 W signal intensity are probably rhabdomyomas.

▶ **Key points.** Fibroma and rhabdomyoma are rare tumors in the pediatric age group. Both entities have an intramural location, but fibromas are solitary whereas rhabdomyomas are multifocal. Rhabdomyomas occur predominantly in patients with tuberous sclerosis.

Thrombi

▶ **Brief definition.** Thrombi are the most common intracardiac "masses." They form on akinetic wall segments due to the stasis of blood in those areas. The atrial appendage is a site of predilection in patients with atrial fibrillation.

▶ **Imaging signs.** Thrombi are usually diagnosed by echocardiography. If findings are equivocal, the modality of choice is MRI. Thrombi appear as signal voids in white-blood sequences such as the cine TrueFISP sequence (▶ Fig. 2.43). They do not enhance after IV injection of contrast medium. In the inversion-recovery GRE sequence used to detect delayed enhancement, thrombi appear as signal voids when long inversion times (> 400 ms) are used.

▶ **Differential diagnosis.** Cardiac tumors generally enhance after IV injection of contrast medium. The presence of akinetic myocardium, indwelling foreign material such as a catheter or port system, or atrial fibrillation is be further evidence of a thrombus.

Malignant Primary Cardiac Tumors

Angiosarcoma

▶ **Brief definition.** Angiosarcomas are the most common malignant primary cardiac tumors (33% of malignant cardiac tumors)

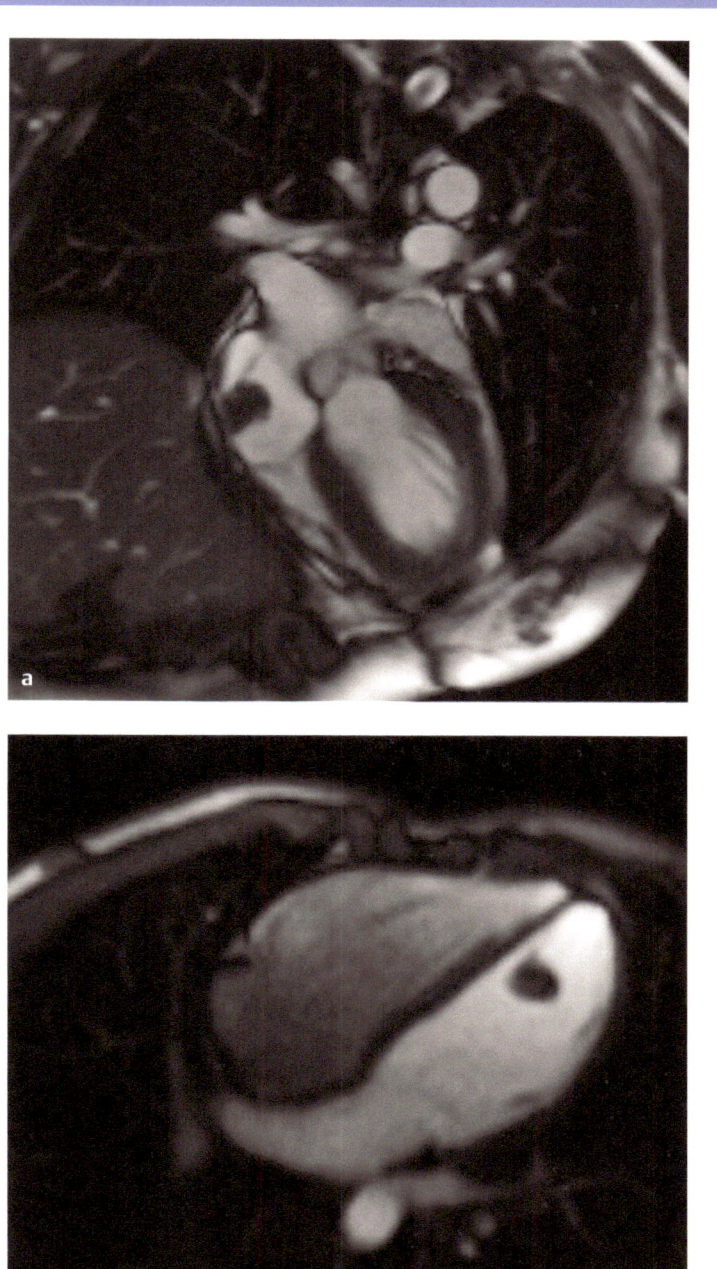

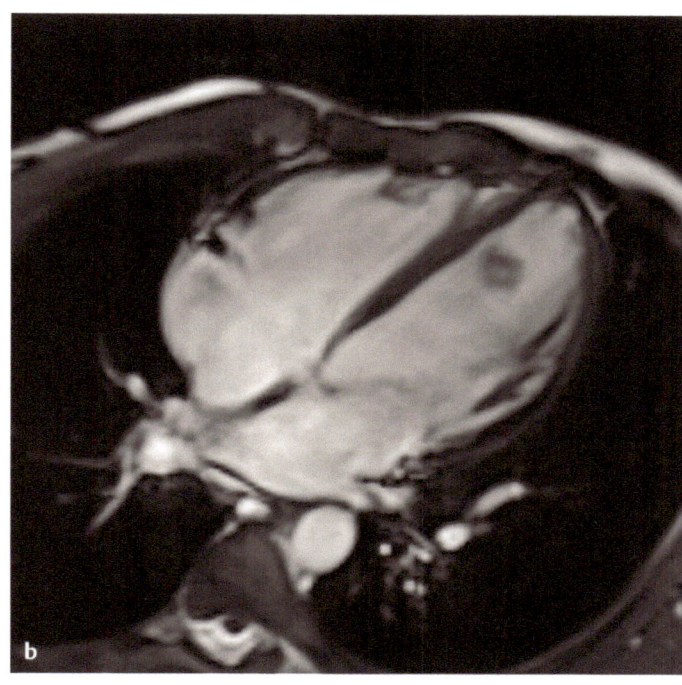

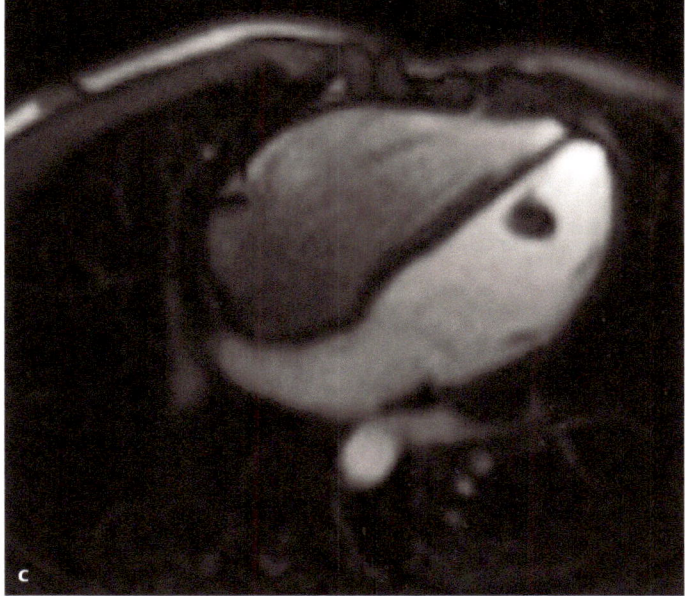

Fig. 2.43 Thrombi. (a) Thrombus in the right atrium at the tip of a port catheter. **(b)** Ventricular thrombus in the left ventricle. **(c)** Frame from a perfusion sequence; the thrombus is nonenhancing even in later sequences.

but are rare in terms of absolute case numbers. The peak incidence age is 20 to 50 years. Two forms are distinguished:
- Angiosarcoma in nonimmunosuppressed patients most commonly occurs in the atrial septum and extends into the right atrium. Up to 80% of patients have distant metastases at the time of diagnosis.
- Angiosarcoma in AIDS patients occur at multifocal sites in the pericardium and epicardium. Most of these tumors are small, asymptomatic lesions. The tumor tissue consists of anastomosing, endothelium-lined vascular spaces embedded in a stroma of pleomorphic spindle cells.

▶ **Clinical features.** Angiosarcoma usually grows at an intramural site, where it may cause conduction disturbances and arrhythmias. It usually takes some time for symptoms to appear, however, so the prognosis is already poor at the time of diagnosis and average life expectancy is only a few months. Because angiosarcomas are soft and bleed easily, hemorrhagic pericardial effusion with pericardial tamponade or acute cardiac rupture is a relatively frequent complication.

▶ **Imaging signs.** Angiosarcoma may show heterogeneous signal intensity on T1 W SE images due to circumscribed areas of intratumoral hemorrhage. The tumor enhances markedly after IV administration of contrast medium due to its rich vascularity. With an intracavitary tumor, this marked enhancement is the main feature differentiating it from a thrombus. The multiple tumor vessels appear as signal voids on T1 W and T2 W SE images and are

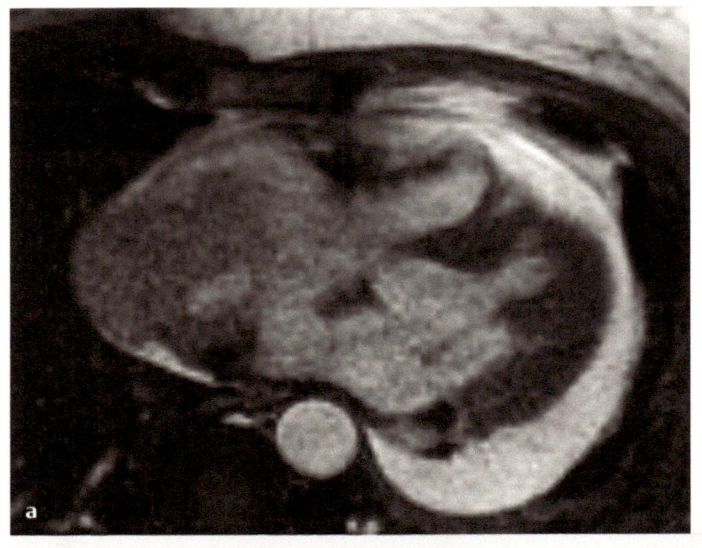

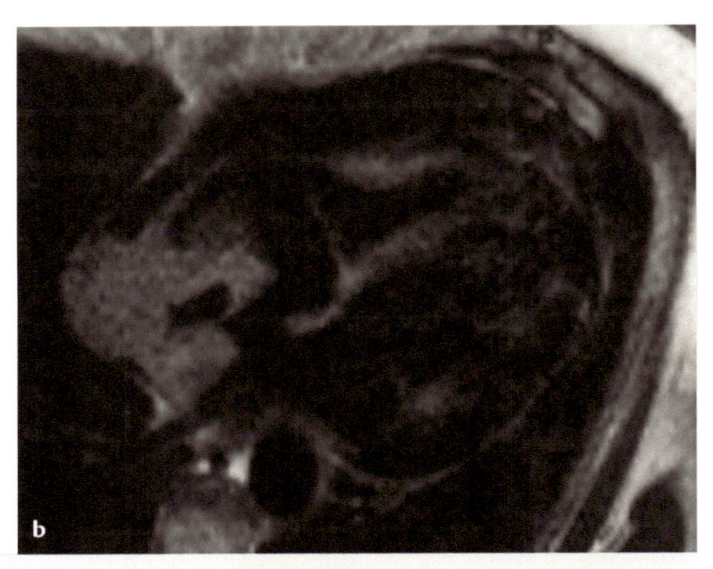

Fig. 2.44 Poorly differentiated angiosarcoma (grade 3). (a) Axial TrueFISP image. The angiosarcoma has infiltrated both atria. The tumor has penetrated the right atrial wall, with an exophytic extension into the pericardial cavity. There is associated pericardial effusion. (b) T2 W TSE sequence with fat suppression. The angiosarcoma has high signal intensity.

hyperintense on GRE images. Poorly differentiated angiosarcomas (grade 3) may have a homogeneous appearance (▶ Fig. 2.44).

Note
Sectional imaging rarely provides a specific diagnosis for malignant primary cardiac tumors in adults. Benign/malignant differentiation and an accurate description of location and infiltrated structures are of prime importance for determining resectability.

▶ **Key points.** The location and extent of the tumor should be described at imaging. Sectional imaging can generally indicate whether an angiosarcoma is benign or malignant. As a rule, however, identification of the lesion is not possible in terms of differentiating the tumor from other types of sarcoma.

Less Common Cardiac Sarcomas

▶ **Brief definition.** Fibrosarcomas, osteosarcomas, leiomyosarcomas, and liposarcomas may also occur in the heart, but together they comprise only 4% of all primary cardiac tumors. Different types of sarcoma have different growth rates and may differ considerably from one another in their prognosis. Life expectancy can be prolonged by tumor excision.[25]

▶ **Imaging signs.** Sarcomas require a histopathologic diagnosis, but an accurate description of tumor extent and the involvement of surrounding structures are important for determining resectability. MRI signal intensity is nonspecific. Most sarcomas are isointense to surrounding myocardium on T1 W images and hyperintense on T2 W images. Most sarcomas enhance after IV injection of contrast medium, making it easier to identify their margins.

▶ **Key points.** See Angiosarcoma above.

Lymphoma

▶ **Brief definition.** Primary cardiac lymphoma is defined as a lymphoma limited to the heart or pericardium at the time of diagnosis. The majority of these lesions are B-cell lymphomas. Primary cardiac lymphomas are much less common than secondary cardiac involvement and occur predominantly in immunosuppressed patients. A 2011 meta-analysis found that the right atrium and ventricle were affected much more frequently than the left cardiac chambers.[26] This observation suggests that the disease begins with occult lymphomas in lymph nodes and spreads to the heart via lymphatic duct drainage into the right cardiac chambers. It is important to include this entity in the differential diagnosis, as early chemotherapy is curative in a high percentage of cases.[27]

▶ **Imaging signs.** Primary cardiac lymphomas may take the form of circumscribed intracavitary lesions or diffuse, infiltrative intramural growth. When the lymphoma tissue reaches a critical mass, a standard chest radiograph may show enlargement of the heart compared with prior films. Lymphomas are hypointense to myocardium on T1 W images and hyperintense on T2 W images. The IV injection of Gd-DTPA may produce homogeneous enhancement (▶ Fig. 2.45) or patchy enhancement if necrosis is present.

▶ **Key points.** Cardiac lymphomas usually involve multiple cardiac chambers by contiguous tumor spread.

Rhabdomyosarcoma

▶ **Brief definition.** Rhabdomyosarcoma is the most common primary cardiac malignancy in children. It is usually multifocal and has no site of predilection within the heart.

▶ **Imaging signs.** Rhabdomyosarcomas are usually isointense to myocardium on T1 W and T2 W SE images. They enhance markedly after IV injection of contrast medium, showing an inhomogeneous pattern of enhancement when there is tumor necrosis. Rhabdomyosarcomas tend to invade the major vessels. These tumor extensions are clearly detectable by MRI.

▶ **Key points.** Rhabdomyosarcoma is the most common malignant cardiac tumor in children. As with malignant tumors in

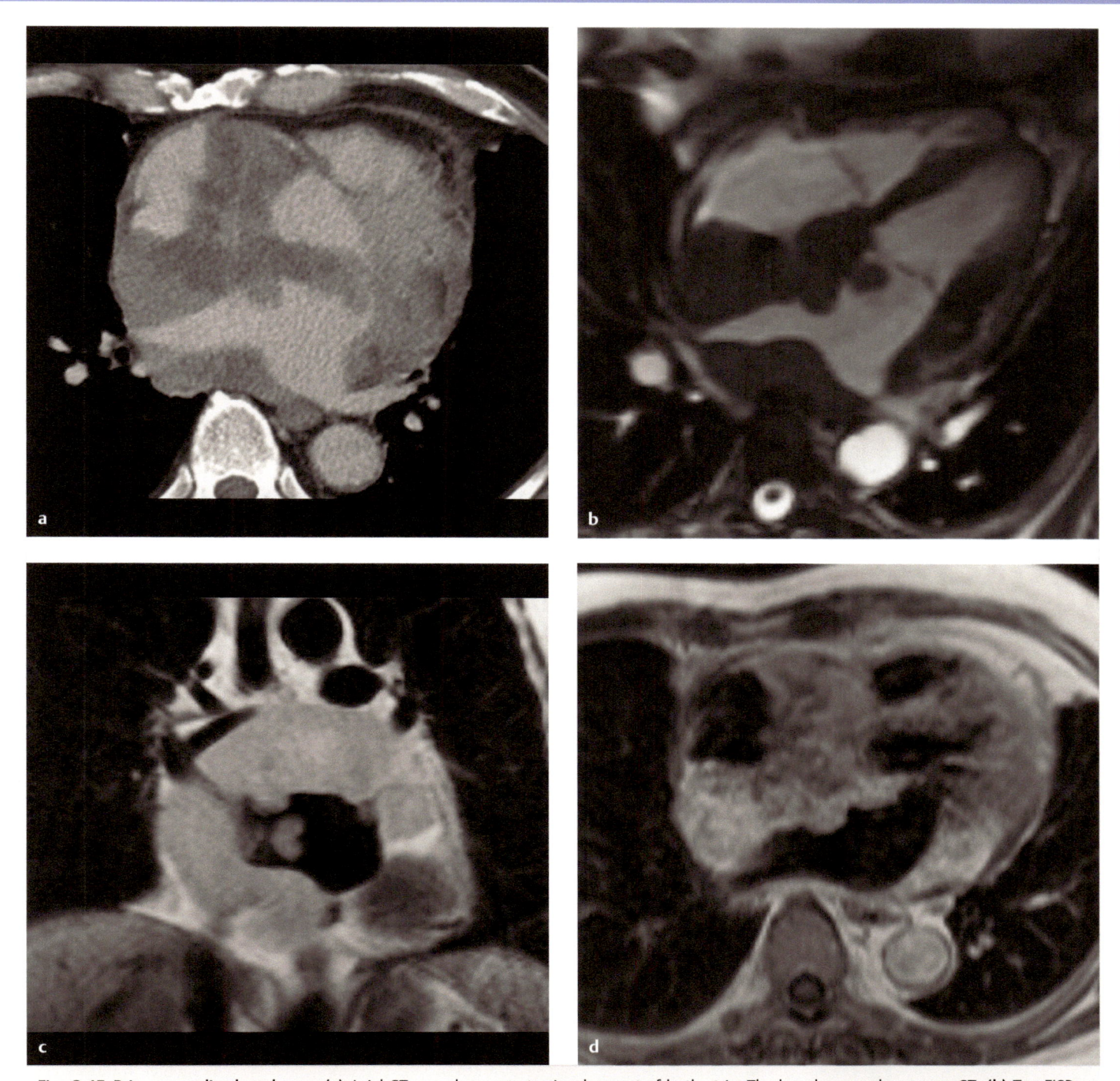

Fig. 2.45 Primary cardiac lymphoma. (a) Axial CT scan demonstrates involvement of both atria. The lymphoma enhances on CT. (b) TrueFISP image from a cine sequence. (c) Coronal T2 W TSE sequence. The lymphoma has high signal intensity. (d) T1 W GRE sequence shows homogeneous enhancement of the lesion after injection of contrast medium.

adults, the main role of imaging is to accurately describe the location of the mass.

Malignant Secondary Cardiac Tumors

Secondary cardiac malignancies include metastases and tumors that invade the heart by contiguous or hematogenous spread.

Invasion of the Heart by Contiguous Spread

The contiguous extension of pulmonary or mediastinal tumors to the heart means that these tumors are nonresectable, and this will affect tumor staging. MRI or CT can define the precise extent of the primary tumor and cardiac invasion and can detect the presence of pericardial effusion.

Transvascular Invasion of the Heart

Transvascular tumor extension into the right atrium via the inferior vena cava occurs with 10% of all renal cell carcinomas but may also be seen with adrenal tumors (p. 385).[28] Malignant thymoma (see Chapter 1, Mediastinum) can invade the heart through the superior vena cava, while bronchial carcinoma (p. 149) can gain access to the heart by infiltrating the pulmonary veins or superior vena cava. The goal of diagnostic imaging is to differentiate noninfiltrating,

Heart and Pericardium

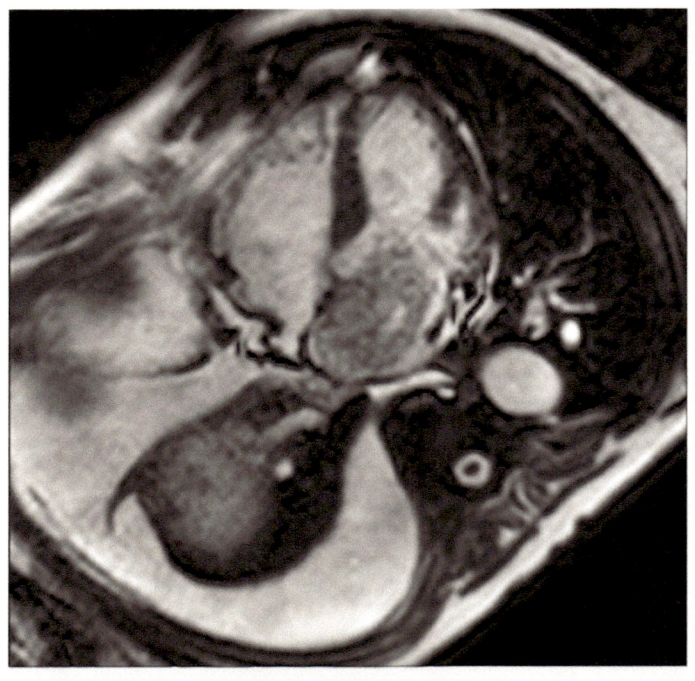

Fig. 2.46 Right bronchial carcinoma. TrueFISP image from a cine sequence. The tumor has invaded the left atrium through a pulmonary vein but has not yet infiltrated the atrial wall.

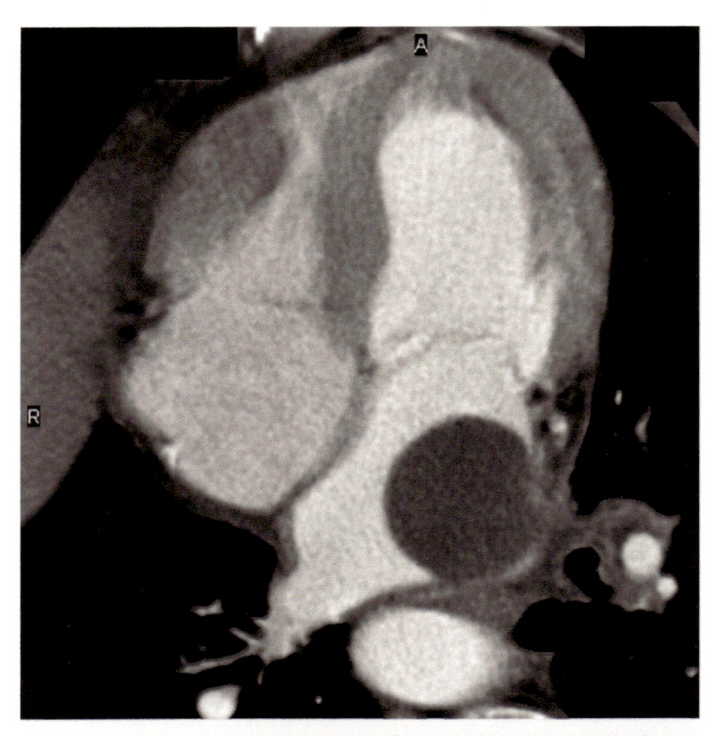

Fig. 2.47 Intracardiac metastases. Reformatted CT image in the four-chamber view. The free wall of the right ventricle is thickened. An intracavitary metastasis is visible in the left atrium.

potentially resectable tumors from tumors that are not resectable because they have infiltrated the atrial wall (▶ Fig. 2.46).

Cardiac Metastases

▶ **Brief definition.** Cardiac metastases occur in 3 to 18% of all patients with malignancies.[29] The myocardium, pericardium, epicardium, and endocardium are affected in descending order of frequency. Metastasis may result from the direct deposition of tumor cells on the endocardium, the hematogenous spread of micrometastases via the coronary arteries, or retrograde flow via bronchomediastinal lymphatics.

▶ **Imaging signs.** Cardiac metastases behave much the same as metastases in other body regions and often show intense contrast enhancement, although some lesions may display central necrosis or show little enhancement due to hypovascularity (▶ Fig. 2.47).

▶ **Clinical features.** Cardiac metastasis usually occurs at a late stage in which the dominant signs and symptoms are those of the advanced primary malignant disease. Depending on the location of the metastases, the clinical findings may include signs of heart failure or valvular dysfunction due to obstructive lesions, conduction abnormalities due to intramural growth, or cardiac enlargement due to pericardial carcinomatosis.

▶ **Key points.** Cardiac metastases generally develop at the end stage of a malignant disease. Staging examinations should include cardiac imaging.

Acquired Valvular Disease

Aortic Stenosis

▶ **Brief definition.** Aortic stenosis is the most common cause of acquired valvular disease, accounting for slightly more than 40% of cases. Degenerative changes are the most common finding at the time of treatment (approximately 80% of cases), followed by postinflammatory changes consistent with an autoimmune response to bacterial infection (rheumatic fever) in the remaining 20%. Other causes such as bacterial endocarditis are rare, accounting for fewer than 1% of cases. Calcium salts are readily deposited in the abnormally thickened valve tissue, so that calcifications are detectable in 90% of all stenotic aortic valves. The opening area of the aortic valve is 3 to 5 cm^2 in healthy individuals. Aortic stenosis is defined as a reduction in the valve opening area to less than 2 cm^2. Aortic stenosis develops gradually over a period of years, and the left ventricle adapts morphologically to the increased pressure by concentric hypertrophy. This myocardial hypertrophy enables the ventricle to keep generating the pressures necessary to maintain a constant stroke volume despite the stenotic valve. This compensatory mechanism is responsible for the radiological and clinical manifestations of aortic stenosis.

> **Note**
>
> Aortic stenosis is classified into three grades based on the valve opening area and pressure gradient:
> - *Grade I*: valve opening area greater than 1.5 cm^2, mean pressure gradient less than 20 mm Hg.
> - *Grade II*: valve opening area between 0.75 and 1.5 cm^2, mean pressure gradient between 20 and 50 mm Hg.
> - *Grade III*: valve opening area less than 0.75 cm^2, mean pressure gradient greater than 50 mm Hg.

▶ **Imaging signs.** Concentric hypertrophy of the myocardium does not cause visible left ventricular enlargement on chest radiographs, so aortic stenosis may go undetected for some time. But once the residual left ventricular blood volume has increased at end systole,

2.1 Heart

the heart assumes the classic "aortic" configuration, also called the "wooden shoe," due to accentuation of the cardiac waist (▶ Fig. 2.48). The lateral radiograph shows increased prominence of the posterior cardiac border. MRI is useful for the quantification of aortic stenosis, as the valve opening area during systole can be measured on cine images. The scan is performed in a small stack of slices parallel to the aortic valve (▶ Fig. 2.49). Cine sequences can also demonstrate an accelerated flow jet in the aorta, which appears as a signal void due to phase dispersion. The degree of phase dispersion depends on factors that include the selection of parameters (repetition time, echo time) and orientation relative to the main field, so the flow jet is not useful for quantifying the stenosis. But the flow jet is still a useful indicator in patients with undiagnosed valvular disease. In aortic stenosis, a flow jet may extend from the valve into the aorta during systole (see ▶ Fig. 2.49a). A second regurgitant jet may be seen from the mitral valve into the atrium during systole, signifying decompensation of the left ventricle and a relative mitral insufficiency caused by the dilatation. The ascending aorta may be dilated in aortic stenosis (see ▶ Fig. 2.49). Hypertrophy of the left ventricular myocardium is measured in the septum at diastole. The pressure gradient in aortic stenosis can be calculated with the modified Bernoulli equation by using phase-contrast MR angiography to determine the maximum flow velocity.

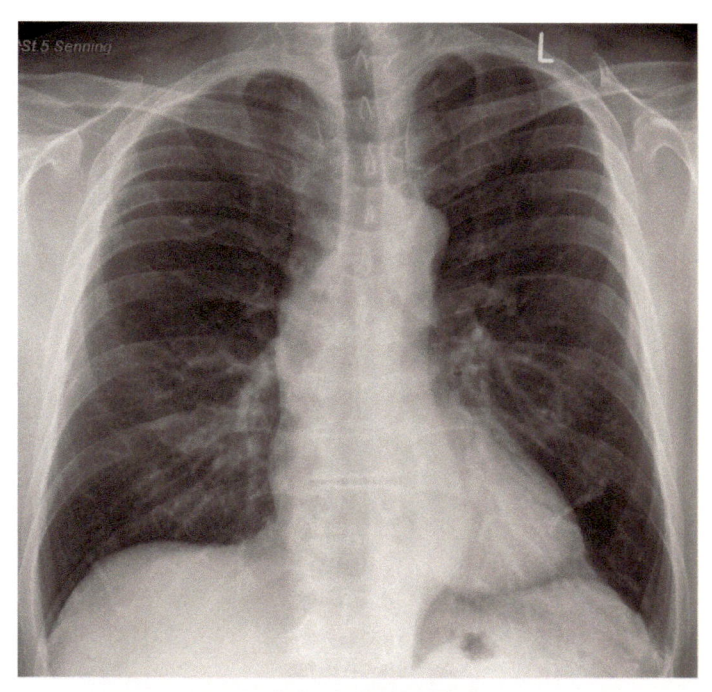

Fig. 2.48 Aortic stenosis. The cardiac waist is deepened due to concentric hypertrophy.

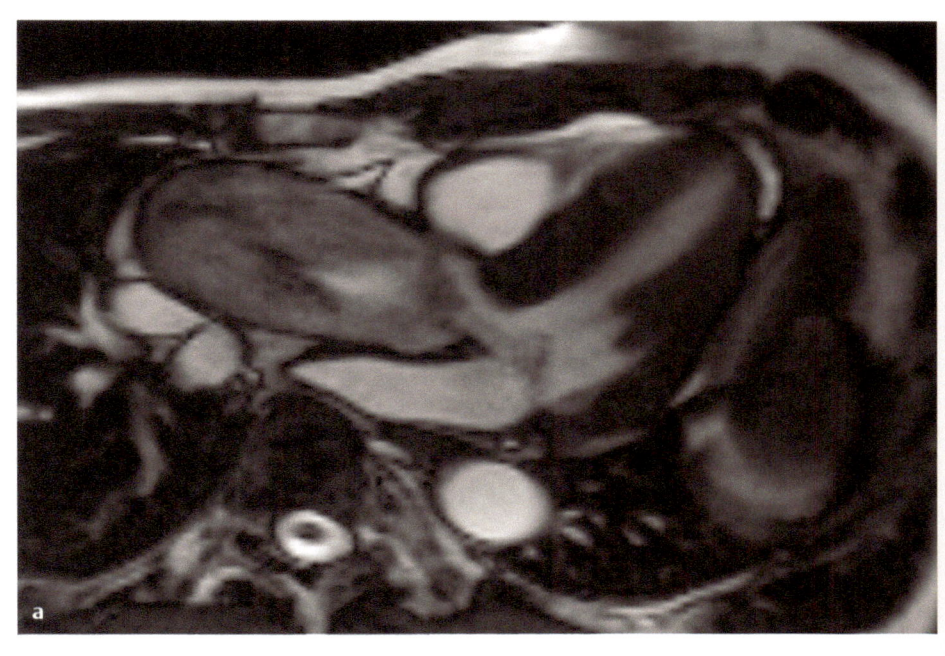

Fig. 2.49 Aortic stenosis. (a) TrueFISP image from a cine sequence. The systolic jet from the aortic valve into the aorta appears as a signal void. The ascending aorta is dilated. **(b)** TrueFISP image at the aortic valve level with the valve closed. **(c)** TrueFISP image at the aortic valve level with the valve open. The valve opening area can be measured.

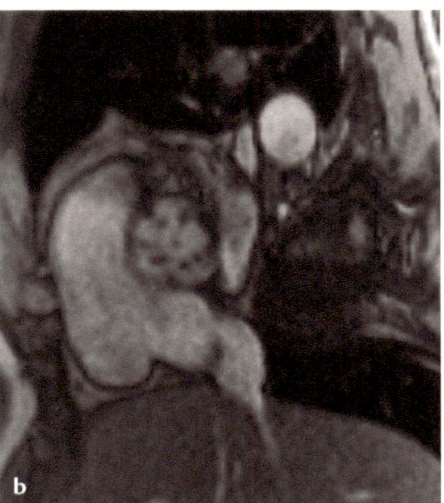

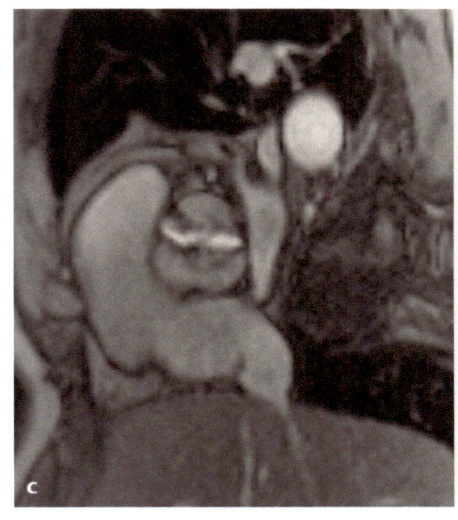

Heart and Pericardium

> **Note**
>
> Modified Bernoulli equation for determining the pressure gradient in aortic stenosis by MRI:
>
> $$\Delta p = 4 \cdot v_{max}^2$$
>
> where Δp = the pressure gradient across the stenotic valve in mm Hg, and v_{max} = maximum flow velocity in meters/second.

Over the last decade, minimally invasive therapy by transcatheter aortic valve implantation (TAVI) through a percutaneous approach in the groin or a transapical mini-thoracotomy has become a routine clinical procedure. This requires an accurate preoperative measurement of the aortic annulus and its distance from the coronary arteries, which is accomplished with CT (▶ Fig. 2.50).

▶ **Clinical features.** Patients with aortic stenosis remain asymptomatic for some time, as concentric hypertrophy of the left ventricular myocardium maintains the stroke volume to provide functional compensation. Eventually, when the myocardium decompensates, the patient experiences decreased exercise tolerance and exertional dyspnea. Angina develops when the perfusion of the hypertrophic myocardium is clinically reduced due to the combination of a raised intracavitary pressure and the increased oxygen demand of the hypertrophic myocardium.

▶ **Key points.** Aortic stenosis is the most common acquired valvular disease. It is characterized by concentric hypertrophy of the left ventricle, which does not enlarge the cardiac silhouette on chest radiographs.

Aortic Insufficiency

▶ **Brief definition.** Aortic insufficiency (aortic regurgitation) is the third most common valvular disease, accounting for 12% of all cases. Its causes are highly diverse but relate mainly to degenerative changes followed by rheumatic changes as a postinflammatory autoimmune response. Due to shrinkage of the valvular tissue, the semilunar valves are unable to create an effective seal, allowing blood to regurgitate into the ventricle during diastole. The amount of diastolic reflux into the ventricle is the regurgitant volume. The magnitude of the regurgitant volume is determined by the size of the closure defect, the heart rate including the duration of diastole, and left ventricular compliance. This diastolic volume load leads to ventricular dilatation and eventual eccentric hypertrophy caused by a compensatory increase in muscle mass. Aortic insufficiency is initially compensated by an increase in stroke volume. Chronic aortic insufficiency can be compensated up to a regurgitant fraction of 80%.

▶ **Imaging signs.** The chest radiograph shows enlargement of the left ventricle (▶ Fig. 2.51). In decompensated cases, signs of left heart decompensation can be seen. On MRI, a flow jet from the aortic valve into the left ventricle during diastole is the hallmark of aortic insufficiency (see ▶ Fig. 2.51). The regurgitant volume can be determined by quantifying the ejection fraction of each ventricle and subtracting the right ventricular ejection fraction from the left ventricular ejection fraction.

▶ **Clinical features.** As in aortic stenosis, patients remain asymptomatic for some time due to functional compensation. When left heart failure supervenes, the patient experiences decreased exercise tolerance and exertional dyspnea.

▶ **Key points.** Aortic insufficiency leads to left ventricular enlargement in response to the increased volume load.

Mitral Stenosis

▶ **Brief definition.** The normal opening area of the mitral valve is 4 to 6 cm². Stenosis becomes hemodynamically significant when the valve opening area is reduced to 1.5 cm² or less. Mitral stenosis is most commonly a result of rheumatic fever. The pathophysiology of the autoimmune-mediated inflammation, characterized by thickening of the valve and hardening and shrinkage of the tissue, usually leads to a combination of valvular stenosis and regurgitation. As a result of the routine antibiotic treatment of bacterial infections, the incidence of this disease in industrialized countries has fallen significantly in recent decades.

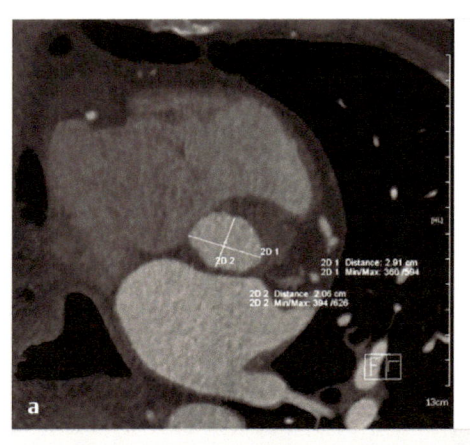

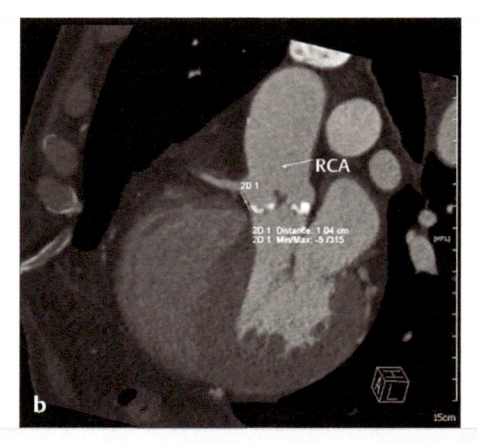

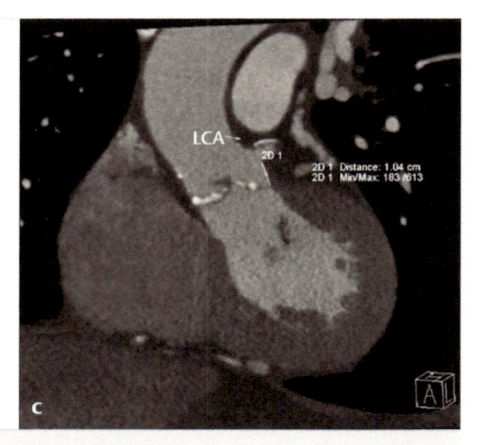

Fig. 2.50 Aortic stenosis. Planning a percutaneous valve implantation. (a) CT shows concentric hypertrophy of the left ventricle in diastole without cardiac enlargement. (b) The dimensions of the aortic annulus are determined. (c) The distance from the right coronary artery and left coronary artery (D) to the annulus is determined. When TAVI is performed through the common femoral artery, the diameters of the external and internal iliac arteries should also be determined.

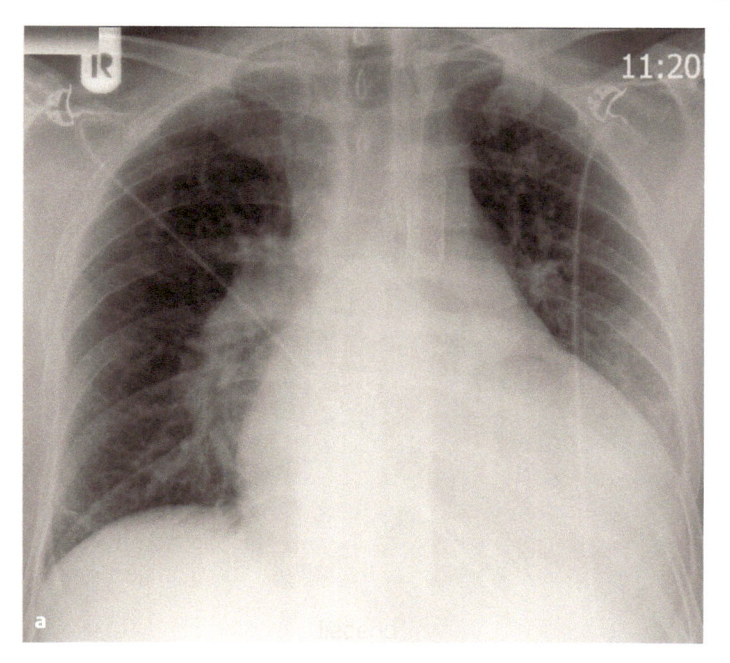

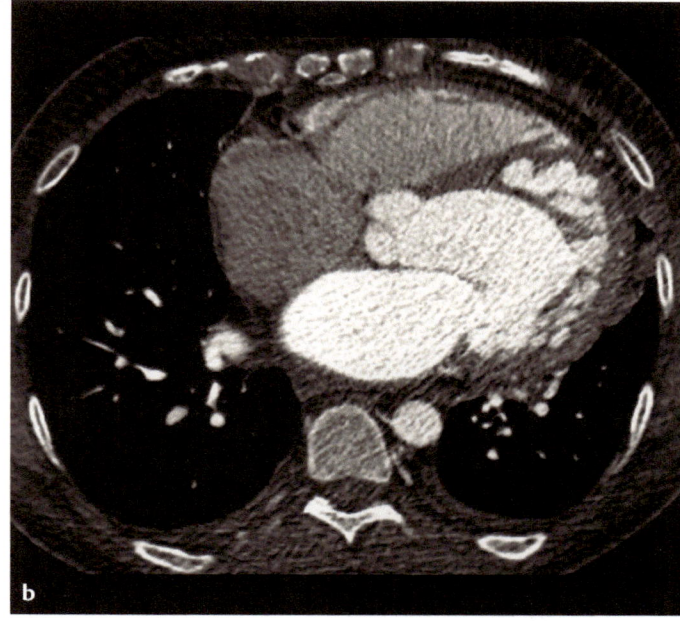

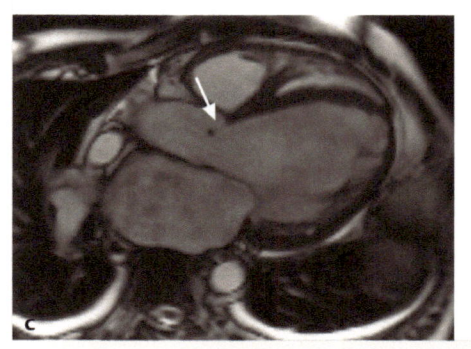

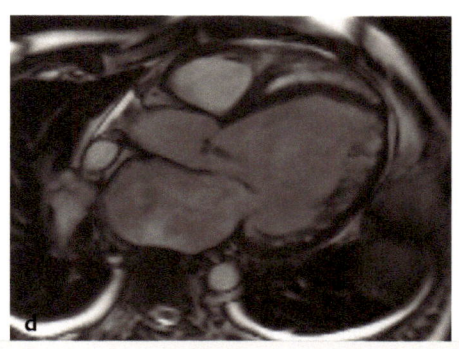

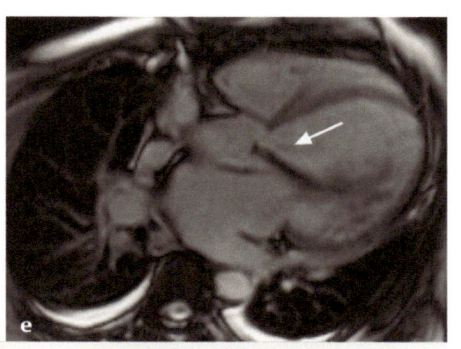

Fig. 2.51 Aortic insufficiency. (a) Chest radiograph shows an enlarged heart with a prominent left ventricle. (b) CT shows left ventricular enlargement. (In addition, the figure shows signs of non-compaction cardiomypathy.) (c) Frame from a trueFISP cine sequence in the three-chamber view documents normal systolic opening of the valve (arrow). (d) Another frame from the trueFISP cine sequence in the three-chamber view. (e) Another frame from the trueFISP cine sequence shows blood regurgitating from the aorta into the left ventricle in diastole. The regurgitant jet appears as a signal void (arrow).

Note

Like aortic stenosis, mitral stenosis is graded according to valve opening area and pressure gradient:
- *Grade I*: valve opening area greater than 1.5 cm^2, mean pressure gradient less than 5 mm Hg.
- *Grade II*: valve opening area 1 to 1.5 cm^2, mean pressure gradient 5 to 10 mm Hg.
- *Grade III*: valve opening area less than 1 cm^2, mean pressure gradient greater than 10 mm Hg.

▶ **Imaging signs.** Decreased blood inflow into the left ventricle leads to dilatation of the left atrium. The left ventricle is small because of the reduced load. The restricted blood flow raises pressures in the pulmonary veins and capillaries proximal to the atrium, leading to pulmonary hypertension and an increased pressure load on the right ventricle. The frontal chest radiograph at this stage shows left atrial enlargement and an effacement of the cardiac waist due to the enlarged left atrial appendage, with a possible double contour sign (see ▶ Fig. 4.3). The lateral radiograph shows enlargement of the left atrium. Signs of pulmonary congestion are seen in decompensated cases. The valve opening area can be determined with MRI.

▶ **Clinical features.** Patients with mild decompensation have exertional dyspnea. An outward manifestation in some patients is a distinctive flushing of the cheeks (mitral facies).

▶ **Key points.** Mitral stenosis is characterized by enlargement of the left atrium.

Mitral Insufficiency

▶ **Brief definition.** In mitral insufficiency left ventricular blood regurgitates into the left atrium during systole. It may be caused by shrinkage of the valvular tissue, or a "relative" insufficiency may result from left ventricular dilatation that prevents the valve leaflets from closing. Acute mitral insufficiency may result from a papillary muscle tear following myocardial infarction. Like aortic insufficiency, mitral insufficiency leads to an increased volume load on the left ventricle, resulting in ventricular dilatation. In patients with chronic mitral insufficiency, the myocardium adapts to the increased volume load with relative hypertrophy. This condition is also known as "eccentric hypertrophy." The left atrium dilates in response to the regurgitant volume. With acute mitral insufficiency, the myocardium has no time to adapt and there is a damming back of blood in the pulmonary circulation, with a rise in pulmonary arterial pressure.

▶ **Imaging signs.** The cardiac silhouette on the chest radiograph is widened to the left as a result of left ventricular enlargement (▶ Fig. 2.52). The left atrium creates a left double contour in the PA radiograph due to its enlarged condition and shows posterior prominence in the lateral radiograph. CT and MRI demonstrate the enlargement of the left atrium and ventricle (▶ Fig. 2.53). The regurgitation volume can be calculated with MRI by determining the difference in stroke volumes between the ventricles. The difference equals the regurgitation volume. A second option is to measure the flow across the mitral and aortic valves by phase contrast angiography. With this method as well, the regurgitation volume is calculated by finding the difference between the two values.

▶ **Clinical features.** Patients with chronic mitral insufficiency remain asymptomatic for a long time because the valvular dysfunction develops slowly and the left ventricle adapts to the increased volume and maintains its stroke volume by dilatation and eccentric hypertrophy. With severe mitral insufficiency, the output to the systemic circulation is decreased and the patient develops exertional dyspnea. Acute mitral insufficiency due to papillary muscle rupture causes an acute rise of the pulmonary arterial pressure, leading to pulmonary edema and dyspnea.

Note
The left atrium is always enlarged in patients with acquired, hemodynamically significant mitral valve dysfunction.

▶ **Key points.** Mitral insufficiency leads to enlargement of the left atrium and ventricle and to a "mitral configuration" of the heart on the chest radiograph.

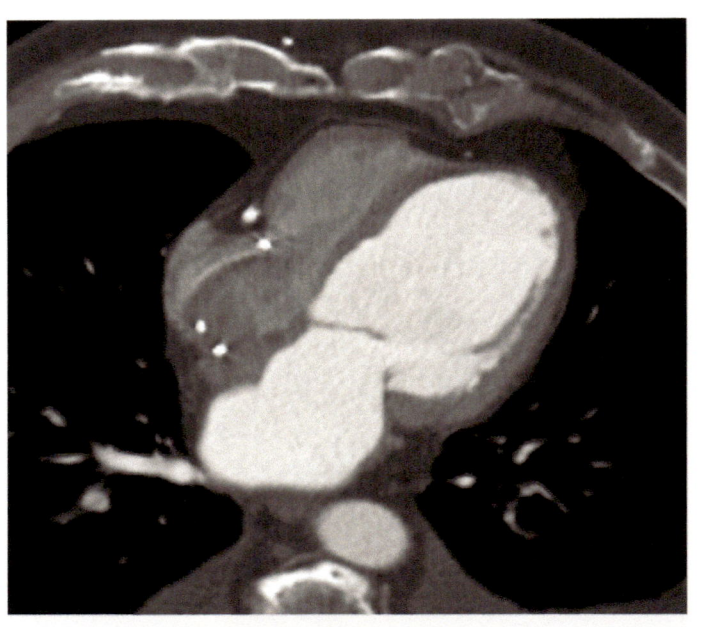

Fig. 2.53 **Mitral insufficiency.** CT scan shows isolated enlargement of the left atrium and ventricle.

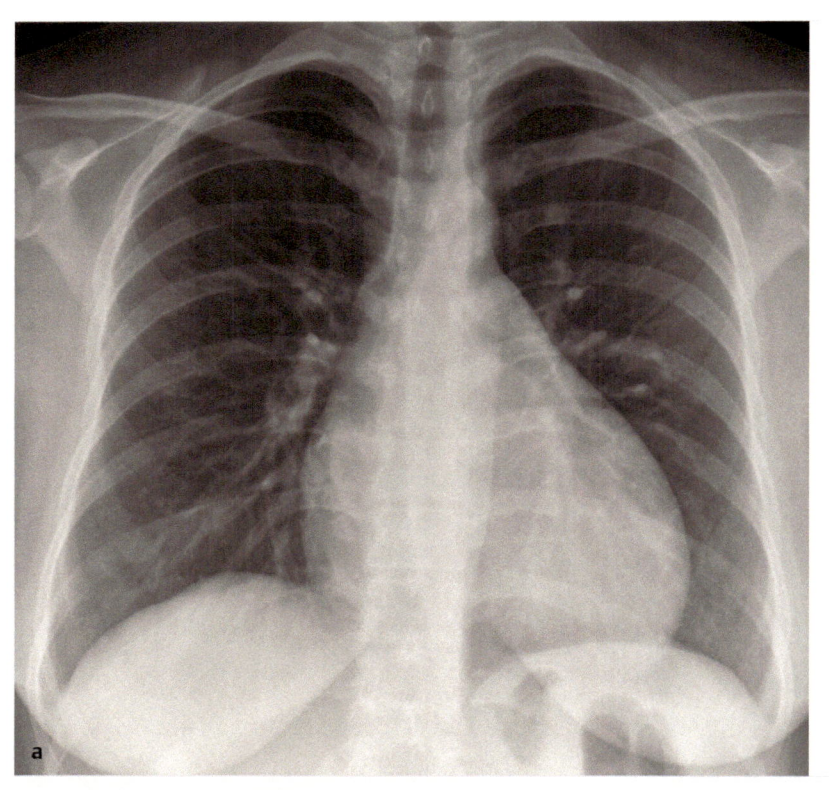

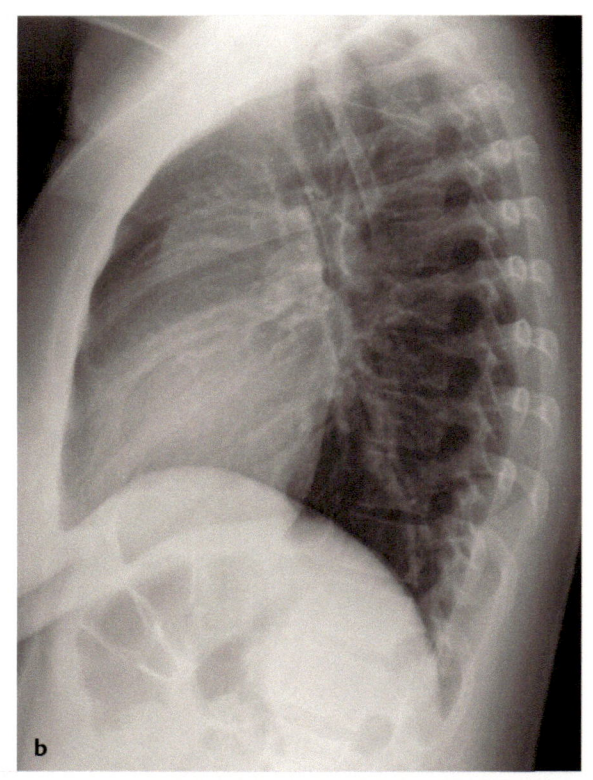

Fig. 2.52 **Grade III mitral insufficiency.** (a) PA chest radiograph. (b) Lateral radiograph. The left ventricle and left atrium are enlarged. The heart shows a mitral configuration.

Tricuspid Stenosis

▶ **Brief definition.** Isolated tricuspid stenosis is rare and most commonly results from rheumatic fever, with the same pathogenic mechanism described for mitral stenosis. Tricuspid stenosis becomes hemodynamically significant when the opening area of the valve is reduced to less than 2 cm². The stenosis is classified as high grade when the pressure gradient between the right atrium and ventricle rises to more than 5 mm Hg.

▶ **Imaging signs.** The characteristic feature of tricuspid stenosis on chest radiographs is enlargement of the right atrium. Diagnosis and follow-up rely on echocardiography.

▶ **Clinical features.** The damming back of blood behind the stenotic valve leads to peripheral edema and possible ascites.

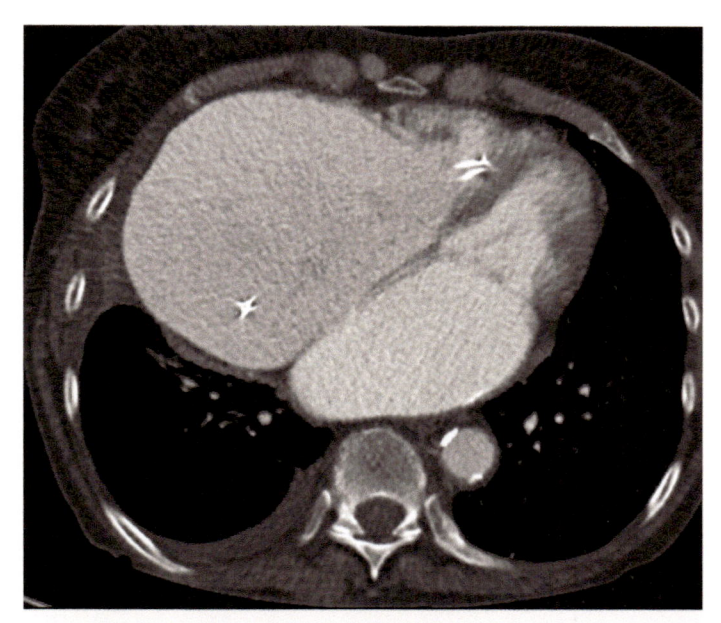

Fig. 2.54 Tricuspid insufficiency. The right atrium is greatly enlarged.

Tricuspid Insufficiency

▶ **Brief definition.** Tricuspid insufficiency is usually a relative insufficiency based on dilatation of the right ventricle. It is less commonly due to structural changes in the valve.

▶ **Imaging signs.** Multivalvular dysfunction with combined tricuspid and mitral insufficiency leads to global cardiac enlargement (▶ Fig. 2.54). MRI demonstrates a regurgitant jet from the tricuspid valve into the right atrium.

▶ **Clinical features.** The clinical presentation is determined by the multivalvular dysfunction. The dominant signs are those of heart failure.

▶ **Key points.** Tricuspid insufficiency is usually one component of acquired multivalvular disease. It most commonly results from global cardiac enlargement in which the leaflets are too small to provide effective closure. The imaging appearance and clinical features are determined by the combination of tricuspid insufficiency with other valvular defects.

2.2 Pericardium

2.2.1 Anatomy

The pericardium encloses the heart with a fibrous parietal layer 1 mm thick. The pericardium contains up to 50 mL of fluid in healthy individuals. The pericardium and epicardium comprise a functional unit that enables the heart to move freely between the two layers. The pericardium extends upward to a level just below the aortic arch, where it forms a superior reflection (▶ Fig. 2.55). Its lower portion is fused medially to the diaphragm in an area called the central tendon. The pericardium is attached anteriorly to the sternum. The pericardium is innervated by the phrenic nerve and vagus nerve.

▶ **Landmarks on CT and MRI.** The pericardium appears as a thin line on CT and MRI (▶ Fig. 2.56). The pericardial reflection at the

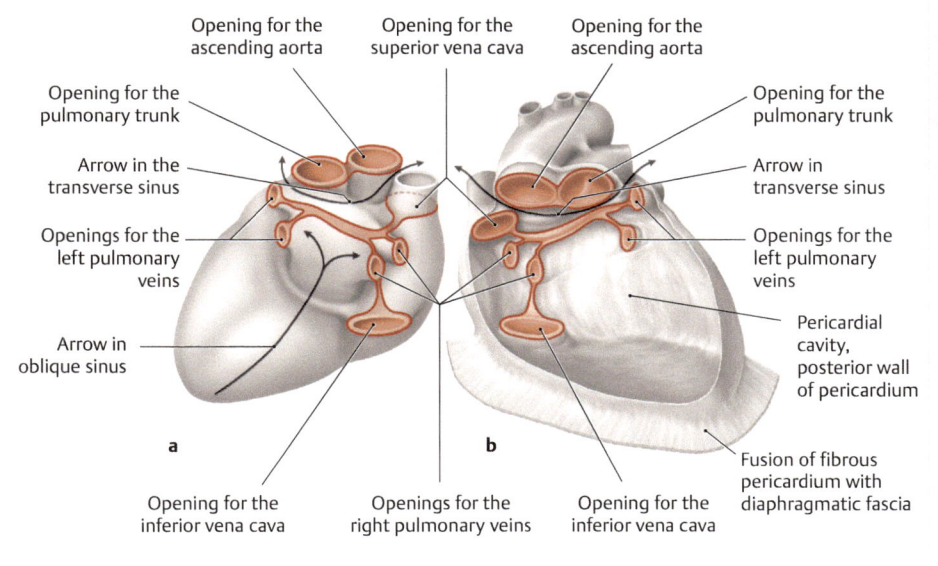

Fig. 2.55 Pericardium with anatomical reflections and openings for the passage of vascular structures. (a) Posterior view of the heart and epicardium. (b) Anterior view into the "empty" pericardial cavity. (Reproduced from Schünke M, Schulte E, Schumacher U. Prometheus. LernAtlas der Anatomie: Innere Organe. Illustrated by M. Voll/K. Wesker. 2nd ed. Stuttgart: Thieme; 2009.)

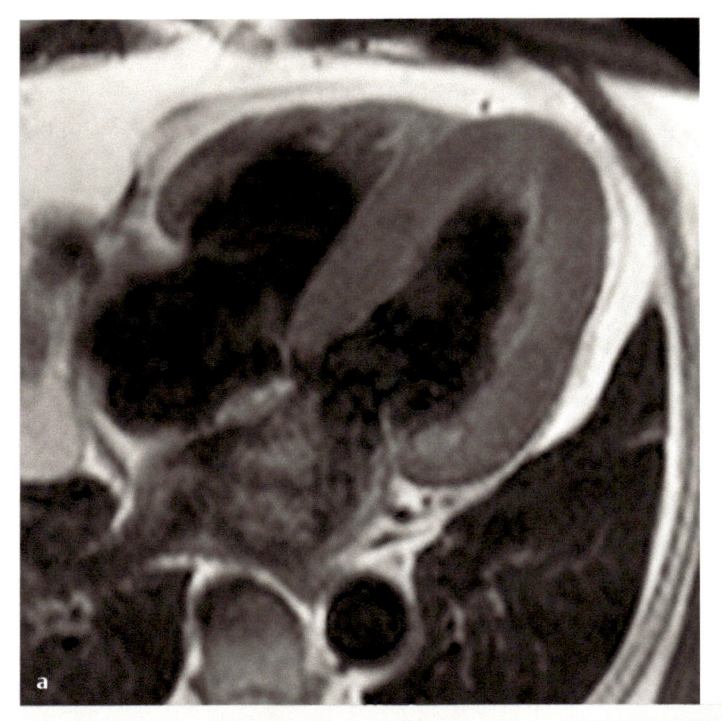

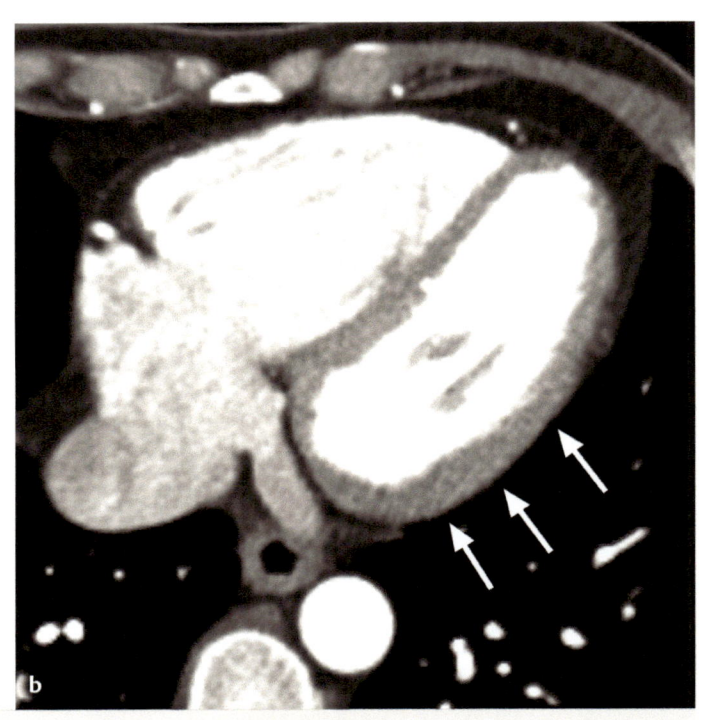

Fig. 2.56 Sectional imaging views of the pericardium. (a) T2 W MRI. The pericardium appears as a fine line. **(b)** The pericardium also appears as a fine line on CT in areas where it contrasts with the myocardium due to the presence of epicardial fat. Healthy pericardium is not defined in areas where the epicardial fat is thin, resulting in low intrinsic contrast (arrows).

level of the junction of the ascending aorta and aortic arch is an important landmark and should not be mistaken for lymph nodes on CT and MRI (▶ Fig. 2.57). The high cranial extent of the pericardium should be considered in cases of catheter malposition. Intrapericardial placement of a central venous catheter may cause a high perforation of the superior vena cava. The question of possible pericardial effusion can be resolved by echocardiography, which is noninvasive and widely available. Its main disadvantage is incomplete visualization of the pericardium. On plain chest radiographs, the pericardium is indistinguishable from other soft tissue structures. When pericardial effusion is present, it enlarges the cardiac silhouette. This differs from an enlarged silhouette due to cardiomegaly as it is not associated with pulmonary venous congestion. The pericardium can be identified as a thin layer on CT and MRI because of its good contrast with surrounding fatty tissue. Both modalities should be used if pericarditis is suspected and it is necessary to image the entire pericardium. CT is superior to MRI for detecting pericardial calcifications and is the modality of choice in patients with suspected constrictive pericarditis.

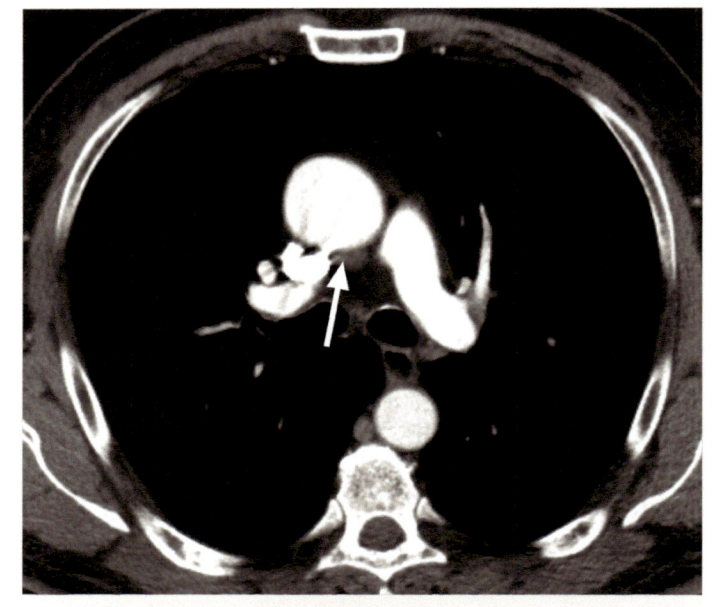

Fig. 2.57 Pericardial reflection (arrow) at the level of the aorta.

2.2.2 Diseases

Pericarditis

▶ **Brief definition.** Pericarditis is an inflammation of the pericardium and is classified by its etiology as infectious or noninfectious.
- *Infectious pericarditis*: This form is caused by viruses (influenza and coxsackievirus) in the great majority of cases. A less frequent cause is bacterial infection (streptococci, staphylococci, Haemophilus, Mycobacterium tuberculosis).
- *Noninfectious pericarditis*: This form may occur in all types of autoimmune disease (including rheumatic diseases), connective tissue diseases, metabolic disorders (uremia), and paraneoplastic conditions, after radiotherapy, and after trauma (including cardiac surgery or myocardial infarction). Pericarditis that follows myocardial damage (trauma, surgery, infarction) is called Dressler's syndrome after the cardiologist who first described it. Dressler's syndrome is an autoimmune pericarditis (with or without myocarditis) that is incited by antibodies against myocardial proteins; it occurs approximately 6 weeks after the initial myocardial injury.

The pathophysiology involves a thickening of the pericardium due to inflammation. The increased capillary permeability resulting from the inflammation leads to pericardial effusion.

▶ **Imaging signs.** The pericardium is thickened and enhances strongly on CT and MRI (▶ Fig. 2.58). Pericarditis is accompanied in most cases by pericardial effusion (exudate or transudate). Chronic pericarditis cannot always be positively differentiated from acute pericarditis on the basis of its imaging characteristics. Irregular thickening of the pericardium may suggest chronicity but is also seen in acute pericarditis caused by *M. tuberculosis* (▶ Fig. 2.59). The only definite sign is the duration of the disease. A large pericardial effusion (volume more than approximately 200 mL) appears on the PA radiograph as a tent-shaped widening of the cardiac silhouette. Provided there is at least a moderate amount of epicardial fat, pericardial effusion appears on the lateral radiograph as a retrosternal, crescent-shaped double contour due to the density differential of the epicardial fat relative to the myocardium and effusion, which both have the same density.

▶ **Clinical features.** The cardinal symptoms of acute pericarditis are retrosternal pain and fever. Echocardiography shows a low-voltage QRS complex due to pericardial effusion. A very large, rapidly developing pericardial effusion may be complicated by pericardial tamponade.

▶ **Differential diagnosis.** Clinical symptoms may also be consistent with myocarditis, which is excluded by MRI.

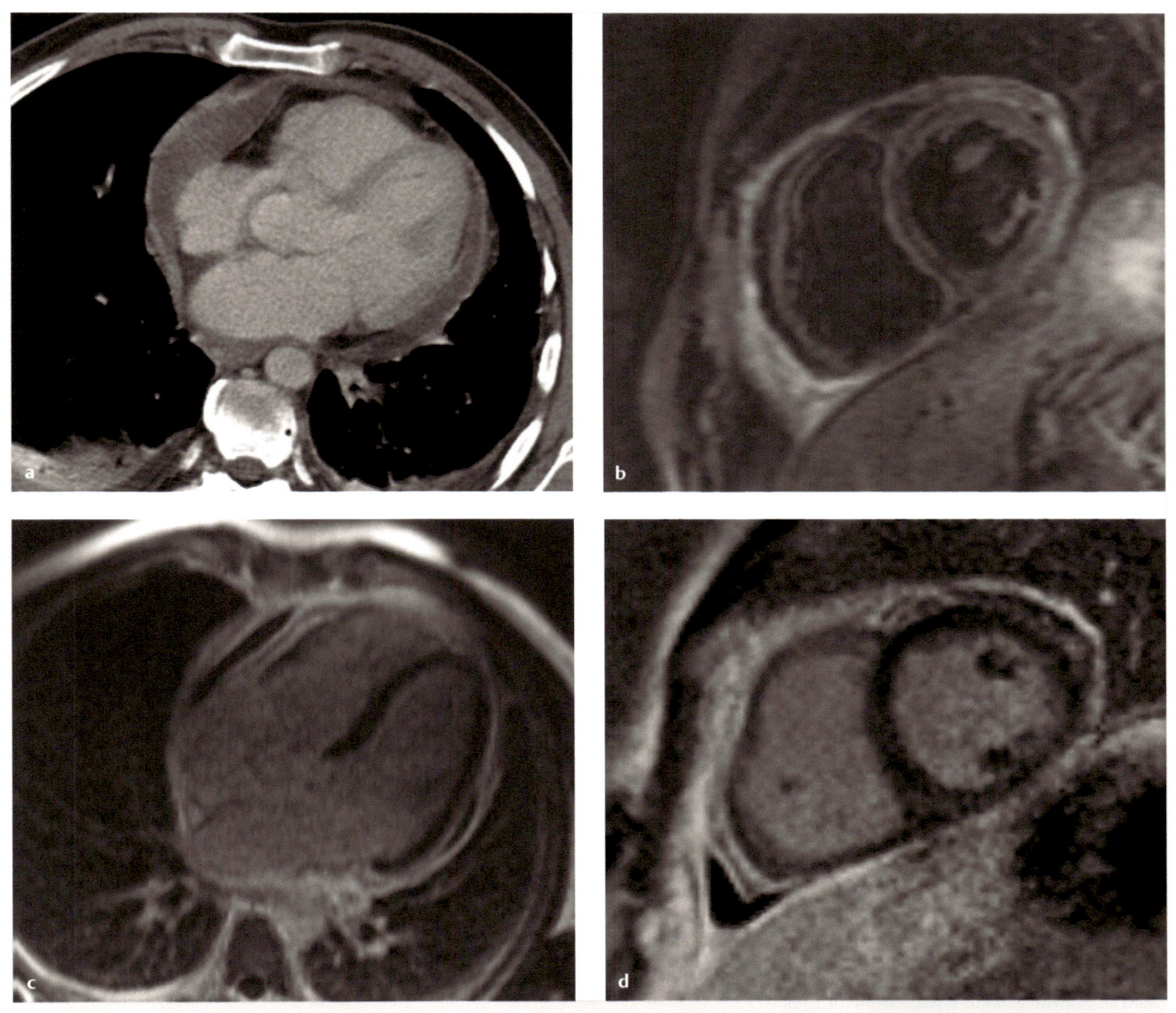

Fig. 2.58 Pericarditis. (a) CT. The pericardium is thickened and shows contrast enhancement. There is a small amount of pericardial effusion. (b) T2 W TSE image. The pericardium is permeated by edema. (c) T1 W inversion recovery GRE sequence after injection of contrast medium, four-chamber view. The pericardium shows marked enhancement. (d) T1 W inversion recovery GRE sequence in the short-axis view also shows marked pericardial enhancement.

Heart and Pericardium

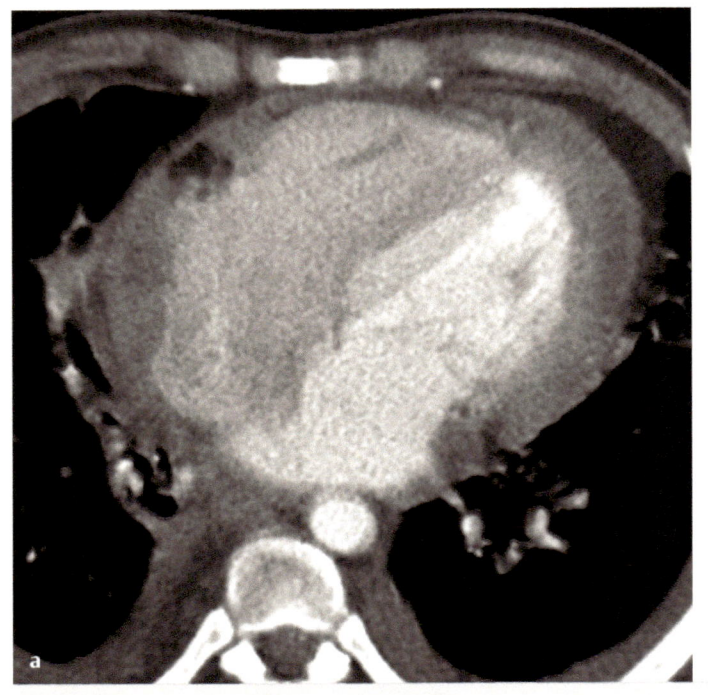

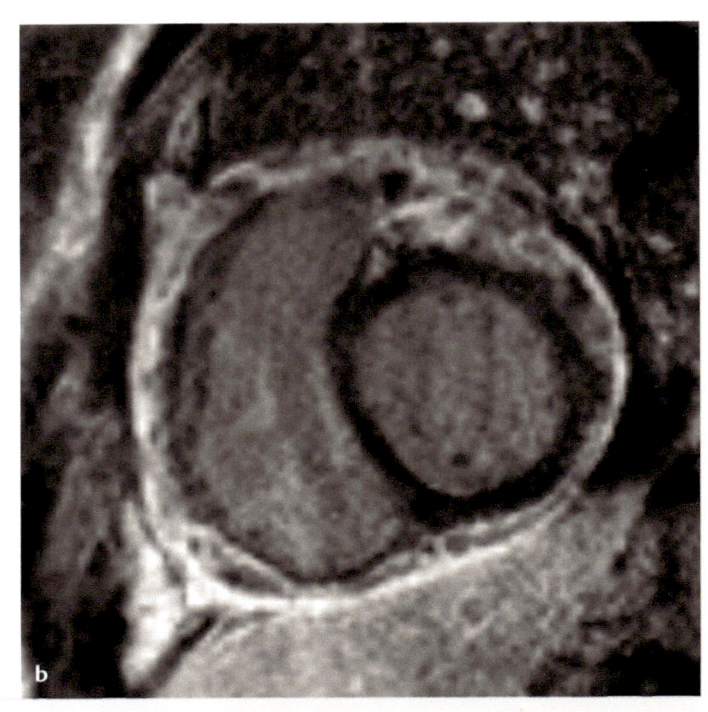

Fig. 2.59 Pericarditis in a tuberculosis patient. (a) CT scan shows thickening of the pericardium. **(b)** T1 W inversion recovery GRE sequence shows prominent enhancement of the irregularly thickened pericardium with enhancing intrapericardial granulomas.

▶ **Key points.** Acute pericarditis is characterized by thickening of the pericardium combined with intense enhancement. Associated pericardial effusion is common.

Constrictive Pericarditis

▶ **Brief definition.** Constrictive pericarditis is thickening and fibrosis of the pericardium that restricts diastolic filling of the cardiac chambers. The atria, ventricles, or the right or left system may be affected, depending on the location of decreased pericardial compliance. Constrictive pericarditis has as many potential causes as acute pericarditis, some of which overlap. The most frequent causes in industrialized countries are previous radiotherapy, surgical procedures, and trauma. The leading cause in developing countries is tuberculosis.

▶ **Imaging signs.** The pericardium is thickened and may be calcified (▶ Fig. 2.60). The atria are enlarged (▶ Fig. 2.61).

> **Note**
>
> A pericardial thickness of 4 mm is taken as the cutoff value for diagnosing constrictive pericarditis.

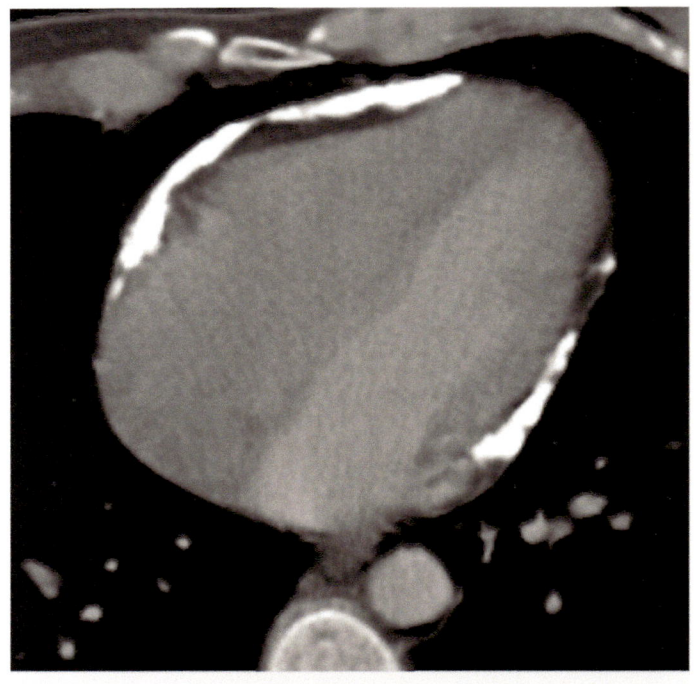

Fig. 2.60 Heavy calcification of the pericardium in constrictive pericarditis ("armored heart").

▶ **Clinical features.** The decrease in cardiac filling and stroke volume leads to a damming back of venous blood, with effects that depend on which chambers are the most severely affected. If right ventricular filling is impaired, the constriction leads to dilatation of the hepatic veins, hepatomegaly, portal hypertension, ascites, and peripheral edema. Restriction of left ventricular filling leads to pulmonary hypertension with the possible development of pulmonary edema. Additional symptoms are dyspnea and decreased exercise tolerance.

▶ **Differential diagnosis.** Constrictive pericarditis mainly requires differentiation from restrictive cardiomyopathy, which is also associated with decreased diastolic filling. These conditions cannot be differentiated by their clinical symptoms, but the distinction is important for treatment and prognosis: while constrictive pericarditis is curable by resection of the pericardium, and thus has an excellent prognosis, restrictive cardiomyopathy is treated medically and has a poor prognosis.

2.2 Pericardium

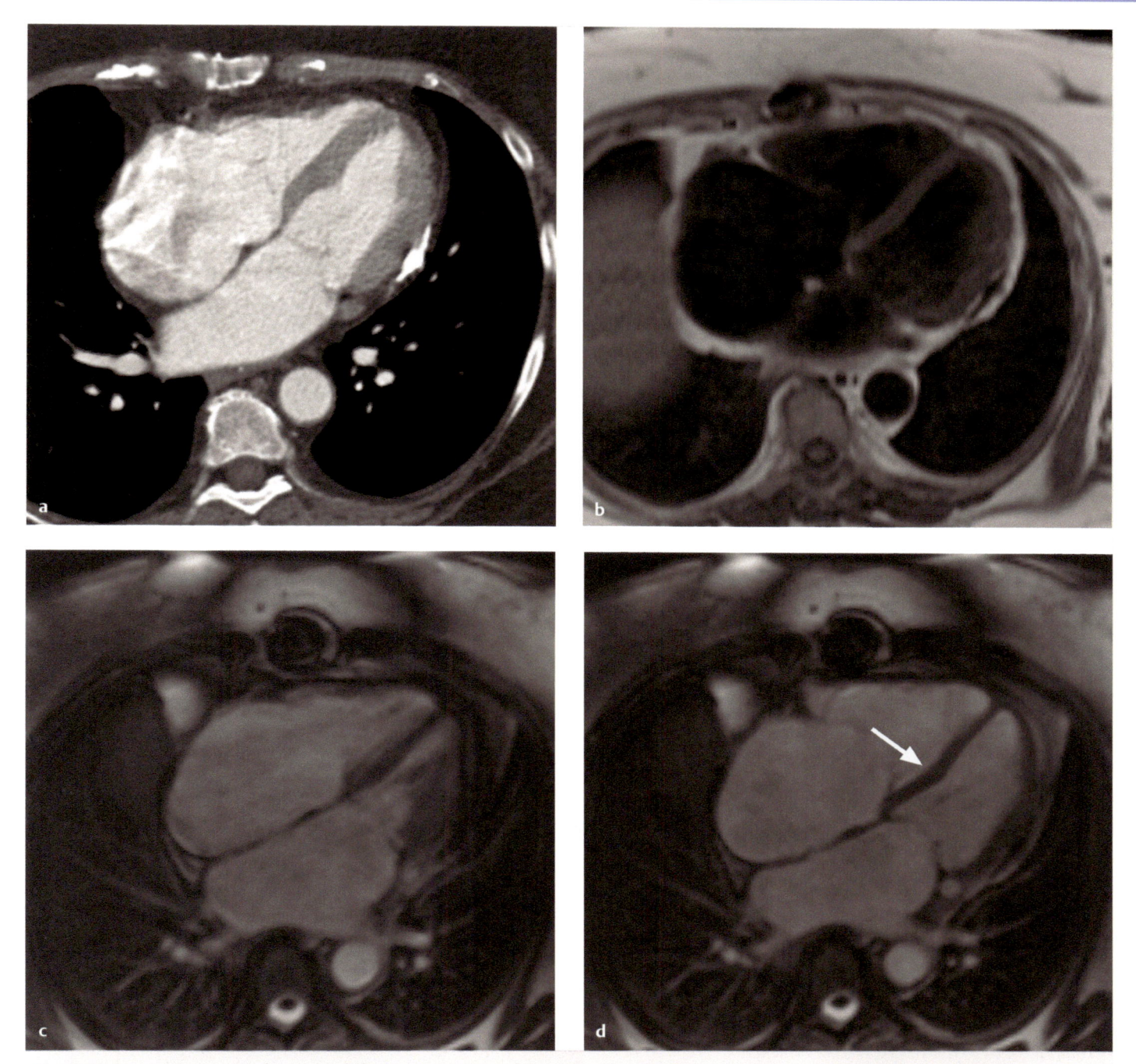

Fig. 2.61 **Constrictive pericarditis.** (a) Calcifications in portions of the pericardium. (b) T2W TSE sequence. The pericardium is thickened. (c) TrueFISP image from a cine sequence in systole, four-chamber view. (d) TrueFISP image from a cine sequence in diastole, four-chamber view. Both atria are enlarged. Diastolic filling of the ventricles is restricted. Paradoxical motion of the septum into the left ventricle (arrow) occurs in diastole.

▶ **Key points.** Constrictive pericarditis is characterized by thickening of the pericardium with loss of distensibility. This restricts diastolic filling of the ventricles, resulting in enlargement of both atria. An important task of MRI is to differentiate constrictive pericarditis from restrictive cardiomyopathy, which is also characterized clinically by decreased diastolic filling.

Pericardial Masses

▶ **Brief definition.** Primary tumors of the pericardium are extremely rare. Possible entities are mesothelioma, sarcoma, teratoma, lymphoma, lipoma, and hemangioma. Secondary tumors of the pericardium may occur by contiguous spread from the mediastinum, myocardium, or lung or by metastasis from a distant primary. With malignant tumors that metastasize to the pericardium, pericardial carcinomatosis may develop as a result of sheetlike tumor growth.

▶ **Imaging signs.** Chest radiographs show no abnormalities in most cases. CT and MRI demonstrate irregular, inhomogeneous thickening of the pericardium (▶ Fig. 2.62).

▶ **Key points.** Pericardial masses may include sarcoma, mesothelioma, lymphoma, or pericardial carcinomatosis. CT and MRI show circumscribed and nodular thickening of the pericardium

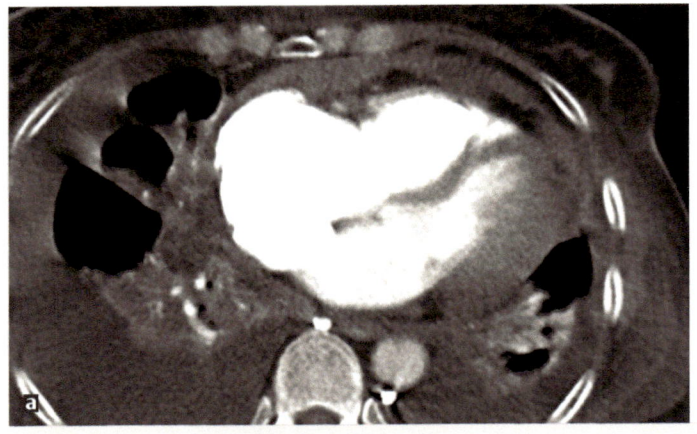

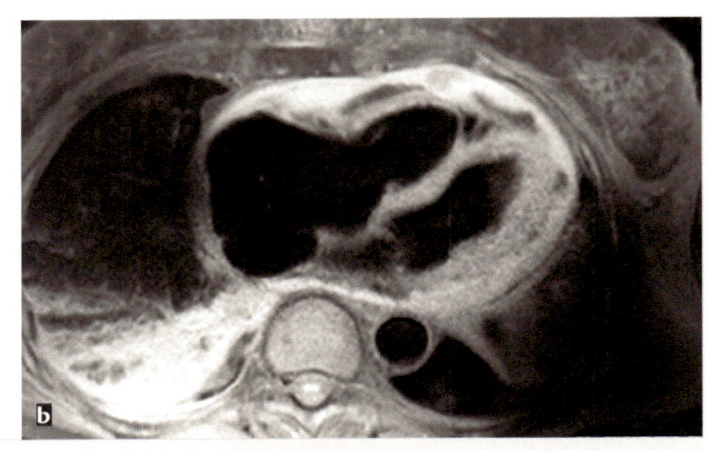

Fig. 2.62 Pericardial carcinomatosis in a lung cancer patient. (**a**) CT shows thickening of the pericardium. The right atrium is enlarged as evidence of decreased pericardial compliance with constriction. (**b**) T1 W GRE sequence. The pericardium shows nodular thickening and intense enhancement.

with intense contrast enhancement. A pericardial effusion is usually present.

Pericardial Mesothelioma

▶ **Brief definition.** Pericardial mesothelioma is very rare and constitutes 1% of all mesotheliomas but 50% of all primary pericardial tumors. It is categorized as an asbestosis and is recognized as an occupational disease, although, unlike the case of pleural mesothelioma, a definite correlation with asbestos exposure has not been established due to the low prevalence of these tumors. Pericardial mesothelioma leads to fusion of the two pericardial layers with the clinical features of constrictive pericarditis. A loculated hemorrhagic pericardial effusion is also present in most cases. Infiltration of the myocardium is rare.

▶ **Imaging signs.** The chest radiograph usually shows an enlarged cardiac silhouette. CT and MRI demonstrate nodular thickening of the pericardium and pericardial effusion.

▶ **Differential diagnosis.** The differential diagnosis includes lymphoma and pericardial carcinomatosis. Another differential diagnosis, fibrinous pericarditis, leads to a more homogeneous and less pronounced thickening of the pericardium.

▶ **Clinical features.** Most patients are asymptomatic. Rarely, patients may describe a feeling of pressure or tightness in the chest.

Pericardial Aplasia

▶ **Brief definition.** With congenital pericardial aplasia, portions of the pericardium are usually absent on the left side. Pericardial defects on the right side are considerably less common. Portions of the heart may herniate through the pericardial defects. If an atrial appendage is present, it may lead to incarceration and thrombus formation.

▶ **Imaging signs.** CT and MRI show complete or partial absence of the pericardial line. In cases of complete pericardial aplasia, lung parenchyma occupies the site of the superior pericardial reflection between the aorta and pulmonary artery. Displacement of the heart into the left hemithorax is a typical finding.

▶ **Clinical features.** Most patients are asymptomatic, but there have been isolated reports of left coronary artery compression at the defect margin, resulting in chest pain and even sudden cardiac death.

▶ **Key points.** Pericardial aplasia is rare. The lack of pericardial fixation may allow the heart to shift into the left hemithorax.

Bibliography

[1] Wolk MJ, Bailey SR, Doherty JU, et al. American College of Cardiology Foundation Appropriate Use Criteria Task Force. ACCF/AHA/ASE/ASNC/HFSA/HRS/SCAI/SCCT/SCMR/STS 2013 multimodality appropriate use criteria for the detection and risk assessment of stable ischemic heart disease: a report of the American College of Cardiology Foundation Appropriate Use Criteria Task Force, American Heart Association, American Society of Echocardiography, American Society of Nuclear Cardiology, Heart Failure Society of America, Heart Rhythm Society, Society for Cardiovascular Angiography and Interventions, Society of Cardiovascular Computed Tomography, Society for Cardiovascular Magnetic Resonance, and Society of Thoracic Surgeons. J Am Coll Cardiol. 2014; 63(4):380–406

[2] Reimer KA, Lowe JE, Rasmussen MM, Jennings RB. The wavefront phenomenon of ischemic cell death. 1. Myocardial infarct size vs duration of coronary occlusion in dogs. Circulation. 1977; 56(5):786–794

[3] Maron BJ, Towbin JA, Thiene G, et al. American Heart Association, Council on Clinical Cardiology, Heart Failure and Transplantation Committee, Quality of Care and Outcomes Research and Functional Genomics and Translational Biology Interdisciplinary Working Groups, Council on Epidemiology and Prevention. Contemporary definitions and classification of the cardiomyopathies: an American Heart Association Scientific Statement from the Council on Clinical Cardiology, Heart Failure and Transplantation Committee; Quality of Care and Outcomes Research and Functional Genomics and Translational Biology Interdisciplinary Working Groups; and Council on Epidemiology and Prevention. Circulation. 2006; 113(14):1807–1816

[4] Richardson P, McKenna W, Bristow M, et al. Report of the 1995 World Health Organization/International Society and Federation of Cardiology Task Force on the Definition and Classification of Cardiomyopathies. Circulation. 1996; 93(5):841–842

[5] Abdel-Aty H, Boyé P, Zagrosek A, et al. Diagnostic performance of cardiovascular magnetic resonance in patients with suspected acute myocarditis: comparison of different approaches. J Am Coll Cardiol. 2005; 45(11):1815–1822

[6] Friedrich MG, Strohm O, Schulz-Menger J, et al. Contrast media-enhanced magnetic resonance imaging visualizes myocardial changes in the course of viral myocarditis. Circulation. 1998; 97:1802–1809

[7] McCrohon JA, Moon JC, Prasad SK, et al. Differentiation of heart failure related to dilated cardiomyopathy and coronary artery disease using gadolinium-enhanced cardiovascular magnetic resonance. Circulation. 2003; 108(1):54–59

[8] Sen-Chowdhry S, Prasad SK, Syrris P, et al. Cardiovascular magnetic resonance in arrhythmogenic right ventricular cardiomyopathy revisited: comparison with task force criteria and genotype. J Am Coll Cardiol. 2006; 48(10):2132–2140

[9] Schünke M, Schulte E, Schumacher U, Cass W. Thieme Atlas of Anatomy. Internal Organs. 2nd ed. Stuttgart: Thieme; 2016. Illustrated by M. Voll/K. Wesker

[10] McKenna WJ, Thiene G, Nava A, et al. Task Force of the Working Group Myocardial and Pericardial Disease of the European Society of Cardiology and of the Scientific Council on Cardiomyopathies of the International Society and Federation of Cardiology. Diagnosis of arrhythmogenic right ventricular dysplasia/cardiomyopathy. Br Heart J. 1994; 71(3):215–218

[11] Marcus FI, McKenna WJ, Sherrill D, et al. Diagnosis of arrhythmogenic right ventricular cardiomyopathy/dysplasia: proposed modification of the Task Force Criteria. Eur Heart J. 2010; 31(7):806–814

[12] Maceira AM, Joshi J, Prasad SK, et al. Cardiovascular magnetic resonance in cardiac amyloidosis. Circulation. 2005; 111(2):186–193

[13] Parsai C, O'Hanlon R, Prasad SK, Mohiaddin RH. Diagnostic and prognostic value of cardiovascular magnetic resonance in non-ischaemic cardiomyopathies. J Cardiovasc Magn Reson. 2012; 14:54

[14] Sekhri V, Sanal S, Delorenzo LJ, Aronow WS, Maguire GP. Cardiac sarcoidosis: a comprehensive review. Arch Med Sci. 2011; 7(4):546–554

[15] Uemura A, Morimoto S, Hiramitsu S, Kato Y, Ito T, Hishida H. Histologic diagnostic rate of cardiac sarcoidosis: evaluation of endomyocardial biopsies. Am Heart J. 1999; 138(2 Pt 1):299–302

[16] Lam KY, Dickens P, Chan AC. Tumors of the heart. A 20-year experience with a review of 12,485 consecutive autopsies. Arch Pathol Lab Med. 1993; 117(10):1027–1031

[17] Lotz J, Kivelitz D, Fischbach R, Beer M, Miller S. [Recommendations for utilizing computerized tomography and magnetic resonance tomography in heart diagnosis. 2—Magnetic resonance tomography]. RoFo Fortschr Geb Rontgenstr Nuklearmed. 2009; 181(8):800–814

[18] Amano J, Kono T, Wada Y, et al. Cardiac myxoma: its origin and tumor characteristics. Ann Thorac Cardiovasc Surg. 2003; 9(4):215–221

[19] Acebo E, Val-Bernal JF, Gómez-Román JJ, Revuelta JM. Clinicopathologic study and DNA analysis of 37 cardiac myxomas: a 28-year experience. Chest. 2003; 123(5):1379–1385

[20] Masui T, Takahashi M, Miura K, Naito M, Tawarahara K. Cardiac myxoma: identification of intratumoral hemorrhage and calcification on MR images. AJR Am J Roentgenol. 1995; 164(4):850–852

[21] Gowda RM, Khan IA, Nair CK, Mehta NJ, Vasavada BC, Sacchi TJ. Cardiac papillary fibroelastoma: a comprehensive analysis of 725 cases. Am Heart J. 2003; 146(3):404–410

[22] Uzun O, Wilson DG, Vujanic GM, Parsons JM, De Giovanni JV. Cardiac tumours in children. Orphanet J Rare Dis. 2007; 2:11

[23] Pruksanusak N, Suntharasaj T, Suwanrath C, Phukaoloun M, Kanjanapradit K. Fetal cardiac rhabdomyoma with hydrops fetalis: report of 2 cases and literature review. J Ultrasound Med. 2012; 31(11):1821–1824

[24] Torimitsu S, Nemoto T, Wakayama M, et al. Literature survey on epidemiology and pathology of cardiac fibroma. Eur J Med Res. 2012; 17:5

[25] Hoffmeier A, Deiters S, Schmidt C, et al. Radical resection of cardiac sarcoma. Thorac Cardiovasc Surg. 2004; 52(2):77–81

[26] Petrich A, Cho SI, Billett H. Primary cardiac lymphoma: an analysis of presentation, treatment, and outcome patterns. Cancer. 2011; 117(3):581–589

[27] Roller FC, Schneider C, Krombach GA. [Rare case of imaging documentation of a rapidly growing primary cardiac lymphoma]. RoFo Fortschr Geb Rontgenstr Nuklearmed. 2013; 185(2):160–162

[28] Mahnken AH, Tacke J. Myocardial heart metastasis in rapidly progressing renal cell carcinoma [in German]. RoFo Fortschr Geb Rontgenstr Nuklearmed. 2000; 172(5):488–490

[29] Reynen K, Köckeritz U, Strasser RH. Metastases to the heart. Ann Oncol. 2004; 15(3):375–381

[30] Krombach GA, Spuentrup E, Buecker A, et al. Herztumoren: Magnetresonanztomographie und Mehrschicht-Spiral-CT. RoFo Fortschr Geb Rontgenstr Nuklearmed. 2005; 177(9):1205–1218

3 Large Vessels

Andreas H. Mahnken

3.1 Aorta

3.1.1 Anatomy

The aorta is the largest arterial vessel in the body. It is divided into several anatomical segments, each of which is subject to specific diseases. The frequency of congenital disorders in particular varies significantly in different aortic segments.

Histologically, the aorta is classified as an elastic artery. As for all vessels in the body, its wall is composed of three layers (from inside to outside):

- *Intima*: The intima consists of endothelium and subendothelial connective tissue with delicate collagen fibers. Endothelial cells are biologically active and secrete vasodilators and vasoconstrictors as required. The aorta has a relatively thick intima, consistent with the mechanical stresses to which the vessel is exposed.
- *Media*: The media consists of concentric layers of smooth muscle cells, collagen fibers, and elastic fibers. The latter form an internal elastic membrane between the intima and media and an external elastic membrane between the media and adventitia. The media absorbs vascular tension and regulates the vascular caliber.
- *Adventitia*: The adventitia surrounds the media with a stabilizing meshwork of collagen fibers and elastic lamellae. The adventitia contains the vasa vasorum, which extend into the outer third of the media and supply blood to the aortic wall.

The principal anatomical segments of the aorta are the aortic root, the ascending aorta, the aortic arch, the descending thoracic aorta, and the abdominal aorta (▶ Fig. 3.1).

- *Aortic root*: The aortic root is the short segment from the aortic valve to the sinotubular junction. The left and right coronary arteries arise from the aortic root.
- *Ascending aorta*: The segment just above the aortic root is the ascending aorta, which extends to the origin of the first supra-aortic branch vessel, the brachiocephalic trunk. The average ascending aorta is approximately 5 cm long and 3.5 cm in diameter.
- *Aortic arch*: The aortic arch extends to the ductus arteriosus or ligamentum arteriosum.[1] It gives off the supra-aortic branch vessels, which are, from proximal to distal, the brachiocephalic trunk, left common carotid artery, and left subclavian artery. Approximately 2 cm from its origin, the brachiocephalic trunk divides into the right subclavian artery and right common carotid artery. The distal segment of the aortic arch from the distal circumference of the left subclavian artery to the ductus arteriosus or ligamentum arteriosum is called the aortic isthmus. The aortic arch is typically located to the left of the midline. It is classified into three types based on the relative position of the brachiocephalic trunk (▶ Fig. 3.2): With a type I aortic arch, the origin of the brachiocephalic trunk is level with the outer curvature (top) of the arch. With a type II aortic arch, the origin of the brachiocephalic trunk is at a level between the outer and inner curvatures of the arch. With a type III arch, the origin is below the level of the inner curvature. This distinction is particularly important for planning interventional therapies, as the interventional approach to the supra-aortic vessels becomes more difficult with increasing complexity of aortic arch anatomy (types II and III), with a corresponding rise in complication rates.
- *Descending thoracic aorta*: The next segment is the descending thoracic aorta, which continues to the diaphragm. The proximal part of this segment, just distal to the ductus arteriosus, may show a slight physiologic expansion. The descending thoracic aorta gives off the segmentally arranged intercostal arteries and the bronchial arteries, which consistently arise at the level of the tracheal bifurcation. Other small-caliber branches are the pericardial, esophageal, and superior phrenic arteries.
- *Abdominal aorta*: The infradiaphragmatic abdominal aorta extends from the diaphragm to the aortic bifurcation at the level of the T4 vertebra, where it divides into the common iliac arteries. The abdominal aorta gives off numerous large vessels to all abdominal structures. The most proximal branch vessel is the celiac trunk, which divides at once into the common hepatic artery, splenic artery, and left gastric artery. Just distal to the celiac trunk (approximately one-half vertebral body height) is the origin of the superior mesenteric artery, which supplies large portions of the small intestine, ascending colon, and proximal two-thirds of the transverse colon. The third unpaired branch vessel is the inferior mesenteric artery, which arises just above

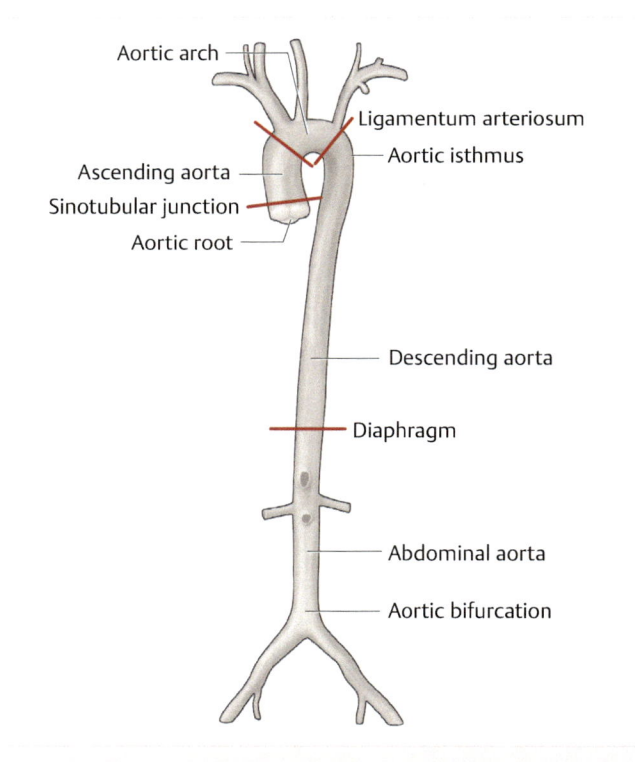

Fig. 3.1 Anatomy of the aorta. Diagrammatic representation of the ascending aorta, aortic arch, descending aorta, abdominal aorta, and the major supra-aortic and abdominal branch vessels. (Reproduced from Schünke M, Schulte E, Schumacher U. Prometheus. LernAtlas der Anatomie: Innere Organe. Illustrated by M. Voll/K. Wesker. 2nd ed. Stuttgart: Thieme; 2009.)

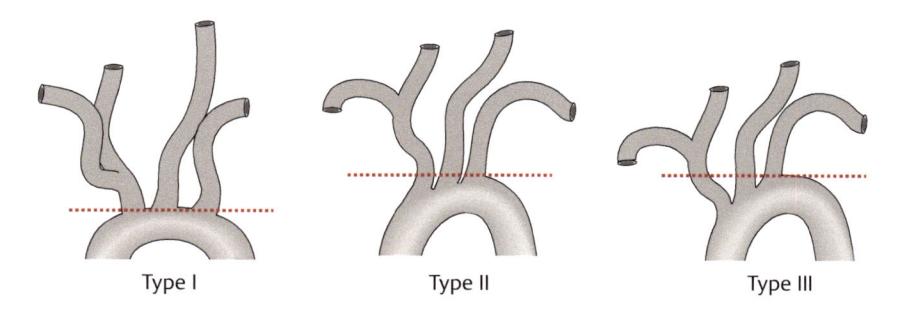

Fig. 3.2 Classification of the aortic arch. Schematic representation. Classification is based on the relationship of the origin of the brachiocephalic trunk to the inner and outer curvatures of the aortic arch.

Type I Type II Type III

the aortic bifurcation and supplies the peripheral colon segments including the sigmoid colon and rectum. These vessel origins are subject to numerous variations, which should be noted in the planning of surgical and interventional procedures. The sacral artery branches from the posterior side of the abdominal aorta to supply the sacrum and coccyx. The largest paired branch vessels are the renal arteries. Proximal to them are the inferior phrenic arteries, which may also arise from one or both sides of the celiac trunk, and small suprarenal arteries, which often arise from the proximal part of the renal arteries. Paired lumbar arteries arise at segmental levels from the back of the aorta to supply the vertebral bodies, back muscles, and spinal cord. The different vascular territories are interconnected by numerous collateral vessels, enabling them to divert blood to other territories that have lost their normal supply. The most familiar of these collaterals is the Riolan anastomosis, which creates a relatively large connection between the territories of the superior and inferior mesenteric arteries in the left upper abdomen.

3.1.2 Development

The development of the aorta and its large branch vessels is a complex, synchronized process. A knowledge of this process is helpful for understanding congenital anomalies and variants. Ontogenetically, the arterial limb of the embryonic circulation begins with the still-undivided truncus arteriosus. This structure is connected with the aortic arch, which carries blood around the gut tube to the paired dorsal aortae. Starting in approximately the third week of gestation, a relatively small right and left ventral aorta is formed along with a larger right and left dorsal aorta. Development of the six branchial arches is paralleled by the development of six aortic arches, which interconnect the ventral and dorsal aortae on each side. The six aortic arches do not all coexist at any one time, however.

The first three aortic arches give rise to the arteries supplying the head and neck region. The first two aortic arches regress while the third one, along with parts of the dorsal aortae, form the major portion of the internal carotid arteries. The latter develop from the ventral aortae. The fourth aortic arch develops asymmetrically, in accordance with the asymmetric development of the heart. The left fourth aortic arch in the embryo persists as the aortic arch, while the right arch forms the brachiocephalic trunk and proximal right subclavian artery. The fifth aortic arch is absent or does not form definitive structures. The sixth aortic arches give rise to the proximal part of the pulmonary trunk, the left arch also forming the ductus arteriosus. Caudal to approximately the T4 vertebral level, the dorsal aortae fuse to form the

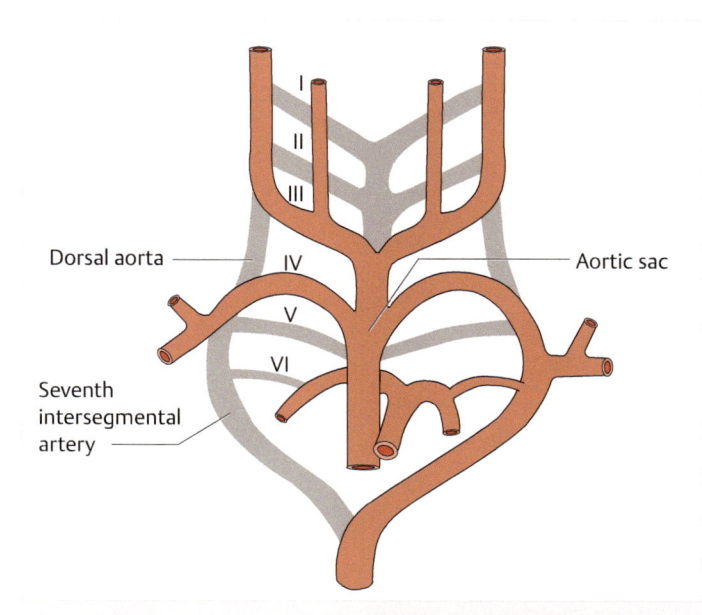

Fig. 3.3 Normal embryological development of the six aortic arches (I–VI). Schematic representation of the results of normal development. Portions of the dorsal aortae that disappear in approximately the seventh week of gestation are shown in gray. (Reproduced from Schünke M, Schulte E, Schumacher U. Prometheus. LernAtlas der Anatomie: Allgemeine Anatomie und Bewegungssystem. Illustrated by M. Voll/K. Wesker. 3rd ed. Stuttgart: Thieme; 2011.)

definitive descending aorta (▶ Fig. 3.3). The originally paired yolk sac arteries fuse during embryonic development and form the unpaired visceral vessels in adults: the celiac trunk and the superior and inferior mesenteric arteries.

3.1.3 Congenital Anomalies

Approximately 20% of all cardiovascular malformations are aortic anomalies.[2] The proximal portions (closest to the heart) are most commonly affected because they undergo the most complex embryological development. The clinical presentation of aortic anomalies is extremely variable and ranges from asymptomatic to life-threatening. The most common anomalies affecting the thoracic aorta distal to the sinotubular junction are as follows:
- Variants in the origins of supra-aortic vessels.
- Aberrant right subclavian artery and Kommerell diverticulum.
- Patent ductus arteriosus.
- Coarctation of the aorta.
- Double aortic arch.
- Right aortic arch.

Variants in the Origins of Supra-aortic Vessels

The normal anatomy described above, with three supra-aortic branch vessels, is present in approximately 70% of the population. The actual arrangement can vary over a very broad range that includes ethnic differences. Possible variants in the origins of the supra-aortic vessels are listed in ▶ Table 3.1. The most frequent variant is a common origin of the brachiocephalic trunk and left common carotid artery (▶ Fig. 3.4). Another common variant is the left common carotid artery arising from the brachiocephalic trunk (▶ Fig. 3.5). Often this is erroneously called a "bovine arch"; by definition, the bovine aorta requires a single origin of all supra-aortic vessels from the aortic arch, a pattern consistently found in cattle.[3] Another variant is illustrated in ▶ Fig. 3.6.

Table 3.1 Variants in the origins of the supra-aortic vessels

Variant	Approximate frequency (%)
Common origin of the brachiocephalic trunk and left common carotid artery	13
Left common carotid artery arising from the brachiocephalic trunk	9
Left vertebral artery arising directly from the aortic arch	5
Left common carotid artery and left subclavian artery arising by a common trunk	1
Aberrant origin of the right subclavian artery from the left side of the aortic arch	0.5

Aberrant Right Subclavian Artery and Kommerell Diverticulum

▶ **Brief definition.** An aberrant origin and course of the right subclavian artery is a clinically significant variant. Also known as a Kommerell diverticulum, it occurs when the right subclavian artery arises from the left side of the descending aorta rather than from the brachiocephalic trunk. Typically the aberrant vessel runs to the right and passes behind the esophagus (▶ Fig. 3.7). Less commonly it may run anterior to the esophagus (15% of cases) or, more rarely, anterior to the trachea (5% of cases). In this variant the recurrent laryngeal nerve does not form a loop around the right subclavian artery but runs directly to the laryngeal muscles. When the aberrant vessel passes behind the esophagus, it may cause "dysphagia lusoria" due to compression of the esophagus. Only about 10% of patients with a retroesophageal right subclavian artery become symptomatic, however, and the aberrant vessel is usually detected incidentally. Dysphagia lusoria is generally treated surgically.

▶ **Imaging signs.** The chest radiograph in patients with an aberrant right subclavian artery may show widening of the superior mediastinum. This is caused by an outpouching of the aorta at the origin of the aberrant vessel. Occasionally the course of an aberrant right subclavian artery is identified on the chest film by vascular calcifications (▶ Fig. 3.8a).[4] A barium esophagogram may show an impression on the posterior esophageal wall. Sectional imaging studies, especially CT angiography (CTA) and MRI, can supply the most definitive results (▶ Fig. 3.8b).

Patent Ductus Arteriosus

▶ **Brief definition.** The ductus arteriosus is the part of the fetal circulation that connects the aorta with the pulmonary arterial

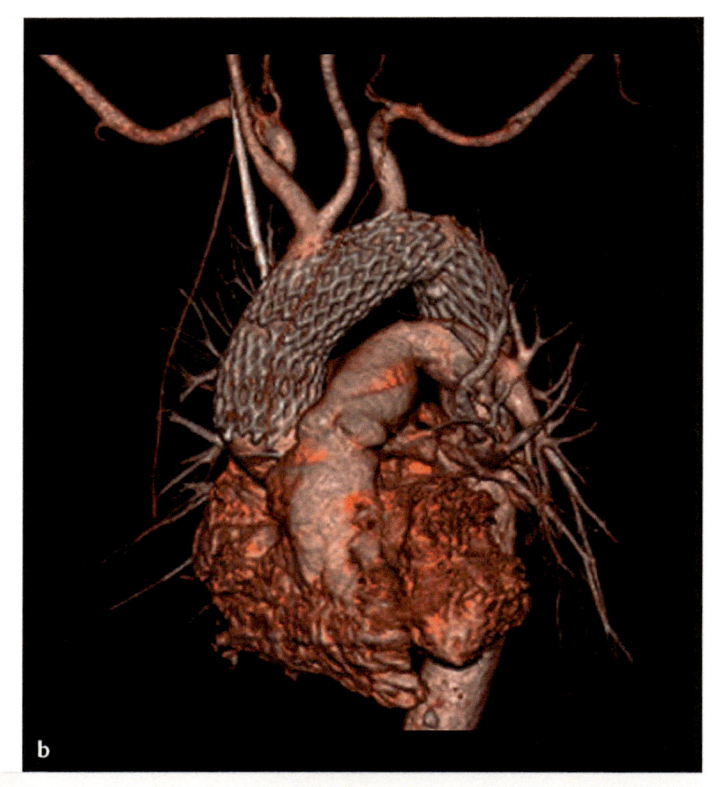

Fig. 3.4 **The most frequent variant in the origin of the supra-aortic vessels.** Common origin of the carotid arteries from the aortic arch. (a) DSA. (b) CT after implantation of a thoracic stent.

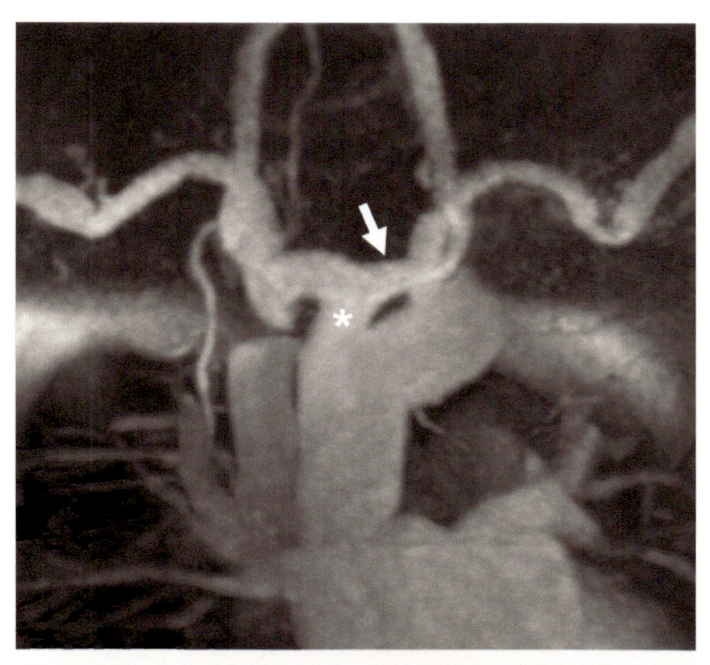

Fig. 3.5 **Variant in the origin of supra-aortic vessels.** The left common carotid artery (arrow) arises from the brachiocephalic trunk (asterisk).

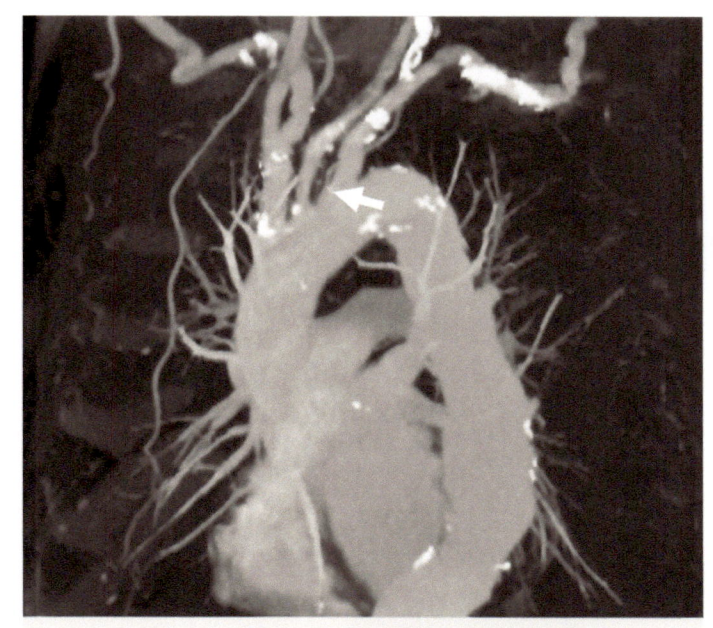

Fig. 3.6 **Variant in the origin of supra-aortic vessels.** The left vertebral artery arises directly from the aortic arch (arrow).

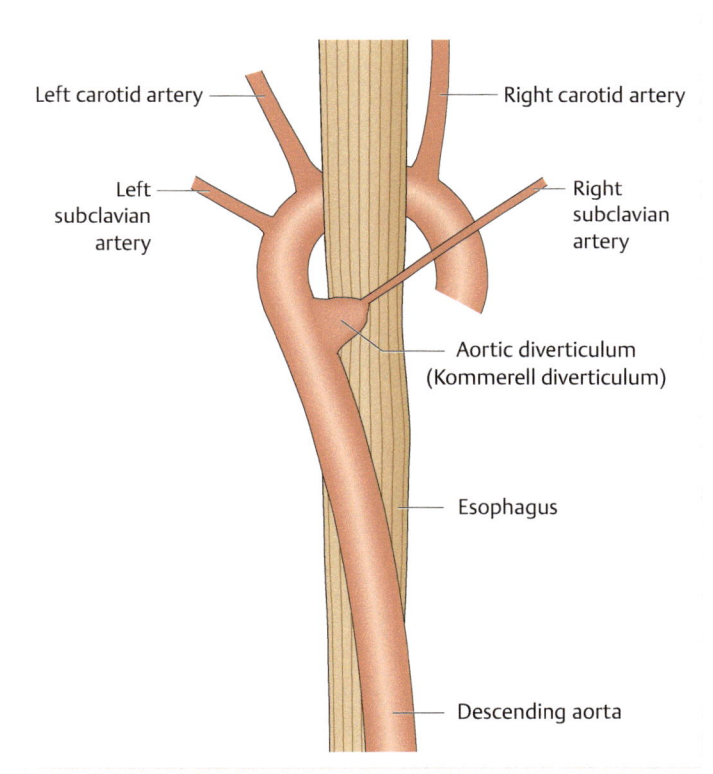

Fig. 3.7 **Kommerell diverticulum.** Diagrammatic posterior view illustrates a Kommerell diverticulum as described by Burckhard Kommerell in the original 1936 publication.

system. The ductus arteriosus runs from the anteromedial circumference of the aortic isthmus to the proximal left pulmonary artery. The ductus arteriosus normally undergoes functional closure within 24 hours after birth and anatomical closure in subsequent days and weeks, leaving behind only a bandlike structure, the ligamentum arteriosum. Patent ductus arteriosus is diagnosed if the ductus is still patent 3 months after birth. This entity is relatively common, with an incidence of 1:2,000 live births. It is particularly common in premature infants.

▶ **Imaging signs.** Echocardiography is the imaging study of choice for the diagnosis of a patent ductus arteriosus. Depending on the shunt volume, the plain chest film may show indirect signs such as an enlarged cardiac silhouette or dilated pulmonary vessels indicative of pulmonary venous hyperemia or pulmonary edema. CT and MRI are excellent for demonstrating the presence of a patent ductus and classifying its morphology.[5]

▶ **Clinical features.** A continuous "machinery murmur" is heard on auscultation. The symptoms depend on the magnitude of the shunt volume and the presence of associated cardiac anomalies. An enlarged left ventricle and pulmonary hypertension are typical manifestations of a patent ductus arteriosus. With some congenital anomalies such as pulmonary atresia, a patent ductus arteriosus is necessary so that lung perfusion, for example, can be maintained by flow across the shunt. Treatment options depend on the timing of diagnosis and the morphology of the patent ductus; they include pharmacologic therapy (indomethacin) as well as surgical and interventional options.

▶ **Differential diagnosis.** Even when the ductus arteriosus closes normally, a localized anteromedial outpouching may be found at the position of the ductus. This variant, called a "ductus bump," is found in up to one-third of newborns and approximately 9% of adults. It can be distinguished clinically from a traumatic aortic rupture, which occurs most commonly at the site of the ligamentum arteriosum.

▶ **Key points.** A patent ductus arteriosus connects the aorta with the pulmonary arterial circulation, running from the aortic isthmus to the left pulmonary artery. It is diagnosed by echocardiography. The chest radiograph shows signs of a shunt defect with an increased volume load on the cardiopulmonary system. Sectional imaging by MRI or CTA allows direct visualization of the patent ductus for planning interventional therapy, etc.

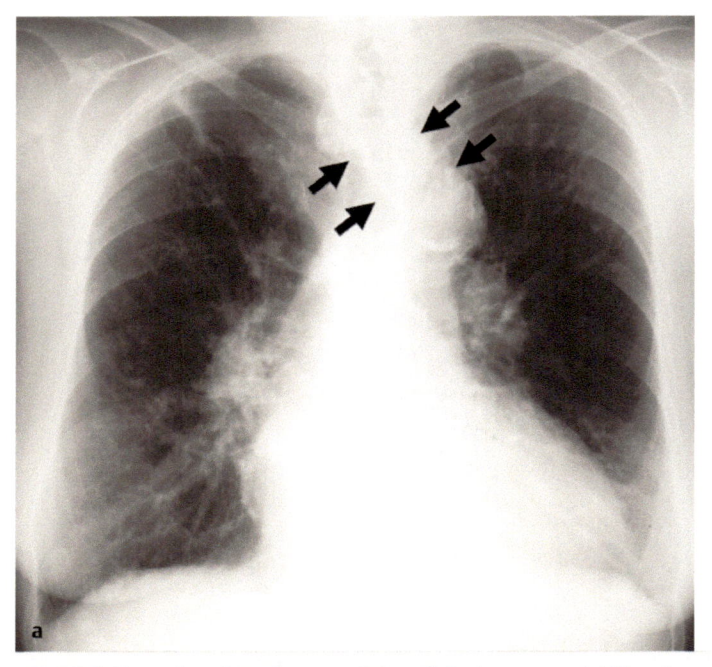

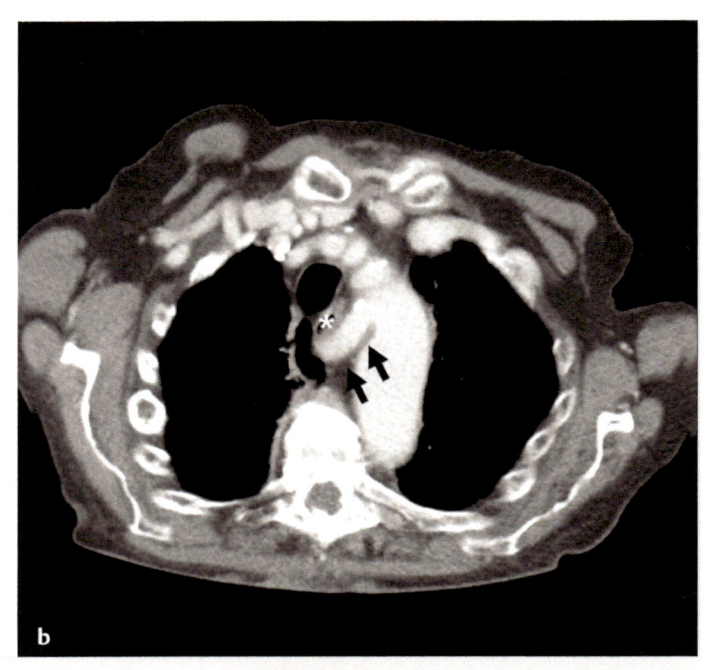

Fig. 3.8 Examples of an aberrant right subclavian artery. (a) The chest radiograph shows widening of the superior mediastinum. In rare cases the course of the vessel is defined by the presence of vascular calcifications (arrows). (b) CT demonstrates the aberrant origin of the right subclavian artery. It arises from the aortic arch as the last supra-aortic vessel and usually runs behind the esophagus (asterisk) to the right side (arrows).

Coarctation of the Aorta

▶ **Brief definition.** Coarctation of the aorta is a congenital narrowing of the thoracic aorta at the level of the aortic isthmus. A preductal (infantile) form is distinguished from a postductal (adult) form based on the relationship of the lesion to the ductus arteriosus. These forms also have different clinical manifestations. Coarctation of the aorta occurs in approximately 0.3% of all live births and comprises 5 to 8% of all congenital cardiac anomalies. It is associated with various syndromic conditions such as Turner's syndrome (20% of cases) and other cardiac anomalies such as a bicuspid aortic valve.

▶ **Imaging signs.** The infantile form of coarctation usually produces nonspecific radiographic changes such as cardiac enlargement and signs of pulmonary venous congestion. A possible direct sign on chest films is the epsilon or figure-3 sign, which reflects the atypical shape of the narrowed aorta. In the adult form, a longstanding coarctation may cause rib notching from enlarged intercostal vessels functioning as collaterals (▶ Fig. 3.9). Notching most commonly affects the fourth through eighth ribs. The first two ribs are always spared, as they are supplied by the costocervical trunk. Direct detection of the lesion, including visualization of the collateral pathways, can be accomplished with CTA (▶ Fig. 3.10) or MRI (▶ Fig. 3.11). MRI also permits flow measurements for assessing hemodynamic significance.

Note

When the dimensions of a coarctation are determined at sectional imaging, it is important to obtain a true cross section for each vascular segment and avoid oblique sections.

▶ **Clinical features.** The clinical presentation depends on the type of aortic coarctation, i.e., whether it is a preductal (infantile) form or a postductal (adult) form:

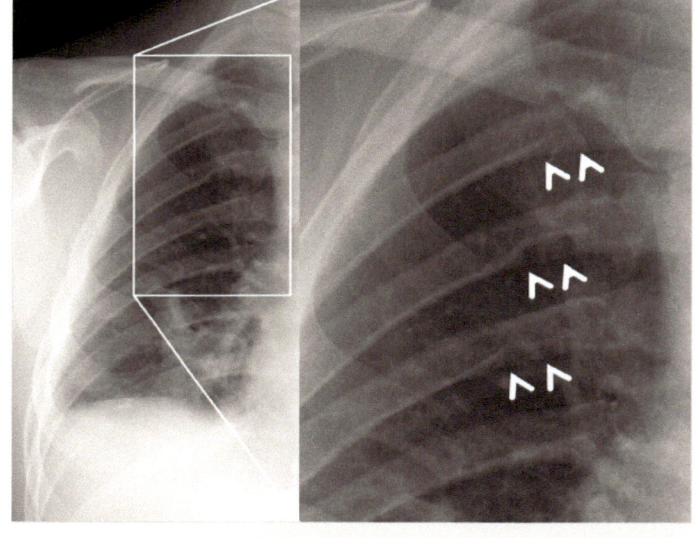

Fig. 3.9 Adult form of coarctation of the aorta. The chest radiograph displays the typical rib notches, seen here predominantly in the fourth through seventh ribs (arrowheads in magnified view).

- *Infantile form*: In this form the stenosis is located proximal to the ductus arteriosus, and the heart pumps against the resistance of the stenosis. Because this proximal type of coarctation is poorly collateralized, patients consistently develop left-sided heart failure and pulmonary venous congestion with dyspnea. The ductus arteriosus typically remains patent, causing venous blood to be shunted to the lower half of the body with resulting cyanosis of the trunk and lower limbs. The poor oxygenation may lead to organ failure.
- *Adult form*: The adult, postductal form of coarctation allows for the compensation of arterial blood flow by collateral vessels. The ductus arteriosus obliterates normally, and cyanosis does not occur; however, physical examination typically reveals

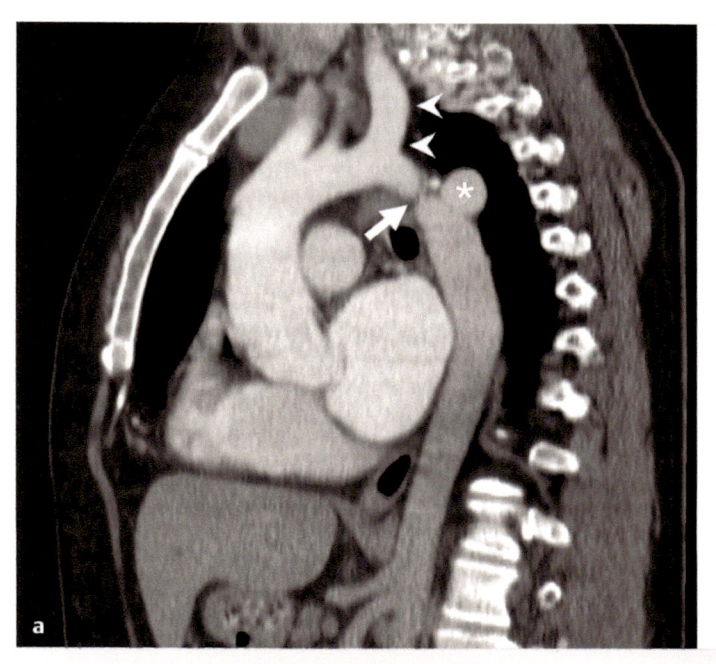

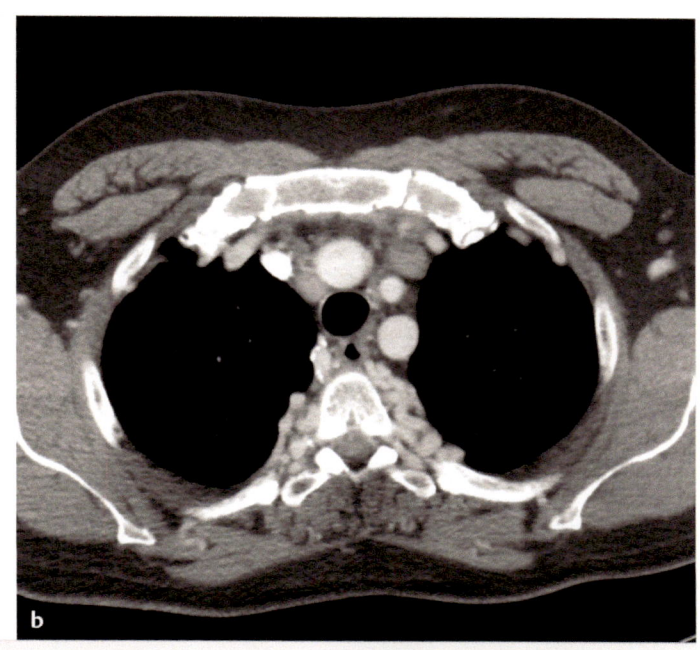

Fig. 3.10 Adult form of coarctation of the aorta. CTA. **(a)** Sagittal reformatted CTA image shows the stenosis (arrow) distal to the origin of the left subclavian artery (arrowheads), which is greatly dilated due to massive collateral flow (asterisk). **(b)** Axial reformatted CTA image displays the numerous collateral vessels.

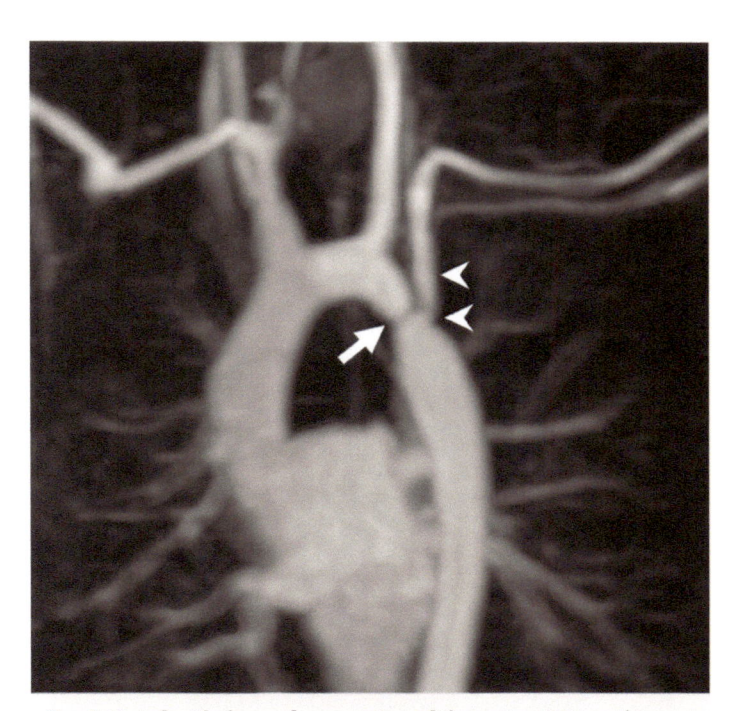

Fig. 3.11 Infantile form of coarctation of the aorta. MRA. In this case the stenosis (arrow) is proximal to the origin of the left subclavian artery (arrowheads) and thus proximal to the ductus arteriosus. This is a moderate coarctation, as indicated by the absence of prominent collaterals.

hypertension in the upper half of the body where the heart must pump against a resistance. This may lead to a pulse and blood pressure discrepancy between the upper and lower halves of the body.

The infantile form has a mortality rate up to 90% in untreated cases. Treatment is urgent, therefore, and usually consists of primary surgery. The adult form should also be corrected in childhood but is an elective indication. Older children or patients with restenosis should be treated by stent implantation or repeated balloon dilatation.

▶ **Differential diagnosis.** The adult form of aortic coarctation must be differentiated from pseudocoarctation due to atypical elongation and kinking of the aorta and from large-vessel arteritis such as Takayasu's arteritis.

▶ **Key points.** Preductal and postductal forms of aortic coarctation are distinguished according to their relationship to the ductus arteriosus as seen on imaging. While the chest radiograph may show specific signs such as the epsilon sign and rib notching, direct visualization by MRI or CTA is state-of-the-art. Assignment of cases to the adult or infantile form is important for directing further treatment and is an essential part of the radiology report.

Double Aortic Arch

▶ **Brief definition.** Double aortic arch is part of a complex group of congenital anomalies that can be collectively referred to as aortic vascular rings:
- Double aortic arch.
- Right aortic arch:
  - With an aberrant left subclavian artery and left ligamentum arteriosum.
  - With mirror-image branching and a retroesophageal ligamentum arteriosum.
- Left aortic arch:
  - With an aberrant right subclavian artery and right ligamentum arteriosum.
  - With a right descending aorta and ligamentum arteriosum.

These anomalies are well explained by the hypothetical model of the double aortic arch postulated by J. E. Edwards in the early

1950s (▶ Fig. 3.12).⁶ In this model, the various possible forms of vascular rings can be traced to different problems in the development and regression of specific structures included in the model. Double aortic arch is the most common vascular ring anomaly, accounting for up to 60% of cases in this group (▶ Fig. 3.13). Embryologically, this variant results from bilateral persistence of the fourth aortic arches. Morphologically, the right aortic arch is the dominant arch in approximately 70% of cases. The left arch is dominant in approximately 25% of cases. Occasionally, both arches are of equal size. With partial atresia of one of the aortic arches, the vascular ring may be completed by fibrotic residues of the atretic vascular segment. This variant of the aortic arch anomaly is rarely associated with congenital heart disease.

▶ **Imaging signs.** The barium esophagogram may show posterior indentation of the trachea or esophagus, depending on the cause of the vascular ring. The sensitivity and specificity of this technique are relatively poor, however. Contrast-enhanced low-dose CT is the modality of choice for initial imaging, while MRI should be used for follow-up. If the vascular ring does not lie in one axial plane of section, then the "four-vessel sign" with the right subclavian artery and right common carotid artery arising from the right arch and the left common carotid and subclavian arteries arising from the left arch will help to identify this anomaly.

▶ **Clinical features.** Patients present clinically with dysphagia or respiratory problems. Respiratory complaints such as stridor are more common in newborns and children, while dysphagia is dominant in older children and undiagnosed adults. Treatment involves surgical division of the smaller aortic arch and ligamentum arteriosum.

Right Aortic Arch

▶ **Brief definition.** A right aortic arch results from involution of the fourth left aortic arch and is found in approximately 0.1% of adults. This variant may occur alone or may be associated with cyanotic congenital heart disease, especially the tetralogy of Fallot. Different types of right aortic arch are distinguished according to the origin of the supra-aortic vessels, and certain configurations may produce a vascular ring (see above).

- The most common form, accounting for 59 to 84% of cases, is a right aortic arch with mirror-image branching relative to normal anatomy.

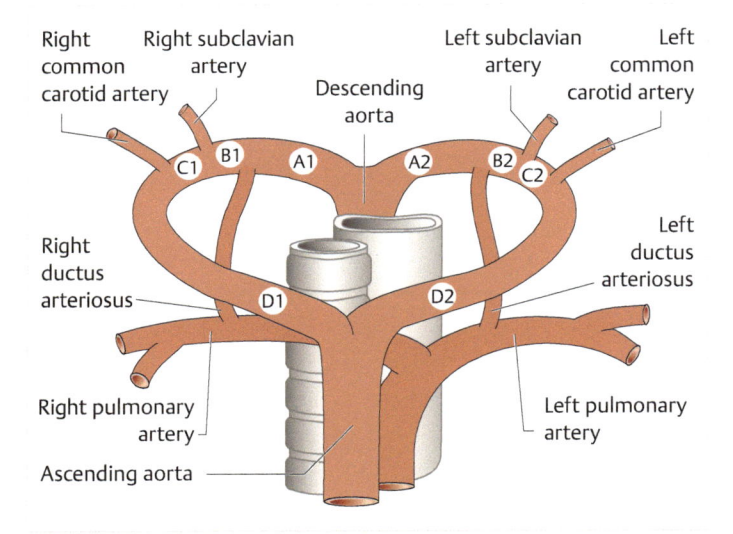

Fig. 3.12 Double aortic arch. Hypothetical model of Edwards. The letters A–D designate potential regression sites for various parts of the aortic arches.

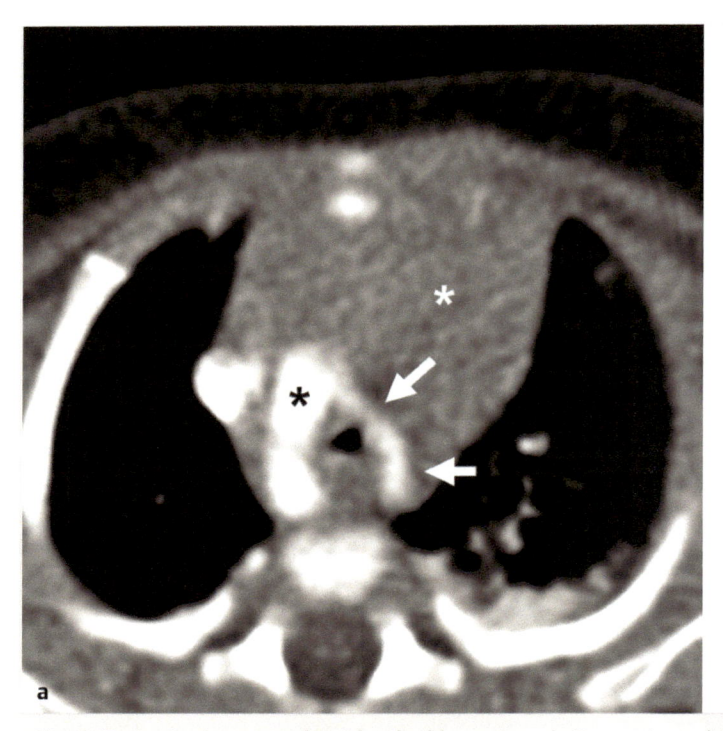

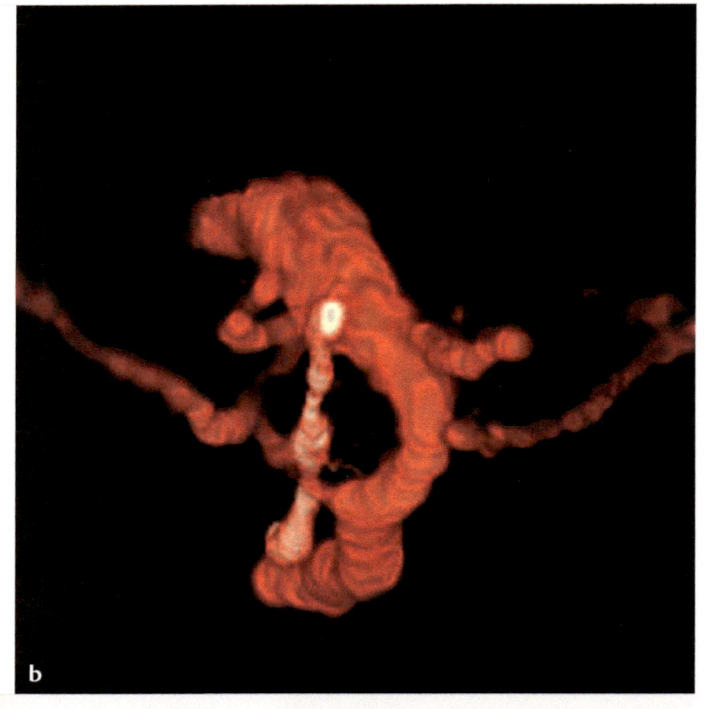

Fig. 3.13 Aortic ring anomaly with a double aortic arch. Two patients. **(a)** Axial CT demonstrates a dominant right aortic arch (black asterisk) and a smaller left aortic arch (arrows). Thymic tissue (white asterisk) is visible in the anterior mediastinum. **(b)** 3D reconstruction of CT data from a different patient shows the four-vessel sign with a subclavian artery and common carotid artery arising from each of the two aortic arches. The left arch is dominant in this patient. A nasogastric tube (white) marks the location of the esophagus.

- The second most common form (14–39% of cases) is a right aortic arch with an aberrant left subclavian artery. This artery is the last branch vessel from the aortic arch and often shows proximal dilatation analogous to a Kommerell diverticulum.
- A very rare form (less than 1% of cases) is a right aortic arch with an isolated left subclavian artery, which may lead to a congenital subclavian steal syndrome and vertebrobasilar insufficiency.

> **Caution**
>
> When describing the finding of a right aortic arch, it is important to be aware that the terminology used in the literature is not uniform, and it is best to provide a verbal description as illustrated above.

▶ **Imaging signs.** The left aortic border is absent in the chest radiograph. The right aortic arch typically appears at a high right paratracheal site, while the aortic border occupies a right paravertebral position (▶ Fig. 3.14). Tracheal indentation may be visible at the level of the aortic arch. Symptomatic patients require sectional imaging evaluation for detection and classification of a vascular ring, for example.

Congenital Abdominal Aortic Stenosis

▶ **Clinical features.** The symptoms of congenital abdominal aortic stenosis are similar to those of the adult form of coarctation of the aorta, with arterial hypertension and a blood-pressure discrepancy between the upper and lower limbs. Blood flow distal to the stenosis may be significantly decreased, leading to peripheral claudication or even renal failure. Treatment is usually surgical. The role of interventional treatments is still greatly limited as a result of numerous setbacks.[7,8]

▶ **Brief definition.** Midaortic syndrome is a variant of congenital aortic stenosis (▶ Table 3.2). Although approximately 98% of cases present as coarctation of the aorta, the stenosis may be located farther distally in 0.5 to 2% of cases and is then termed "midaortic syndrome." Many other names have also been applied to this condition such as "hypoplasia of the abdominal aorta," "congenital abdominal aortic stenosis," and "coarctation of the abdominal aorta." Midaortic syndrome may occur in the descending thoracic aorta or in the abdominal aorta. The site of occurrence is highly variable and has also been described as suprarenal or infrarenal.

3.1.4 Diseases

Aortic Aneurysms

▶ **Brief definition.** An aneurysm is defined as the permanent dilatation of a vessel by at least 50% of its normal diameter.[9] Given that the diameter of the aorta, especially its thoracic portion, increases with aging, it is reasonable to assume that the midportion diameter of the ascending aorta should not exceed 4 cm while the diameter of the descending aorta should not exceed 3 cm.

A basic distinction is made between true and false aneurysms. A true aneurysm involves all three layers of the vessel wall (intima, media, adventitia) while a false aneurysm, also called a pseudoaneurysm, does not. Many pseudoaneurysms involve only the adventitia and periadventitial tissue. Typical causes of pseudoaneurysms include aortic dissection and posttraumatic aneurysms. The causes of true aortic aneurysms are extremely diverse, the most common being degenerative changes in the aortic wall due to atherosclerosis. This mechanism is responsible for 30% to more than 80% of aortic aneurysms in different studies. Other relatively frequent causes of aortic aneurysms are aortic dissection,

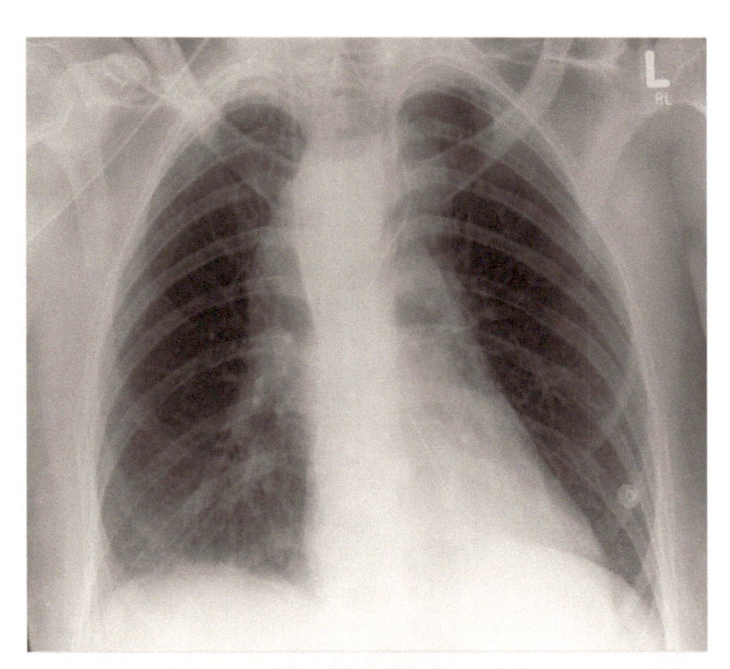

Fig. 3.14 Right aortic arch and a right descending aorta in a 47-year-old woman. The right descending aorta is clearly visualized in its right paravertebral location. The trachea and esophagus are displaced to the left by the right aortic arch. The esophagus is identified by a nasogastric tube.

Table 3.2 Congenital anomalies of the aorta by vascular segments

Ascending thoracic aorta	Aortic arch	Descending aorta
• Supravalvular aortic stenosis • Aortoventricular tunnel • Sinus of Valsalva aneurysm • Aortopulmonary window • Truncus arteriosus • Hemitruncus	• Aberrant right subclavian artery, Kommerell diverticulum • Patent ductus arteriosus • Hypoplasia of the aortic arch • Double aortic arch • Right aortic arch • Interrupted aortic arch • Branch vessels arising from the pulmonary artery • Cervical aortic arch	• Congenital abdominal aortic stenosis (midaortic syndrome)

Table 3.3 Causes of aortic aneurysms

Cause	Frequency (%)
Common	
Atherosclerosis	ca. 70 (30–80)
Aortic dissection	<50
Aortitis (infectious)	12
Media degeneration	6
Marfan's syndrome	5–10
Rare	
Ehlers–Danlos syndrome	
Turner's syndrome	
Bicuspid aortic valve	
Trauma	
Noninfectious aortitis: • Rheumatic fever • Rheumatoid arthritis • Reiter's disease • Giant cell arteritis • Takayasu's arteritis • Systemic lupus erythematosus • Ulcerative colitis • Behçet's disease	
Scleroderma	
Osteogenesis imperfecta	
Radiation-induced	

inflammatory changes, and congenital disorders (▶ Table 3.3), most notably Marfan's syndrome and Ehlers–Danlos syndrome. Marfan's syndrome in particular leads to early, significant aneurysmal growth.

▶ **Imaging signs.** Asymptomatic aortic aneurysms, unlike symptomatic lesions, are generally detected incidentally in imaging studies ordered for a different indication. Aortic aneurysms most commonly involve the abdominal aorta (31%), followed by the ascending aorta (22%), the aortic arch (11%), and the descending aorta (7.5%). Thoracoabdominal aortic aneurysms are relatively rare, comprising approximately 3% of cases.

Caution

The diagnostic work-up of an aneurysm should include imaging of the entire aorta because, for example, 28% of patients diagnosed with a thoracic aortic aneurysm are also found to have an abdominal aneurysm (▶ Fig. 3.15).

The chest radiograph shows widening of the aortic contour. Calcifications in the aortic wall can be very helpful in determining vessel diameter and are often seen most clearly in the lateral chest film. In extreme cases an aneurysm of the ascending aorta may occupy all of the retrosternal space (▶ Fig. 3.16). The abdominal plain film can clearly demonstrate the presence and size of an aneurysm when conspicuous calcifications are present, but the sensitivity of this technique is very low. In some cases an abdominal aortic aneurysm is also indicated by its displacement of intestinal structures. Ultrasound, CT, and MRI can generally provide a definitive diagnosis by showing aortic enlargement to more than 4 cm in the ascending aorta and more than 3 cm in the descending and abdominal aorta.

Note

Especially in patients with a presumed aneurysm of the ascending aorta, ECG-gated imaging should be done to eliminate motion artifacts. The aortic valve should also be evaluated because of the strong association of ascending aortic aneurysm with a bicuspid aortic valve.

Besides making the diagnosis, important imaging goals with an aortic aneurysm are the determination of its size, follow-up, and treatment planning. Another purpose in high-risk groups is screening for the presence of an aortic aneurysm. While this should rely mainly on ultrasound, CTA has become the current clinical standard for detecting aneurysm extension and planning treatment. The follow-up of abdominal aneurysms can be done with ultrasound in patients under age 65 years; CT is the accepted clinical standard in older patients. In comparing imaging measurements, it is important to note that ultrasound underestimates vascular diameters by approximately 4 mm compared with CT. MRI is also effective for detecting aneurysm extension but is less widely used for this indication due to factors such as high cost and limited availability. Aortic aneurysms are classified on the basis of sectional imaging findings. Classification is useful for directing treatment and predicting outcomes. The Estrera classification is used for thoracic aneurysms (▶ Fig. 3.17),[10] the Crawford classification for thoracoabdominal aortic aneurysms (▶ Fig. 3.18, ▶ Fig. 3.19).[11]

Note

It is important to follow a uniform measurement standard for aortic aneurysms to ensure accurate follow-up. The measurement of aortic diameter is based on well-defined reference points in a true short-axis view of the vessel (see ▶ Fig. 3.16).

Use of the following reference points is recommended:
- Sinotubular junction.
- Proximal aortic arch.
- Proximal descending aorta.
- Aorta at the level of the diaphragm.
- Infrarenal aorta (approximately 2 cm below the renal arteries).
- Aortic bifurcation.
- Maximum sectional diameter of any aortic aneurysms that are present.

The recommended intervals for follow-up imaging are based on the size of the aneurysm (▶ Table 3.4). It is also important to note typical postoperative changes such as elephant trunk, graft kinking, and foreign materials as well as typical complications such as perigraft hematoma and abscess, fistulas, and pseudoaneurysms.[12,13]

▶ **Clinical features.** Most aortic aneurysms are clinically silent and are detected incidentally. Symptomatic aneurysms usually

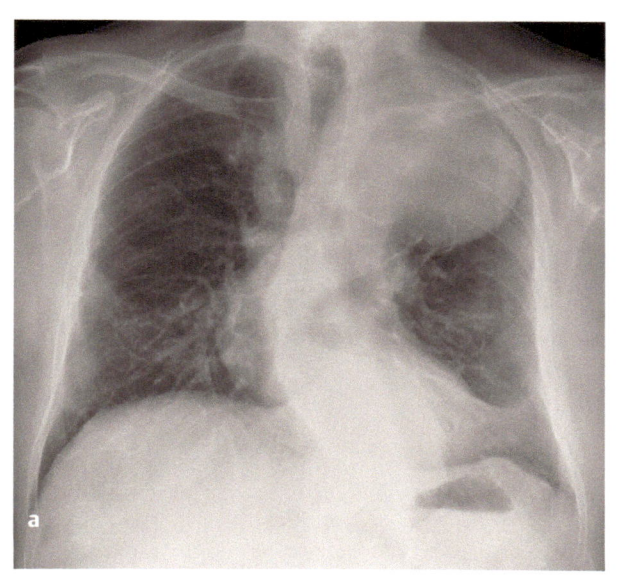

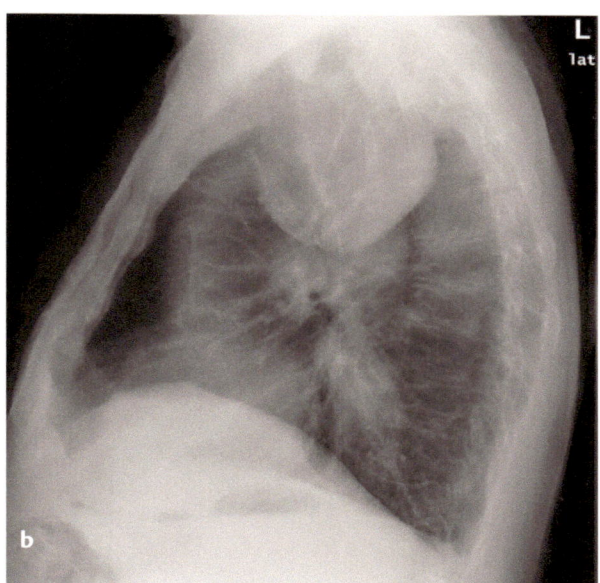

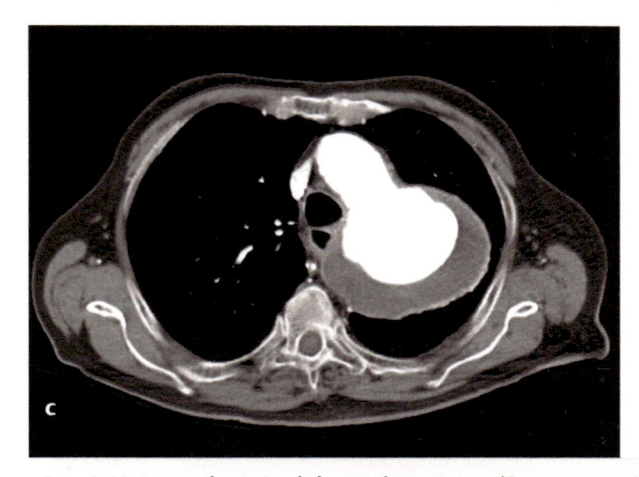

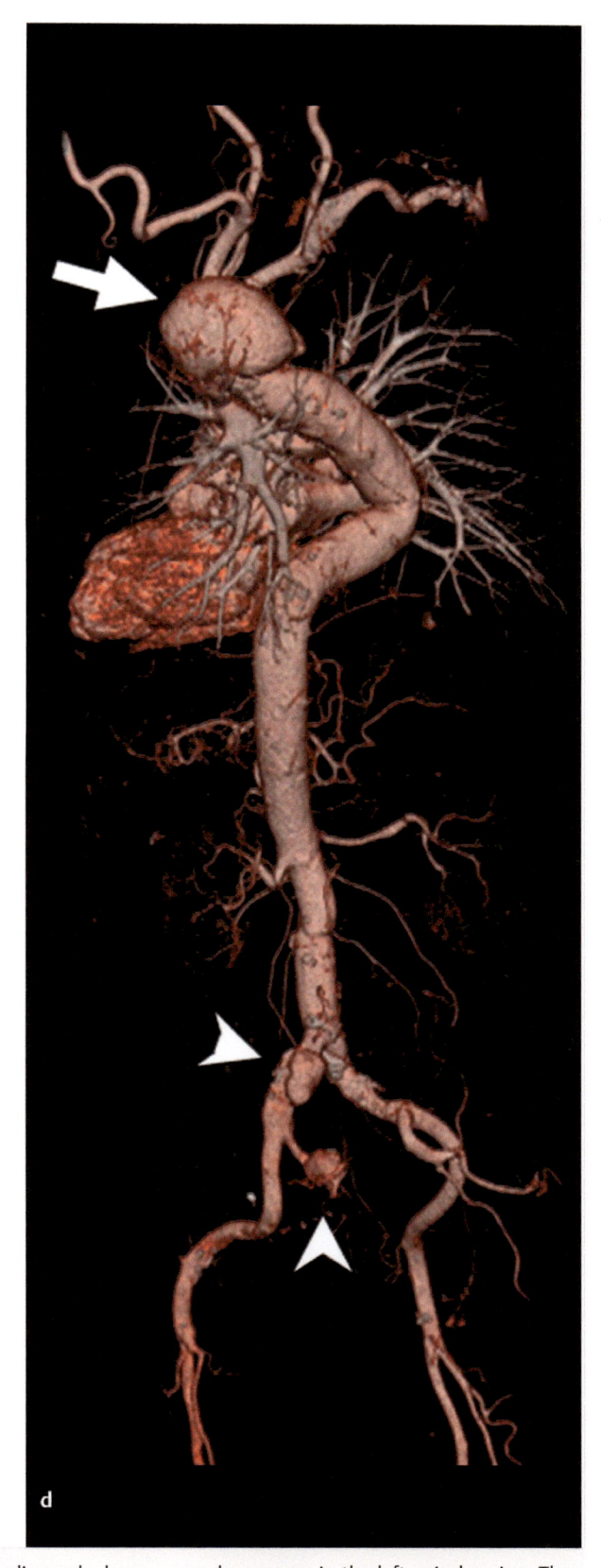

Fig. 3.15 Large thoracic abdominal aneurysm (Estrera type A).[10] (a) PA chest radiograph shows a very large mass in the left apical region. The lesion is distinguishable from a malignant tumor by its relationship to the aorta, its pushing margins, and the absence of local destructive changes in the chest wall, for example. (b) Lateral chest radiograph. (c) CTA accurately localizes the aneurysm and also demonstrates a mural thrombus. (d) The entire aorta should be imaged at initial work-up, as one-third of patients with a thoracic aortic aneurysm have additional aneurysms. In the case shown, the thoracic aneurysm (arrow) coexists with other aneurysms of the right common iliac artery and internal iliac artery (arrowheads).

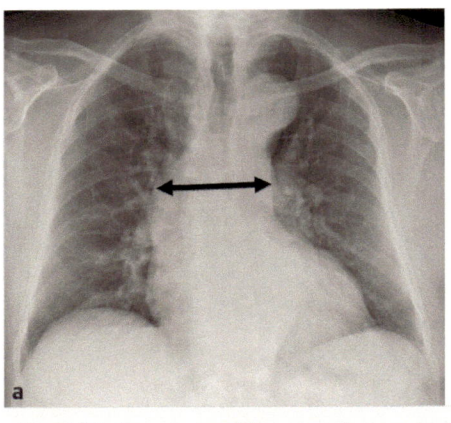

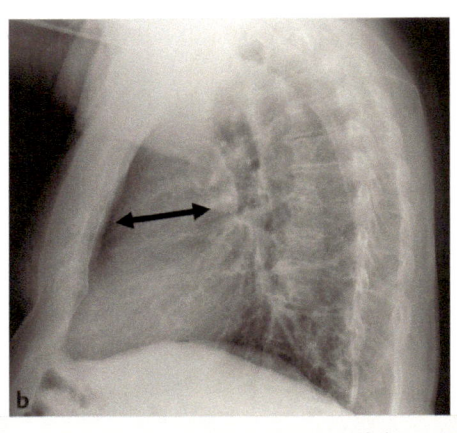

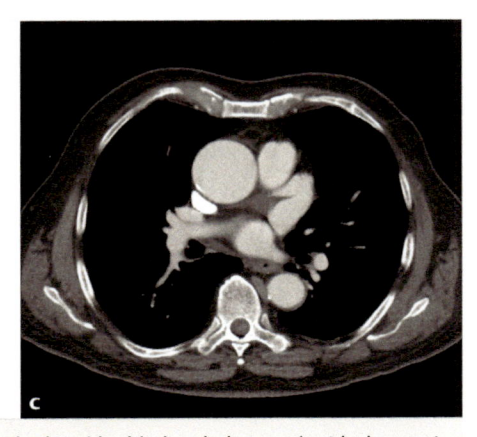

Fig. 3.16 Aneurysm of the ascending aorta. Chest radiographs **(a, b)** show widening of the aortic shadow (double-headed arrows) with the aortic contour normalizing toward the aortic arch. Axial CT scan at right angles to the vessel **(c)** permits an accurate measurement of the vascular diameter (e.g., for preoperative planning). **(a)** PA chest radiograph. **(b)** Lateral chest radiograph. **(c)** CT, axial.

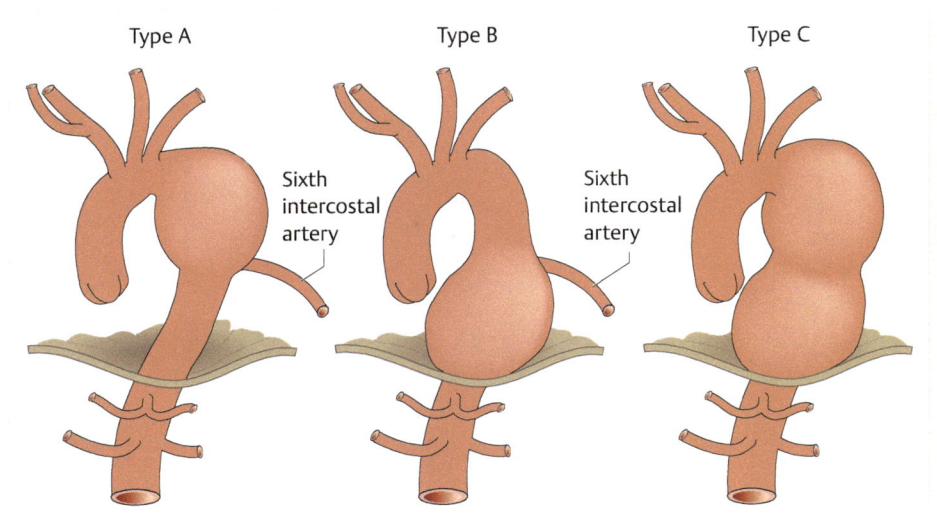

Fig. 3.17 Estrera classification of thoracic aortic aneurysms.[10] The Estrera classification identifies three types of aneurysm as involving the upper or lower aorta (proximal or distal to the sixth intercostal artery) or the entire thoracic aorta. Types A and B aneurysms have a much lower risk of spinal complications than type C in surgical and interventional procedures.[10]

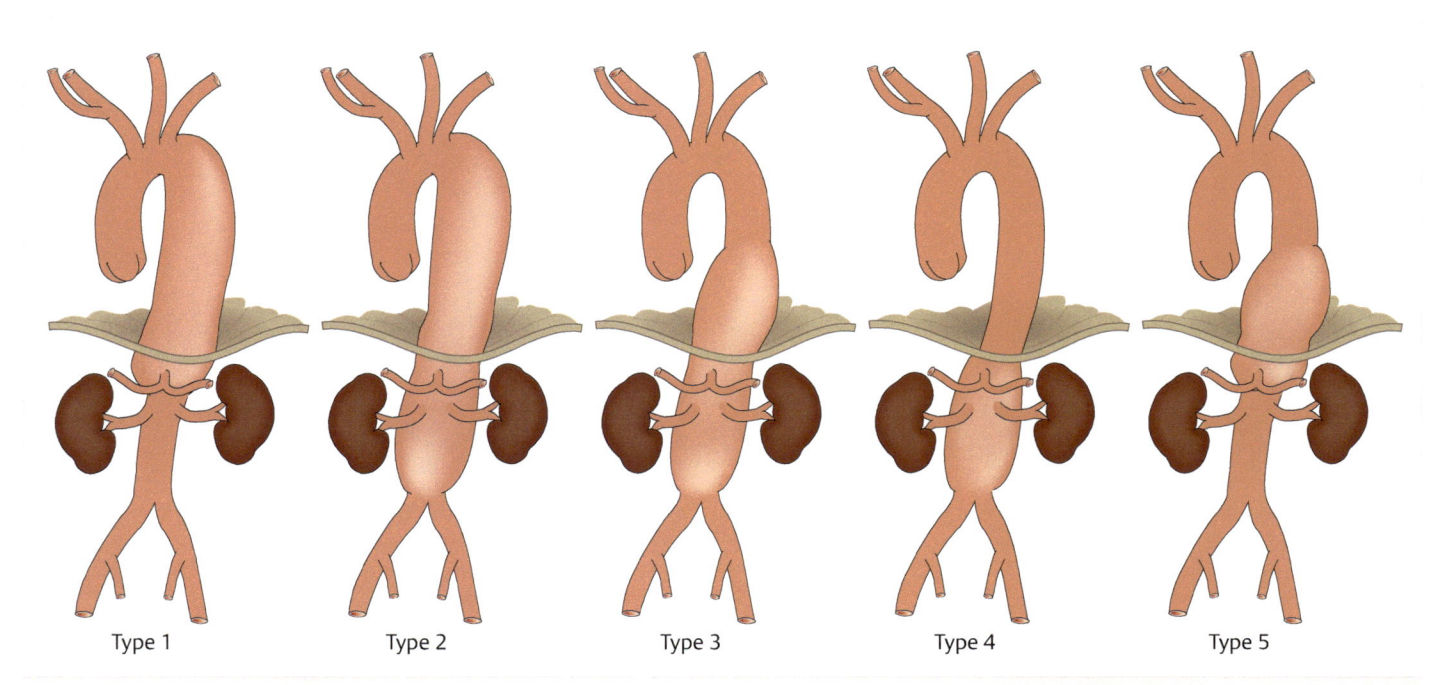

Fig. 3.18 Crawford classification of thoracoabdominal aortic aneurysms. Type 1 extends from the left subclavian artery to a level above the renal arteries and type 2 from the left subclavian artery to a level below the renal arteries. Type 3 extends from below the sixth intercostal artery to a level below the renal arteries, type 4 from below the 12th intercostal artery to a level below the renal arteries. Type 5 was added later to denote an aneurysm starting below the sixth intercostal artery and extending to a level above the renal arteries.

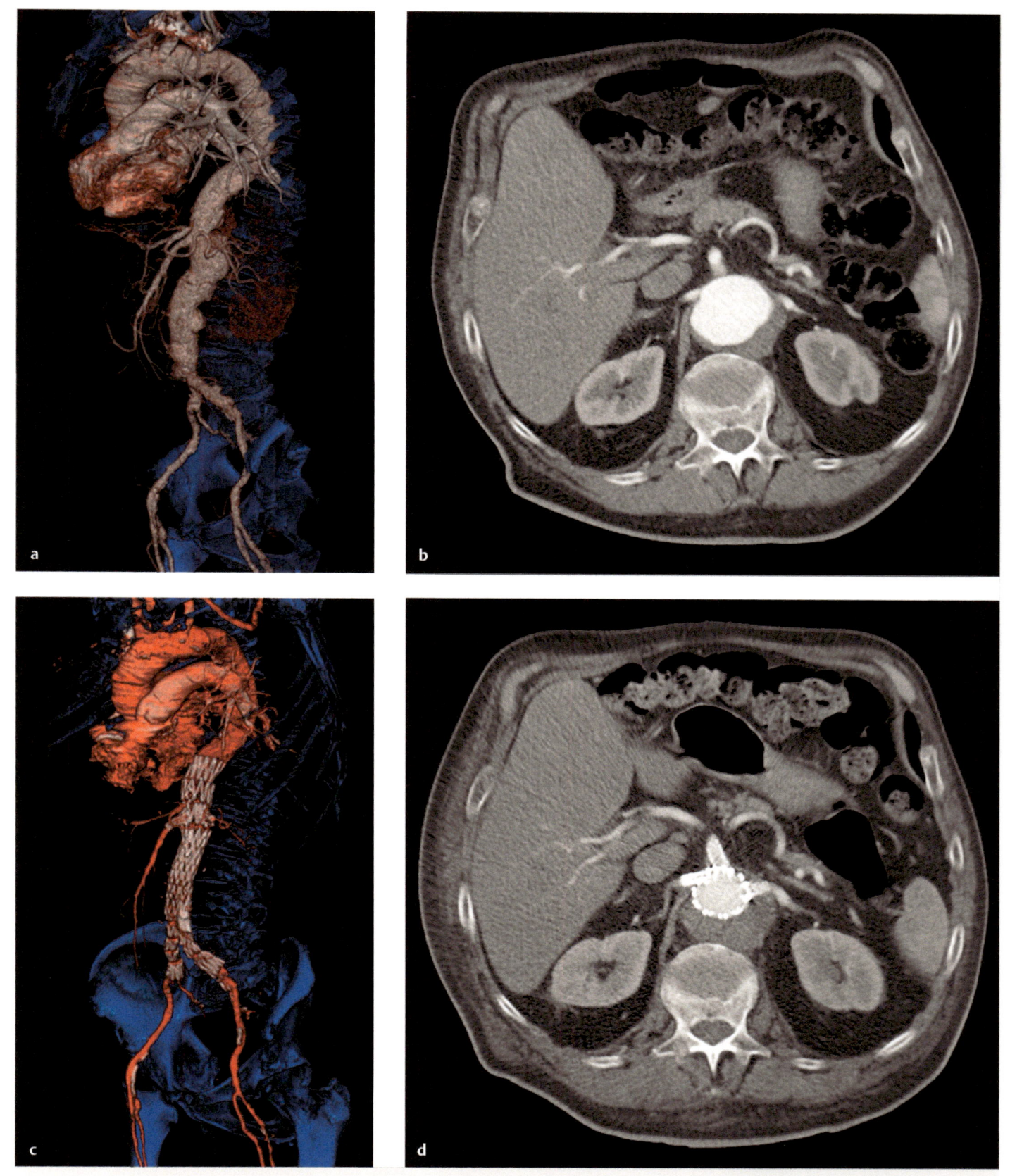

Fig. 3.19 Thoracoabdominal aortic aneurysm (Crawford type 4). (a) 3D reconstruction displays the infrarenal extent of the aneurysm. **(b)** Axial CT scans demonstrate involvement of the visceral vascular segment. **(c)** 3D reconstruction after interventional therapy with a quadruple fenestrated aortic stent. At this point the aneurysm is excluded from the circulation and the visceral vessels are well perfused. **(d)** Axial CT scan after interventional therapy. The aneurysm sac is completely thrombosed.

Table 3.4 Follow-up recommendations for spontaneous abdominal aortic aneurysms. Closer follow-up intervals and earlier initiation of vascular therapy should be considered in patients with rapidly progressive aneurysm growth (> 5 mm/year) or known underlying disease such as Marfan's syndrome

Maximum aneurysm size (cm)	Follow-up interval
< 3.0	None
3.0–4.0	Once a year
4.0–4.9	Every 6 months
5.0 or larger	Initiate treatment

Table 3.5 Relationship between thoracic aortic diameter and complication rates[14]

Risk (%/year)	Complication rate (%)		
	Diameter > 4 cm	Diameter > 5 cm	Diameter > 6 cm
Rupture	0.3	1.7	3.6
Dissection	1.5	2.5	3.7
Death	4.6	4.8	10.8
At least 1 complication	5.3	6.5	14.1

present with thoracic, abdominal, or back pain, depending on their location, or become symptomatic only when they rupture. In rare cases thrombotic material from the aneurysm wall may cause a peripheral embolism with associated symptoms. The complication rate correlates with aneurysm size (▶ Table 3.5). Moreover, thoracic aortic aneurysms in particular may cause compression-related symptoms such as hoarseness due to compression of the recurrent laryngeal nerve, stridor or dyspnea due to airway compression, and a superior or inferior vena cava syndrome.

▶ **Differential diagnosis.** Elongation of the aorta and aortic dissection are the most common differential diagnoses on radiographs. Motion artifacts in the ascending aorta can mimic aortic dissection on non-ECG-gated CT. Rarely, tumors or congenital anomalies such as a Kommerell diverticulum can mimic an aneurysm. Similarly, the left superior intercostal vein may simulate an outpouching of the aortic arch ("aortic nipple"; ▶ Fig. 3.20). This variant may be found in approximately 5% of the population. The differential diagnosis on sectional imaging includes a penetrating aortic ulcer and ductus diverticulum.

▶ **Key points.** A distinction is made between true and false aortic aneurysms. Diagnostic imaging should cover the entire aorta, at least initially, because aneurysms are often multifocal. Both CTA and MR angiography (MRA) are suitable as diagnostic modalities. An aneurysm is present if the midportion diameter of the ascending aorta is greater than 4 cm or the diameter of the descending or abdominal aorta is greater than 3 cm. Follow-up should employ standardized measurements and is important because the risk of aneurysm rupture rises sharply with increasing absolute diameter and rate of enlargement.

Subgroup: Mycotic Aneurysms

▶ **Brief definition.** Mycotic aneurysms are a subgroup of aortic aneurysm caused by bacterial infection of the vessel wall. The name, which erroneously implies a fungal infection, refers to the typical "mushroom" shape of mycotic aneurysms. Risk factors include atherosclerosis, arterial grafts and catheters, joint replacement, alcoholism, IV drug abuse, steroid therapy, chemotherapy, and diabetes mellitus. Mycotic aneurysms account for 0.5 to 3.0% of all aortic aneurysms. The aorta is most commonly affected, followed by the femoral artery and brachial artery. Mycotic aneurysms are rare in the intracerebral and mesenteric vessels, but essentially any vessel may be affected.

▶ **Imaging signs.** Mycotic aneurysms usually show a mixed pattern of fusiform and saccular aortic dilatation with regular wall thickening. Rarely, intramural or perianeurysmal gas inclusions may be detected. Surrounding fat imbibition and fluid inclusions may occur. An enhancing periaortic soft tissue component may be present. Sites of vertebral body erosion, abscesses (especially psoas abscess), or embolic organ infarction may occur, depending on the location of the aneurysm. Mycotic aneurysms are relatively dynamic and may undergo rapid changes in their shape and size.

▶ **Clinical features.** Nonspecific symptoms such as fever and local inflammatory signs may be suggestive in patients with peripheral mycotic aneurysms. Abdominal, back or flank pain may occur, depending on the site of occurrence. Paresthesias or neurologic symptoms have also been described. Approximately 7% of all mycotic aneurysms are asymptomatic. Mycotic aneurysms of peripheral arteries are associated with a palpable, pulsating mass. Untreated cases have a poor prognosis, with an approximately 50% rate of spontaneous rupture or uncontrolled septic complications. Even with treatment, mycotic aortic aneurysms have a reported mortality rate as high as 75%. Peripheral aneurysms have a single-digit mortality rate, with an amputation rate as high as 20%.

▶ **Differential diagnosis.** The differential diagnosis includes all other forms of spontaneous aortic aneurysm, penetrating aortic ulcer, and Kommerell diverticulum.

▶ **Key points.** Mycotic aneurysms result from bacterial inflammation and have a very poor prognosis without treatment. At imaging, the presence of a lobulated or mixed fusiform-saccular aneurysm with associated periaortic fluid or soft tissue component should suggest the correct diagnosis.

Acute Aortic Syndrome

▶ **Brief definition.** "Acute aortic syndrome" is a collective term for a group of etiologically diverse diseases of the thoracic aorta, aortic dissection, intramural hematoma, and penetrating aortic ulcer. The incidence is approximately 3:100,000 population per year.

▶ **Imaging signs.** The basic imaging tool is the plain chest radiograph. Possible findings are mediastinal widening, opacity of the aortopulmonary window, widening of the mediastinal silhouette, and displaced intimal calcifications, especially

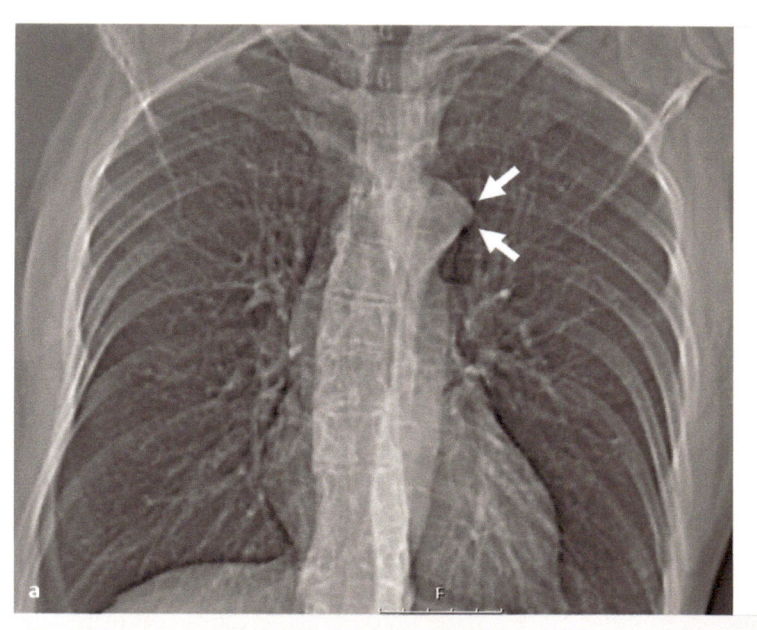

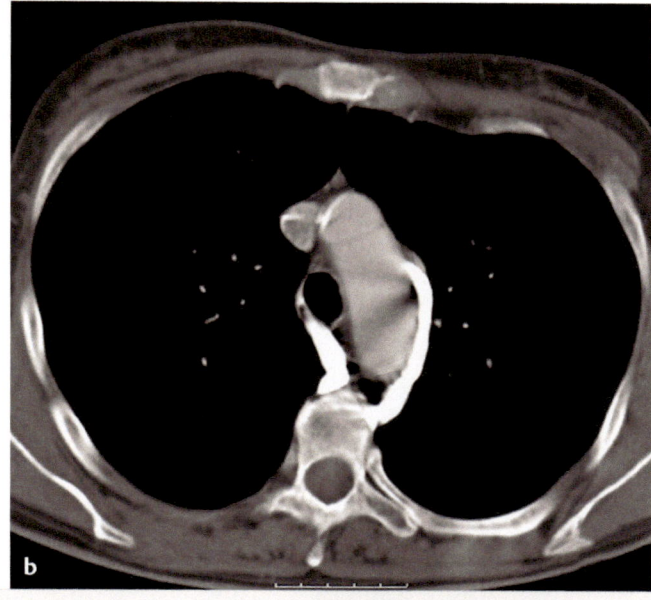

Fig. 3.20 Aortic nipple. (a) The aortic nipple (arrows), visible on the PA chest radiograph, should be included in the differential diagnosis of thoracic aortic aneurysms and penetrating aortic ulcer. **(b)** CT identifies the feature as a projection effect caused by the left superior intercostal vein.

with an aortic dissection. More than 20% of patients have a normal chest film, however, and symptomatic cases will require further investigation. With the high spatial resolution of modern CT scanners and the capability for ECG gating, even the coronary arteries can be evaluated along with other structures, eliminating the need for invasive tests such as coronary angiography. MRA also provides a high level of accuracy in the diagnosis of acute aortic syndrome.

▶ **Clinical features.** The cardinal symptom of acute aortic syndrome is acute chest pain, which is usually projected posteriorly between the scapulae. It is typically perceived as a severe tearing or shearing pain that is maximal within seconds or minutes. Two or more peaks are known to occur, especially in patients with an aortic dissection. In this case the location of the pain will shift with the advancement of the dissection flap in the aorta and its side branches. A pulsating pain has also been described in patients with a penetrating aortic ulcer, for example. Atypical pain or a complete absence of pain have also been reported in acute aortic syndrome. Physical examination may reveal pulse and blood pressure discrepancies between the upper and lower limbs, depending on the cause. Acute aortic syndrome may also be manifested by its complications. Diagnosis may be delayed in cases that present as an acute myocardial infarction due to dissection-related displacement of the coronary arteries, for example; or as acute left heart failure due to aortic insufficiency; or as syncope due to carotid involvement, dissection, or pericardial tamponade; or even as acute abdomen due to mesenteric ischemia.

▶ **Differential diagnosis.** In the differential diagnosis of acute chest pain, acute aortic syndrome is the most common acutely life-threatening condition after acute coronary syndrome. Differentiation is particularly required from myocardial infarction and pulmonary embolism. The complete differential diagnosis of acute aortic syndrome should include all conditions that present with acute chest pain (or occasionally with lumbar pain). Spontaneous aortic rupture is also an important differential diagnosis.

▶ **Key points.** In the differential diagnosis of acute chest pain, acute aortic syndrome is the most common acutely life-threatening condition after acute coronary syndrome, ranking ahead of pulmonary embolism. Because the plain chest radiograph is normal in more than 20% of cases, swift and definitive imaging, preferentially by ECG-gated CT, provides the basis for effective patient management.

Aortic Dissection

▶ **Brief definition.** Aortic dissection occurs when a tear in the intima allows blood between the wall layers, causing a longitudinal separation of the intima from the media. This creates a new, false vascular lumen. The separation of the wall layers may spread in an antegrade or retrograde direction. This may lead to involvement of the aortic branch vessels, although vessels that are perfused entirely from the true lumen are rarely affected. The pressure in the false lumen may equal or exceed the pressure in the true lumen. In principle, the false lumen may remain patent, it may thrombose, it may recommunicate with the true lumen, or it may rupture into adjacent spaces such as the pericardial, pleural, or peritoneal cavity. Classification is based on the location of the reentry point or the primary intimal tear. The most widely used system is the Stanford classification, which distinguishes between type A and type B dissections (▶ Fig. 3.21). In a Stanford type A dissection, the primary intimal lesion is located in the ascending aorta (60–70% of cases); in a type B dissection, it is located distal to the origin of the left subclavian artery (30–40% of cases). In type B dissections the aortic arch and ascending

Large Vessels

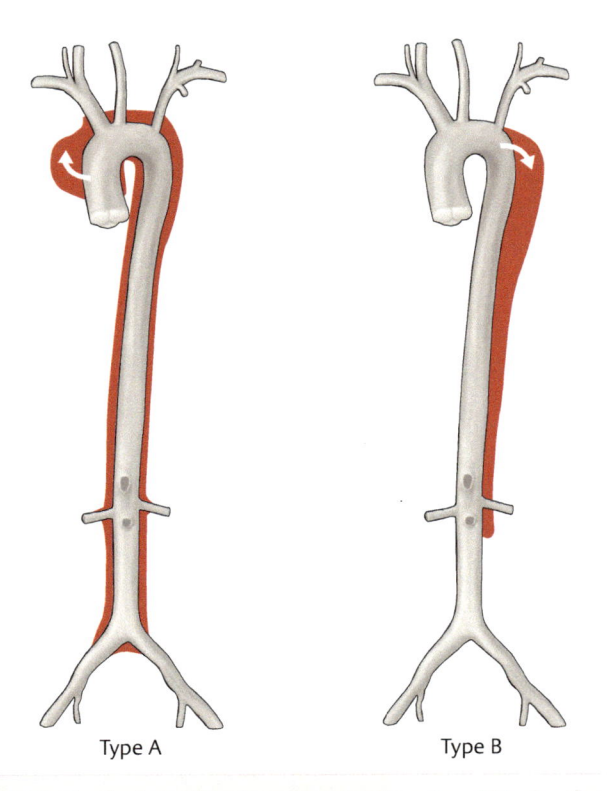

Fig. 3.21 Stanford classification of aortic dissection. This classification is based on the location of the primary intimal lesion. With a type A dissection it is located in the ascending aorta; with a type B dissection it is distal to the left subclavian artery. (Reproduced from Schünke M et al. Prometheus. Lernatlas der Anatomie: Innere Organe. Illustrated by M. Voll and K. Wesker. 2nd ed. Stuttgart: Thieme; 2009.)

Caution

When using CTA or MRA, especially with a type A dissection, note that motion artifacts at the aortic root and in the proximal ascending aorta can mimic a dissection. It is therefore best to use ECG gating. This technique is also very helpful for detecting possible involvement of the coronary arteries.

Sectional imaging typically shows a membranelike flap separating the true lumen from the false lumen (▶ Fig. 3.22). The thickness of the intimal flap increases over time, but the flap in an acute dissection may be relatively thin. The true lumen can usually be traced owing to its continuity with the undissected portion of the aorta. An intraluminal thrombus may identify the false lumen. Because of pressure differences, the true lumen is smaller than the false lumen in approximately 90% of cases. Delayed imaging at 90 seconds may show delayed enhancement of the false lumen. Additionally, even unenhanced CT will consistently show calcifications that are displaced inward from the vessel wall. Unlike intramural hematoma, these calcifications may be arranged in a straight line if they lie on the intimal axis. Sectional imaging may also identify an entry point into the false lumen and perhaps a reentry point into the true lumen, as well as the involvement of aortic branch vessels. The sensitivity and specificity of CT and MRI in the diagnosis of an aortic dissection are reported as approximately 95% and 100%, respectively.

Note

Besides confirming the diagnosis and providing a classification, imaging should also document the precise extent of the aortic dissection. It is also important to document the involvement and perfusion of the side branches (see ▶ Fig. 3.22), as this will have therapeutic implications.

In treatment planning, it is important to distinguish a dynamic obstruction due to collapse of the true aortic lumen or obstruction by an intimal flap from a static obstruction in which the intimal flap enters a branch-vessel origin without a reentry point. Dynamic obstruction is treated by interventional aortic fenestration, while static obstruction is treated by placement of an intravascular stent.

▶ **Clinical features.** The clinical presentation of an acute aortic dissection is the same as in acute aortic syndrome. Syncope occurs in 5 to 10% of patients with an aortic dissection. This is more common in patients with a type A dissection than patients with a type B. Syncope points to complications of the dissection such as pericardial tamponade or the involvement of supra-aortic arteries. Spinal cord ischemia may also occur (2–10% of cases), especially in type B dissections, due to the interruption of essential intercostal arteries. Other possible manifestations are pulse deficits and nerve lesions. The spontaneous course of a symptomatic type A dissection is associated with a mortality rate of 1 to 2%, which is increased by complications such as pericardial tamponade or involvement of supra-aortic branch vessels. An acute, symptomatic type B dissection has a 2-week mortality rate of approximately 10%. Advanced age, aortic rupture, shock, and decreased blood flow to dependent areas are independent

aorta are not involved in the aneurysm. The reported incidence is approximately 3 per 100,000 per year in Germany and the Western World. Type A dissections have a peak age of incidence in the fifth and sixth decades, while type B dissections are most common in the seventh decade. Risk factors for the development of an aortic dissection are arterial hypertension, cystic medial necrosis, vessel wall diseases such as Marfan's syndrome, and preexisting aortic aneurysms. Iatrogenic dissections after catheter-based procedures or aortic surgery have also been described. An acute, usually symptomatic dissection is distinguished from a chronic dissection (lasting longer than 8 weeks), which is usually asymptomatic.

▶ **Imaging signs.** The chest radiograph often shows mediastinal widening with a widened aortic silhouette. The PA radiograph in aortic dissection may occasionally show a separation of aortic-wall calcifications from the outer aortic silhouette by more than 1 cm in the aortic arch. Pleural effusion is a consistent radiographic finding. The chest film may also show no abnormalities at all. Transthoracic and transesophageal echocardiography can visualize the dissection, although the sensitivity of transthoracic echocardiography is no better than 83% in various studies. Moreover, neither of these echocardiographic techniques can define total extent or detect involvement of the major branch vessels. Thus, CTA and MRA are the modalities of choice for a presumed aortic dissection and have replaced invasive angiography as the gold standard.

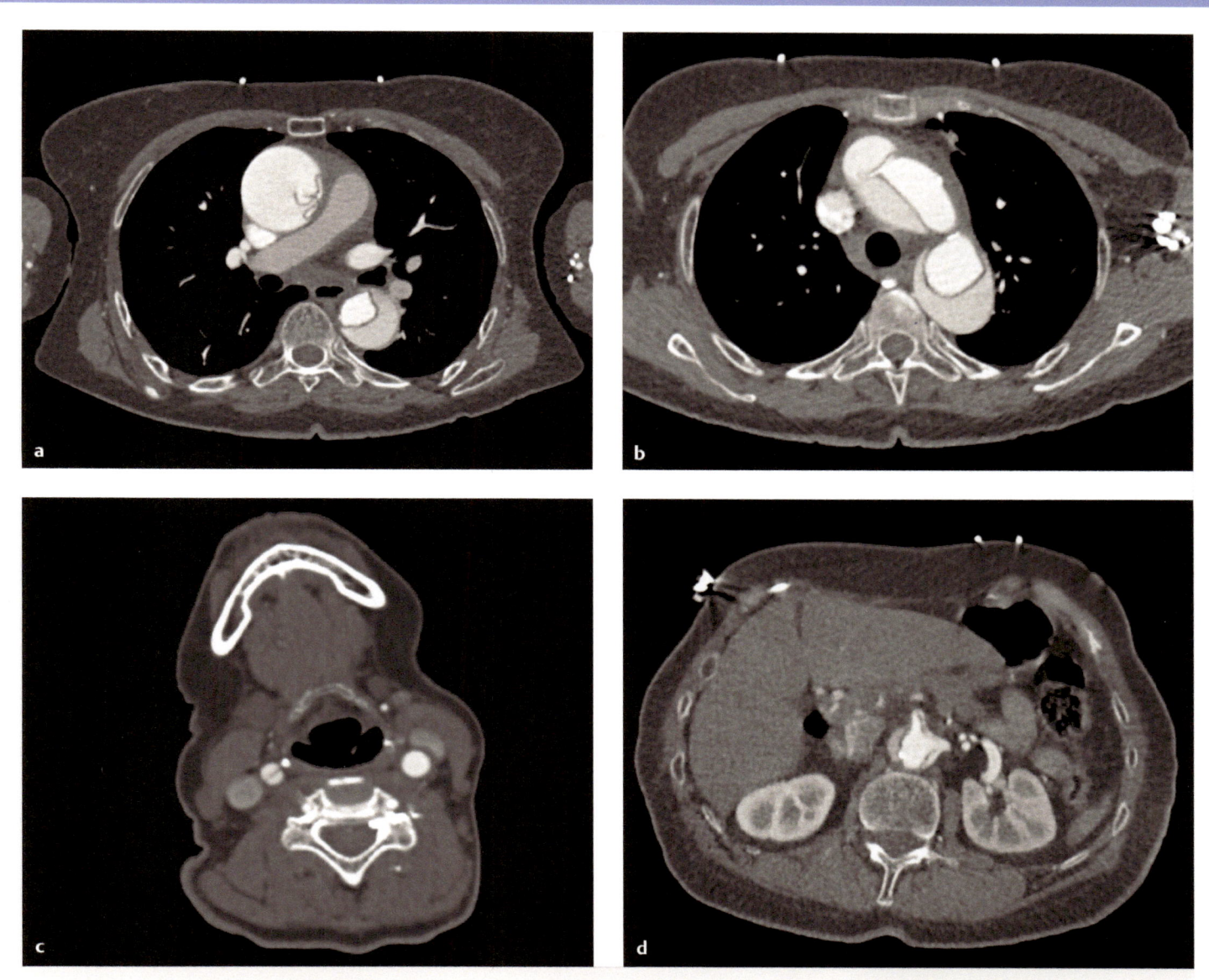

Fig. 3.22 Stanford type A aortic dissection. CTA can diagnose an aortic dissection and also define its extent. (a) The intimal flap starts in the ascending aorta and separates the true lumen from the false lumen. (b) The false lumen is somewhat less opacified than the true lumen, particularly in the descending thoracic aorta. (c) The dissection extends into the right common carotid artery. (d) Involvement of the visceral arteries is also clearly displayed.

predictors of increased early mortality. If the patient survives the acute phase, the dissection may resolve spontaneously with some residual wall thickening, or the false lumen may undergo complete thrombosis. However, the majority of dissections show persistent (partial) perfusion of the false lumen with or without aneurysmal dilatation of the false lumen. Over time, up to 20% of dissections may undergo progressive dilation and rupture even in the chronic stage. Type A dissections are treated by open surgery, while acute type B dissections can be treated interventionally. A chronic dissection is generally treated surgically or with a stent graft if it shows aneurysmal progression (1 cm growth/year) or if the aneurysm diameter is greater than 5.5 cm.

▶ **Differential diagnosis.** Differentiation is mainly required from intramural hematoma and penetrating aortic ulcer. Additionally, motion artifacts in the aortic root and ascending aorta or a high pericardial reflection site can mimic a type A dissection (pseudodissection). A mural thrombus in a fusiform aortic aneurysm may also be misinterpreted as an aortic dissection with a thrombosed lumen.

▶ **Key points.** Symptomatic aortic dissection is a condition with a high mortality. According to the entry point of blood into the false lumen, aortic dissections are classified as type A (involvement of the ascending aorta or aortic arch) or type B (distal to the left subclavian artery). Imaging tasks are confirmation of diagnosis, classification with identification of the entry point and possible reentry point, determination of extent, and detection of complications.

Intramural Hematoma

▶ **Brief definition.** Aortic intramural hematoma, also known by the erroneous term "atypical dissection," results from a spontaneous rupture of the vasa vasorum of the aortic media with subsequent bleeding into the vessel wall (▶ Fig. 3.23). Unlike an aortic dissection, which is considered a precursor of this condition, an intramural hematoma forms without disrupting the intima. An intramural hematoma may extend over the complete length of the aorta. The Stanford classification distinguishes type A,

Large Vessels

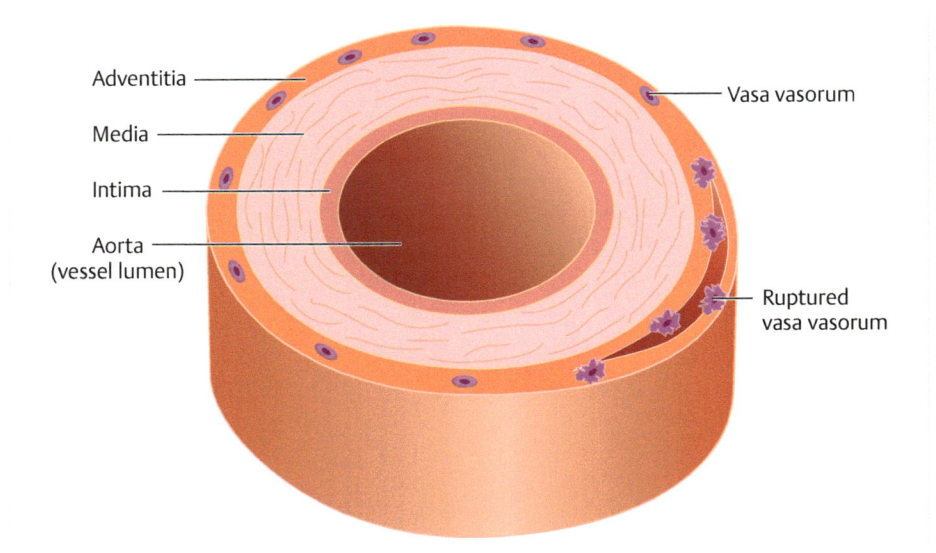

Fig. 3.23 Intramural hematoma. Schematic representation. An intramural hematoma results from a spontaneous rupture of the vasa vasorum. This leads to intramural bleeding that weakens the aortic wall and increases the vascular diameter. In contrast to a dissection, the intima remains largely intact.

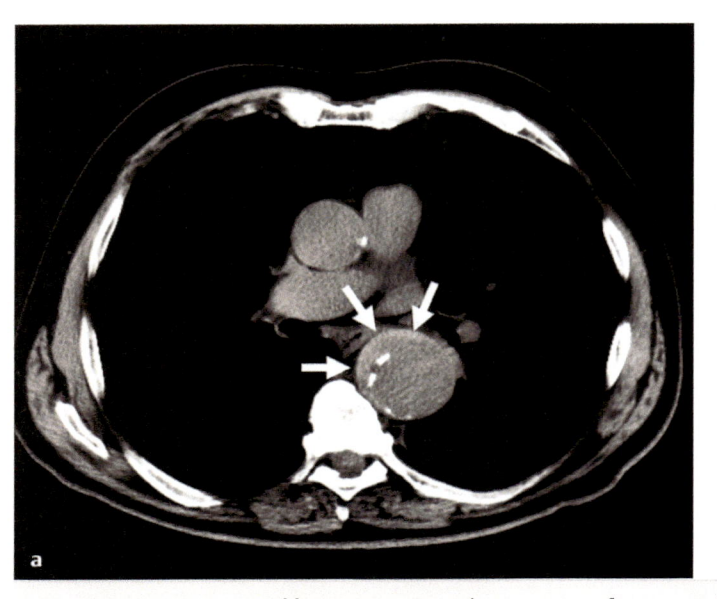

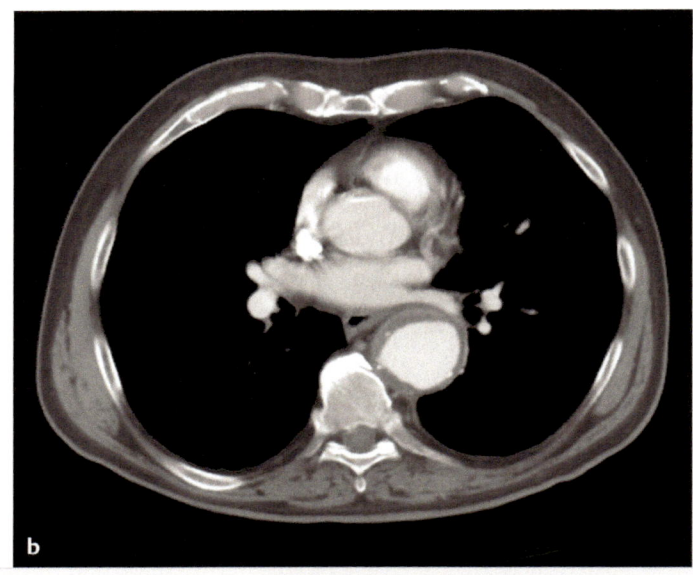

Fig. 3.24 Acute intramural hematoma. Typical appearance of eccentric thickening of the aortic wall with separation of the calcified plaques from the outer aortic contour. A hyperdense crescent-shaped component ([a], arrows) is a characteristic finding on unenhanced scans in the acute phase. It represents the fresh intramural hematoma. **(a)** Unenhanced CTA. **(b)** Contrast-enhanced CTA. (Reproduced with kind permission of R. Fischbach, Hamburg, Germany.)

which involves the ascending aorta, from type B, which does not; 60% of intramural hematomas are assigned to type A.[15] Starting from an intramural vascular rupture, the process may spread and progress to an aneurysm by weakening the aortic wall or to a dissection by tearing the intima. The thickness of the intramural hematoma appears to be a predictor of the likelihood of progression to a dissection: hematomas thicker than 11 mm are more likely to form a dissection. The hematoma may also resolve spontaneously over a period of months, especially if it involves only the descending aorta.

▶ **Imaging signs.** The chest film findings of intramural hematoma, like those of aortic dissection, are nonspecific and unrewarding. Unenhanced CT in the acute phase shows eccentric thickening of the aortic wall with a crescent-shaped, acutely hyperdense area corresponding to the intramural hematoma (▶ Fig. 3.24). The hematoma shows fading density over time, and by one week it may already be isodense or even slightly hypodense to the aortic lumen. Wall calcifications may be displaced inward but retain their circumferential structure. On CTA, an intramural hematoma is distinguished from a dissection or penetrating aortic ulcer by the absence of a visible intimal tear, dissection flap, or outpouching of the aortic wall. Intramural hematoma is also clearly visualized by MRI, which displays the typical morphological changes described above. The age of an intramural hematoma can estimated from the signal intensity of the intramural hemorrhage:

- The blood in a fresh intramural hematoma appears hyperintense in T2 W GRE sequences and isointense in T1 W sequences.
- The signal intensity changes if the hematoma is more than 7 days old: T2 W images show intermediate signal intensity while the blood appears hyperintense in T1 W images due to the presence of methemoglobin.

Absence of change in signal characteristics may indicate active bleeding.

Note

Besides a change in density or signal intensity, intramural hematoma may exhibit a number of other changes over time: the hematoma may become thinner, and it may dissolve completely over a period of several months. In complicated cases, the hematoma may progress to a frank dissection or an aortic aneurysm, each of which is associated with typical complications. Regular follow-up imaging is essential, therefore.

▶ **Clinical features.** The clinical presentation of an intramural hematoma resembles that of an acute aortic dissection. Chest pain is more common with an intramural hematoma of the ascending aorta, whereas back pain is more suggestive of an intramural hematoma of the descending aorta. An important clinical distinction is that malperfusion syndromes are less common with aortic intramural hematoma than with aortic dissection. Syncope, anterior spinal artery syndrome, hoarseness, and diminished pulses are also uncommon. Pericardial or pleural effusion may occur but is not typical. The diagnosis of intramural hematoma cannot be excluded from clinical findings alone, however, and 5 to 20% of all patients with a clinically suspected dissection are found to have an intramural hematoma. Consequently, sectional imaging of the entire aorta should be performed in all suspected cases. The clinical course is highly variable and difficult to predict. Treatment is controversial; type A intramural hematomas are usually treated surgically, while type B hematomas are managed conservatively whenever possible.

▶ **Differential diagnosis.** The first differential diagnosis to be considered is aortic dissection. Also, the layering phenomenon in an intramural thrombus in an aortic aneurysm is easily mistaken for chronic intramural hematoma, which may also be associated with aortic dilatation. In most cases, however, chronic hematoma can be diagnosed from the history and clinical presentation. Aortitis is also associated with wall thickening but, unlike an intramural hematoma, does not enhance after IV contrast medium administration.

▶ **Key points.** Intramural hematoma results from a spontaneous rupture of the vasa vasorum in the aortic wall with subsequent intramural hemorrhage. In contrast to a classic dissection, the intima remains intact. The two entities cannot be distinguished from each other clinically and require sectional imaging, usually by CT imaging of the entire aorta. CT typically shows crescent-shaped wall thickening, which is hyperdense to the aortic lumen in the acute phase and becomes isodense over time. Given the potential for complications in the form of dissection or aneurysm formation, regular imaging follow-up is essential.

Penetrating Aortic Ulcer

▶ **Brief definition.** A penetrating aortic ulcer is defined as an ulceration that has penetrated through the internal elastic lamina into the media of the aorta. It is associated with a variable amount of hematoma in the aortic wall.[15] A penetrating aortic ulcer typically results from the ulceration of atherosclerotic plaque in patients with severe aortic sclerosis. In the early phase the lesion is confined to the intima and is usually painless. A penetrating aortic ulcer may lead to erosion of the vasa vasorum by the ulcer, forming a painful intramural hematoma. This condition has a poorer prognosis than a simple penetrating aortic ulcer. The descending thoracic aorta and abdominal aorta are predominantly affected. Patients with a penetrating aortic ulcer are typically over 70 years of age.

▶ **Imaging signs.** Penetrating aortic ulcers appear on sectional imaging and invasive angiography as a circumscribed, crater-like outpouching in the aortic wall. They may be accompanied by local intramural hematoma but, unlike a typical intramural hematoma, a penetrating aortic ulcer appears as a localized lesion that is generally confined to the descending or abdominal aorta. Variable thrombus deposition may be found on the wall of a penetrating aortic ulcer. As a general rule, penetrating aortic ulcers are associated with severe atherosclerosis (▶ Fig. 3.25).

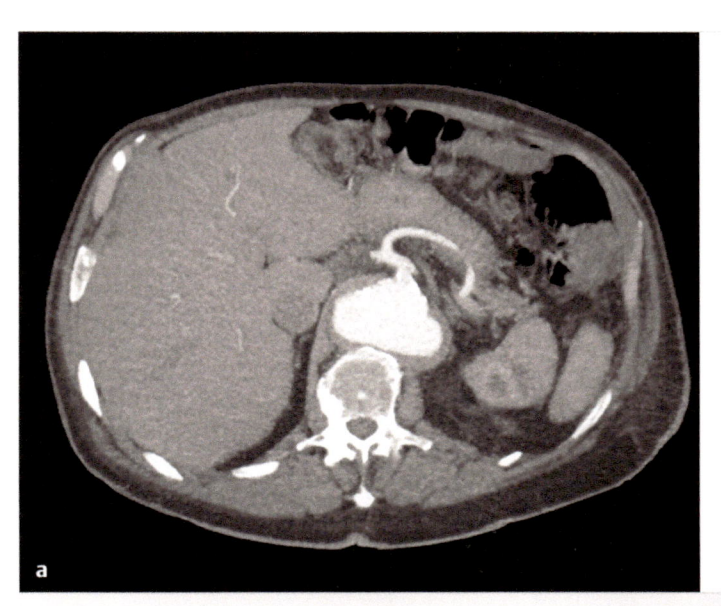

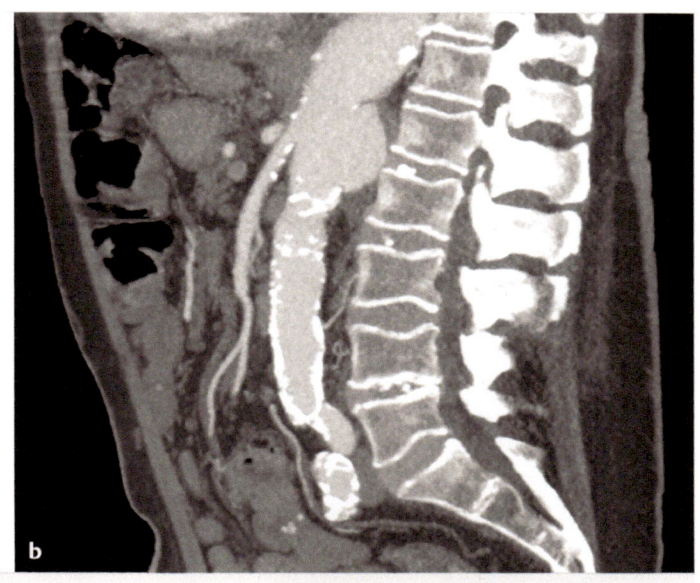

Fig. 3.25 Penetrating aortic ulcer in a 75-year-old man presenting clinically with back pain. (a) CTA. A large ulceration, disrupted posteriorly, with a small amount of mural thrombus is demonstrated in the visceral segment of the abdominal aorta. (b) Sagittal reformatted image shows the mushroomlike appearance of the penetrating aortic ulcer and the underlying atherosclerosis.

▶ **Clinical features.** The clinical presentation is variable. A penetrating aortic ulcer may be an incidental finding but is usually noted during the investigation of an acute aortic syndrome. The finding is usually associated with thoracic back pain or lumbar pain, depending on its location. Symptomatic penetrating aortic ulcers, like penetrating aortic ulcers that lead to intramural hematoma, have a poorer prognosis than uncomplicated or asymptomatic lesions. Penetrating aortic ulcers have a reported short-term rupture rate (within 12 months) of up to 40%.[16] Penetrating aortic ulcer is generally treated by the interventional placement of a stent graft. Hybrid procedures that combine debranching and stenting may also be necessary, depending on the site of occurrence.

▶ **Differential diagnosis.** Penetrating aortic ulcer mainly requires differentiation from intramural hematoma, aortic dissection, and pseudoaneurysm. While classic dissection and intramural hematoma are most prevalent in the fifth and sixth decades of life, most patients with a penetrating aortic ulcer are considerably older. The site of occurrence is also different. Unlike a dissection or intramural hematoma, penetrating aortic ulcers almost never involve the ascending aorta or proximal aortic arch. "Aortic nipple" is a less common entity included in the differential diagnosis of penetrating aortic ulcer (see ▶ Fig. 3.20).

▶ **Key points.** Penetrating aortic ulcer results from the ulceration of atherosclerotic plaque. It may be a precursor to intramural hematoma or aortic dissection. These conditions are clinically indistinguishable from one another, and clinical suspicion requires prompt sectional imaging of the entire aorta. Treatment is interventional or a combination of surgery and interventional therapy.

Aortic Rupture

▶ **Brief definition.** Aortic rupture is characterized by a complete discontinuity in the aortic wall with the disruption of all three wall layers. This distinguishes an aortic rupture from aortic dissection or a pseudoaneurysm, in which typically the intima is injured while the outer wall layers remain intact. A traumatic aortic rupture, also called a "transection" and usually caused by high-velocity trauma, is distinguished from the spontaneous rupture of a preexisting aortic aneurysm. The distribution of spontaneous ruptures follows the frequency distribution of aortic aneurysms. A traumatic aortic rupture typically occurs in the aortic isthmus but may also occur occasionally in the ascending aorta and at the level of the aortic hiatus in the diaphragm. Additionally, a faulty suture line after surgery may give rise to a pseudoaneurysm with a potential for subsequent rupture.

▶ **Imaging signs.** The chest radiograph may show typical signs such as mediastinal widening, displacement of the trachea and esophagus, or blurring of the aortic border (▶ Fig. 3.26). Often these findings do not differ from the features of an uncomplicated aortic aneurysm. A classic aortic rupture is often accompanied by pleural effusion, usually on the left side. In addition, the cardiac silhouette may be enlarged to a globular shape due to pericardial effusion. These signs are nonspecific, however, and sectional imaging should be initiated as soon as possible for further investigation. CTA, which may include delayed scans, is the imaging technique most commonly used for this indication. Both types of aortic rupture may be associated with a large periaortic hematoma, with or without extravasation of contrast medium (▶ Fig. 3.27). Delayed scans may be helpful in this case for detecting contrast medium extravasation. The distribution of the hematoma varies with the site of the rupture:

- Hemopericardium may be found with an aneurysm of the ascending thoracic aorta.
- Rupture of the descending thoracic aorta typically causes a hemothorax, usually on the left side.
- Rupture of the abdominal aorta leads to a retroperitoneal hematoma but may also have intraperitoneal components depending on the size and location of the underlying aneurysm.

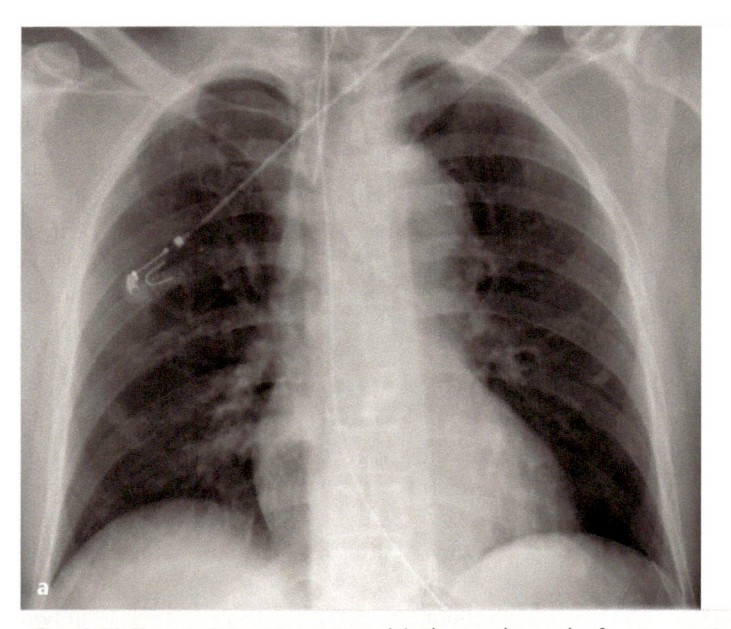

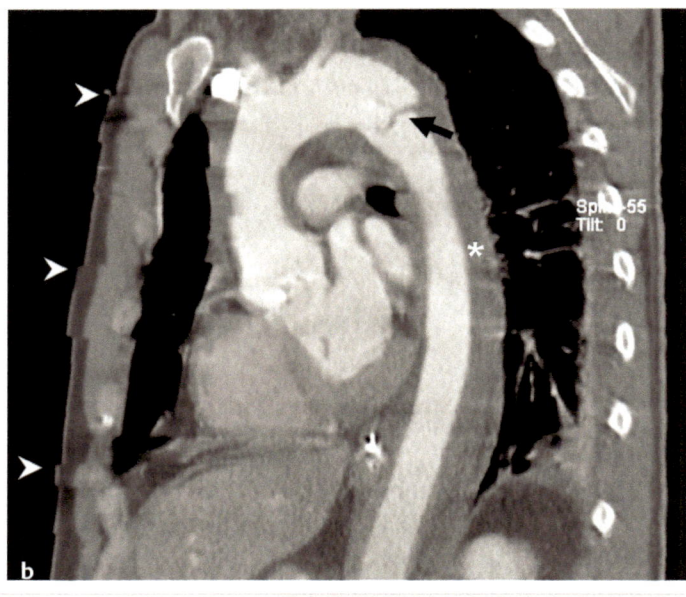

Fig. 3.26 Traumatic aortic rupture. (a) Chest radiograph after traumatic aortic rupture due to deceleration trauma in a motor vehicle accident shows indistinct widening of the mediastinum. (b) Sagittal reformatted CT image identifies the typical rupture site at the aortic isthmus (black arrow). A large mural hematoma (asterisk) is also seen. CTA is the study of choice in these critically ill patients because it almost always provides diagnostic image quality even with poor imaging conditions (here: significant respiratory artifacts [arrowheads]).

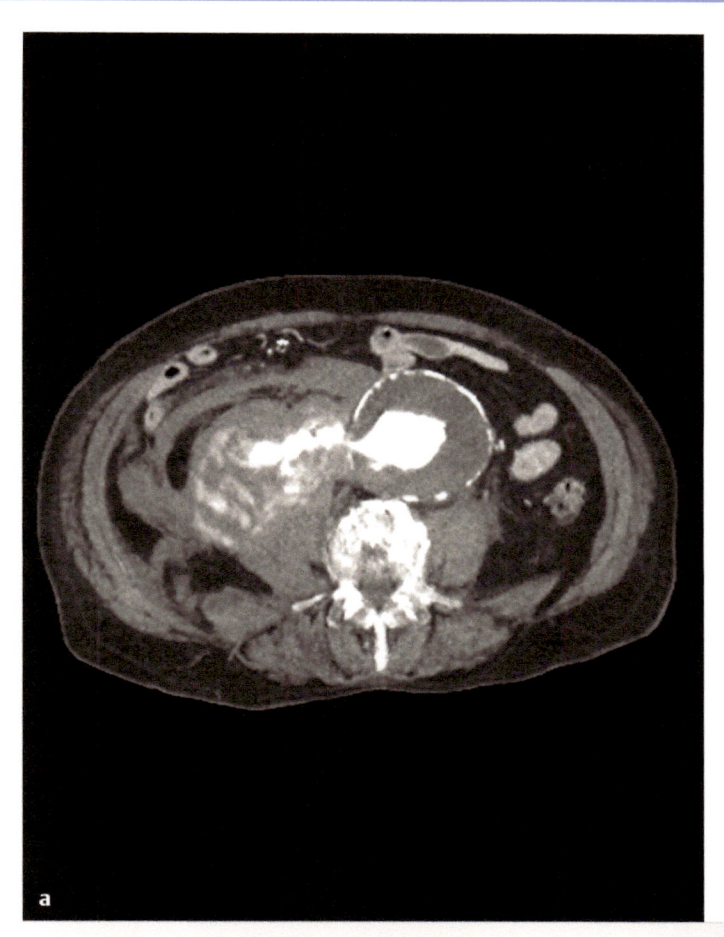

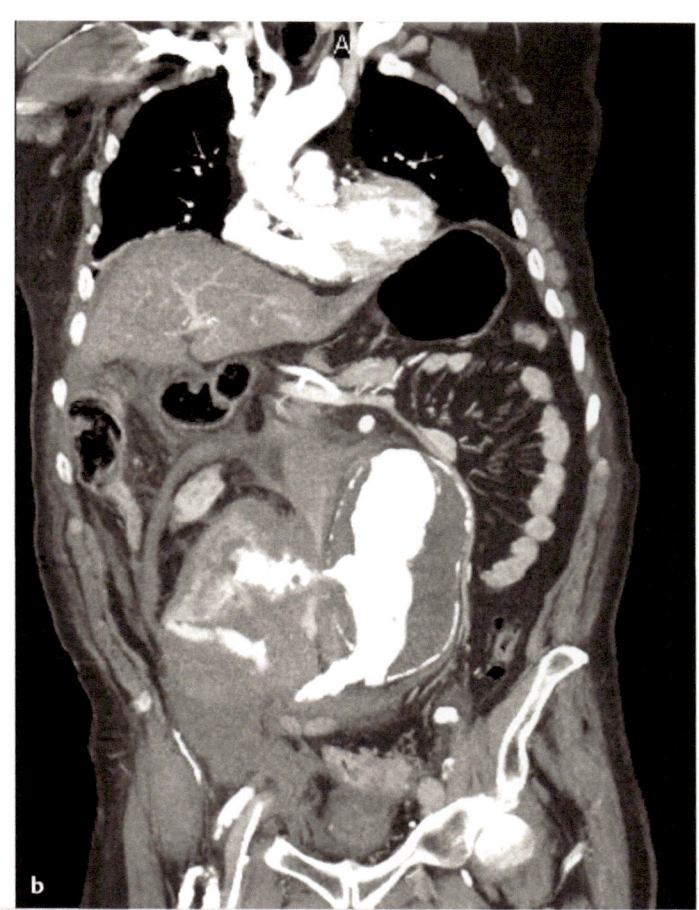

Fig. 3.27 Acute aortic rupture. (a) CTA reveals the exact site of extravasation of contrast from the abdominal aorta with an underlying aortic aneurysm. (b) Coronal reformatted image also displays the extent of the retroperitoneal hematoma.

There are also significant differences in the pattern of findings, depending on whether the aortic rupture is traumatic or spontaneous:
- *Spontaneous rupture*: Spontaneous rupture occurs in a preexisting aneurysm and is most common at the abdominal level, conforming to the frequency distribution of aortic aneurysms. Imminent rupture may be signaled by layering of the thrombus in the aneurysm with crescent-shaped hyperdense components. Often this is most clearly appreciated on unenhanced CT scans. The contained rupture of an abdominal aortic aneurysm may present the "draped aorta sign," in which the posterior wall of the aorta is undefined and follows the vertebral contour.
- *Traumatic aortic rupture*: Up to 90% of traumatic ruptures occur at the aortic isthmus. In patients who reach the hospital alive, imaging typically reveals a saccular type of contained aortic rupture and a hemomediastinum. The findings may be very subtle in some cases and should not be mistaken for a harmless ductus diverticulum.

▶ **Clinical features.** A spontaneous rupture, like acute aortic syndrome, presents with acute, severe pain in the chest or abdomen. This may be associated with signs and symptoms of cardiovascular shock, with a fall in blood pressure, tachycardia, centralization of blood flow with limb ischemia, and respiratory distress. With a contained rupture where bleeding is confined by an external structure such as the peritoneum, the clinical manifestations may progress for several days, leading to a "two-stage" aortic rupture. Surgical treatment is increasingly being superseded by the interventional placement of a stent graft.

▶ **Differential diagnosis.** While the clinical differential diagnosis of a spontaneous rupture is very difficult and conditions such as myocardial infarction, pulmonary embolism, or an acute peripheral vascular occlusion may produce similar complaints, a traumatic aortic rupture is often preceded and characterized by a massive deceleration trauma. The radiological differential diagnosis of a spontaneous aortic rupture is usually a simple matter; but especially in cases where a bleeding site is not directly visualized, other vascular regions should also be considered as potential rupture sites. The hematoma distribution is usually suggestive in cases of this kind. The diagnosis of a traumatic aortic rupture may be difficult because the site of predilection is identical to that of a ductus diverticulum, and confusion of the two entities should be avoided.

▶ **Key points.** A traumatic aortic rupture is distinguished from a spontaneous rupture. Traumatic rupture is a result of deceleration trauma, whereas spontaneous ruptures occur in a preexisting aneurysm. The clinical presentation is nonspecific, featuring pain and possible shock symptoms. An aortic rupture may progress from a contained rupture to an open rupture in two stages separated by an interval of hours or days. A prompt imaging evaluation, usually by CT, is necessary for confirming the diagnosis and planning treatment. A traumatic aortic rupture at the level of the isthmus should not be confused with a ductus diverticulum.

Leriche Syndrome

▶ **Brief definition.** Leriche syndrome, also called aortoiliac occlusive disease, refers to an occlusion of the aortic bifurcation and distal aorta. The extent of the occlusion is variable; it may range from the infrarenal level to the iliac bifurcation. Secondary involvement of the visceral vessels may occur, especially of the renal arteries. Leriche syndrome may be acute or chronic:
- *Acute Leriche syndrome* usually results from an embolic occlusion of the distal aorta or iliac bifurcation; it is a life-threatening emergency due to the absence of collateral pathways.
- *Chronic Leriche syndrome* generally results from an atherosclerotic vascular stenosis or occlusion. Rarely, arteritis or a dissection may be causative. Chronic Leriche syndrome is distinguished by its gradual progression, allowing time for collaterals to develop.

An awareness of potential and actual collateral pathways (▶ Fig. 3.28) is important in the evaluation of Leriche syndrome, as they will influence treatment options.[17]

▶ **Imaging signs.** The occlusion can be identified by ultrasound and often its extent can be defined. CTA and MRA are the standard techniques for the imaging of aortoiliac occlusive vascular disease (▶ Fig. 3.29). Therapeutic decisions are still guided by the Transatlantic Intersociety Consensus Document on Management of Peripheral Arterial Disease (TASC II)[18] (▶ Table 3.6, ▶ Fig. 3.30).

▶ **Clinical features.** The diagnosis of chronic Leriche syndrome is based on the triad of intermittent claudication of the buttocks and thighs, impotence, and diminished pulses due to aortoiliac occlusion.[19] Pallor and coldness of the lower extremities are also consistently present. Acute Leriche syndrome generally begins with ischemic pain and neurologic symptoms such as paresthesia, paralysis, or even circulatory shock.

▶ **Differential diagnosis.** The differential diagnosis centers on considerations of cause, particularly the identification of an embolic source or arteritis as a possible underlying disease. The differential diagnosis should also include coral reef aorta and mid-aortic syndrome.

▶ **Key points.** Leriche syndrome results from occlusion of the aortic bifurcation. The acute form usually results from an embolic occlusion and is a life-threatening emergency that requires immediate interventional or surgical treatment. Chronic Leriche syndrome is distinguished by the development of extensive collaterals. The goals of imaging are to define extent and, with acute Leriche syndrome, to identify the cause.

Coral Reef Aorta

▶ **Brief definition.** "Coral reef aorta" refers to aortic stenosis caused by massive, eccentric intravascular calcification with a polypoid surface resembling a coral reef.[20] The pararenal segment of the abdominal aorta is typically affected. There are also case reports of coral reef aorta occurring in the infrarenal aorta and, uncommonly, in the thoracic aorta. This form of aortic stenosis

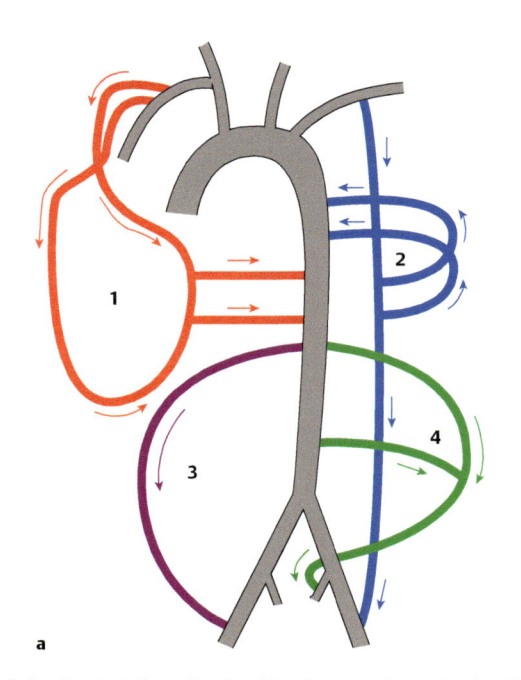

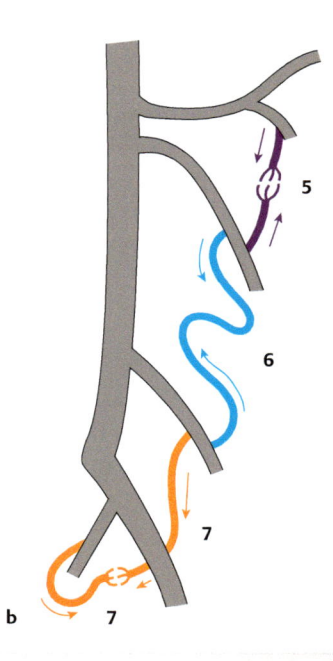

Fig. 3.28 Schematic diagram of the collateral pathways described by Sebastiá. (a) Thoracic and abdominal collateral pathways. (b) Visceral collateral pathways. 1, The thoracoacromial artery (arising from the axillary artery) and posterior scapular artery supply the thoracic aorta via the intercostal arteries. 2, The internal mammary arteries (arising from the subclavian arteries) connect with the descending thoracic aorta via the intercostal arteries and with the external iliac arteries via the superior and inferior abdominal epigastric arteries. 3, The intercostal arteries supply the external iliac arteries via the superficial and deep iliac circumflex arteries. 4, The lumbar arteries supply the internal iliac arteries via the inferior gluteal arteries. 5, The celiac trunk and superior mesenteric artery connect with each other via the gastroduodenal artery and the anterior and posterior pancreaticoduodenal arteries. 6, The superior and inferior mesenteric arteries can supply each other bidirectionally through the Riolan anastomosis. 7, The inferior mesenteric artery can supply blood to the middle and inferior rectal arteries, and thus to the internal iliac arteries, via the superior rectal artery.

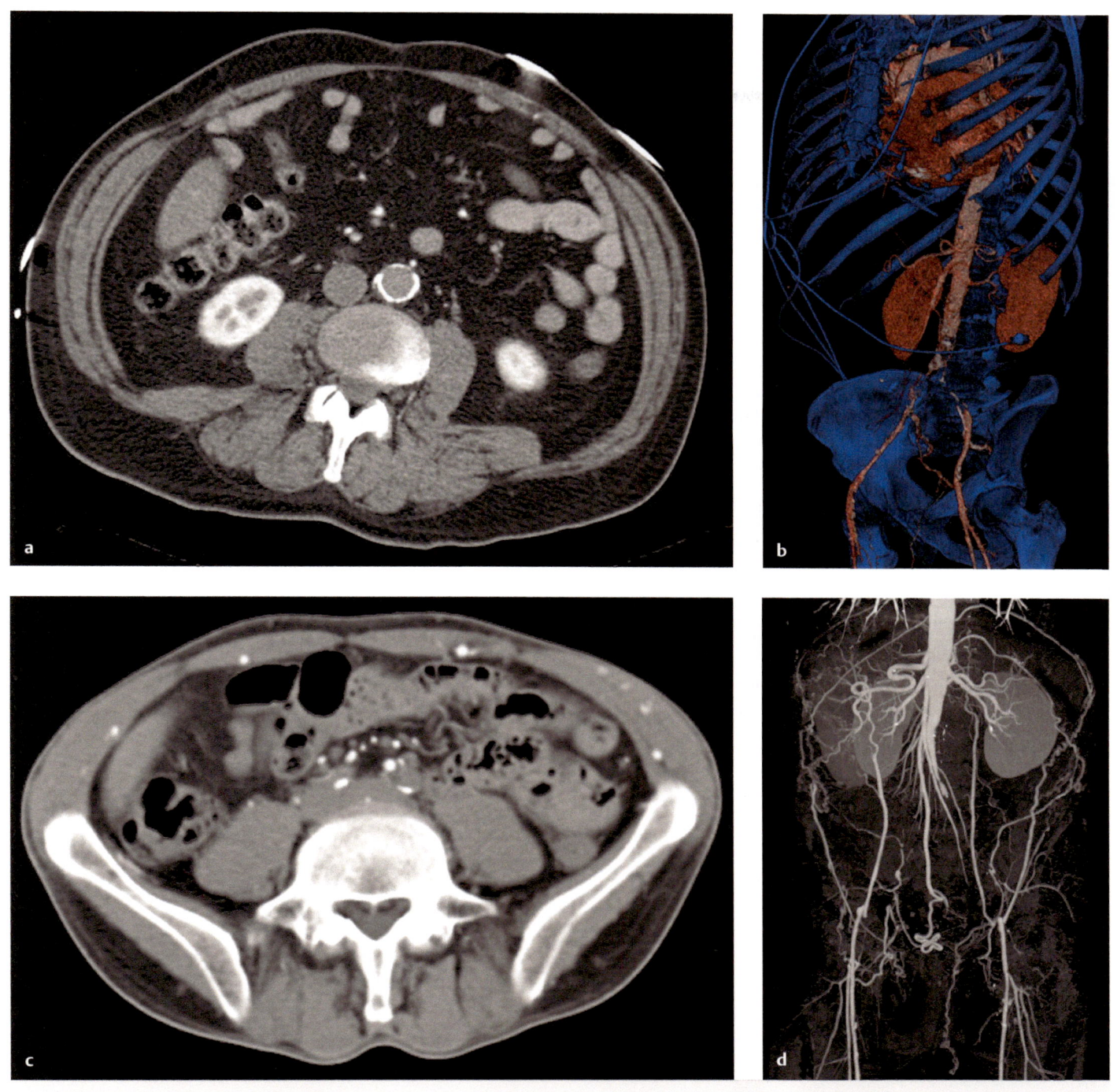

Fig. 3.29 Acute and chronic Leriche syndrome. In acute Leriche syndrome (**a, b**), CTA shows occlusion of the distal aorta and common iliac artery with no collateral flow. In chronic Leriche syndrome (**c, d**), in contrast, an effective collateral supply is developed via visceral and epigastric vessels. *Acute Leriche syndrome*: (**a**) Axial CT shows an absence of contrast medium in the aorta accompanied by good arterial inflow in the renal cortex. (**b**) 3D reconstruction demonstrates the absence of collaterals. *Chronic Leriche syndrome*: (**c**) The large epigastric vessels appear markedly thickened on axial CT. (**d**) 3D reconstruction in chronic Leriche syndrome.

generally affects patients approximately 20 years younger than typical atherosclerotic aortic stenosis.

▶ **Imaging signs.** Coral reef aorta is clearly depicted on the abdomen plain film as a dense, intraluminal aortic calcification. Doppler and duplex ultrasound can also demonstrate the flow acceleration and turbulence associated with the aortic stenosis. The tasks of imaging, especially CT, are to identify the attachment site of the calcification to the aortic wall prior to surgical or interventional therapy (▶ Fig. 3.31) and determine the clamping points for surgical treatment or provide essential vascular measurements for planning endovascular therapy.

▶ **Clinical features.** Coral reef aorta may present clinically with lower limb ischemia, depending on the site of occurrence. Pararenal stenosis often provokes arterial hypertension that is refractory to medical therapy. Abdominal pain may also occur due to involvement of the mesenteric arteries. Open endarterectomy is the most widely used surgical technique, but aortic bypass and interventional therapies are also employed.

Large Vessels

Table 3.6 TASC II classification of aortoiliac stenoses

Lesion type	Description
A	• Unilateral or bilateral stenoses of the common iliac artery • Unilateral or bilateral short-segment stenoses of the external iliac artery
B	• Short-segment stenosis of the infrarenal aorta • Unilateral occlusion of the common iliac artery • Single or multiple stenosis of the external iliac artery totaling 3–10 cm in length not extending into the common femoral artery • Unilateral occlusion of the external iliac artery not involving the origins of the internal iliac artery or common femoral artery
C	• Bilateral occlusion of the common iliac artery • Bilateral stenosis of the external iliac artery 3–10 cm long not extending into the common femoral artery • Unilateral stenosis of the external iliac artery extending into the common femoral artery • Unilateral occlusion of the external iliac artery that involves the origins of the internal iliac or common femoral artery • Heavily calcified unilateral occlusion of the external iliac artery with or without internal iliac and/or common femoral artery origin involvement
D	• Infrarenal aortoiliac occlusion • Diffuse disease involving the aorta and both iliac arteries requiring treatment • Diffuse multiple unilateral stenoses involving the common iliac artery, external iliac artery, and common femoral artery • Unilateral occlusion of the common iliac artery and external iliac artery • Bilateral occlusion of the external iliac artery • Iliac stenoses in patients requiring treatment for abdominal aortic aneurysm who are poor candidates for endovascular treatment or who have other lesions requiring open surgical repair of the aorta or iliac arteries

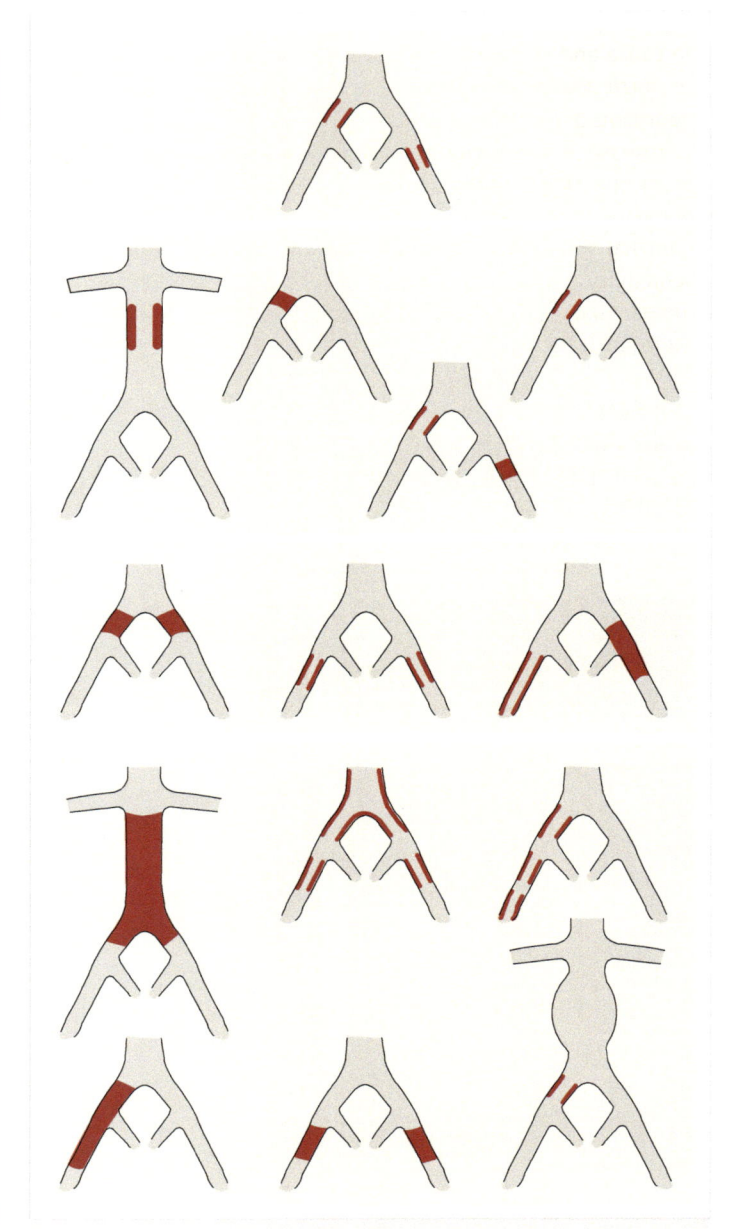

Fig. 3.30 TASC II classification of aortoiliac vascular stenoses. The Leriche syndrome is classified as a type D lesion.

▶ **Differential diagnosis.** Differentiation is required from uncomplicated atherosclerotic aortic stenosis and congenital abdominal aortic stenosis. Although the same aortic segment is affected, the patient's age and the pathognomonic calcifications with coral reef aorta allow for the confident differentiation of these entities.

▶ **Key points.** Coral reef aorta is a rare type of aortic stenosis caused by massive intravascular calcification. The symptoms depend on the affected aortic segment. The entity can be recognized on plain radiographs by the presence of massive intra-aortic calcifications. Sectional imaging serves mainly as a basis for treatment planning.

Aortitis

▶ **Brief definition.** Aortitis refers to a group of conditions that cause inflammatory changes in the aortic wall. This group of diseases has two main etiologies: infectious and noninfectious (▶ Table 3.7). The principal causative organisms of infectious aortitis, accounting for more than 40% of cases, are *Staphylococcus aureus* and salmonellae. Other pathogenic mechanisms have also been discussed:
- Hematogenous seeding with colonization of atherosclerotic plaques or intimal lesions.
- Septic emboli into the vasa vasorum of the aortic wall.
- Contiguous spread of a nearby inflammatory focus.
- Direct colonization by infectious organisms (e.g., after surgical procedures).

Risk factors are atherosclerosis, preexisting aneurysms, diabetes mellitus, cystic medial necrosis, and surgery of the aorta, which is also the basis for graft infection, a special type of aortitis. The principal noninfectious causes are Takayasu's arteritis, giant cell arteritis, rheumatoid diseases, and a number of rarer causes.

▶ **Imaging signs.** As the screening modality, ultrasonography consistently shows a hyperechoic halo around the vessel lumen. A common finding is thickening of the aortic wall, ideally with associated fat stranding (▶ Fig. 3.32). Late-phase CTA after administration of contrast medium may show a double-ring sign formed by a hyperdense (intensely enhancing) ring around the less enhancing inner layers of the aortic wall. Vascular stenosis ranging up to (sub)total occlusion may be found, depending on the cause and stage of the disease. In rare cases air is present in the aortic wall. The relatively rapid development of vessel-wall aneurysms and calcifications may be evident during the course of the disease. Besides wall thickening, fluid-sensitive MRI sequences in the florid phase of the disease may also demonstrate edema of the vessel wall. MRI is superior to CT in detecting abnormal wall enhancement, which can be quantified to assess the activity of the inflammation. Alternatively, nuclear medicine studies, especially ^{18}F-FDG PET, can be used for the evaluation of a florid inflammation.

▶ **Clinical features.** The clinical features are nonspecific and are usually characterized by the underlying disease. Prolonged fever and back pain are a typical but nonspecific presentation. The presence of risk factors facilitates diagnosis. Treatment is oriented toward the cause of the disease. A key aspect of therapy is the restoration of perfusion across a stenosis. In cases with an infectious cause, long-term antibiotic therapy and the removal of inflammatory tissue are integral components of therapy.

Note
Especially in patients with a graft or perigraft infection with abscess formation, image-guided drain insertion is recommended before surgery as the results of this two-stage approach are superior to those of primary surgery alone.

Table 3.7 Selected causes of aortitis

Etiologic categories	Causative organism or disease
Infectious	
Bacterial	• Staphylococcus aureus • Salmonellae • Streptococci • Enterococci, etc.
Mycobacterial	
Syphilitic	
Viral	HIV
Noninfectious	
Vasculitides	• Takayasu's arteritis • Giant cell arteritis • Wegener's disease • Polyarteritis nodosa • Behçet's disease
Other rheumatic diseases	• Long-standing ankylosing spondylitis • Reiter's disease • Systemic lupus erythematosus • Relapsing polychondritis • Cogan's syndrome • Rheumatoid arthritis
Radiation-induced aortitis	
Idiopathic	

Fig. 3.31 "Coral reef" aorta in a 46-year-old man with massive intraluminal calcification of the abdominal aorta. CT shows the attachment site of the calcifications to the anterior aortic wall.

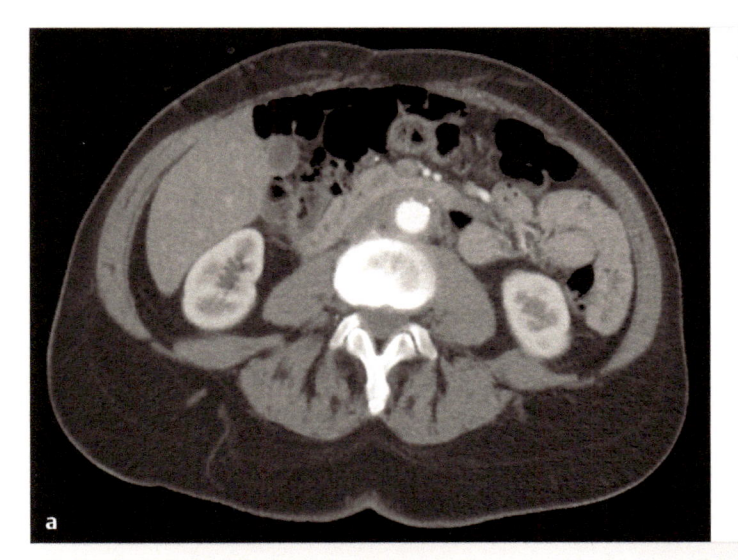

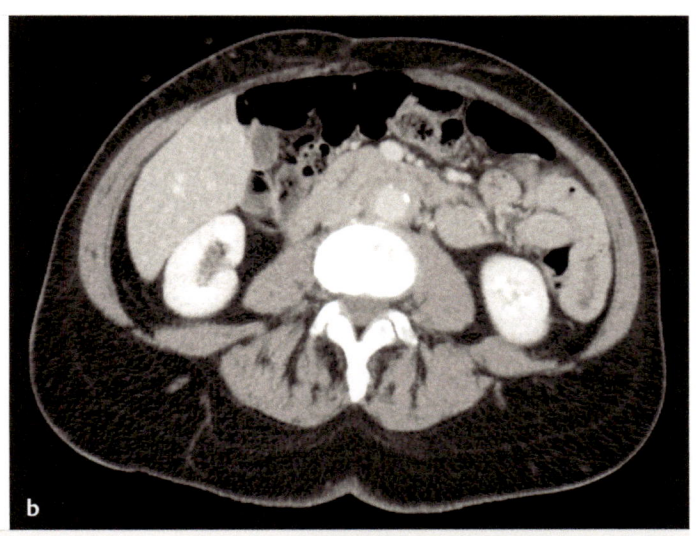

Fig. 3.32 Salmonella aortitis in a 39-year-old woman. Thickening and increased enhancement of the abdominal aortic wall are typical findings. (a) CTA. (b) Delayed phase.

▶ **Differential diagnosis.** The radiological differential diagnosis mainly includes intramural hematoma, spontaneous aortic aneurysm, retroperitoneal fibrosis (periaortitis) and, less commonly, periaortic lymphoma.

▶ **Key points.** Aortitis denotes inflammatory changes in the aortic wall, which may result from a heterogeneous group of infectious and noninfectious causes. Imaging plays a key role in the diagnosis of patients with nonspecific clinical findings. Pivotal signs include vessel wall thickening and edema with perivascular edema and abnormal enhancement of the aortic wall. Interventional restoration of perfusion across hemodynamically significant stenoses and interventional drainage in cases with abscess formation are major components of therapy.

Vasculitis

▶ **Brief definition.** "Vasculitis" is a collective term for diseases that involve inflammatory vascular changes with a potential for ischemic injury to dependent organs. The 2012 revision of the Chapel Hill Consensus Conference established a uniform nomenclature system for vasculitides (▶ Table 3.8).[21] The large-vessel vasculitides, most notably giant cell arteritis and Takayasu's arteritis, are particularly relevant in large-vessel imaging:

- *Giant cell arteritis*: Giant cell arteritis is a granulomatous vasculitis that predominantly affects the large and medium arteries of the head, especially the temporal artery. The aortic arch and large supra-aortic vessels are involved in approximately 15% of patients. The disease most commonly affects patients over 70 years of age.
- *Takayasu's arteritis*: Takayasu's arteritis is a necrotizing, granulomatous inflammation that predominantly affects the media of large arteries such as the aorta and its branches but may also occur in the pulmonary artery, for example (15% of cases). Progression leads to fibrotic changes in the vessel wall, usually with associated stenosis and eventual aneurysm formation. Takayasu's arteritis predominantly affects young women, especially those of Asian descent.

▶ **Imaging signs.** Ultrasonography is the primary imaging study for the diagnosis of arteritis. It is particularly accurate for giant cell arteritis, with a sensitivity of 68% and specificity of 91% in cases where a halo is seen in one temporal artery. These rates increase to 100% when a halo is found in both arteries.[22] Sectional imaging demonstrates luminal and extraluminal changes with typical sites of vessel-wall thickening and stenosis. The aorta is most commonly affected (65% of cases). Other potentially affected vessels, in descending order of frequency, are the brachiocephalic trunk, left subclavian artery, left carotid artery, femoral arteries, mesenteric arteries, iliac arteries, and renal arteries. Besides typical wall thickening and stenosis, affected vessels may also show abnormal dilatation. Dilatation of the thoracic aorta is seen in approximately 15% of patients. Delayed CT scans may additionally show a contrast halo localized to the media (▶ Fig. 3.33). MRI findings are similar to those in aortitis, consisting of vessel wall edema and abnormal enhancement that correlates with disease activity. One advantage of MRI over CT is that, when suitable surface coils are used, MRI can also detect these changes in medium and small vessels. CT is useful for defining the overall extent of the disease.

Table 3.8 Classification of vasculitides based on the 2012 Chapel Hill nomenclature.[21]

Groups of vasculitis	Diseases
Large-vessel vasculitis	• Takayasu's arteritis • Giant cell arteritis
Medium-vessel vasculitis	• Polyarteritis nodosa • Kawasaki's disease
Small-vessel vasculitis	• ANCA-associated vasculitis: • Microscopic polyangiitis • Granulomatosis with polyangiitis (Wegener's granulomatosis) • Eosinophilic granulomatosis with polyangiitis (Churg–Strauss syndrome) • Immune complex vasculitis • Anti-GBM disease • Cryoglobulinemic vasculitis • IgA vasculitis (Henoch–Schönlein) • Hypocomplementemic urticarial vasculitis (anti-C1q vasculitis)
Variable-vessel vasculitis	• Behçet's disease • Cogan's syndrome
Single-organ vasculitis	• Cutaneous leukocytoclastic angiitis • Cutaneous arteritis • Primary central nervous system vasculitis • Isolated aortitis • Others
Vasculitis associated with systemic disease	• Lupus vasculitis • Rheumatoid vasculitis • Sarcoid vasculitis • Others
Vasculitis associated with probable etiology	• Hepatitis C virus-associated cryoglobulinemic vasculitis • Hepatitis B virus-associated vasculitis • Syphilis-associated aortitis • Drug-associated immune complex vasculitis

Abbreviations: ANCA, antineutrophil cytoplasmic antibody; GBM, glomerular basement membrane; IgA, immunoglobulin A

▶ **Clinical features.** Systemic signs of infection such as fever, night sweats, limb pain, and weight loss are nonspecific and may even give rise to a long delay in diagnosis. Later symptoms are more suggestive and may include decreased blood flow to the extremities and neurologic problems such as dizziness, impaired vision, stroke, or blood pressure elevation under 40 years of age. A large percentage of patients with giant cell arteritis report a stabbing headache as the initial symptom. A diagnosis of Takayasu's arteritis is suggested by upper limb claudication with a diminished brachial artery pulse, leading to the clinical classification of pulseless or pre-pulseless disease.

▶ **Differential diagnosis.** Similar imaging patterns may be seen in any form of aortitis. In contrast to infectious aortitis, for example, the large-vessel arthritides also affect the large supra-aortic vessels and visceral vessels. Very severe large-vessel atherosclerosis and intramural hematoma are potential mimics of vasculitis.

▶ **Key points.** Large-vessel arteritis predominantly affects the aorta and the supra-aortic and visceral vessels. The clinical manifestations are nonspecific. A number of features, most notably a halo around the temporal artery on ultrasound, segmental wall

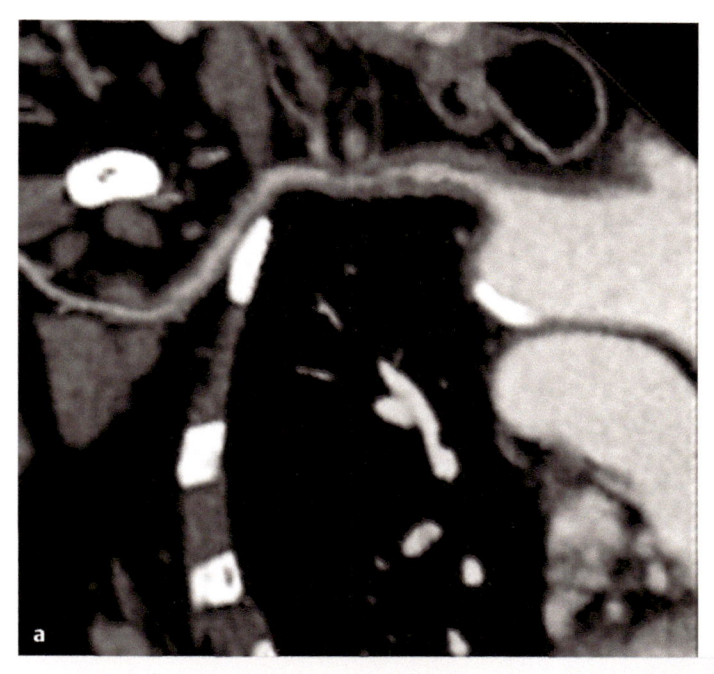

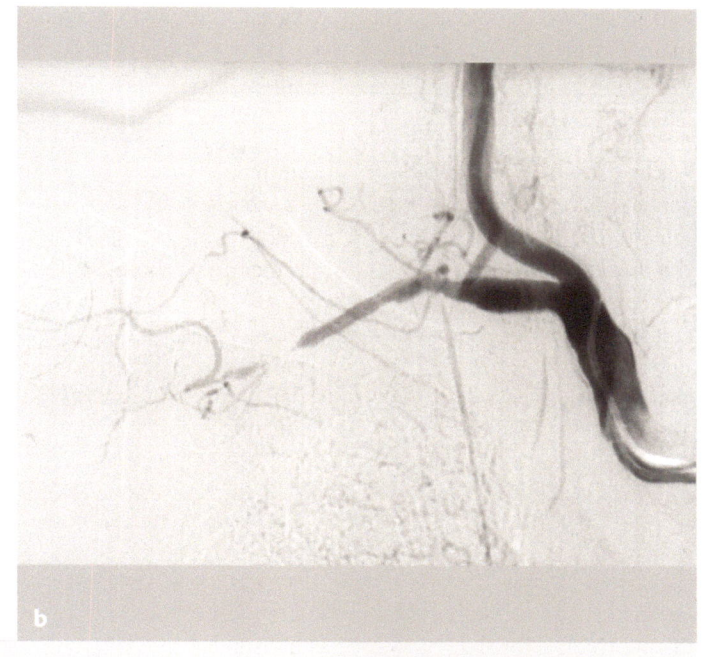

Fig. 3.33 **Takayasu's arteritis** in a 59-year-old woman. (a) CTA, performed to investigate a cold extremity, shows irregular halolike wall thickening of the brachiocephalic trunk and right subclavian artery. (b) Angiography confirms the finding and shows a typical pattern of large-vessel vasculitis. Peripheral vascular cutoff is also seen.

thickening and vascular dilatation on CT, and abnormal vessel wall enhancement on MRI suggest the correct diagnosis. The distribution pattern is helpful in differentiating large-vessel arteritis from aortitis due to other causes.

Malignant Vascular Tumors

▶ **Brief definition**
- *Primary large-vessel malignancies*: These extremely rare lesions affect, in descending order of frequency, the inferior vena cava, pulmonary arteries, and (thoracic) aorta. Primary sarcomas of the aorta are generally angiosarcomas arising from the intima, while sarcomas of the venous angioma cava are mostly leiomyosarcomas arising from the media or adventitia. They most commonly affect the inferior vena cava; less than 5% of these rare tumors are found in the superior vena cava. Angiosarcomas and leiomyosarcomas may also occur in the pulmonary artery. These tumors that primarily involve the large vessels are distinguished from lymphangiosarcoma, malignant epithelioid hemangioendothelioma, and malignant hemangiopericytoma, which may occur anywhere in the body.
- *Secondary large-vessel malignancies*: Malignancies that invade the large vessels secondarily, particularly the large veins, are far more common than primary tumors; see Tumor Thrombi in the Vena Cava. A typical example is a tumor thrombus from renal cell carcinoma extending into the inferior vena cava from the renal vein. Reports indicate that this type of invasion is also seen with other entities and may occur in all venous territories.

▶ **Imaging signs.** Ultrasound and other sectional imaging modalities show an intraluminal filling defect that may have smooth or polypoid margins. Unlike a simple thrombus, malignant vascular tumors have a blood supply and therefore enhance after IV injection of contrast medium (▶ Fig. 3.34). This provides differentiation from the typically hypodense appositional thrombus demonstrated by CT. Unlike secondary tumors of large vessels, primary tumors do not display an extravascular component. MRI shows enhancement in T1W sequences and will generally show increased signal intensity on T2W images. The depth of wall invasion can be determined with transesophageal ultrasound, provided the tumor is within the acoustic window. In addition to this growth pattern, mural angiosarcomas may also extend beyond the vessel wall and invade surrounding structures.

▶ **Clinical features.** Patients often remain asymptomatic for a long time. The symptoms vary with the affected vascular territory and range from signs of lower extremity venous congestion (e.g., a tumor occluding the inferior vena cava) to dyspnea (e.g., pulmonary artery sarcoma). Systemic signs of a malignant disease such as lethargy and weight loss are typical. Often these rare tumors go undetected for some time. The prognosis is unfavorable and ranges from a mean survival of 37 months with leiomyosarcoma to approximately 9 months with angiosarcoma.[23,24] Embolic complications from appositional thrombi also play a significant role.

▶ **Differential diagnosis.** The diagnosis of vascular malignancies is difficult because of their rarity, and many are diagnosed only at postmortem examination. There have also been numerous reports of initial misdiagnosis followed by a postoperative histological diagnosis. Angiosarcoma of the pulmonary arteries and leiomyosarcoma of the vena cava are frequently mistaken for pulmonary embolism or spontaneous vena cava thrombosis. If the intrahepatic segment of the vena cava is involved, the tumor may be mistaken for hepatic metastasis or primary hepatocellular carcinoma. Primary large-vessel tumors require differentiation from tumors that invade the vascular system secondarily, such as renal cell carcinoma with extension of tumor thrombus into the vena cava.

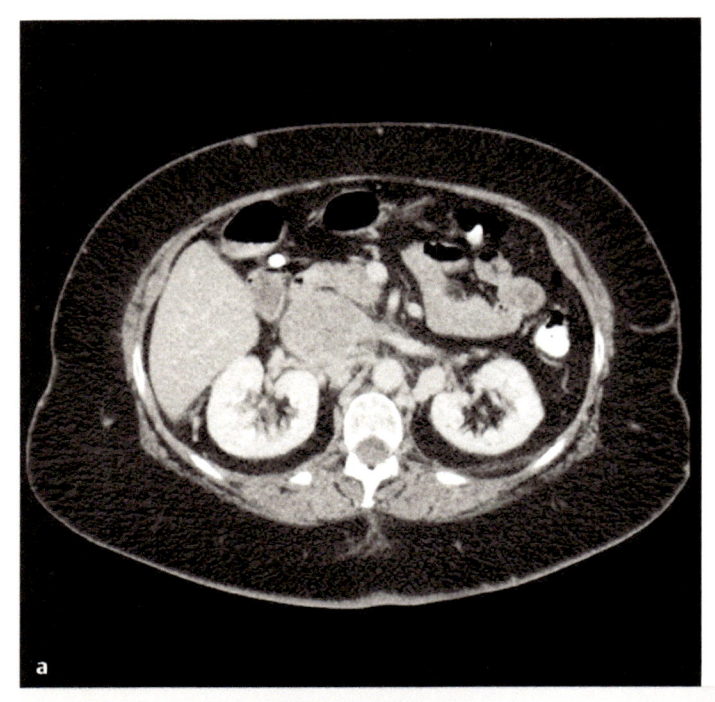

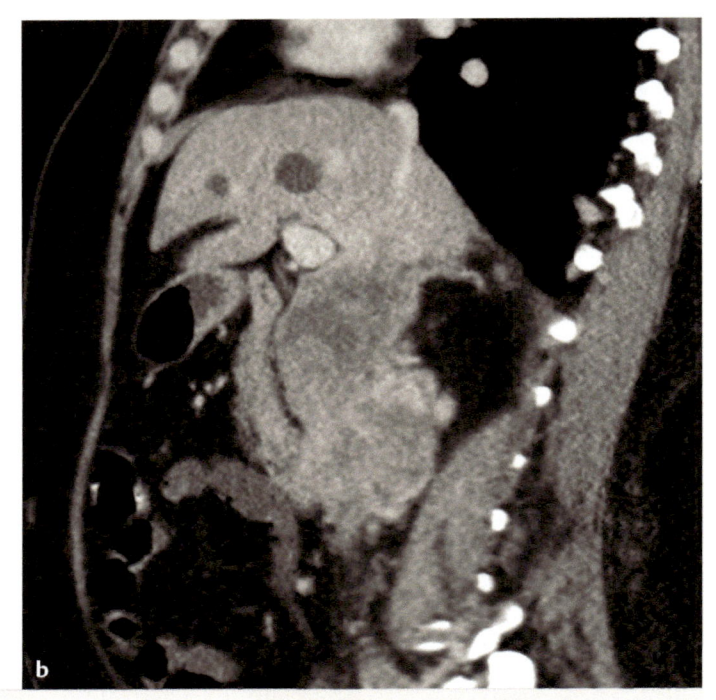

Fig. 3.34 Primary angiosarcoma of the inferior vena cava. Venous-phase CT shows a well-circumscribed, inhomogeneously enhancing tumor of the inferior vena cava. The lesion does not transcend the boundaries of the vessel. The differential diagnosis would include a tumor thrombus, but there is no evidence of a tumor originating from hepatic or renal veins, for example. Postoperative histology after vena cava replacement confirmed a primary angiosarcoma of the inferior vena cava. **(a)** Axial reformatted CT. **(b)** Sagittal reformatted CT.

▶ **Key points.** Primary sarcomas of large vessels are rare and have a poor prognosis. Diagnosis is commonly delayed. A typical sign on imaging is an enhancing intraluminal mass with no evidence of an extraluminal component or a separate primary tumor.

Aortic Fistulas

▶ **Brief definition.** Aortic fistulas are a rare complication of aortic pathology, especially aortic aneurysms. These primary fistulas are very rare. Secondary aortic fistulas are more common and generally occur as a postoperative or postinflammatory lesion following treatment for an aortic aneurysm (up to 0.6% of patients after aortic surgery). Tumor-induced, posttraumatic, and radiation-induced fistulas have also been reported. Aortoenteric or aortopulmonary fistulas may develop within several days or up to 10 years after aortic surgery. These fistulas can be classified into three broad categories:
- *Aortoenteric fistulas* (aortoesophageal, aortoduodenal): from 60 to 80% involve the duodenum, but virtually any part of the gastrointestinal tract may be affected.
- *Aortopulmonary fistulas* (aortobronchial, aortotracheal): approximately 90% involve the bronchi of the left lung. Aortotracheal fistulas are the rarest form.
- *Aortocaval fistulas* (p.99)

▶ **Imaging signs.** The diagnostic modality of choice is CT with arterial and late-phase imaging. Positive oral contrast medium is not used. CT has a reported sensitivity of 40 to 90% with a specificity of 33 to 100%.
- *Aortoenteric fistula*: nonspecific signs of an aortoenteric fistula, besides immediate proximity of the vessel and bowel, are a periaortic or periprosthetic fluid collection and local fat stranding (▶ Fig. 3.35). These signs are often found in association with local and prosthetic infections, however. More specific signs are thickening and retraction of adjacent bowel structures, ectopic gas collections (more than 2 weeks after surgery), and, as a pathognomonic sign, direct contrast extravasation from the aorta into the bowel.
- *Aortopulmonary fistula*: almost never visualized directly but usually evidenced by aortic pathology accompanied by peribronchial infiltrates. Additionally, the bronchial wall may be thickened at the fistula site, and ipsilateral material of blood attenuation may be found in the bronchial system.

Caution

Ultrasound and MRI are not considered reliable modalities in the diagnosis of aortic fistula. With an aortoenteric fistula, they could at most show limited indirect signs such as a periaortic fluid collection. Small ectopic gas collections are easily missed. Invasive angiography is of limited diagnostic value due to the frequently small volume of the fistulas.

▶ **Clinical features.** The clinical presentation of aortoenteric and aortopulmonary fistulas is highly variable and includes acute and chronic, mild or severe hematochezia or hematemesis. Other possible manifestations are back pain or prolonged, often subacute signs of infection (prosthetic infection). Aortopulmonary fistulas are distinguished by varying degrees of hematemesis and hemoptysis. Massive hemoptysis at a rate of 300 to 400 mL of blood/24 hours is strongly suspicious for an aortopulmonary fistula. Apart from previous surgery, malignancies are a particularly frequent cause of aortopulmonary fistulas, in which case the symptoms of

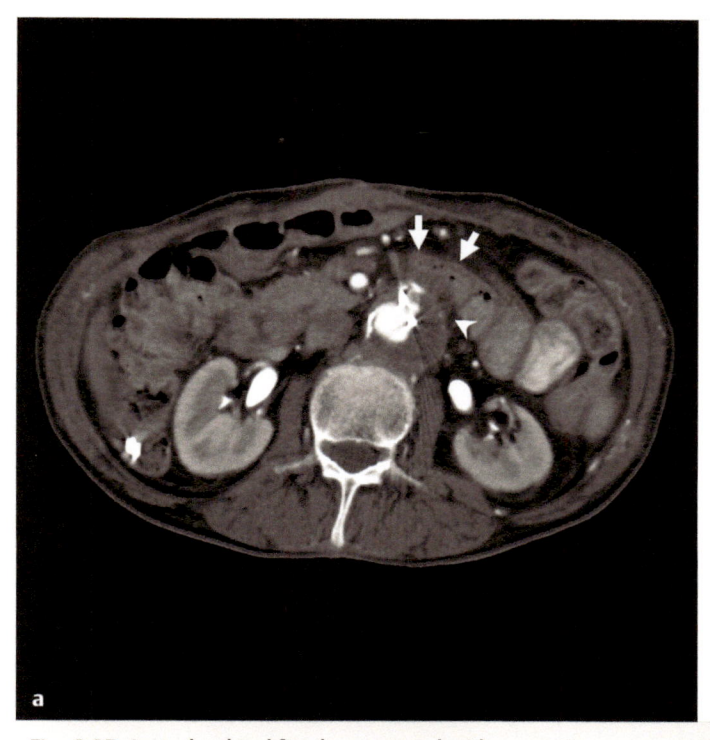

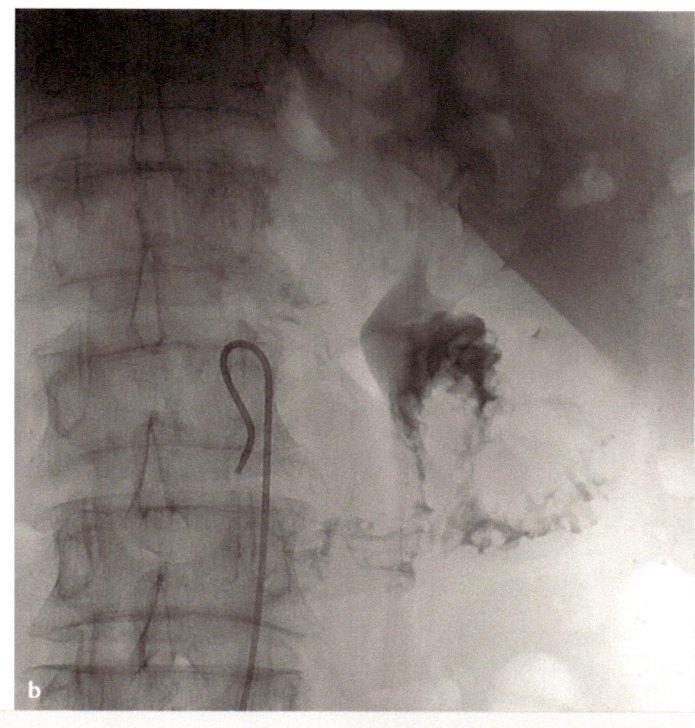

Fig. 3.35 Aortoduodenal fistula associated with an aortic aneurysm. (a) CTA shows local fat stranding (arrowhead) plus distortion and retraction of the horizontal part of the duodenum toward an abdominal aortic aneurysm (arrows). This finding is suggestive of an aortoduodenal fistula associated with an aortic aneurysm. **(b)** The finding was confirmed by angiography, which shows extravasation of contrast medium into the duodenum.

the malignancy may be dominant. In some cases hemoptysis may even be falsely attributed to a fistula rather than an underlying tumor. All aortic fistulas present with episodes of reduced hemoglobin levels and low blood pressure. Immediate treatment, which is usually surgical and rarely interventional, is necessary due to the very high mortality in untreated cases. Aortoesophageal and aortotracheal fistulas have a particularly poor prognosis.

▶ **Differential diagnosis.** The differential diagnosis of aortoenteric fistula includes simple aortitis, prosthetic infection, mycotic aneurysm, retroperitoneal abscess, and retroperitoneal fibrosis. The differential diagnosis of aortopulmonary fistulas includes primary and secondary lung malignancies and granulomatous inflammations, especially tuberculosis.

▶ **Key points.** Aortoenteric and aortopulmonary fistulas are a rare and difficult diagnosis on imaging. Most cases are acquired as a result of aortic surgery. The diagnostic imaging modality of choice is CT, which can show direct contact between the aorta and bowel or bronchial system. Suggestive signs are local wall thickening and possible ectopic gas collections.

Subgroup: Aortocaval Fistulas

▶ **Brief definition.** Aortocaval fistulas are rare lesions that have two possible etiologies. The more frequent cause is the contained rupture of an aortic aneurysm into the inferior vena cava. Less commonly, an aortocaval fistula may develop due to trauma.

▶ **Imaging signs.** Both arteriography and contrast-enhanced CT show very early entry of contrast medium into the inferior vena cava and its tributaries, creating a level of enhancement approaching that of the arterial circulation. Ultrasound can demonstrate turbulent flow at the level of the fistula. All imaging modalities show marked dilatation of the inferior vena cava.

▶ **Clinical features.** Typical clinical signs result from the arteriovenous shunt and its generally high flow volume and present with right heart failure and possible lower extremity edema. A bruit is typically noted on auscultation. Hematuria and crossed embolism may also occur. The prognosis is fatal without prompt treatment. Besides surgical ligation, the implantation of stent grafts has become a first-line treatment option.

▶ **Key points.** Aortocaval fistula is a rare complication that results predominantly from the confined perforation of an aortic aneurysm. It requires immediate treatment, usually by interventional means.

Subclavian Steal Syndrome

▶ **Brief definition.** Subclavian steal syndrome is the result of a a stenotic or occlusive lesion of the proximal subclavian artery or brachiocephalic trunk (▶ Fig. 3.36). This leads to retrograde flow in the vertebral artery on the affected side, which diverts blood away from the brain to the ipsilateral arm. The left side is affected four times more frequently than the right side. In 90% of cases the syndrome results from atherosclerotic disease. Other cases are attributable to postoperative changes, postirradiation changes, trauma, arteritis, or a thoracic outlet syndrome. Because most patients are asymptomatic, the true prevalence of the disease is unknown but is believed to be in the range 0.6 to 6.0%.

Coexisting coronary steal syndrome has also been described as a variant; it arises from the same pathology but causes retrograde flow in an ipsilateral internal mammary artery bypass graft.

▶ **Imaging signs.** The principal finding on ultrasound, CTA, or MRA is a stenotic or occlusive lesion of one or both subclavian arteries or the brachiocephalic trunk. Retrograde flow in the ipsilateral vertebral artery can be directly visualized by ultrasound or dynamic MRA (▶ Fig. 3.37). Conventional angiography, while still the diagnostic gold standard, has been almost completely discontinued in routine settings due to its inherent complications. It may still be used in the setting of interventional therapy, which has become the established clinical standard.

Note

In patients with an internal mammary artery bypass on the affected side, stress cardiac imaging can be added to exclude a coexisting coronary steal syndrome.

▶ **Clinical features.** Most patients are asymptomatic, but clinical examination may reveal a typical blood pressure discrepancy between the arms. Classic symptoms involve the posterior cerebral circulation and consist of dizziness, ataxia, nystagmus, syncopal attacks, or visual disturbances. An inadequate collateral supply may lead to atypical symptoms such as arm and hand weakness and coldness and paresthesias in the affected limb. In patients with a coexisting coronary steal syndrome, signs of cardiac ischemia or angina pectoris may be the only finding. Symptoms may be evoked by stress maneuvers such as turning the head to the opposite side or elevation of the arm.

▶ **Differential diagnosis.** The main differential diagnosis is stroke as a potential cause of neurologic symptoms. Other neurologic diseases such as cerebellar tumors or multiple sclerosis may have similar manifestations. The differential diagnosis should also include aortic dissection and vasculitides, which may additionally cause a subclavian steal syndrome in rare cases.

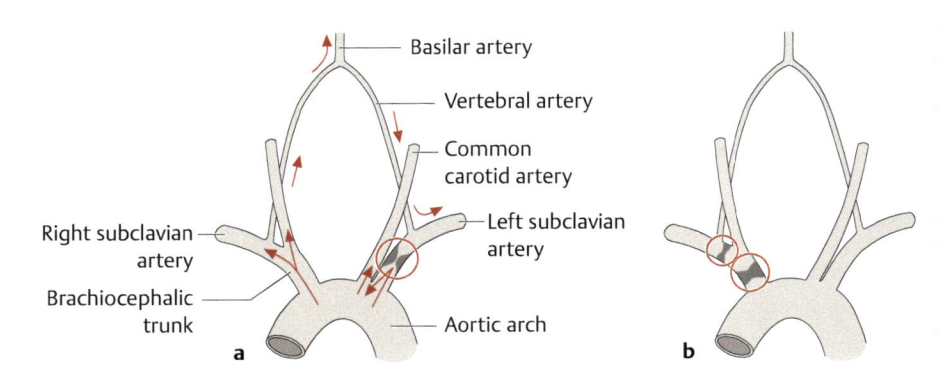

Fig. 3.36 Subclavian steal syndrome, characterized by flow reversal in the vertebral artery on the affected side. Schematic representation. (a) The subclavian steal syndrome in this case results from a stenotic or occlusive lesion of the proximal subclavian artery. (b) In this case the lesion may involve the brachiocephalic trunk as well as the proximal right subclavian artery. (Reproduced from Schünke M, Schulte E, Schumacher U. Prometheus. LernAtlas der Anatomie: Kopf, Hals und Neuroanatomie. Illustrated by M. Voll/K. Wesker. 2nd ed. Stuttgart: Thieme; 2009.)

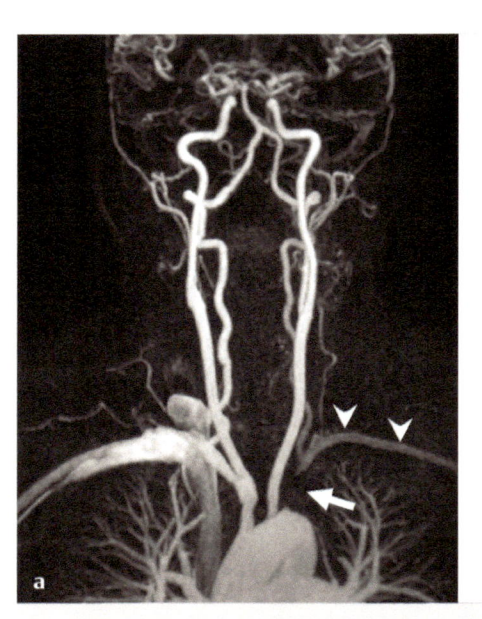

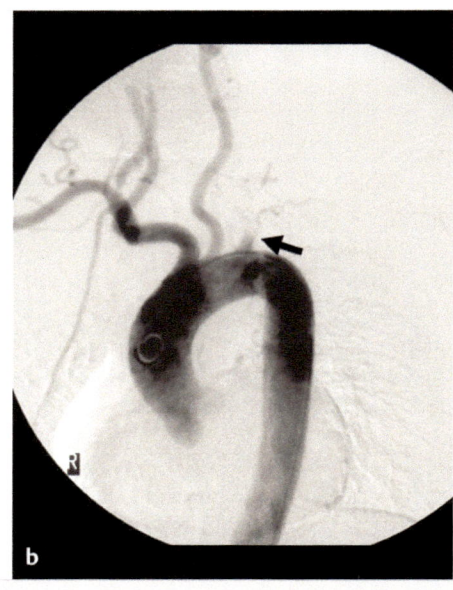

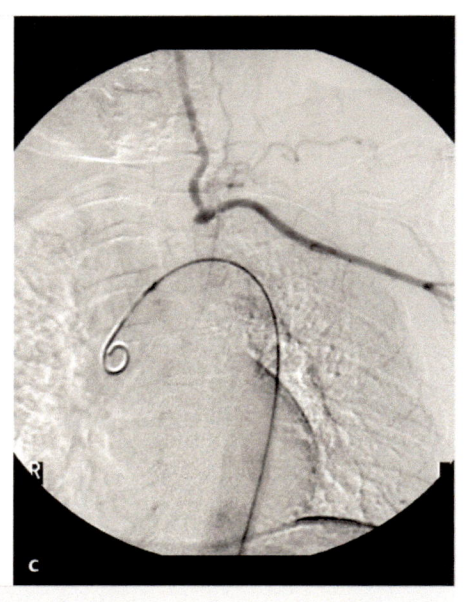

Fig. 3.37 Subclavian steal syndrome. (a) MRA in a patient with an occlusion of the left subclavian artery (arrow). The lesion has caused retrograde flow in the left vertebral artery, which is perfusing the left arm distal to the occlusion. This accounts for the fainter enhancement of the left vertebral artery and left axillary artery (arrowheads). (b) Sequence of conventional angiograms (b, c) shows that the left subclavian artery is occluded ([b], arrow) while the other supra-aortic branches are normally perfused. (c) A later image documents blood flow to the left arm from the vertebral artery.

▶ **Key points.** Subclavian steal syndrome results from a stenotic or occlusive lesion of the proximal subclavian artery, usually on the left side. Most patients are asymptomatic. When symptoms arise, they are typically neurologic although a subclavian steal syndrome may also produce atypical complaints such as arm weakness or angina pectoris. Ultrasound is diagnostic as a rule, but clinical findings plus the detection of arterial stenosis or occlusion by CTA or MRA can also establish the syndrome. Treatment is usually interventional by stent angioplasty.

Thoracic Outlet and Thoracic Inlet Syndrome

▶ **Brief definition.** Thoracic outlet syndrome is a neurovascular compression syndrome involving the superior thoracic aperture. It is a collective term for various disorders that lead to the compression of neurovascular structures in the upper thorax. The term *thoracic outlet syndrome* refers to arterial compression, while *thoracic inlet syndrome* refers to impaired venous return due to the compression of large veins. Four specific syndromes are distinguished:

- *Cervical rib syndrome*: compression of the subclavian artery and/or the brachial plexus not involving the subclavian vein (▶ Fig. 3.38a).
- *Scalenus syndrome*: compression of the neurovascular bundle between the scalenus anterior and medius muscles (scalenus anterior syndrome). If the interscalene triangle is narrowed by the scalenus minimus, the term *scalenus minimus syndrome* is also used (▶ Fig. 3.38b).
- *Costoclavicular syndrome*: compression of the neurovascular bundle between the clavicle and first rib. This is the most common type of pure thoracic inlet syndrome (▶ Fig. 3.38c).
- *Pectoralis minor syndrome*: compression of the neurovascular bundle by the pectoralis minor tendon attachment to the coracoid process. This occurs on elevation of the arm and is also known as hyperabduction syndrome (▶ Fig. 3.38d).

Additionally, fused ribs, malunited clavicular fractures, or exostoses on the ribs or clavicle may also cause an (atypical) compression syndrome.

▶ **Imaging signs.** The chest radiograph can establish the presence of cervical ribs and also reveal the cause of an atypical compression syndrome due to exostoses or old fractures. If arterial or venous symptoms are predominant, then angiography or venography in the neutral position and with provocative arm abduction (placing the hand on the back of the neck) can confirm a thoracic outlet or thoracic inlet syndrome (▶ Fig. 3.39). Thrombosis can be

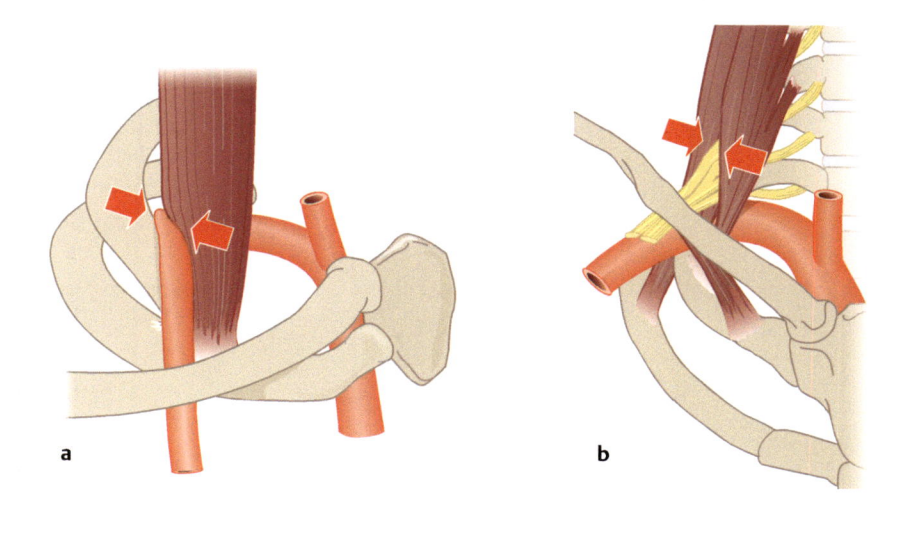

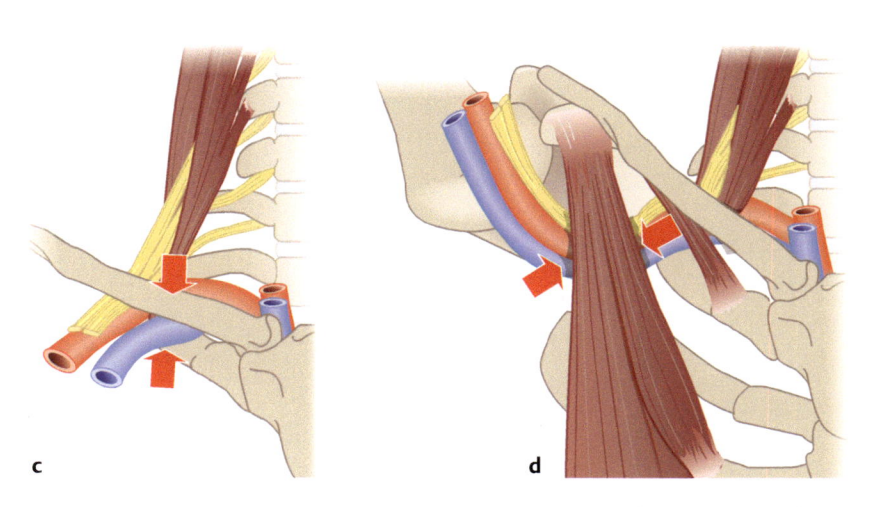

Fig. 3.38 Neurovascular compression at the superior thoracic aperture. Schematic representation of various potential causes. (a) Cervical rib syndrome with compression of the subclavian artery by a cervical rib and the scalenus anterior muscle. (b) Scalenus anterior syndrome with compression of the neurovascular bundle between the scalenus anterior and medius muscles. (c) Costoclavicular compression between the first rib and clavicle. (d) Pectoralis minor or hyperabduction syndrome with compression of the neurovascular bundle by the pectoral muscle attachment to the coracoid process. (Reproduced from Schünke M, Schulte E, Schumacher U. Prometheus. LernAtlas der Anatomie: Allgemeine Anatomie und Bewegungssystem. Illustrated by M. Voll/K. Wesker. 3rd ed. Stuttgart: Thieme; 2011.)

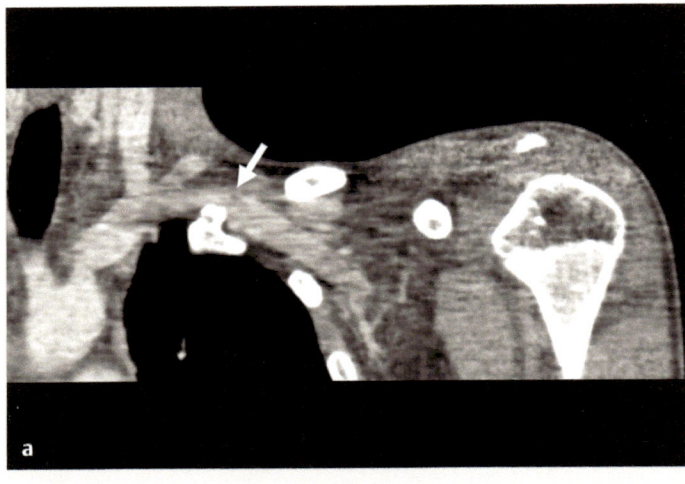

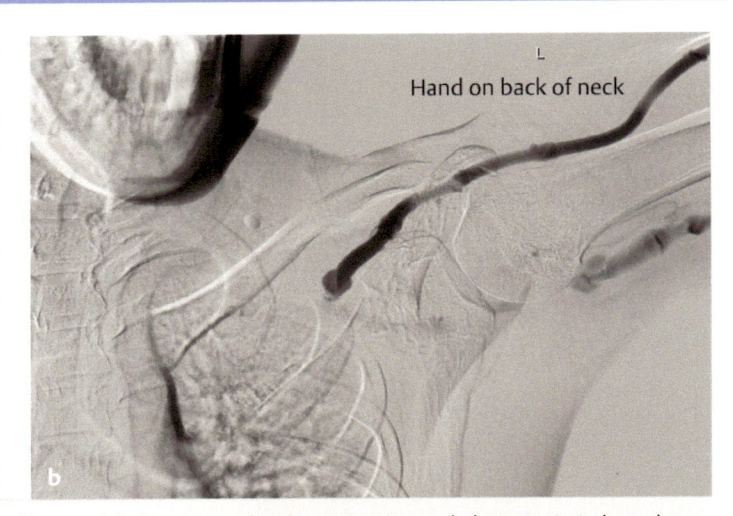

Fig. 3.39 Thoracic outlet syndrome in a clinically symptomatic 18-year-old man. **(a)** CT venography shows a patent subclavian vein indented caudally by an exostosis on the first rib (arrow). **(b)** Provocation test during venography confirms the functional effect of the exostosis, which causes complete occlusion of the subclavian vein.

directly visualized with ultrasound. MRA and CTA are also used, but provocative positioning is difficult with these techniques so they are used mainly for anatomical correlation.

▶ **Clinical features.** Signs and symptoms depend on the compression mechanism. A pure thoracic inlet syndrome with thrombosis of the subclavian vein and possible involvement of the tributary axillary and brachial veins almost invariably results from costoclavicular compression, while a pure thoracic outlet syndrome is due to compression by a cervical rib. All other forms usually cause mixed neurologic and vascular symptoms with pain, dysesthesia, and muscle weakness or even paralysis as the neurologic component. In patients with thoracic outlet syndrome, elevation of the arm leads to ipsilateral cold sensation, weakness, and loss of the peripheral radial artery pulse. Venous compression leads to venous congestion problems marked by pain, heavy sensation, and possible venous thrombosis.

▶ **Differential diagnosis.** The differential diagnosis is complex and includes focal neurologic causes such as radiculopathy or plexopathy, ulnar groove syndrome, and carpal tunnel syndrome as well as systemic neurologic diseases such as multiple sclerosis. Combinations may also be encountered, such as a *double crush syndrome* in which thoracic outlet or inlet syndrome is combined with carpal tunnel syndrome.[25] Arterial symptoms may be confused with a subclavian steal syndrome, while venous symptoms should prompt consideration of possible lymphedema or paraneoplastic thrombosis.

▶ **Key points.** A thoracic outlet or inlet syndrome due to neurovascular compression at the superior thoracic aperture can have various causes. Diagnosis relies on chest radiographs and on invasive angiography or venography with provocative hyperabduction, depending on whether arterial or venous symptoms are present.

3.2 Vena Cava and Large Veins

3.2.1 Anatomy

The normal anatomy of the large thoracic veins includes the bilateral subclavian and jugular veins, which unite to form the brachiocephalic veins (or innominate veins) that drain into the superior vena cava on the right side. The left brachiocephalic vein passes behind the sternum and is considerably longer than the right brachiocephalic vein. The azygos vein runs a considerable right paravertebral course before opening into the superior vena cava, draining the posterior portions of the chest and abdomen. Its counterpart on the left side is the hemiazygos vein, which drains into the azygos vein at a variable intrathoracic level.

The venous anatomy of the abdomen is formed by the bilateral iliac veins; both drain into the inferior vena cava, which ascends just to the right of the vertebral column. The renal and hepatic veins are also major tributaries of the inferior vena cava. Other clinically relevant tributaries are the ovarian veins (female) and spermatic veins (male), which open directly into the inferior vena cava on the right side and typically open into the renal vein on the left side (▶ Fig. 3.40). The normal diameter of the inferior vena cava is approximately 24 mm. The term megacava is applied when the caval diameter is 28 mm or more.

3.2.2 Development

The embryonic development of the veins is complex, involving the formation of a series of anastomoses between three sets of large, paired embryonic veins: the vitelline veins, umbilical veins, and cardinal veins. This development is typically completed in the eighth week of gestation. Venous anatomy is variable, depending on the persistence or regression of these large embryonic veins. Numerous variants may occur, especially with regard to the inferior vena cava.

Development of the veins proceeds as follows:
- The *vitelline veins* give rise to the portal venous system and the posthepatic segment of the inferior vena cava.
- The initially paired *umbilical veins* form early connections with hepatic sinusoids. While the right umbilical vein regresses at an early stage, the ductus venosus develops to form a connection between the left umbilical vein and right heart. At birth this channel is obliterated and forms the hepatic round ligament and ligamentum venosum.
- The paired anterior *cardinal veins* form the systemic veins for the upper half of the body. In addition to the cardinal veins, the paired subcardinal veins are formed between the fifth and

3.2 Vena Cava and Large Veins

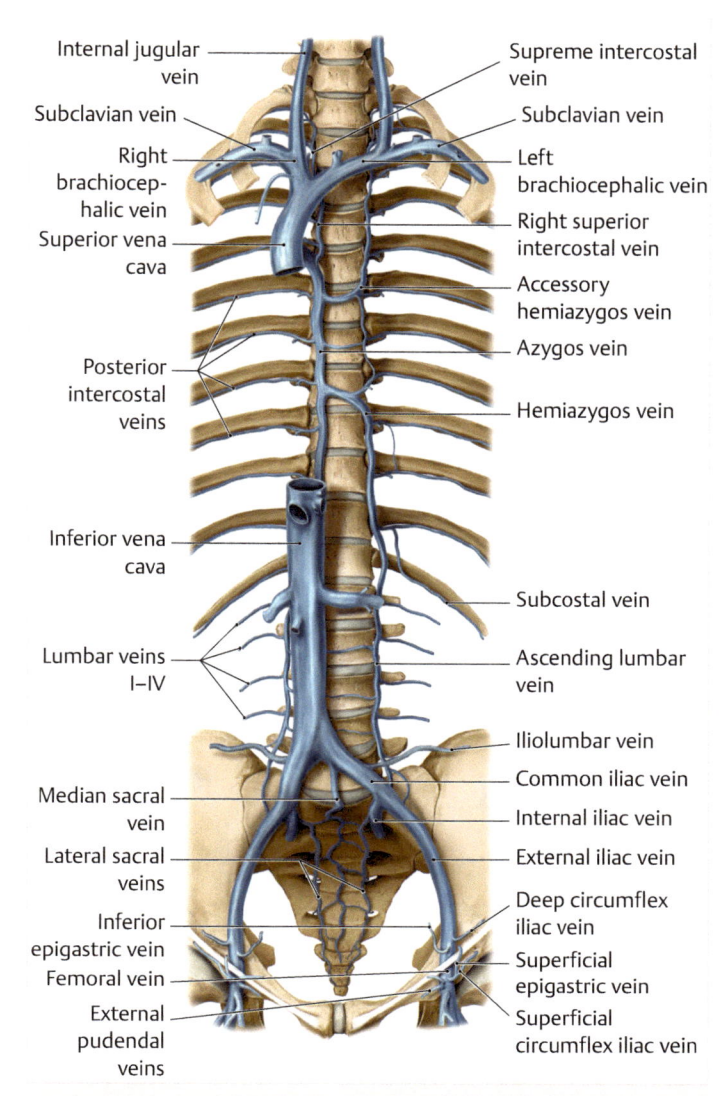

Fig. 3.40 Anatomy of the venous system. (Reproduced from Schünke M, Schulte E, Schumacher U. Prometheus. LernAtlas der Anatomie: Allgemeine Anatomie und Bewegungssystem. Illustrated by M. Voll/K. Wesker. 3rd ed. Stuttgart: Thieme; 2011.)

seventh weeks to drain the embryonic kidneys, the sacrocardinal veins to drain the lower extremity, and the supracardinal veins to drain the body wall. The right subcardinal vein ultimately forms the renal segment of the inferior vena cava, while the left subcardinal vein largely regresses. The right subcardinal vein forms the rest of the inferior vena cava, while the anastomosis between the subcardinal veins forms the left common iliac vein. As the cardinal veins are obliterated, the supracardinal veins assume greater importance and eventually form the major portions of the azygos and hemiazygos veins (▶ Fig. 3.41).

3.2.3 Congenital Anomalies

Consistently with this complex and largely symmetrical developmental process, vascular anatomy is subject to a number of possible variants (▶ Table 3.9).[26] In addition to actual anomalies of the inferior vena cava, the renal arteries can give rise to variants such as a retroaortic course of the left renal vein or the presence of anterior and posterior left renal veins forming a ring around the aorta.

These variants are clinically silent as a rule but may have important implications prior to a surgical or interventional procedure.

Persistent Left Superior Vena Cava

▶ **Brief definition.** Embryologically, a persistent left superior vena cava results from persistence of the left anterior cardinal vein. This vein generally drains through the coronary sinus (▶ Fig. 3.42), but very rarely it may drain into the left atrium. The left brachiocephalic vein often forms a communication between the left and right superior vena cava. A persistent left superior vena cava has a prevalence up to 0.5%. This increases to as much as 5% when other congenital cardiac anomalies are present.

Left-Sided and Duplicated Inferior Vena Cava

▶ **Brief definition.** An isolated left-sided inferior vena cava occurs in up to 0.5% of the population; duplication of the inferior vena cava may occur in up to 3%. The left-sided inferior vena cava ascends in the retroperitoneum on the left side and ends at the left renal vein. Above that level the vena cava occupies a normal position on the right side. With a duplicated inferior vena cava, there is a left-sided inferior vena cava and a persistent inferior vena cava on the right side. The crossing site of the left inferior vena cava is typically at the left renal vein but may be lower in unusual cases.

▶ **Imaging signs.** Venography shows a vessel ascending to the left of the vertebral column. With duplication of the inferior vena cava, this may occasionally be misinterpreted as a long iliac vein with a high iliac bifurcation, for example. Sectional imaging aids diagnosis by demonstrating a large, left retroperitoneal vein that terminates at the left renal vein.

▶ **Clinical features.** These variants are generally asymptomatic; they become significant when complications arise. There are reports of pulmonary embolism occurring despite the placement of a vena cava filter in patients with a duplicated inferior vena cava, as thrombi are still able to escape through the left-sided inferior vena cava.[27] Also, these variants produce abnormal flow conditions that constitute a risk factor for thrombosis, especially in young adults.

▶ **Differential diagnosis**

> **Note**
>
> Retroperitoneal lymphadenopathy is the most important clinical differential diagnosis for an inferior vena cava variant. The latter condition is an absolute contraindication for biopsy, while biopsy is often needed in retroperitoneal lymphadenopathy.

The differential diagnosis also includes other variants of the inferior vena cava such as a double right inferior vena cava.

▶ **Key points.** Variants of the inferior vena cava are relatively common. Although they are usually clinically silent, it is important to be aware of them prior to surgery and interventional procedures.

103

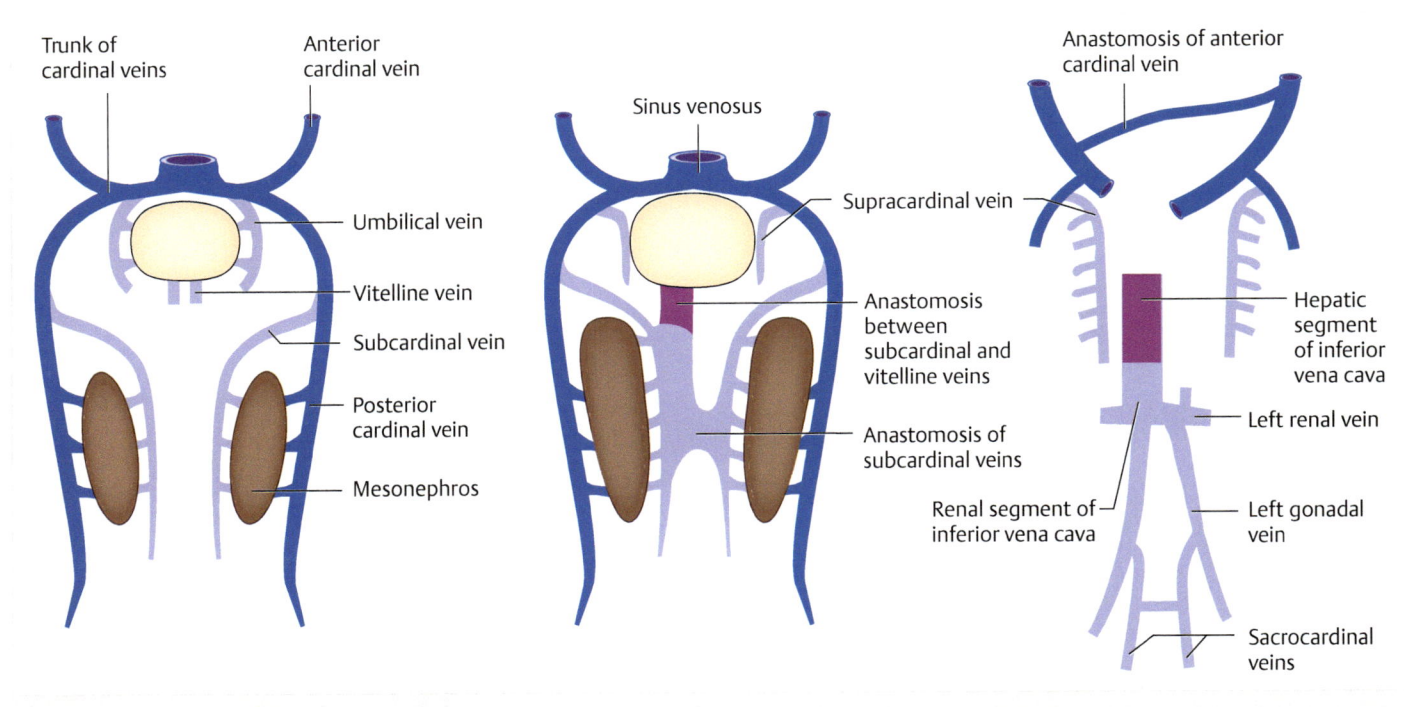

Fig. 3.41 Embryological development of the principal body veins. Schematic representation.

Table 3.9 Overview of typical congenital variants and anomalies of the vena cava

Superior vena cava	Inferior vena cava
• Persistent left superior vena cava • Mirror-image superior vena cava anatomy • Retroaortic left brachiocephalic vein	• Left inferior vena cava • Double inferior vena cava • Agenesis of the infrarenal inferior vena cava • Azygos or hemiazygos continuation • Congenital portocaval shunts • Membranous vena cava obstruction • Retrocaval ureter

Azygos or Hemiazygos Continuation

In this anomaly the infrahepatic segment of the inferior vena cava fails to form at the level of the anastomosis of the subcardinal veins. As a result, the renal veins and more peripheral venous segments drain directly into the azygos vein, while the hepatic veins drain normally to the right atrium via the suprahepatic segment of the inferior vena cava. With a left-sided inferior vena cava, the renal veins drain into the hemiazygos vein. The azygos and hemiazygos veins are markedly dilated due to the increased blood flow. This variant is present in up to 0.6% of the population.

▶ **Imaging signs.** This continuity syndrome is manifested on chest films by widening of the mediastinum, especially at the level of the azygos vein termination. Axial CT typically shows large vessels on the left and right sides of the aorta (the azygos and hemiazygos veins), whose diameters may be comparable to that of the aorta (see ▶ Fig. 3.45b).

▶ **Clinical features.** Generally this variant is asymptomatic. Its association with situs anomalies, asplenia, polysplenia, and congenital heart disease has been described in the literature. The variant assumes major importance prior to gastrointestinal surgery that requires azygos vein ligation, for example, or cardiopulmonary bypass surgery. An awareness of this variant also aids in the planning of right-heart catheterization or pulmonary angiography.

▶ **Differential diagnosis.** The widened azygos vein termination may be mistaken for a paratracheal tumor on chest radiographs. Confusion with retrocrural lymphadenopathy is possible at the level of the diaphragm. The differential diagnosis also includes collateral circulation in response to extrinsic vena cava compression. Differential diagnosis has become much easier, however, owing to the ubiquitous availability of CT.

▶ **Key points.** Due to absence of the infrahepatic segment of the inferior vena cava, the renal veins and more peripheral vascular segments drain into the azygos vein. This leads to marked dilatation of the azygos and hemiazygos veins, which is particularly well demonstrated by sectional imaging. Awareness of this variant is essential before surgical and interventional procedures to ensure that the draining vessels are preserved.

3.2.4 Diseases

Nutcracker Syndrome

▶ **Brief definition.** "Nutcracker syndrome" refers to the compression of the left renal vein between the superior mesenteric artery and aorta or, rarely, the compression of a left renal vein that passes behind the aorta. The compression causes a venous pressure gradient to develop between the inferior vena cava and peripheral renal vein.

3.2 Vena Cava and Large Veins

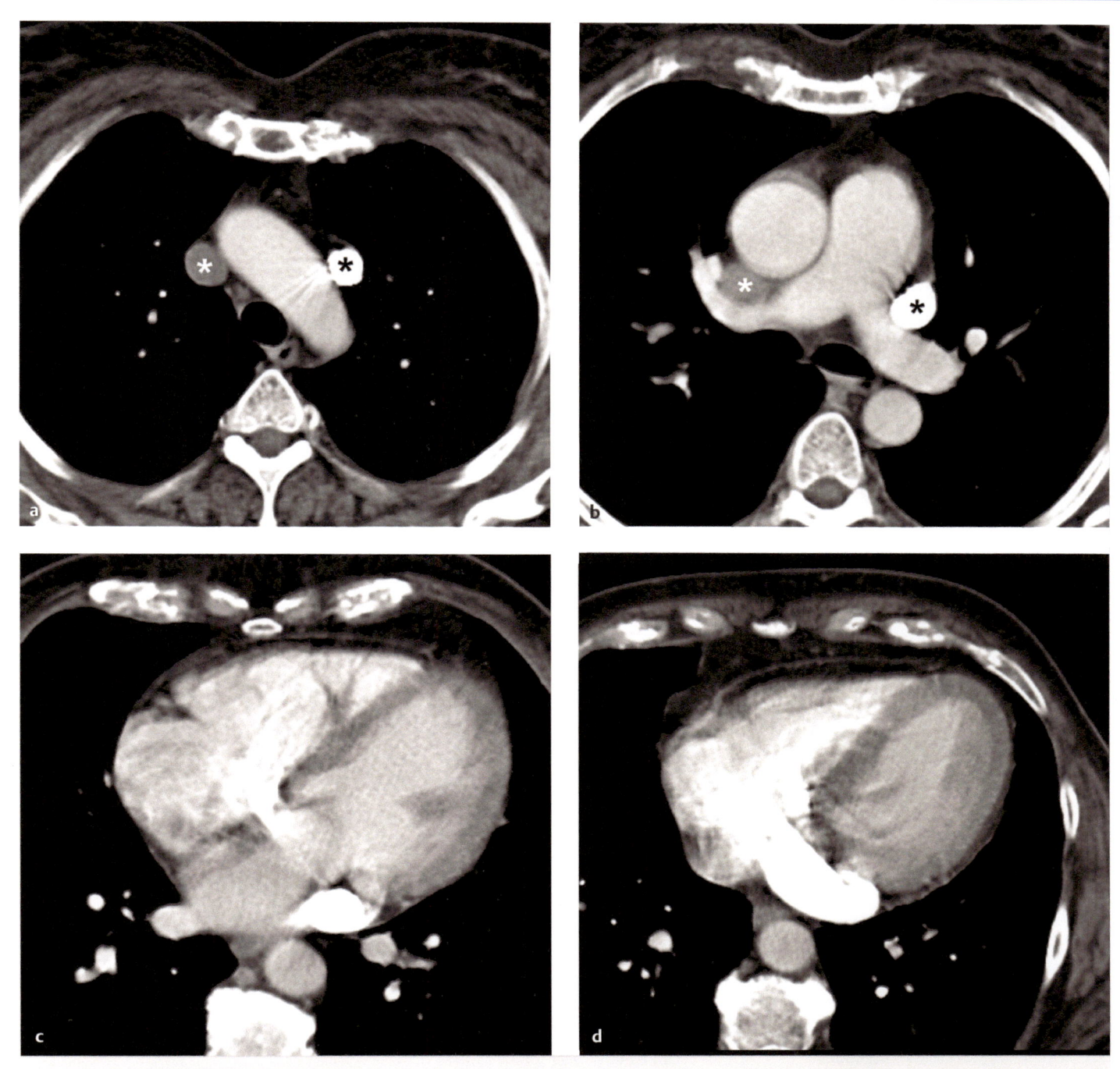

Fig. 3.42 Persistent left superior vena cava. (a) CT with venous injection of contrast medium via the left arm illustrates the course of the opacified persistent left superior vena cava (black asterisk). The right superior vena cava, also present, is not opacified (white asterisk). (b) The right superior vena cava (white asterisk) occupies a normal position, while the persistent left superior vena cava (black asterisk) runs on the left side of the pulmonary arteries. (c) Scan at a lower level shows the persistent left superior vena cava coursing in the left interventricular groove. (d) The persistent left superior vena cava finally drains into the coronary sinus.

▶ **Imaging signs.** Ultrasound has a sensitivity of 78% and specificity of up to 100% in the diagnosis of this condition. Compression of the left renal vein is also well displayed by other sectional modalities. A left-sided varicocele may also be apparent. An established parameter is the diameter of the left renal vein at the renal hilum and at the point of maximum compression. A 3:1 ratio in the supine patient is considered abnormal. Additionally, collaterals may develop in the renal pelvis, and ectasia of the prestenotic renal vein may be noted. The diagnosis is established by an IV pressure measurement showing a pressure differential of at least 3 mm Hg across the stenosis.

▶ **Clinical features.** The clinical presentation is characterized by flank pain or back pain, hematuria, and orthostatic proteinuria. Due to drainage of the left spermatic or ovarian vein into the left renal vein, a left-sided varicocele or pelvic congestion syndrome (pelvic tenderness, dysmenorrhea, dysuria, and dyspareunia) may also be symptomatic of nutcracker syndrome. The spontaneous resolution of symptoms has been reported, especially in children and adolescents. Treatment traditionally consists of surgical transposition of the left renal vein, but the successful use of stents has increasingly been reported.

105

▶ **Differential diagnosis.** The differential diagnosis includes uncomplicated varicoceles, lithiasis, and, less commonly, tumors or pyelonephritis. Nephrotic syndrome and various gastrointestinal disorders may also have a similar clinical presentation.

▶ **Key points.** The nutcracker syndrome involves compression of the left renal vein, leading to a painful pressure rise in the prestenotic segment. In patients with nonspecific imaging findings, invasive pressure measurement can establish the diagnosis after other causes have been excluded.

May–Thurner Syndrome

▶ **Brief definition.** Classic May–Thurner syndrome results from compression of the left common iliac vein between the common iliac artery and L5 vertebral body. Less common variants have been described. The combination of venous compression and pulsatile stress leads to endothelial damage in the compressed vein. Repair mechanisms give rise to the formation of intraluminal webs, canals, or prominences ("venous spurs"). This can cause flow changes that culminate in iliofemoral venous thrombosis. Between 20 and 50% of all patients with left-sided deep vein thrombosis have May–Thurner syndrome as the underlying pathology.

▶ **Imaging signs.** This entity usually presents initially with deep vein thrombosis, which can be accurately diagnosed with ultrasound, MRI, or CT (▶ Fig. 3.43). Typical collateral vessels are the ascending lumbar vein as well as presacral, lumbar, and abdominal-wall veins. Venography should always be performed at multiple levels to ensure detection of the compression site.

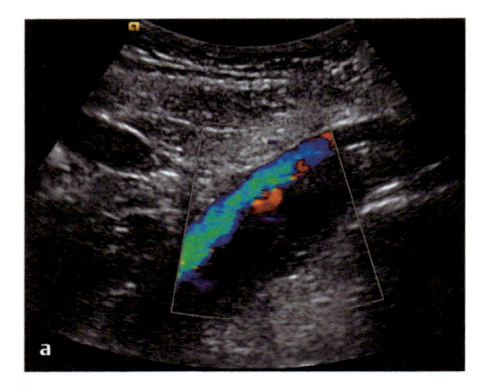

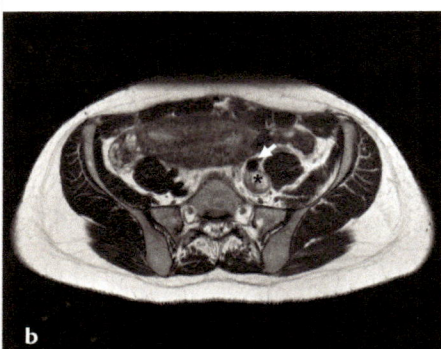

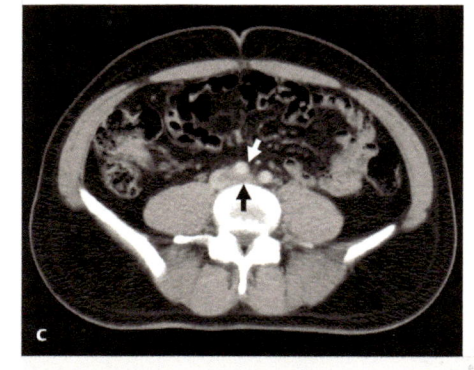

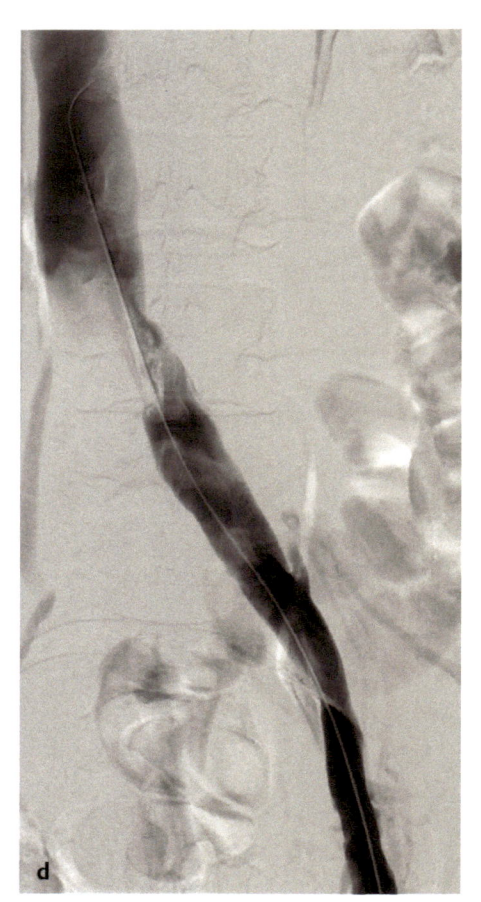

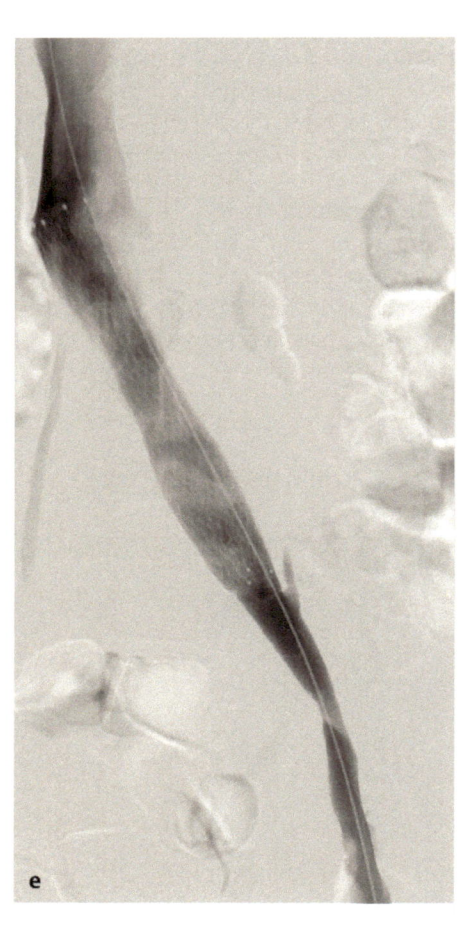

Fig. 3.43 May–Thurner syndrome. (a) May–Thurner syndrome is usually manifested by deep iliac vein thrombosis on the left side, pictured here by ultrasound as a thickened, unperfused vessel closely adjacent to the iliac artery. (b) On T2 W MRI the vein is thickened and shows inhomogeneous increased signal intensity (asterisk), while the adjacent artery appears hypointense owing to its normal high flow (arrow). The artery and vein on the contralateral side had normal hypointense signal. (c) At the site where the common iliac artery (white arrow) crosses over the thickened common iliac vein (black arrow), CT shows narrowing of the vein between the artery and the promontory of the L5 vertebra. The head of the thrombus protrudes into the superior vena cava, which is otherwise patent. (d) Angiogram after thrombolysis shows the typical appearance of a left-sided venous spur. (e) The venous spur was treated interventionally by stent angioplasty.

> **Note**
>
> The IV webs and canals in May–Thurner syndrome can be directly visualized with intravascular ultrasound. A pressure differential of at least 2 mm Hg across the lesion is considered proof of hemodynamic significance and an indication for treatment.

▶ **Clinical features.** May–Thurner syndrome typically presents as acute iliofemoral thrombosis with pain and swelling of the leg. A less common initial presentation is pulmonary embolism. Cases in the chronic stage may develop features of chronic venous insufficiency with varices and skin changes, including possible venous ulceration. Modern treatment options consist mainly of interventional procedures using pharmacomechanical thrombolysis and stent angioplasty.

▶ **Differential diagnosis.** Differentiation is mainly required from spontaneous iliofemoral venous thrombosis. Another possible underlying cause may be extrinsic venous compression by lymph nodes, for example, or a pelvic tumor.

▶ **Key points.** May–Thurner syndrome results from iliocaval compression that leads to deep vein thrombosis. Imaging can demonstrate the iliofemoral thrombosis and underlying compression of the left common iliac vein between the right common iliac artery and the spinal column with high sensitivity and specificity. Treatment is generally interventional.

Superior Vena Cava Syndrome

▶ **Brief definition.** Superior vena cava syndrome results from impaired venous return through the superior vena cava. It may have a variety of malignant and nonmalignant causes.

▶ **Imaging signs.** The imaging modality of choice is CT, as it can quickly demonstrate the entire superior vena cava and collateral pathways. MRI is a good alternative. The extrinsic compression of the superior vena cava and its residual lumen can be directly visualized and quantified with both modalities (▶ Fig. 3.44). The most important indirect sign is the dilatation of collateral vessels, which are not directly visualized by CT or MRI in healthy individuals. Collateral vessels also give an indication of the hemodynamic significance of a stenosis. The presence of dilated collaterals that drain via the azygos and hemiazygos system has a sensitivity of 96% and specificity of 92% in the diagnosis of superior vena cava syndrome. This is important when we consider that a discrepancy often exists between clinical manifestations and the morphological grade of superior vena cava stenosis. Besides the dilatation of collateral veins in the thoracic and abdominal wall, for example, decreased hepatic blood flow may also occur in the early stage, predominantly affecting the quadrate lobe and reflecting a communication between the left portal vein and systemic veins.

▶ **Clinical features.** Typical clinical manifestations of superior vena cava syndrome are neck and facial swelling, dyspnea, and headaches due to brain edema, which may lead to decreased alertness in severe cases. These symptoms are more pronounced when the obstruction also involves the azygos vein, making it unavailable as a collateral vessel.

▶ **Differential diagnosis.** Differential diagnosis centers on identifying the cause of the superior vena cava syndrome. The most common malignant cause is extrinsic compression of the superior vena cava by bronchogenic carcinoma or lymphoma. Mediastinal lymph node metastases are a less frequent cause. Nonmalignant causes include compression by benign tumors such as teratoma, thymoma, a large thoracic aortic aneurysm, or sarcoidosis. A rare benign cause is vena cava compression due to displacement and kinking of that vessel by a tension pneumothorax or by postoperative changes following the repair of a congenital heart defect in children. A special subgroup consists of vascular strictures due to

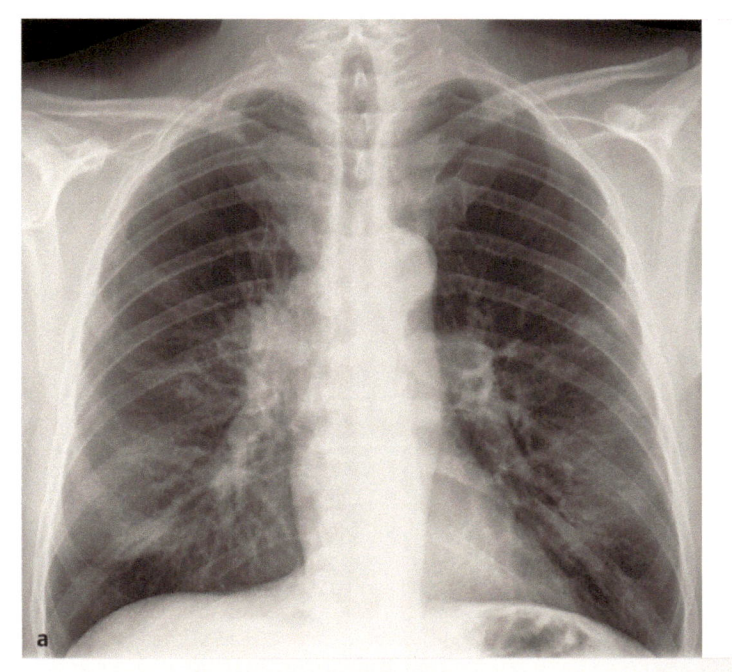

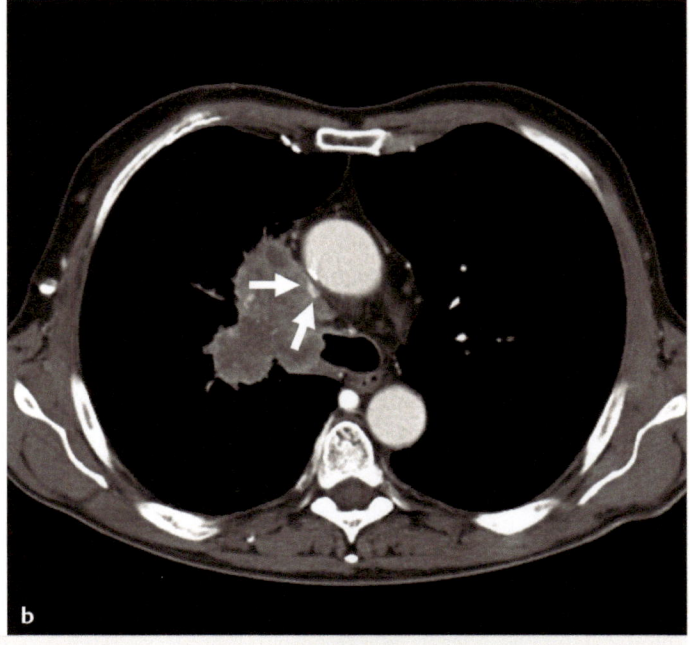

Fig. 3.44 Superior vena cava syndrome. (a) A 63-year-old man with clinical superior vena cava syndrome. Right hilar lung cancer was previously identified in his chest radiograph. (b) CT reveals a filiform stenosis of the superior vena cava (arrows) adjacent to the tumor as the cause of the central venous obstruction.

radiotherapy or chronic catheter placement (repeated central venous catheterization, dialysis access, etc.).

▶ **Key points.** Superior vena cava syndrome results from obstruction of the superior vena cava by extrinsic malignant compression or, less commonly, a variety of nonmalignant causes. Superior vena cava syndrome is generally detectable by CT. The detection of collateral drainage via the azygos vein provides high diagnostic accuracy.

Vena Cava Thrombosis

▶ **Brief definition.** The term *vena cava thrombosis* refers to thrombosis of the superior vena cava or, much more commonly, the inferior vena cava. It belongs to the category of deep vein thrombosis and has an incidence of 4 to 15% in patients with known deep vein thrombosis. Typical risk factors are immobility, right heart failure, dehydration, sepsis, coagulopathies, and malignant disease. Blood flow changes that are due to congenital anomalies, extrinsic compression, or permanent inferior vena cava filters are other known risk factors for vena cava thrombosis. Moreover, tumor thrombus in the vena cava is consistently associated with appositional thrombus formation. Thrombi may become superinfected, producing the features of septic thrombosis. Typical causative organisms are *Staphylococcus aureus*, streptococci, and enterobacteria. Yeasts may cause thrombus infection in the inferior vena cava.

▶ **Imaging signs.** Ultrasound may demonstrate a mass within the vena cava lumen. CT and MRI show a nonenhancing lesion in the vessel lumen or a filling defect in the vein. The absence of enhancement is best appreciated in delayed contrast enhanced imaging obtained approximately 90 to 120 seconds after injection of contrast medium. The intraluminal thrombus may be outlined by contrast medium. Complete obstruction of the vena cava is associated with edematous imbibition of the surrounding fat as an expression of venous congestion. With acute thrombosis, the vascular diameter is initially enlarged and returns to normal over time. Chronic vena cava thrombosis may lead to complete obliteration of the vena cava, leaving only a filiform residual structure in extreme cases (▶ Fig. 3.45). Concomitant involvement of the iliofemoral tributaries is often found. Septic thrombosis is typically associated with the presence of gas inclusions.

▶ **Clinical features.** The clinical hallmarks of acute vena cava thrombosis are superior and inferior vena cava syndrome. Depending on its location, the thrombosis may cause headaches and swelling of the arms or neck, palpebral edema, bilateral lower limb swelling, and possible anasarca. Other possible symptoms are low back pain and a feeling of tension. Phlegmasia cerulea dolens may develop in patients with concomitant iliac vein involvement and insufficient collateral flow. Involvement of the renal veins may lead to flank pain, hematuria, and possible oliguria. With septic thrombosis, the dominant clinical features are those of infection or even septic shock.

▶ **Differential diagnosis.** The most common filling defect in the inferior vena cava is a pseudolesion caused by the inflow of contrast material from the renal veins into the inferior vena cava. This phenomenon produces two columns of opacified blood from the renal veins around a central column of nonopacified blood returning from the lower body. The pseudolesion disappears over time due to mixing and is not seen on delayed images; this distinguishes it from true thrombosis. Primary and secondary malignancies of the inferior vena cava should also be included in the differential diagnosis.

▶ **Key points.** Thrombosis of the inferior vena cava can be confidently diagnosed by imaging. Particularly with isolated vena cava thrombosis, it is important to consider potential causes such as extrinsic compression or the presence of a tumor as this type of thrombosis often has a paraneoplastic cause.

Tumor Thrombi in the Vena Cava

▶ **Brief definition.** A distinction is made between primary and secondary tumors of the vena cava that present as tumor thrombi. Primary tumors are rare; most are leiomyosarcomas arising from the media; see Malignant Vascular Tumors. Tumor thrombi of the vena cava most commonly involve the inferior vena cava and usually result from its invasion by a malignant tumor. Extension of benign tumors into the vena cava is extremely rare (▶ Table 3.10). Appositional thrombi may form on tumor thrombi. Tumor invasion and primary venous tumors from other vascular territories have been reported. For example, tumor thrombi of the portal vein are consistently found in patients with hepatocellular carcinoma.

▶ **Imaging signs.** The imaging findings are similar to those of primary vascular malignancies. All imaging modalities show a filling defect in the vena cava (▶ Fig. 3.46, ▶ Fig. 3.47). In contrast to an uncomplicated thrombus, malignant vascular tumors have a blood supply and therefore enhance after IV injection of contrast medium. This also provides a differentiating criterion from appositional thrombus. Secondary tumor extension into the vena cava shows structural continuity with an extravascular tumor component, thus distinguishing it from other entities. MRI shows enhancement in T1 W sequences and generally shows high signal intensity on T2 W images.

▶ **Clinical features.** Patients usually become symptomatic from the primary tumor, whereas the tumor thrombus is noted as an ancillary finding during investigation of the primary tumor. Possible symptoms range from signs of lower extremity venous congestion to dyspnea (e.g., pulmonary embolism from appositional thrombus). Complications arising from embolized fragments of appositional thrombi are particularly significant.

▶ **Differential diagnosis.** The differential diagnosis includes an artifactual filling defect, uncomplicated vena cava thrombus, and extrinsic compression of the vena cava. Tumor thrombosis in the intrahepatic segment of the inferior vena cava may be mistaken for a hepatic mass.

▶ **Key points.** Tumor thrombi in the vena cava may arise from various benign and malignant diseases. They are generally diagnosed during staging of the primary tumor. A typical imaging sign is an enhancing intraluminal tumor that is in continuity with an extraluminal tumor component.

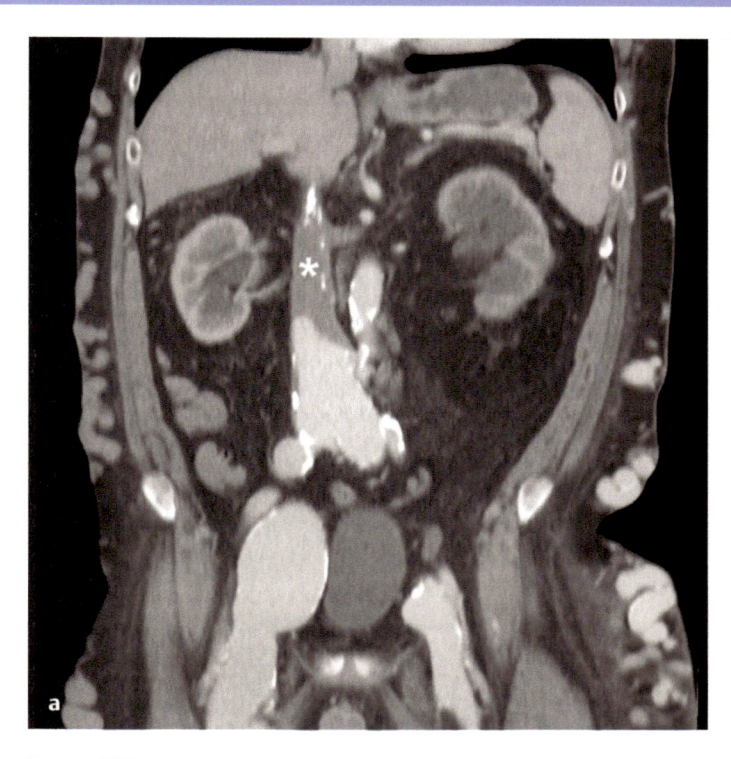

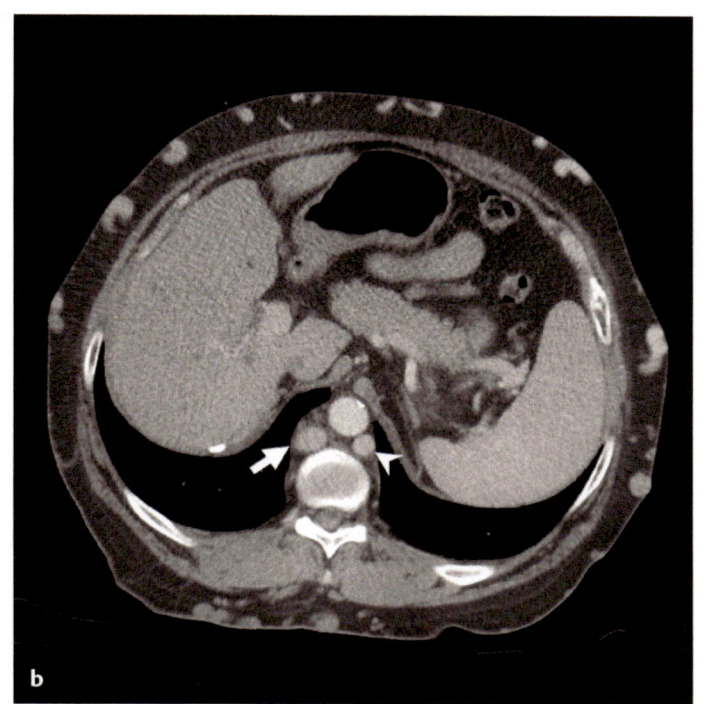

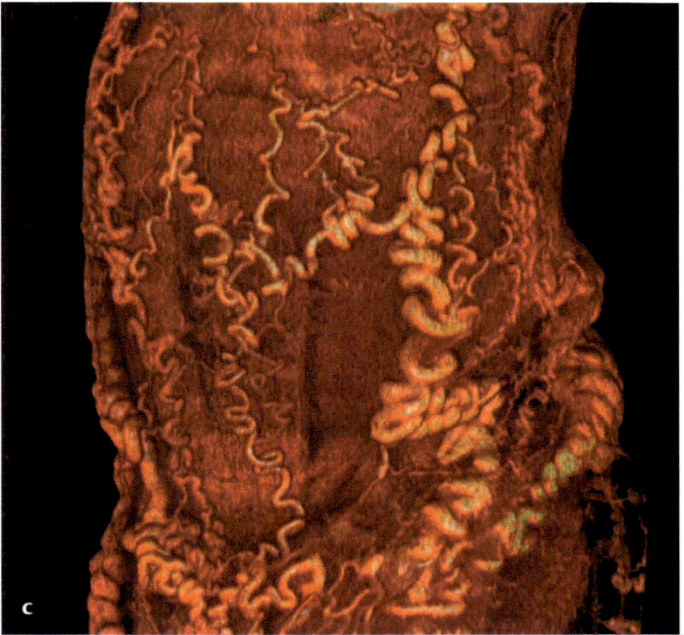

Fig. 3.45 Vena cava thrombosis. (a) Chronic thrombosis of the inferior vena cava (asterisk) in this patient led to severe ectasia of the iliofemoral tributaries with the development of extensive collateral pathways. (b) The deep collaterals drain via the azygos vein (arrow) and hemiazygos (arrowhead) vein, which are markedly dilated. (c) 3D surface-rendered image displays the extent of the superficial collateral veins.

3.3 Pulmonary Vessels

3.3.1 Anatomy

The pulmonary arteries arise from the pulmonary trunk as a continuation of the right ventricular outflow tract. Rule of thumb: The maximum normal diameter of the pulmonary trunk is 3 mm, which is approximately twice that of the pulmonary arteries. The right pulmonary artery generally has a slightly larger caliber than the left. It runs through the aortic arch, passing behind the ascending thoracic aorta, superior vena cava, and right superior pulmonary vein to the hilum of the lung. The left pulmonary artery is shorter and is directed more vertically and posteriorly than the right pulmonary artery. It runs to the left beneath the aortic arch, passing in front of the descending thoracic aorta. It is connected to the aortic isthmus by the ligamentum arteriosum. On reaching the pulmonary hilum, both pulmonary arteries divide in accordance with the segmental anatomy of the lungs. They follow the distribution of the bronchi and bronchioles, continuing as functional end arteries to the alveolar capillary bed. Blood oxygenated in the alveolar capillary bed is received by the pulmonary veins, which converge toward the hilum in the interlobar septa and later the intersegmental septa. Finally, one superior and one inferior venous trunk from each lung—the

Large Vessels

Table 3.10 Causes of tumor thrombi in the vena cava

Primary/secondary causes	Entities
Primary	Leiomyosarcoma
Secondary	
• Benign	Angiomyolipoma
	Pheochromocytoma
	Intravenous leiomyomatosis
• Malignant	Renal cell carcinoma
	Wilms's tumor
	Hepatocellular carcinoma
	Thymoma, thymic carcinoma
	Thyroid carcinoma
	Adrenocortical carcinoma
	Pancreatic carcinoma
	Retroperitoneal lymph node metastases

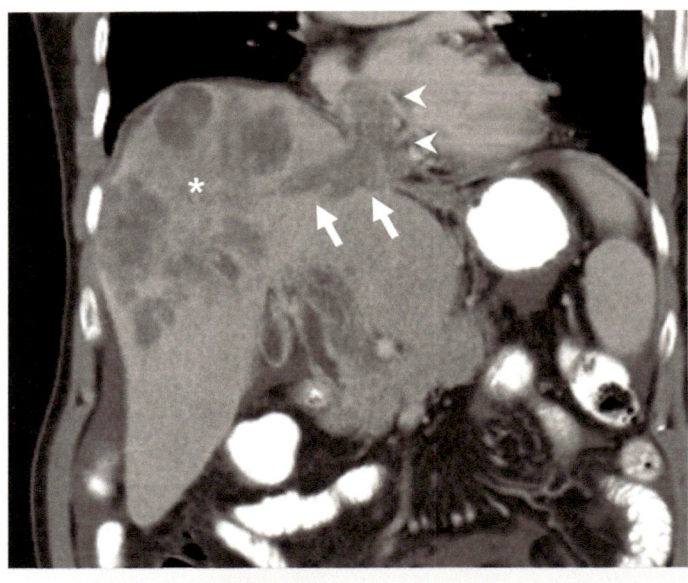

Fig. 3.46 **Malignant tumor thrombus in the inferior vena cava.** Large hepatocellular carcinoma (asterisk) has invaded the hepatic veins (arrows), from which an enhancing tumor thrombus has extended into the right atrium (arrowheads).

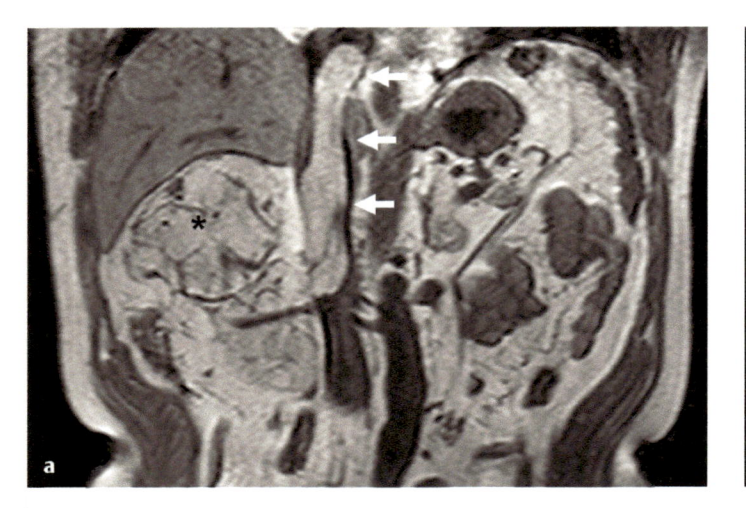

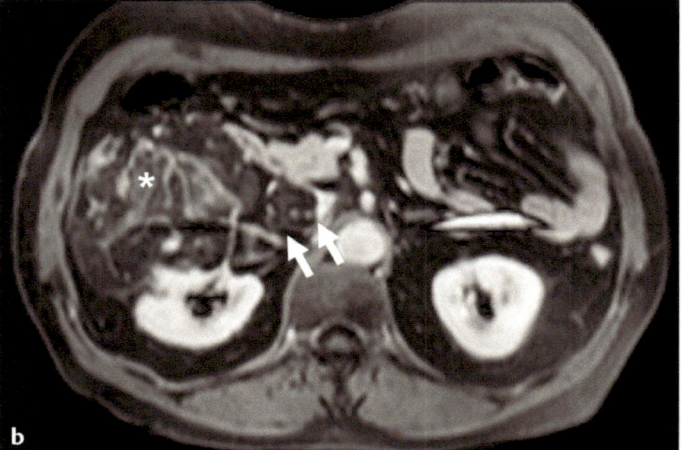

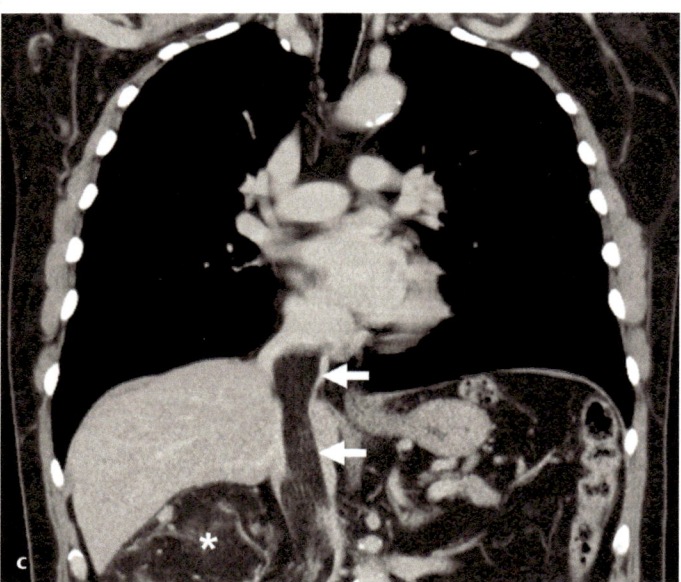

Fig. 3.47 **Benign tumor thrombus of the inferior vena cava.** (a) T2 W image shows a large, inhomogeneous angiomyolipoma of the right kidney, predominantly isointense to fat (asterisk), with extension into the inferior vena cava (arrows). (b) Fat-suppressed image shows analogous findings with a corresponding loss of fat signal (asterisk: angiomyolipoma; arrows: tumor thrombus). (c) CT confirms the finding by showing a tumor of fat attenuation (asterisk) and the tumor thrombus, which is also isodense to fat (arrows).

pulmonary veins—drain into the left atrium from the posterior side. The venous anatomy is somewhat variable, however, and additional veins, especially from the pulmonary middle lobe and lingula, are frequently found. The bronchial arteries and pleurosystemic collaterals complete the pulmonary circulation. These vessels have an important role as *major aortopulmonary collaterals* in patients with congenital disorders.

3.3.2 Development

The proximal pulmonary arteries and ductus arteriosus develop from the proximal segments of the left and right sixth embryonic aortic arch. Buds from the arteries of the sixth branchial arch grow into the primitive lungs and anastomose with the primitive pulmonary circulation. The pulmonary veins develop at the site where the lung bud arises from the gut tube. The intrapulmonary vascular segment subsequently loses its connection with the systemic venous circulation and then can drain only through the pulmonary veins. Flow in the pulmonary veins is very limited during the embryonic period, however.

3.3.3 Congenital Anomalies

Most congenital anomalies of pulmonary vessels occur in conjunction with other cardiovascular anomalies such as pulmonary artery stenosis, pulmonary artery agenesis, or the tetralogy of Fallot (▶ Table 3.11).

Table 3.11 Summary of possible congenital anomalies of the pulmonary circulation

Pulmonary arteries	Pulmonary veins
• Agenesis (main trunk, right pulmonary artery, left pulmonary artery) • Hypoplasia • Congenital stenosis • Pulmonary artery sling • Pulmonary artery arising from the ascending aorta	• Partial anomalous pulmonary venous return • Scimitar syndrome • Total anomalous pulmonary venous return

Pulmonary Artery Agenesis

▶ **Brief definition.** Pulmonary artery agenesis refers to congenital absence of either the pulmonary trunk or the right or left pulmonary artery. This rare anomaly results from abnormal regression of the sixth primitive aortic arch on the affected side. The lung on that side receives its blood supply from the bronchial arteries (major aortopulmonary collaterals) or through a patent ductus arteriosus. While agenesis of the right pulmonary artery may occur in isolation, absence of the left pulmonary artery is typically associated with other cardiac anomalies.

▶ **Imaging signs.** Pulmonary artery agenesis is typically manifested on chest radiographs by an ipsilateral small lung with decreased pulmonary vascular markings. Sectional imaging may show cystic lung changes and major aortopulmonary collaterals, functioning chiefly via the bronchial arteries but also involving the subclavian artery (▶ Fig. 3.48).[28]

▶ **Clinical features.** Left-sided pulmonary artery agenesis usually becomes symptomatic due to associated cardiac anomalies. Otherwise the clinical presentation is variable, with dyspnea as a possible symptom. Hemoptysis has also been reported as an initial finding.

Pulmonary Artery Sling

▶ **Brief definition.** Pulmonary artery sling refers to an anomalous origin of the left pulmonary artery from the distal portion of the right pulmonary artery, proximal to the origin of the right upper lobar artery. The left pulmonary artery then runs behind the trachea to the left, passing anterior to the esophagus. This creates a functional sling around the trachea while also compressing the esophagus from the anterior side (▶ Fig. 3.49). The anomaly is typically associated with localized tracheomalacia. Two types are distinguished on the basis of bronchial anatomy: type I with normal bronchial anatomy and type II with a low position of the carina and an abnormal bronchial bridging segment.

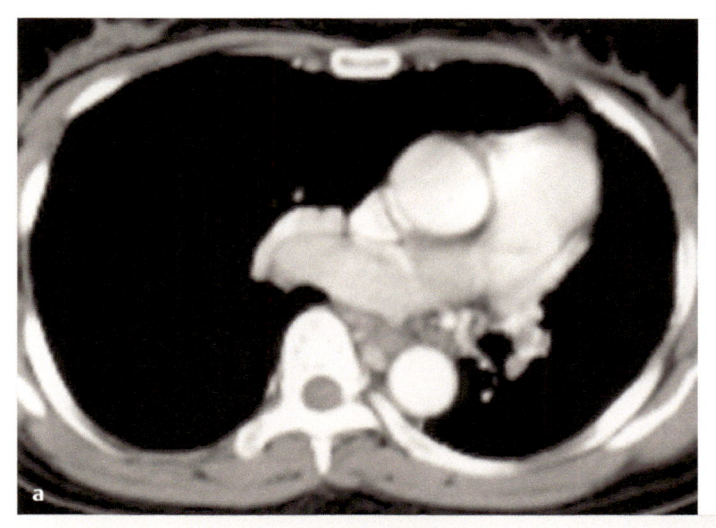

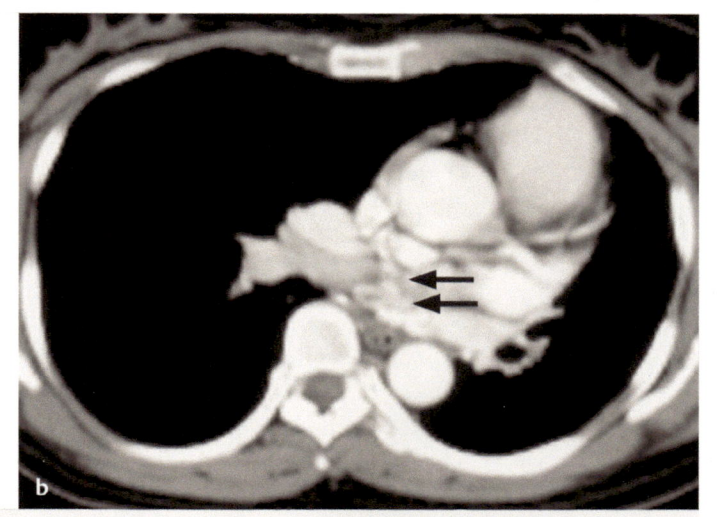

Fig. 3.48 Unilateral pulmonary artery agenesis. (a) Contrast-enhanced CT in this woman documents congenital absence of the left pulmonary artery. (b) Accordingly, the left lung is perfused by large bronchial arteries (arrows).

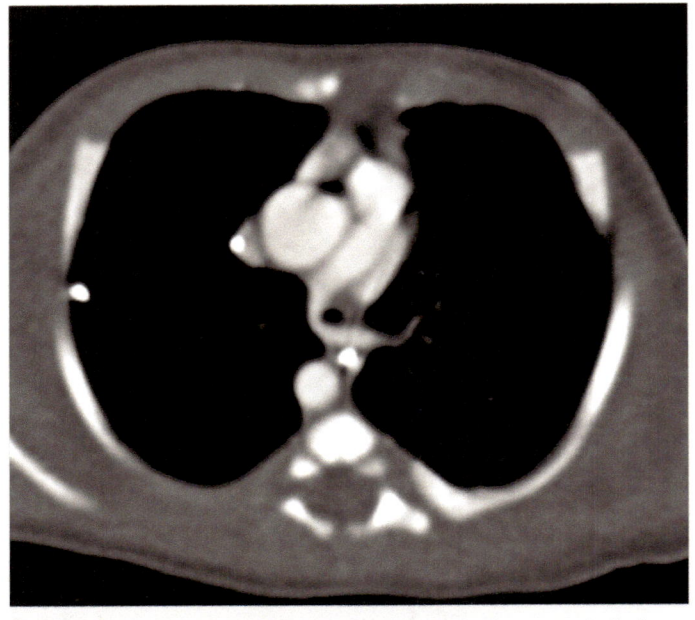

Fig. 3.49 Pulmonary artery sling. Typical arrangement in which the left pulmonary artery runs between the trachea and esophagus. The esophagus is clearly identified in this image by the presence of a gastric tube. This child presented clinically with stridor and frequent vomiting.

▶ **Imaging signs.** A barium esophagogram in the lateral projection may demonstrate anterior compression of the esophagus by a pulmonary artery running posterior to the trachea. This is sometimes visible in the plain chest film. There may also be circumscribed displacement of the trachea toward the right side. CT, MRI, and echocardiography can also aid the diagnosis. MRI has emerged as the modality of choice in the pediatric age group.

▶ **Clinical features.** The clinical presentation is marked by cough, stridor, and frequent vomiting. Recurrent pulmonary infections may also occur.

Anomalous Pulmonary Venous Return

▶ **Brief definition.** Abnormalities in the development of the pulmonary veins are rare and usually involve the proximal embryonic connection to the systemic veins and a failure to establish drainage to the cardinal venous system during embryonic life. This can lead to an anomalous pattern of pulmonary venous drainage that is either complete (total anomalous pulmonary venous return) or incomplete (partial anomalous pulmonary venous return). The most common patterns are anomalous drainage of the pulmonary veins into the superior vena cava, right atrium, or inferior vena cava. With partial anomalous pulmonary venous return, an atrial septal defect is generally present. A significant variant of partial anomalous pulmonary venous return is the scimitar syndrome, in which all or some of the pulmonary veins of the right lung drain into the inferior vena cava, forming the curved shape of a Turkish sword ("scimitar"). Besides the pulmonary veins, the lung itself is often affected in scimitar syndrome, and the anomalous pulmonary venous drainage may be accompanied by sequestration of the right lung.

▶ **Imaging signs.** Prenatal ultrasound has a sensitivity of approximately 85% in the detection of anomalous pulmonary venous return. The main limitation of this technique is a potentially inadequate acoustic window. Scimitar syndrome, as a subtype of partial anomalous pulmonary venous return, is detectable on chest radiographs, appearing as a curved collecting vessel running from the right lung to the inferior vena cava (▶ Fig. 3.50). Most other types of anomalous pulmonary venous return can be directly visualized only by sectional imaging. The choice between high-resolution MRA or CTA depends on the clinical status of the patient. In infants with presumed total anomalous pulmonary venous return, CT is preferred owing to the faster scan time and better access for patient monitoring. Contrast-enhanced MRI is the modality of choice for older children with partial anomalous pulmonary venous return.

▶ **Clinical features.** Total anomalous pulmonary venous return is incompatible with life in children who do not have an associated left-to-right shunt, so early corrective surgery is required. Partial anomalous pulmonary venous return is often asymptomatic. The increased blood flow to the right heart may lead to pulmonary hypertension. These patients also have heightened susceptibility to bronchitis and other infections.

3.3.4 Diseases
Pulmonary Artery Aneurysm

▶ **Brief definition.** An aneurysm denotes the enlargement of a vessel by more than 50% of its normal diameter. Thus, the dilatation of pulmonary vessels as large as a main pulmonary artery trunk to more than 4.5 cm, or the dilatation of central pulmonary arteries to more than 3 cm, is considered to be a (pseudo)aneurysm. Aneurysms and pseudoaneurysms of the pulmonary vessels are rare; the reported prevalence in autopsy series is 1:14,000. The most common causes of pseudoaneurysms are infection, trauma, and malignant tumors. True aneurysms, which by definition involve all layers of the vessel wall, are particularly common in patients with pulmonary arterial hypertension (▶ Table 3.12).

▶ **Imaging signs.** The imaging appearance of pulmonary artery aneurysm is variable, depending on the cause. When the aneurysm is caused by pulmonary arterial hypertension, the chest radiograph will generally show a widened mediastinum and dilated central pulmonary arteries with marked distal pruning. CT identifies the mediastinal widening as a dilated pulmonary artery trunk. In contrast, scans in patients with Behçet's disease will generally show multiple bilateral, perihilar or peripheral circumscribed aneurysms. Iatrogenic or posttraumatic aneurysms typically occur as solitary lesions in the region affected by the trauma or surgery (▶ Fig. 3.51, ▶ Fig. 3.52). Complications such as adjacent bronchial compression, atelectasis, hemorrhage, or postinfarction pneumonia may also be identified. CT typically displays the aneurysms as enhancing fusiform or saccular structures, often with an associated mural thrombus.

▶ **Clinical features.** The clinical presentation frequently includes dyspnea and chest pain. Otherwise there are specific symptoms relating to the underlying disease. Typical aneurysm-associated complications are aneurysmal thrombosis, pulmonary embolism, and compression atelectasis. Larger aneurysms are at greater risk for rupture and require appropriate surgical or interventional treatment.

3.3 Pulmonary Vessels

▶ **Differential diagnosis.** The differential diagnosis includes all types of benign and malignant tumors. Bronchogenic carcinoma, peripheral postinfarction pneumonia, or pulmonary arteriovenous malformations may be misinterpreted as pulmonary artery aneurysms. The differential diagnosis also includes less common infectious lung diseases such as cryptococcosis or aspergillosis. The differential diagnosis of aneurysms of the pulmonary artery trunk should include other central vascular diseases such as aortic aneurysm.

▶ **Key points.** Pulmonary artery aneurysm is a rare disease of the large pulmonary vessels that has a variety of potential underlying causes. Although the aneurysm is often visible on chest radiographs, sectional imaging, especially with CTA, is the diagnostic procedure of choice. The initial imaging work-up should include a detailed investigation of the cause. Larger aneurysms have a particularly high risk of rupture and require prompt surgical or interventional treatment.

Pulmonary Embolism

▶ **Brief definition.** Pulmonary embolism refers to the partial or complete obstruction of a central or peripheral (segmental or subsegmental) pulmonary artery by material that has embolized to the site via the bloodstream. In approximately 90% of cases the embolus is a blood clot, and in approximately 80% of those cases

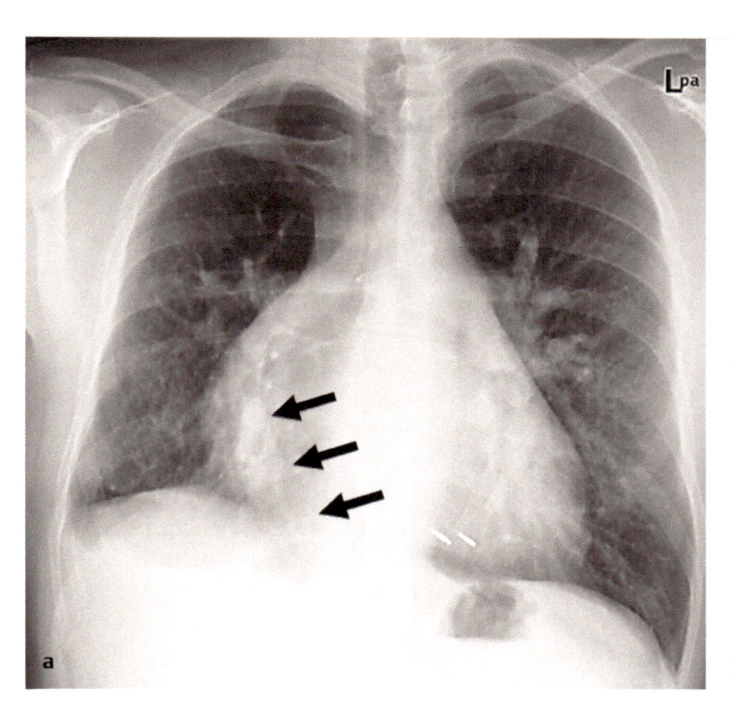

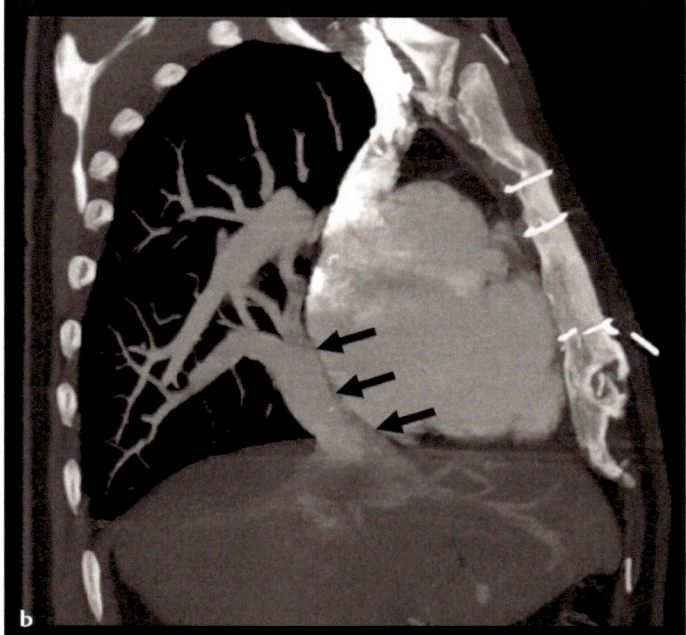

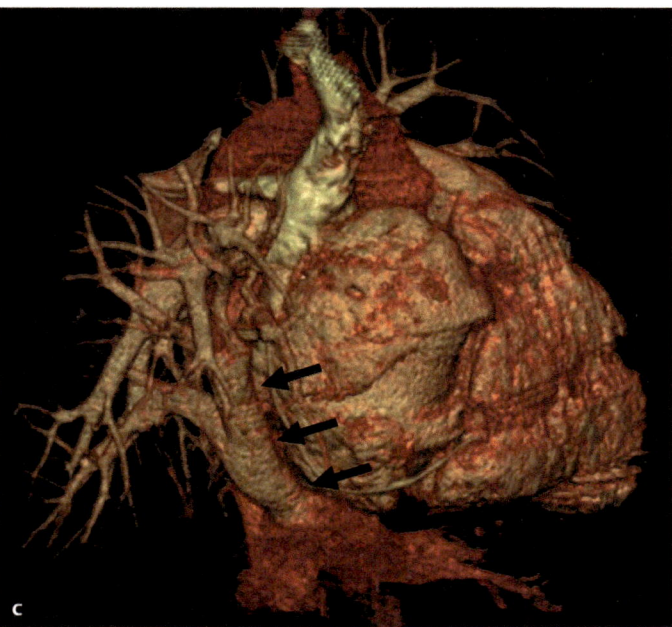

Fig. 3.50 Scimitar syndrome. Scimitar syndrome is a variant of partial anomalous pulmonary venous return. The chest radiograph (a) already shows a saber-shaped pulmonary vein (arrows) running to the inferior vena cava from the lower lobe of the right lung. The maximum intensity projection (b) and 3D reconstruction (c) of CT data confirm the finding and show the abnormal lower lobe vein draining into the inferior vena cava at the confluence of the hepatic veins. (a) PA chest radiograph. (b) Maximum intensity projection of CT data. (c) 3D reconstruction of CT data.

Large Vessels

Table 3.12 Classification of aneurysms of the pulmonary arteries and veins[29]

Pulmonary arterial aneurysms	Pulmonary venous aneurysms
Congenital: • Valvular/postvalvular stenosis • Left-to-right shunt with increased pulmonary arterial flow • Connective tissue diseases (e.g., Marfan's syndrome, Ehlers–Danlos syndrome, Williams–Beuren syndrome) *Acquired*: • Pulmonary arterial hypertension • Cystic medial necrosis • Vasculitis (e.g., Behçet's disease, Hughes–Stovin syndrome) • Infection (e.g., tuberculosis with Rasmussen's aneurysm, purulent inflammations, syphilis) • Endocarditis • Malignant neoplasms • Trauma • Iatrogenic • Idiopathic	• Varices • Arteriovenous malformation (especially Rendu-Osler-Weber disease) • Mitral valve diseases

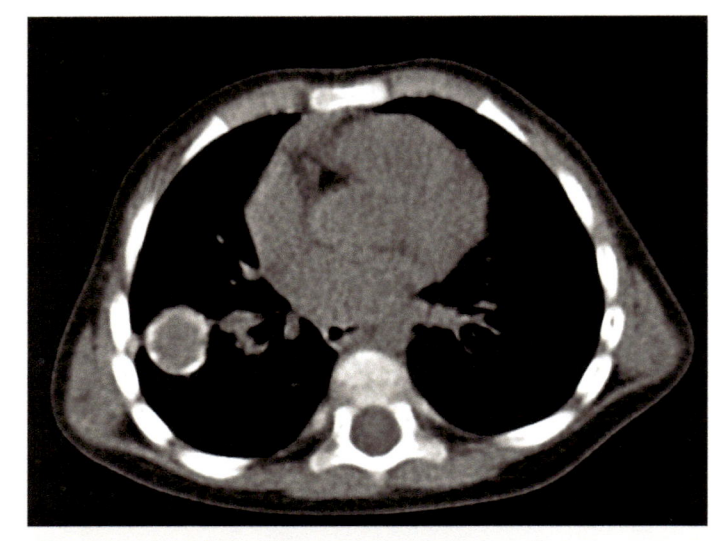

Fig. 3.51 Idiopathic pulmonary artery aneurysm. The aneurysm appears on unenhanced CT as a peripheral round mass with residual rim enhancement after previous pulmonary angiography. The central isodense portions represent a thrombus within the aneurysm.

the clot has originated from a site of deep venous thrombosis in the iliac or lower extremity veins. There are a number of other, rare causes of embolism that should be considered in the differential diagnosis. They include septic embolism, gas embolism, fat embolism, tumor embolism, and amniotic fluid embolism. The prevalence of pulmonary embolism is approximately 0.4%.[30] With a mortality rate of up to 30%, pulmonary embolism is the third leading cause of cardiovascular death after myocardial infarction and stroke. Typical risk factors are age, obesity, prior pulmonary embolism, malignancy, recent surgery, prolonged bed rest or paresis, and thrombophilia. Chronic pulmonary embolism is a condition in which residual thrombi persist despite the high thrombolytic capacity of the lung.

▶ **Imaging signs.** The chest radiograph is relatively insensitive and nonspecific, although predominantly right-sided cardiomegaly and increased lucency in peripheral lung zones (Westermark sign) may be suggestive (▶ Fig. 3.53). Chronic pulmonary embolism is associated with signs of pulmonary arterial hypertension, including dilated central pulmonary arteries. The ventilation/perfusion scan, once considered the gold standard, shows perfusion defects with normal ventilation in the affected area (▶ Fig. 3.54). This ventilation/perfusion mismatch is indicative of pulmonary embolism. Important differential diagnoses such as acute aortic pathology, pneumothorax, or neoplasms are not directly detectable by this technique, however. For this reason, CTA of the pulmonary arteries has become the established clinical gold standard and is included in current diagnostic algorithms.[31] CTA can directly visualize the partial or complete occlusion of one or more pulmonary arterial segments (▶ Fig. 3.55, ▶ Fig. 3.56). With a complete occlusion, the vascular diameter is often larger than the diameter of the accompanying bronchus. A partial obstruction may be peripheral or central and exhibit a central target pattern. Indirect signs are subpleural, wedge-shaped areas of consolidation due to postinfarction pneumonia. Acute signs of right heart overload are enlargement of the right ventricle (ratio of right to left ventricle > 1), paradoxical bowing of the ventricular septum to the left, and reflux of contrast medium into the hepatic veins due to functional tricuspid insufficiency. MRA has not come into wide clinical use. A multicenter study found an average sensitivity of 78% and sensitivity of 99%, with 25% of cases excluded due to technically inadequate results.[32] Direct signs of chronic pulmonary embolism (in contrast to acute pulmonary embolism) are partial recanalization of the vessel with residual mural filling defects that appear as wall thickening or with residual intravascular webs. Chronic thrombi may exhibit calcifications. Local stenosis and poststenotic vascular dilatation may be found; complete vascular occlusion is rare. Possible indirect signs are scars or wedge-shaped subpleural defects secondary to lung infarction. There may also be a mosaic perfusion pattern with sharply circumscribed lung areas of increased and decreased density.

▶ **Clinical features.** The clinical manifestations of pulmonary embolism are variable. The acute stage is characterized by chest pain, hypotension, hemoptysis, cough, tachycardia, tachypnea, cardiac arrhythmia, lower limb swelling (as evidence of deep vein thrombosis due to venous thromboembolism), and lower limb

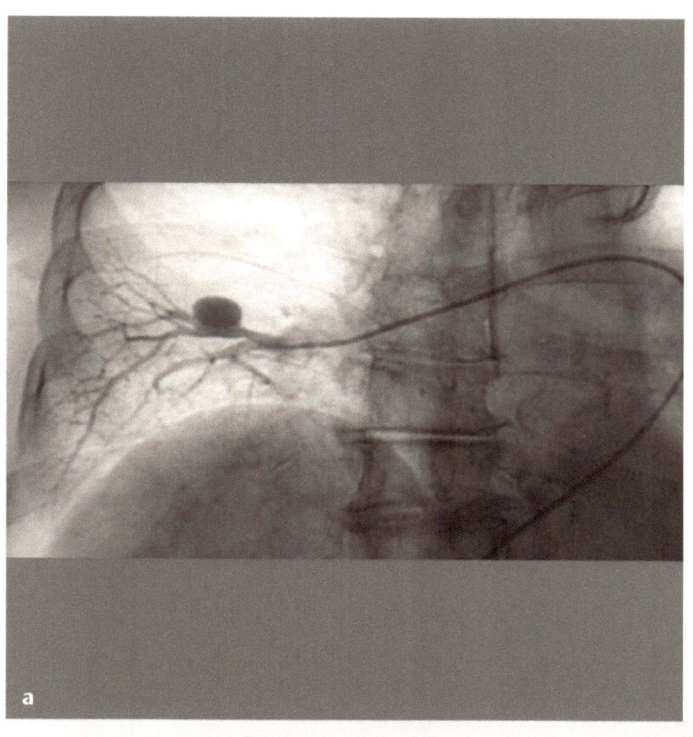

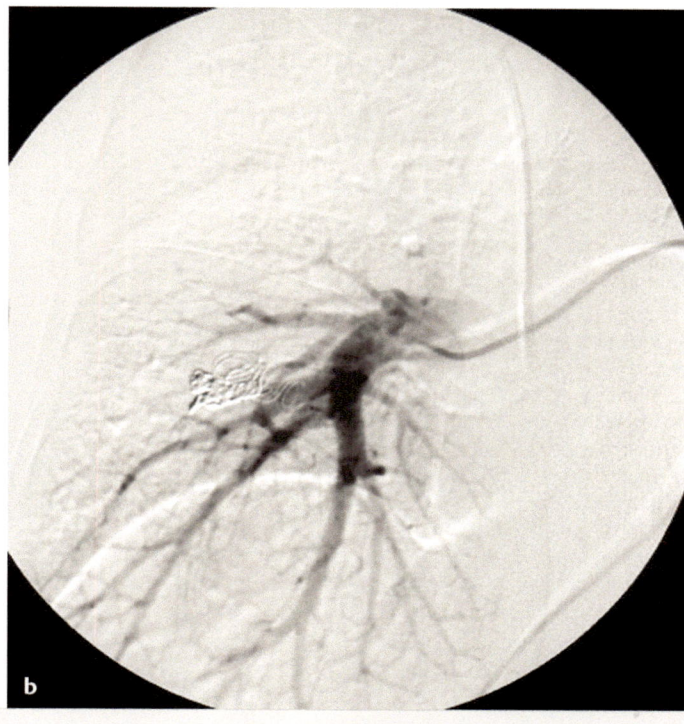

Fig. 3.52 Iatrogenic pulmonary artery aneurysm. Pulmonary angiography 6 months after lung biopsy. **(a)** Vessel feeding the aneurysm. **(b)** Image after interventional embolization confirms that the aneurysm has been obliterated.

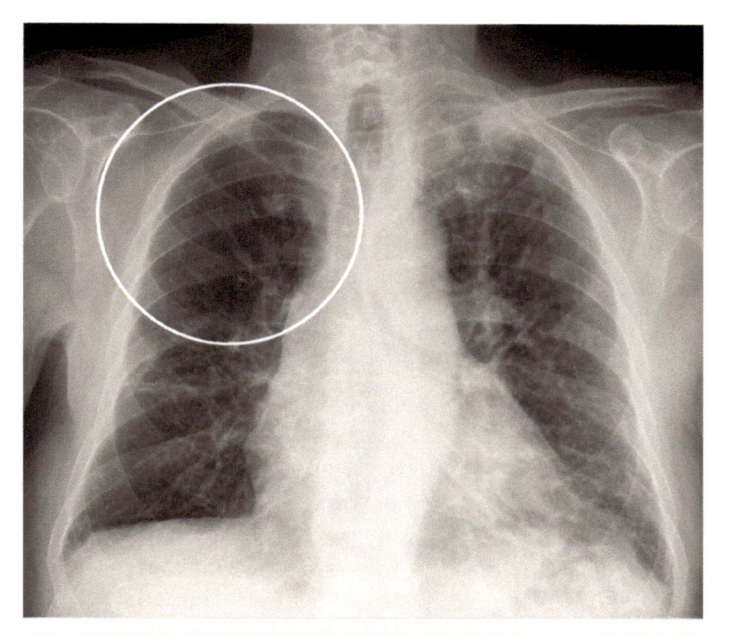

Fig. 3.53 Pulmonary embolism. In rare cases pulmonary embolism is manifested on the plain chest radiograph by predominantly right-sided cardiac enlargement and decreased pulmonary vascular markings, or increased lucency, peripheral to the embolus (circle). This is called the Westermark sign.

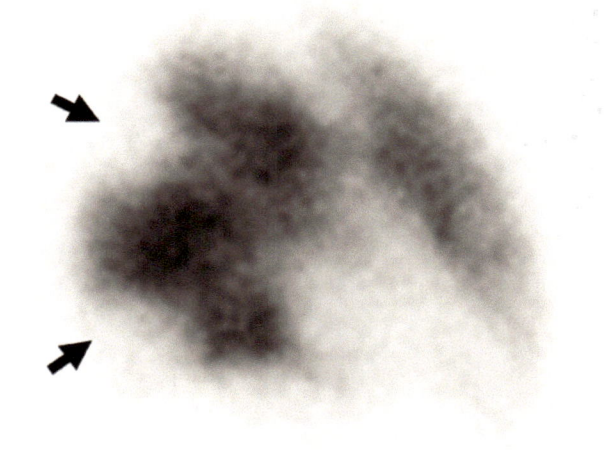

Fig. 3.54 Pulmonary embolism. Perfusion lung scan in a 29-year-old man with known resistance to activated protein C and a presumed pulmonary embolism. Ventilation scan was normal (not shown). The perfusion scan demonstrates multiple (sub)segmental perfusion defects as a result of the embolism. (Reproduced with kind permission of Dr. A. Pfestroff, Department of Nuclear Medicine, University Hospital of Giessen and Marburg, Germany.)

pain. Other common symptoms are chest pain with respiratory excursions and hypotension ranging to shock. The embolism compromises the oxygen supply to dependent lung areas, which may lead to (partial) pulmonary infarction as well as postinfarction pneumonia if superinfection occurs. Especially with recurrent embolisms (also called chronic pulmonary embolism), chronic pulmonary arterial hypertension may develop over time.

▶ **Differential diagnosis.** The differential diagnosis of pulmonary embolism is based on the cardinal symptoms of chest pain, dyspnea, and hemodynamic instability. Accordingly, the

Large Vessels

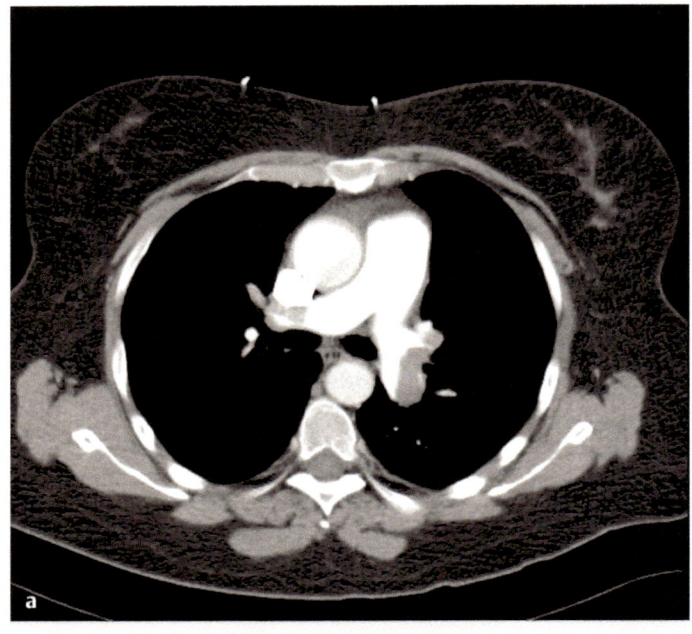

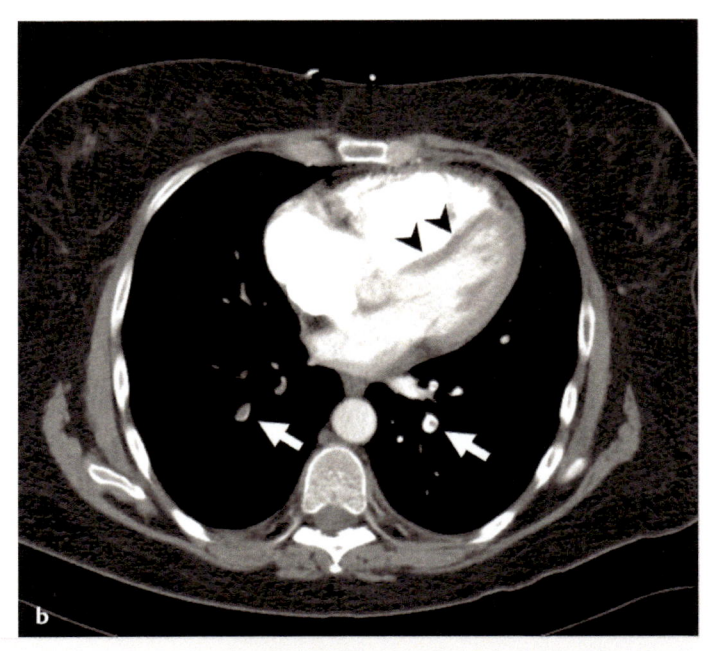

Fig. 3.55 Central pulmonary embolism with subsegmental vascular occlusions. (a) Acute pulmonary embolism with a central embolus. (b) Subsegmental vascular occlusions are also present (arrows). The scan additionally shows an enlarged right ventricle with paradoxical bowing of the septum to the left (arrowheads) as a sign of right heart overload.

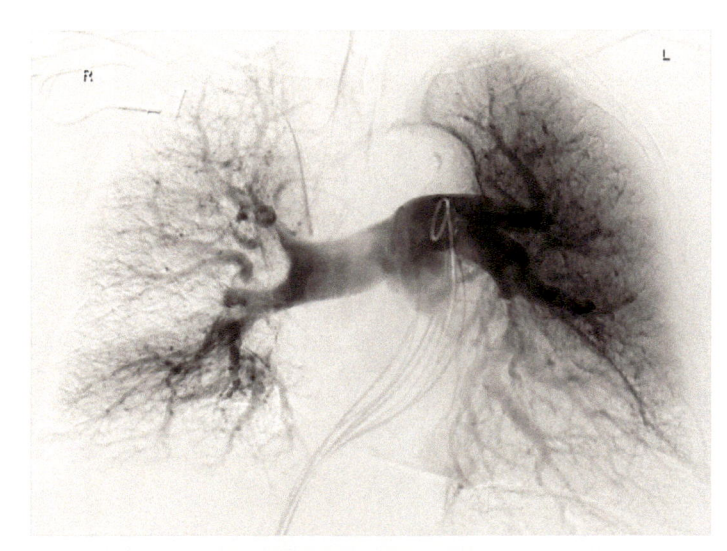

Fig. 3.56 Central pulmonary embolism with subsegmental vascular occlusions in a different patient from that in ▶ Fig. 3.55. Pulmonary angiogram shows filling defects and marked hypoperfusion of the right lung and the lower lobe of the left lung. The left upper lobe and portions of the right lower lobe show normal perfusion.

most important clinical differential diagnoses are myocardial infarction, acute aortic syndrome, pneumonia, and pneumothorax, which require imaging studies for differentiation. The radiological differential diagnosis should include primary tumors (sarcoma) of the pulmonary arteries, vasculitis, idiopathic arterial hypertension, and fibrosing mediastinitis. As well as confirming pulmonary embolism, an important imaging task is to differentiate its causes whenever possible and exclude nonthromboembolic causes such as septic embolism, gas embolism, fat embolism, tumor embolism, and amniotic fluid embolism.[33]

▶ Key points. Acute pulmonary embolism is a common emergency diagnosis with a high mortality rate. Prompt diagnosis is essential, with CTA of the pulmonary arteries being the diagnostic modality of choice. Typical signs of acute pulmonary embolism are unifocal or multifocal filling defects in the pulmonary vessels. Incomplete resolution of the thrombi leads to chronic pulmonary embolism.

Pulmonary Hypertension

▶ Brief definition. Pulmonary hypertension and pulmonary arterial hypertension constitute a group of disorders that are associated with elevation of blood pressure in the pulmonary circulation. Pulmonary hypertension is present if the mean pulmonary artery pressure is greater than 25 mm Hg at rest or greater than 30 mm Hg during exercise. In addition to the rare idiopathic pulmonary hypertension, there are numerous causes of secondary pulmonary hypertension. The most common causes include chronic pulmonary embolism (chronic thromboembolic pulmonary hypertension) and chronic obstructive pulmonary disease (COPD). The classification of pulmonary hypertension is based on its causes (▶ Table 3.13).

▶ Imaging signs. The basic imaging workup of presumed pulmonary hypertension includes echocardiography and plain chest radiography (▶ Fig. 3.57). Pulmonary hypertension can be diagnosed by echocardiography with a high degree of confidence. The chest radiograph can reveal signs of pulmonary hypertension as

Table 3.13 Simplified Nice classification of pulmonary hypertension[34]

Group	Subgroup	Description
1		Pulmonary arterial hypertension
	1.1	Idiopathic pulmonary arterial hypertension
	1.2	Heritable pulmonary arterial hypertension
	1.3	Drug- and toxin-induced pulmonary arterial hypertension
	1.4	Pulmonary arterial hypertension associated with: • Connective tissue diseases • HIV infection • Portal hypertension • Congenital heart disease • Schistosomiasis • Chronic hemolytic anemia
1'		Pulmonary veno-occlusive disease and/or pulmonary capillary hemangiomatosis
1"		Persistent pulmonary hypertension of the newborn
2		Pulmonary hypertension due to left heart diseases
3		Pulmonary hypertension due to lung diseases and/or hypoxemia
	3.1	COPD
	3.2	Interstitial lung disease, etc.
4		Chronic thromboembolic pulmonary hypertension
5		Pulmonary hypertension with unclear multifactorial mechanisms
	5.1	Hematologic disorders: • Chronic hemolytic anemia • Myeloproliferative disorders • Splenectomy
	5.2	Systemic disorders: • Sarcoidosis • Pulmonary histiocytosis • Lymphangioleiomyomatosis
	5.3	Metabolic disorders: • Glycogen storage disease • Gaucher's disease • Thyroid disorders
	5.4	Others: • Tumoral obstruction • Fibrosing mediastinitis • Chronic renal failure • Segmental pulmonary hypertension

well as the underlying disease. Important potential underlying diseases are interstitial lung disease, COPD, and pulmonary emphysema, as well as cardiac causes of pulmonary hypertension. The classic signs of pulmonary hypertension (dilatation of the interlobar segment of the right pulmonary artery to at least 16 mm and right ventricular enlargement) are detectable only in advanced stages of the disease. CTA of the pulmonary arteries is more sensitive and, as well as showing direct vascular signs, supplies more information on cardiac and parenchymal lung changes. Dilatation of the central pulmonary arteries to at least 29 mm, together with enlargement of the segmental pulmonary arteries to exceed the bronchial diameter (ratio of arterial to bronchial diameter > 1:1), is 100% specific for a diagnosis of pulmonary hypertension in patients without concomitant interstitial lung disease. A ratio of the pulmonary artery trunk and ascending aortic diameters greater than 1:1 likewise has a sensitivity and specificity greater than 90% in the detection of pulmonary hypertension. Signs of chronic pulmonary embolism may indicate chronic thromboembolic pulmonary hypertension.

Cardiac signs are:
- Thickening of the right ventricular wall to more than 4 mm.
- Right ventricular enlargement (ratio of right to left ventricle greater than 1:1).
- In extreme cases, abnormal left convex bowing of the ventricular septum.

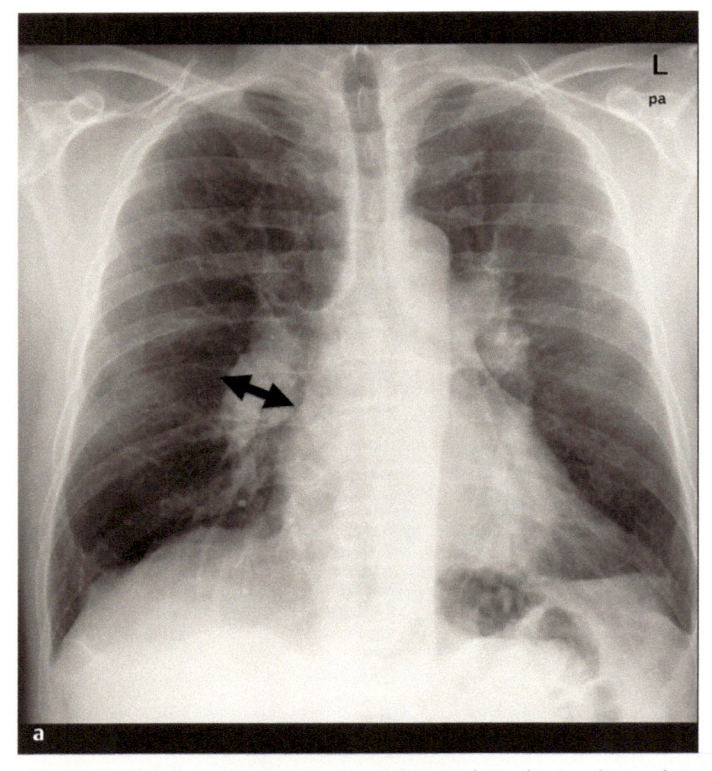

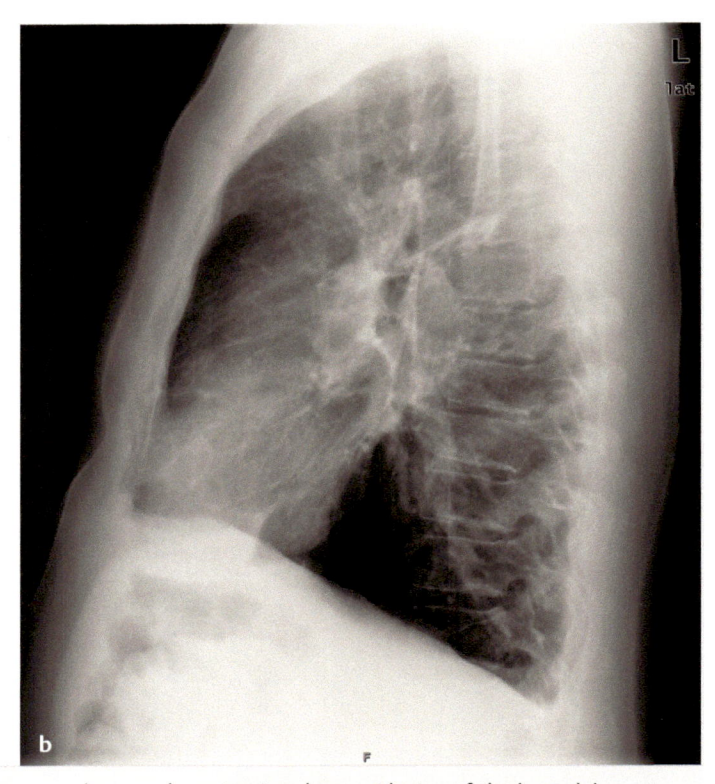

Fig. 3.57 Pulmonary hypertension. (a) Typical PA chest radiograph in severe pulmonary hypertension shows widening of the lower lobar artery (here 2.4 cm, double-headed arrow) and distal pruning of the pulmonary vessels. (b) Lateral radiograph shows marked flattening of the diaphragm and hyperlucency of the retrocardiac space as a sign of pulmonary emphysema, considered to be the cause of pulmonary hypertension in this patient.

Dilatation of the inferior vena cava and hepatic veins is also indicative of right heart overload. The reduced ejection fraction of the right ventricle can be quantitatively evaluated by cardiac MRI or ECG-gated CT. Ventilation/perfusion scanning can confirm a presumptive diagnosis of chronic thromboembolic pulmonary hypertension; nowadays it is usually supplemented by CTA. Additionally, cardiac MRI can provide a direct quantitative approach by permitting the evaluation of right ventricular function and noninvasive measurements of pulmonary arterial pressure and flow. A significant right ventricular pressure load also leads to the characteristic pattern of delayed myocardial enhancement at the junction of the right and left ventricles.

▶ **Clinical features.** The clinical presentation is extremely variable. In mild pulmonary hypertension, symptoms usually appear only during exercise. At pressures of approximately 50 mm Hg or more, symptoms are also present at rest and may consist of fatigue, reduced exercise tolerance, syncope, angina pectoris, Raynaud's phenomenon, and peripheral edema. These symptoms result from a steady decline in cardiac output due to disease-related right heart failure.

▶ **Differential diagnosis.** Differential diagnosis is based on the classification of pulmonary hypertension. The Nice classification forms the basis for the radiological differential diagnosis, which covers almost all organ systems (see ▶ Table 3.13).

▶ **Key points.** "Pulmonary hypertension" is a collective term for a complex array of diseases in various organ systems that lead to pressure elevation in the pulmonary circulation. Chronic thromboembolic pulmonary hypertension, COPD, and interstitial lung diseases are particularly relevant to imaging. But hematologic and metabolic disorders are also detectable by imaging and may underlie pulmonary hypertension.

Arteriovenous Malformations

▶ **Brief definition.** Pulmonary arteriovenous malformation is defined as an abnormal connection (shunt) between the pulmonary arterial and pulmonary venous systems. Arteriovenous malformations may be congenital or acquired (trauma, infection, surgery). More than 80% of arteriovenous malformations are congenital, and most of these are associated with hereditary hemorrhagic telangiectasia (Rendu-Osler-Weber disease). Pulmonary arteriovenous malformations have a predilection for the lower lobes. Multiple lesions can usually be detected, especially in patients with hereditary hemorrhagic telangiectasia. It is important clinically to distinguish a simple shunt connection fed by a pulmonary artery branch from a complex form with more than one feeding or draining vessel.

▶ **Imaging signs.** Contrast echocardiography can be used for screening, although it provides information only on the presence

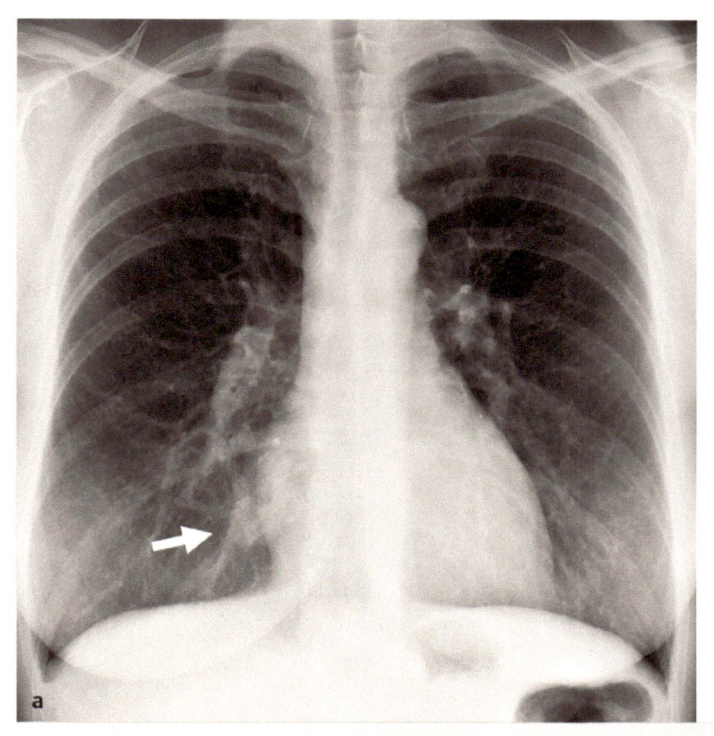

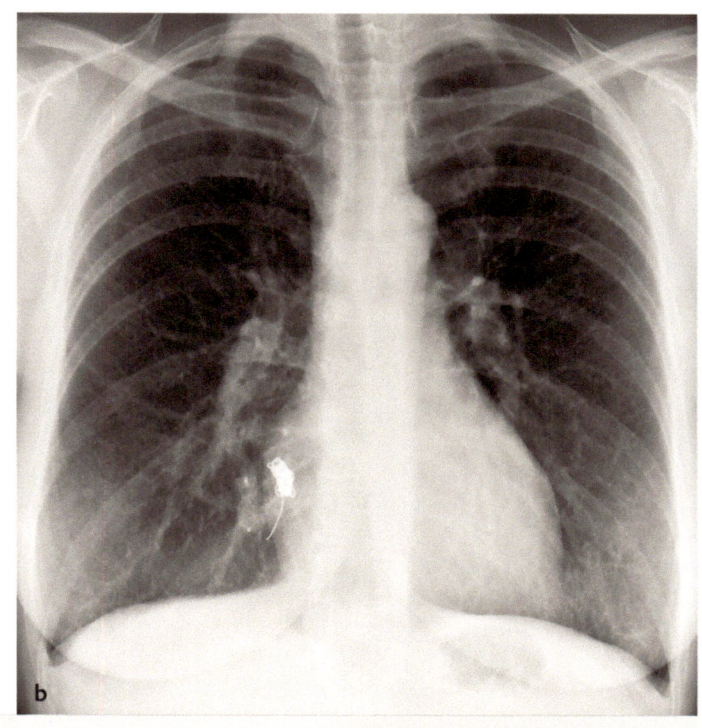

Fig. 3.58 Pulmonary arteriovenous malformation. (a) Chest radiograph of a pulmonary arteriovenous malformation prior to embolization. The large arteriovenous malformation appears only as a paracardiac nodule (arrow) in the radiograph. **(b)** Chest radiograph of the pulmonary arteriovenous malformation after embolization. The embolic material (Amplatzer plug and metal coils) used to occlude the two feeding vessels is clearly visualized. The radiograph confirms that the material has not been dislodged.

of shunts, not on their location or morphology. Chest radiographs can demonstrate arteriovenous malformations as pulmonary nodules, often with an associated feeding and draining vessel (▶ Fig. 3.58). Lesions smaller than 1 cm are consistently missed on chest radiographs, so early sectional imaging is advised. The modality of choice is thin-slice CT supplemented by maximum intensity projections (▶ Fig. 3.59). Unenhanced CT is adequate if only pulmonary arteriovenous malformations are being sought, but because arteriovenous malformations may also occur in other organs, especially in hereditary hemorrhagic telangiectasia, the study should include IV injection of contrast medium with evaluation of the upper abdominal organs, especially the liver. The former gold standard of diagnostic digital subtraction angiography (DSA) is no longer necessary and today has a role only in treatment. Contrast-enhanced MRI can be used for follow-up.

▶ **Clinical features.** The typical symptoms of pulmonary arteriovenous malformations are dyspnea, cyanosis, hemoptysis and, very rarely, hemothorax. The arteriovenous shunt may give rise to paradoxical emboli with cerebral infarction and brain abscess. The dominant features in these cases are neurologic symptoms such as headaches, fever, seizures, altered mental status, and focal neurologic symptoms. On the whole, the clinical manifestations are highly variable.

▶ **Differential diagnosis.** Besides malignancies, differentiation is mainly required from other diseases that may cause peripheral pulmonary aneurysms such as Behçet's disease, Hughes–Stovin syndrome, and infections, most notably tuberculosis (Rasmussen aneurysm). The differential diagnosis should also include other diseases that are associated with peripheral pulmonary nodules on radiographs, although sectional imaging can usually exclude these disorders through the characteristic appearance of arteriovenous malformations with feeding and draining vessels.

▶ **Key points.** Pulmonary arteriovenous malformations are most commonly observed in patients with hereditary hemorrhagic telangiectasia. They are easily diagnosed at CT. Besides the diagnosis of arteriovenous malformations, imaging is also used to determine the number of feeding and draining vessels and direct the planning of interventional or surgical treatment.

> **Caution**
>
> Remember that arteriovenous malformations may also occur in other organ regions (e.g., the liver), especially in patients with hereditary hemorrhagic telangiectasia. Moreover, new arteriovenous malformations may become apparent after treatment. Arteriovenous malformations that are already embolized may recanalize, underscoring the need for regular follow-up that includes imaging.

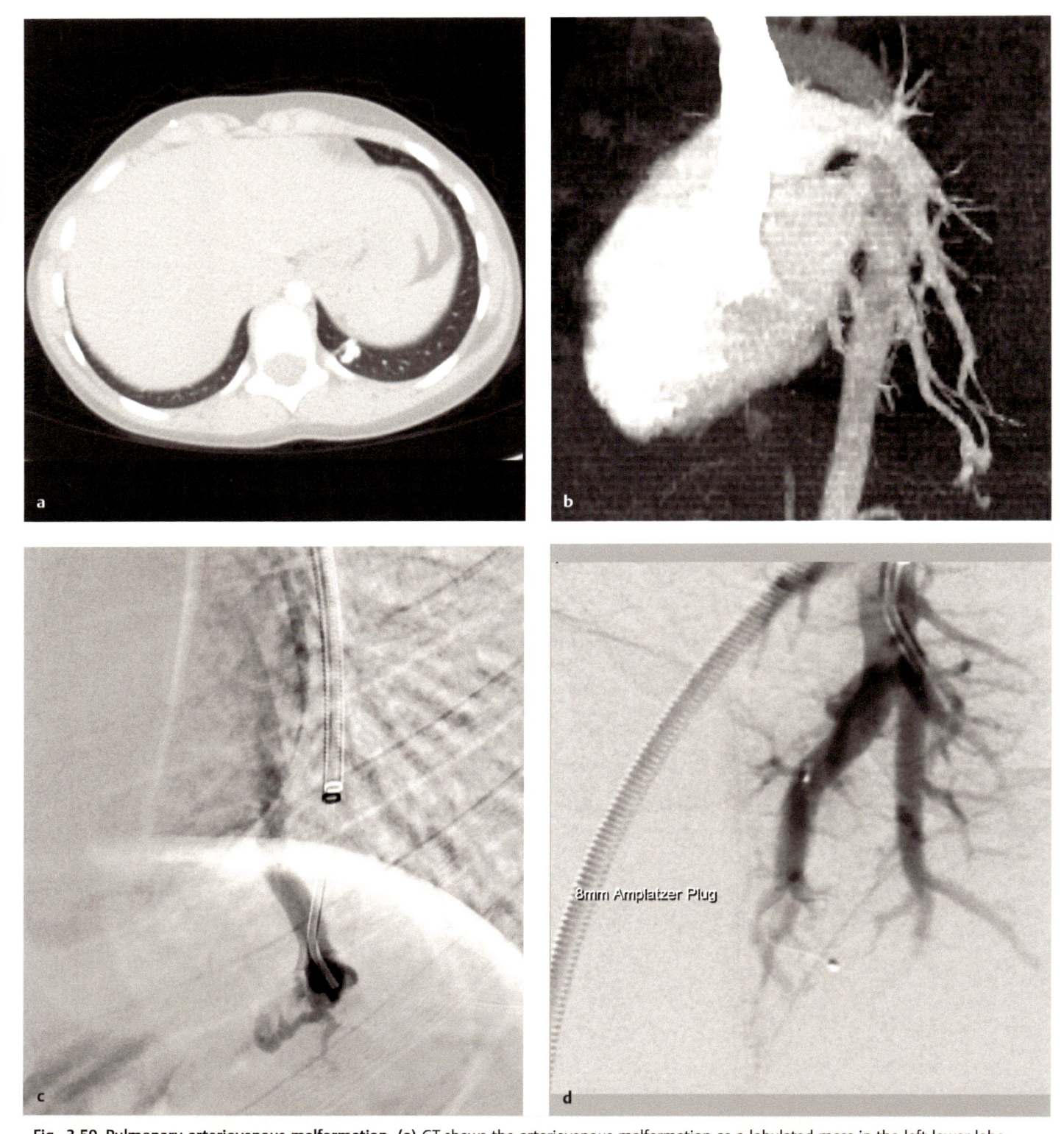

Fig. 3.59 Pulmonary arteriovenous malformation. (a) CT shows the arteriovenous malformation as a lobulated mass in the left lower lobe. (b) Maximum intensity projection of CTA demonstrates one feeding and one draining vessel. (c) This is confirmed by pulmonary angiography before embolization of the arteriovenous malformation. (d) Postembolization image shows that the arteriovenous malformation has been excluded from the circulation.

Bibliography

[1] Goo HW, Park IS, Ko JK, et al. CT of congenital heart disease: normal anatomy and typical pathologic conditions. Radiographics. 2003; 23(Spec No):S147-S165

[2] Goldmuntz E. The epidemiology and genetics of congenital heart disease. Clin Perinatol. 2001; 28(1):1-10

[3] Layton KF, Kallmes DF, Cloft HJ, Lindell EP, Cox VS. Bovine aortic arch variant in humans: clarification of a common misnomer. AJNR Am J Neuroradiol. 2006; 27(7):1541-1542

[4] van Son JA, Konstantinov IE, Burckhard F. Kommerell and Kommerell's diverticulum. Tex Heart Inst J. 2002; 29(2):109-112

[5] Krichenko A, Benson LN, Burrows P, Möes CA, McLaughlin P, Freedom RM. Angiographic classification of the isolated, persistently patent ductus arteriosus and implications for percutaneous catheter occlusion. Am J Cardiol. 1989; 63(12):877-880

[6] Edwards JE. Malformations of the aortic arch system manifested as vascular rings. Lab Invest. 1953; 2(1):56-75

[7] Delis KT, Gloviczki P. Middle aortic syndrome: from presentation to contemporary open surgical and endovascular treatment. Perspect Vasc Surg Endovasc Ther. 2005; 17(3):187-203

[8] Lewis VD, III, Meranze SG, McLean GK, O'Neill JA, Jr, Berkowitz HD, Burke DR. The midaortic syndrome: diagnosis and treatment. Radiology. 1988; 167(1):111-113

[9] Johnston KW, Rutherford RB, Tilson MD, Shah DM, Hollier L, Stanley JC. Suggested standards for reporting on arterial aneurysms. Subcommittee on Reporting Standards for Arterial Aneurysms, Ad Hoc Committee on Reporting Standards, Society for Vascular Surgery and North American Chapter, International Society for Cardiovascular Surgery. J Vasc Surg. 1991; 13(3):452-458

[10] Estrera AL, Miller CC, III, Chen EP, et al. Descending thoracic aortic aneurysm repair: 12-year experience using distal aortic perfusion and cerebrospinal fluid drainage. Ann Thorac Surg. 2005; 80(4):1290-1296, discussion 1296

[11] Crawford ES, Crawford JL, Safi HJ, et al. Thoracoabdominal aortic aneurysms: preoperative and intraoperative factors determining immediate and long-term results of operations in 605 patients. J Vasc Surg. 1986; 3(3):389-404

[12] Prescott-Focht JA, Martinez-Jimenez S, Hurwitz LM, et al. Ascending thoracic aorta: postoperative imaging evaluation. Radiographics. 2013; 33(1):73-85

[13] Sundaram B, Quint LE, Patel HJ, Deeb GM. CT findings following thoracic aortic surgery. Radiographics. 2007; 27(6):1583-1594

[14] Elefteriades JA. Natural history of thoracic aortic aneurysms: indications for surgery, and surgical versus nonsurgical risks. Ann Thorac Surg. 2002; 74(5) Suppl.:S1877-S1880, discussion S1892-S1898

[15] Maraj R, Rerkpattanapipat P, Jacobs LE, Makornwattana P, Kotler MN. Meta-analysis of 143 reported cases of aortic intramural hematoma. Am J Cardiol. 2000; 86(6):664-668

[16] Coady MA, Rizzo JA, Hammond GL, Pierce JG, Kopf GS, Elefteriades JA. Penetrating ulcer of the thoracic aorta: what is it? How do we recognize it? How do we manage it? J Vasc Surg. 1998; 27(6):1006-1015, -discussion 1015-1016

[17] Schünke M, Schulte E, Schumacher U. Prometheus. LernAtlas der Anatomie: Innere Organe. 2nd ed. Stuttgart: Thieme; 2009. Illustrated by M. Voll/K. Wesker

[18] Norgren L, Hiatt WR, Dormandy JA, Nehler MR, Harris KA, Fowkes FG, TASC II Working Group. Inter-society consensus for the management of peripheral arterial disease (TASC 11). J Vasc Surg. 2007; 45 Suppl S:S5-S67

[19] Leriche R, Morel A. The syndrome of thrombotic obliteration of the aortic bifurcation. Ann Surg. 1948; 127(2):193-206

[20] Qvarfordt PG, Reilly LM, Sedwitz MM, Ehrenfeld WK, Stoney RJ. "Coral reef" atherosclerosis of the suprarenal aorta: a unique clinical entity. J Vasc Surg. 1984; 1(6):903-909

[21] Jennette JC, Falk RJ, Bacon PA, et al. 2012 revised International Chapel Hill Consensus Conference nomenclature of vasculitides. Arthritis Rheum. 2013; 65(1):1-11

[22] Arida A, Kyprianou M, Kanakis M, Sfikakis PP. The diagnostic value of ultrasonography-derived edema of the temporal artery wall in giant cell arteritis: a second meta-analysis. BMC Musculoskelet Disord. 2010; 11:44

[23] Burke AP, Virmani R. Sarcomas of the great vessels. A clinicopathologic study. Cancer. 1993; 71(5):1761-1773

[24] Penel N, Taieb S, Ceugnart L, et al. Report of eight recent cases of locally advanced primary pulmonary artery sarcomas: failure of Doxorubicin-based chemotherapy. J Thorac Oncol. 2008; 3(8):907-911

[25] Lo SF, Chou LW, Meng NH, et al. Clinical characteristics and electrodiagnostic features in patients with carpal tunnel syndrome, double crush syndrome, and cervical radiculopathy. Rheumatol Int. 2012; 32(5):1257-1263

[26] Bass JE, Redwine MD, Kramer LA, Huynh PT, Harris JH, Jr. Spectrum of congenital anomalies of the inferior vena cava: cross-sectional imaging findings. Radiographics. 2000; 20(3):639-652

[27] Kouroukis C, Leclerc JR. Pulmonary embolism with duplicated inferior vena cava. Chest. 1996; 109(4):1111-1113

[28] Mahnken AH, Wildberger JE, Spüntrup E, Hübner D. Unilateral absence of the left pulmonary artery associated with coronary-to-bronchial artery anastomosis. J Thorac Imaging. 2000; 15(3):187-190

[29] Restrepo CS, Carswell AP. Aneurysms and pseudoaneurysms of the pulmonary vasculature. Semin Ultrasound CT MR. 2012; 33(6):552-566

[30] Torbicki A, Perrier A, Konstantinides S, et al. ESC Committee for Practice Guidelines (CPG). Guidelines on the diagnosis and management of acute pulmonary embolism: the Task Force for the Diagnosis and Management of Acute Pulmonary Embolism of the European Society of Cardiology (ESC). Eur Heart J. 2008; 29(18):2276-2315

[31] Agnelli G, Becattini C. Acute pulmonary embolism. N Engl J Med. 2010; 363(3):266-274

[32] Stein PD, Chenevert TL, Fowler SE, et al. PIOPED III (Prospective Investigation of Pulmonary Embolism Diagnosis III) Investigators. Gadolinium-enhanced magnetic resonance angiography for pulmonary embolism: a multicenter prospective study (PIOPED III). Ann Intern Med. 2010; 152(7):434-443, W142-3

[33] Pena E, Dennie C, Franquet T, Milroy C. Nonthrombotic pulmonary embolism: a radiological perspective. Semin Ultrasound CT MR. 2012; 33(6):522-534

[34] Simonneau G, Gatzoulis MA, Adatia I, et al. Updated clinical classification of pulmonary hypertension. J Am Coll Cardiol. 2013; 62(25) Suppl:D34-D41

[35] Schünke M, Schulte E, Schumacher U. Prometheus. LernAtlas der Anatomie: Kopf, Hals und Neuroanatomie. 2nd ed. Stuttgart: Thieme; 2009. Illustrated by M. Voll/K. Wesker

[36] Schünke M, Schulte E, Schumacher U. Prometheus. LernAtlas der Anatomie: Allgemeine Anatomie und Bewegungssystem. 3rd ed. Stuttgart: Thieme; 2011. Illustrated by M. Voll/K. Wesker

[37] Sebastià C, Quiroga S, Boyé R, Perez-Lafuente M, Castellà E, Alvarez-Castells A. Aortic stenosis: spectrum of diseases depicted at multisection CT. Radiographics. 2003; 23(Spec No):S79-S91

[38] Stanson AW, Kazmier FJ, Hollier LH, et al. Penetrating atherosclerotic ulcers of the thoracic aorta: natural history and clinicopathologic correlations. Ann Vasc Surg. 1986; 1(1):15-23

4 Lung and Pleura

Gabriele A. Krombach

4.1 Anatomy

4.1.1 Pleura and Interlobar Fissures

The outer surfaces of both lungs are covered by visceral pleura, which also surrounds the lobes and is reflected into the interlobar fissures, where it forms a double layer. The interlobar fissures are visible on chest radiographs when they are tangential to the X-ray beam. The chest cavity is lined by parietal pleura. The space between the visceral and parietal pleura contains a thin fluid film that facilitates relative movement between the pleural layers during respiratory excursions. The pleural cavity is normally at a negative pressure of approximately 5 mm H_2O on expiration and as low as −20 mm H_2O on inspiration. This enables the lung to remain expanded and apposed to the chest wall.

> **Caution**
>
> In the percutaneous needle biopsy of lung nodules, the likelihood of pneumothorax increases with the number of passes through the pleura. For this reason it is best to avoid passing the needle through the interlobar fissures, even if this may necessitate a longer pathway from skin to lesion.

The minor fissure separates the upper lobe of the right lung from the middle lobe. It is visible in PA and lateral radiographs because it has a partial tangential orientation in both projections (▶ Fig. 4.1). The major fissure of the right lung separates the lower lobe from the upper and middle lobes (see ▶ Fig. 4.1). The left lung has one major fissure separating the upper and lower lobes. The major fissure on each side is visible only in the lateral radiograph, as that is the only projection in which it is tangential to the X-ray beam.

▶ **Imaging landmarks.** Lung changes seen in the frontal radiograph cannot be localized to a specific lobe because the lobes are superimposed. Instead, findings are assigned to any of three lung zones: the upper zone (extending from the apex to the upper pole of the hilum), middle zone (from the upper to lower poles of the hilum), and lower zone (inferior to the hilar lower pole; ▶ Fig. 4.2a). Additionally, the outer 4 cm of lung parenchyma is called the peripheral lung and the perihilar tissue is called the central lung (▶ Fig. 4.2b).

4.1.2 Trachea and Pulmonary Segments

The trachea extends from the larynx to the two main bronchi. It is located along the midline, anterior to the esophagus. It

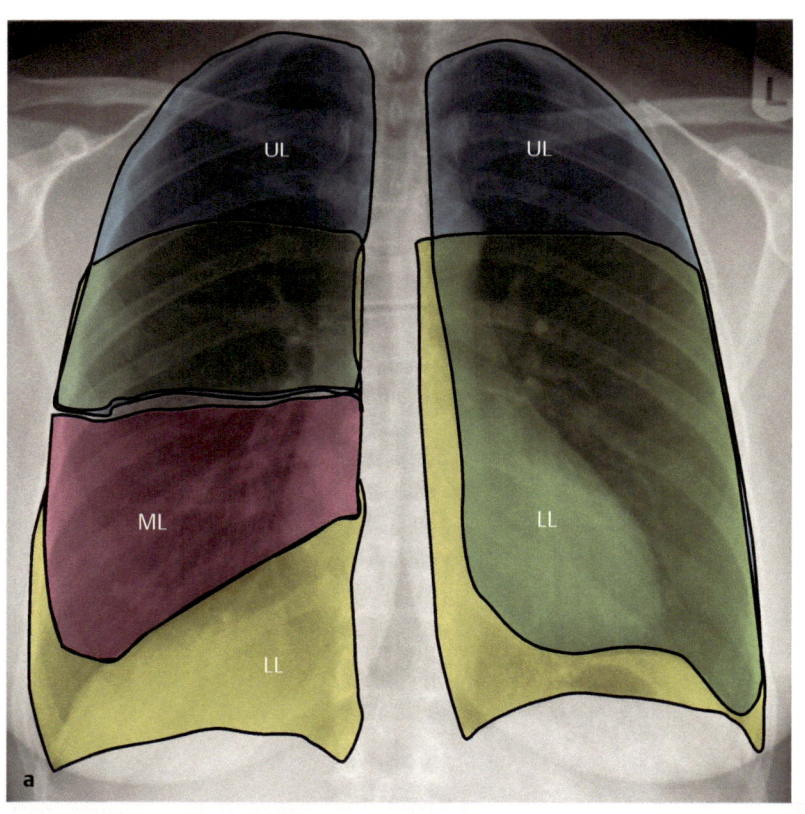

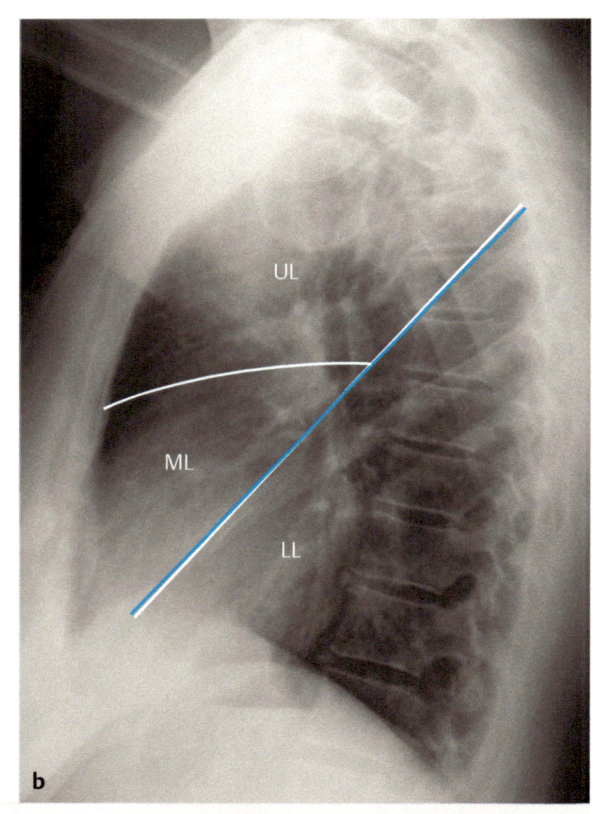

Fig. 4.1 Standard radiographic views of the chest. (a) The pulmonary lobes are partially superimposed in the PA projection. The interlobar fissures are not visible except for a peripheral portion of the minor fissure. (b) Lateral radiograph. The interlobar fissures are visible in this projection because of their horizontal orientation relative to the X-ray beam (white lines: indicate interlobar fissures of the right lung; blue line indicates interlobar fissure of the left lung). UL, upper lobe; ML, middle lobe; LL, lower lobe.

4.1 Anatomy

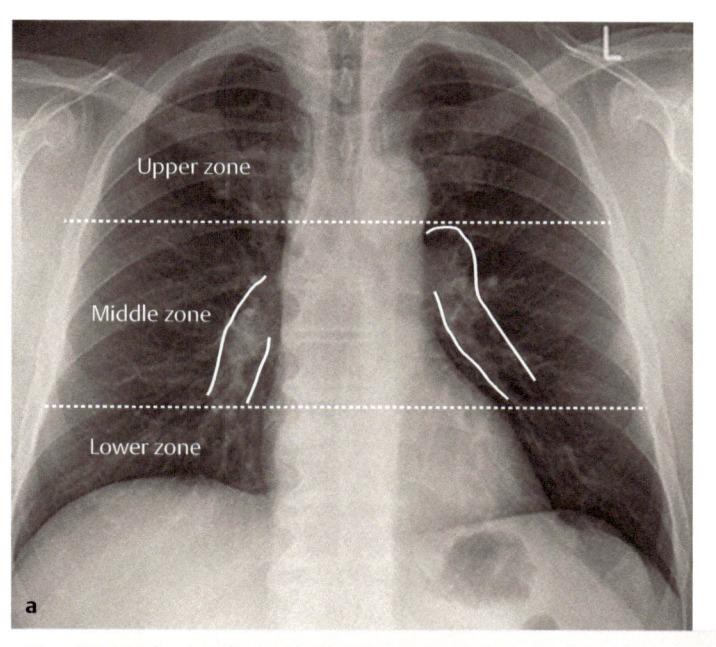

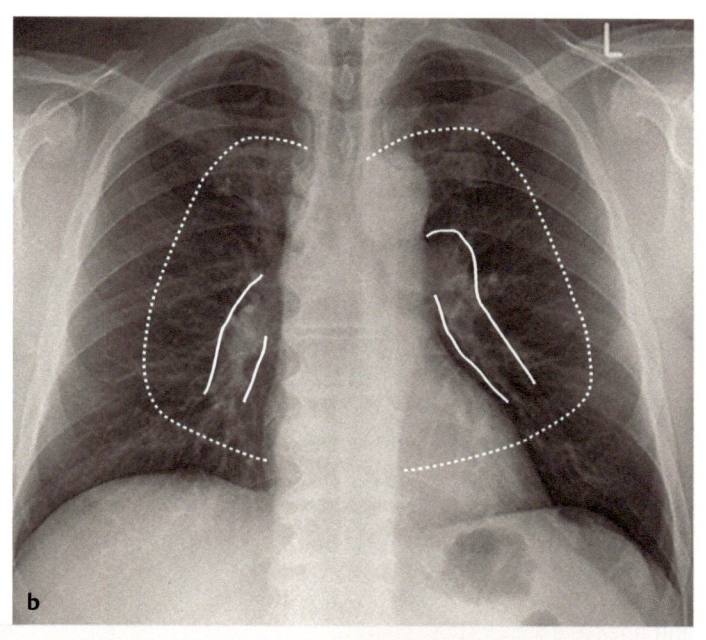

Fig. 4.2 PA chest radiograph. (a) Changes visible in the frontal view are assigned to any of three lung zones: upper, middle, and lower. The hila serve as landmarks for defining the lung zones. **(b)** The lung parenchyma is divided into the central (perihilar) lung and the peripheral lung.

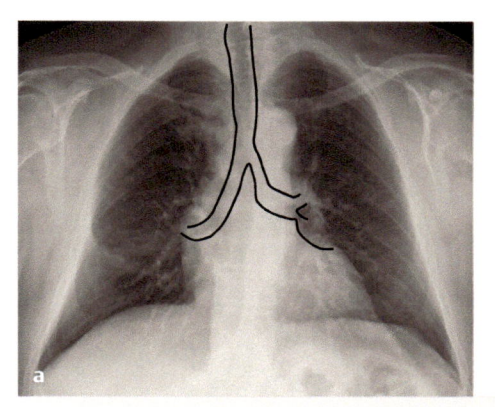

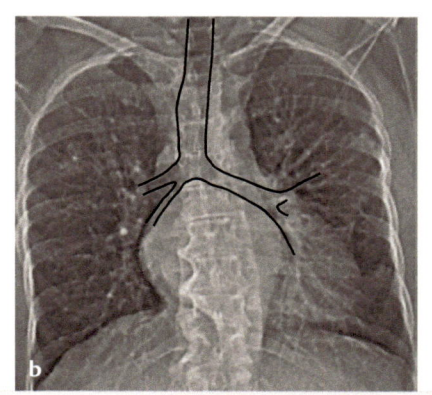

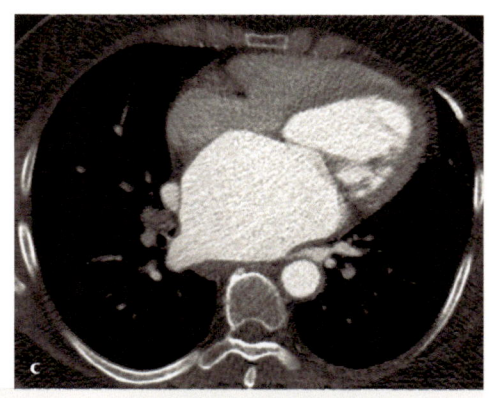

Fig. 4.3 Normal and abnormal bifurcation angles. (a) The normal bifurcation angle at the carina is less than 70°. The right main bronchus in adults is more vertical than the left, which is why aspiration is more common on the right side. **(b)** The bifurcation angle is abnormally increased to more than 90°, due in this case to an enlarged left atrium. **(c)** CT (same patient as in [b]) demonstrates enlargement of the left atrium. The other cardiac chambers are not dilated.

begins at the cricoid cartilage and ends at the carina approximately at the level of the T4 vertebra. Its walls are reinforced by horseshoe-shaped cartilage rings that are interconnected by the anular ligaments and stabilize the trachea so that it does not collapse. The posterior membranous part of the trachea, called the pars membranacea, is stretched between the two ends of the incomplete cartilage rings; it contains elastic connective tissue and smooth muscle cells. The cartilage rings are continued inferiorly into the main bronchi. In the segmental bronchi they are replaced by cartilage plates, which diminish in size and number in the smaller bronchial branches and are finally absent in the bronchioles.

The right main bronchus is steeper than the left. The angle between the two main bronchi measures 60 to 75°. Splaying of the carina is most commonly caused by an enlarged left atrium (▶ Fig. 4.3) but may also result from enlarged infracarinal lymph nodes.

Note
The more vertical orientation of the right main bronchus, present by the age of about 12 years, explains why aspiration is more common on the right side in adults.

▶ Fig. 4.4 illustrates the segmental anatomy of the lung. When isolated pulmonary nodules are found, the affected lung segment should be identified in the radiology report whenever possible.

4.1.3 Vessels

The lung oxygenates blood delivered to it by the pulmonary arteries. Similarly to the liver, the lung also has a second vascular system: the bronchial arteries. These vessels arise from the descending aorta at the level of the T4 vertebra (▶ Fig. 4.5a), and

Lung and Pleura

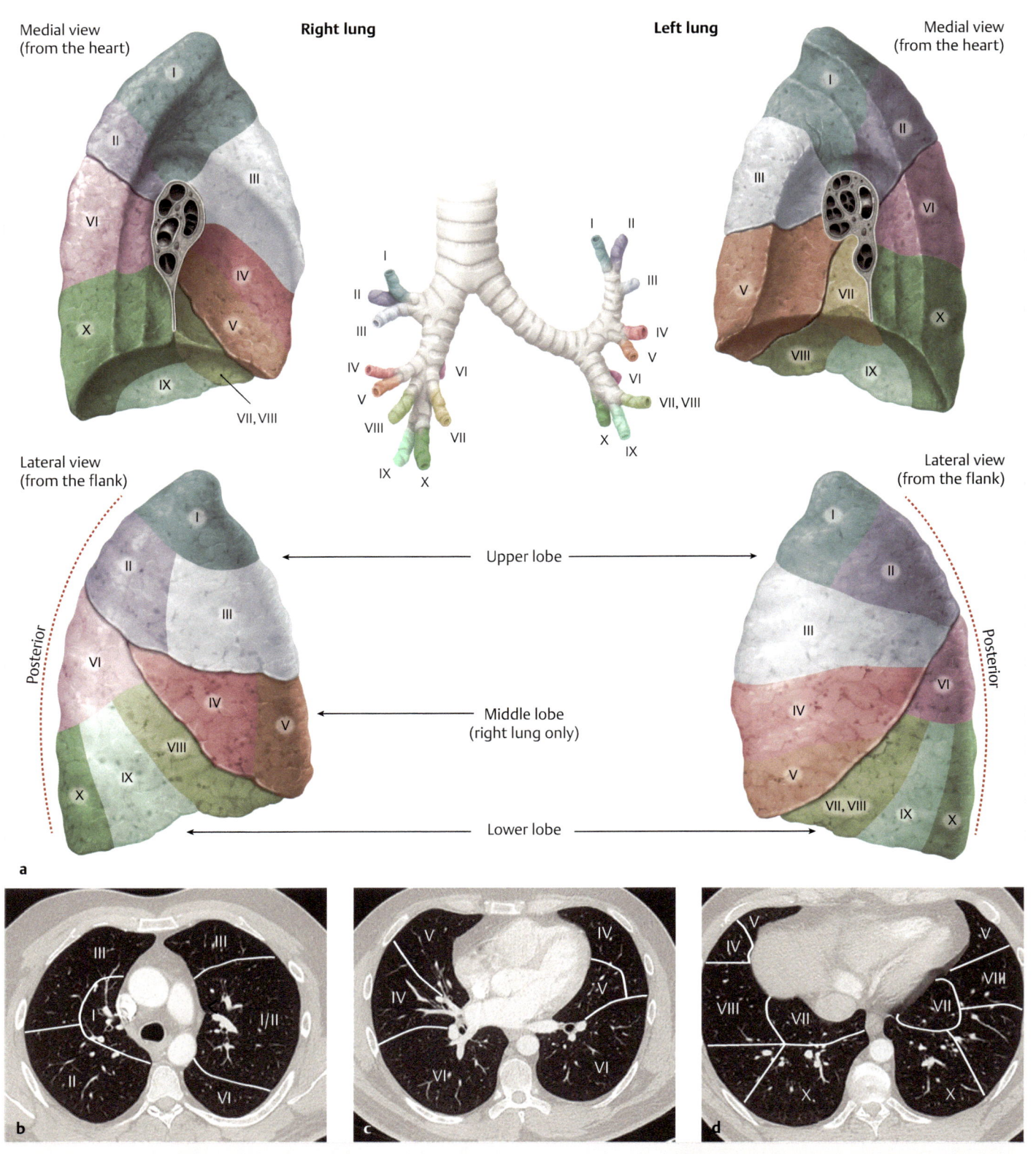

Fig. 4.4 Segmental bronchi and pulmonary segments. (a) Segmental anatomy of the lung. (b) Axial CT scan with lung window setting at the level of the upper lobes. (c) Axial CT scan with lung window setting at the level of the middle lobe. (d) Axial CT scan with lung window setting at the level of the lower lobes. **Right:** I, apical upper lobe segment; II, posterior upper lobe segment; III, anterior upper lobe segment; IV, lateral middle lobe segment; V, medial middle lobe segment; VI, apical lower lobe segment; VII, mediobasal lower lobe segment; VIII, anterobasal lower lobe segment; IX, laterobasal lower lobe segment; X, posterobasal lower lobe segment. **Left:** I and II, apicoposterior upper lobe segment; III, anterior upper lobe segment; IV, superior lingular segment; V, inferior lingular segment; VI–X, same as on the right. (Reproduced from Schünke M, Schulte E, Schumacher U. Prometheus. LernAtlas der Anatomie: Innere Organe. Illustrated by M. Voll/K. Wesker. 2nd ed. Stuttgart: Thieme; 2009.)

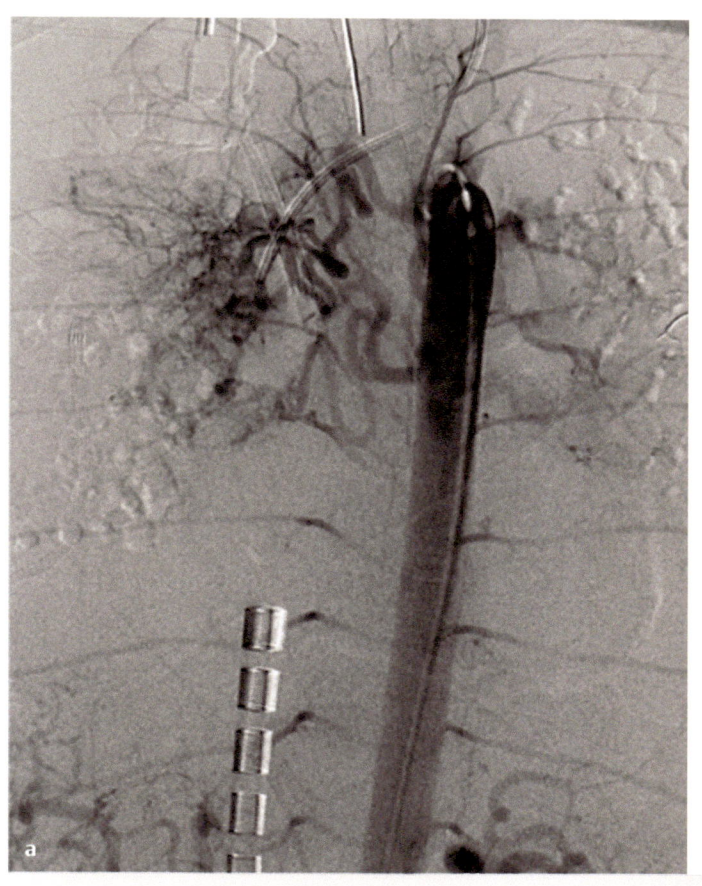

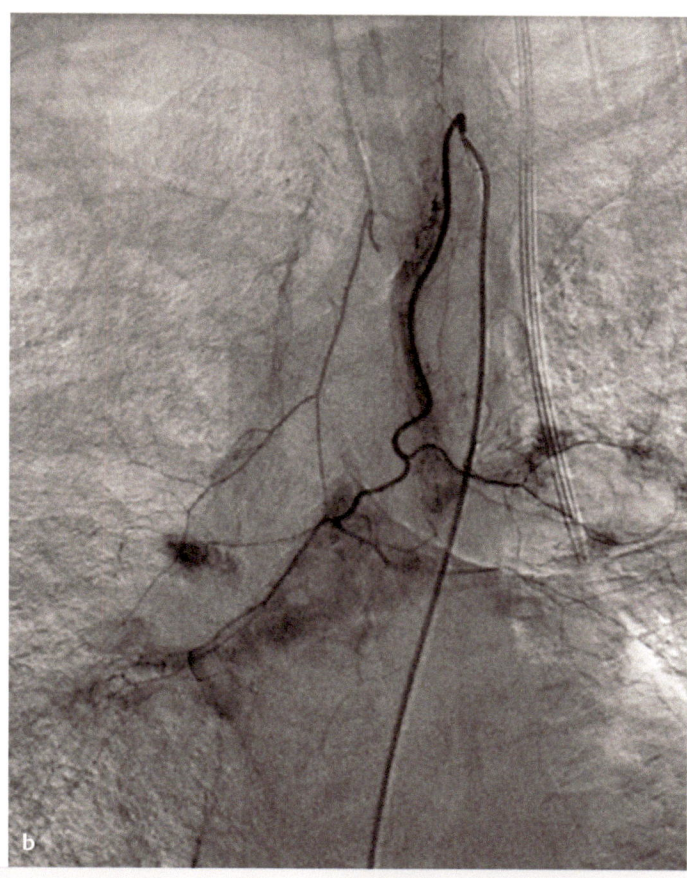

Fig. 4.5 Origin of the bronchial arteries. (a) Typical origin from the descending aorta at the level of the T4 vertebra. Marked hypertrophy of the bronchial arteries is noted due to chronic infection. **(b)** Variant in which the bronchial arteries arise from the left subclavian artery.

their origins are subject to variation (▶ Fig. 4.5b). The bronchial arteries accompany the bronchi as nutrient vessels. Some of the bronchial arteries in the peripheral lung open into the perialveolar capillaries, forming anastomoses by which the bronchial and pulmonary vessels communicate. These connections may protect the lung tissue from infarction following a pulmonary embolism. The rest of the blood in the bronchial arteries drains through the bronchial veils to the pulmonary veins and also to the azygos and hemiazygos veins.

The pulmonary arteries run parallel to the bronchi and branch with them into the segmental arteries.

Note

The normal pulmonary arterial pressure is less than 25 mm Hg at rest and less than 30 mm Hg during exercise.

The pulmonary arteries, being a low-pressure system, are highly distensible. Only one-fourth of the pulmonary capillaries are perfused at rest. When the cardiac output rises during exercise, the large vessels dilate and the percentage of perfused capillaries increases. Given the normal pressure gradients that exist in the lung, the vessels in the basal lung regions are more dilated than in the apical regions when the individual is in an upright position. This relationship is altered when pulmonary venous congestion is present (see ▶ Fig. 2.11).

▶ **Imaging landmarks.** The right pulmonary artery runs horizontally through the mediastinum and thus appears as an oval figure in the lateral chest radiograph (see ▶ Fig. 1.2). The left pulmonary artery forms a more linear, cane-shaped figure that arches over the left main bronchus (see ▶ Fig. 1.2). The pulmonary arteries and lymph nodes form the hilar shadow in the PA or AP radiograph.

Note

The lower lobe artery on the right side is considered dilated if its diameter exceeds 12 mm in women or 15 mm in men.

The diameter of the pulmonary trunk is measurable on CT or MRI. It should not exceed 2.8 cm. The ascending aorta provides a reference standard that is independent of body size: The diameter of the pulmonary trunk should not exceed the diameter of the ascending aorta. In patients with ectasia of the ascending aorta, the descending aorta can be used instead.

4.1.4 Pulmonary Veins

The lung is drained by four pulmonary veins, which open at a steep angle into the left atrium (▶ Fig. 4.6, ▶ Fig. 4.7). The upper lobe veins drain the upper lobes plus the middle lobe of the right lung; the lower lobe veins drain the lower lobes.

▶ **Imaging landmarks.** The pulmonary veins and arteries form vascular markings that are visible on chest radiographs. Generally the two vascular systems cannot be differentiated in the peripheral lung, although the pulmonary veins, which open into

Lung and Pleura

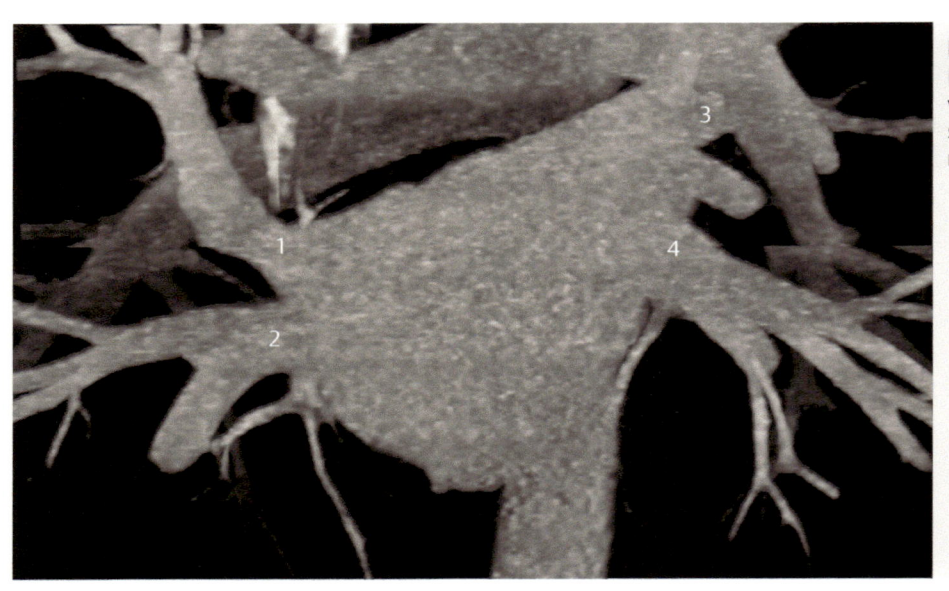

Fig. 4.6 Pulmonary veins. Coronal reformatted MP RAGE image. 1, Right superior pulmonary vein; 2, right inferior pulmonary vein; 3, left superior pulmonary vein; 4, left inferior pulmonary vein.

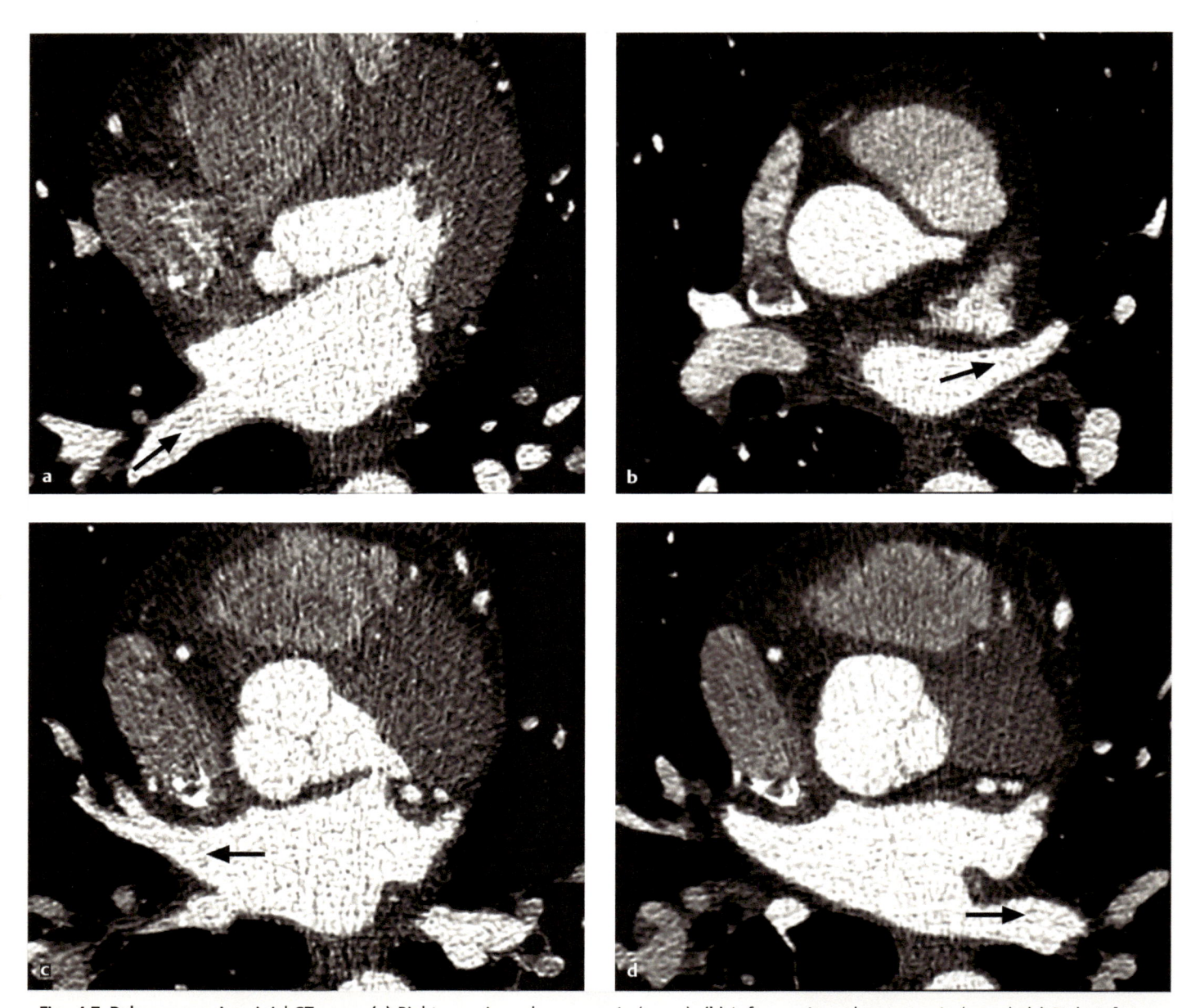

Fig. 4.7 Pulmonary veins. Axial CT scans. **(a)** Right superior pulmonary vein (arrow). **(b)** Left superior pulmonary vein (arrow). **(c)** Right inferior pulmonary vein (arrow). **(d)** Left inferior pulmonary vein (arrow).

the left atrium, are more horizontal than the pulmonary arteries, which arise at a more caudal level and have a steeper orientation. The pulmonary arteries form the hilar silhouette.

4.1.5 Lung Parenchyma

The alveoli are the site where gas exchange takes place and are also the smallest functional unit of the lung parenchyma.[1] They fluctuate in size during respiration: their individual diameters are approximately 50 µm during expiration and 250 µm during inspiration. There are approximately 400 million alveoli, which provide a total gas-exchange surface area of up to 120 m². Their histological structure is optimized for gas exchange: The alveoli have a thin basement membrane covered by squamous type I pneumocytes. Cellular thickness may be as little as 0.1 µm in places to keep the diffusion pathway short. The cells have an elongated shape, with each cell covering a relatively large surface area. Type II pneumocytes, which are more compact and have a somewhat oval shape, are interspersed among the type I cells. They form surfactant, which reduces surface tension and keeps the alveoli from collapsing during expiration. While type II pneumocytes cover only about 20% of the alveolar surface area, they comprise almost 90% of the pneumocyte population. The capillaries are embedded in the interstitium, which is extremely thin so as to shorten the diffusion pathway. The alveoli are interconnected by the pores of Kohn.

One pulmonary acinus is supplied by one terminal bronchiole (▶ Fig. 4.8). The acinus measures 6 to 10 mm in diameter. Up to 12 acini form the secondary lobule, which ranges from 1.0 to 2.5 cm in diameter, depending on its location, and is the smallest unit visible on high-resolution (HR) CT. The secondary lobules are surrounded by connective tissue septa, which are traversed by veins and lymphatics. Each encloses approximately 12 acini, the exact number ranging from a minimum of 3 to a maximum of 24 (▶ Fig. 4.9). The secondary lobules are largest in the peripheral lung, where they have a relatively uniform cuboid shape. The septa are thicker in this region (approximately 100 µm). The secondary lobules become smaller toward the center of the lung, the acini fewer in number, and the connective tissue septa thinner. The connective tissue septa in most healthy individuals cannot be defined by imaging.

> **Note**
>
> The secondary lobule is the smallest unit enclosed by connective tissue in the lung. It is the most important anatomical landmark for the interpretation of high-resolution pulmonary CT.

The interlobular septa in the secondary lobule are the principal anatomical landmarks for the interpretation of high-resolution CT data sets.[1] They are composed of connective tissue and separate the secondary lobules from one another. They arise from the pleura and are part of the "peripheral connective-tissue framework" that covers the exterior of the lung and permeates it in the form of interlobar septa. These septa transmit the lymphatic vessels of the lung and the pulmonary veins. Thickening of the interlobular septa is a feature of many interstitial lung diseases and occurs in lymphangitic carcinomatosis

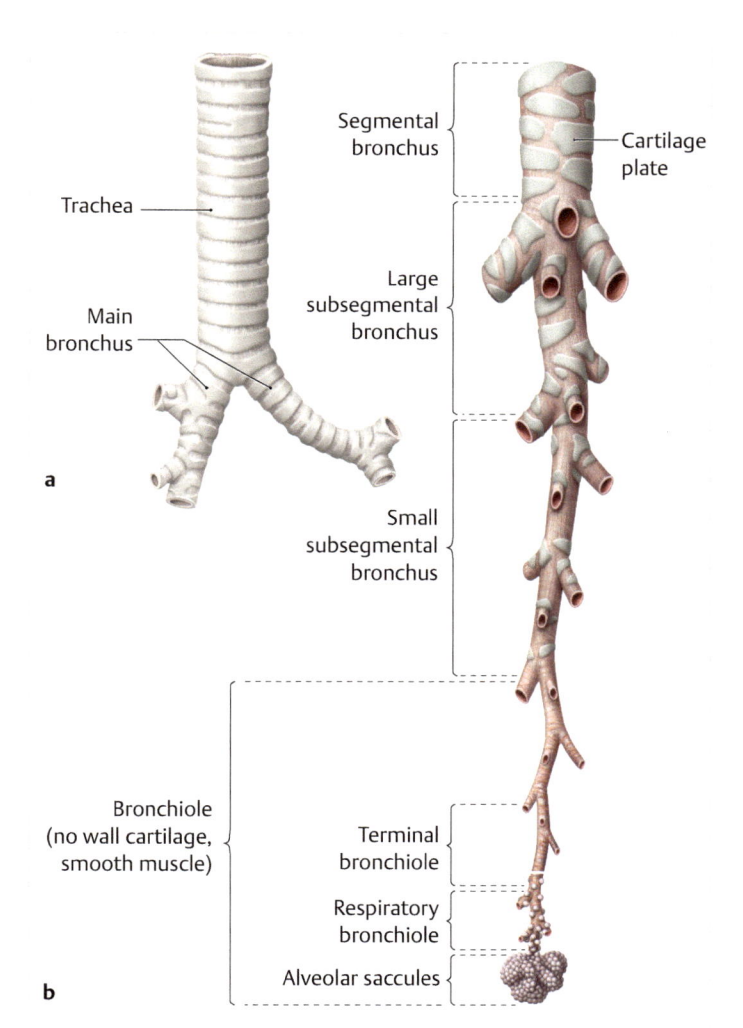

Fig. 4.8 Bronchial tree. The number of bronchial divisions varies with location and ranges from approximately 10 in the perihilar region to 25 in the peripheral lung. (a) Trachea and main bronchi. (b) Segmental bronchi and alveoli. (Reproduced from Schünke M, Schulte E, Schumacher U. Prometheus. LernAtlas der Anatomie: Innere Organe. Illustrated by M. Voll/K. Wesker. 2nd ed. Stuttgart: Thieme; 2009.)

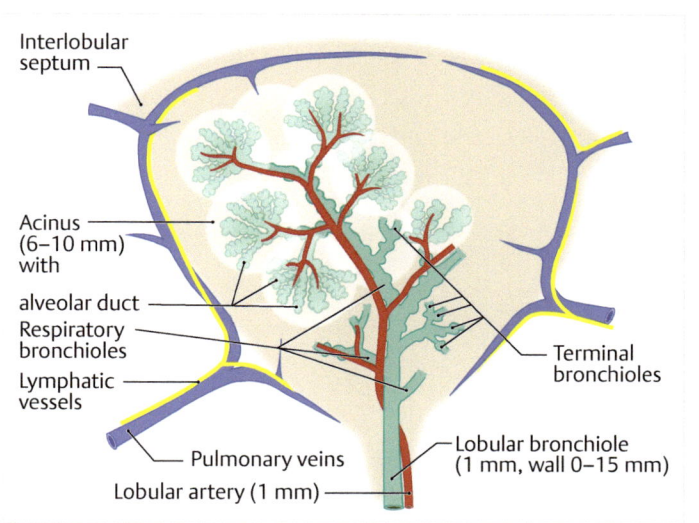

Fig. 4.9 Secondary lobule. Diagrammatic representation. The bronchiole and artery run together through the center of the lobule while the veins follow the interlobular septa.

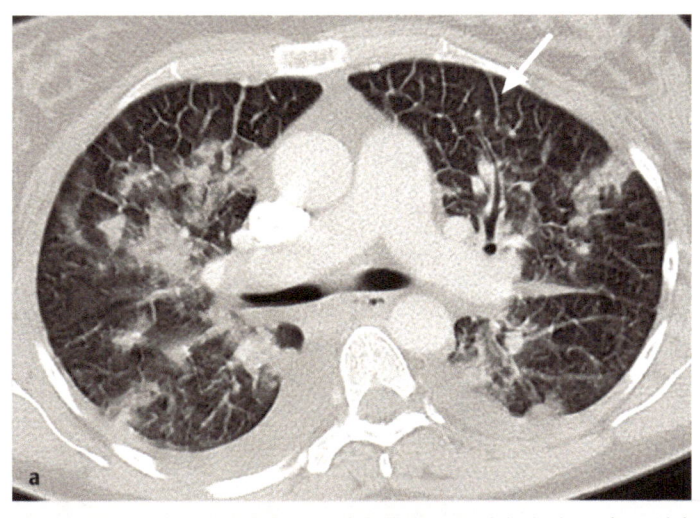

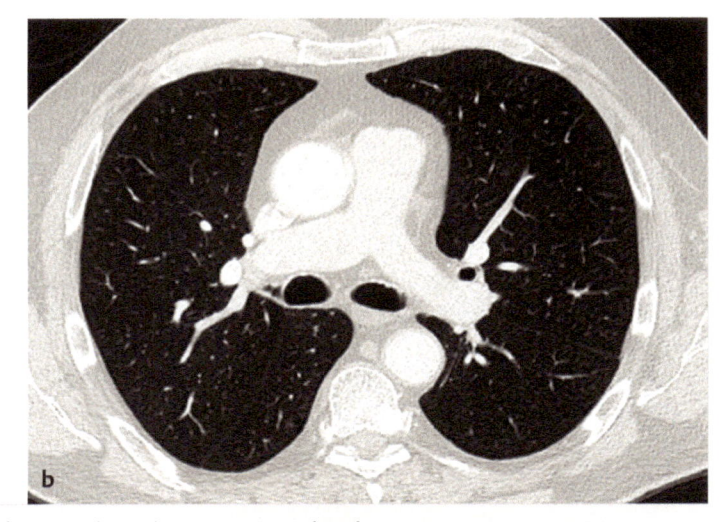

Fig. 4.10 Thickening of the interlobular septa. (a) Thickened interlobular septa (arrow) in a patient with pulmonary venous congestion. The thickened septa are especially prominent in the subpleural lung. **(b)** The interlobular septa are not visualized in a healthy lung.

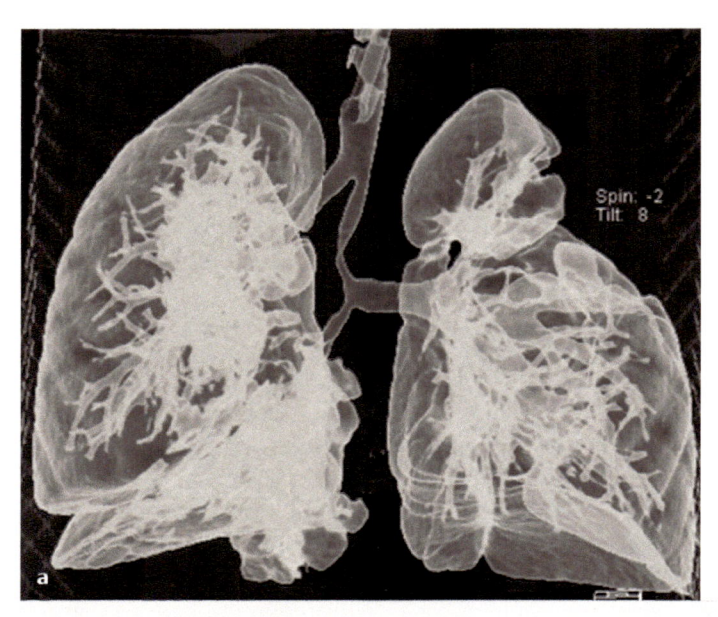

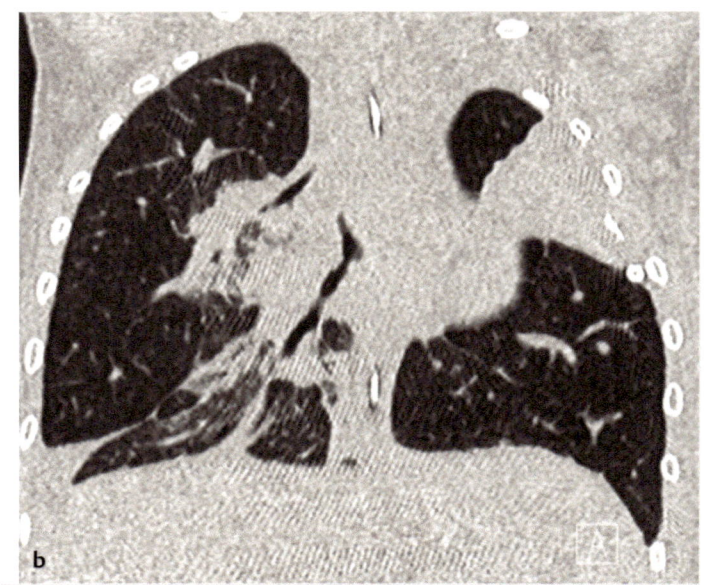

Fig. 4.11 Tracheal bronchus. (a) 3D reconstruction from a CT data set displays the high origin of the right upper lobe bronchus from the supracarinal trachea. **(b)** Multiple stenotic sites are visible in the lower trachea, the right main bronchus, and in the bronchus of the anterior upper lobe segment, leading to hypoventilation and atelectasis.

as well as pulmonary venous congestion (▶ Fig. 4.10). Two other important structures in the secondary lobule are the artery and bronchus, but they are visible only in pathologic states. At the center of each secondary lobule is one artery and one bronchus, each approximately 1 mm in diameter. The bronchus at this level is called a preterminal bronchiole. Because of the great variability in the size of the secondary lobule it is not possible to identify the generation of the bronchus.[2] Bronchi and arteries divide in an irregular dichotomous pattern, i.e., they always divide into two vessels of different diameters. A centrilobular bronchus 1 mm in diameter has a wall thickness of approximately 0.15 mm, which is below the resolution limit of HRCT. Bronchi and arteries are embedded in a connective tissue framework that originates from the hila and permeates the lung. The central arteries and bronchi in the secondary lobule are surrounded by functional lung parenchyma.

4.2 Tracheobronchial System

4.2.1 Normal Variant: Tracheal Bronchus

▶ **Brief definition.** A tracheal bronchus is an accessory bronchus that arises directly from the supracarinal trachea. A tracheal bronchus that supplies the entire upper lobe is also called a "pig bronchus" or bronchus suis. The incidence of this variant is low, at approximately 1%.

▶ **Imaging signs.** CT directly visualizes the accessory bronchus and can identify the lung parenchyma supplied by it (▶ Fig. 4.11).

▶ **Clinical features.** Most patients with a tracheal bronchus are asymptomatic. Recurrent episodes of pneumonia may occur if there is stenosis or obstruction.

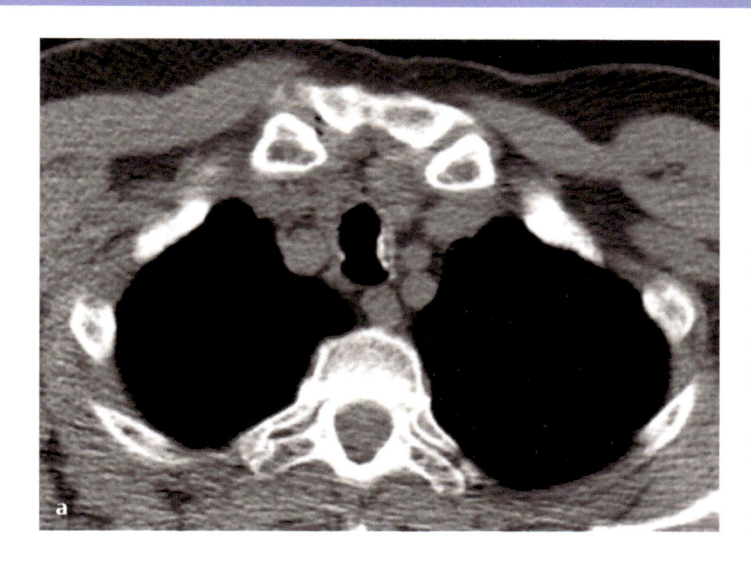

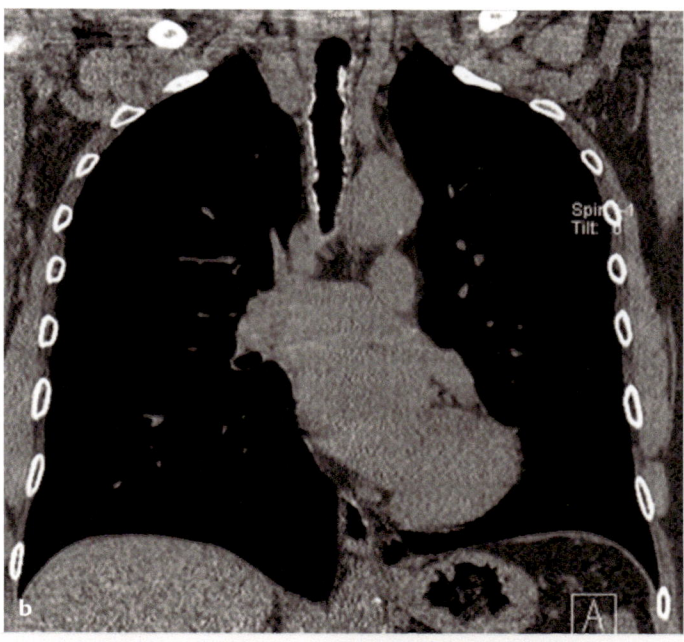

Fig. 4.12 Tracheopathia osteochondroplastica. (a) Axial CT scan shows ossifications with typical sparing of the pars membranacea. **(b)** Coronal reformatted image defines the craniocaudal extent of the process.

▶ **Key points.** CT can define the location and extent of the tracheal bronchus and detect possible sites of tracheal stenosis.

4.2.2 Tracheal Stenosis and Tracheopathia Osteochondroplastica

▶ **Brief definition.** Acquired tracheal stenosis may result from long-term mechanical ventilation, inflammation, or intra- or extraluminal tumors. Tracheopathia osteochondroplastica is characterized by the formation of osseous or cartilaginous nodules in the submucosa, which in some cases may cause tracheal stenosis. The peak age of incidence is after the fifth decade, with a predilection for males.

▶ **Imaging signs.** CT can differentiate compression by an extraluminal mass from stenosis due to scarring. The location and extent of the stenosis can also be evaluated with CT. The location of the osseous or cartilaginous nodules can be determined in tracheopathia osteochondroplastica (▶ Fig. 4.12).

▶ **Clinical features.** The cardinal symptoms of tracheal stenosis are dyspnea and stridor. Tracheopathia osteochondroplastica may be asymptomatic when not associated with tracheal stenosis.

4.2.3 Bronchiectasis

▶ **Brief definition.** Bronchiectasis is an abnormal dilatation of bronchi. Most commonly it is caused by weakening of the bronchial walls due to recurrent inflammation combined with raised intraluminal pressure like that caused by mucous plugging with a check-valve mechanism that restricts expiration. This combination may occur as a result of recurrent bronchopneumonia, cystic fibrosis, alpha$_1$-antitrypsin deficiency, ciliary dyskinesia syndrome, chronic aspiration of gastric juice, and other diseases giving rise to the described pathogenic mechanism. In turn, sites of bronchiectasis create microbial reservoirs with a potential for recurrent infections.

▶ **Imaging signs.** Areas of bronchiectasis appear on chest radiographs as bandlike structures of increased lucency that are often framed by thickened bronchial walls (▶ Fig. 4.13). This finding is called the "tram-track sign." Bronchi that are completely filled with mucus appear as dense bands (▶ Fig. 4.14). On CT, the bronchi are dilated to a diameter larger than the accompanying artery. If the ratio of bronchial to arterial diameter is greater than 1.5, there is bronchiectasis (see ▶ Fig. 4.13b). Bronchiectasis is classified by its morphology as cylindrical, saccular, or cystic. There may be mucus retention due to impaired clearance of secretions.

▶ **Clinical features.** A common symptom of bronchiectasis is a morning cough productive of sputum. Patients suffer from recurrent bronchopulmonary infections.

▶ **Differential diagnosis.** As a rule, bronchiectasis is easily diagnosed on CT scans. In rare cases bronchiectasis with mucus retention may be mistaken for an abscess or cavitating mass.

▶ **Key points.** Bronchiectasis is an abnormal dilatation of bronchi caused by recurrent inflammation and weakening of the bronchial walls combined with raised intraluminal pressure due to plugging by mucus or debris. The chest radiograph typically shows parallel "tram-track" structures. CT permits direct visualization of the dilated bronchi.

4.2.4 Bronchiolitis

▶ **Brief definition.** Bronchiolitis is an inflammation of the bronchioles that may have various causes. Acute infectious bronchiolitis in infants and small children may be caused by adenoviruses, respiratory syncytial virus, chlamydiae, or *Mycoplasma pneumoniae*. Due to the small diameters of the bronchioles in children

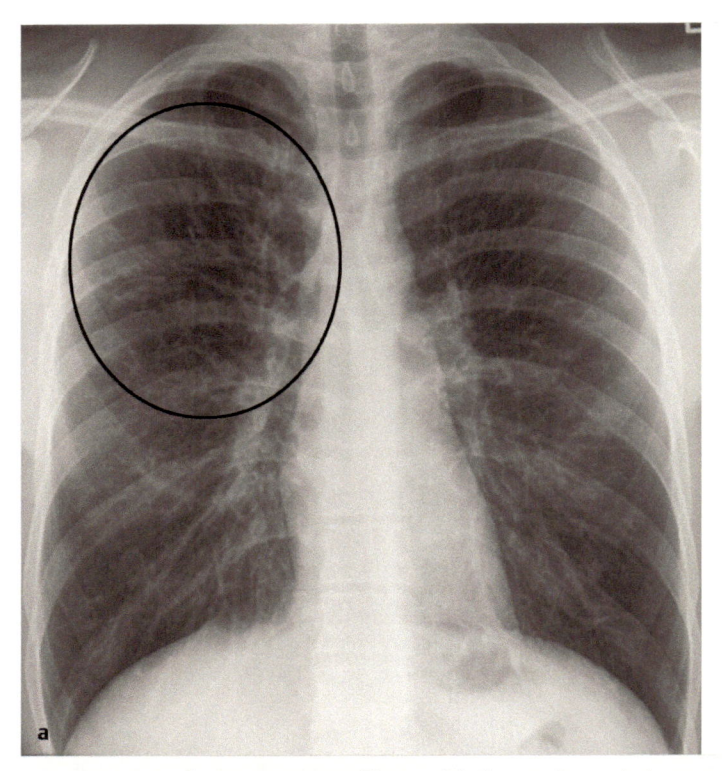

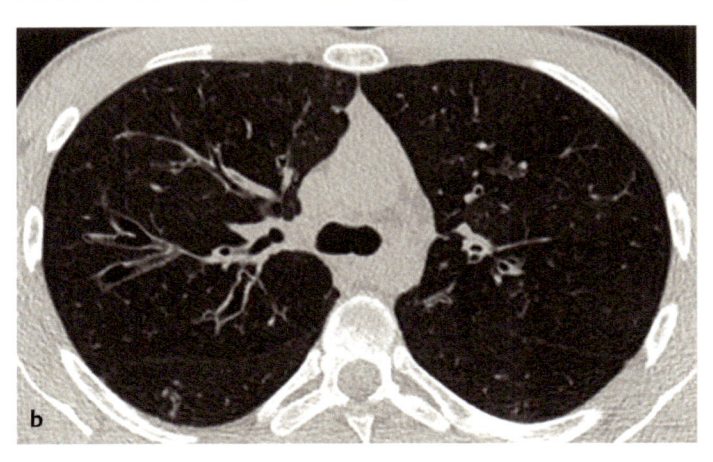

Fig. 4.13 **Bronchiectasis in cystic fibrosis.** (a) Chest radiograph shows a positive tram-track sign in the right upper lobe (circle). (b) Axial CT shows bronchial dilatation.

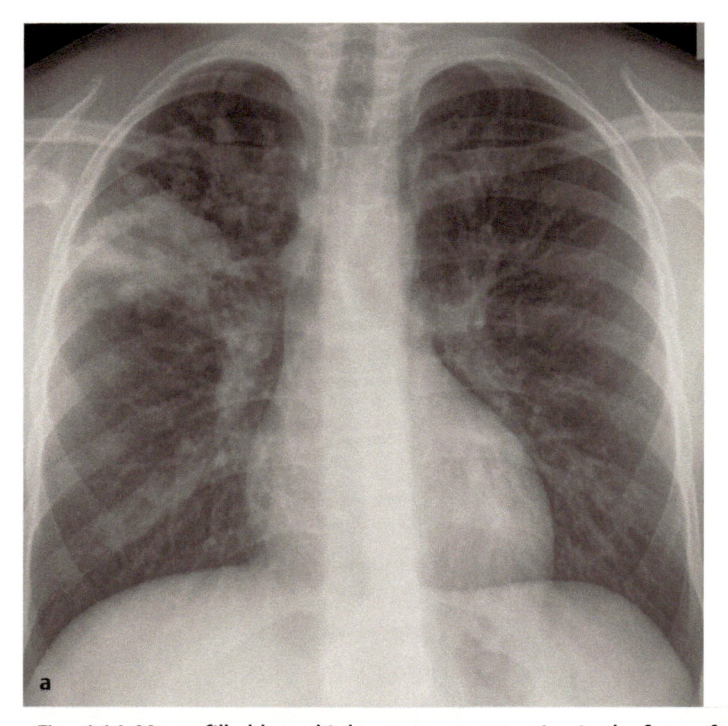

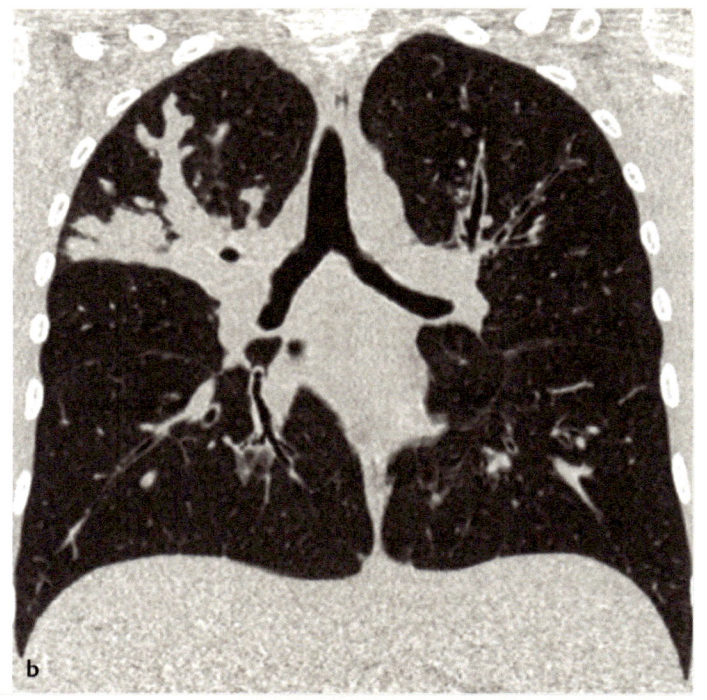

Fig. 4.14 **Mucus-filled bronchi due to mucus retention in the form of a mucocele.** (a) Chest radiograph shows bandlike opacities pointing toward the hilum in a V-shaped pattern. (b) Coronal reformatted CT image shows mucus-filled bronchi in the right upper lobe and bronchiectasis on the left side.

under 3 years of age, the inflammation typically causes bronchiolar obstruction with a check-valve mechanism and overinflation of the lungs. Bronchiolitis in older children and adults may be caused by the organisms mentioned in addition to bacteria (*Haemophilus influenzae*, atypical mycobacteria, *Mycobacterium tuberculosis*) and fungi such as *Aspergillus* species.

▶ **Imaging signs.** Affected bronchial walls appear blurred and thickened on the plain chest radiograph. The lung is overinflated in children under 3 years of age (▶ Fig. 4.15); this feature is absent in older children and adults. HRCT shows centrilobular nodules and a characteristic "tree-in-bud" pattern. The latter is caused by plugging of the terminal and respiratory bronchioles

4.2 Tracheobronchial System

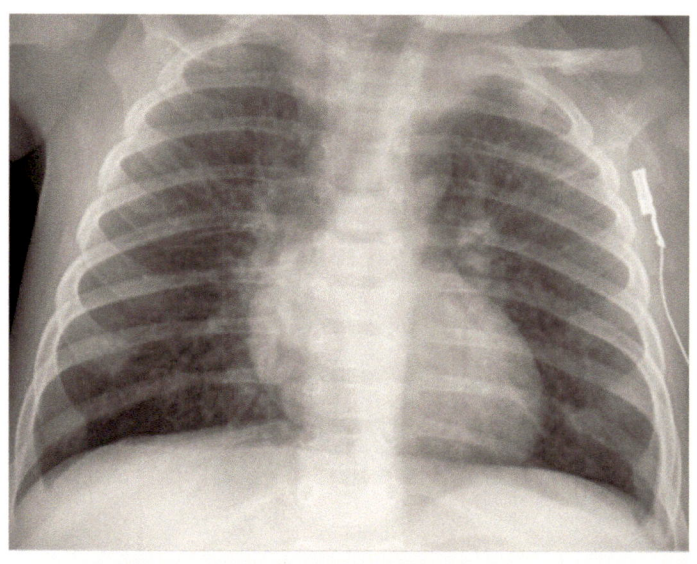

Fig. 4.15 Bronchiolitis in a 5-month-old child. Chest radiograph demonstrates overinflation of the lung. Bilateral perihilar ringlike structures are end-on views of wall-thickened bronchi. The tram-track signs in both upper lobes are from wall-thickened bronchi viewed in longitudinal projection. The blurred appearance of the bronchi is due to infiltration of the peribronchial connective tissue. Hilar enlargement is caused by associated lymphadenopathy.

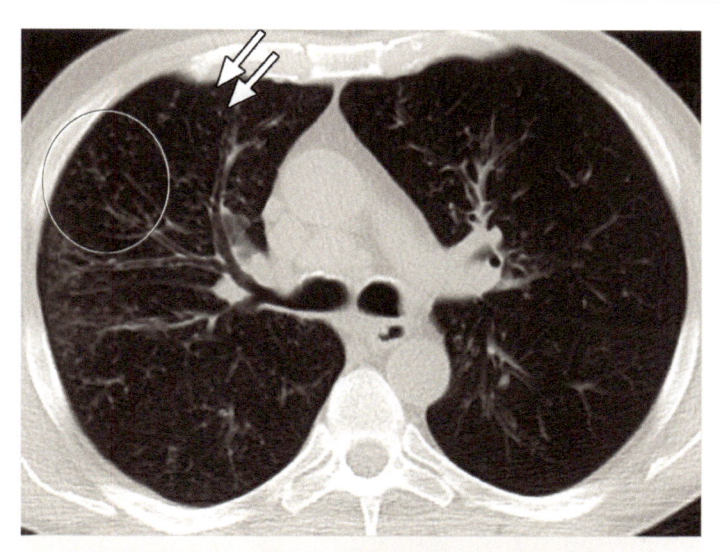

Fig. 4.16 Bronchitis and bronchiolitis. The bronchial walls on the right side are thickened. Sharply circumscribed centrilobular nodules (arrows) correspond to bronchioles filled with mucus, cells, and debris. The tree-in-bud pattern (circled area) visible at the periphery and near the interlobar fissure is caused by obstructed bronchioles sectioned by the CT slice. Centrilobular densities with blurred margins represent peribronchial alveolar infiltrates.

by cells, mucus, and debris. As a result, the bronchioles create an arborizing pattern that resembles a budding tree, which is most pronounced in the outer third of the lung parenchyma (▶ Fig. 4.16).

> **Note**
> The tree-in-bud sign is typical of cellular infiltrates in response to infection and is virtually pathognomonic for an infection.

▶ **Clinical features.** Small children present with acute dyspnea, tachypnea, and occasional cyanosis. The symptoms improve over a period of several days. Adults complain of dry cough and dyspnea.

▶ **Differential diagnosis.** Bronchiolitis due to other causes can be differentiated by careful history taking (allergen exposure in sensitized patients, dysphagia suggesting aspiration, and so on) and laboratory tests.

▶ **Key points.** Infectious bronchiolitis leads to overinflation of the lungs in children under 3 years of age. The tree-in-bud sign is the hallmark of infection on CT scans, which are obtained principally in adult patients.

4.2.5 Constrictive Bronchiolitis

▶ **Brief definition.** Constrictive bronchiolitis is characterized by a peribronchial fibrosis that causes luminal narrowing of the bronchioles. This creates a check-valve mechanism, leading to overinflation of affected lung areas. Constrictive bronchiolitis can have a variety of causes that include infection, connective tissue diseases, drug toxicity, graft-versus-host disease after bone marrow transplantation, or a chronic rejection response after heart or lung transplantation.

▶ **Imaging signs.** The chest radiograph is usually normal. A mosaic density pattern is characteristically present on CT scans. Images at end-expiration show increased density in unaffected areas and regional air trapping in affected areas, which differs from the homogeneous expiratory density increase seen in the lung parenchyma of healthy individuals (▶ Fig. 4.17). Perfusion in these hypoventilated regions is reduced by the Euler–Liljestrand mechanism, causing a compensatory increase of perfusion in the unaffected areas with an accentuated mosaic pattern. The bronchial walls may be thickened. The involvement of small bronchi leads to the appearance of sharply circumscribed centrilobular nodules.

> **Caution**
> The tree-in-bud pattern is not characteristic of constrictive bronchiolitis.

▶ **Clinical features.** The cardinal symptoms are dyspnea and dry cough.

▶ **Differential diagnosis.** Differentiation is required mainly from cryptogenic organizing pneumonia (COP) and acute bronchiolitis.

▶ **Key points.** Constrictive bronchiolitis may be caused by various diseases. The common end point is fibrotic narrowing of the small airways. Many patients have a normal chest radiograph. CT shows regional overinflation with expiratory air trapping as a characteristic sign.

4.2.6 Emphysema, Alpha$_1$-Antitrypsin Deficiency, and Chronic Obstructive Pulmonary Disease

▶ **Brief definition.** Emphysema is defined as enlargement of the alveolar air space due to destruction of the alveolar septa.

Lung and Pleura

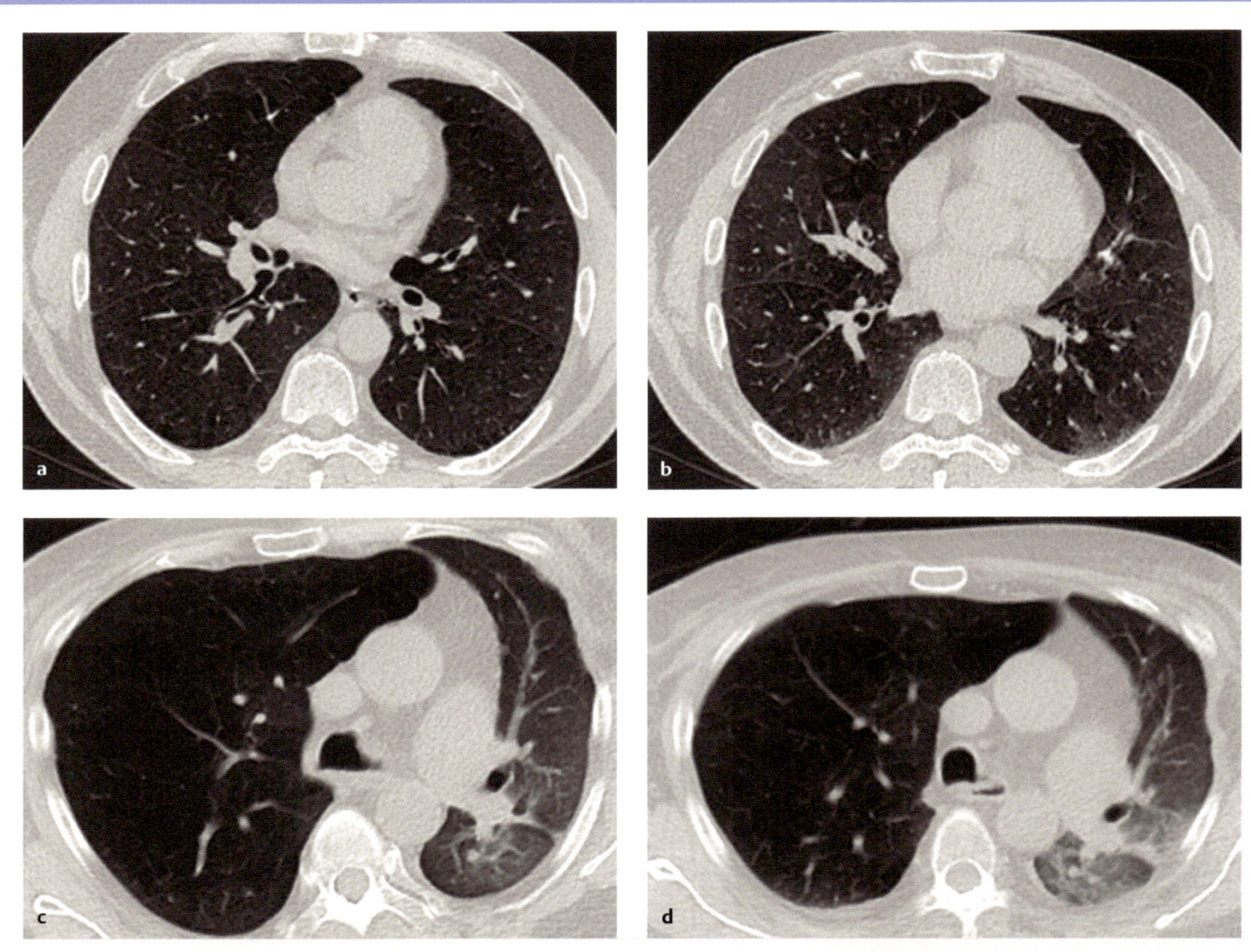

Fig. 4.17 Axial CT scans after lung transplantation in patients with and without constrictive bronchiolitis. (a) Image at end-inspiration in a patient with constrictive bronchiolitis, in rejection after bilateral lung transplantation. (b) Image at end-expiration in the same patient as in (a) shows patchy areas of decreased density. (c) Image at end-inspiration in a patient without constrictive bronchiolitis after left lung transplantation. (d) Image at end-expiration in the same patient as in (c) shows homogeneous increased density of the lung parenchyma.

A homogeneous distribution across the secondary lobules is called panlobular emphysema and occurs in patients with alpha$_1$-antitrypsin deficiency. Centrilobular emphysema, on the other hand, shows an asymmetrical distribution around the terminal bronchus at the center of the secondary lobule. This type of emphysema is smoking-related and occurs in the setting of COPD. The upper lobes and apical lower lobes are most severely affected as a rule. Advanced stages of centrilobular emphysema may progress to panlobular emphysema. Subtypes are paraseptal emphysema, which spreads beneath the pleura and may be complicated by spontaneous pneumothorax, and paracicatricial emphysema caused by retraction due to scarring of adjacent parenchyma. Alpha$_1$-antitrypsin inhibits trypsin and other elastases that are acutely released from inflammatory cells such as neutrophilic granulocytes and alveolar macrophages in response to inflammation. The function of elastases is to enable inflammatory cells to migrate rapidly through the tissue to an inflammatory focus. An alpha$_1$-antitrypsin deficiency or chronic inflammation creates an imbalance which culminates in destruction of the alveolar walls.

▶ **Imaging signs.** The upright chest radiograph shows flattening of the diaphragm due to overinflation of the lungs; this is the most sensitive and often earliest sign of pulmonary emphysema (▶ Fig. 4.18). The retrosternal airspace is increased to more than 2.5 cm, and the distance between the sternum and spinal column is also increased. The retrosternal contact area of the right ventricle is decreased to less than 3 cm. The lateral radiograph shows bulging of lung parenchyma into the intercostal spaces. The costophrenic angles are increased to more than 90° in both projections. Lung lucency is markedly increased in the advanced stage. Emphysematous bullae may be visible as hyperlucent areas. The threshold attenuation value for diagnosing emphysema on CT scans is > 950 HU. The heart remains small, and pulmonary vascularity is decreased due to parenchymal destruction. Centrilobular and panlobular emphysema can be differentiated by HRCT (▶ Fig. 4.19).

▶ **Clinical features.** The main symptom is slowly progressive dyspnea.

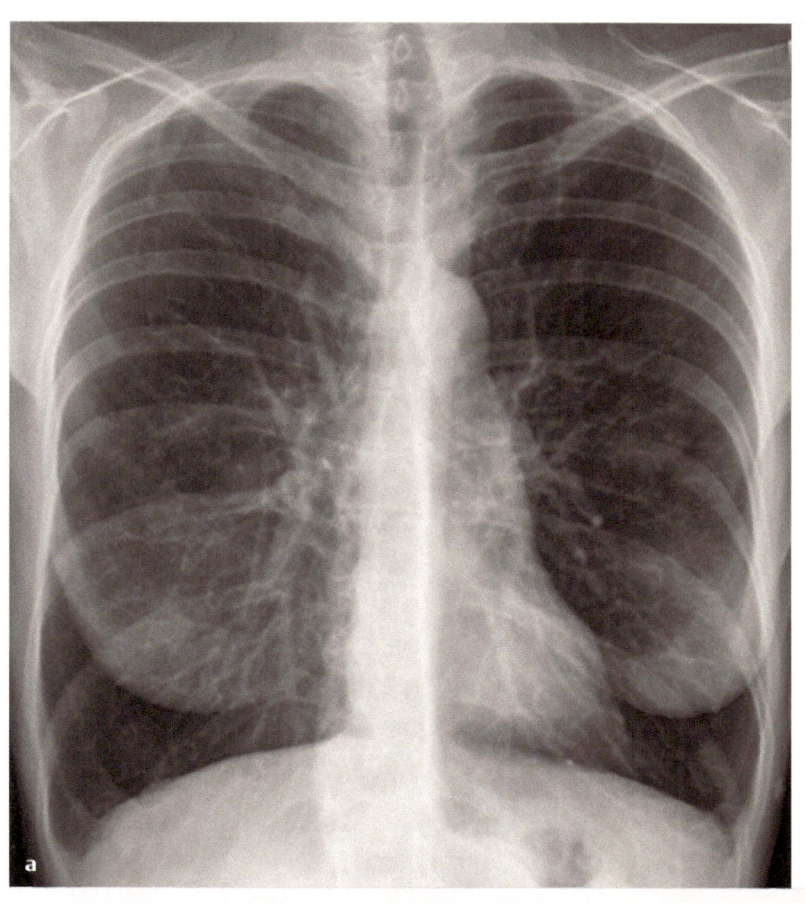

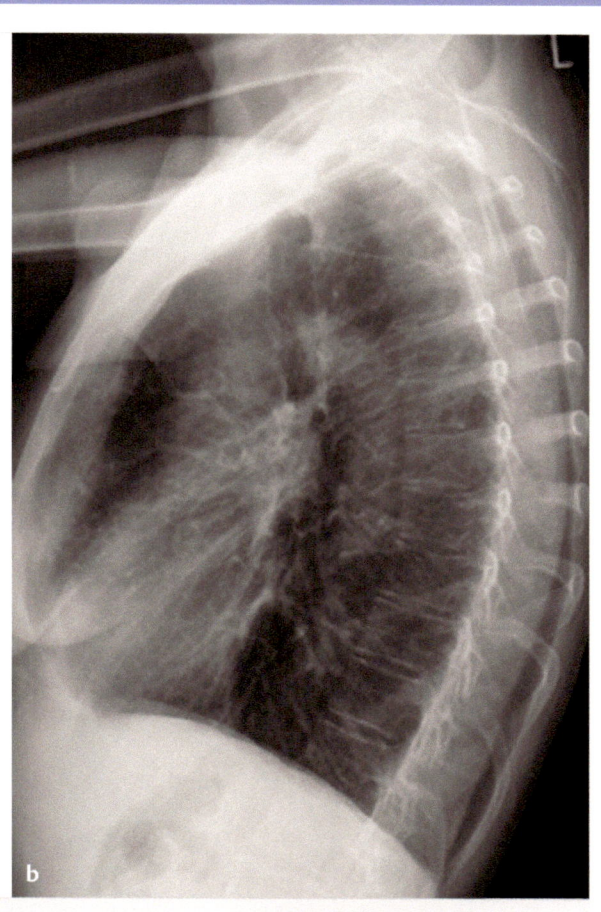

Fig. 4.18 Pulmonary emphysema. Chest radiographs show hyperlucent lungs with marked flattening and depression of the diaphragm. The retrosternal contact area is decreased. **(a)** PA radiograph. **(b)** Lateral radiograph.

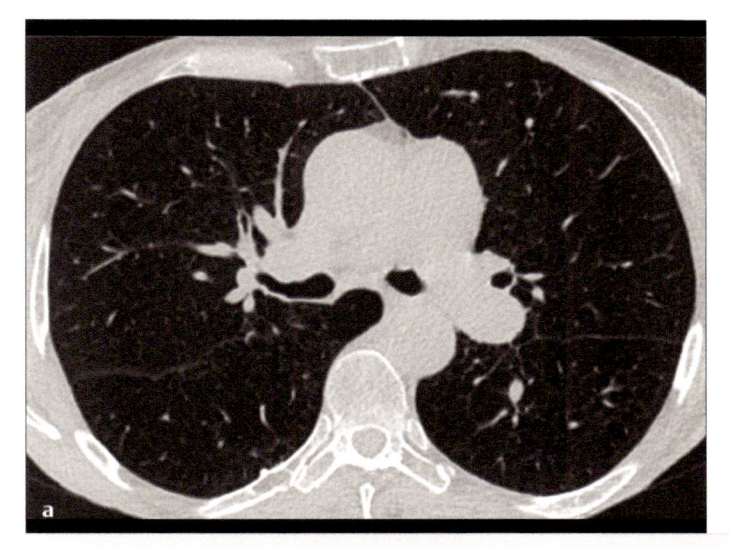

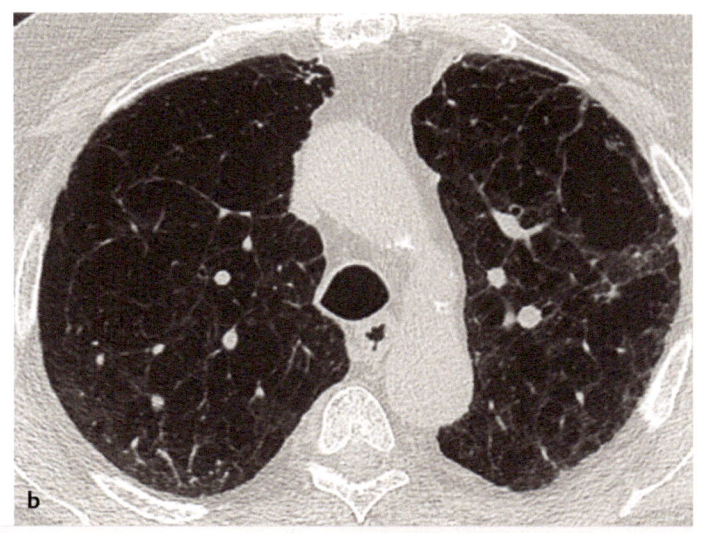

Fig. 4.19 Centrilobular and panlobular pulmonary emphysema. HRCT. **(a)** Centrilobular pulmonary emphysema. **(b)** Panlobular pulmonary emphysema.

▶ **Key points.** Pulmonary emphysema is characterized by parenchymal destruction beyond the terminal bronchioles and results from an imbalance between elastases and inhibitory enzymes. Pulmonary overinflation is marked by flattening and depression of the diaphragm and hyperlucency of the lung. Cor pulmonale is present due to the rarefaction of vessels in the pulmonary circulation.

4.2.7 Atelectasis

▶ **Brief definition.** Atelectatic lung areas are hypoventilated but perfused, with the result that blood is shunted to the arterialized side. The term "atelectasis" comes from the Greek *ateles* meaning "incomplete" and *ektasis* meaning "expansion." Four types are distinguished by their pathogenic mechanism:

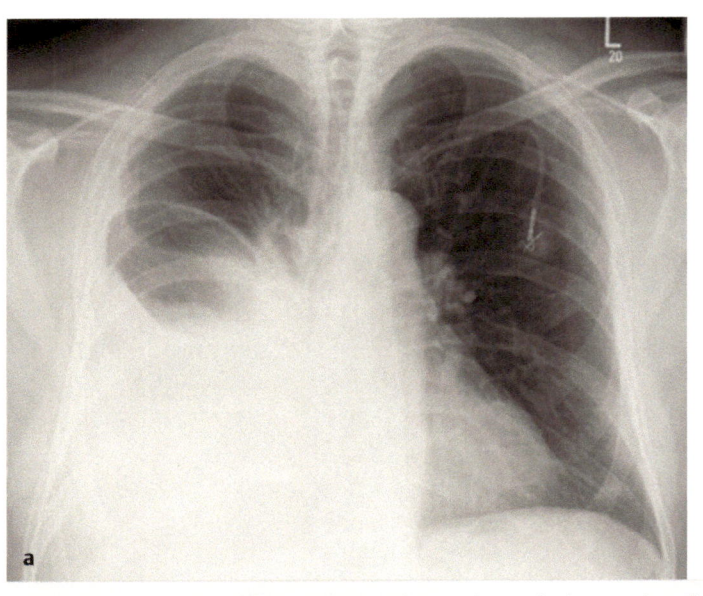

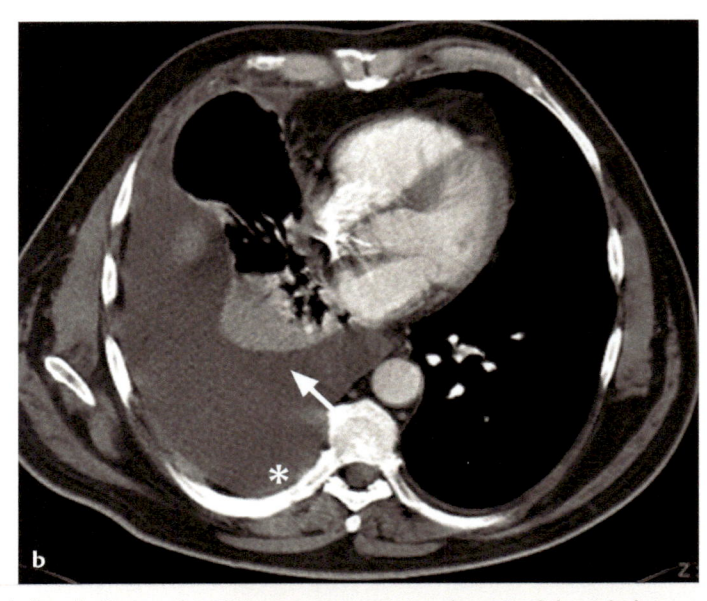

Fig. 4.20 Compression atelectasis. (a) Chest radiograph shows right-sided pleural effusion. **(b)** CT shows compression atelectasis of the right lower lobe (arrow) with a unilateral pleural effusion (asterisk). The mediastinum is not shifted because the mass effects of the pleural effusion and atelectasis cancel out.

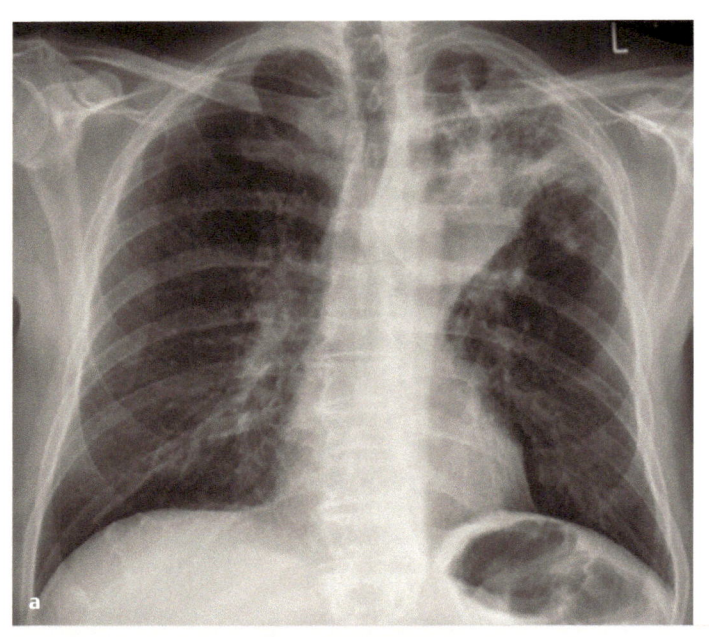

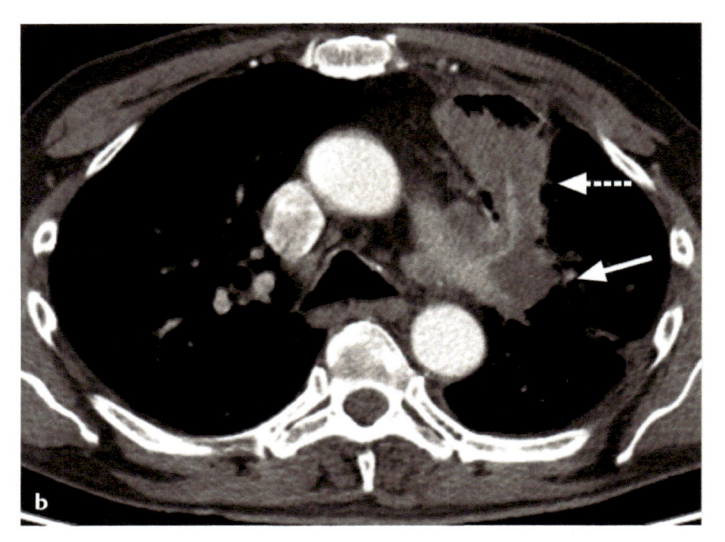

Fig. 4.21 Absorption atelectasis associated with a bronchogenic carcinoma in the central left lung. The segmental bronchus of the anterior lower lobe segment is obstructed. **(a)** Chest radiograph shows the borders typical of atelectasis. **(b)** Left central mass (arrow) shows little contrast with the atelectasis (dashed arrow). Vessels are defined within the atelectatic segment.

- *Compression atelectasis*: This type results from extrinsic compression of the lung parenchyma and is almost always present in patients with pleural effusions (▶ Fig. 4.20). Compression by a chest-wall tumor is a less common cause.
- *Absorption atelectasis*: This type results from the obstruction of a bronchus. The most common cause in intensive care patients is mucous plugging. In ambulatory patients, it is necessary to exclude tumors that obstruct the bronchial lumen by extrinsic pressure or occlude it due to endobronchial growth (▶ Fig. 4.21). Absorption atelectasis takes 24 hours to develop in patients breathing room air; room air consists of approximately 78% nitrogen, which has low solubility in the blood and is absorbed very slowly. Atelectasis develops more rapidly in patients ventilated with oxygen-enriched air due to the higher solubility of oxygen.
- *Adhesive atelectasis*: Adhesive atelectasis results from surfactant deficiency. This type of atelectasis is rarer than the first two and may occur, for example, in pulmonary embolism patients with deficient surfactant formation in the affected areas. It is also encountered in premature infants: surfactant formation begins in the 24th week of gestation.
- *Contraction atelectasis* occurs in areas that border scars.

> **Caution**
>
> Atelectasis in different pulmonary lobes leads to characteristic patterns of opacity and to displacement of the diaphragm and mediastinum (▶ Fig. 4.22). Awareness of these patterns is important in the diagnosis of atelectasis, which may be the initial sign of a pulmonary mass.

▶ **Imaging signs.** Atelectases appear as opacities on chest radiographs, usually without an air bronchogram. In absorption atelectasis, the mediastinum is generally shifted toward the affected side, occupying the space vacated by atelectatic lung. Lower lobe atelectasis may also be associated with elevation of the ipsilateral hemidiaphragm. The borders of the atelectasis are sharply defined, and the opacity pattern typical of a particular lobe can be identified (see ▶ Fig. 4.22). Atelectatic lung parenchyma shows marked contrast enhancement on CT. The pulmonary vessels are crowded together and enhance with IV contrast medium due to continued perfusion of the atelectatic lobe.

▶ **Clinical features.** The clinical presentation is determined by the disease underlying the atelectasis. In patients with absorption atelectasis caused by a tumor, the main clinical findings are B symptoms (undesired weight loss, fever, night sweats) and cough. Intensive care patients with atelectasis may show decreased oxygenation due to intrapulmonary shunting. Patients with significant pleural effusion present mainly with dyspnea.

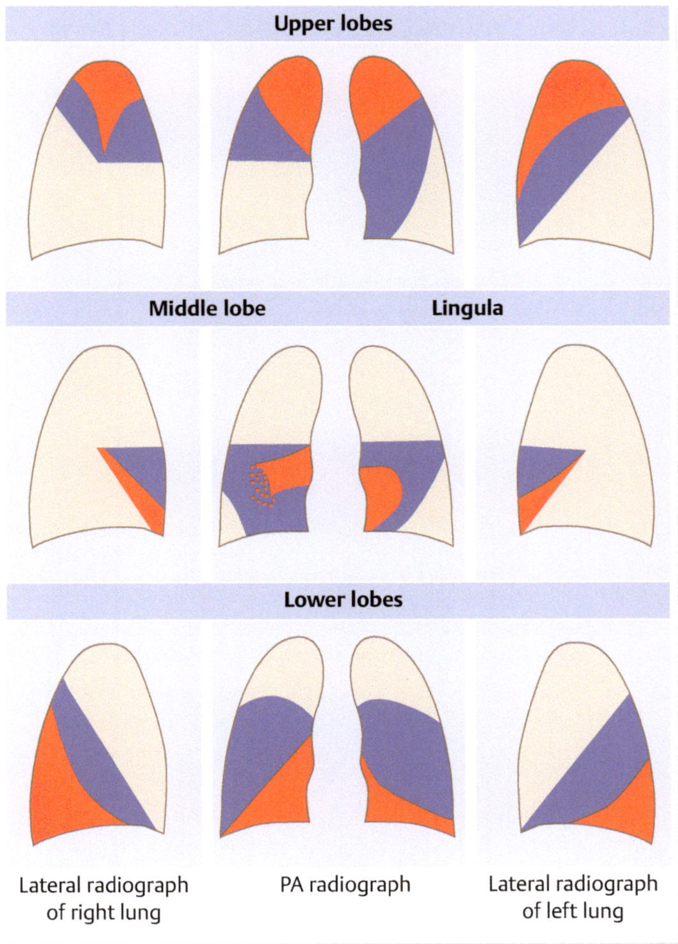

▶ **Differential diagnosis.** Pneumonic infiltrates are an important differential diagnosis but are more likely to produce a mass effect and a positive air bronchogram extending farther into the peripheral lung.

▶ **Key points.** Partial pulmonary atelectasis is common in intensive care patients as a result of retention of mucus (absorption atelectasis) or pleural effusion (compression atelectasis). Areas of atelectasis appear as sharply circumscribed opacities on the chest radiograph, and CT shows marked enhancement of the atelectatic lung parenchyma. Atelectasis in ambulatory patients requires exclusion of bronchial compression by an endoluminal or extraluminal tumor. Atelectasis in different lobes produces characteristic radiographic patterns with the displacement of adjacent structures.

4.3 Lung

4.3.1 Congenital Malformations

Malformations of the lung can be classified according to site of involvement as malformations of the lung parenchyma, bronchi, or vessels. Malformations and variants of the pulmonary vessels can in turn be classified by the affected vessels and type of anomaly (▶ Fig. 4.23). The entities overlap in diseases such as pulmonary sequestration and pulmonary artery aplasia.

Malformations of the Lung

Symptoms common to lung malformations are dyspnea, cyanosis, failure to thrive, recurrent pneumonia, and hemoptysis. The clinical spectrum depends on the severity of disease and can range from onset of symptoms in adulthood to respiratory distress in the newborn.

Pulmonary Aplasia and Agenesis

▶ **Brief definition.** Pulmonary agenesis is a rare anomaly in which there is unilateral or bilateral absence of the lungs. Bilateral pulmonary agenesis is incompatible with postnatal life, but the majority of cases are unilateral. There is compensatory overinflation of the existing lung. The pulmonary artery is absent on the affected side. Associated cardiac anomalies are common, and tracheoesophageal fistula may be present.

▶ **Imaging signs.** The ipsilateral bronchus and pulmonary artery are absent. The mediastinum and heart prolapse toward the affected side. The affected hemithorax is smaller than the contralateral side, and many children will develop scoliosis. The chest radiograph shows opacity of the affected hemithorax with overinflation of the contralateral lung. CT or MRI can demonstrate the pulmonary agenesis (▶ Fig. 4.24, ▶ Fig. 4.25).

▶ **Clinical features.** Patients may be asymptomatic. Infants with a tracheoesophageal fistula exhibit dyspnea after nursing. Pulmonary arterial hypertension may develop and will determine the prognosis. Treatment is symptomatic. Fistulas are surgically repaired.

Fig. 4.22 Typical patterns of opacity produced by atelectasis and pulmonary infiltrates. Diagrammatic representation. Atelectases are shown in red, infiltrates in blue.

Lung and Pleura

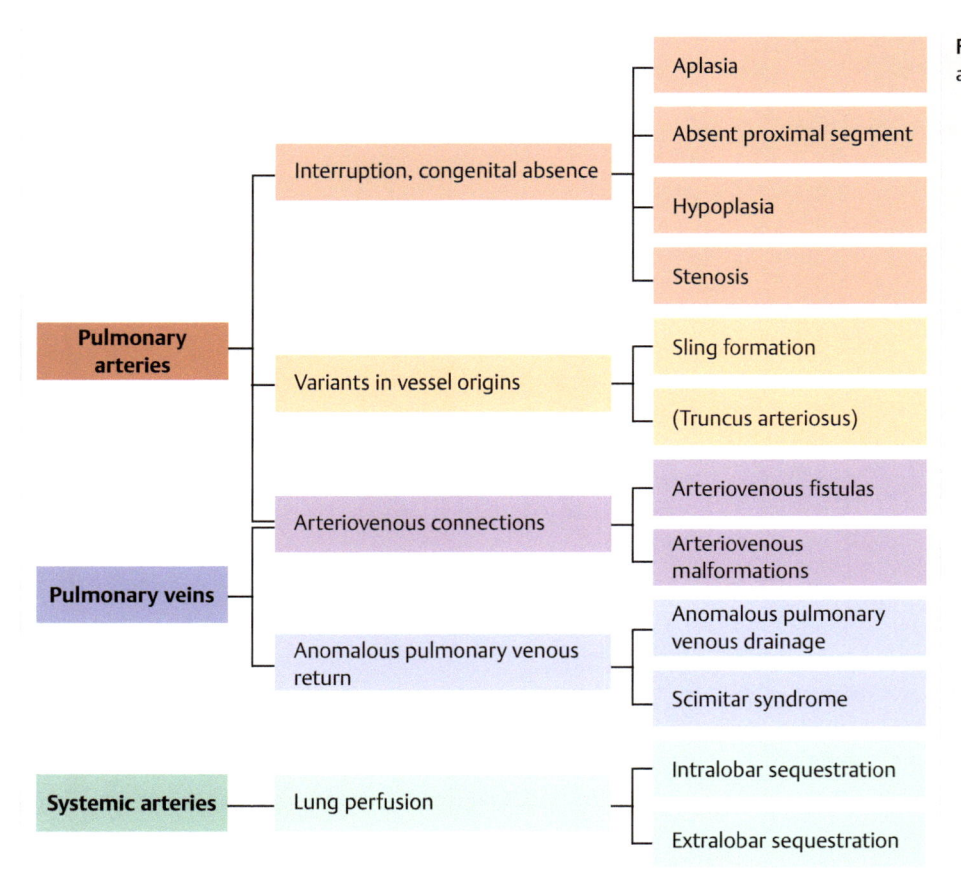

Fig. 4.23 The spectrum of pulmonary vascular anomalies.

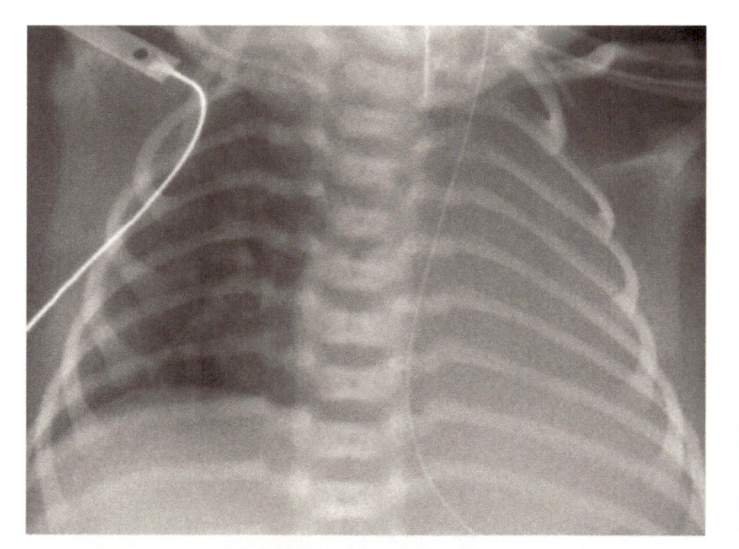

- **Pulmonary arteries**
  - Interruption, congenital absence
    - Aplasia
    - Absent proximal segment
    - Hypoplasia
    - Stenosis
  - Variants in vessel origins
    - Sling formation
    - (Truncus arteriosus)
- **Pulmonary veins**
  - Arteriovenous connections
    - Arteriovenous fistulas
    - Arteriovenous malformations
  - Anomalous pulmonary venous return
    - Anomalous pulmonary venous drainage
    - Scimitar syndrome
- **Systemic arteries**
  - Lung perfusion
    - Intralobar sequestration
    - Extralobar sequestration

Fig. 4.24 Agenesis of the left lung. Chest radiograph shows complete opacity of the left hemithorax.

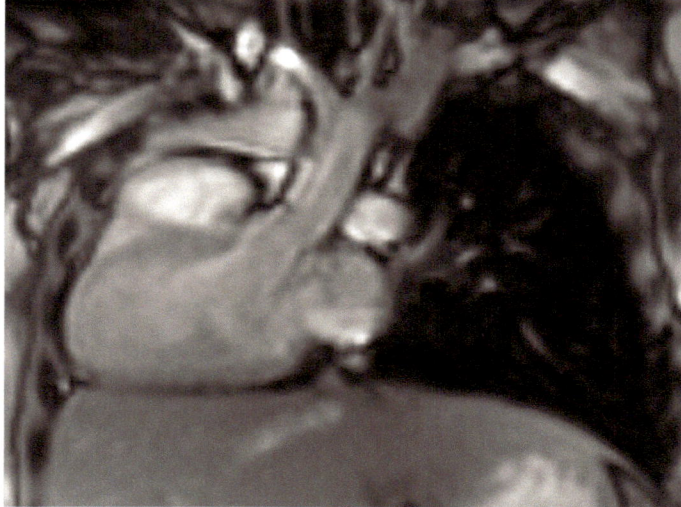

Fig. 4.25 Agenesis of the right lung. MRI shows the heart occupying the right hemithorax in a patient with right pulmonary agenesis.

▶ **Key points.** Pulmonary agenesis or aplasia is a rare anomaly. Bilateral agenesis is incompatible with postnatal life. In unilateral cases, possible pulmonary hypertension will determine the prognosis. The chest radiograph allows a presumptive diagnosis, which is confirmed by CT or MRI. The affected hemithorax is occupied by the heart and mediastinum. There is compensatory overinflation of the contralateral lung.

Cystic Adenomatoid Malformation of the Lung

▶ **Brief definition.** Cystic adenomatoid malformation of the lung results from abnormal budding of the terminal bronchi early in the first trimester of pregnancy. This leads to an overgrowth of bronchial tissue, which, being derived from the terminal bronchioles, is devoid of cartilage. Alveoli are absent in the affected regions, which are occupied by cysts. There is no predilection for a particular lobe.

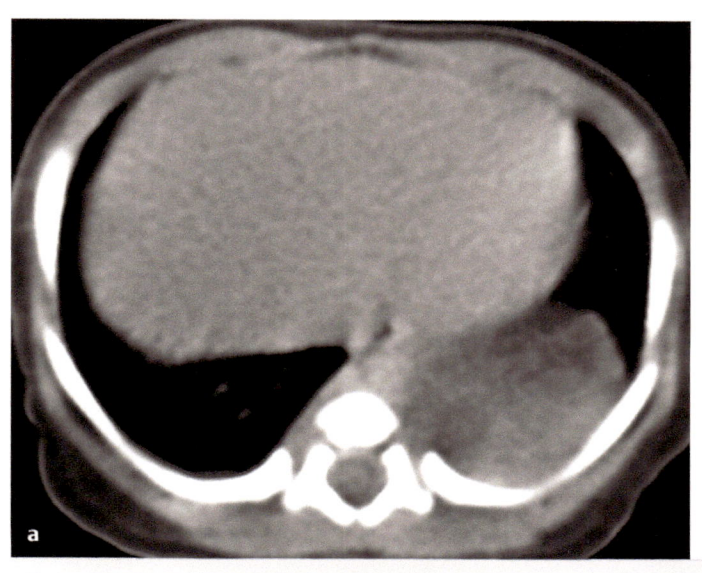

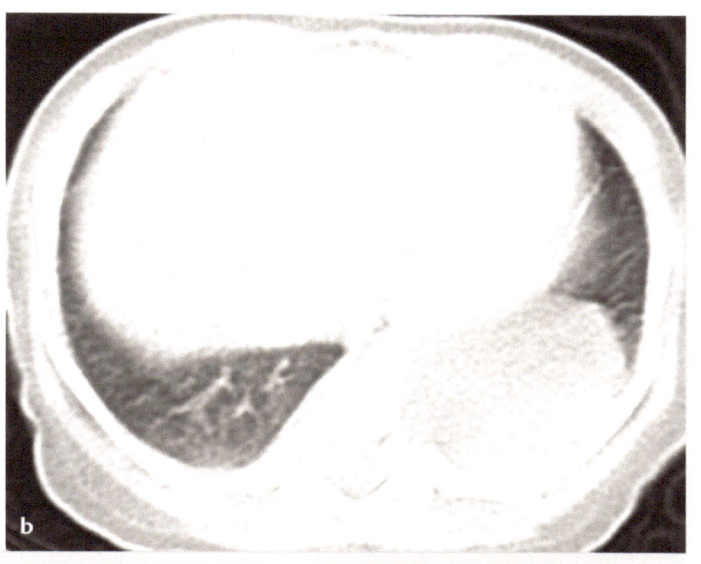

Fig. 4.26 **Cystic adenomatoid malformation of the left lower lobe.** (a) Axial CT with a soft tissue window shows homogeneous opacity with smooth borders. (b) Lung window setting shows absence of an air bronchogram.

The malformed tissue is usually confined to one lobe and may produce a mass effect causing compression of the esophagus and trachea and a mediastinal shift. Cystic adenomatoid malformation is frequently diagnosed at prenatal ultrasound. Malignant transformation with the formation of various types of sarcoma or bronchoalveolar carcinoma is known to occur, and therefore resection is the treatment of choice even for smaller lesions.

▶ **Imaging signs.** Cystic adenomatoid malformation of the lung appears on chest radiographs as a homogeneous opacity with smooth margins and no air bronchogram (▶ Fig. 4.26). Mediastinal shift may be apparent. The dysplastic bronchial structures may have a connection to the tracheobronchial tree, in which case the cysts can drain and may appear as ring shadows on chest radiographs. CT and MRI can demonstrate the cystic nature of the lesions. The ipsilateral lung may be hypoplastic.

▶ **Clinical features.** Compression of the fetal esophagus may occur, leading to polyhydramnios. Compression of the ipsilateral lung leads to hypoplasia of that lung. Approximately 50% of affected newborns exhibit respiratory distress. Recurrent infections may be the only symptom in children with smaller lesions.

▶ **Differential diagnosis**
- *Lymphangioma* additionally affects the neck as a rule. It can be traced in continuity from that region to the pulmonary apex, with extension into the mediastinum.
- With a *congenital diaphragmatic hernia*, the diaphragm is not visualized and the gastric bubble is not found at its typical location.
- *Bronchogenic cysts* can be very difficult to distinguish from cystic adenomatoid lung malformation and, when large, may produce the same set of symptoms. Resection is the treatment of choice for both entities.

▶ **Key points.** Cystic adenomatoid malformation of the lung results from abnormal budding and overgrowth of terminal bronchioles and leads to the formation of cystic dysplastic tissue that is usually confined to one lobe. The malformation may compress

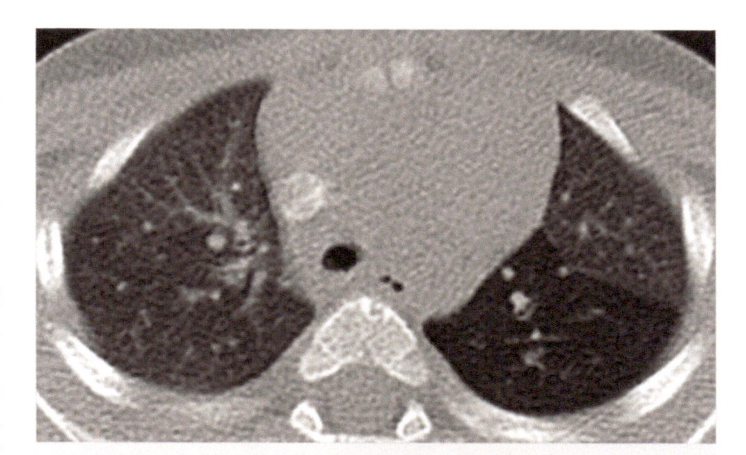

Fig. 4.27 Congenital pulmonary emphysema in the apicoposterior segment of the left upper lobe.

the ipsilateral lung parenchyma, leading to pulmonary dysplasia on that side. Compression of the trachea and esophagus may occur. Half of affected newborns exhibit respiratory distress. Imaging can demonstrate the cystic tissue and associated mass effect. The differential diagnosis should include congenital diaphragmatic hernia. The treatment of choice is resection.

Congenital Lobar Emphysema

▶ **Brief definition.** Congenital lobar emphysema refers to the overinflation of one pulmonary lobe or segment. Possible causes are a check-valve mechanism due to circumscribed bronchomalacia (a wall cartilage defect may lead to expiratory collapse with an obstructive check-valve mechanism), bronchial stenosis, or presence of a mass, or may be idiopathic. The left upper lobe is affected in 50% of cases, while the right upper and middle lobes each account for approximately 20% of cases.

▶ **Imaging signs.** The affected lung area is hyperlucent on the chest radiograph. Vascular markings are decreased (▶ Fig. 4.27). Pronounced overinflation may cause mediastinal shift and the atelectasis of adjacent, unaffected pulmonary segments.

▶ **Clinical features.** Due to the pathogenic mechanism described above, the disease becomes clinically apparent only with the onset of respiration after birth. In 25% of cases, dyspnea manifests postnatally with the onset of respiration. Approximately 50% of children manifest dyspnea and cyanosis during the first month of life. In milder forms of the anomaly, the diagnosis may be suggested by recurrent episodes of pneumonia during the first months of life. The treatment of choice is segmentectomy or lobectomy.

▶ **Differential diagnosis.** The identification of vascular markings in congenital lobar emphysema permits differentiation from pneumothorax and congenital cysts. Another important differential diagnosis is Swyer–James syndrome.

▶ **Key points.** Congenital lobar emphysema may result from a check-valve mechanism with inspiratory overinflation of the affected lobe or segment. The left upper lobe is affected in one-half of cases, and the right upper and middle lobes are each affected in 20%. The cause is usually a circumscribed cartilage defect in the bronchus to the affected lobe, destabilizing the bronchial lumen and leading to circumscribed bronchomalacia. Affected children show early symptom onset with dyspnea and cyanosis, generally enabling the condition to be diagnosed during the first months of life. Only a small percentage of patients have recurrent episodes of pneumonia as their dominant symptom. The treatment of choice is resection of the affected lobe.

Congenital Diaphragmatic Hernia or Diaphragmatic Defect

▶ **Brief definition.** Congenital diaphragmatic hernia refers to partial or complete congenital absence of the diaphragm. The left hemidiaphragm is affected in more than 90% of cases. The herniation of intestinal organs into the chest leads to pulmonary hypoplasia, which may also affect the contralateral side if the mediastinum is displaced and the right lung is also compressed. Today almost 70% of affected children survive the condition as a result of early treatment. If the lung volume is very small prenatally, the placement of a tracheal balloon by fetal surgery in the 26th week of gestation can raise the intrapulmonary pressure and stimulate lung growth. The balloon is removed a few weeks later. Reportedly, this procedure can increase survival rates by 30 to 40%. The incidence of the disease is approximately 1:4,000 births. The cause is still unknown but presumably involves a failure of closure of the pleuroperitoneal folds in the sixth week of gestation. Almost 50% of cases are diagnosed by prenatal ultrasound. The prognosis depends on the degree of pulmonary hypoplasia and the persistence of pulmonary hypertension in the newborn.

▶ **Imaging signs.** The herniation is detectable sonographically by approximately the 18th week of gestation. The ultrasound-determined ratio of head circumference to lung volume is useful in making a prognosis: The longest lung diameters are measured at the level of the cardiac four-chamber view. The two values are multiplied together and divided by the head circumference. If the result is less than 1, the prognosis for survival is poor (survival rate < 30%) and current best practice is to proceed with fetal tracheal balloon occlusion. Prenatal MRI also enables volumetry of

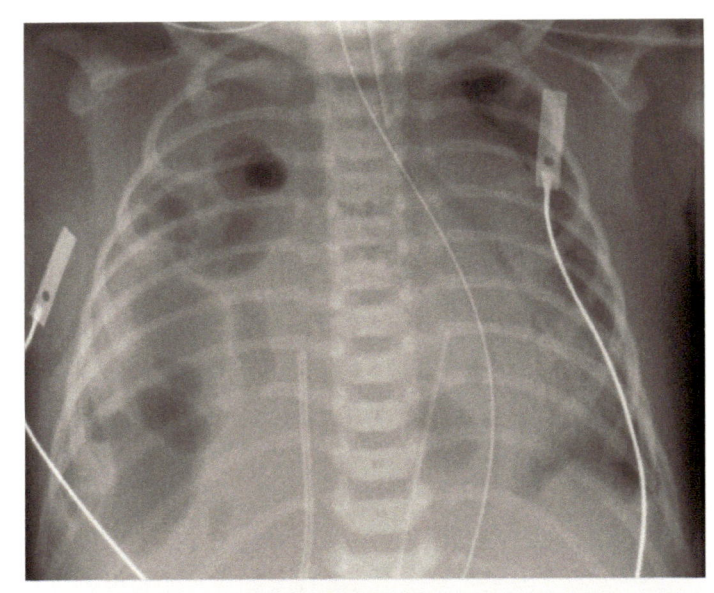

Fig. 4.28 Congenital diaphragmatic hernia on the right side. The right hemithorax is filled with bowel loops.

the lung. Postnatal chest radiography shows the presence of herniated abdominal viscera within the thorax (▶ Fig. 4.28).

▶ **Clinical features.** The degree of pulmonary hypoplasia determines the severity of postnatal respiratory distress. Because one-half of affected children have coexisting congenital heart disease, heart failure is common. The abdomen is scaphoid. Auscultation reveals absence of breath sounds in the left hemithorax, but intestinal sounds are audible in that region. Children with a small diaphragmatic defect may be initially asymptomatic.

▶ **Differential diagnosis.** With hypoplasia or aplasia of the lung, the diaphragm is intact. Postnatal chest radiography displays the gastric bubble below the diaphragm.

▶ **Key points.** Congenital diaphragmatic hernia is generally diagnosed by prenatal ultrasound and is detectable by the 18th week of gestation. The prognosis depends on the severity of pulmonary hypoplasia.

Pulmonary Sequestration

▶ **Brief definition.** Pulmonary sequestration results from an accessory lung bud and consists of aberrant lung tissue that lacks a normal connection with the bronchial tree. The sequestrum receives its blood supply from a systemic artery that usually arises from the descending aorta. Intralobar sequestrations, which account for 75% of all pulmonary sequestrations and do not have a separate pleura, are distinguished from extralobar sequestrations, which are enclosed within their own pleura. Extralobar sequestrations may also be infradiaphragmatic. Fistulas may be present between the esophagus and sequestered lung.

▶ **Imaging signs.** Sequestra are most commonly located in the left basal lung. The chest radiograph may show a well-circumscribed, partially lobulated opacity in the affected segment. CT or MRI can demonstrate the arterial supply. The sequestered parenchyma is usually not aerated, and fluid-filled cysts are typically

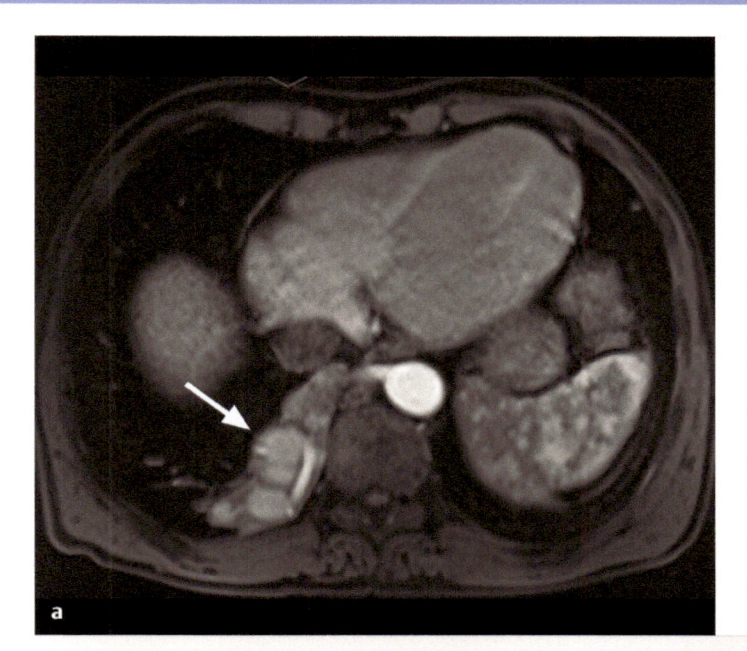

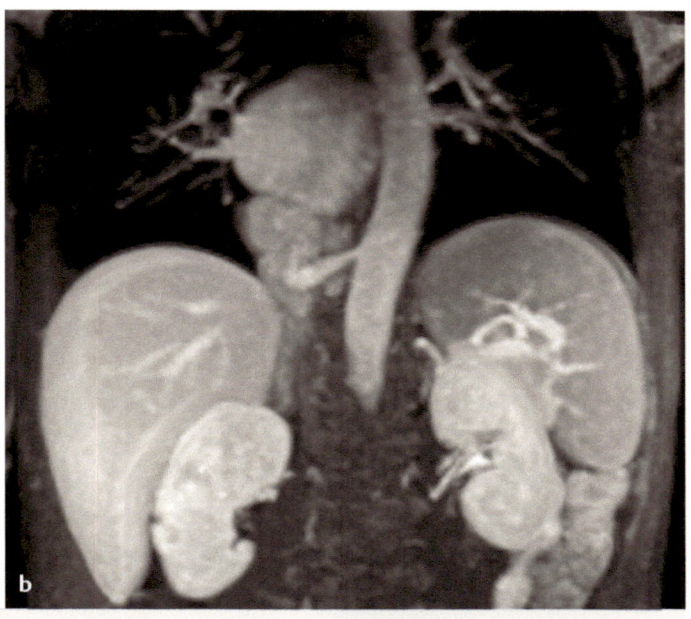

Fig. 4.29 **Intralobar pulmonary sequestration on the right side.** (a) Axial T1 W image shows cysts filled with protein-rich fluid in the anomalous lung tissue (arrow). (b) Maximum intensity projection shows the large-caliber artery arising from the aorta.

present (▶ Fig. 4.29). The venous drainage of an intralobar sequestration usually occurs via the pulmonary veins. An extralobar sequestration drains via the azygos–hemiazygos system.

▶ **Clinical features.** Pulmonary sequestrations often contain cysts that gradually fill with mucus and may perforate into the tracheobronchial tree. This connection may then form a pathway for superinfection of the sequestered lung, manifested clinically by recurrent episodes of pneumonia. Due to the systemic arterial supply to the hypofunctioning tissue, recurrent hemoptysis may also occur. The treatment of choice is resection.

▶ **Differential diagnosis**
- *Infradiaphragmatic sequestra* may be impossible to differentiate from other masses. Diagnosis in these cases must rely on postoperative histology.
- A *paravertebral sequestration* requires mainly differentiation from neuroblastoma. The large-caliber supply artery is a key differentiating feature.

▶ **Key points.** Pulmonary sequestration is most commonly located in the posterior portion of the left lower lobe. The hallmark of pulmonary sequestration is a large supply artery arising from the aorta, which differentiates it from other masses. Resection is the treatment of choice for symptomatic cases with recurrent pneumonia and hemoptysis.

4.3.2 Infections

Pneumonia

▶ **Brief definition.** Pneumonia may be caused by a broad spectrum of infectious organisms that includes fungi and viruses in addition to classic bacterial pathogens. While viral pneumonias show an interstitial pattern of involvement, bacterial pneumonias spread in the alveolar air spaces and generally do not permit a specific diagnosis based on morphological imaging findings. A definitive diagnosis requires isolation of the causative organism from sputum or blood cultures. Pneumonias have three, somewhat different pathogenic mechanisms that involve different routes of spread:
- *Lobar pneumonia*: This form is characterized by the spread of inflammation in the alveoli, to the alveolar duct, and to the terminal bronchioles as well as between alveoli through the pores of Kohn. Lobar pneumonia spreads in stages, all of which are rarely seen nowadays or occur in a mild form due to the early initiation of antibiotic therapy:
  - *Congestion*: The initial response is an exudation of protein-rich fluid into the alveolar space and an influx of monocytes.
    – *Red hepatization*: Capillary damage allows extravasation of red cells and fibrin into the alveoli; the parenchyma becomes heavy and grossly resembles liver tissue in its color and consistency.
    – *Gray hepatization*: Within a few days the red cells are phagocytosed; the lung tissue becomes dry and grayish, and gray hepatization is achieved. Perfusion is maintained during these stages and is not diminished. Because the alveolar space is filled with inflammatory cells and debris and can no longer participate in gas exchange, nonoxygenated blood is shunted into the systemic circulation, and hypoxemia develops.
    – *Yellow hepatization*: In the last stage the phagocytosing granulocytes undergo purulent transformation and the tissue inflammation resolves.
- *Bronchopneumonia*: The inflammation in bronchopneumonia spreads along terminal and respiratory bronchioles to the alveoli. This leads to the multifocal spread of infiltrates, creating a patchy pattern of involvement. There is no lobar predilection.
- *Interstitial/atypical pneumonia*: This type of pneumonia is caused by viruses, the fungus *Pneumocystis jiroveci*, or *Rickettsia* bacteria and involves the interstitium. Because the alveoli are spared, the infiltrate does not follow a typical pattern, hence the alternate term "atypical pneumonia."

Note

Classic lobar pneumonia is very rare today owing to early antibiotic therapy. *Streptococcus pneumoniae* and *Haemophilus influenzae* are the principal causative organisms of lobar pneumonia.

The differentiation between community-acquired pneumonia and nosocomial pneumonia is clinically relevant:
- *Nosocomial pneumonia*: This term is applied to pneumonia that was not incubating on admission and develops more than 48 hours after hospitalization. Pneumonia that develops several weeks or months after hospitalization is also classified as nosocomial because colonization by hospital organisms is still demonstrable at that time. Current guidelines do not specify a time limit, but 4 to 6 weeks is generally accepted. Nosocomial infections are usually mixed infections, the most common organisms being *Pseudomonas aeruginosa*, Enterobacteriaceae (*Escherichia coli*, *Klebsiella* spp., *Enterobacter* spp.), *Haemophilus influenzae*, *Acinetobacter baumannii*, and *Stenotrophomonas maltophilia*. Foremost among the gram-positive organisms that cause nosocomial pneumonia are *Staphylococcus aureus* and *Streptococcus pneumoniae*. The incidence of nosocomial pneumonia is 5 to 15 per 1000 ventilation days.[3] The mortality rate in ventilated patients is 20%.
- *Community-acquired pneumonia*: This refers to pneumonia occurring in immunocompetent patients who have not been hospitalized. The main causative organisms are *Streptococcus pneumoniae*, *Mycoplasma pneumoniae*, and *Haemophilus influenzae*.
- *Pneumonia in immunocompromised patients*: This is a separate category with a different spectrum of causative organisms. Opportunistic organisms such as *Pneumocystis jiroveci* and cytomegalovirus are predominant. Immunocompromised status may result from chemotherapy for solid or hematological malignancies, HIV infection in the AIDS stage, previous organ or bone marrow transplantation, immunosuppressant therapy for autoimmune disease, or at least 4 weeks of corticosteroid therapy at a maintenance dose of at least 10 mg/day.

▶ **Selection of imaging modalities.** Chest radiography is sensitive in the diagnosis of clinically suspected pneumonia because of the sharp contrast between pneumonic infiltrates and healthy lung, and it provides reasonable confidence in the assessment of therapeutic response.

Note

One of the most common indications for chest radiography is for evaluating the presence and extent of infiltrates in patients with suspected pneumonia. Chest radiography detects infiltrates with a sensitivity of 70% but is inferior to CT in patients with subtle findings (sensitivity 100%).

Low-dose CT can be used in cases where it is necessary to detect subtle findings or incipient infiltrates, as in immunocompromised patients. "Positive air bronchogram" refers to the visualization of still-aerated bronchi within an infiltrated region. MRI has proved equivalent to CT in several studies, as infiltrates visualized with T2W sequences are very hyperintense to unaffected tissue, which is almost devoid of signal due to its aeration. Additionally, MRI can detect interstitial edema and ground-glass opacity with the same sensitivity as CT. MRI has not yet become established in routine clinical settings, however, due to its longer scan times and more limited availability.

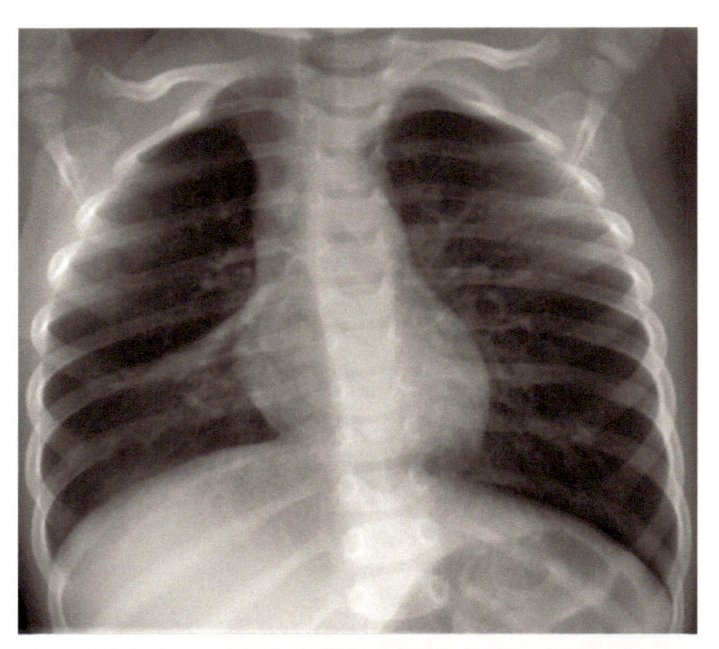

Fig. 4.30 **Lobar pneumonia of the right lower lobe.** Positive air bronchogram.

▶ **Imaging signs.** Imaging findings for specific types of pneumonia:
- *Lobar pneumonia*: homogeneous opacity of the affected lobe or segment. Bronchi that are still aerated appear as well-defined lucencies within the opacity (▶ Fig. 4.30).
- *Bronchopneumonia*: focal opacities that coalesce in severe cases. The bronchial walls are thickened, as demonstrated particularly well by bronchi viewed end-on in the frontal radiograph and on CT (▶ Fig. 4.31). CT in bronchopneumonia shows centrilobular opacities, which may also coalesce. Vessels are no longer visible in areas with confluent infiltrates.
- *Interstitial pneumonia*: the intralobar septa are thickened in this type of pneumonia. Enlargement of hilar lymph nodes is very rarely seen. With proper antibiotic therapy, the infiltrates will regress in 50% of patients within 2 weeks, in approximately 70% of patients by 4 weeks, and in 80% by 6 weeks. Infection with the fungus *Pneumocystis jiroveci* is characterized by ground-glass opacities (▶ Fig. 4.32), which often spare a narrow strip beneath the pleura. Generally the lymph nodes are not enlarged. Thickening of the interlobular septa is evident in up to 40% of patients.

Bacterial pneumonia as well as bronchial stenosis may be associated with abscess formation. Extrapulmonary abscesses may also spread contiguously to the lung. The abscess can be seen on chest radiographs only if it communicates with the tracheobronchial tree and an air crescent is visible in the abscess cavity. As in other organs, CT shows a nonenhancing area of liquefaction (▶ Fig. 4.33).

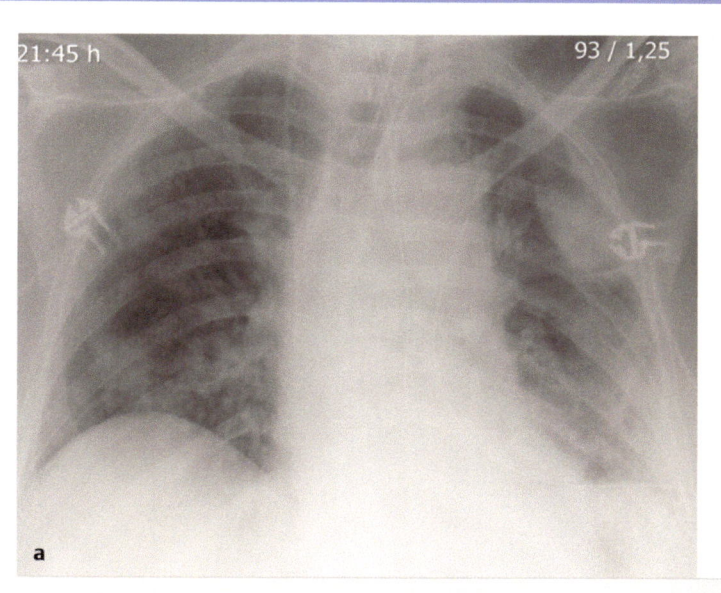

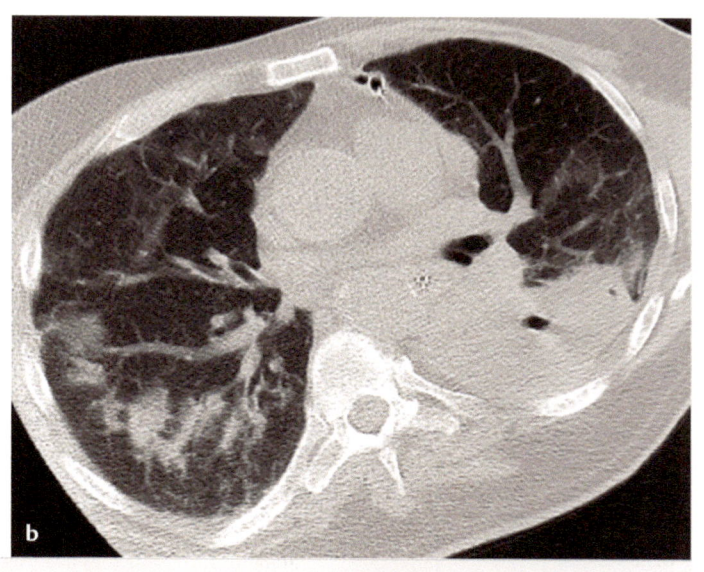

Fig. 4.31 **Bronchopneumonia.** (a) Chest radiograph shows patchy infiltrates. (b) CT shows thickening of the bronchial walls. The infiltrates are distributed around the bronchi as evidence of bronchogenic spread.

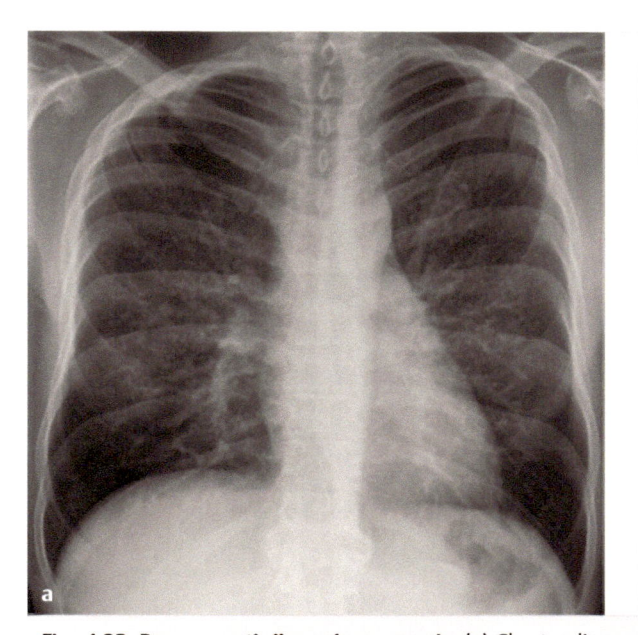

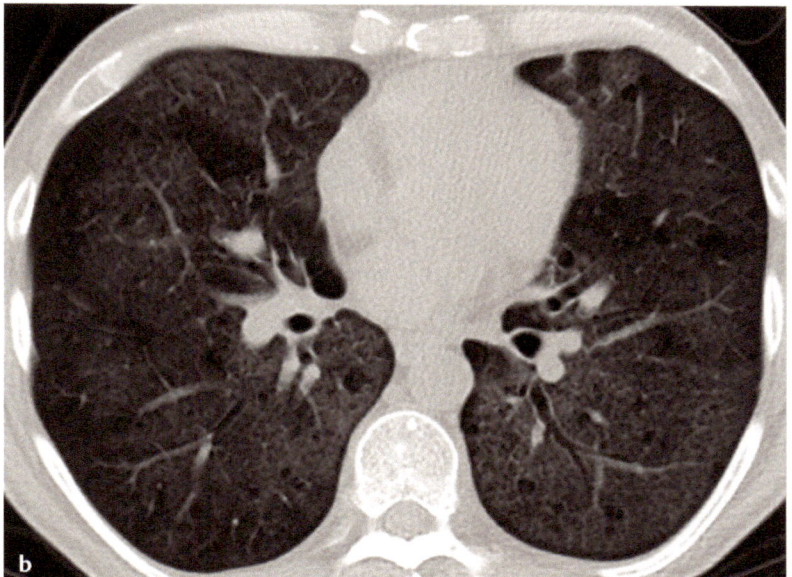

Fig. 4.32 *Pneumocystis jiroveci* pneumonia. (a) Chest radiograph shows low-density infiltrates. (b) CT shows ground-glass opacities with subpleural sparing.

▶ **Clinical features.** Typical symptoms are fever, productive cough, and audible crackles. Laboratory tests show a left shift, elevated C-reactive protein, and leukocytosis.

▶ **Differential diagnosis.** Pulmonary venous congestion is the most important radiological differential diagnosis, especially in supine radiographs obtained in ICU patients.

Septic Emboli

▶ **Brief definition.** Septic pulmonary embolism refers to the hematogenous spread into the lungs of thrombi that contain microorganisms (usually *Staphylococcus aureus*). The infectious particles may originate from sources such as valvular endocarditis, a superinfected central venous catheter or port system, or IV drug abuse. The thrombi remain lodged in the peripheral vessels.

An infiltrate forms initially, which then liquefies within a few days to form a small cavity. Treatment consists of IV antibiotics and eradication of the source.

▶ **Imaging signs.** The chest radiograph shows multiple faint, rounded opacities with or without cavitation. They occur predominantly in the peripheral and basal lung. CT can often reveal the relationship of the emboli to blood vessels (▶ Fig. 4.34).

▶ **Clinical features.** Patients are febrile and show laboratory signs of inflammation.

▶ **Key points.** Septic pulmonary emboli most commonly occur in the peripheral lung. The foci cavitate within a short time. CT can document proximity to vessels.

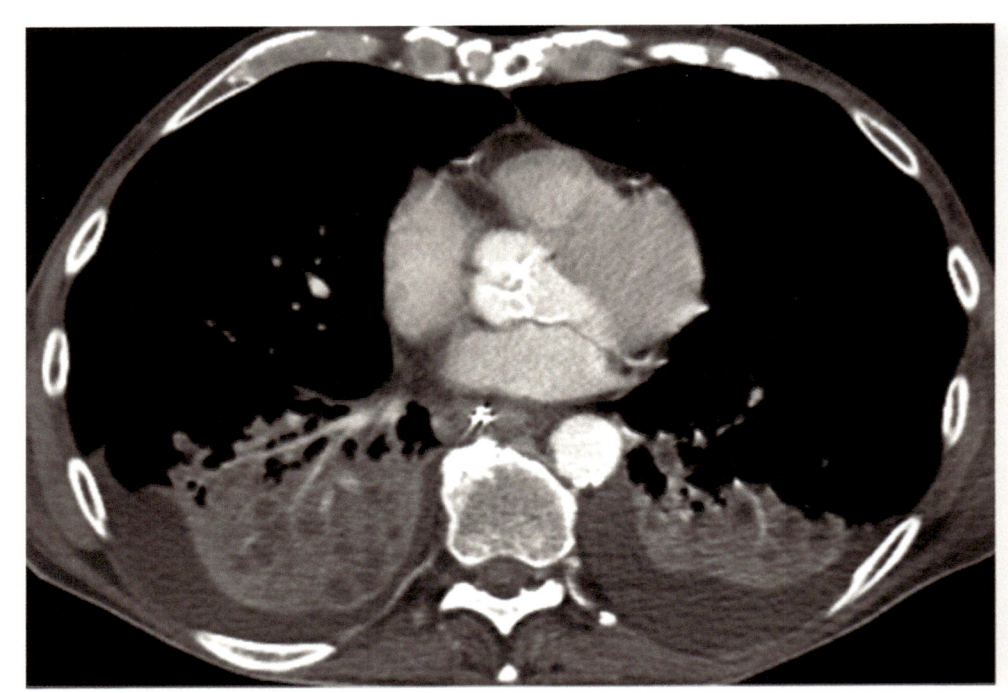

Fig. 4.33 Lung abscesses in pneumonia.

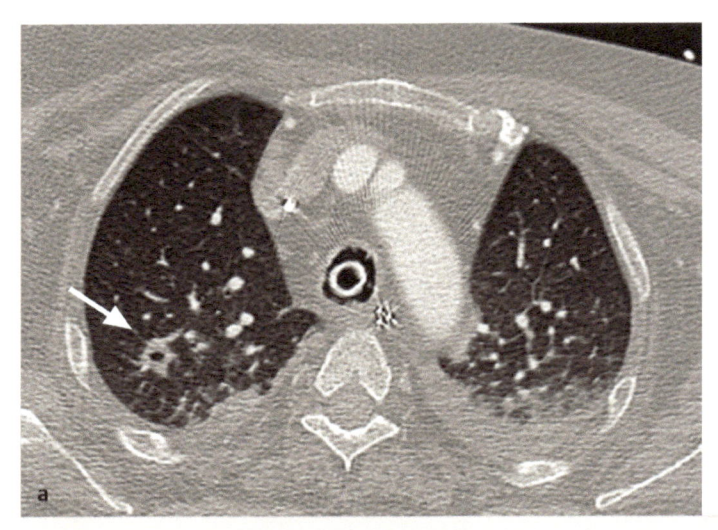

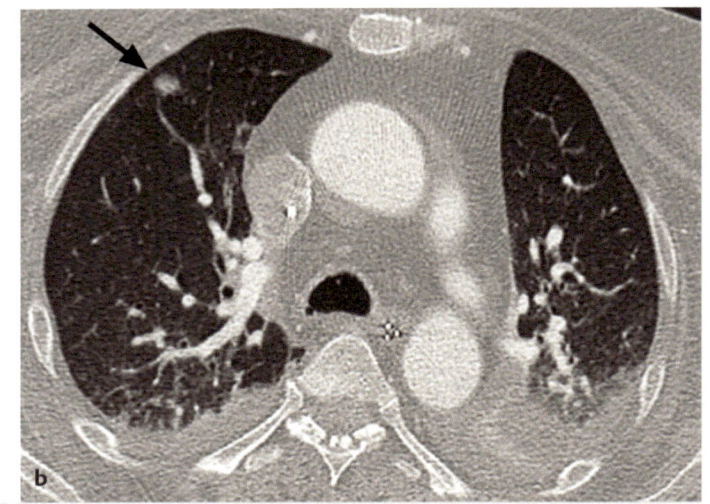

Fig. 4.34 Septic pulmonary emboli. (a) Solitary foci show central liquefaction (arrow). (b) The peripheral location of the emboli (arrow) in proximity to blood vessels is typical.

Tuberculosis

Primary Tuberculosis

▶ **Brief definition.** Tuberculosis is an infection with aerobic gram-positive organisms of the genus *Mycobacterium*. The causative organisms are, in descending order of frequency, *M. tuberculosis*, *M. bovis* (transmissible by cattle, especially in countries without compulsory pasteurization of milk, such as Asia), *M. africanum* (lymph node involvement), and *M. microti*. The 2013 WHO report states that in 2012 an estimated 8.6 million people worldwide developed tuberculosis and 1.3 million died from the disease. Endemic regions are Asia, Africa, and the countries of the former Soviet Union. Multidrug-resistant strains no longer sensitive to the standard antibiotics rifampicin and isoniazid are becoming more widespread in these regions. In extremely drug-resistant (XDR) tuberculosis, the bacteria are also resistant to many second-line antibiotics. Initial diagnosis is by light microscopic examination with Ziehl–Neelsen stain. If this does not detect acid-fast rods (i.e., rods that retain stain after washing in an acid solution), a bacterial culture should be grown. Culture takes approximately 4 weeks due to the slow replication of mycobacteria. A primary infection denotes initial contact with tuberculosis before antibodies have been developed. Pulmonary tuberculosis is acquired by droplet inhalation, which often occurs in childhood. This stage is asymptomatic in immunocompetent patients or may present with symptoms of a mild cold. The mycobacteria are phagocytosed in the alveolar space to form a Ghon focus, a caseating granuloma that contains mycobacteria at its center. Transport to the regional (hilar) lymph nodes leads to hilar lymphadenopathy with enlargement of the hilar nodes. The Ghon focus and associated lymphadenitis are called the *primary complex* (also called the Ranke complex). In immunocompetent individuals, the primary complex heals by fibrosis and may calcify. Viable bacteria remain walled-off within the healed focus and may be reactivated years or even decades later due to a weakened immune status. This can lead to bronchogenic spread of the infectious organisms and the development of pneumonia.

> **Caution**
> Primary pulmonary tuberculosis is very rarely detected due to its mild clinical presentation in immunocompetent individuals (absence of symptoms, or symptoms of a slight cold).

▶ **Imaging signs.** Imaging findings consist of a faint infiltrate in the lower or middle lobe or, less commonly, in the perihilar portions of the upper lobe and hilar lymphadenopathy on the ipsilateral side (▶ Fig. 4.35).

Postprimary Tuberculosis

▶ **Brief definition.** Postprimary tuberculosis may follow the primary infection and is based on hematogenous dissemination of the causal organisms, which may spread to almost all organs in the body including the lung.

▶ **Imaging signs.** Postprimary tuberculosis commonly affects the upper lobe or the apical segment of the lower lobe (▶ Fig. 4.36), where ventilation is good and there is less perfusion than in other lung areas. Hilar lymphadenopathy is absent in immunocompetent patients but is generally present in AIDS. Cavitation is typical and occurs in half of all patients. The tree-in-bud pattern on CT is characteristic of bronchogenic spread. Tuberculosis may also be manifested as pleurisy; this condition is unilateral, it is not associated with infiltrates or lymphadenopathy, and its imaging appearance is indistinguishable from that of pleural effusion due to other causes. Postprimary tuberculosis often heals by scarring with upward retraction of the hila (▶ Fig. 4.37).

▶ **Clinical features.** Patients may present with B symptoms, chronic cough, chest pain, and hemoptysis.

▶ **Differential diagnosis.** Postprimary tuberculosis with cavitation requires differentiation from adenocarcinoma and lung abscess. Miliary tuberculosis is a subtype of postprimary tuberculosis that occurs in immunocompromised patients. It is characterized by innumerable fine nodules 1 to 2 mm in diameter distributed throughout the lung (▶ Fig. 4.38).

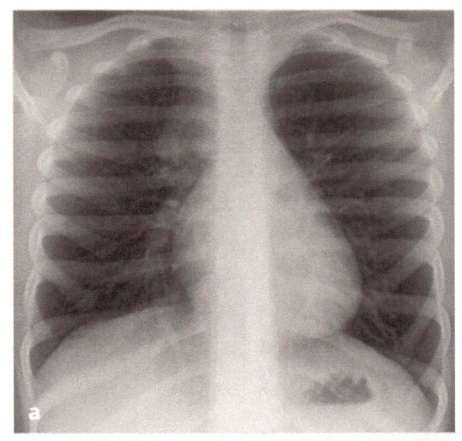

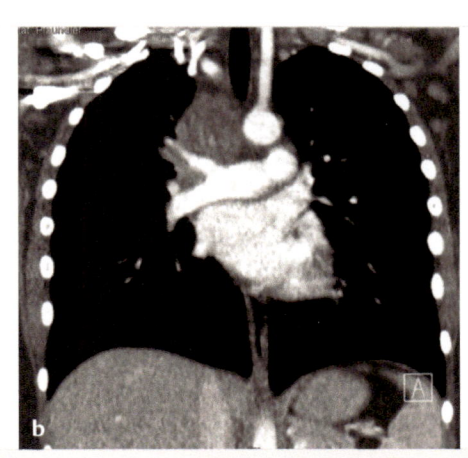

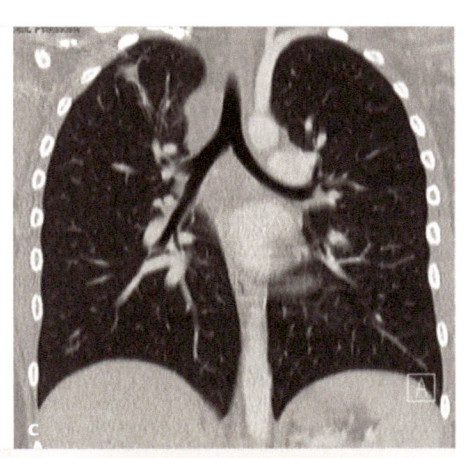

Fig. 4.35 **Primary tuberculosis** in a 7-year-old girl. **(a)** Frontal chest radiograph shows enlarged lymph nodes. **(b)** Hilar and mediastinal lymphadenopathy. **(c)** Primary infiltrate in the upper lobe.

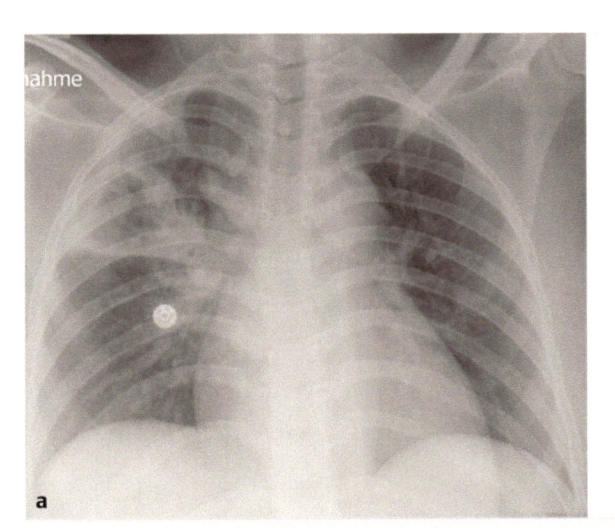

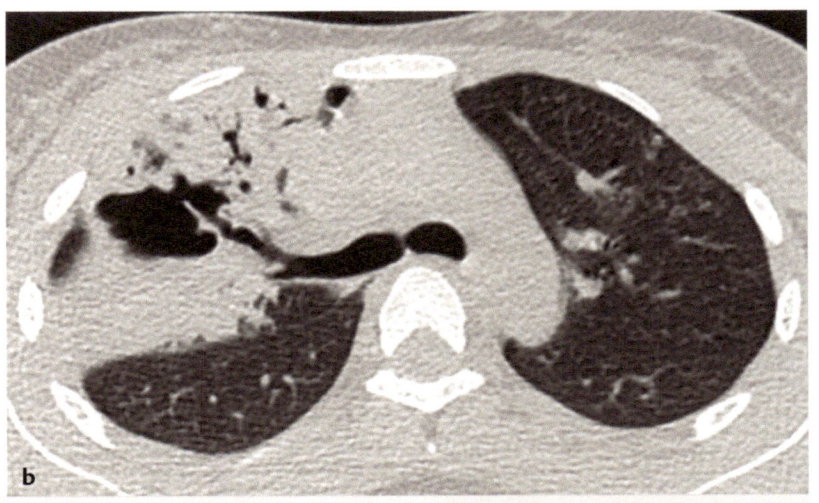

Fig. 4.36 **Postprimary tuberculosis with typical upper lobe involvement. (a)** Chest radiograph demonstrates a cavity in the infiltrated upper lobe. **(b)** CT shows communication with the tracheobronchial tree.

Lung and Pleura

Note

Tuberculosis is a notifiable disease in the European Union and the United States.

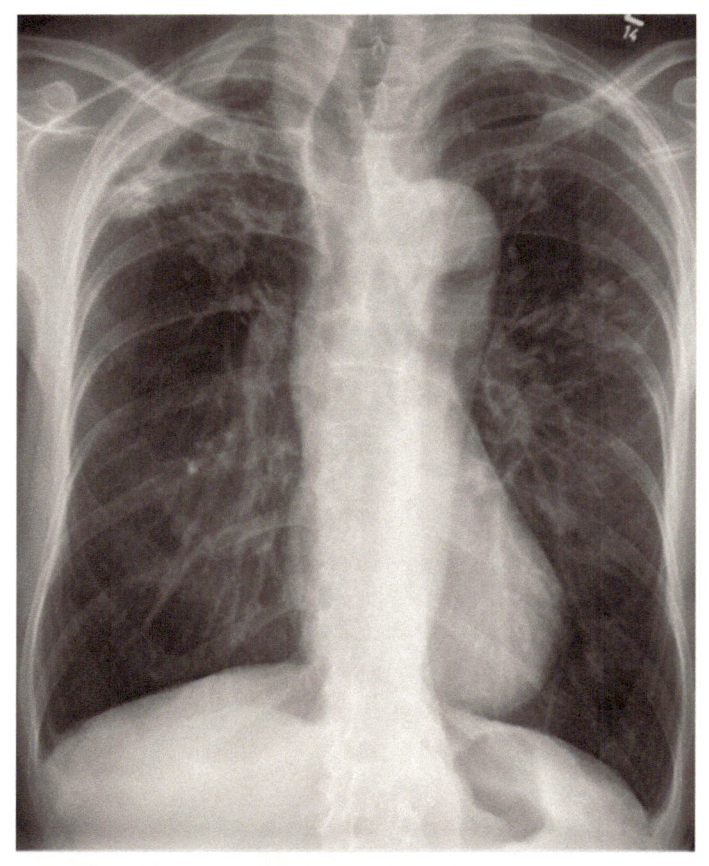

Fig. 4.37 **Healed tuberculosis.** Chest radiograph shows typical upward retraction of the hila.

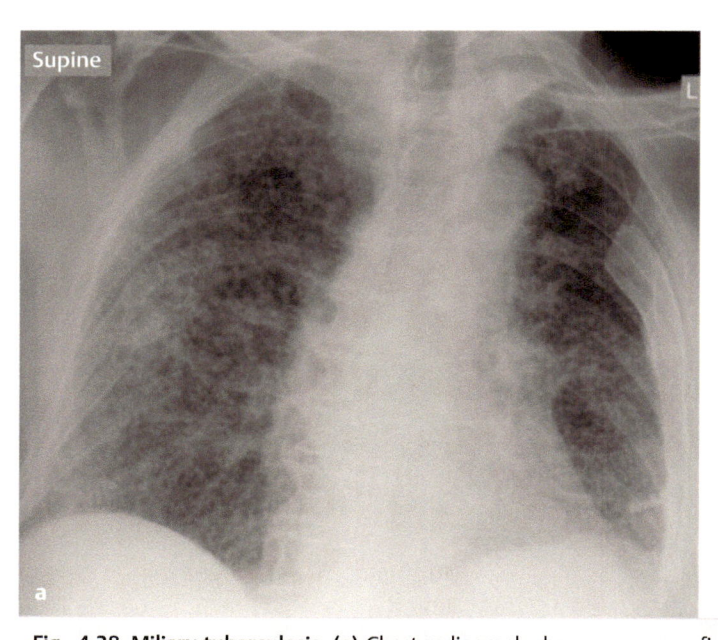

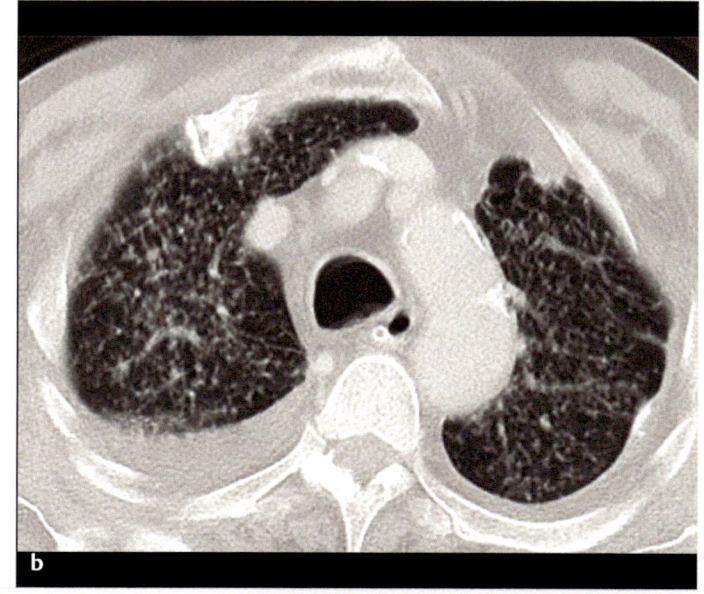

Fig. 4.38 **Miliary tuberculosis.** (a) Chest radiograph shows numerous fine nodules distributed throughout the lung. (b) Centrilobular nodules on axial CT.

Aspergillosis

▶ **Brief definition.** Fungi of the genus *Aspergillus* include molds and occur ubiquitously in the environment. Species pathogenic to humans are *Aspergillus fumigatus*, which alone is responsible for 80% of all *Aspergillus* infections, as well as *A. flavus* and *A. niger*. Aspergilli are dimorphic and may occur as spores (conidia) or hyphae, which can sprout to form mycelia. *Aspergillus fumigatus* can often be isolated from the nasopharynx of healthy individuals. The colonization rate is 50% in cystic fibrosis patients and 20% in patients with pulmonary fibrosis. Three different types of aspergillosis are known:

- *Aspergilloma*: This refers to fungal involvement of a preexisting cavity in the lung, forming a fungus ball composed of mycelia and cellular debris.
- *Allergic bronchopulmonary aspergillosis*: This type occurs as an allergic response to fungal spores in an asthma patient, leading to the destruction of lung parenchyma and the development of bronchiectasis. The cellular immune response plus a type I (immunoglobulin E) and type II hypersensitivity (complement system) response incite an inflammatory reaction with destruction of the bronchial walls. The pathophysiology involves granuloma formation in the bronchial lumen, causing obstruction of the bronchus and retained secretions (endobronchial mucoid impaction). With inadequate treatment, these processes lead to multifocal bronchiectasis.
- *Angioinvasive aspergillosis*: This type, with the subtype of bronchoinvasive (semi-invasive) aspergillosis, occurs in immunocompromised patients. Since phagocytosis is impaired in the immunocompromised host, inhaled fungal spores can develop into hyphae that infiltrate the lung tissue and vessels, causing occlusions. Invasion of the bronchial walls causes bronchiolitis and bronchopneumonia.

▶ **Imaging signs**
- *Aspergilloma*: The conglomeration of fungal hyphae appears as a rounded opacity within a cavity. Because it does not

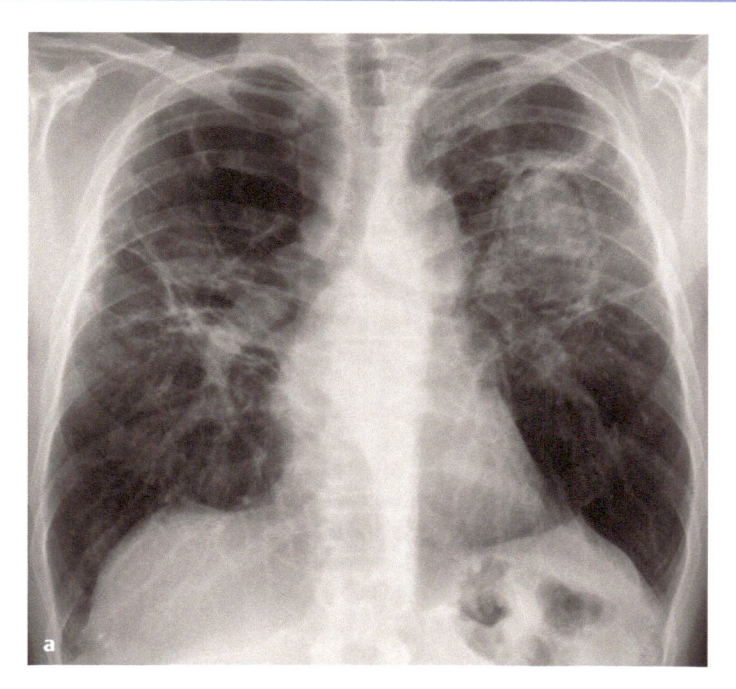

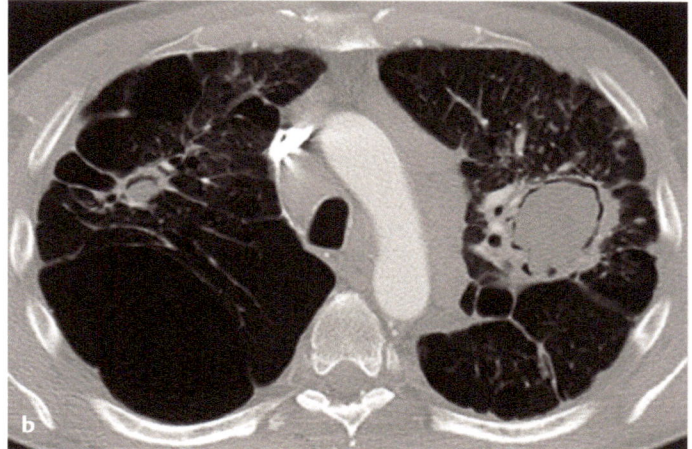

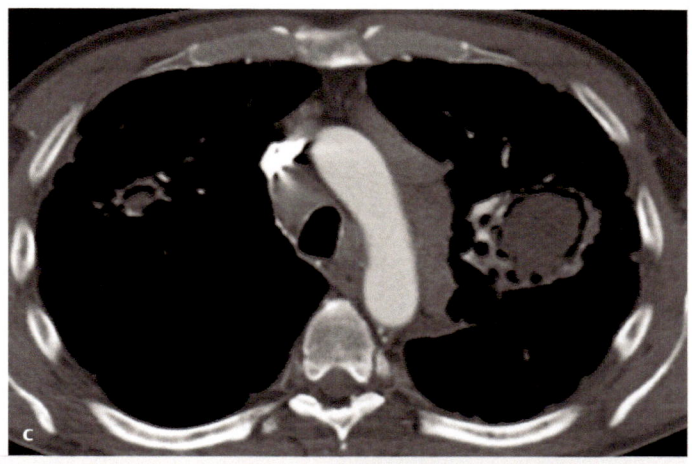

Fig. 4.39 Aspergilloma in an emphysematous bulla. The patient has traction emphysema due to stage IV sarcoidosis. **(a)** Air crescent sign on the chest radiograph. **(b)** CT shows another aspergilloma in the right lung. **(c)** The fungus ball remains hypodense after administration of contrast medium.

completely fill the cavity, an air crescent is visible between the fungus ball and cavity walls (air crescent sign, ▶ Fig. 4.39). The fungus ball may initially contain air inclusions, similar to a sponge, but may later be very dense and contain calcifications. Usually the fungus ball is freely mobile within the cavity and will move with changes in the patient's position. Typically the cavity wall is not infiltrated. Local pleural thickening may be noted at the level of the cavity.
- *Invasive aspergillosis*: This form is characterized by rapidly progressive opacities in the chest radiographs. CT shows surrounding ground-glass opacity due to hemorrhage (the halo sign). Peripheral wedge-shaped densities may develop due to vascular invasion and tissue infarction. These densities may subsequently clear, leaving cavities in which aspergillomas may form (▶ Fig. 4.40). Semi-invasive aspergillosis is marked by the development of slowly progressive opacities or nodules in the apical region.
- *Allergic bronchopulmonary aspergillosis*: This entity is characterized by opacities that migrate over a period of several days. Central foci of bronchiectasis with mucus retention determine the typical imaging appearance (▶ Fig. 4.41). The mucus may show high density on CT due to its high content of *Aspergillus* hyphae and eosinophilic granulocytes. The inflammation may eventually progress to pulmonary fibrosis (▶ Fig. 4.42).

▶ **Differential diagnosis.** Other fungal infections such as Wegener granulomatosis should be considered in the differential diagnosis. Pulmonary embolism with infarction can usually be positively distinguished from angioinvasive aspergillosis based on the clinical presentation.

▶ **Clinical features.** Cough, fever, chills, and chest pain are the dominant clinical symptoms, making it difficult to distinguish aspergillosis from bacterial pneumonia. Differentiation is aided by correlation with laboratory findings (neutropenia) and imaging signs. The clinical aspects of various forms of aspergillosis are reviewed below:
- *Aspergilloma* occurs in immunocompetent patients; it requires a preexisting cavity.
- *Invasive aspergillosis* is a disease of severely immunocompromised patients, occurring in approximately 20% of patients with acute leukemia and 20% of patients after chemotherapy or transplantation. Neutropenia is the crucial risk factor and should suggest angioinvasive aspergillosis when combined with fever and lung opacities. Even with appropriate therapy, invasive aspergillosis has a high mortality rate, at 40%. Approximately 40% of patients develop hemoptysis from the erosion of bronchial arteries at some time during the course of the disease. These

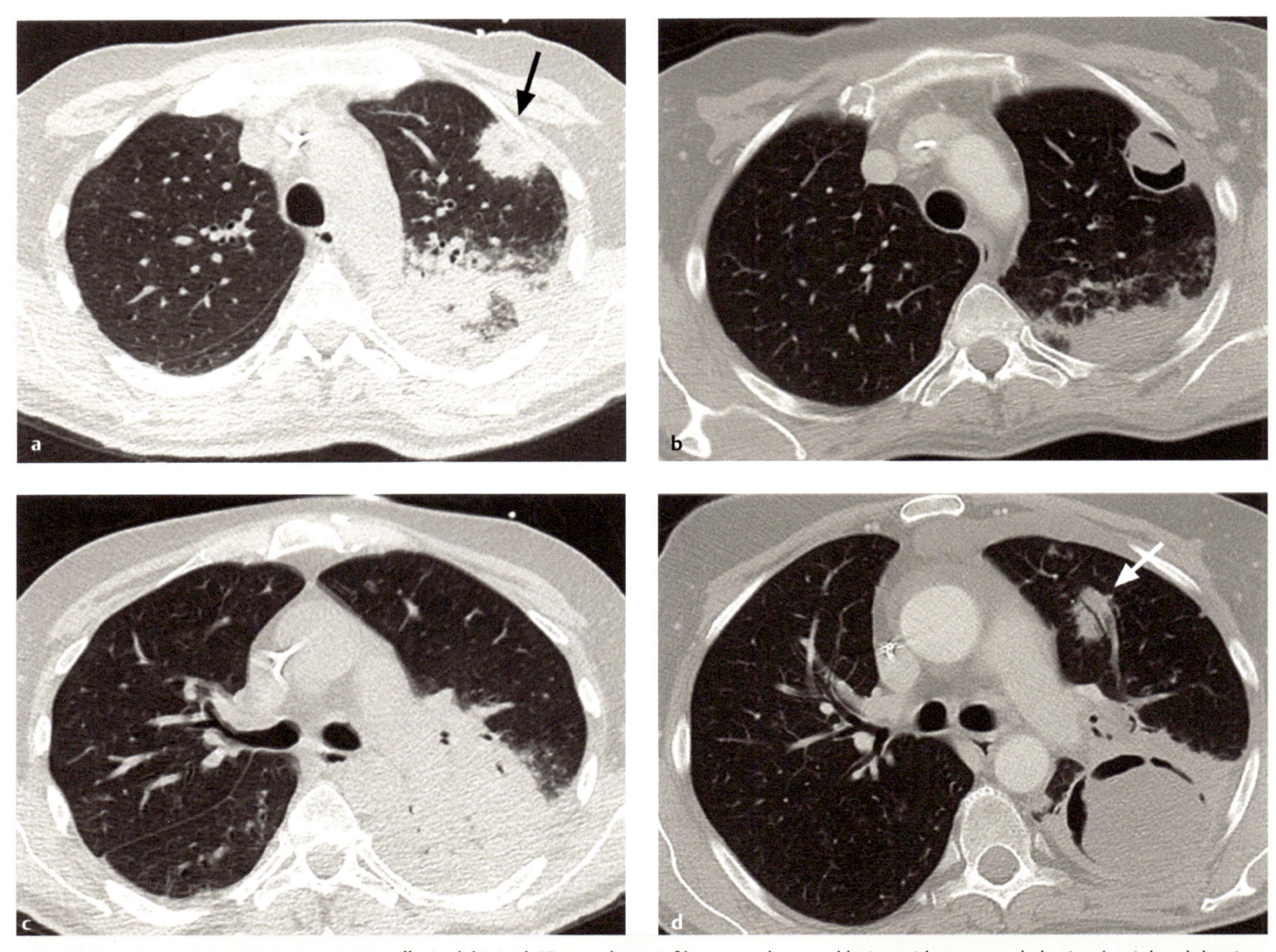

Fig. 4.40 Angioinvasive necrotizing aspergillosis. (a) Initial CT scan shows infiltrates and a round lesion with a reverse halo sign (peripheral density greater than central density, arrow). (b) Dense infiltrate. (c) Scan 2 weeks later shows transformation of the round lesion to a cavity with central density. (d) New infiltrate (arrow). Cavitation is also noted in the area of the preexisting infiltrate. The central density consists mostly of infarcted necrotic lung tissue permeated by fungi.

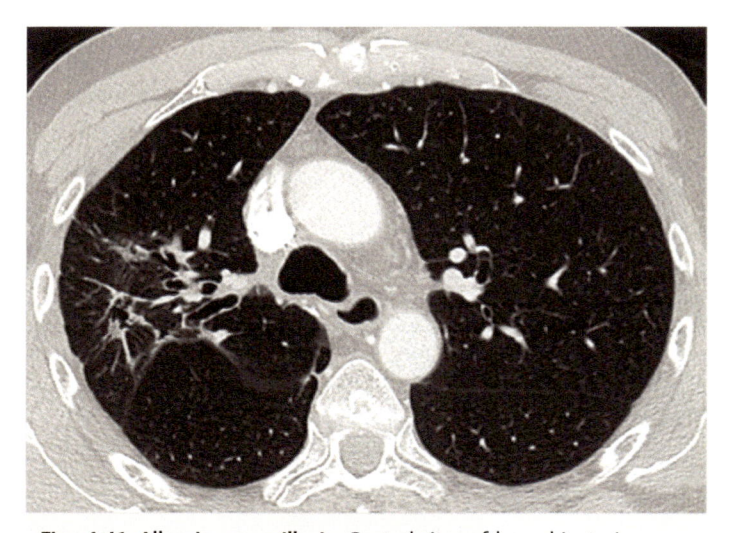

Fig. 4.41 Allergic aspergillosis. Central sites of bronchiectasis are a typical sign.

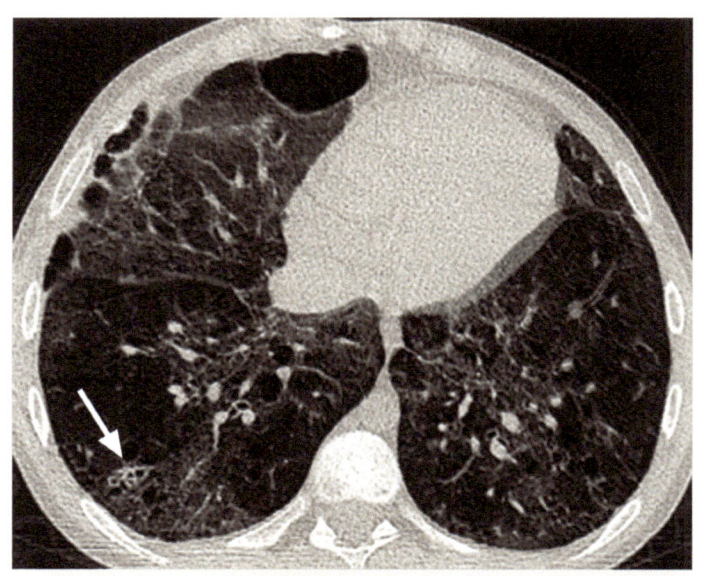

Fig. 4.42 Allergic aspergillosis in a different patient with end-stage pulmonary fibrosis and individual foci of bronchiectasis (arrow).

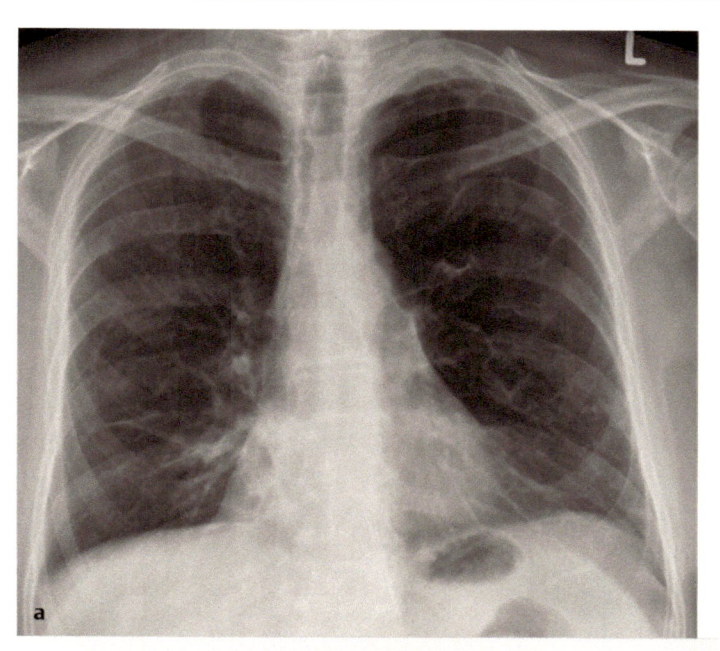

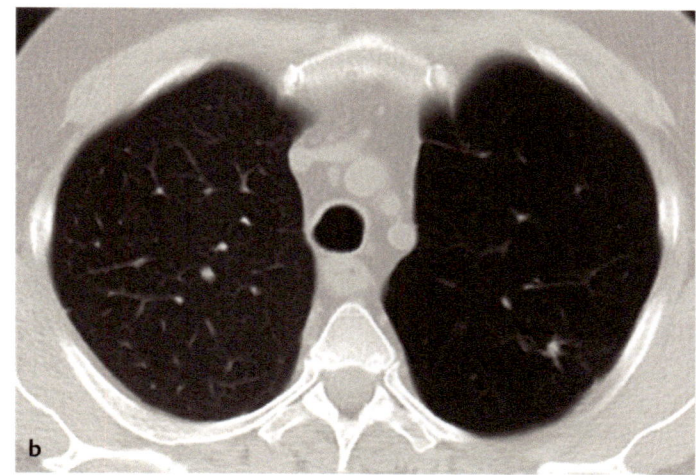

Fig. 4.43 Swyer–James–MacLeod syndrome. (a) Chest radiograph shows hyperlucency of the left upper lobe. The left hilum is small. (b) CT shows decreased pulmonary markings.

patients may require endovascular embolization. Semi-invasive aspergillosis may develop in patients with slight immunodeficiency (due to corticosteroid therapy, diabetes mellitus, alcoholism, etc.) and runs a protracted course in many cases.
- *Allergic bronchopulmonary aspergillosis* is rare in otherwise healthy individuals. Patients with cystic fibrosis or bronchial asthma are at high risk, with an incidence of 20%. Most patients are asymptomatic. On average, exacerbation with fever and viscous sputum occurs once yearly.

Swyer–James–MacLeod Syndrome

▶ **Brief definition.** Swyer–James–MacLeod syndrome is the result of obliterative bronchiolitis in early childhood with the destruction of lung parenchyma. Adenoviruses, respiratory syncytial virus, and *Mycoplasma* bacteria have been identified as causative agents.

▶ **Imaging signs.** A characteristic finding on chest radiographs is a unilateral hyperlucent lung. The hilum is small, vascularity is decreased, and the affected hemithorax may be small in relation to the contralateral side (▶ Fig. 4.43). Air trapping is an important characteristic of the disease. The degree of air trapping can be determined by CT scanning at end-expiration. Individual lobes may be affected.

▶ **Clinical features.** Chronic cough or dyspnea may already be present in childhood. Some patients present with recurrent episodes of pneumonia. Approximately 50% of patients are asymptomatic.

▶ **Differential diagnosis.** Differentiation is required mainly from hypoplastic lung (aplasia or hypoplasia of the pulmonary artery) and congenital emphysema. With congenital emphysema, often only one lobe is affected and the affected lobe is overinflated and not diminished in volume as in Swyer–James–MacLeod syndrome.

4.3.3 Neoplasms

Pulmonary Nodules

Pulmonary nodules are defined as rounded opacities 3 cm or less in diameter with absence of atelectasis in the same lobe and without enlargement of hilar or mediastinal lymph nodes.[4] A circumscribed opacity larger than 3 cm in diameter is classified as a mass. Focal ground-glass opacities with either sharp or hazy margins are termed "ground-glass nodules."[4]

Imaging has two major roles with regard to pulmonary masses: In patients with a known malignancy, screening should include the exclusion of pulmonary metastases; and once a pulmonary nodule has been detected, it should be determined whether the lesion is benign or malignant. A possible third role for imaging is the use of CT for screening patients deemed to be at high risk. Pulmonary nodules that are detected incidentally on thoracic CT performed for a different reason present a challenge. On the one hand, a great many patients are found to have small nodules, and the percentage of patients with nodules detected incidentally in reconstructed thin slices is nearly 50%. On the other hand, the level of follow-up should be commensurate with the risk that the detected lesions are actually malignant. With these considerations in mind, the Fleischner Society has published recommendations on the follow-up of pulmonary nodules.[5] The Fleischner Society for Thoracic Imaging and Diagnosis is an international medical society with approximately 60 active members that was founded in 1969 with the goal of improving diagnostic thoracic radiology. Its recommendations are based on international studies published until 2005 dealing with screening for the early detection of lung cancer.

Solid Nodules

With solid pulmonary nodules, the risk of malignancy increases with lesion size and the presence of risk factors:

Lung and Pleura

- *Solid nodule less than 5 mm in diameter*: there is less than a 1% risk that these nodules are malignant, even in smokers.
- *Solid nodule 8 mm in diameter*: the risk of malignancy is 20%.

To avoid unnecessary follow-ups with the disadvantages of radiation exposure, high cost, and psychosocial stress to the patient, the Fleischner Society has devised a staged approach to follow-up that takes into account nodule size and patient risk factors (▶ Table 4.1). Smoking is the greatest risk factor and increases the risk for smokers by a factor of 10 to 35 compared with nonsmokers.

Table 4.1 Recommendations of the Fleischner Society for the follow-up of incidentally detected solid nodules in patients aged over 35 years with no prior history of malignancy

Nodule size (mm)	Low-risk patient	High-risk patient
≤4	No follow-up needed	Follow-up CT at 12 months; if unchanged, no further follow-up
>4 and ≤6	Follow-up CT at 12 months; if unchanged, no further follow-up	Initial follow-up CT at 6–12 months, then at 18–24 months if no change
>6 and ≤8	Initial follow-up CT at 6–12 months, then at 18–24 months if no change	Initial follow-up CT at 3–6 months, then at 9–12 and 24 months if no change
>8	Follow-up CT at 3, 9, and 24 months, dynamic contrast-enhanced CT, PET, and/or biopsy	
>10	Biopsy or resection	

Other risk factors are exposure to asbestos or uranium and the inhalation of radon. Pulmonary fibrosis is associated with a 10-fold increase in risk. Intrapulmonary scarring is another risk factor that often creates a starting point for lung cancer. Patients' age is also significant risk factor, as lung cancer is extremely rare before 40 years of age.

Subsolid Nodules

Because solid nodules differ from subsolid nodules in their growth and malignancy rates, in 2013 the Fleischner Society published new recommendations for the CT follow-up of subsolid pulmonary nodules that supplement the 2005 recommendations, being based on data from more recent studies (▶ Table 4.2).[6]

Note

Subsolid pulmonary nodules, especially those with a part-solid component, are less common than solid nodules but are more likely to be malignant. On the other hand, they have a much slower growth rate than malignant solid nodules. In a screening study of 233 patients with positive findings on baseline scans, 7% of the incidentally detected solid nodules were malignant compared with 63% of subsolid nodules and 18% of ground-glass (nonsolid) nodules.[7]

In the case of incidentally detected subsolid nodules, the key difference compared with the follow-up recommendations for solid incidental nodules is that no distinction is made between high-risk patients and other risk groups.

Table 4.2 Recommendations of the Fleischner Society for the follow-up of subsolid pulmonary nodules

Nodule morphology	Recommendations	Additional remarks
Solitary pure ground-glass nodules		
≤5 mm	No CT follow-up required	Obtain contiguous 1-mm-thick sections to confirm that the nodule is really a pure ground-glass nodule
>5 mm	Initial follow-up CT at 3 months to confirm persistence, then annual surveillance CT for a minimum of 3 years[a]	FDG PET is potentially misleading and therefore not recommended
Solitary part-solid nodules		
Solid component <5 mm	Initial follow-up CT at 3 months to confirm persistence, then yearly surveillance CT for a minimum of 3 years	Consider PET-CT for part-solid nodules >10 mm
Solid component ≥5 mm	Initial follow-up CT at 3 months; biopsy or resection if no change	
Multiple subsolid nodules		
Pure ground-glass nodules ≤5 mm	Obtain follow-up CT at 2 and 4 years	Consider alternate causes for nodules
>5 mm	Initial follow-up CT at 3 months to confirm persistence, then annual surveillance CT for a minimum of 3 years	FDG PET is potentially misleading and therefore not recommended
Dominant nodule(s) with part-solid or solid component	Initial follow-up CT at 3 months to confirm persistence. If persistent, biopsy or resection is recommended, especially for lesions with >5 mm solid component	Consider lung-sparing surgery for patients with dominant lesion(s) suspicious for lung cancer

[a]The differential diagnosis of solitary pure ground-glass nodules includes focal inflammation, organizing pneumonia, hemorrhage, and focal interstitial fibrosis. These changes are reversible and will generally clear by 3 months.

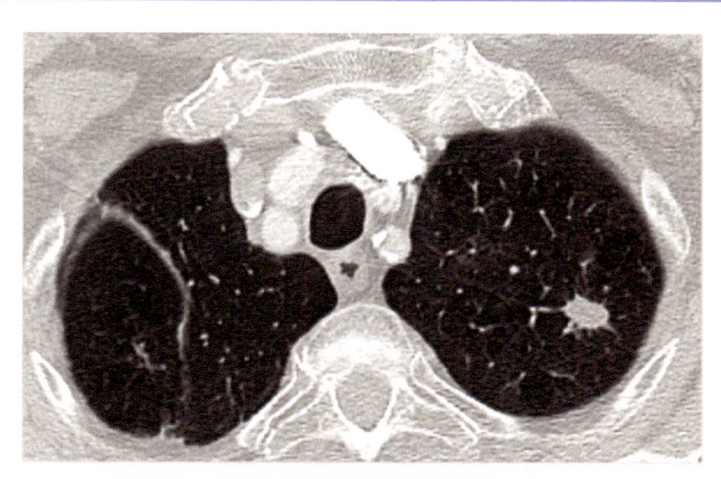

Fig. 4.44 **Bronchogenic carcinoma** appears as a pulmonary nodule with typical spiculated margins.

The size of pulmonary nodules is determined on CT scans reconstructed with a lung window setting. Contrast enhancement by more than 15 HU is suggestive of malignancy. Spiculated margins (corona radiata sign) also indicate a high index of suspicion (▶ Fig. 4.44). Bubblelike air inclusions within a nodule are also suggestive of malignancy. For enhancement to be quantified, the same parameters should be used for the unenhanced and contrast-enhanced scans. A 25% increase in the diameter of a nodule indicates a doubling of its volume, although that increase in nodules smaller than 10 mm would be within the range of measurement error. This suggests that, at the very least, the same examiner should determine nodule size in both the initial and follow-up examinations; however, computer volumetry with suitable software is superior to manual measurements.

The most common benign intrapulmonary masses are granulomas, intrapulmonary lymph nodes (mainly in the lower lobes), and hamartomas. Granulomas often contain flocculent calcification.

Based on the results of the National Lung Screening Trials,[8] some societies, e.g., the American College of Radiology (ACR) or the Radiological Society of North America (RSNA), currently recommend screening patients at high risk for lung cancer with low-dose CT. This study found that screening could reduce lung cancer mortality by 20%. Because similar studies in Europe have been unable to reproduce these results, and the results of further large European studies will not be available for several years, screening for early lung cancer detection is not currently recommended in Europe.

Lung Cancer

▶ **Brief definition.** Lung cancer, or bronchogenic carcinoma, is the most common malignant tumor in males and the leading cause of death. The 5-year survival rate is only 15%. Small cell lung cancer, which has a particularly poor prognosis, is distinguished histologically from all other lung cancers, known collectively as non–small cell lung carcinomas. This category includes squamous cell carcinoma, large cell carcinomas, and adenocarcinoma. At present, adenocarcinoma accounts for the largest percentage of lung cancers. In 2011 the International Association for the Study of Lung Cancer (IASLC), the American Thoracic Society (ATS), and the European Respiratory Society (ERS) published a classification that divides adenocarcinoma into five subtypes (▶ Table 4.3).[2] The new classification eliminated the older term "bronchoalveolar carcinoma," which refers to an array of lesions that differ in their prognosis and CT manifestations. The new classification of lung adenocarcinoma takes into account the prognostic differences among the subtypes. Pancoast tumor (named for the American radiologist Henry Pancoast, 1875–1939) is the term applied to lung cancers located in the superior sulcus (synonym: superior sulcus tumor) regardless of their histology. Invasion of the stellate ganglion, located above the head of the first rib and medial to the vertebral artery, may lead to Horner's syndrome, characterized by miosis, ptosis, and enophthalmos. Lymphangitic carcinomatosis is tumor growth in the lymphatics of the lung, which course in the interlobar septa. This process is characterized by smooth or nodular thickening of the interlobar septa. Lymphangitic carcinomatosis may occur in association with lung cancer as well as other tumors.

Note

The term "lepidic growth" describes tumor growth that lines the alveoli without completely filling them. The stroma is not invaded, and the alveolar septa are not destroyed.[9] Adenocarcinomas with lepidic growth may become smaller over the course of CT follow-ups due to alveolar collapse and interstitial fibrosis, even without treatment.

▶ **Imaging signs.** The goals of imaging include the earliest possible diagnosis of lung cancer. Spiculations extending into the area around the tumor are a typical feature of histologically diverse lung cancers, including adenocarcinoma (see ▶ Fig. 4.44). Fine spiculations from subpleural lesions may extend to the pleura, with associated pleural retraction toward the tumor ("pleural fingers," ▶ Fig. 4.45). Lung cancers may contain fine calcifications. Flocculent, popcornlike calcifications within a mass are more suggestive of hamartoma than carcinoma. Central, nonenhancing necrotic foci are most commonly seen in squamous cell carcinoma (▶ Fig. 4.46). This may also occur in lymph node metastases from squamous cell carcinoma. If the necrotic component communicates with the bronchial tree, the necrotic material may be coughed up with sputum, and the tumor appears as a thick-walled cavity with a nodular wall. With the subtotal occlusion of a bronchus, "retention pneumonia" may develop in the lung parenchyma. A total occlusion leads to atelectasis; both features are typical of bronchogenic carcinoma. Lymphangitic carcinomatosis may occur at the periphery of lung cancers (see ▶ Fig. 4.46). Central lung cancers may narrow or occlude vessels and bronchi (▶ Fig. 4.47). This distinguishes them from lymphoma, which generally encases the vessels without narrowing them. Compression or infiltration of the phrenic nerve leads to elevation of the ipsilateral hemidiaphragm (▶ Fig. 4.48). All lung cancers, regardless of their histology, are uniformly classified according to the 7th edition of the TNM classification (▶ Table 4.4).[10] ▶ Table 4.5 shows the staging system for lung cancer.

Table 4.3 Classification of lung cancer[2]

Entities	Pathology	CT morphology	5-year survival rate (%)
Small-cell lung cancer (ca. 20% of all lung cancers; frequent central location)			
Non–small cell lung cancer (ca. 80–85% of all lung cancers)			
Squamous cell carcinoma (30% of all non–small cell lung cancers)		Arises from main, lobar or segmental bronchi, so it usually occurs in the central lung. Central necrosis in the tumor or lymph node metastases is a typical feature	
Large-cell carcinoma (10% of all non–small cell lung cancers)		Frequent peripheral location	
Neuroendocrine carcinoma		Often endobronchial, only 20% occur as pulmonary nodules	90
Adenocarcinoma (ca. 45% of all non–small cell lung cancers)			100
• Adenocarcinoma in situ	<3 cm in diameter, pure lepidic growth, generally nonmucinous	Usually appears as a pure ground-glass nodule	100
• Minimally invasive adenocarcinoma	<3 cm in diameter, invasive component <5 mm, generally nonmucinous	Semisolid nodule <3 cm, solid component <5 mm	100
• Lepidic predominant adenocarcinoma	Invasive, nonmucinous adenocarcinoma, predominant lepidic growth	Semisolid nodule, solid component >5 mm or pure solid	
• Predominantly invasive adenocarcinoma (acinous, papillary, micropapillary) with nonmucinous lepidic components	Nonmucinous adenocarcinoma, predominantly invasive (acinar, papillary, micropapillary or solid) with small lepidic component	Solid, may diminish in size, contains a nonsolid component	
• Invasive mucinous adenocarcinoma	Invasive mucinous adenocarcinoma (completely fills alveoli) with lepidic growth	Variable features (solid or part-solid), with or without an air bronchogram, may also be multifocal	

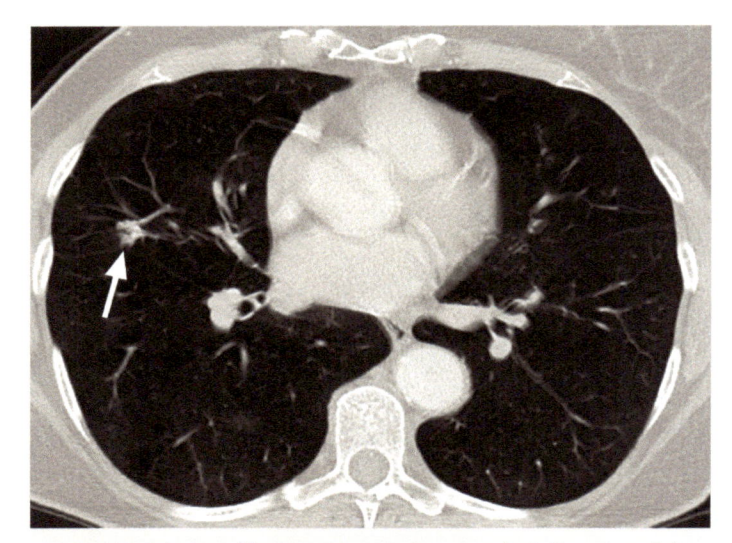

Fig. 4.45 **Subpleural lung cancer.** CT shows marked distortion of the interlobar fissure by the small tumor (arrow).

Caution

When a lung cancer touches the wall of a major vessel (aorta or pulmonary artery) with no evidence of invasion or luminal narrowing, only surgery can establish whether the wall is actually infiltrated or the tumor merely abuts it, meaning that the tumor is resectable.

▶ **Clinical features.** The clinical manifestation of lung cancer in descending order of frequency are cough, weight loss, dyspnea, chest pain, and hemoptysis. The likelihood of cerebral metastasis from invasive adenocarcinoma increases with tumor size. With a tumor 2 cm in diameter, the incidence of cerebral metastasis is 14% and increases linearly with tumor size. With a tumor 6 cm in diameter, the incidence of cerebral metastasis is 64%. Small cell lung cancers are of neuroendocrine origin, so they often produce hormones or hormonelike peptides leading to paraneoplastic syndromes. Most small cell lung cancers have already metastasized by the time they are diagnosed.

Hamartoma

▶ **Brief definition.** Hamartomas are mesenchymal mixed tumors composed of fat, cartilage, epithelium, smooth muscle cells, and connective tissue. They account for 75% of all benign lung tumors but only 6% of all nodules. The peak age of incidence is the sixth decade. Pulmonary hamartomas have an approximately 3:1 predilection for males. Hamartomas grow very slowly and do not undergo malignant change, so treatment is not required.

▶ **Imaging signs.** Areas of fat density are typically present and exclude a malignant tumor with reasonable confidence. When combined with popcorn calcifications, they are pathognomonic for hamartoma (▶ Fig. 4.49). Hamartomas occur predominantly in the lower lobes and have smooth or lobulated margins.

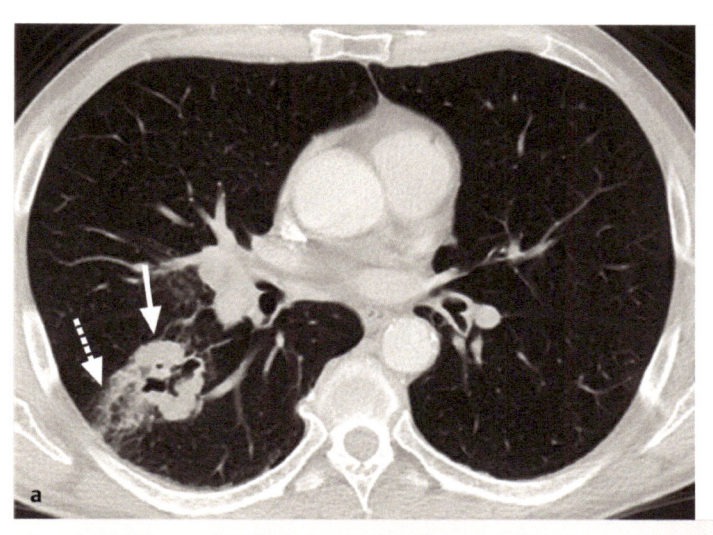

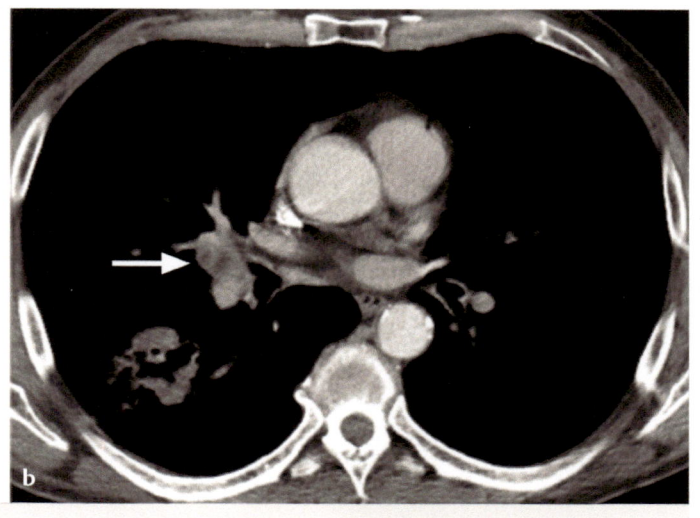

Fig. 4.46 Squamous cell carcinoma. (a) The tumor shows central liquefaction. Necrotic material that communicates with the bronchial tree may be coughed up, and air inclusions are visible within the lesion (arrow). Local widening of the surrounding interlobular septa reflects lymphangitic carcinomatosis (dashed arrow). **(b)** Scan with a soft tissue window demonstrates hilar lymph node metastases, which remain hypointense after IV injection of contrast medium due to central necrosis (arrow).

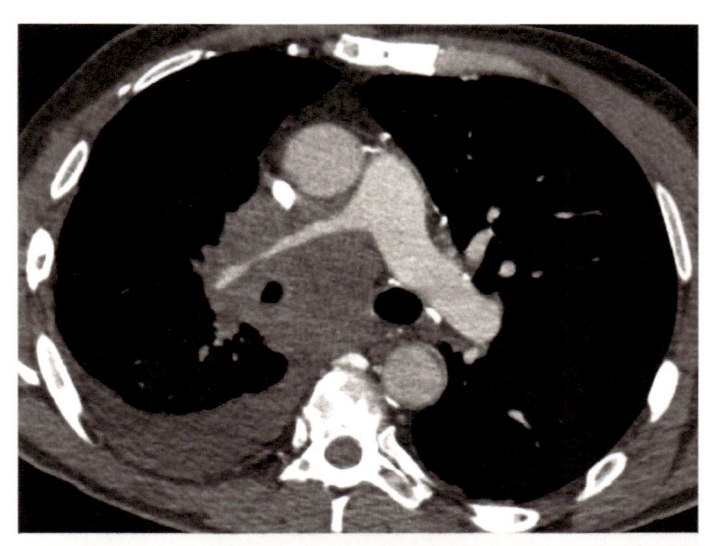

Fig. 4.47 Central lung cancer. The right pulmonary artery, right main bronchus, and superior vena cava are narrowed by the tumor.

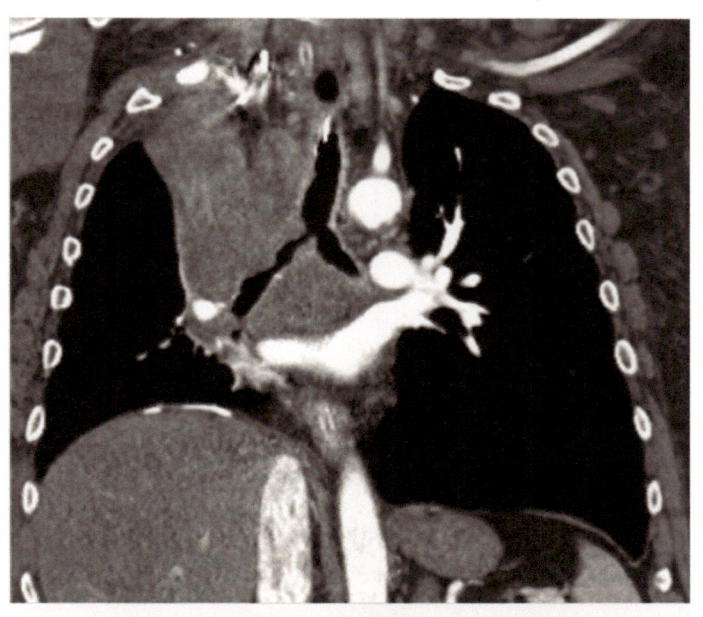

Fig. 4.48 Mediastinal lung cancer. Elevation of the right hemidiaphragm due to phrenic nerve damage by the tumor.

▶ **Clinical features.** Hamartomas are almost always asymptomatic and are detected incidentally in examinations performed for other indications.

▶ **Key points.** Hamartomas are benign mesenchymal mixed tumors, with 95% occurring after 40 years of age. They are asymptomatic and thus represent incidental findings. The detection of fat and calcifications in the lesion eliminates any other differential diagnosis.

4.3.4 Diffuse Lung Diseases

Interstitial Lung Diseases: Idiopathic Interstitial Pneumonias

At the start of the 21st century, the ATS worked jointly with the ERS to develop a classification for idiopathic interstitial pneumonia (IIP),[11] which was revised in 2013 on the basis of discoveries in more recent studies.[12] The classification covers eight entities, which are differentiated by their clinical features, course, prognosis, histology, and imaging features on HRCT. The diagnosis is made on an interdisciplinary basis with correlation of all findings, but a histological workup is not required for all entities if the symptoms and imaging features are considered definitive. This particularly applies to the most common form of IIP, idiopathic interstitial fibrosis.[13] The updated 2013 classification differentiates IIPs into common and rare forms. The common entities are further subdivided into chronic fibrosing IIP, smoking-related IIP, and acute or subacute IIP (▶ Table 4.6).

Table 4.4 TNM classification of lung cancer[10]

Designation	Characteristics
Primary tumor	
Tx	Malignant cells in bronchial washings, but tumor not visualized by imaging or bronchoscopy
T0	No evidence of primary tumor
T1	Tumor ≤ 3 cm in greatest dimension, surrounded by lung or visceral pleura or Endobronchial tumor proximal to a lobar bronchus, does not invade the carina or pleura
• T1a	Tumor ≤ 2 cm in greatest dimension
• T1b	Tumor > 2 cm but ≤ 3 cm in greatest dimension
T2	Tumor > 3 cm but ≤ 7 cm or Involves main bronchus, > 2 cm distal to the carina or Invades visceral pleura or Associated with atelectasis
• T2 a	Tumor > 3 cm but ≤ 5 cm in greatest dimension
• T2 b	Tumor > 5 cm but ≤ 7 cm in greatest dimension
T3	Tumor > 7 cm in greatest dimension or Directly invades the chest wall, diaphragm, mediastinal pleura, parietal pericardium or Associated atelectasis of the entire lung or Tumor in the main bronchus < 2 cm distal to the carina or Separate tumor nodule(s) in the same lobe
T4	Tumor of any size that invades any of the following: mediastinum, heart, great vessels, trachea, recurrent laryngeal nerve, esophagus, vertebral body, carina or Separate tumor nodule(s) in a different ipsilateral lobe
Lymph nodes	
N0	No regional lymph node metastasis
N1	Metastasis in ipsilateral peribronchial and/or ipsilateral hilar lymph nodes
N2	Metastasis in ipsilateral mediastinal and/or subcarinal lymph node(s)
N3	Metastasis in contralateral mediastinal, contralateral hilar, ipsilateral or contralateral scalene, or supraclavicular lymph node(s)
Distant metastasis	
M0	No distant metastasis
M1	Distant metastasis, including separate tumor nodule(s) in a contralateral lobe

Table 4.5 Staging of lung cancer

Stage	Designation
0	Tis N0 M0
IA	T1a/b N0 M0
IB	T2a N0 M0
IIA	T2b N0 M0 T1a/b N1 M0 T2a N1 M0
IIB	T2b N1 M0 T3 N0 M0
IIIA	T1a/b N2 M0 T2a/b N2 M0 T3 N1/2 M0 T4 N0/1 M0
IIIB	T4 N2 M0 Any T N3 M0
IV	Any T any N M1a Any T any N M1b

Note

It is common practice to use acronyms for the various IIPs (see ▶ Table 4.6). HRCT with spiral acquisition of a data set covering the entire lung is the standard technique for imaging patients with suspected IIP. Different IIPs are individually characterized by a combination of multiple imaging features.

The lung has only a limited potential for pathophysiologic response patterns. Most notably, this includes the influx of inflammatory cells or fibroblasts and myofibroblasts and the formation of connective tissue matrix. The IIPs are associated with different pathophysiologic response patterns, although these patterns are also seen in other disorders such as connective tissue diseases, vasculitides, sarcoidosis, extrinsic allergic alveolitis, and drug toxicity. Specific laboratory tests diagnose a connective tissue disease or rheumatoid arthritis in up to 15% of patients with initial suspicion of an IIP, and the diagnosis of IIP must be revised accordingly. An IIP should be diagnosed only when other diseases have been confidently excluded.

Chronic Fibrosing Idiopathic Interstitial Pneumonias

Idiopathic Pulmonary Fibrosis

▶ **Brief definition.** Idiopathic pulmonary fibrosis (IPF) is the most common form of IIP, with an incidence of approximately 8:100,000 population per year. It has a male predilection and typically occurs during and after the fifth decade. Currently the pathogenic mechanism is believed to involve a disordered regenerative process following damage to the alveolar epithelium and the apoptosis of type I pneumocytes induced by an external agent. Cytokines activate the release of myofibroblasts, which

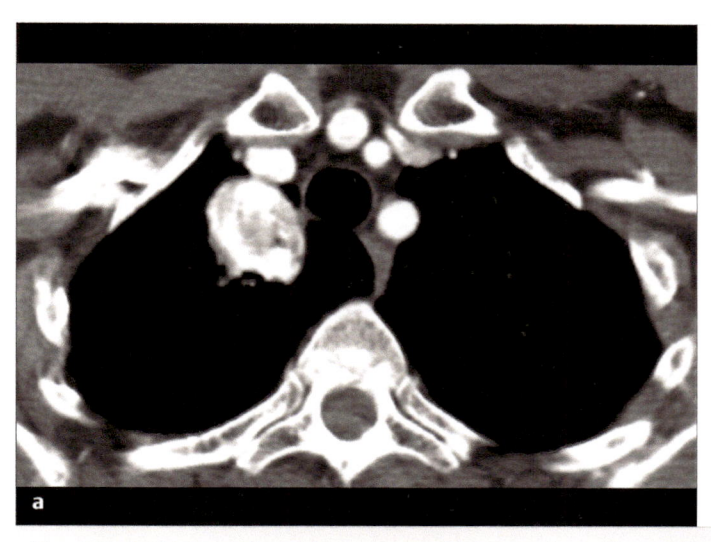

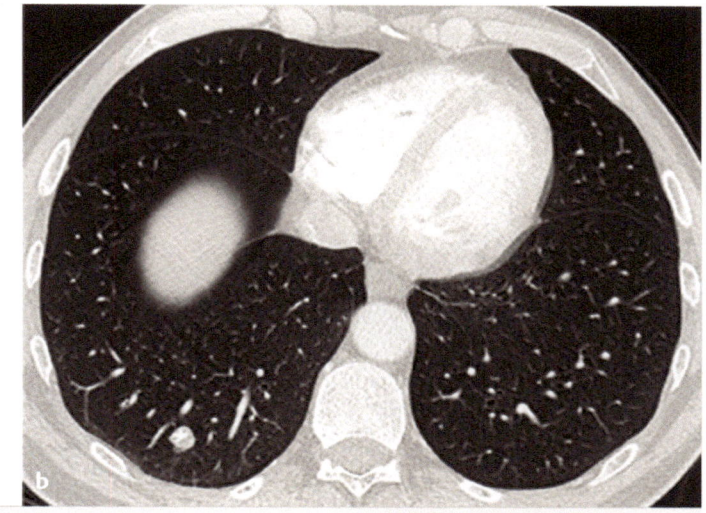

Fig. 4.49 (a, b) **Examples of hamartomas.** The smooth margins and popcorn calcifications in the tumor matrix are typical of hamartoma.

Table 4.6 Classification of idiopathic interstitial pneumonia (IIP) based on the updated classification of the ATS and ERS[12]

Classification		Acronym	Designation
Common IIPs	Chronic fibrosing IIP	IPF (UIP)	Idiopathic pulmonary fibrosis (usual interstitial pneumonia)
		NSIP	Nonspecific interstitial pneumonia
	Smoking-related IIP	RB-ILD	Respiratory bronchiolitis with interstitial lung disease
		DIP	Desquamative interstitial pneumonia
	Acute/subacute IIP	COP	Cryptogenic organizing pneumonia
		AIP	Acute interstitial pneumonia
Rare IIPs		LIP	Lymphoid interstitial pneumonia
		PPFE	Pleuroparenchymal fibroelastosis

form extracellular matrix to provide a scaffold for tissue regeneration. In the setting of normal tissue regeneration, the myofibroblasts would eventually become apoptotic after serving their function. This does not occur in IPF, however, as the myofibroblasts and extracellular matrix persist to form fibrotic foci. This process is known histologically as *usual interstitial pneumonia* (UIP). IIP is refractory to corticosteroid therapy and even worsens in response to cortisone. It is treated with proliferation-inhibiting drugs. The prognosis is very poor, with a mean survival of 2 to 4 years, so that early consideration of lung transplantation is recommended.

▶ **Imaging signs.** The changes show an inhomogeneous distribution with a marked gradient from the central to peripheral lung and from base to apex. The changes are found predominantly in the basal and subpleural regions. Thickened subpleural septa create a reticular pattern of opacities. This is accompanied by subpleural parenchymal destruction creating a honeycomb pattern of cystic structures that are typically 3 to 10 mm in diameter but may reach 2.5 cm (▶ Fig. 4.50). The intrapulmonary fibrotic foci lead to traction bronchiectasis, and overall lung volume is reduced. Ground-glass opacities may occur.

Caution

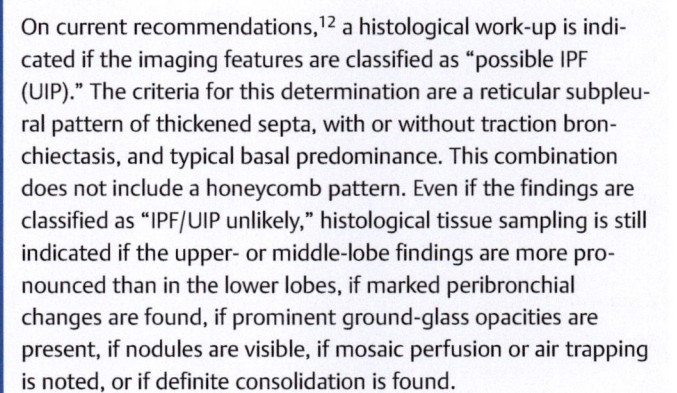

On current recommendations,[12] a histological work-up is indicated if the imaging features are classified as "possible IPF (UIP)." The criteria for this determination are a reticular subpleural pattern of thickened septa, with or without traction bronchiectasis, and typical basal predominance. This combination does not include a honeycomb pattern. Even if the findings are classified as "IPF/UIP unlikely," histological tissue sampling is still indicated if the upper- or middle-lobe findings are more pronounced than in the lower lobes, if marked peribronchial changes are found, if prominent ground-glass opacities are present, if nodules are visible, if mosaic perfusion or air trapping is noted, or if definite consolidation is found.

▶ **Clinical features.** The clinical symptoms of IPF are dyspnea and a nonproductive cough.

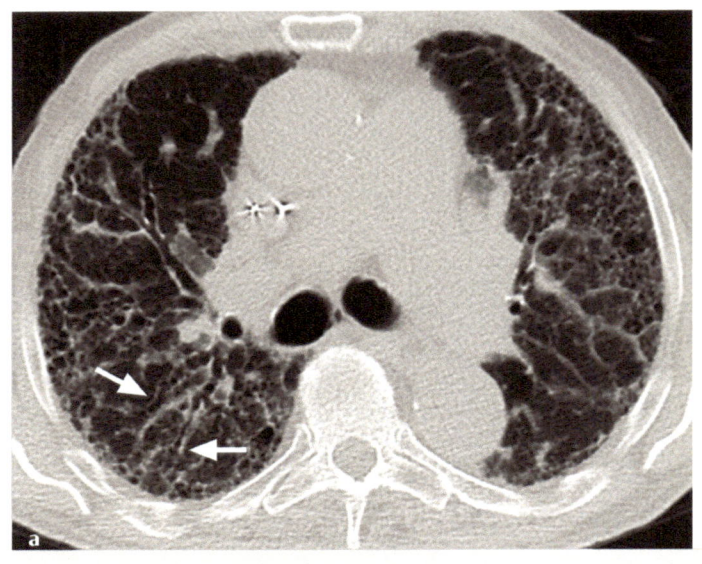

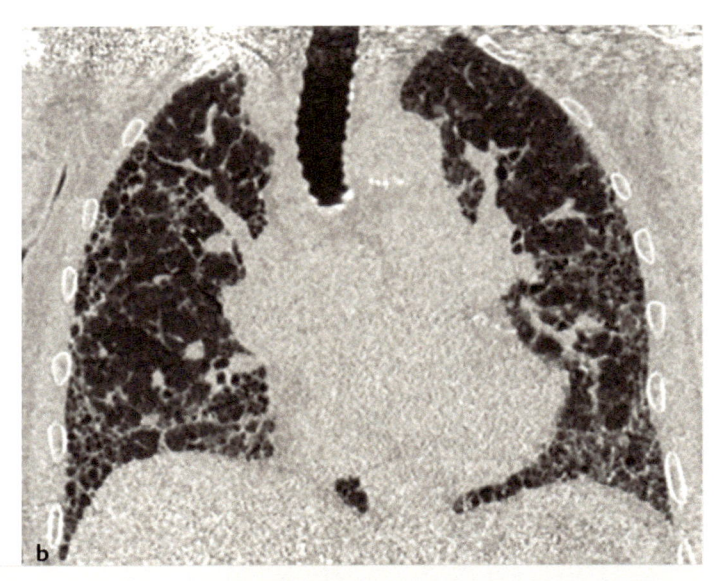

Fig. 4.50 IPF. (a) CT demonstrates a subpleural honeycomb pattern. Sites of traction bronchiectasis (arrows) are visualized. (b) The fibrosis shows a predominantly basal and peripheral distribution.

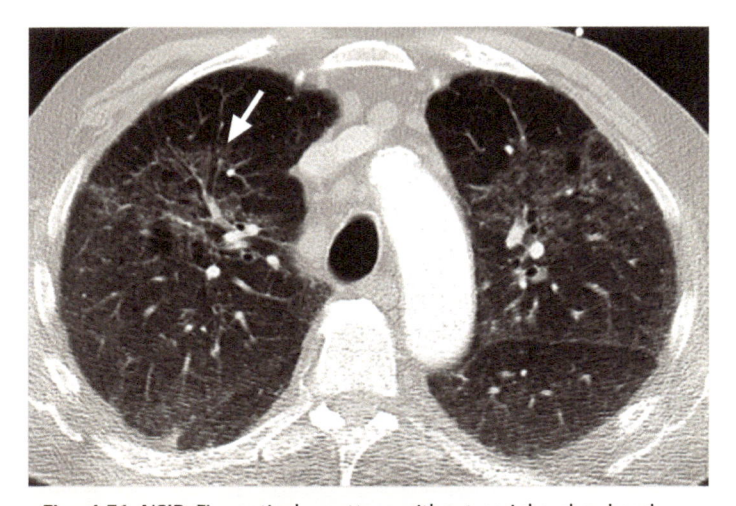

Fig. 4.51 NSIP. Fine reticular pattern without peripheral or basal predominance (arrow).

Note

In patients with typical imaging features that include thickened septa with basal and subpleural predominance, a honeycomb pattern, traction bronchiectasis, and agreement with clinical presentation (dyspnea and nonproductive cough), IPF can be diagnosed without a biopsy.

▶ **Differential diagnosis.** Differentiation is required mainly from stage IV sarcoidosis, chronic extrinsic allergic alveolitis, nonspecific interstitial pneumonia, asbestosis, connective tissue diseases, and rheumatoid arthritis.

Nonspecific Interstitial Pneumonia

▶ **Brief definition.** Nonspecific interstitial pneumonia (NSIP) has a poorer prognosis than IPF but is responsive to cortisone therapy, so the differentiation of the two entities has major clinical implications. NSIP occurs approximately one decade earlier than IPF, with a peak incidence around age 40 years. The main histological finding is thickening of the alveolar septa. Recently a distinction has been made between a fibrotic form of NSIP and a cellular form. The cellular form is characterized by the histological predominance of an interstitial cellular inflammatory response and has a somewhat better prognosis.

▶ **Imaging signs.** NSIP shows a homogeneous distribution in the pulmonary lobes with a concomitant basal accentuation, which often leads to volume loss in the lower lobes.[14] Prominent bilateral ground-glass opacities are found in one-third of patients. Reticular changes are also present but a honeycomb pattern is not seen. Cysts smaller than 3 mm may occur, creating a microcystic pattern (▶ Fig. 4.51, ▶ Fig. 4.52).

▶ **Clinical features.** Patients with NSIP develop dyspnea and a nonproductive cough, similar to IPF.

▶ **Differential diagnosis.** Given the variable features of NSIP, the differential diagnosis is broad and includes several other IIPs: UIP/IPF, desquamative interstitial pneumonia (DIP), COP, and chronic extrinsic allergic alveolitis.

Smoking-Related Idiopathic Interstitial Pneumonias

Bronchiolitis-Associated Interstitial Lung Disease

▶ **Brief definition.** Respiratory bronchiolitis-associated interstitial lung disease (RB-ILD) is a specific response of the bronchioles to smoking and is characterized histologically by the accumulation of pigmented alveolar macrophages in the respiratory bronchioles. The pigmentation is caused by granular inclusions from compounds present in cigarette smoke. RB-ILD is characterized by infiltration of the bronchial walls and adjacent alveoli. Histology reveals peribronchial fibrosis. The peak age of incidence is 30

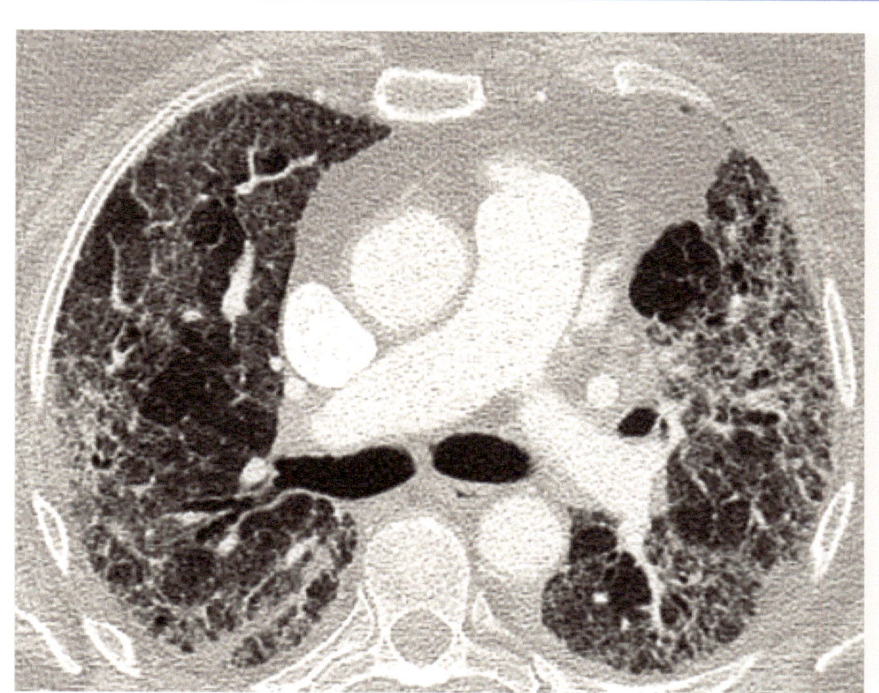

Fig. 4.52 NSIP. Even the advanced stage shows no honeycomb pattern and minimal traction bronchiectasis.

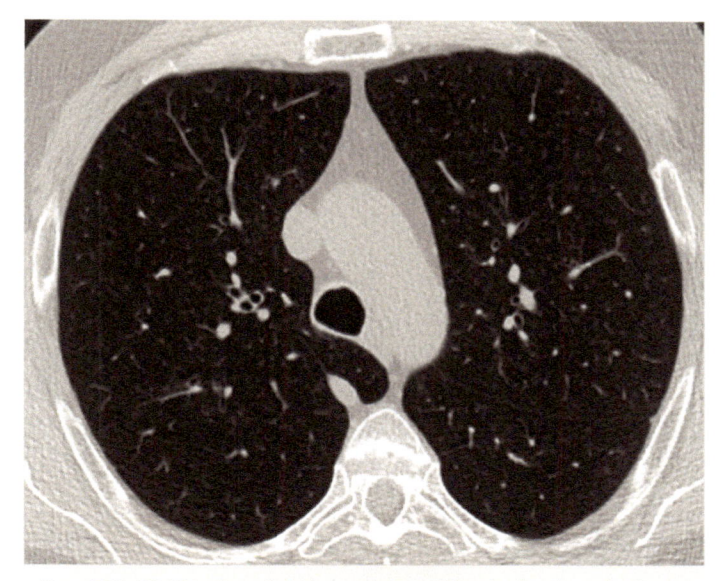

Fig. 4.53 RB-ILD. Centrilobular nodules, diffusely distributed. The bronchial walls are slightly thickened.

to 40 years, with an average of 30 pack years (number of cigarette packs smoked per day multiplied by the number of years the patient has smoked). Smoking cessation is the most effective therapy, and that measure alone will lead to clinical and radiological improvement. Corticosteroids are also effective and are frequently prescribed as an adjunct.

▶ **Imaging signs.** HRCT shows ground-glass opacities caused by alveoli filled with pigmented alveolar cells. Other findings are thickened bronchial walls and centrilobular nodules corresponding to peribronchial infiltrates and fibrosis (▶ Fig. 4.53). The upper lobes are predominantly affected. Because RB-ILD occurs in smokers, centrilobular emphysema is also present in many cases.

Note
Centrilobular nodules are characteristic of RB-ILD and are caused by peribronchial infiltrates and fibrotic changes. A tree-in-bud pattern is not observed.

▶ **Clinical features.** The main symptoms are cough, dyspnea, and rapid fatigability.

▶ **Differential diagnosis.** The differential diagnosis includes DIP, NSIP, and acute extrinsic allergic alveolitis.

Desquamative Interstitial Pneumonia

▶ **Brief definition.** Desquamative interstitial pneumonia (DIP) and RB-ILD are interpreted as different degrees of change based on the same pathogenic mechanism. Approximately 90% of all DIP patients are smokers with an average smoking history of 18 pack years. The peak age of incidence is 30 to 40 years. In DIP, the alveoli are partially filled with pigmented alveolar macrophages. The alveolar walls are thickened due to infiltration by inflammatory cells (eosinophilic granulocytes and lymphocytes). Desquamated alveolar cells (type I pneumocytes) are also found in the alveolar space.

▶ **Imaging signs.** HRCT shows diffuse ground-glass opacities, usually confluent over a large area, that result from thickening of the alveolar septa and consolidation of the alveoli. Irregular linear opacities are characteristic. Microcysts are observed in one-half of patients (▶ Fig. 4.54).

▶ **Clinical features.** As in other IIPs, the principal symptoms of DIP are dyspnea and nonproductive cough.

▶ **Differential diagnosis.** The differential diagnosis includes NSIP, RB-ILD, extrinsic allergic alveolitis, sarcoidosis, and *Pneumocystis jiroveci* pneumonia.

Lung and Pleura

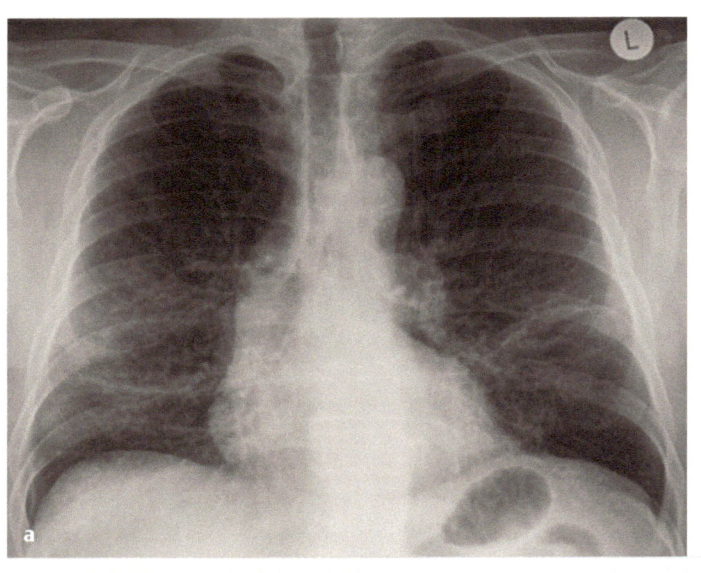

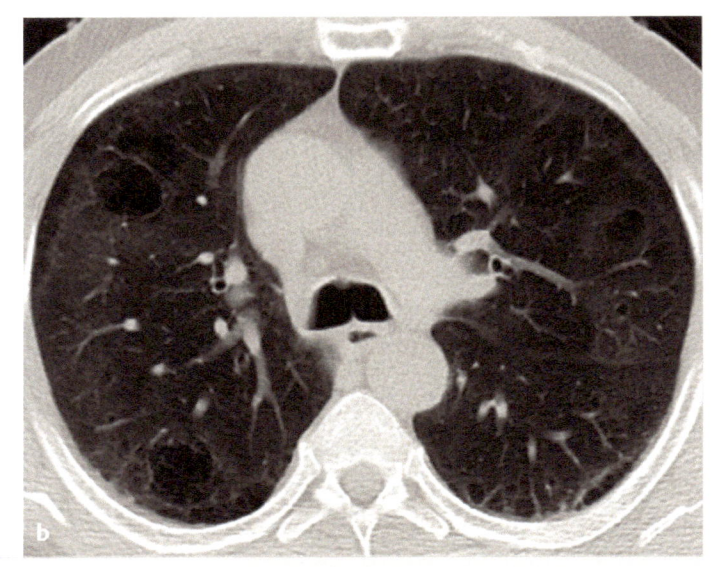

Fig. 4.54 **DIP.** Both images show ground-glass opacities. (a) Chest radiograph. (b) CT.

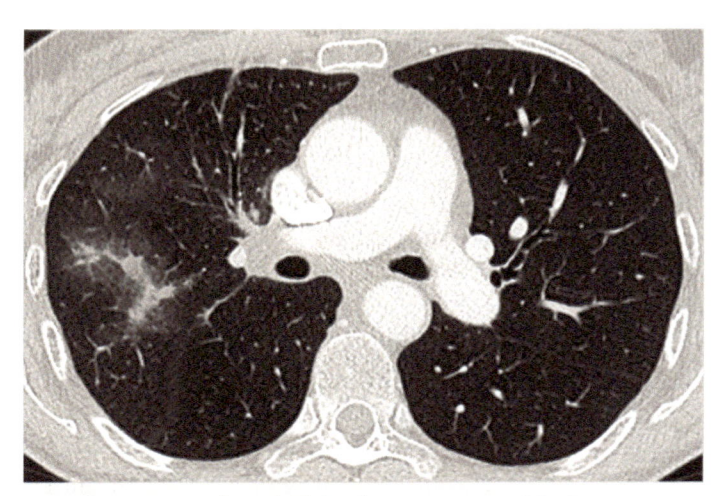

Fig. 4.55 **COP.** Peribronchial distribution is a typical finding.

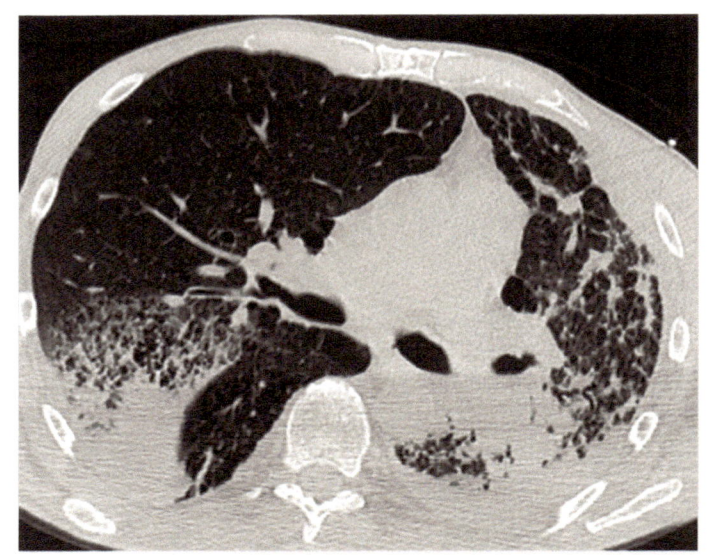

Fig. 4.56 **More severe COP** with marked areas of consolidation.

Acute and Subacute Idiopathic Interstitial Pneumonias

Cryptogenic Organizing Pneumonia

▶ **Brief definition.** Cryptogenic organizing pneumonia (COP) usually develops after an infection of the tracheobronchial system. It is characterized histologically by buds of granulation tissue with myofibroblasts and fibrocytes along with intercellular matrix in the alveolar airspace. The peak age of incidence of the disease is 55 years. The prognosis is very good, and most cases will resolve completely with corticosteroid therapy.

▶ **Imaging signs.** HRCT shows peribronchial opacities (▶ Fig. 4.55). The bronchi may be mildly ectatic. Ground-glass opacities are seen when there is incomplete filling of the alveoli with granulation tissue. Consolidation (▶ Fig. 4.56) as well as ground-glass opacities may regress on follow-up and reappear at different sites. Rarely, imaging reveals nodules that may undergo central liquefaction. A special feature is the "reverse halo sign," which may be seen in 20% of patients. It is produced by a ringlike, slightly ragged opacity that surrounds normal tissue or parenchyma of ground-glass opacity.

▶ **Clinical features.** Typical symptoms are mild dyspnea, cough, and fever lasting for several weeks.

▶ **Differential diagnosis.** Differentiation is required mainly from infections. Other diseases to be considered are vasculitis, stage III sarcoidosis, adenocarcinoma, lymphoma, eosinophilic pneumonia, and NSIP.

Acute Interstitial Pneumonia

▶ **Brief definition.** Acute interstitial pneumonia (AIP) is characterized histologically by damage to type II pneumocytes. Because AIP has the same histological and clinical features as acute respiratory distress syndrome (ARDS) in adults, it is considered to be an idiopathic form of ARDS—see Chapter 4.3.15— which in turn occurs in a setting of sepsis or shock. The precipitating event is believed to be destruction of the surfactant film. Analogously to ARDS, the initial histological finding is interstitial edema, followed swiftly by intra-alveolar edema and the subsequent

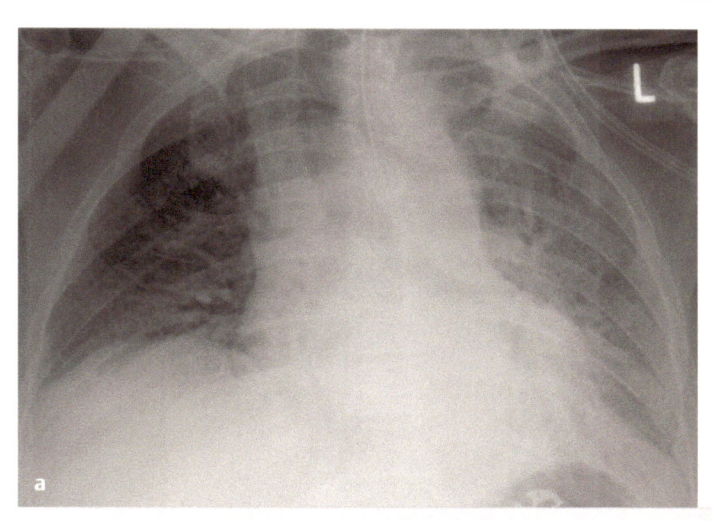

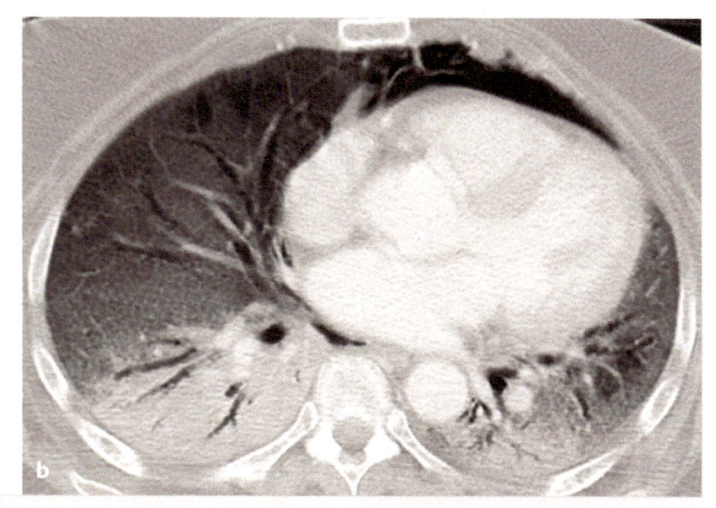

Fig. 4.57 AIP. Ground-glass opacities and consolidation in dependent lung areas. (a) Chest radiograph. (b) CT.

formation of hyaline membranes. The acute stage is followed by the development of pulmonary fibrosis. If the acute stage is survived, this late stage is variable and ranges from good recovery of pulmonary structure to honeycombing and fibrosis with high cellularity and a small proportion of collagen fibers. The peak age of incidence is the fifth decade. The mortality rate is high; 50% of patients die in the acute stage.

▶ **Imaging signs.** Given their almost identical histological characteristics, the imaging features of AIP are the same as for ARDS. The chest radiograph shows bilateral opacities. The costophrenic angles are often spared. HRCT initially shows ground-glass opacities as a correlate for the interstitial edema and formation of hyaline membranes (▶ Fig. 4.57). Early consolidation develops in dependent lung areas. In the late stage, pulmonary fibrosis leads to traction bronchiectasis and the formation of a honeycomb pattern. Typically these findings are most pronounced in nondependent lung areas.

▶ **Clinical features.** Severe dyspnea develops over a period of several weeks in a previously healthy patient or following a viral infection. The dyspnea progresses rapidly to respiratory failure requiring mechanical ventilation.

▶ **Differential diagnosis.** The disease is distinguishable from ARDS only by the absence of an identifiable precipitating cause. The acute stage of AIP is differentiated from cardiogenic pulmonary edema by typical signs of pulmonary venous congestion. Pulmonary edema due to other causes should also be considered. Atypical pneumonia may have similar manifestations.

Rare Idiopathic Interstitial Pneumonias
Lymphoid Interstitial Pneumonia

▶ **Brief definition.** Lymphoid interstitial pneumonia (LIP) is characterized histologically by infiltration of the pulmonary interstitium by lymphocytes, plasma cells, and histiocytes with associated thickening of the alveolar septa. The perilymphatic tissue is predominantly affected. There may be a secondary accumulation of macrophages and protein-rich fluid in the alveoli. LIP is more common in females than males, with a peak age of incidence in the fifth decade. Symptomatic patients are treated with corticosteroids. Approximately one-third of patients eventually develop pulmonary fibrosis.

Note

The extremely rare idiopathic form of LIP is less common than a secondary form with identical histology that may develop in Sjögren's syndrome or HIV and AIDS, especially in children.

▶ **Imaging signs.** The predominance of infiltrates in the perilymphatic tissue leads to thickening of the interlobar septa and bronchovascular bundle. Bilateral ground-glass opacities are also typically present. In approximately 80% of patients, thin-walled perivascular cysts from a few millimeters to 30 mm in diameter are found in the central lung.

Note

The combination of both features—ground-glass opacities and perivascular cysts—is typical of LIP.

▶ **Clinical features.** Patients develop cough and dyspnea over a period of several years. Accompanying weight loss and night sweats are less common. Approximately 80% of patients show a monoclonal rise in immunoglobulins G or M.

▶ **Differential diagnosis.** Lymphangitic carcinomatosis is an important differential diagnosis. LIP also requires differentiation from stage III sarcoidosis and histiocytosis.

Pleuroparenchymal Fibroelastosis

▶ **Brief definition.** Pleuroparenchymal fibroelastosis (PPFE) was added to the classification of IIPs as an eighth entity in the 2013 update. The hallmark of the disease is the development of fibrosis along the pleural surface including the interlobar fissures. The upper lobes are predominantly affected.

▶ **Imaging signs.** Predominantly apical pleural thickening is found along with subpleural opacities. Accompanying fibrosis may lead to bronchiectasis.

▶ **Differential diagnosis.** Differentiation is mainly required from prior tuberculosis with apical pleural caps. Upward retraction of the hila may also be a feature of PPFE.

Summary

The seven IIPs are prototypes of pathophysiologic response patterns in the lung and also occur in secondary interstitial pneumonias in the form described. The diagnosis of an IIP requires interdisciplinary consideration of the clinical presentation, HRCT findings, possible histological findings, and the exclusion of a different cause. Histology is unnecessary in IPF (UIP) if typical signs are present on HRCT.

Sarcoidosis

▶ **Brief definition.** Sarcoidosis is a systemic disease of unknown etiology characterized by the formation of noncaseating granulomas in multiple organs. The lung is affected in 90% of all patients, either alone or combined with other sites of involvement. Two-thirds of patients develop typical pulmonary changes with bihilar lymphadenopathy and/or perilymphatic nodules 2 to 4 mm in diameter. One-third of patients show atypical changes such as larger solitary nodules or patchy opacities. Sarcoidosis has two age peaks, one between the second and fourth decades and another between the sixth and seventh decades. There is a marked female predominance. Treatment consists of steroid medication. Up to 20% of patients develop irreversible pulmonary fibrosis.

▶ **Imaging signs.** A traditional four-stage system is still followed in the radiological classification of sarcoidosis (▶ Table 4.7). The stages are generally identified on chest radiographs.[15,16] HRCT provides higher sensitivity in the evaluation of parenchymal changes.

The stages do not necessarily follow one another in orderly succession. They are mainly useful for describing morphological findings and—with the exception of stage IV (fibrosis)—correlate poorly with treatment response and prognosis. Lymphadenopathy in sarcoidosis is generally bihilar and symmetrical. The paratracheal and mediastinal lymph nodes are also commonly involved. The enlarged lymph nodes assume an oval shape. Manifestations in the lung parenchyma can have a variety of CT appearances. Upper and middle lobe predominance is typically seen. Common findings include nodular opacities 2 to 4 mm in diameter distributed along the bronchovascular bundles, interlobular septa, interlobar fissures, and subpleural lung in a string-of-beads pattern (▶ Fig. 4.58). Bilateral ground-glass opacities

Table 4.7 Stages of sarcoidosis. All patients do not progress from one stage to the next

Stage	Findings	Frequency on initial diagnosis (%)	Spontaneous regression (% of cases)
0	Extrapulmonary manifestations without lung involvement	10	
I	Lymphadenopathy	50	60–90
II	Lymphadenopathy and involvement of lung parenchyma	25	40–70
III	Involvement of lung parenchyma	10	10–20
IV	Pulmonary fibrosis	5 (20 thereafter)	Irreversible

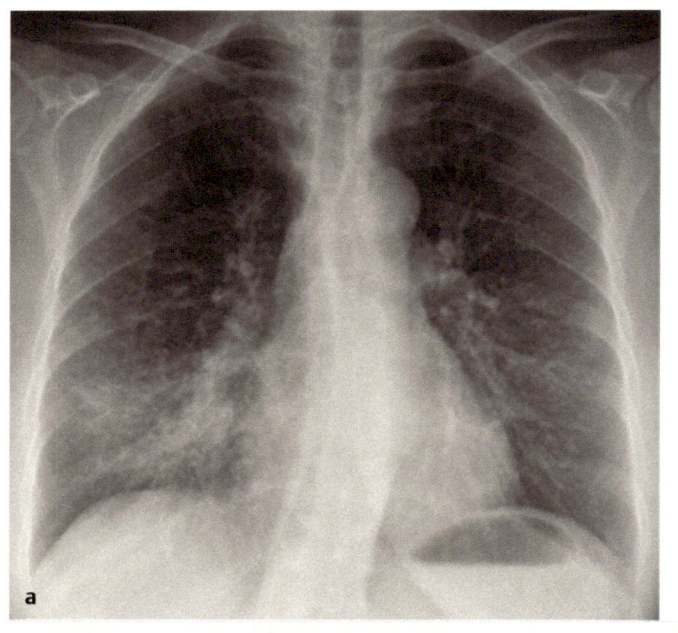

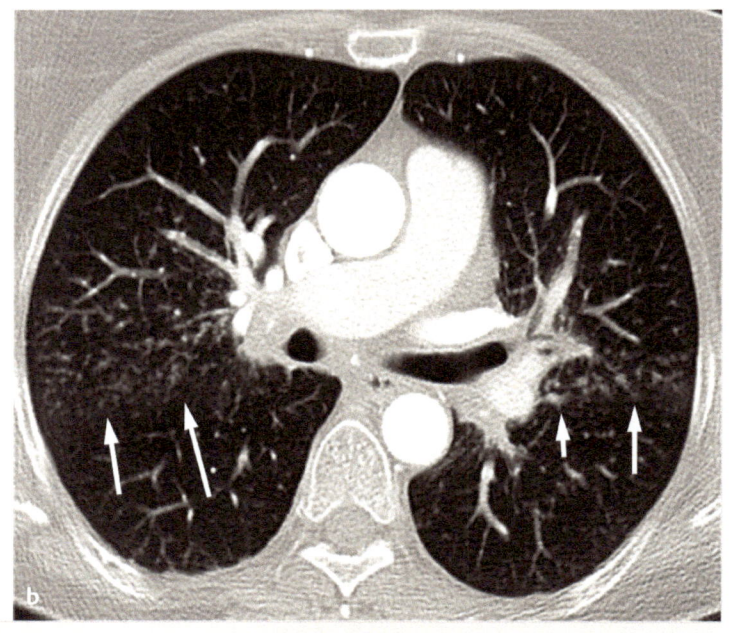

Fig. 4.58 Stage IIIA sarcoidosis. (a) Chest radiograph shows nodular opacities that are confluent in the lower right lung. (b) The nodules are distributed along bronchovascular bundles, interlobar septa, and interlobar fissures (arrows).

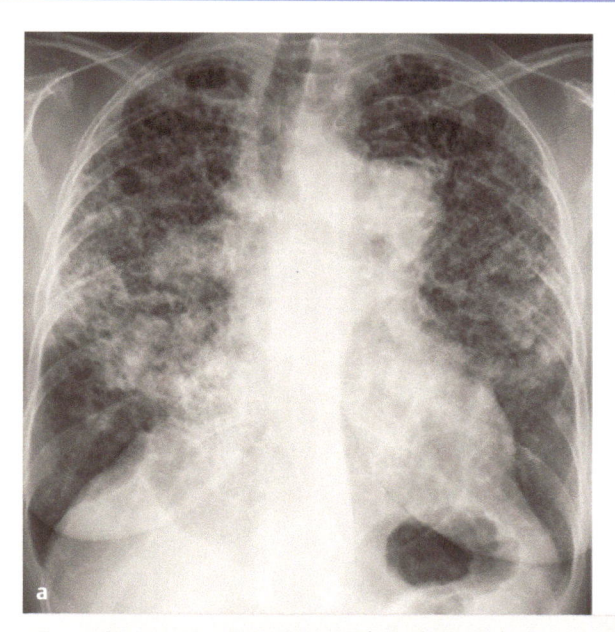

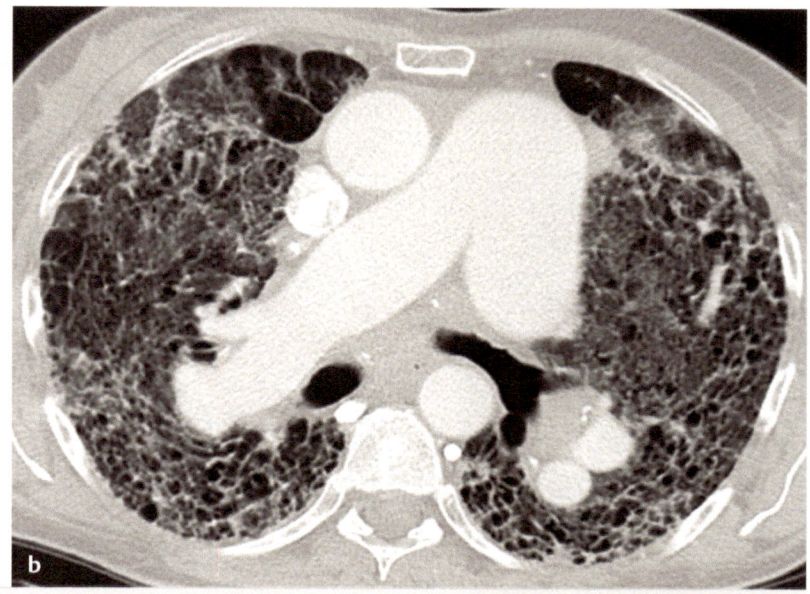

Fig. 4.59 **Images in stage IV sarcoidosis** show marked pulmonary fibrosis with a typical reticular pattern in both modalities. **(a)** Chest radiograph. **(b)** CT.

may also develop due to alveolar involvement. Nodular or patchy opacities with or without cavitation are less typical of sarcoidosis but may occur. In stage IV disease, pulmonary fibrosis, sites of traction bronchiectasis develop in addition to the fibrotic changes (▶ Fig. 4.59). The upper lobe predominance leads to upward retraction of the hila, similar to that found in tuberculosis. Aspergillomas may form in bullae.

▶ **Clinical features.** Almost half of patients are asymptomatic; the rest complain of cough and dyspnea. Night sweats, weight loss, and fever may occur.

▶ **Differential diagnosis.** Given the variable presentation of sarcoidosis and the potential for atypical changes, the differential diagnosis covers a broad spectrum, depending on the presentation. The most important differential diagnoses are lymphoma and tuberculosis. Lung cancer should be excluded in patients with solitary nodules.

▶ **Key points.** Sarcoidosis is a systemic disease of unknown etiology characterized by the formation of noncaseating granulomas. Up to 95% of all patients have symmetrical bihilar lymphadenopathy with associated enlargement of mediastinal lymph nodes. Lung imaging typically shows a perilymphatic distribution of nodules along the bronchovascular bundle, interlobar fissures, subpleural areas and, to a lesser degree, along the interlobular septa.

Langerhans Cell Histiocytosis, Histiocytosis X

▶ **Brief definition.** Langerhans cell histiocytosis is a granulomatosis of unknown cause that occurs predominantly in children and young adults. The juvenile form is based on a clonal cellular proliferation. The lung is seldom affected in the juvenile form, which predominantly involves the bones, followed by the skin. In adults, the disease is associated with smoking (95% of adult patients are smokers). It is postulated that the etiology involves an allergic response to substances contained in cigarette smoke. The lung is invariably affected. Granulomas with Langerhans cells form around the respiratory and terminal bronchioles.

▶ **Imaging signs.** Granulomas appear as stellate densities on CT. Reticular thickenings and thin-walled cysts develop rapidly during the course of the disease. In contrast to lymphangioleiomyomatosis, the cysts in Langerhans cell histiocytosis are elongated and noncircular (▶ Fig. 4.60).

▶ **Clinical features.** Children usually present with osseous involvement and bone pain. Adults complain of dyspnea and cough. Approximately 25% of patients are asymptomatic.

▶ **Differential diagnosis.** One possible differential diagnosis is lymphangioleiomyomatosis, but nodules do not occur in that disease. Cysts are not present in sarcoidosis.

▶ **Key points.** Langerhans cell histiocytosis is a granulomatous disease that is manifested in the lung by nodules and accompanying cysts.

Lymphangioleiomyomatosis and Pulmonary Involvement by Tuberous Sclerosis

▶ **Brief definition.** Lymphangioleiomyomatosis is a very rare disease characterized by the uncontrolled proliferation of immature smooth muscle cells in the small vessels, bronchi, alveoli, and lymphatics based on a defect in the TSC genes. The mTOR signal pathway is not inhibited, which allows excessive cellular proliferation to occur. There is a sporadic form that almost exclusively affects women of childbearing age, and an inherited form that presents as tuberous sclerosis with benign cellular proliferation in the brain, skin, and kidneys. Interestingly, most patients with the sporadic form are strongly symptomatic as against just 1% of patients with tuberous sclerosis; this results from different degrees of

Lung and Pleura

pulmonary involvement in each form. The occlusion of small airways leads to the formation of thin-walled cysts of variable size (up to 3 cm) throughout the lungs. Cyst rupture may cause a spontaneous pneumothorax. The prognosis of lymphangioleiomyomatosis is not good, with a 5-year survival rate of 70%. Treatment is symptomatic and includes long-term oxygen therapy in advanced cases. The only curative option is lung transplantation.

▶ **Imaging signs.** Thin-walled cysts at least 5 to 10 mm in diameter, some as large as 3 cm, are the radiological hallmark of lymphangioleiomyomatosis (▶ Fig. 4.61). Thickened interlobular septa are also found.

▶ **Clinical features.** The main symptoms are dyspnea and cough. Many patients present with a spontaneous pneumothorax with chest pain and dyspnea.

▶ **Differential diagnosis.** Differentiation is required mainly from pulmonary emphysema, Langerhans cell histiocytosis, and IPF.

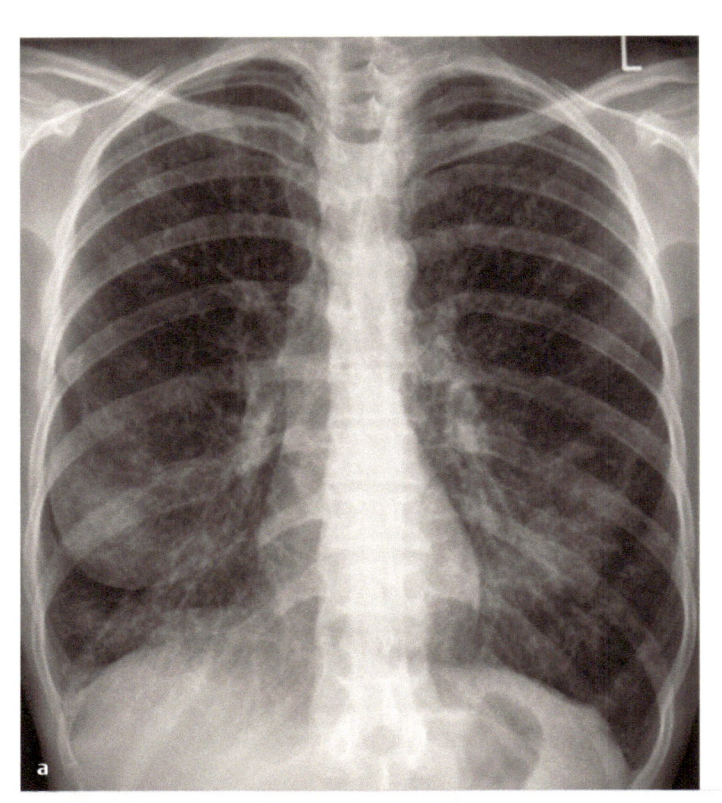

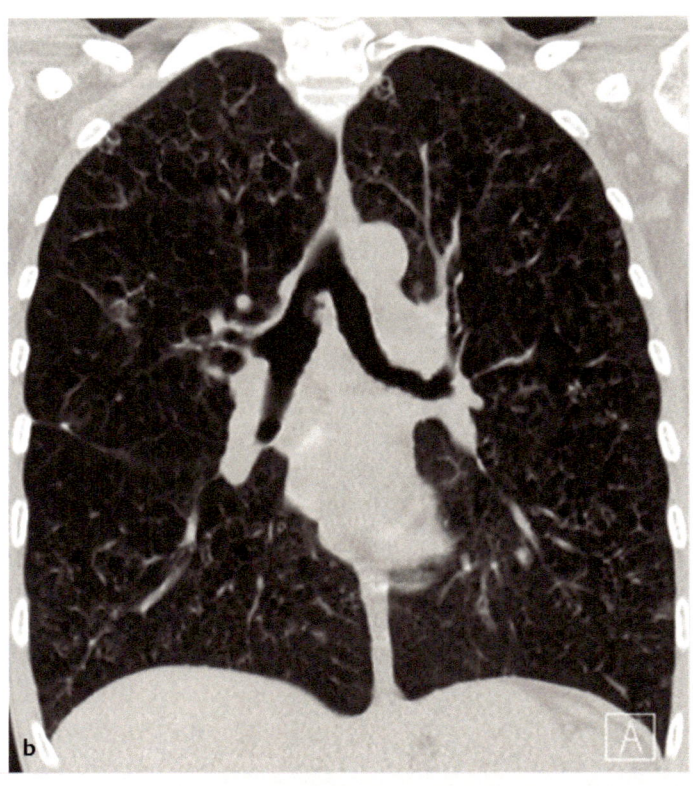

Fig. 4.60 Langerhans cell histiocytosis. (a) Hyperlucency of the lungs. (b) The lungs are permeated by contiguous, irregularly shaped cysts with upper-zone predominance of findings.

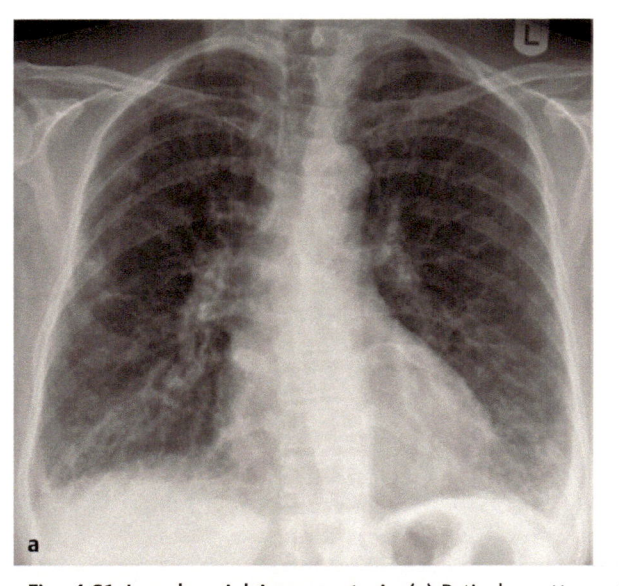

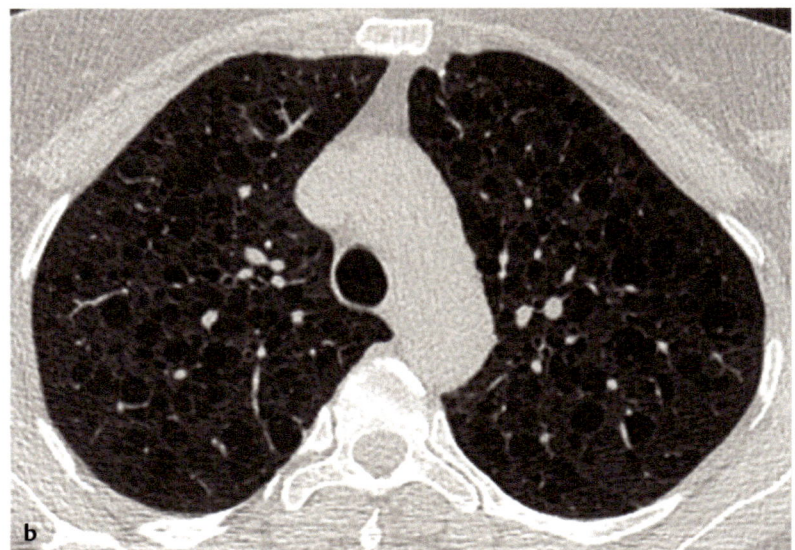

Fig. 4.61 Lymphangioleiomyomatosis. (a) Reticular pattern with unchanged lung volume. (b) Thin-walled round cysts with no zonal predominance.

▶ **Key points.** Lymphangioleiomyomatosis is characterized by a genetic defect leading to the uncontrolled proliferation of atypical smooth muscle cells in vessels, lymphatics, and airways.

There are patients with tuberous sclerosis, 30% of whom present the phenotype of lymphangioleiomyomatosis, and there is a sporadic form that almost exclusively affects women of childbearing age. Imaging shows thin-walled cysts approximately 5 to 10 cm in diameter, with some up to 3 cm, and thickening of the interlobular septa.

Cystic Fibrosis

▶ **Brief definition.** Cystic fibrosis is an autosomal recessive disease based on a genetic defect in the chloride channels in the cell membrane. Chloride ions accumulate within cells while less chloride is eliminated in glandular secretions. This disables the osmotic mechanism that would normally draw water from the interior of the cell into the secretions, with the result that the secretions from all exocrine glands have greatly increased viscosity. In the lung, this impairs mucociliary clearance, leading to mucous plugging of bronchi and bronchioles and to obstructive ventilatory impairment. The decreased clearance promotes colonization by microbes, leading to recurrent episodes of pneumonia and peribronchial infections. Many cases show chronic colonization by *Pseudomonas aeruginosa*. The combination of mucus retention and inflammatory reactions with activation of elastases leads to bronchiectasis, peribronchial fibrosis, and emphysema. Cystic fibrosis is one of the most common genetically transmitted diseases, with an incidence of 1:2,000 live births. The prognosis has improved significantly in recent decades owing to improvements in symptomatic therapy and infection prophylaxis, and most patients now live to 50 years of age.

▶ **Imaging signs.** Even in infants, chest radiographs show marked evidence of the disease with pulmonary hyperinflation and depression of the diaphragm. Over time, patients develop a barrel chest characterized by an increased distance between the sternum and spinal column and increased kyphosis. The bronchial walls are thickened due to peribronchial inflammation. Sites of bronchiectasis develop predominantly in the upper lobes and appear as "tram tracks" (see ▶ Fig. 4.13) or bandlike opacities due to mucous plugging (▶ Fig. 4.62). Small infiltrates appear as focal opacities. There may also be atelectasis. Pulmonary hyperinflation causes the heart to appear very small in children and adolescents; the cardiothoracic ratio (see ▶ Fig. 2.8) is typically less than 0.35 initially (see ▶ Fig. 4.13). Cor pulmonale develops in later stages of the disease, and the heart enlarges. CT is more sensitive in the detection of early and subtle changes and shows a mosaic pattern due to air trapping by a check-valve mechanism. Mucus retention in smaller bronchi creates a tree-in-bud pattern. Reactive lymphadenopathy is a common feature due to recurrent infection. The bronchial arteries are hypertrophic as a result of recurrent infections.

Note

Strategies to reduce radiation exposure in cystic fibrosis patients are strongly recommended because of the need for life-long imaging follow-ups.

MRI is very promising due to its ability to give detailed images of the bronchial walls and lymph nodes, evaluate lung perfusion, and provide information on disease activity based on edema and contrast enhancement. Currently MRI is being tested in large multicenter studies for its suitability for diagnostic and follow-up applications in cystic fibrosis patients.

▶ **Clinical features.** Meconium ileus occurs in up to 15% of patients due to increased viscosity of the meconium. Affected infants fail to thrive due to malabsorption resulting from exocrine pancreatic insufficiency. They are prone to recurrent pulmonary infections. Over time the symptoms and disease course are determined by pulmonary involvement and pancreatic insufficiency with malabsorption and weight loss. Hemoptysis may occur and, in patients with a significant fall in hemoglobin levels, can be managed by embolization. In adolescents the rupture of

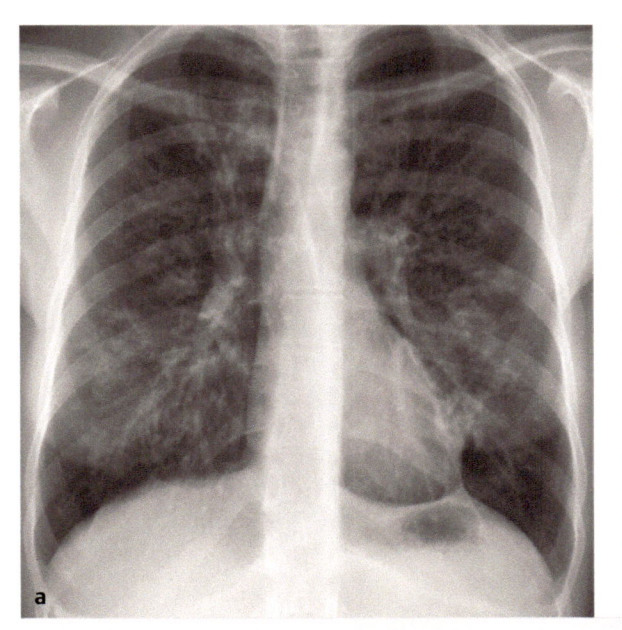

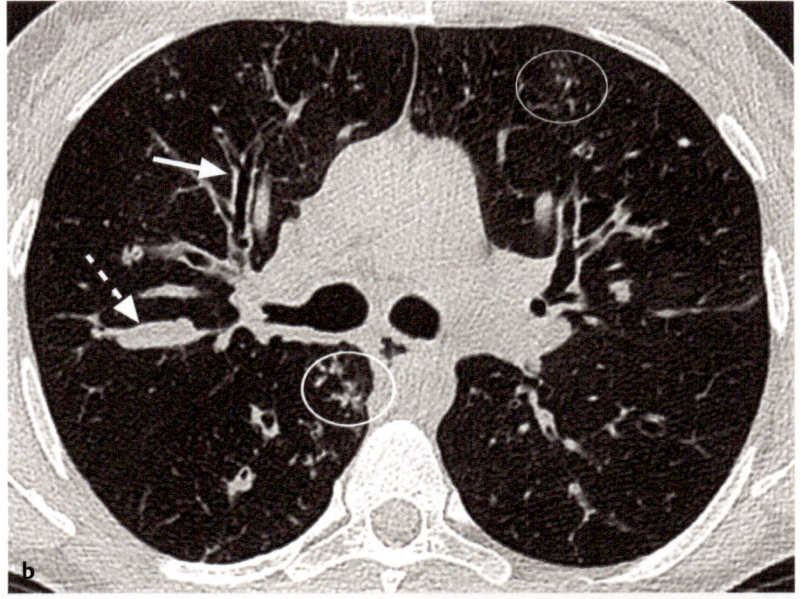

Fig. 4.62 Cystic fibrosis. (a) Chest radiograph shows patchy infiltrates along with extensive bronchiectasis. (b) CT shows bronchiectasis (arrow), thickened bronchial walls, mucous plugging in bronchiectatic areas (dashed arrow), and the tree-in-bud sign (circles).

subpleural emphysematous bullae may lead to spontaneous pneumothorax. The prognosis for survival is determined by the progression of lung involvement. Systematic inhalation therapy with saline and N-acetylcysteine, respiratory exercises, and bronchial hygiene can decrease the frequency of infections and reduce lung damage. Together with improved replacement therapies for pancreatic insufficiency, these measures have significantly improved the life expectancy of cystic fibrosis patients in recent decades.

▶ **Differential diagnosis.** From the combination of typical symptoms and early onset, cystic fibrosis can generally be diagnosed by laboratory tests (sweat test) without the need for imaging studies. Imaging is used mainly for follow-up and making a prognosis.

▶ **Key points.** Cystic fibrosis is an autosomal recessive disease caused by a genetic chloride-channel defect that increases the viscosity of exocrine gland secretions. Pulmonary effects include impaired ciliary clearance and retention of mucus; this promotes obstructive ventilatory impairment and colonization by infectious organisms. Later changes include bronchiectasis with upper lobe predominance, peribronchial fibrosis, and pulmonary emphysema.

4.3.5 Pneumoconioses

Pneumoconioses are lung diseases caused by the inhalation of respirable dust particles small enough to reach the alveoli. Respirable dust has a particle size less than 5 μm; larger particles are trapped in the upper airways before reaching the alveoli and are eliminated from the body by various mechanisms. The pulmonary reaction depends on the type of material inhaled. Collagenous pneumoconiosis, characterized by interstitial fibrosis and caused by inhaling quartz dust or asbestos, is distinguished from noncollagenous pneumoconiosis caused by the inhalation of inert substances such as iron oxide (siderosis), carbon, or aluminum. The changes in noncollagenous pneumoconiosis may be reversible after exposure is discontinued. In all pneumoconioses, the duration of exposure and dust volume correlate with the severity of disease. Most pneumoconioses occur as a result of occupational exposure.

Note
Occupationally acquired pneumoconioses are classified as notifiable occupational diseases.

The evaluation of disability claims is based on the patient's occupational history, PA chest radiograph, and pulmonary function tests. The International Labor Organization (ILO) has developed a classification system for interpreting chest radiographs that includes standard sets of radiographs for comparison with a patient's own films. The ILO classification system starts by grading the technical quality of the chest radiographs. Pulmonary opacities are evaluated according to their size, shape, location, and profusion category. Pleural abnormalities are also evaluated along with the presence of calcifications and ancillary findings such as pleural effusion, pulmonary emphysema, lymph node calcifications, and atherosclerosis.

Silicosis

▶ **Brief definition.** Silicosis is caused by the inhalation of quartz dust (silicate). Mine workers, stonemasons, and sandblasters are at greatest risk. Effective occupational safety measures plus cutbacks in mining operations have contributed to a significant decline in silicosis during recent decades. Quartz dust is phagocytosed by alveolar macrophages that migrate along lymphatic pathways. Because they cannot break down the silicate, they disintegrate and release the silicate, which is then phagocytosed by other macrophages. This process releases cytokines that promote the migration of fibroblasts. First, small nodules forms, which later fuse to form larger plaques. Due to the mechanisms described, these plaques undergo a dynamic process of gradual hilar migration over time, even if exposure to dust is discontinued. Paracicatricial emphysema develops at the periphery of the plaques.

▶ **Imaging signs.** The earliest imaging change is the appearance of multiple, equal-sized focal opacities up to approximately 4 mm in diameter, predominantly in the upper lung zones (▶ Fig. 4.63). Later they coalesce to form larger plaques. The hila may be distorted. Eggshell calcification of the hilar lymph nodes is virtually pathognomonic and results from silicate deposition in the hilar notch of the nodes (▶ Fig. 4.64). Pulmonary fibrosis develops over time and is accompanied by centrilobular emphysema.

▶ **Clinical features.** Silicosis generally runs a gradual course over a period of decades without becoming symptomatic. Patients eventually develop dyspnea. The dyspnea worsens with the development of cor pulmonale in the late stage. A subtype of the

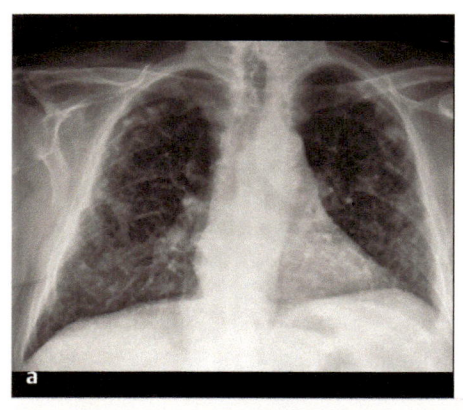

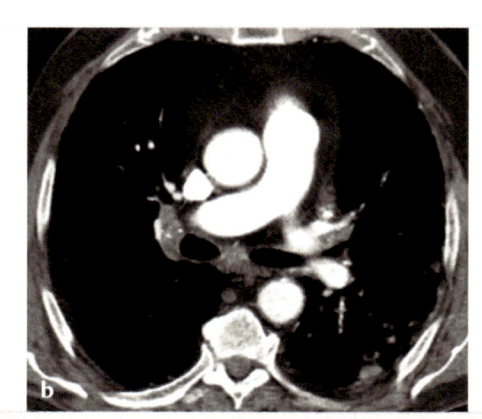

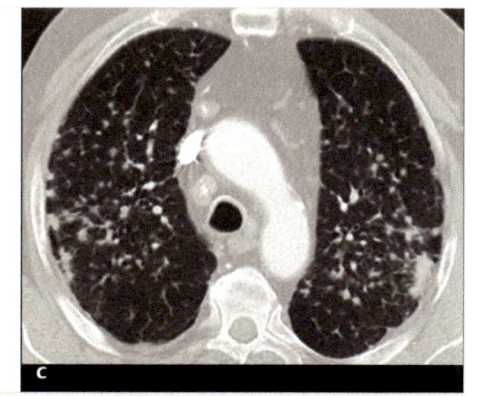

Fig. 4.63 Silicosis. (a) Nodular opacities. **(b)** Hilar lymph nodes show focal calcifications. **(c)** The nodules are diffusely distributed. In this case nodules have already coalesced to form a larger fibrotic mass on the left side.

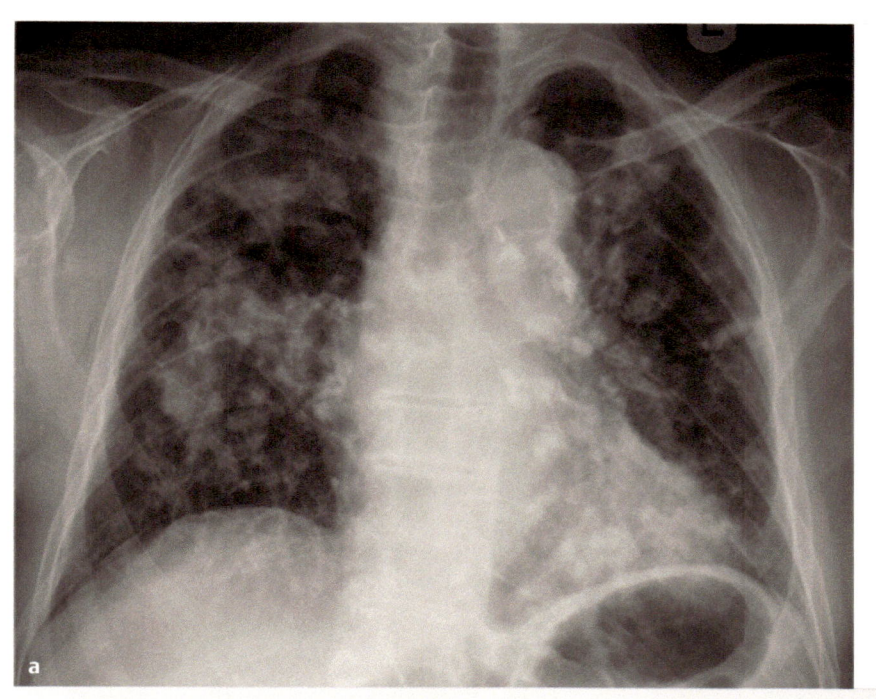

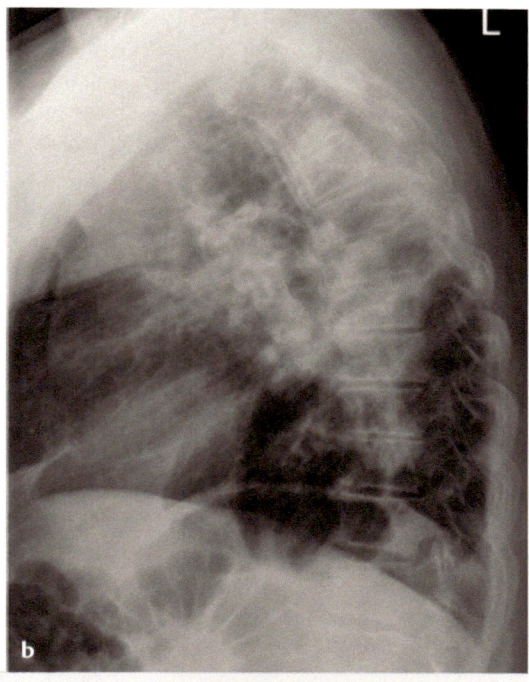

Fig. 4.64 Silicosis. Intrapulmonary nodules and eggshell calcification of hilar and mediastinal lymph nodes on the left side. (a) AP radiograph. (b) Lateral radiograph.

disease is acute silicosis, which may develop within months in response to brief, heavy exposure and is characterized by proteinosis. "Silicon tuberculosis" refers to a tuberculous infection of the lung and silicon plaques.

> **Caution**
> A subtype of silicosis called Caplan's syndrome has been described in rheumatoid patients. It is characterized by the more rapid formation of multiple pulmonary nodules approximately 1 cm in diameter.

Asbestosis

▶ **Brief definition.** Asbestos is a naturally occurring, fine fibrous mineral that was widely used in industry, construction, and automaking (for brake linings) in the 20th century because of its fire resistance and durability. Numerous countries throughout the world have adopted national asbestos bans. But given the long lifespan of building materials, asbestos-containing parts are still widely distributed in the environment and must be safely disposed of during renovations and demolitions. Different types of asbestos differ in their fiber geometry and associated health risks. Blue asbestos (crocidolite) is more carcinogenic than white asbestos (chrysotile). From 10 to 20% of occupationally exposed persons will develop lung cancer or mesothelioma (also in the pericardium or peritoneum), depending on their "fiber years" of exposure. It should be noted, however, that the latent period is 30 to 40 years for carcinogenesis and approximately 20 years for pulmonary fibrosis; thus it is reasonable to expect a rise in the incidence of asbestosis and its sequelae in the coming years.

> **Caution**
> Asbestos exposure may also cause pericardial or peritoneal mesothelioma.

Lung macrophages can phagocytize asbestos fibers but they cannot retain them and are killed, releasing the fibers. Release of macrophage cytokines induces fibrosis. Meanwhile the asbestos fibers can be ingested by new macrophages, setting a destructive cycle into motion. Fibers that are not phagocytosed can pierce the alveolar walls and migrate by this route to the pleura. The pleural irritation incites plaque formation, and the plaques may subsequently calcify.

▶ **Imaging signs.** Small, irregular focal opacities may occur, appearing predominantly in the lower and middle lung zones. Costophrenic angle effusion may develop as an early sign. Areas of pleural thickening may be visible on radiographs, but HRCT is much more sensitive in depicting the changes of asbestosis. Hyaline plaques typically appear on CT as elevated flat lesions (▶ Fig. 4.65). These plaques occur predominantly in the basal region and may calcify. The interlobular septa and bronchovascular bundles appear thickened. Scar thickenings termed parenchymal bands may extend at right angles from the pleural surface into the lung parenchyma. Rounded atelectasis is a common finding.

> **Note**
> Pleural plaques with a linear pattern of fibrous thickening are typical of prior asbestos exposure and are considered a key indicator of asbestos-related disease. The fibrotic changes that characterize asbestosis are nonspecific, however, and may have other causes (▶ Fig. 4.66; see also ▶ Fig. 4.65).

Lung and Pleura

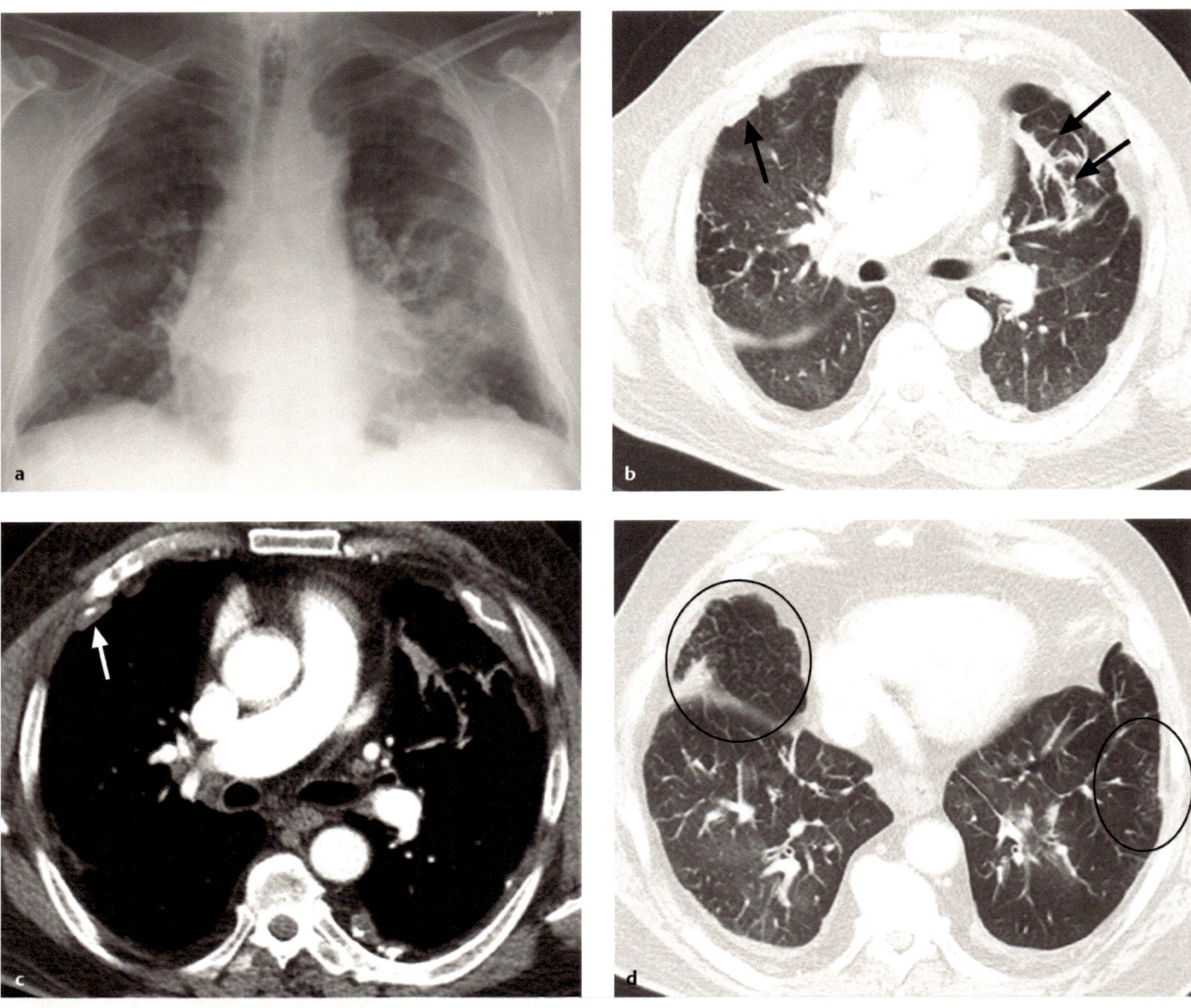

Fig. 4.65 Asbestosis. (a) Chest radiograph demonstrates pleural plaques. **(b)** The pleural plaques appear on CT as elevated flat lesions. Areas of atelectasis (arrows) are also identified. **(c)** The pleural plaques contain calcifications (arrow). **(d)** The interlobular septa are thickened (circles).

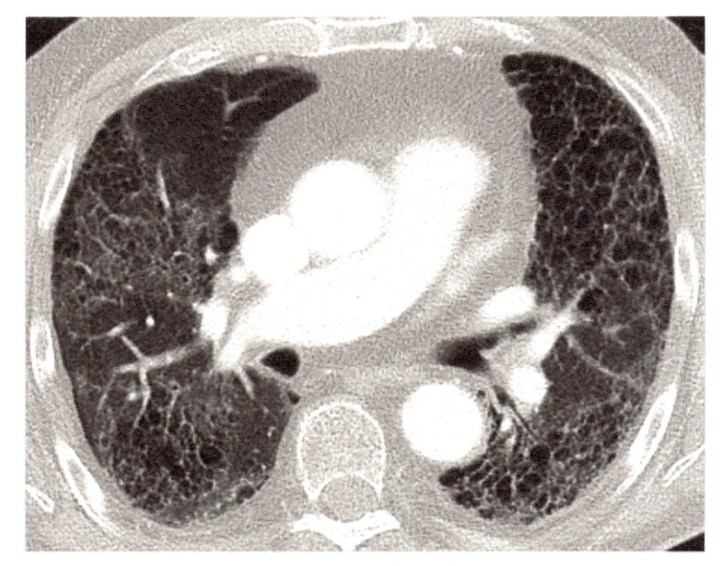

Fig. 4.66 Pulmonary fibrosis in asbestosis. Differentiation is required mainly from IPF/UIP.

▶ **Clinical features.** Dyspnea is preceded by a very long latent period. Patients with mesothelioma also complain of chest pain.

Other Pneumoconioses

▶ **Brief definition**
- *Anthracosis*: Pure anthracosis is a noncollagenous pneumoconiosis. It does not generally occur in isolation, however. Coal miners are also exposed to silicate, resulting in the development of silicoanthracosis with the added features of silicosis. Anthracosis alone does not have an imaging correlate.
- *Siderosis*: Siderosis results from the inhalation of iron oxide dust and may be found in welders and steel workers. Alveolar macrophages phagocytize the dust, which is then deposited in the interstitium and on bronchovascular bundles. Since the particles do not provoke fibrosis, changes regress after the cessation of exposure through elimination by expectoration and other mechanisms.

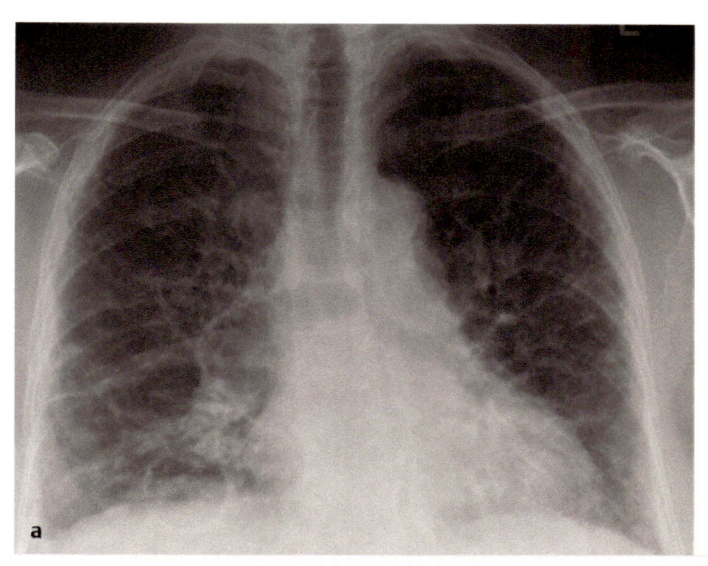

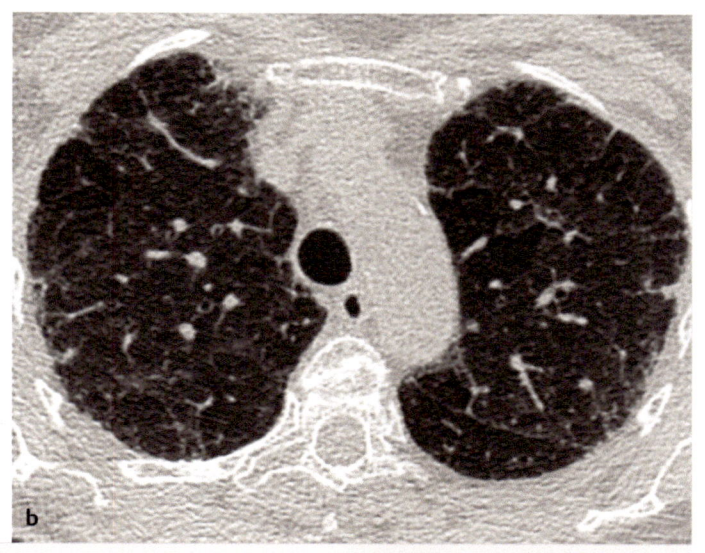

Fig. 4.67 Extrinsic allergic alveolitis. (a) Opacities in the chest radiograph. **(b)** CT shows areas of air trapping and increased density. Subpleural fibrosis is characteristic of long-standing disease.

▶ **Imaging signs.** Very dense focal opacities are typically found. They may clear gradually after the cessation of exposure.

▶ **Clinical features.** Siderosis is almost asymptomatic.

Summary

Pneumoconioses may develop after years of inhaling respirable dust (particle size < 5 μm) and are classified as notifiable occupational diseases. Collagenous pneumoconiosis is distinguished from noncollagenous pneumoconiosis:
- *Collagenous pneumoconiosis* is considered the pathophysiologic endpoint of exposure-induced fibrotic changes. Imaging patterns depend on the type of dust inhaled. Siderosis is characterized by the development of nodules that are most numerous in the upper and middle zones. Later the nodules coalesce to form fibrotic masses, and the hila may show eggshell calcifications. Prior asbestos exposure leads to the formation of elevated flat hyaline and/or calcified plaques, predominantly in the basal region. Interstitial fibrotic changes are characteristic of asbestosis. Mesothelioma or lung cancer develops in up to 20% of patients.
- *Noncollagenous pneumoconiosis* may be caused by the inhalation of iron oxide dust. The inhaled particles cause the formation of dense focal opacities, which may be cleared by phagocytosis and eliminated from the lung once exposure has ceased, resulting in a complete resolution of findings.

4.3.6 Extrinsic Allergic Alveolitis

▶ **Brief definition.** Extrinsic allergic alveolitis is often found in settings of occupational exposure. It may be caused by various inhalable organic allergens or chemical compounds that combine with endogenous proteins to form haptens. Less than 1% of exposed individuals develop extrinsic allergic alveolitis, and most of these patients contract the disease only after years of exposure. Perhaps the most familiar form is "bird fancier's lung," in which proteins from bird excrement and feather particles are the precipitating allergens. The precipitating agents in farmer's lung are the thermophilic actinomycetes that occur in damp hay. Molds are the causative agent of extrinsic allergic alveolitis in people who work in fruit processing, mushroom growing, or dairy farming. Immunoglobulin G incites type III and type IV immune responses in the alveoli. Histopathologic features consist of cellular infiltrates in the bronchiolar walls, interstitial inflammatory reactions with cellular infiltrate, and alveolitis with intraalveolar giant cells and noncaseating granulomas. Over time, recurring cytokine secretion leads to irreversible fibrosis unless allergen exposure is discontinued.[17]

▶ **Imaging signs.** The hallmark of extrinsic allergic alveolitis on HRCT is a combination of ground-glass opacities, centrilobular ground-glass densities, normal-appearing lung areas, and air trapping. The chronic stage is characterized by signs of pulmonary fibrosis with increased reticular markings. Air trapping is also demonstrable in these cases (▶ Fig. 4.67).

▶ **Clinical features.** In most patients, extrinsic allergic alveolitis develops only after years of antigen exposure. In the acute stage, allergen exposure is followed within 3 to 6 hours by flulike complaints with fever, chills, dyspnea, and a feeling of weakness. The symptoms begin to subside in just 1 to 2 days. Chronic cases are characterized by an insidious onset of symptoms. The first-line treatment is the cessation of exposure. Steroids can shorten the inflammatory response and reduce the severity of complaints.

▶ **Differential diagnosis.** Other diffuse lung diseases such as IPF and NSIP can be excluded by the history and the distribution pattern of the changes.

▶ **Key points.** Extrinsic allergic alveolitis is caused by type III and IV immune response to organic allergens or substances that bind with endogenous proteins to form haptens. The principal features on HRCT are ground-glass opacities accompanied by air trapping and centrilobular ground-glass densities.

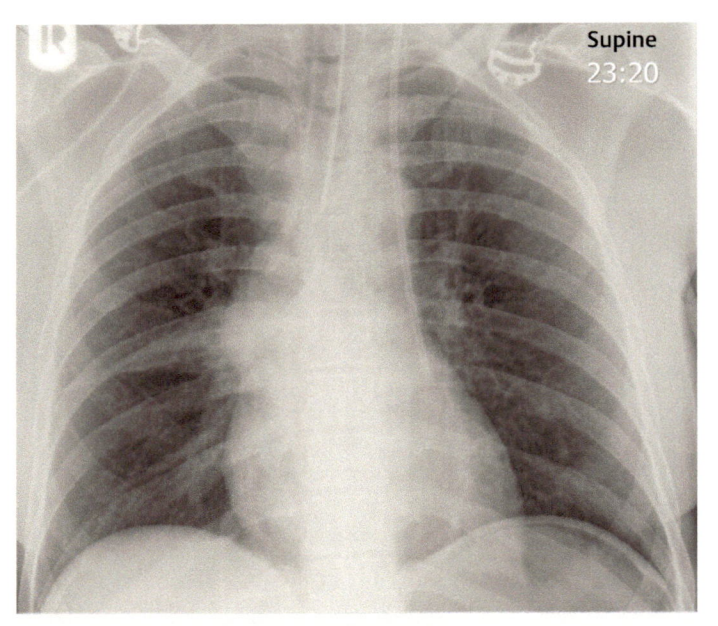

Fig. 4.68 Inhalation trauma from a house fire. Peribronchial opacities are visible in the right lung.

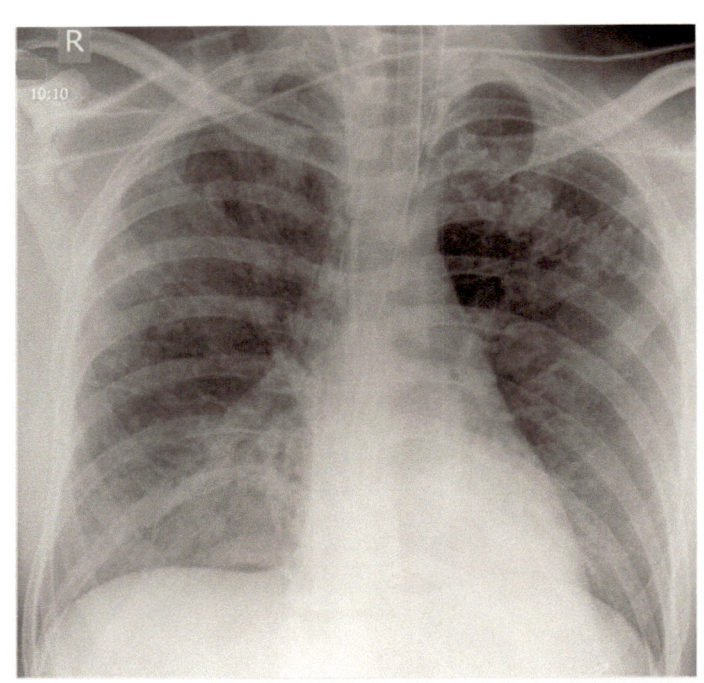

Fig. 4.69 Chest radiograph in a near-drowning victim shows bilateral pulmonary edema.

4.3.7 Pulmonary Trauma

Trauma Due to Smoke Inhalation, Fire, or Toxic Gases

▶ **Brief definition.** Fire generates a mixture of various toxic gases in hot air. Inhalational lung injury occurs in approximately 25% of burn victims. Most cases involve concomitant injury to the tracheobronchial mucosa and alveoli. The bronchial walls are thickened due to edema and cellular infiltration. Damage to type II pneumocytes and the surfactant film leads to pulmonary edema.

▶ **Imaging signs.** Chest radiographs obtained shortly after exposure to the fire may show no abnormalities. Initial changes may take 24 hours to appear and range from opacities to lung edema, depending on the severity of the inhalational injury (▶ Fig. 4.68). CT demonstrates thickened bronchial walls and ground-glass opacities. Dense consolidation is found in severely affected areas and may be accompanied by intraparenchymal hemorrhage. Severe injury may also lead to irreversible pulmonary fibrosis.

▶ **Clinical features.** Smoke inhalation is associated with dyspnea. The mortality rate of severe inhalational lung injury after a fire is very high, at 70 to 90%, and depends on the degree of injury, on associated injuries, and especially on the severity of skin burns.

▶ **Differential diagnosis.** Pulmonary changes may result from ARDS secondary to severe skin burns and also from direct injury by smoke inhalation.

Mixed Aspiration Events

▶ **Brief definition.** A variety of aspiration events may cause lung injury. Examples include near-drowning with pulmonary edema and possible ARDS, the aspiration of gastric juice with low pH (Mendelson's syndrome), the effects of pulmonary infiltrates, and foreign body aspiration, especially in small children, causing the occlusion of a bronchus and mediastinal flutter.

▶ **Imaging signs**
- *Near-drowning*: This is characterized by the development of bilateral pulmonary edema (▶ Fig. 4.69). Similarly to smoke inhalation, the injury often takes 1 to 2 days to produce visible radiological changes.
- *Aspiration of gastric juice or orally ingested substances*: This leads to infiltrates in dependent lung areas (▶ Fig. 4.70).
- *Aspiration of a foreign body (such as a peanut) in a small child*: Mediastinal flutter is noted on fluoroscopy. The aspirated foreign body creates a check-valve mechanism that blocks air expiration from the affected lung, causing the mediastinum to shift toward the normal side during exhalation (▶ Fig. 4.71). A complete occlusion leads to atelectasis. If the foreign body is not extracted by bronchoscopy, pressure necrosis may develop in the bronchus and heal to form a scar stricture.

4.3.8 Vasculitides

Vasculitides are vessel wall inflammations that usually have an autoimmune cause. The lung is affected in most cases due to its extensive vascular bed.

Wegener's Granulomatosis

▶ **Brief definition.** Wegener's granulomatosis is a necrotizing granulomatous vasculitis with manifestations in the respiratory tract including the paranasal sinuses and lung (90% of all cases) and the kidney (85% of cases). Possible sites of pulmonary involvement are the arteries, arterioles, capillaries, and veins.

▶ **Imaging signs.** Imaging reveals nodular or confluent opacities 1 to 10 cm in diameter (▶ Fig. 4.72). Liquefaction is typical and

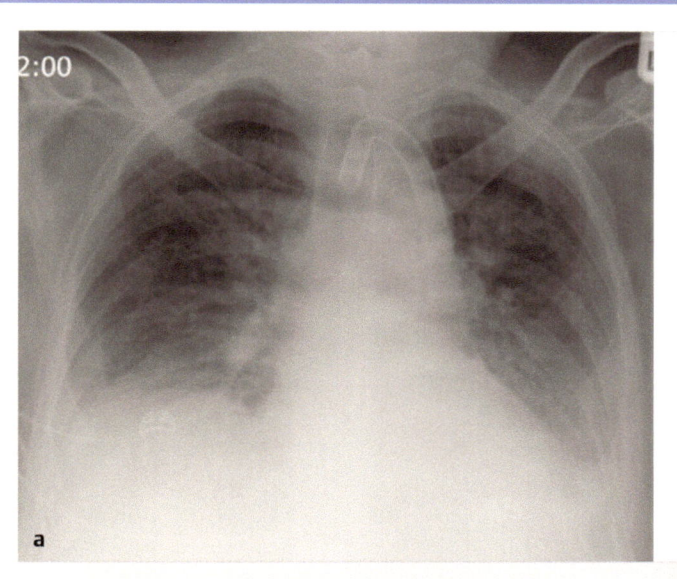

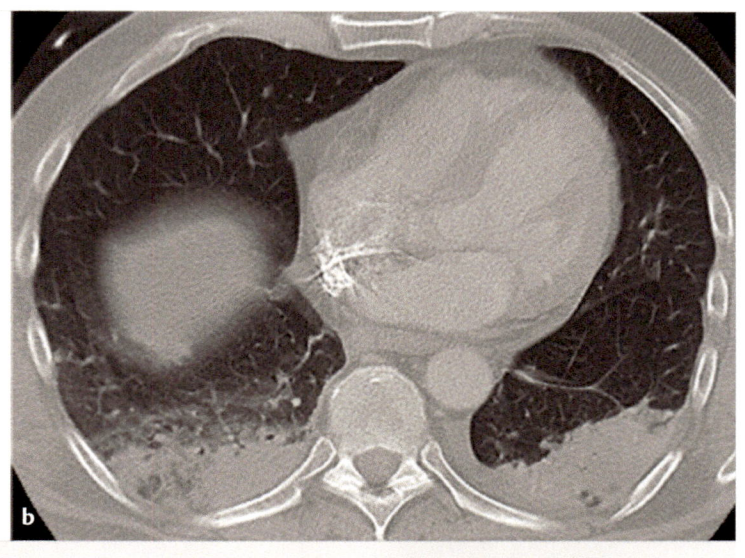

Fig. 4.70 Aspiration pneumonia after ingestion of lye. Bilateral infiltrates in the posterobasal lower lobes. (a) Chest radiograph. (b) CT.

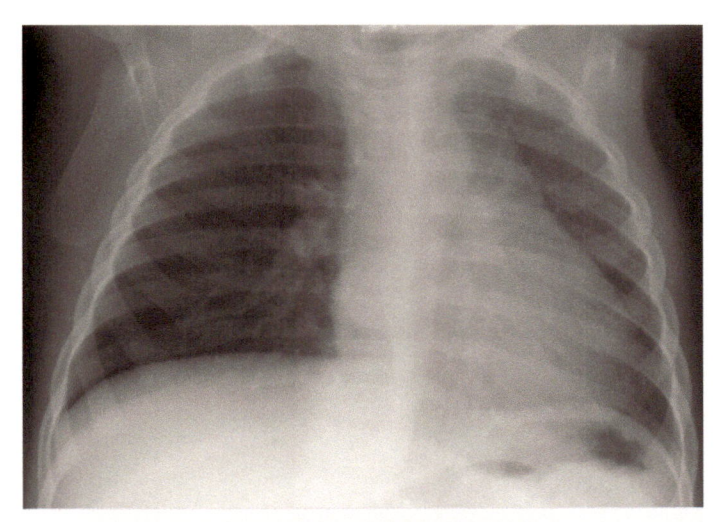

Fig. 4.71 Aspiration of a peanut into the right main bronchus of a 4-year-old boy. The right lung is overinflated due to a check-valve mechanism.

occurs in one-half of cases, especially in larger foci. Intralesional hemorrhage leads to ground-glass opacities and thickened interlobular septa.

▶ **Clinical features.** Typical features are sinusitis, cough, and dyspnea. Involvement of the lower respiratory tract may lead to tracheal stenosis. Some patients exhibit hemoptysis. Laboratory tests show elevated titers of cytoplasmic antineutrophil cytoplasmic antibodies (cANCA). Glomerulonephritis is present in approximately 20% of patients at the start of the disease and develops subsequently in up to 85%.

> **Note**
> The combination of sinusitis, cough, and hematuria is a typical symptom complex in Wegener's granulomatosis. Biopsy from the lung or respiratory tract shows typical granulomas. Glomerulonephritis, on the other hand, is histologically nonspecific, so renal biopsy does not contribute to the diagnosis.

▶ **Key points.** Wegener's granulomatosis is a granulomatous vasculitis with manifestations in the respiratory tract, lungs, and kidneys. Lung imaging shows confluent or nodular opacities, which may show liquefaction.

Churg–Strauss Syndrome

▶ **Brief definition.** Churg–Strauss syndrome is a small-vessel vasculitis. Patients almost invariably suffer from bronchial asthma and have increased numbers of eosinophilic granulocytes and elevated titers of perinuclear antineutrophil cytoplasmic antibodies (pANCA).

▶ **Imaging signs.** Imaging shows predominantly peripheral infiltrates and ground-glass opacities (caused by eosinophilic granulocytes; ▶ Fig. 4.73), which may migrate within the lung. The interlobular septa may be thickened due to infiltration with eosinophilic granulocytes. There is no liquefaction. The bronchial walls are thickened.

▶ **Clinical features.** Churg–Strauss syndrome has three phases, each of which may last for several years:
- *Phase 1*: bronchial asthma and allergic rhinosinusitis.
- *Phase 2*: eosinophilic vasculitis in the lung and gastrointestinal tract with hemorrhage and associated abdominal pain and weight loss.
- *Phase 3*: systemic small-vessel vasculitis. Cardiac involvement leads to myocardial infarction and determines the prognosis. The involvement of vessels that supply nerves causes neuritis with neuropathic pain. Renal involvement may lead to renal hypertension.

▶ **Differential diagnosis.** The differential diagnosis includes Wegeners' granulomatosis, especially due to paranasal sinus involvement in both diseases, as well as COP and pneumonia including allergic bronchopulmonary aspergillosis.

▶ **Key points.** Churg–Strauss syndrome is a small-vessel vasculitis characterized by infiltration with eosinophilic granulocytes. It

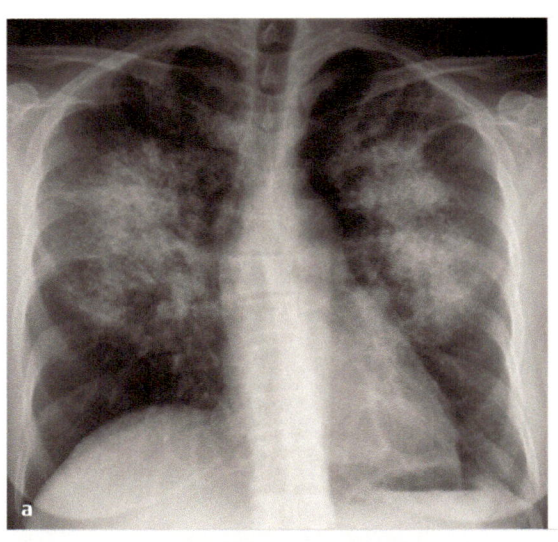

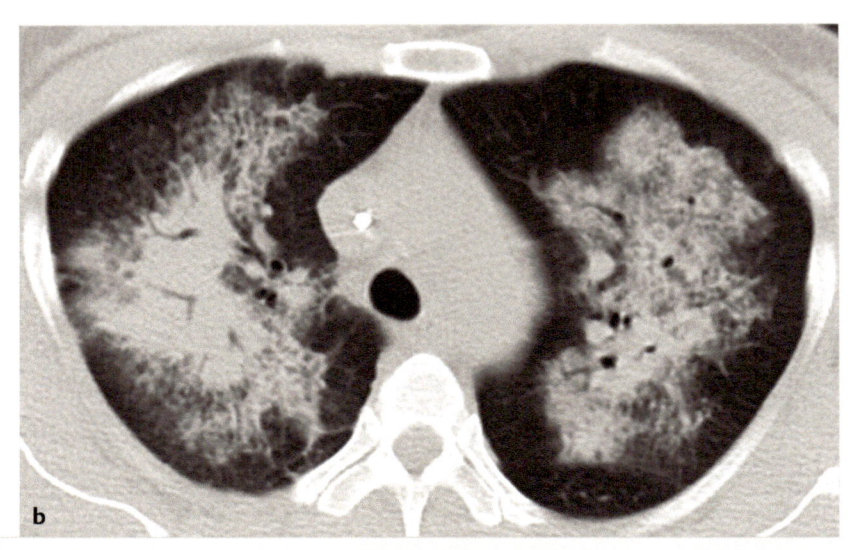

Fig. 4.72 Wegener's granulomatosis. (a) Confluent reticular opacities are visible in both upper and middle zones. (b) Dense consolidations are accompanied by thickening of the interlobar septa and ground-glass opacities.

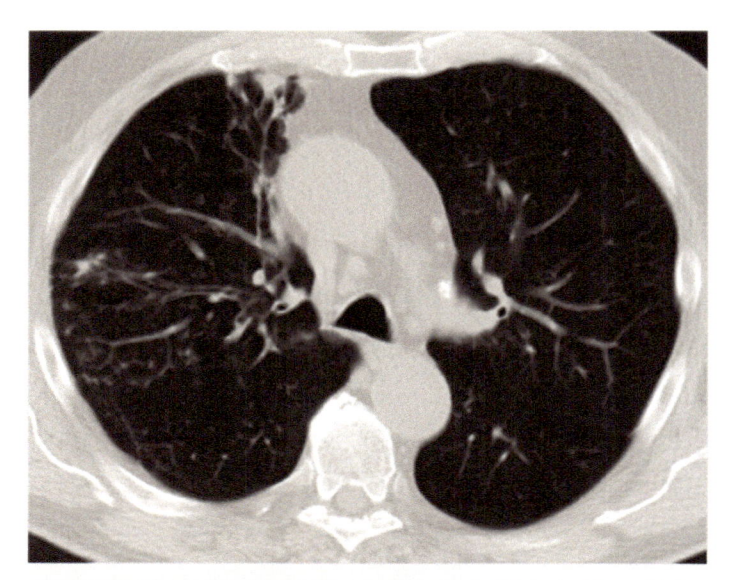

Fig. 4.73 Churg–Strauss syndrome. CT reveals thickened bronchial walls, peripheral consolidations, and ground-glass opacities.

has three clinical phases, the first consisting of bronchial asthma and allergic rhinosinusitis. Phase 2 is eosinophilic infiltrative disease in the lung and gastrointestinal tract. Phase 3 is systemic vasculitis with cardiac involvement and risk of myocardial infarction plus renal involvement and neuritis. Lung imaging shows migratory infiltrates and ground-glass opacities with a peripheral predominance.

4.3.9 Connective Tissue Diseases

▶ **Brief definition.** Connective tissue diseases are a diverse group of autoimmune disorders that affect the connective tissue. They encompass the diseases listed in ▶ Table 4.8. The lung is affected in varying degrees. Pulmonary involvement is most pronounced in scleroderma, polymyositis, dermatomyositis, and rheumatoid arthritis, with a pattern resembling NSIP or IPF. The common end point is fibrosis. Connective tissue diseases may also lead to constrictive bronchiolitis, pleurisy, or vasculitis resulting in pulmonary hypertension. The most common findings in various diseases are reviewed in ▶ Table 4.8. Pulmonary imaging is done to determine the extent of lung involvement and for follow-up. Bronchoalveolar lavage is also used in routine clinical settings to confirm the radiological findings. Pulmonary function tests are also performed. The diagnosis of connective tissue diseases themselves requires the correlation of history, clinical findings, and laboratory values. CREST syndrome (an acronym for calcinosis, Raynaud phenomenon, esophageal dysmotility, sclerodactyly, and telangiectasia) is included among the connective tissue diseases but is defined as scleroderma without parenchymal organ involvement, and therefore the lung is not affected.

> **Caution**
>
> If a connective tissue disease or rheumatoid arthritis is present in a patient with interstitial lung disease, do not attribute the lung findings to the underlying disease without further investigation. Always consider the possibility of a separate interstitial lung disease. Moreover, immunosuppressant therapy for the underlying disease will predispose to pneumonia, and several therapeutically applied medications have the potential to incite drug-induced pneumonitis. The rate with methotrexate use is 3%, regardless of the dose or duration of therapy.

> **Note**
>
> Interstitial lung diseases that are due to connective tissue disease are typically bilateral and show peripheral and basal predominance. The pattern of findings is the same as in NSIP or IPF.

▶ **Imaging signs**
- *Lupus erythematosus*: The most common manifestation is dry pleurisy, characterized by pleural thickening with little or no pleural effusion. All other changes are rare.
- *Polymyositis and dermatomyositis*: The dominant patterns are like those in IPF and COP, with reticular densities, ground-glass opacities, or consolidation. Lung volume is reduced due to weakness of the respiratory muscles.

- *Sjögren's syndrome*: Initial findings are often analogous to those in LIP, with later progression to the pattern seen in IPF.
- *Scleroderma and CREST syndrome*: Up to 90% of scleroderma patients have interstitial lung disease with the features of IPF. Approximately 30% of patients have pleural thickening. Some 60% of patients with CREST syndrome have interstitial lung disease with the features of IPF.
- *Sharp's syndrome*: The predominant change in Sharp's syndrome is interstitial fibrosis.
- *Rheumatoid arthritis*: The most common finding is the pattern seen in IPF. Most patients also have pleural thickening and there may also be features of COP. Approximately 20% of all patients develop bronchiectasis. Intrapulmonary rheumatoid nodules occur only in rare cases (less than 5%). Typically they are 8 mm or less in diameter, are located in the subpleural lung, and cavitate in one-half of cases.

4.3.10 Amyloidosis

▶ **Brief definition.** Amyloidosis is characterized by the deposition of glycoproteins in the extracellular space. In primary amyloidosis these changes are idiopathic, i.e., they occur without an identifiable causal disease. The lung is usually affected in this form. Plasmacytoma is commonly associated with amyloid deposition. "Reactive" amyloidosis may occur in chronic inflammatory diseases such as osteomyelitis, Crohn's disease, or rheumatoid arthritis. The lung is very rarely affected in these patients. Age-related amyloidosis almost always affects the heart but not the lung. Three sites of pulmonary involvement in amyloidosis are known: amyloid may be deposited in the tracheal and bronchial walls with associated bronchial-wall thickening, in the interstitium, or in the form of small nodules.

▶ **Imaging signs.** In accordance with the deposition sites, imaging may show circumscribed or ubiquitous thickening of the tracheal wall. There may also be demonstrable thickening of the interlobular septa with features of pulmonary fibrosis. Intrapulmonary nodules ranging in size from 0.5 to 5.0 cm may occur. These nodules contain calcifications in up to 40% of cases and occur predominantly in the lower zones (▶ Fig. 4.74). Deposition in the pleura leads to marked pleural thickening.

Table 4.8 Manifestations of connective tissue diseases and rheumatoid arthritis

Disease	Tracheobronchial tree	Interstitial lung changes	Pleural thickening or effusion	Vasculitis, possibly resulting in pulmonary hypertension
Lupus erythematosus	+	+	+++	+
Polymyositis and dermatomyositis	–	+++	–	+
Sjögren syndrome	++	++	+	–
Scleroderma and CREST syndrome	–	+++	++	+++
Sharp syndrome	+	++	+	++
Rheumatoid arthritis	++	++	++	–

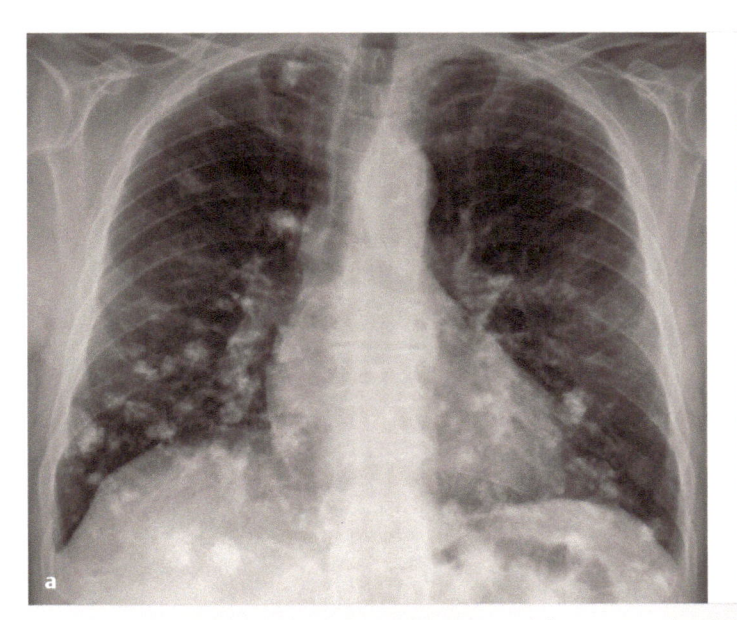

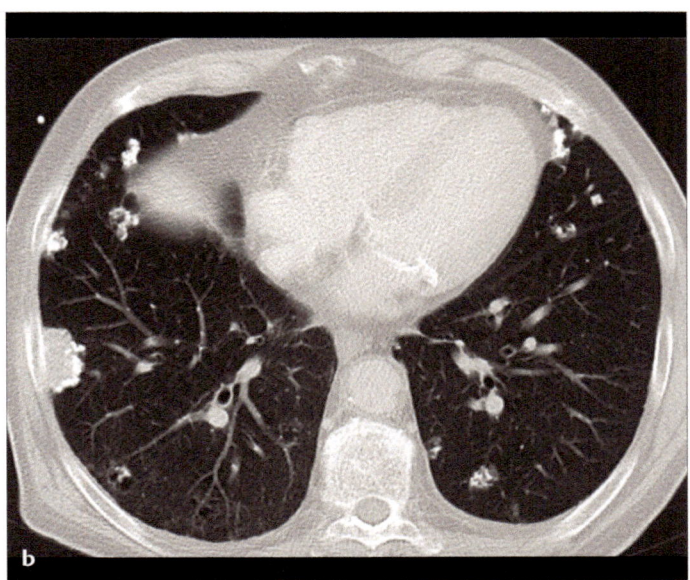

Fig. 4.74 Amyloidosis. (a) Basally predominant nodules, some with calcification. (b) The nodules are sharply circumscribed. The parenchyma is otherwise normal.

▶ **Differential diagnosis.** If the dominant findings are nodular changes, the differential diagnosis should include silicosis and sarcoidosis. Metastases or lung cancer should be considered in patients with larger pulmonary nodules. Mesothelioma should be excluded if pleural thickening is present.

▶ **Key points.** Amyloidosis is characterized by the extracellular deposition of abnormal glycoproteins called amyloid fibrils. In the lung, this material may be deposited in the tracheobronchial tree, the interstitium, and the pleura, and in the form of nodules, resulting in a range of possible imaging findings.

4.3.11 Goodpasture's Syndrome, Intrapulmonary Hemorrhage

▶ **Brief definition.** Goodpasture's syndrome is an autoimmune disease in which antibodies attack the basement membrane in the lungs and kidneys. Renal involvement leads to rapidly progressive glomerulonephritis, while recurrent hemorrhages occur within the lung. Treatment consists of plasmapheresis and immunosuppressant therapy.

▶ **Imaging signs.** Intra-alveolar hemorrhage appears as focal opacities on the chest radiograph (▶ Fig. 4.75). CT shows nodular ground-glass opacities, some of which may coalesce. These findings change within a few days due to clearance of the extravasated blood. As blood breakdown occurs, there may be transient thickening of the interlobular septa (see ▶ Fig. 4.75). As hemorrhagic episodes recur over time, pulmonary fibrosis develops.

> **Caution**
>
> Intrapulmonary hemorrhage may occur in a number of different diseases such as rheumatoid arthritis, connective tissue diseases, and Henoch–Schönlein purpura. The imaging signs in each case are identical.

▶ **Clinical features.** Patients with Goodpasture's syndrome complain of acute-onset dyspnea, hemoptysis (in up to 90% of cases), and cough. Iron deficiency anemia may lead to weakness and decreased exercise tolerance. Glomerulonephritis may culminate in renal failure.

▶ **Differential diagnosis.** Differentiation is required from Wegener's granulomatosis, Churg–Strauss syndrome, polyangiitis, and systemic lupus erythematosus. Diffuse idiopathic hemosiderosis should also be excluded.

> **Note**
>
> In diffuse idiopathic hemosiderosis, recurrent intra-alveolar bleeding occurs due to an unknown cause. The imaging findings are the same as in Goodpasture's syndrome.

▶ **Key points.** Intrapulmonary hemorrhage due to various causes leads to ground-glass opacities and, with clearance, transient thickening of the interlobular septa. Recurrent alveolar hemorrhages eventually lead to pulmonary fibrosis.

4.3.12 Alveolar Microlithiasis

▶ **Brief definition.** Alveolar microlithiasis is a rare, autosomal recessive disease characterized by the precipitation of calcium phosphate in the alveoli. Approximately 15% of all reported cases have been observed in Turkey. There is a familial occurrence pattern suggesting a genetic etiology. As there is no treatment, lung transplantation is the only option available for patients in respiratory failure.

▶ **Imaging signs.** Both lungs are very dense in the chest radiograph, contrasting sharply with the less dense mediastinum. The dense micronodules create the appearance of a sandstorm, giving rise to the term "sandstorm lung," which is widely used in the literature (▶ Fig. 4.76). CT shows ground-glass opacities and multiple dense micronodules, which coalesce in the subpleural lung, in the interlobar fissures, and along bronchovascular bundles.

▶ **Clinical features.** Most patients (70%) are asymptomatic, so the disease is detected incidentally. The remaining patients

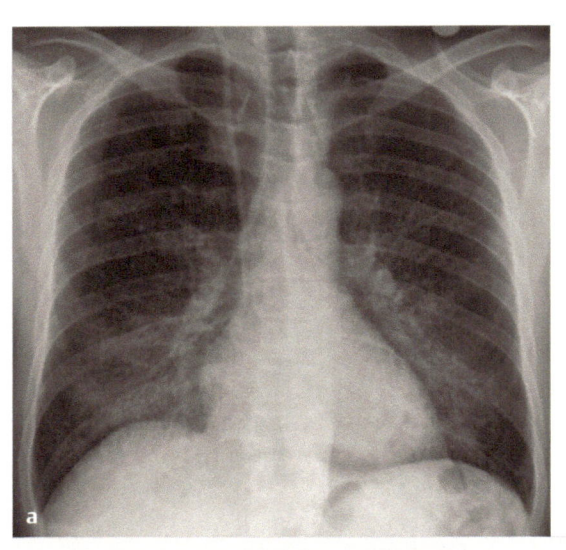

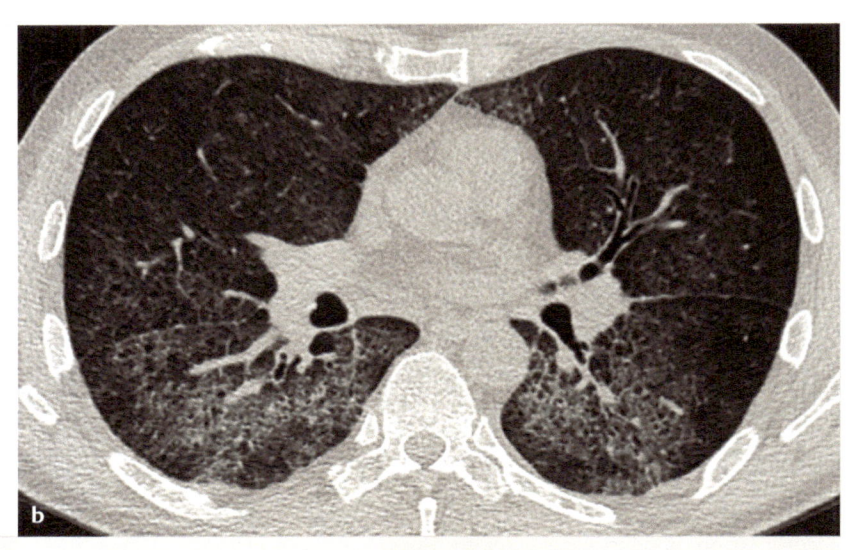

Fig. 4.75 Goodpasture's syndrome. (a) Basal opacity following acute intrapulmonary hemorrhage. **(b)** Ground-glass opacities and thickening of interlobar septa.

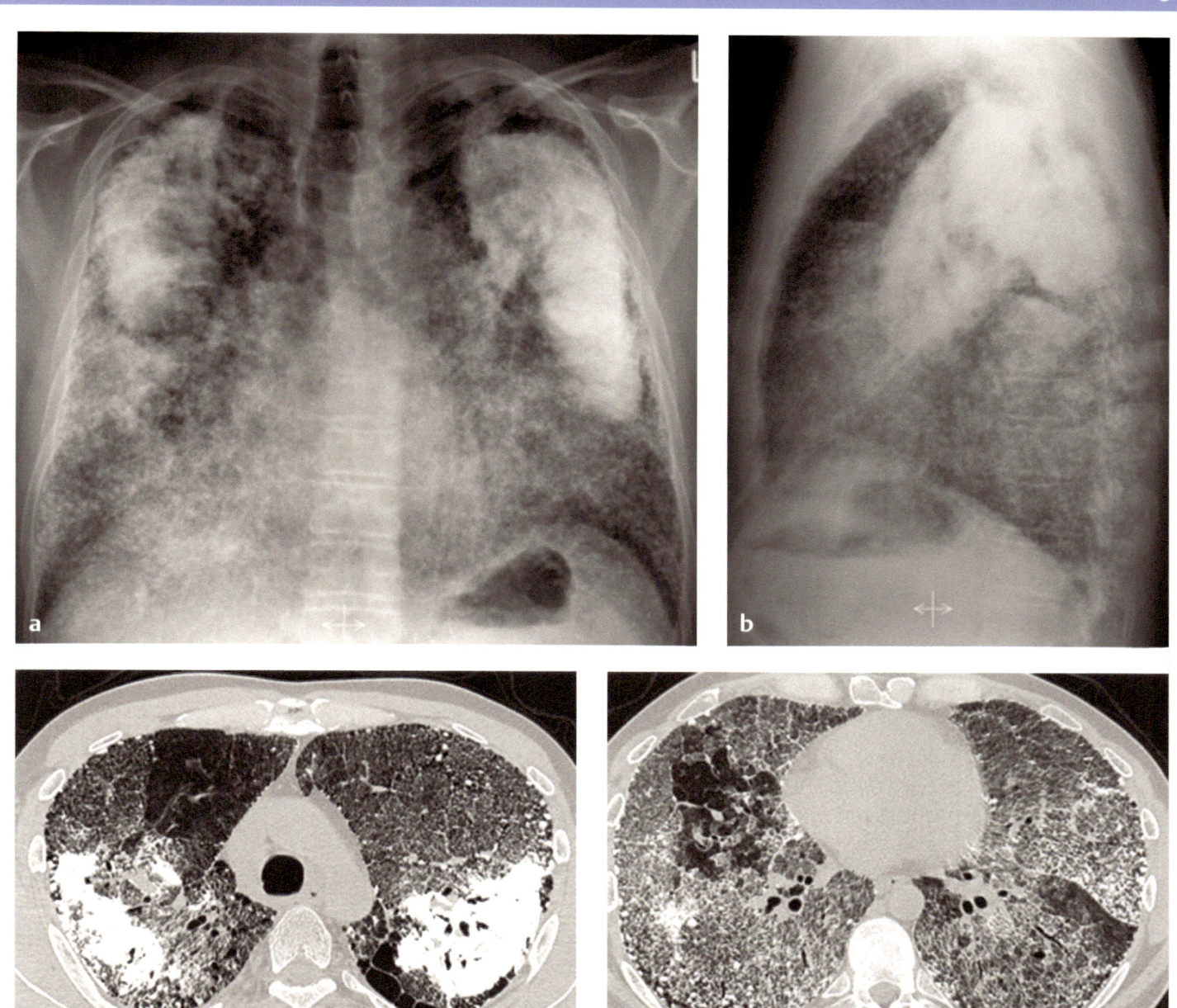

Fig. 4.76 Alveolar microlithiasis. (a) Chest radiograph shows a "sandstorm lung." (b) Confluent opacities in the lateral view. (c) Confluent calcifications on CT. (d) Alveolar calcifications on CT.

develop dyspnea or, in more severe cases, respiratory insufficiency and right heart failure.

▶ **Differential diagnosis.** Differentiation is required from silicosis and sarcoidosis.

▶ **Key points.** Alveolar microlithiasis is a rare congenital disease in which calcium phosphate is deposited in the alveoli. The chest radiograph shows a characteristic dense lung accompanied by few or no symptoms.

4.3.13 Alveolar Proteinosis

▶ **Brief definition.** Alveolar proteinosis is characterized by an accumulation of viscous surfactant with a high protein and lipid content in the alveoli due to an imbalance between production and clearance by alveolar macrophages. A very rare congenital form is known and is characterized by a genetic defect in macrophage colony-stimulating factor and surfactant-transporting proteins. The congenital form is a new mutation that is fatal in infancy. Almost 90% of all adult cases are an acquired autoimmune disease. Alveolar proteinosis can also be caused by dust inhalation, hematologic malignancy, and pulmonary infection. In these cases the condition is called secondary alveolar proteinosis. There is no causal treatment, but the proteinaceous material can be washed out of the alveoli by lavage. Many patients remain asymptomatic for many years after a single pulmonary lavage and require no further treatment. Superinfection is a critical problem that occurs in approximately 13% of patients.

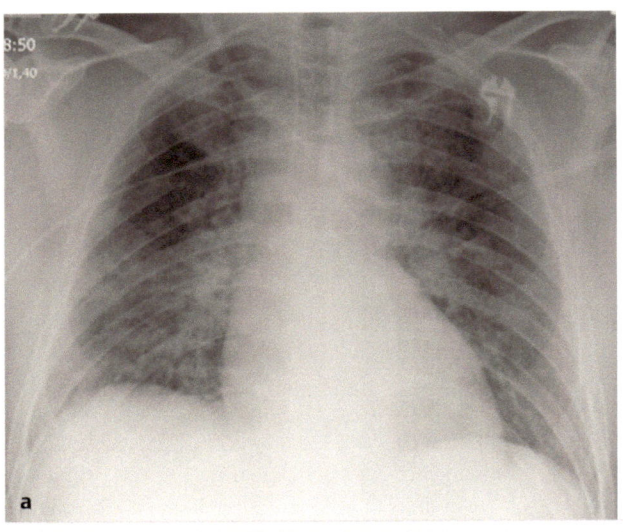

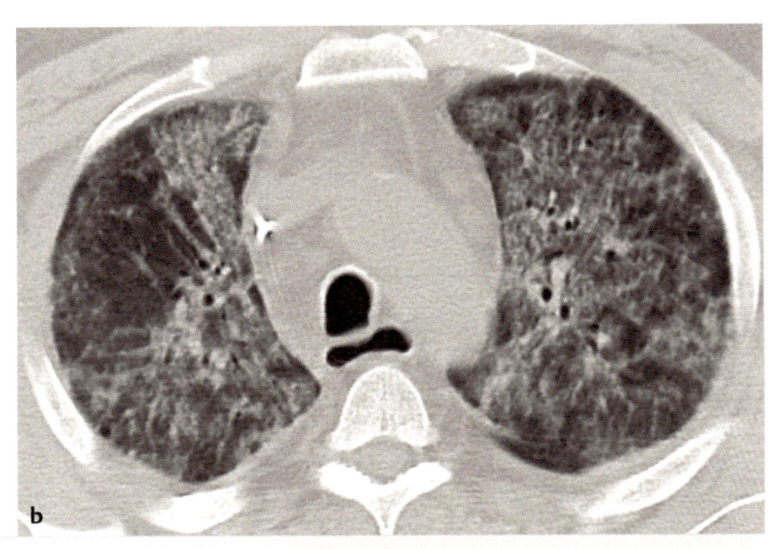

Fig. 4.77 Alveolar proteinosis. (a) Increased reticular markings and hyperlucency. **(b)** The most striking CT features are ground-glass opacities and thickened alveolar septa.

▶ **Imaging signs.** The chest radiograph shows a predominantly central, geographic reticular pattern with ground-glass opacities (▶ Fig. 4.77). Only portions of the lung are affected, and normal-appearing areas alternate with affected areas. The mediastinal lymph nodes may be slightly enlarged.

Caution

Imaging findings in alveolar proteinosis are often more severe than the clinical presentation would suggest.

▶ **Clinical features.** The dominant signs and symptoms are dyspnea and increased alveolar obstruction accompanied by fatigue and reduced exercise tolerance. Approximately one-third of patients are asymptomatic.

▶ **Differential diagnosis.** The imaging features of alveolar proteinosis may require differentiation from alveolar hemorrhage, infection with *Pneumocystis jiroveci*, and pulmonary edema.

▶ **Key points.** Alveolar proteinosis is characterized by the alveolar accumulation of lipoproteinaceous surfactant and is based in an imbalance between production and clearance. Typical CT findings are ground-glass opacities and thickened interlobular septa. The changes show a predominantly central distribution. Affected lung areas alternate with unaffected areas.

4.3.14 Pulmonary Infarction

▶ **Brief definition.** A pulmonary infarct consists of blood-saturated lung tissue that has undergone ischemic infarction. Because the lung has a dual blood supply from the pulmonary and bronchial arteries, pulmonary infarction is very rare. It occurs only if left heart function is so impaired that the pressure in the bronchial arteries is no longer high enough to adequately perfuse the peripheral lung vessels.

▶ **Imaging signs.** Infarctions generally occur in the peripheral lung and exhibit a rounded or wedge shape with the apex pointing toward the hilum. Pulmonary infarction most commonly occurs in the lower lobe. The chest radiograph shows a corresponding opacity, CT a density, often containing foci of liquefaction. There may also be cavitation (▶ Fig. 4.78).

▶ **Clinical features.** The cardinal symptom is chest pain due to associated pleurisy.

▶ **Differential diagnosis.** Lung infarction mainly requires differentiation from pulmonary infiltrates and cavitated lung cancer.

▶ **Key points.** Pulmonary infarction may result from pulmonary embolism with coexisting heart failure and appears as a peripheral opacity or density due to hemorrhage in the infarcted area.

4.3.15 Respiratory Distress Syndrome

Adult Respiratory Distress Syndrome

▶ **Brief definition.** Known also as "shock lung" and "acute lung failure," adult respiratory distress syndrome (ARDS) may be caused by a direct insult to the lung such as contusion, aspiration, or inhalation trauma but is most commonly caused by indirect injury due to sepsis, multiple trauma, burns, head trauma, and so on. The syndrome is diagnosed clinically on the basis of the definition of the American–European Consensus Conference (AECC), which was formulated in 1994,[18] was later refined by a panel of experts, and has since been supported by empirical studies.[19]

Note

Diagnostic criteria for ARDS:
- Hypoxia requiring mechanical ventilation, with a PaO_2/FiO_2 (arterial oxygen partial pressure/fraction of oxygen in the inspired air) less than 200.
- Pulmonary capillary wedge pressure less than 18 mmHg.
- Bilateral pulmonary infiltrates on the chest radiograph.

According to the revised definition, three grades of severity are recognized for ARDS,[19] each of which has prognostic implications:
- *Severe*: PaO_2/FiO_2 = 100 or less, with a positive end-expiratory pressure (PEEP) of at least 5 cm H_2O.
- *Moderate*: PaO_2/FiO_2 = 101–200 with a PEEP of at least 5 cm H_2O.
- *Mild*: PaO_2/FiO_2 = 201–300 with a PEEP of at least 5 cm H_2O.

The mortality rate is 45% for severe ARDS, 32% for moderate ARDS, and 27% for mild ARDS. All categories have the same pathogenic mechanism.

▶ **Imaging signs.** ARDS has three stages:
- *Exudative stage* is characterized by increased capillary permeability during the first 24 hours, with the development of interstitial edema followed by alveolar edema. The chest radiograph is still normal when interstitial edema is present, but the patient is strongly symptomatic. This discrepancy is an important aid to differential diagnosis and is not seen in patients with cardiogenic edema. By the end of the exudative stage, CT shows ground-glass opacities and thickening of the interlobar septa.
- *Intermediate stage* lasts from approximately days 2 to 7, characterized by the destruction of type I and type II pneumocytes. The histological picture is described as "diffuse alveolar injury." A protein-rich alveolar exudate forms, and hyaline membranes are formed from a mixture of cellular debris, exudate, and infiltrating inflammatory cells. The chest radiograph shows bilateral opacities that become denser over time and obscure the borders of the heart and diaphragm, creating a "white lung" appearance (▶ Fig. 4.79). This is associated with a positive air bronchogram. In subsequent days these densities partially regress, and ventilation therapy leads to areas of increased lucency. Later the lung acquires a reticular pattern, but the changes are still reversible. CT shows a typical density gradient with consolidation predominantly in dependent lung areas, ground-glass opacities in the middle zone, and normal density

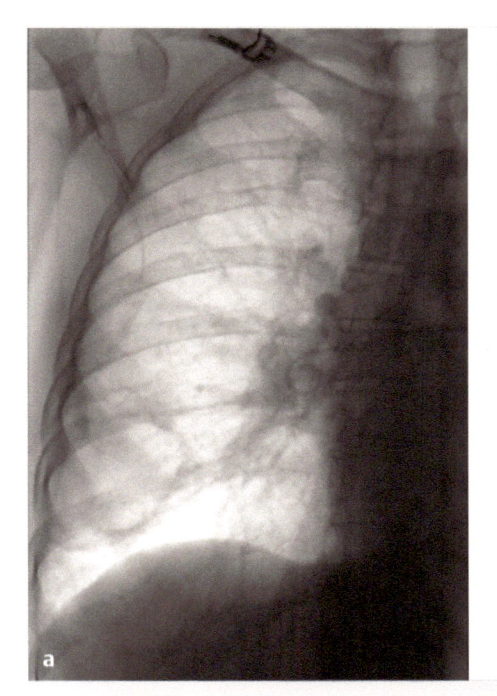

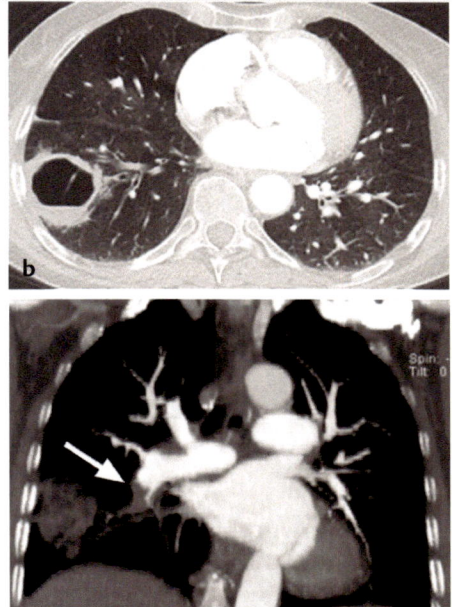

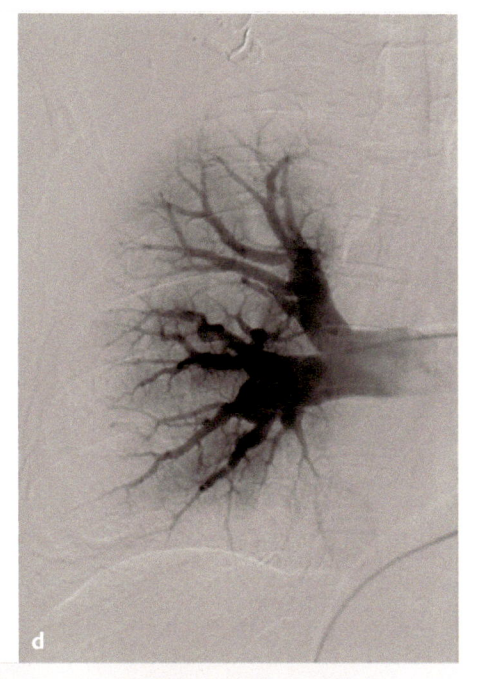

Fig. 4.78 Pulmonary infarction. (a) Chest radiograph shows a peripheral cavity. (b) CT defines the thin cavity walls. (c) Maximum intensity projection demonstrates a thrombus in the lower lobe artery (arrow). (d) Pulmonary angiogram shows vascular changes typical of chronic thromboembolic pulmonary hypertension, with bandlike stenoses and vascular cutoffs.

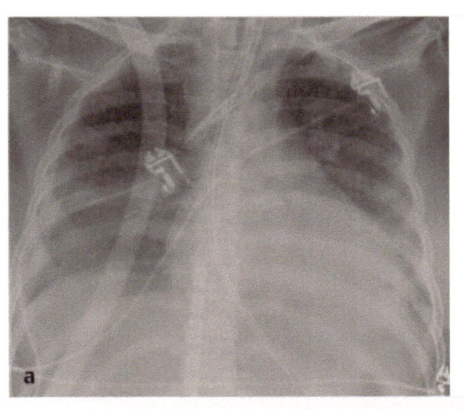

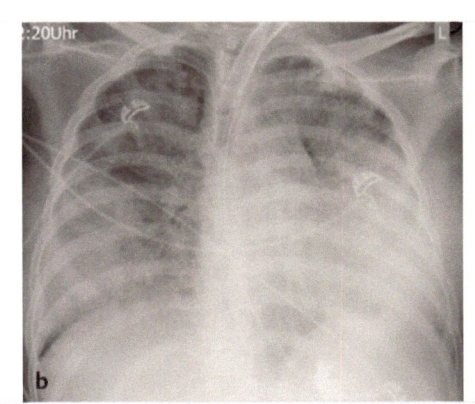

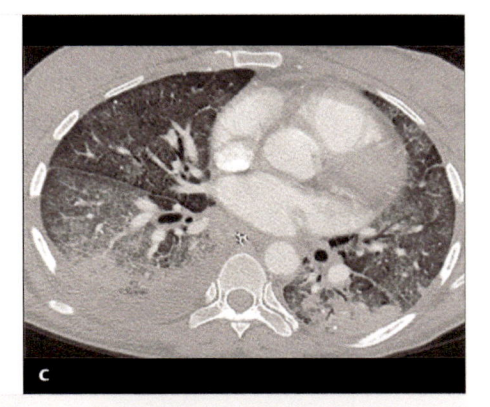

Fig. 4.79 ARDS. Rapid development of a white lung (from [a] to [b]) and (c) typical gradient. (a) Chest radiograph at time 1. (b) Chest radiograph at time 2. (c) CT.

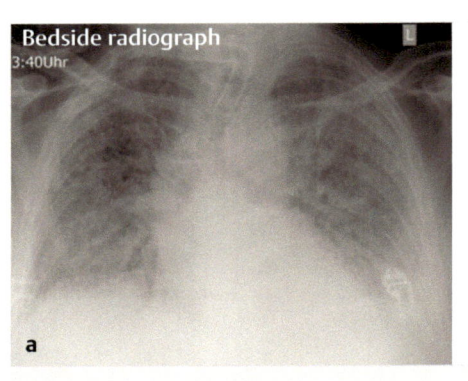

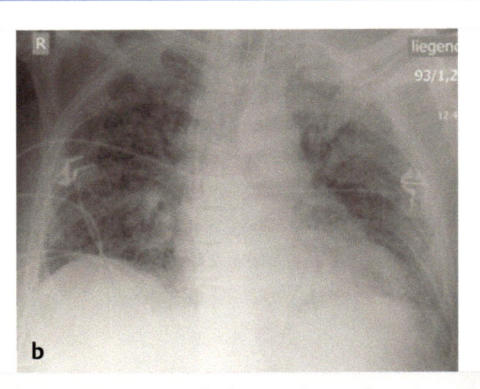

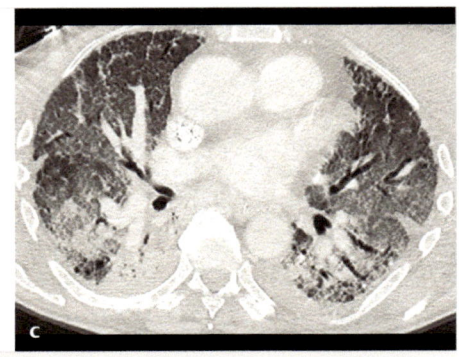

Fig. 4.80 ARDS. Typical increase of reticular markings in stage III. (a) Chest radiograph at time 1. (b) Chest radiograph at time 2. (c) CT.

in the upper zone. These changes are position-dependent. The areas with ground-glass opacities are considered recruitable for PEEP ventilation. The density gradient on CT scans is typical of ARDS due to extrapulmonary causes and does not occur in ARDS caused by direct lung injury.
- *Proliferative stage* occurs from 1 week to 1 month after onset, characterized by the proliferation of fibroblasts and myofibroblasts in the alveolar space and interstitium. The chest radiograph shows increased reticular markings (▶ Fig. 4.80). The condition may resolve with pulmonary fibrosis. The fibrosis is usually accentuated in the anterior portions of the lung, a fact that is attributed to barotrauma during ventilation. CT shows features of pulmonary fibrosis with thickening of the interlobar septa and traction bronchiectasis.

> **Caution**
>
> The classic stages of ARDS are no longer manifested in every patient owing to significant improvements in the intensive care of ARDS patients.

▶ **Clinical features.** ARDS occurs during the first week after the injury and leads to hypoxia requiring mechanical ventilation.

▶ **Differential diagnosis.** Differentiation is mainly required from cardiogenic edema, in which the heart is enlarged, the vessels are dilated, and there is pleural effusion.

▶ **Key points.** ARDS is an acute lung injury that has three stages in its acute form. The diagnosis is based on correlation of clinical and radiographic findings. The disease may resolve with pulmonary fibrosis as an end stage.

Infant Respiratory Distress Syndrome

▶ **Brief definition.** Premature infants younger than 33 weeks' gestation with a birthweight less than 2500 g are at high risk for infant respiratory distress syndrome (IRDS) due to a relative surfactant deficiency. IRDS, also called hyaline membrane disease, is present in 60% of infants born before 29 weeks. Surfactant is a surface-active agent that consists of 90% lipids and 10% proteins and is rich in calcium ions. The lung begins to form surfactant in about the 24th week of gestation, but this process is not complete until about the 36th week. In IRDS, incomplete expansion of the

Table 4.9 Stages of IRDS

Stage	Radiographic signs
I	Fine granular opacities
II	Positive air bronchograms extending over the cardiac border
III	Increasing opacity with blurring of the diaphragm and cardiac silhouette
IV	White lung; the heart is completely obscured

alveoli leads to microatelectasis. IRDS is classified into four radiographic stages (▶ Table 4.9). Infants with milder disease are treated with a nasal mask and CPAP ventilation. Infants with more severe IRDS are intubated and surfactant is administered through the endotracheal tube. In premature infants younger than 27 weeks' gestation, surfactant is administered prophylactically through an endotracheal tube placed for that purpose. Potential complications of ventilation are pneumothorax and interstitial pulmonary emphysema.

> **Caution**
>
> Ventilation may be complicated by the development of interstitial pulmonary emphysema. This condition is characterized by rounded lucencies a few millimeters in diameter, which should not be misinterpreted as improvement of IRDS. It is the precursor of a pneumothorax.

▶ **Imaging signs.** Both lungs show decreased lucency and volume due to alveolar atelectasis. Micronodular densities are also present (▶ Fig. 4.81).

▶ **Clinical features.** IRDS usually presents immediately after birth. Respiratory distress is manifested by nasal flaring and indrawing of the sternum and intercostal spaces. Breath sounds are diminished, and the infant may be cyanotic.

▶ **Differential diagnosis.** Congenital pneumonia is the main condition requiring differentiation from IRDS. But up to 60% of newborns with pneumonia have pleural effusion, which is absent in IRDS. Treatment with surfactant may give rise to an inhomogeneous pattern with well-ventilated areas, and this may prompt a misdiagnosis of meconium aspiration.

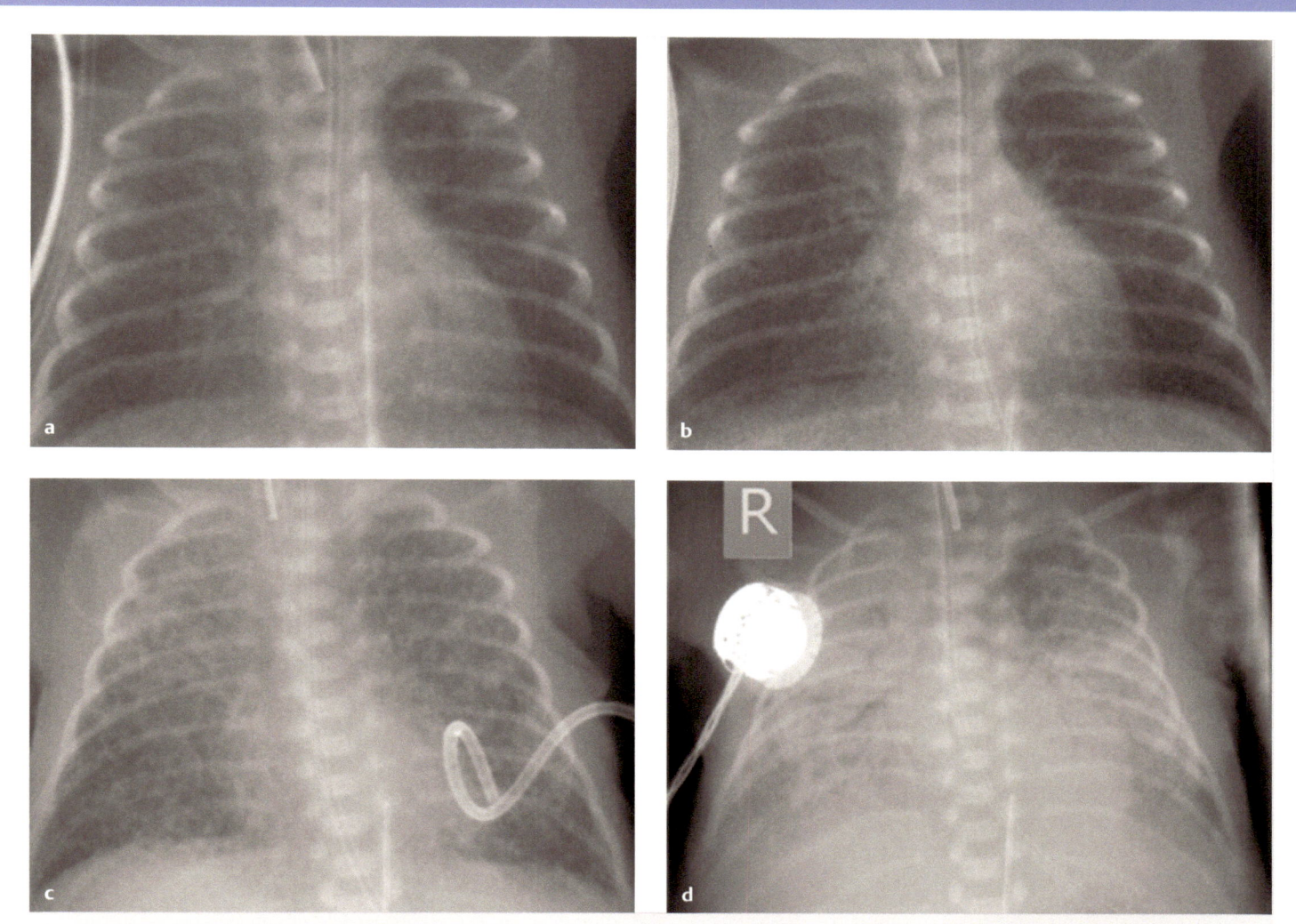

Fig. 4.81 Respiratory distress syndrome (stages II–IV) in a premature infant born at 23 weeks' gestation. (a) Plain chest radiograph on the first day of life. (b) Radiograph on day 7 shows increased fine nodular opacity in the lungs. (c) Development of interstitial emphysema. (d) Progression to stage IV disease.

▶ **Key points.** IRDS results from a surfactant deficiency in the immature lungs of premature infants. Four radiographic stages are distinguished, based on degree of severity. Interstitial pulmonary emphysema and pneumothorax are possible complications.

4.4 Pleura

4.4.1 Pneumothorax

▶ **Brief definition.** Pneumothorax is defined as the presence of air between the two pleural layers. It may result from trauma or may be iatrogenic due to lung biopsy or the placement of a central venous catheter. Spontaneous pneumothorax is caused by the rupture of a subpleural bulla. This often occurs in thin adolescent males. The elastic fibers in the lung cause the lung to retract. A tension pneumothorax develops when air enters the pleural space on inspiration but cannot escape on expiration due to a check-valve mechanism. The mediastinum is shifted toward the unaffected side, with associated compression of the superior and inferior vena cava. A tension pneumothorax quickly becomes life-threatening due to impaired venous return to the heart via the superior and inferior vena cava.

▶ **Imaging signs.** The chest radiograph in full expiration demonstrates a pneumothorax with higher sensitivity than a radiograph at full inspiration. In most cases the pleura is visible as a fine line due to the edge-on effect (▶ Fig. 4.82). No vascular markings are seen peripheral to the pleural line. With a tension pneumothorax, the mediastinum is shifted toward the healthy side and the hemidiaphragm on the affected side is flattened and depressed (▶ Fig. 4.83). The intercostal spaces are widened on the affected side. The costophrenic angle may be deepened with an extensive pneumothorax. The pleural air collects anteriorly in the supine patient; the pleura may even be apposed laterally to the chest wall, causing the pneumothorax to appear as a round or oval area of increased lucency ("black oval"). Usually the diaphragm is sharply outlined.

▶ **Clinical features.** Pneumothorax is usually associated with chest pain. With a tension pneumothorax, the dominant symptoms are those of shock (cold sweats, pallor, weakness) due to a decrease in cardiac stroke volume. The immediate placement of a chest tube (Heimlich valve with the advantage of small size) is life-saving.

▶ **Key points.** A pneumothorax may result from trauma or iatrogenic pleural injury, or it may be spontaneous. The chest radiograph at full expiration is very sensitive in the detection of

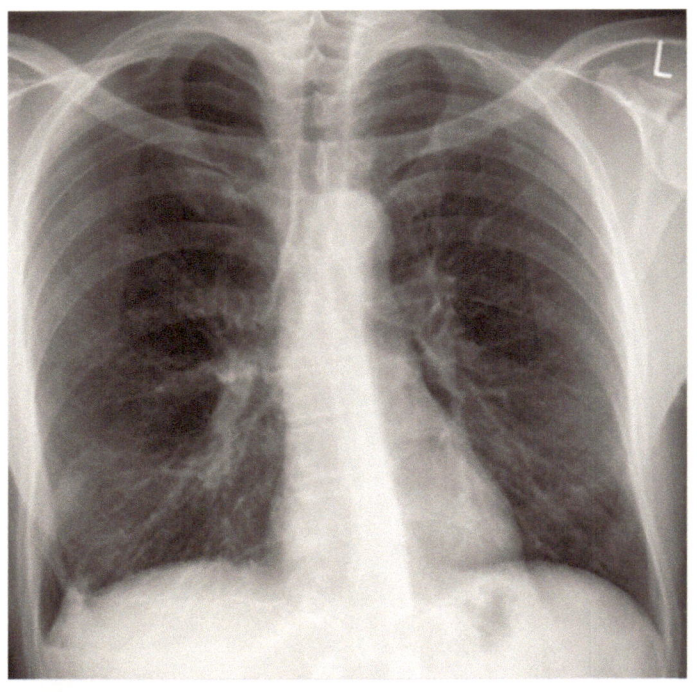

Fig. 4.82 Pneumothorax. The pleura appears as a fine line in the apical region because it is tangential to the X-ray beam. Vascular markings are not visible in peripheral lung areas.

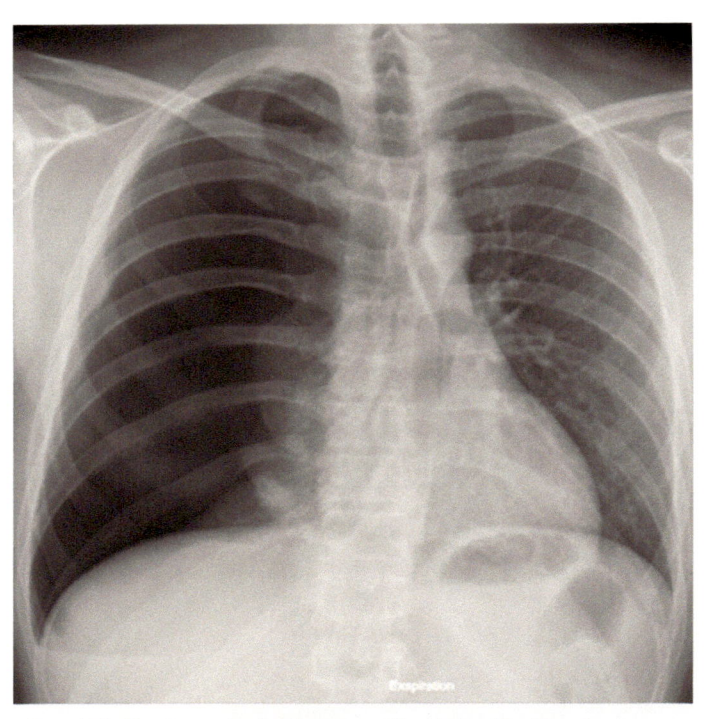

Fig. 4.83 Tension pneumothorax on the right side. The chest radiograph shows almost complete atelectasis of the right lung. The mediastinum is shifted to the left. The intercostal spaces are widened on the right side.

pneumothorax. The pleura may appear as a fine line where it is tangential to the X-ray beam. Absence of peripheral vascular markings is another important sign. In the supine radiograph, an anterior pneumothorax may appear as an area of increased lucency.

4.4.2 Pleural Effusion

▶ **Brief definition.** Pleural effusion, defined as a fluid collection between the pleural layers, can have many causes. A *transudate* may result from reduced oncotic pressure in the serum due to a protein deficiency (e.g., in hepatic cirrhosis) or protein loss (e.g., in nephrotic syndrome or renal failure) or from increased hydrostatic pressure in the vessels due to heart failure or pulmonary embolism. An *exudate*, which is more cellular and contains more protein, results from altered capillary permeability due, for example, to inflammation or a tumor.

▶ **Clinical features.** The dominant symptoms are those of the underlying disease. Large effusions cause dyspnea due to compression atelectasis.

▶ **Imaging signs.** A free pleural effusion of 150 mL or more is detectable on the upright lateral chest radiograph as blunting of the costophrenic angle (see ▶ Fig. 4.18). Effusions trapped in the interlobar fissure typically appears in the lateral radiograph as lentiform opacities (▶ Fig. 4.84). A free pleural effusion of approximately 500 mL or more appears in the supine radiograph as opacity that decreases along a caudocranial gradient. On axial CT, free pleural effusion appears as a posterior collection that typically causes compression atelectasis of adjacent lung areas.

▶ **Differential diagnosis.** Pleural empyema is an important differential diagnosis that can be recognized clinically by fever and laboratory changes and on CT by pleural thickening and possible gas inclusions.

▶ **Key points.** Pleural effusions of 150 mL or more are detectable on upright chest radiographs, and effusions of 500 mL or more on supine radiographs.

4.4.3 Pleural Empyema

▶ **Brief definition.** Pleural empyema is a bacterial inflammation characterized by pus formation between the pleural layers. A pleurocutaneous fistula may develop in tuberculosis or fungal infections.

▶ **Imaging signs.** The pleura is thickened and enhancing (▶ Fig. 4.85). CT cannot differentiate pus from serous fluid. Air inclusions indicate gas-forming bacteria, unless air has previously entered the chest during needle aspiration of the pleural empyema.

▶ **Clinical features.** Bacterial empyema presents clinically with fever and chills. Tuberculosis may be associated with B symptoms.

▶ **Differential diagnosis.** The differential diagnosis includes a free or loculated pleural effusion.

4.4.4 Pleural Mesothelioma

▶ **Brief definition.** Pleural mesothelioma is a malignant mass of the pleura. Exposure to asbestos is a risk factor, and 77% of all mesothelioma patients have a prior history of asbestos exposure. The latent period is long—25 to 40 years—so the peak age of incidence is from 40 to 60 years of age. Asbestos-exposed individuals have an 8% risk of developing mesothelioma. The prognosis is

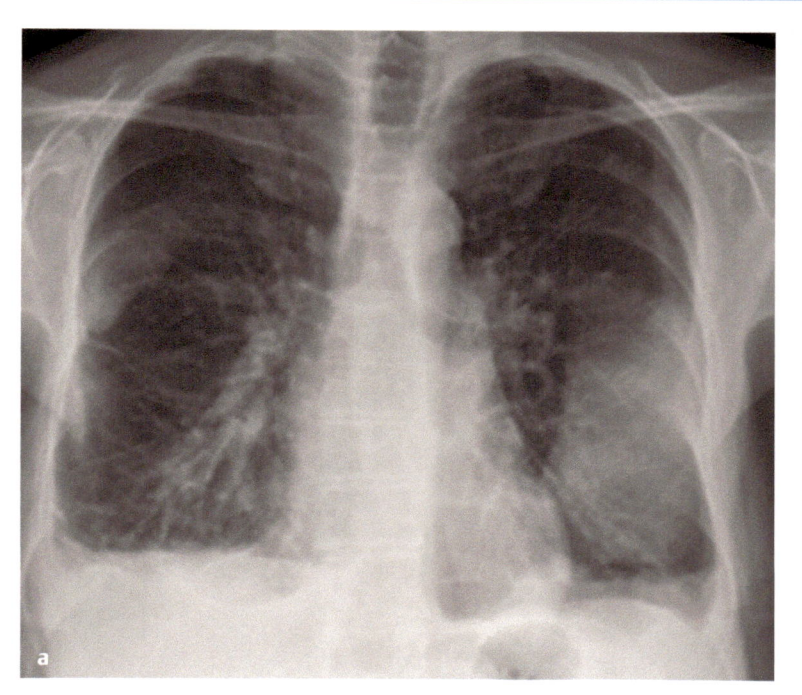

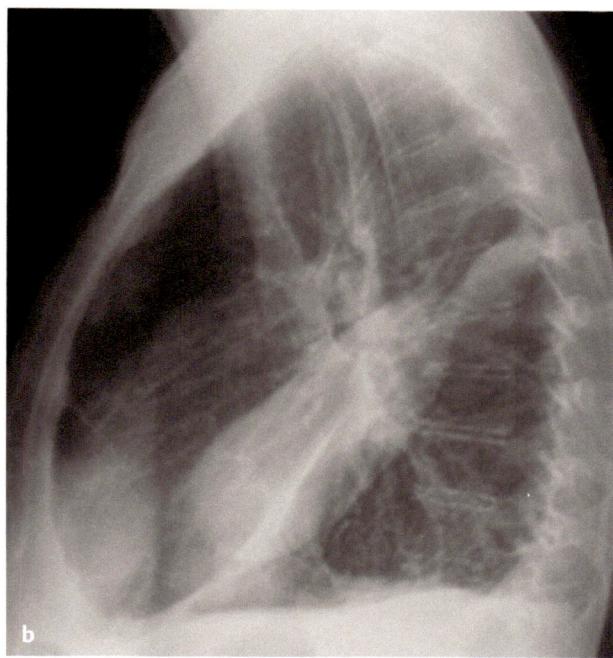

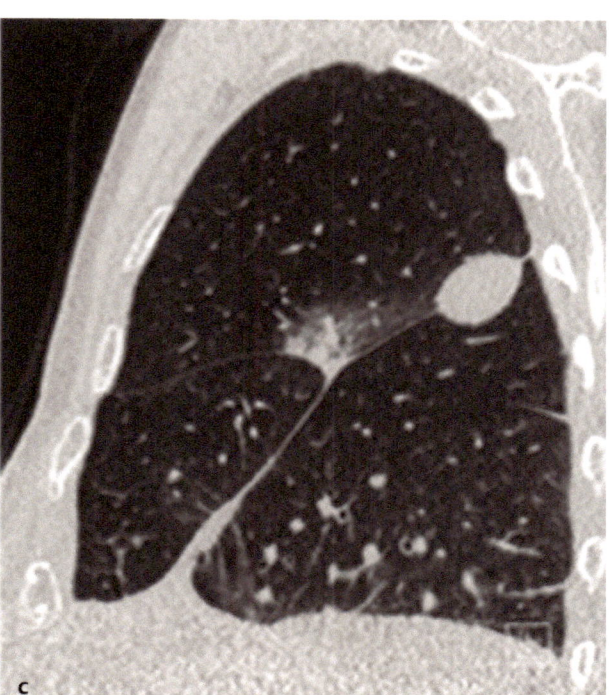

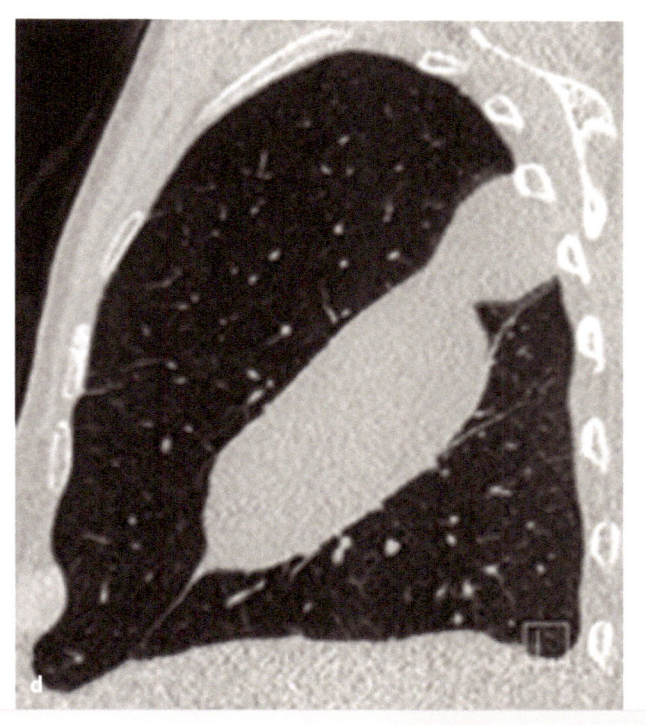

Fig. 4.84 Pleural effusion. (a) Chest radiograph shows effusion trapped in the interlobar fissures on both sides. (b) Lateral radiograph shows a typical ellipsoid appearance. (c) Sagittal reformatted CT image demonstrates the effusion trapped in the interlobar fissures on both sides. (d) Sagittal reformatted image in a different plane.

very guarded, with a 1-year-survival rate of 25%, because mesotheliomas respond poorly to chemotherapy and distant metastases in the pleura often reduce the efficacy of pleural resection.

▶ **Imaging signs.** The chest radiograph shows pleural thickening. With larger lesions, the affected side is reduced in volume. CT shows nodular thickening of the pleura (▶ Fig. 4.86). Mesotheliomas enhance after IV injection of contrast medium. Pleural mesotheliomas may be accompanied by extensive pleural effusion.

▶ **Clinical features.** The dominant features are dyspnea, night sweats, weight loss, and fatigue.

▶ **Differential diagnosis.** Fibrous pleural thickening after asbestos exposure is an important differential diagnosis. Generally, however, these lesions are no more than 1 cm thick. Extension to the mediastinal pleura is also suggestive of mesothelioma. If there is doubt, CT-guided biopsy should be undertaken.

▶ **Key points.** Mesothelioma occurs in 8% of all individuals with long-term asbestos exposure, forming tumors that line the chest cavity like a carpet. Imaging shows nodular thickening of the pleura, which may spread to the mediastinal pleura in the late stage, causing extensive pleural effusion.

Lung and Pleura

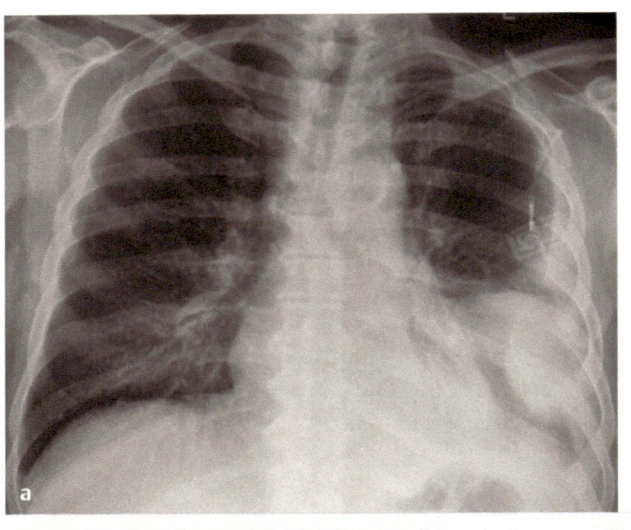

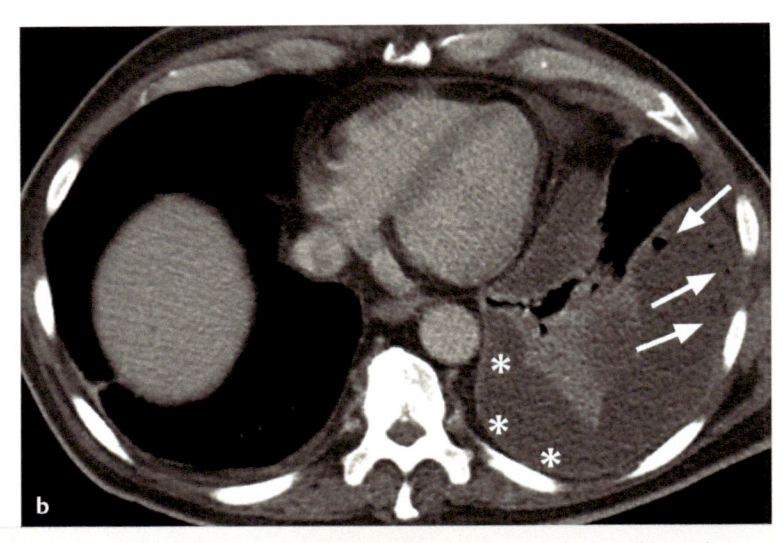

Fig. 4.85 **Pleural empyema.** (a) Chest radiograph shows an effusion that can be differentiated from pleural empyema only by CT. (b) CT shows thickened, enhancing pleura in the affected area (asterisks) and air inclusions in the fluid (arrows).

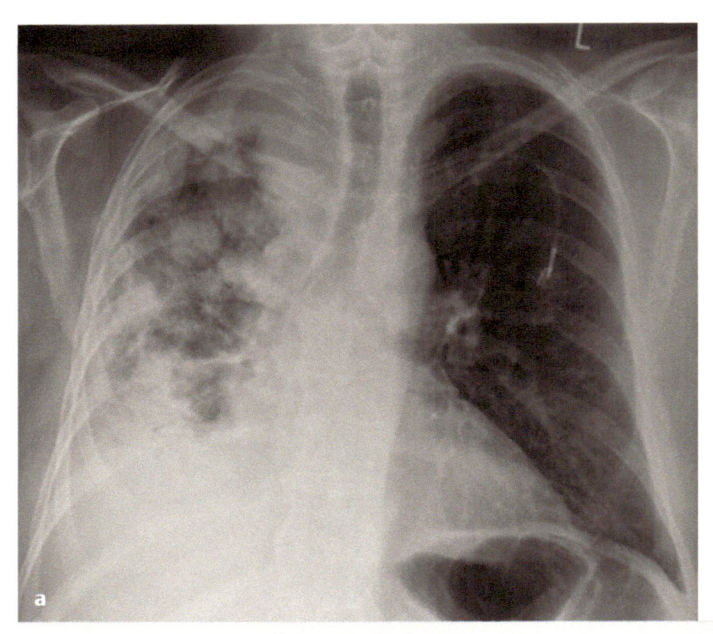

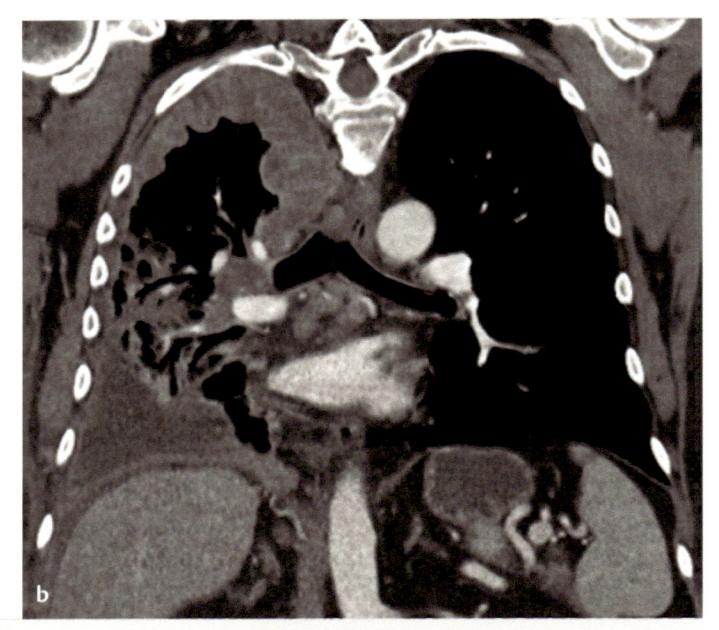

Fig. 4.86 **Pleural mesothelioma.** (a) Chest radiograph shows pleural thickening that extends around the lung. (b) Coronal reformatted CT image shows nodular pleural thickening and a malignant pleural effusion.

Bibliography

[1] Webb WR. Thin-section CT of the secondary pulmonary lobule: anatomy and the image—the 2004 Fleischner lecture. Radiology. 2006; 239(2):322–338

[2] Travis WD, Brambilla E, Noguchi M, et al. International Association for the Study of Lung Cancer/American Thoracic Society/European Respiratory Society International Multidisciplinary Classification of Lung Adenocarcinoma. J Thorac Oncol. 2011; 6:244–285

[3] Barbier F, Andremont A, Wolff M, Bouadma L. Hospital-acquired pneumonia and ventilator-associated pneumonia: recent advances in epidemiology and management. Curr Opin Pulm Med. 2013; 19(3):216–228

[4] Hansell DM, Bankier AA, MacMahon H, McLoud TC, Müller NL, Remy J. Fleischner Society: glossary of terms for thoracic imaging. Radiology. 2008; 246(3):697–722

[5] MacMahon H, Austin JH, Gamsu G, et al. Fleischner Society. Guidelines for management of small pulmonary nodules detected on CT scans: a statement from the Fleischner Society. Radiology. 2005; 237(2):395–400

[6] Naidich DP, Bankier AA, MacMahon H, et al. Recommendations for the management of subsolid pulmonary nodules detected at CT: a statement from the Fleischner Society. Radiology. 2013; 266(1):304–317

[7] Henschke CI, Yankelevitz DF, Mirtcheva R, McGuinness G, McCauley D, Miettinen OS, ELCAP Group. CT screening for lung cancer: frequency and significance of part-solid and nonsolid nodules. AJR Am J Roentgenol. 2002; 178(5):1053–1057

[8] Aberle DR, Adams AM, Berg CD, et al. National Lung Screening Trial Research Team. Reduced lung-cancer mortality with low-dose computed tomographic screening. N Engl J Med. 2011; 365(5):395–409

[9] Jones KD. Whence lepidic?: the history of a Canadian neologism. Arch Pathol Lab Med. 2013; 137(12):1822–1824

[10] Rami-Porta R, Crowley JJ, Goldstraw P. The revised TNM staging system for lung cancer. Ann Thorac Cardiovasc Surg. 2009; 15(1):4–9

[11] American Thoracic Society, European Respiratory Society. American Thoracic Society/European Respiratory Society international multidisciplinary consensus Classification of the Idiopathic Interstitial Pneumonias. This joint

statement of the American Thoracic Society (ATS) and the European Respiratory Society (ERS) was adopted by the ATS board of directors, June 2001, and by the ERS Executive Committee, June 2001. Am J Respir Crit Care Med. 2002; 165(2):277–304
[12] Travis WD, Costabel U, Hansell DM, et al. ATS/ERS Committee on Idiopathic Interstitial Pneumonias. An official American Thoracic Society/European Respiratory Society statement: Update of the international multidisciplinary classification of the idiopathic interstitial pneumonias. Am J Respir Crit Care Med. 2013; 188(6):733–748
[13] Raghu G, Collard HR, Egan JJ, et al. ATS/ERS/JRS/ALAT Committee on Idiopathic Pulmonary Fibrosis. An official ATS/ERS/JRS/ALAT statement: idiopathic pulmonary fibrosis: evidence-based guidelines for diagnosis and management. Am J Respir Crit Care Med. 2011; 183(6):788–824
[14] Travis WD, Hunninghake G, King TE, Jr, et al. Idiopathic nonspecific interstitial pneumonia: report of an American Thoracic Society project. Am J Respir Crit Care Med. 2008; 177(12):1338–1347
[15] Scadding JG. Prognosis of intrathoracic sarcoidosis in England. A review of 136 cases after five years' observation. BMJ. 1961; 2(5261):1165–1172
[16] Schünke M, Schulte E, Schumacher U. Prometheus. LernAtlas der Anatomie: Innere Organe. 2nd ed. Stuttgart: Thieme; 2009. Illustrated by M. Voll/ K. Wesker
[17] Hirschmann JV, Pipavath SN, Godwin JD. Hypersensitivity pneumonitis: a historical, clinical, and radiologic review. Radiographics. 2009; 29(7):1921–1938
[18] Bernard GR, Artigas A, Brigham KL, et al. The American-European Consensus Conference on ARDS. Definitions, mechanisms, relevant outcomes, and clinical trial coordination. Am J Respir Crit Care Med. 1994; 149(3 Pt 1):818–824
[19] Ranieri VM, Rubenfeld GD, Thompson BT, et al. ARDS Definition Task Force. Acute respiratory distress syndrome: the Berlin Definition. JAMA. 2012; 307 (23):2526–2533
[20] Amorosa JK, Bramwit MP, Mohammed TL, et al. ACR appropriateness criteria routine chest radiographs in intensive care unit patients. J Am Coll Radiol. 2013; 10(3):170–174
[21] Lange S. Radiologische Diagnostik der Thoraxerkrankungen. 2nd ed. Stuttgart: Thieme; 2005:18
[22] Siltzbach LE. Sarcoidosis: clinical features and management. Med Clin North Am. 1967; 51(2):483–502

Part 2
Abdomen

5	Liver	*182*
6	Gallbladder and Biliary Tract	*242*
7	Pancreas	*295*
8	Gastrointestinal Tract	*322*
9	Spleen and Lymphatic System	*355*
10	Adrenal Glands	*374*
11	Kidney and Urinary Tract	*393*
12	Female Pelvis	*430*
13	Male Pelvis	*467*

5 Liver

Guenther Schneider and Gabriele A. Krombach

5.1 Anatomy

Local surgical and radiological procedures such as tumor ablation, transarterial chemoembolization (TACE), and selective internal radiotherapy (SIRT) require the highly sensitive detection of all existing lesions and their localization to a specific hepatic segment.

The liver is intraperitoneal in its location and is firmly attached to the diaphragm in the bare area on its superior surface. The liver is divided into nine segments.[1,2,3] Each of the hepatic segments can be resected individually or in association with other segments. The liver is subdivided by the hepatic veins and portal vein, which run along the segmental boundaries: The main branches of the portal vein divide the liver into upper and lower segments (including segments IVa and IVb), while the hepatic veins define vertical planes of segmental division. The site of portal vein entry into the liver defines the "portal plane" for identifying the upper and lower segments (▶ Fig. 5.1, ▶ Fig. 5.2; see also ▶ Fig. 6.1c).

Venous drainage to the hepatic veins occurs between the hepatic segments and lobes, while branches of the hepatic artery, portal vein, and biliary ducts course together at the center of each segment.

5.2 Anatomical Variants

An anomalous location of the liver is found in patients with complete situs inversus or abdominal situs inversus. A more common congenital anomaly is the presence of accessory hepatic lobes. They are often found on the undersurface of the liver, such as an accessory Riedel's lobe, which is a small inferior projection of the hepatic right lobe.

Rare anatomical anomalies of the liver take the form of agenesis of the left lobe or hypoplasia of the right lobe. It is more common to find hypoplasia of individual segments, however. Segmental hypoplasia is sometimes found in association with diffuse liver diseases such as primary sclerosing cholangitis.

The liver typically derives its arterial supply from the celiac trunk, which divides into the splenic artery, common hepatic artery, and left gastric artery. The common hepatic artery past the origin of the gastroduodenal artery is called the "proper hepatic artery" (▶ Fig. 5.3). It gives rise to the cystic artery and the right and left hepatic arteries, but into the left and right hepatic arteries is found in only about 50% of the population; the remaining 50% show variants in this pattern. Common anatomical variants in the arterial supply of the liver involve the right hepatic artery arising from the superior mesenteric artery, or the left lobe of the liver receiving its supply from a side branch of the left hepatic artery. There are other variants in which the hepatic artery arises directly from the aorta, or the liver is supplied entirely by the superior mesenteric artery.

> **Note**
>
> The liver parenchyma receives approximately 75% of its blood supply from the portal venous system and 25% from the hepatic artery.

The dual vascular supply to the liver determines the imaging appearance of the liver after IV injection of contrast medium in all modalities.

5.3 Imaging

5.3.1 Landmarks

Segment I corresponds to the caudate lobe. The falciform ligament divides the left lobe of the liver into a lateral and medial segment. Segments II and III represent the lateral segments of the left lobe, the left portal vein branch separating segment II above from segment III below. The medial segment of the left lobe lies between the left and middle hepatic veins. Occasionally it forms a complete unit, segment IV, but it may also be subdivided into an upper part, designated as segment IVa, and a lower part, designated as segment IVb.

The right lobe of the liver is subdivided into anterior and posterior segments. The right hepatic vein serves as the anatomical landmark that separates the anterior and posterior segments. The right lobe is also subdivided into upper and lower segments, again defined by the portal plane. The anterior superior segment is segment VIII, and the posterior superior segment is segment VII. The lower segments are formed anteriorly by segment V and posteriorly by segment VI.

An easy way to distinguish the right and left lobes of the liver is to imagine a line running from the middle hepatic vein to the gallbladder fossa. Assuming normal liver anatomy, this line defines the boundary between the right and left lobes. It is useful for differentiating the lobes and for quickly assessing the distribution of hepatic lesions as involving just one lobe or both lobes.

The liver is attached to the abdominal wall by the falciform ligament, whose lower portion is called the round ligament of the liver. Embedded in the round ligament is the umbilical vein, which may reopen in response to portal hypertension and hepatic cirrhosis, providing a collateral pathway for blood drainage to subcutaneous veins. The dilated subcutaneous veins in this case are visible externally as the "caput medusae." The hepatogastric ligament extends broadly from the liver to the lesser curvature of the stomach and constitutes the lesser omentum. The hepatoduodenal ligament extends from the porta hepatis of the liver to the pancreas.

5.3.2 Imaging Techniques

Ultrasonography

Ultrasound is used throughout the world for screening and as the initial modality in the diagnostic algorithm for suspected liver disease because it is noninvasive, widely available, and economical. The liver is easily accessible to ultrasound scanning in almost all patients. The posterior and subdiaphragmatic segments may be difficult to scan, and this limitation reduces the sensitivity of ultrasound imaging in the liver.

Ultrasound contrast agents can be used for the more precise classification of hepatic lesions. They consist of tiny bubbles of a

5.3 Imaging

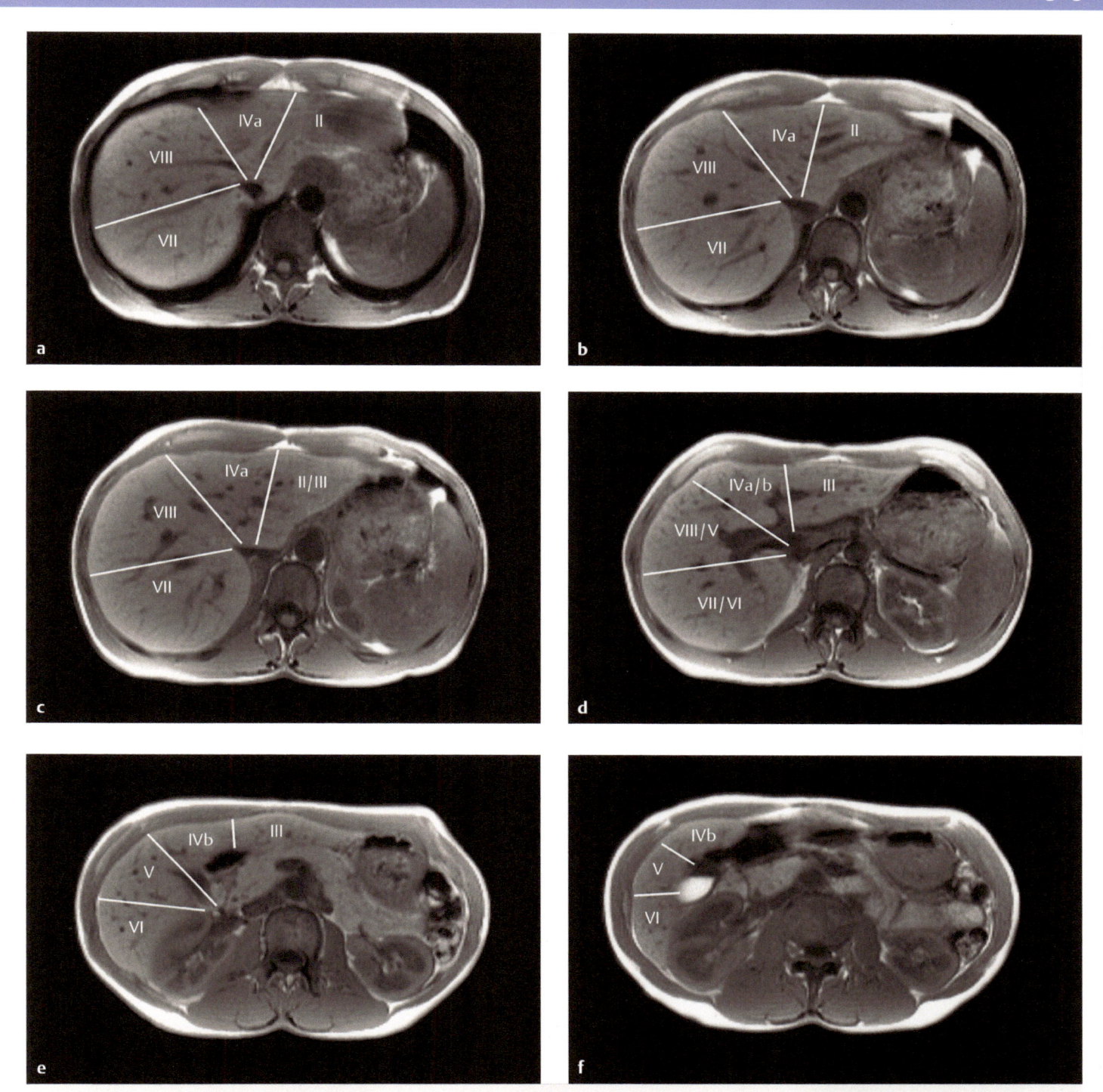

Fig. 5.1 Segmental anatomy of the liver after Couinaud and Bismuth. (a) Cranial image slice. (b) Axial slices at progressively lower level. Segmental boundaries are defined by the hepatic veins and portal vein branches. (c) Axial slices starting from the liver dome (a) and progressively more caudal levels. Segmental boundaries are defined by the hepatic veins and portal vein branches. (d) Axial slices at progressively higher levels. Segmental boundaries are defined by the hepatic veins and portal vein branches. (e) Axial slices at progressively higher levels. Segmental boundaries are defined by the hepatic veins and portal vein branches. (f) Axial slices at progressively higher levels. Segmental boundaries are defined by the hepatic veins and portal vein branches.

stable, water-insoluble gas. The microbubbles are contained within a delivery material and are 1 to 4 µm in diameter. They oscillate when impinged by an ultrasound pulse, which differentiates them from tissue. Hepatic malignancies are characterized by rapid wash-in and early washout of the contrast agent.

Computed Tomography

Computed tomography (CT) has the advantage of a short examination time and is the modality of choice for staging. Contrast-enhanced CT scanning of the liver employs a biphasic protocol with an arterial phase 25 seconds after injection of contrast medium and a portal venous phase 60 to 90 seconds after injection (▶ Fig. 5.4). When administration of contrast medium is adjusted for body weight (BW), the administered dose is 0.6 g iodine/kg BW. There is no need to add images without contrast, since calcifications are also visualized in the portal venous phase. Hypervascular and hypovascular lesions can be distinguished by this method (▶ Fig. 5.5). The number of additional lesions detectable on images without contrast is negligibly small. However,

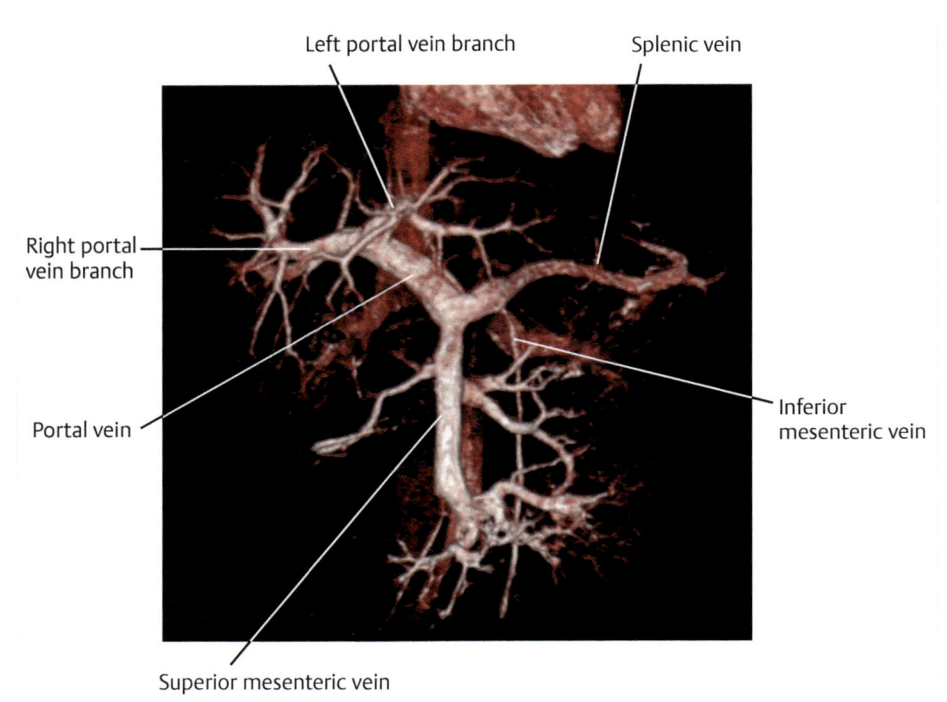

Fig. 5.2 Portal venous vessels. Maximum intensity projection of 3D MRA.

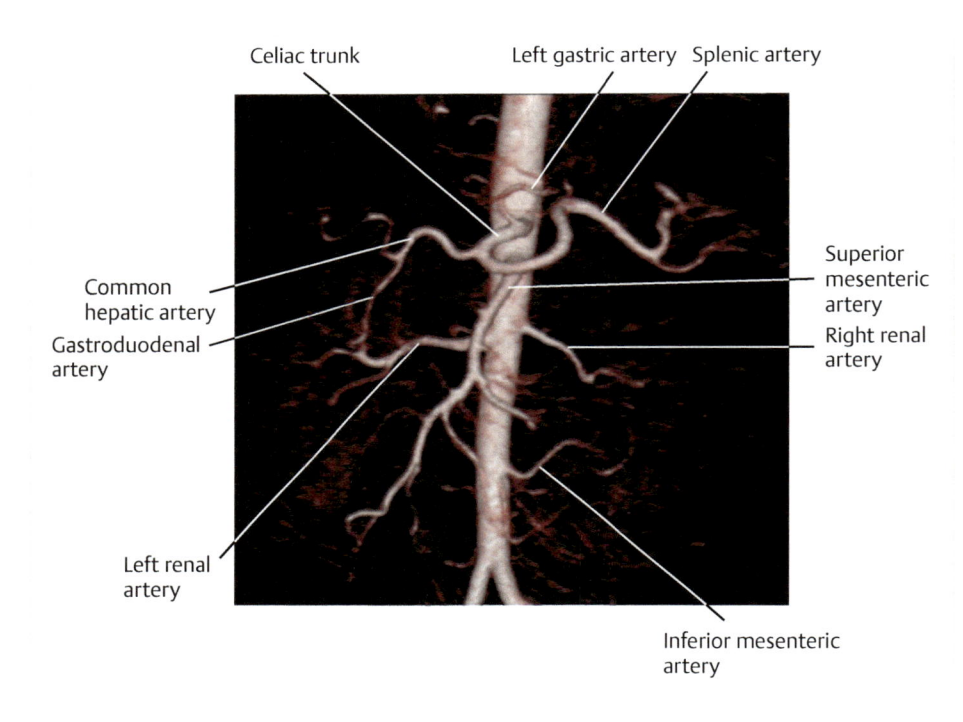

Fig. 5.3 Visceral arteries. Maximum intensity projection of 3D MRA.

unenhanced liver imaging still has a role in patients with a suspected acute hemorrhage.

If equivocal findings warrant further investigation or if an elective examination of the liver is required then MRI is used, but CT is still the first-line modality for acute disorders ranging from liver injuries and hemorrhage to sepsis with abscess formation.

Magnetic Resonance Imaging

When used electively, magnetic resonance imaging (MRI) permits a detailed analysis of hepatic lesions. MRI without contrast permits the detection of blood, fat, or an inhomogeneous cellular structure; or the upper abdomen can be investigated by dynamic contrast-enhanced MRI. This technique can differentiate between arterial hypervascular and hypovascular lesions and can identify lesions that show persistent delayed enhancement ▶ Fig. 5.4 and ▶ Fig. 5.5. Hepatobiliary contrast agents have provided a new tool for the characterization of hepatic lesions. This technique can supply information on the presence of functional hepatocytes within a lesion from 20 to 60 minutes after injection of the contrast agent (see Liver-Specific Contrast Agents). This cannot be done with CT.[4]

Contrast-enhanced MRA is also excellent for evaluating vascular anatomy. The arterial, venous, and portal venous anatomy of the liver can be visualized with this technique (▶ Fig. 5.4, ▶ Fig. 5.5).

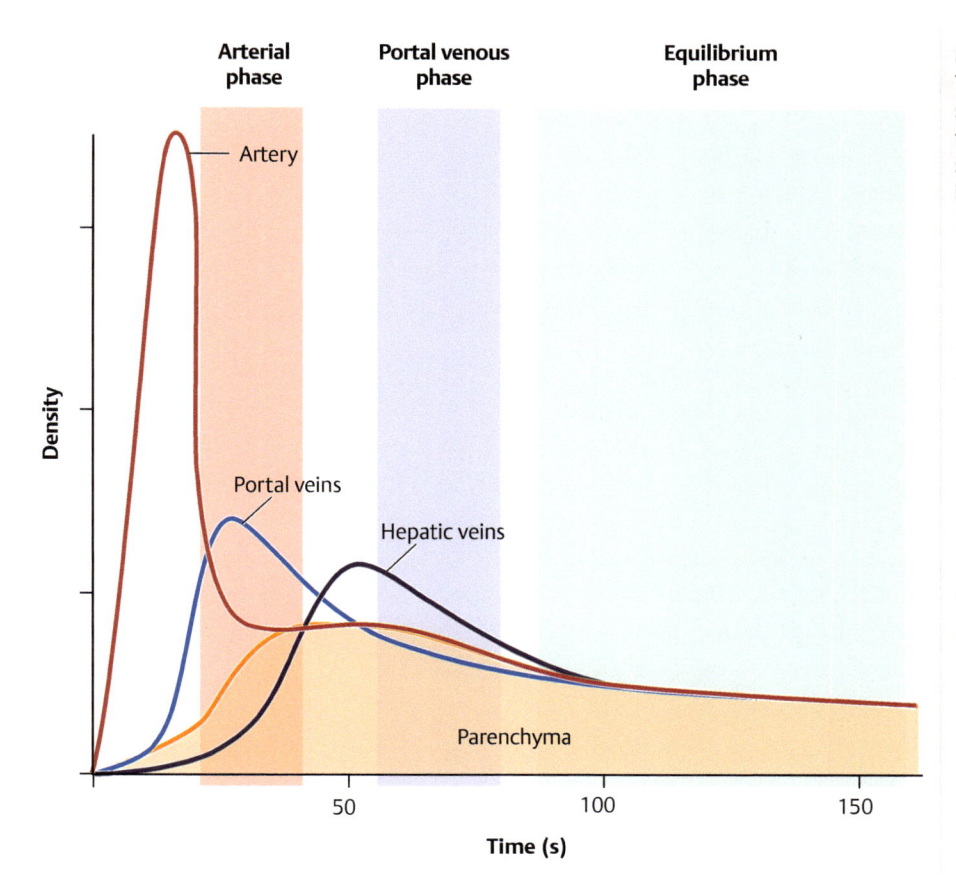

Fig. 5.4 Phases of liver enhancement in CT. The arterial phase starts approximately 25 seconds after IV injection of contrast medium, the portal venous phase at approximately 60–90 seconds. Equilibrium is established at approximately 3 minutes.

Unenhanced Imaging Techniques

MRI of the liver without the use of contrast medium is based on T1 W and T2 W sequences. The standard sequences are supplemented by chemical shift techniques such as the opposed-phase sequence and fat-suppressed sequences.[5] These sequences are used to detect or exclude fatty infiltration of the liver and to evaluate the proportion of fat within focal hepatic lesions (▶ Fig. 5.6).

Diffusion-weighted imaging (DWI) is a noncontrast technique that is used increasingly in the characterization of hepatic lesions. The b values in DWI can be varied to supply information on the restriction of proton diffusion.[5] Simply put, restricted diffusion within a focal liver lesion is suggestive of malignancy, whereas focal liver lesions that do not show restricted diffusion are likely to be benign. Additional computation of the apparent diffusion coefficient (ADC) values improves the accuracy of characterization of lesions, since benign lesions may also show restricted diffusion at higher b values (▶ Fig. 5.7).

Contrast-Enhanced Imaging Techniques

In dynamic contrast-enhanced T1 W imaging of the liver, just as in CT, images are acquired during various phases of hepatic perfusion. Normal liver tissue, as mentioned, receives up to 75% of its blood flow from the portal vein and only about 25% from the hepatic artery. These percentages are often reversed in primary and secondary liver tumors. The predominantly arterial blood supply to liver tumors is exploited in transarterial chemoembolization (TACE), in which the tumor is selectively treated by advancing angiographic catheters directly to the lesion via the hepatic artery and hepatic segmental arteries.

Note

For the most accurate lesion characterization, the liver MRI protocol should include at least one acquisition each in the arterial phase, portal venous phase, and equilibrium phase (▶ Fig. 5.8). Each of the dynamic sequences should require no more than a 20-second breath hold.[6,7]

During the equilibrium phase, the T1 W sequences should be supplemented by the acquisition of fat-suppressed T1 W sequences to detect special phenomena such as a pseudocapsule or delayed enhancement in tumor areas that have undergone desmoplastic change.

Liver-Specific Contrast Agents

Modern hepatobiliary contrast agents permit liver evaluation in a "hepatocyte-specific" phase.[8,9] During this phase the contrast agent is taken up by functioning hepatocytes and excreted in the bile. Thus, hepatobiliary agents can be used to detect the presence of functional hepatocytes within a lesion and also to assess the biliary tract. Liver lesions that do not contain hepatocytes, such as metastases, typically are not enhanced by hepatobiliary agents; liver masses of primary hepatocellular origin, such as focal nodular hyperplasia, take up more contrast agent than normal liver parenchyma.[10,11]

Both T1 W and fat-suppressed T1 W sequences can be acquired during the hepatobiliary phase of contrast excretion. As in the noncontrast sequences, there is no need for rapid acquisition, so sequences with high contrast and high resolution can be acquired (▶ Fig. 5.9).

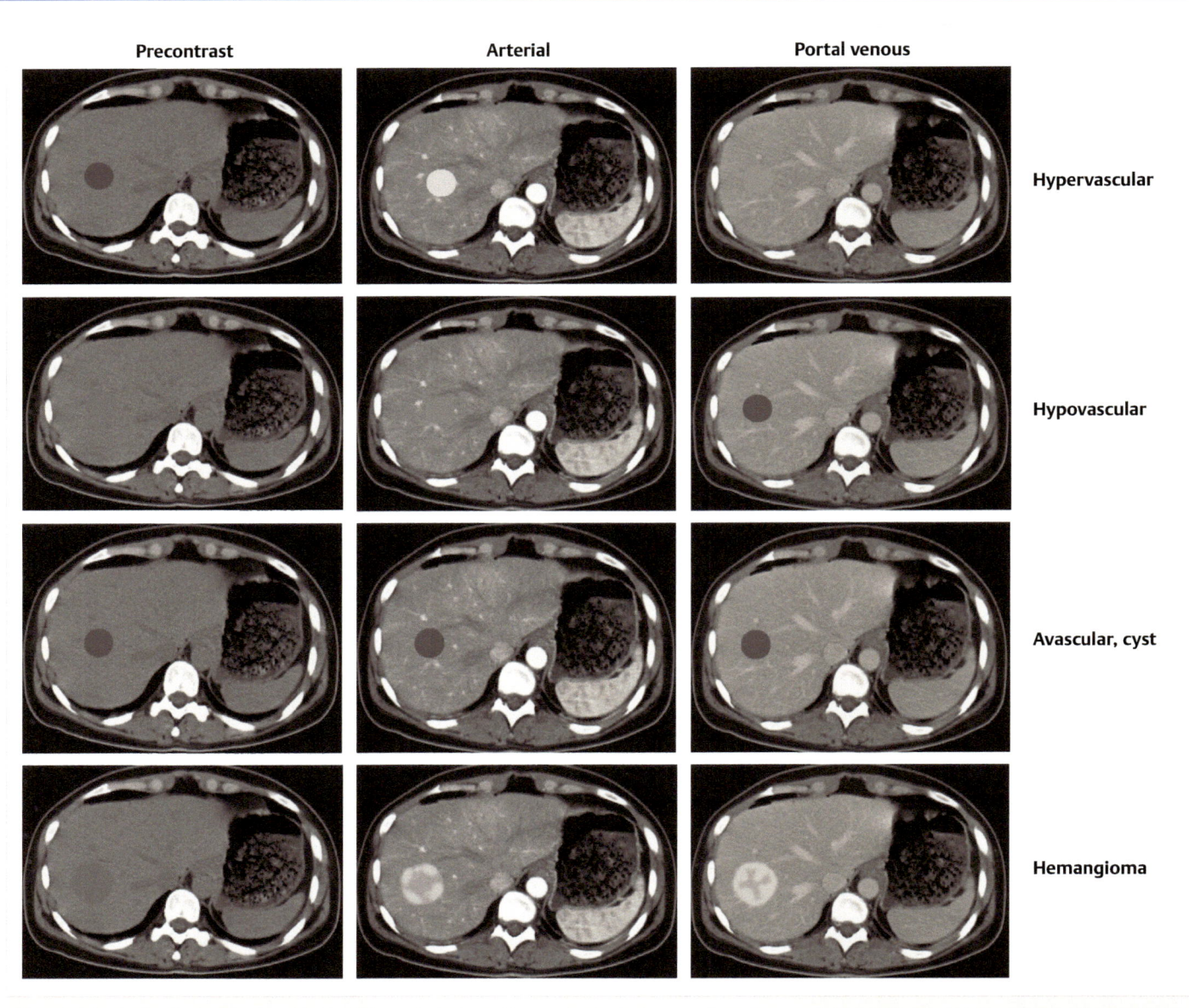

Fig. 5.5 Typical enhancement patterns of hepatic lesions. Hypervascular lesions are hypodense to surrounding parenchyma on unenhanced images. Nevertheless, even large studies indicate that acquisition without contrast medium can detect only an additional 5% of lesions. Hypovascular hepatic lesions are generally indistinguishable from surrounding parenchyma on unenhanced images. Hemangiomas have a pathognomonic enhancement pattern that spreads from the periphery of the lesion toward its center ("iris diaphragm sign").

Hepatobiliary contrast agents in current use include Gd-BOPTA and Gd-EOB-DTPA (gadoxetalate).[4,12] Gd-BOPTA is administered at a dose of 0.05 to 0.10 mmol/kg BW, Gd-EOB-DTPA at a dose of 0.025 mmol/kg BW. Both agents are partially taken up by hepatocytes and excreted in the bile. Gd-EOB-DTPA provides a higher percentage uptake, at approximately 50% of the injected dose, and it undergoes faster biliary excretion than Gd-BOPTA.[13] With Gd-EOB-DTPA, hepatobiliary phase images can be acquired just 10 to 15 minutes after injection of contrast medium. When Gd-BOPTA is used, much less of the contrast agent is eliminated with the bile (only 3–5%), and it takes at least 45 minutes until hepatobiliary phase images can be acquired.[9]

Both Gd-BOPTA and Gd-EOB-DTPA permit dynamic imaging studies of the liver, similar to extracellular contrast agents, and the liver can additionally be evaluated in the hepatobiliary phase during excretion of the contrast agent with the bile.

Extracellular Contrast Agents

Besides liver-specific agents, extracellular contrast agents are also available. Typically they are administered at a dose of 0.1 mmol/kg BW. Examples are Gd-DTPA, gadoterate meglumine, gadoteridol, and gadobutrol. These agents can be used for dynamic contrast-enhanced imaging of the liver in the arterial, portal venous, and equilibrium phases.[14]

5.4 Vascular Diseases

5.4.1 Portal Vein Thrombosis

▶ **Brief definition.** The etiology of portal vein thrombosis is described by the classic Virchow's triad, i.e., decreased blood flow within the vessel, an alteration in the viscosity or cellularity of

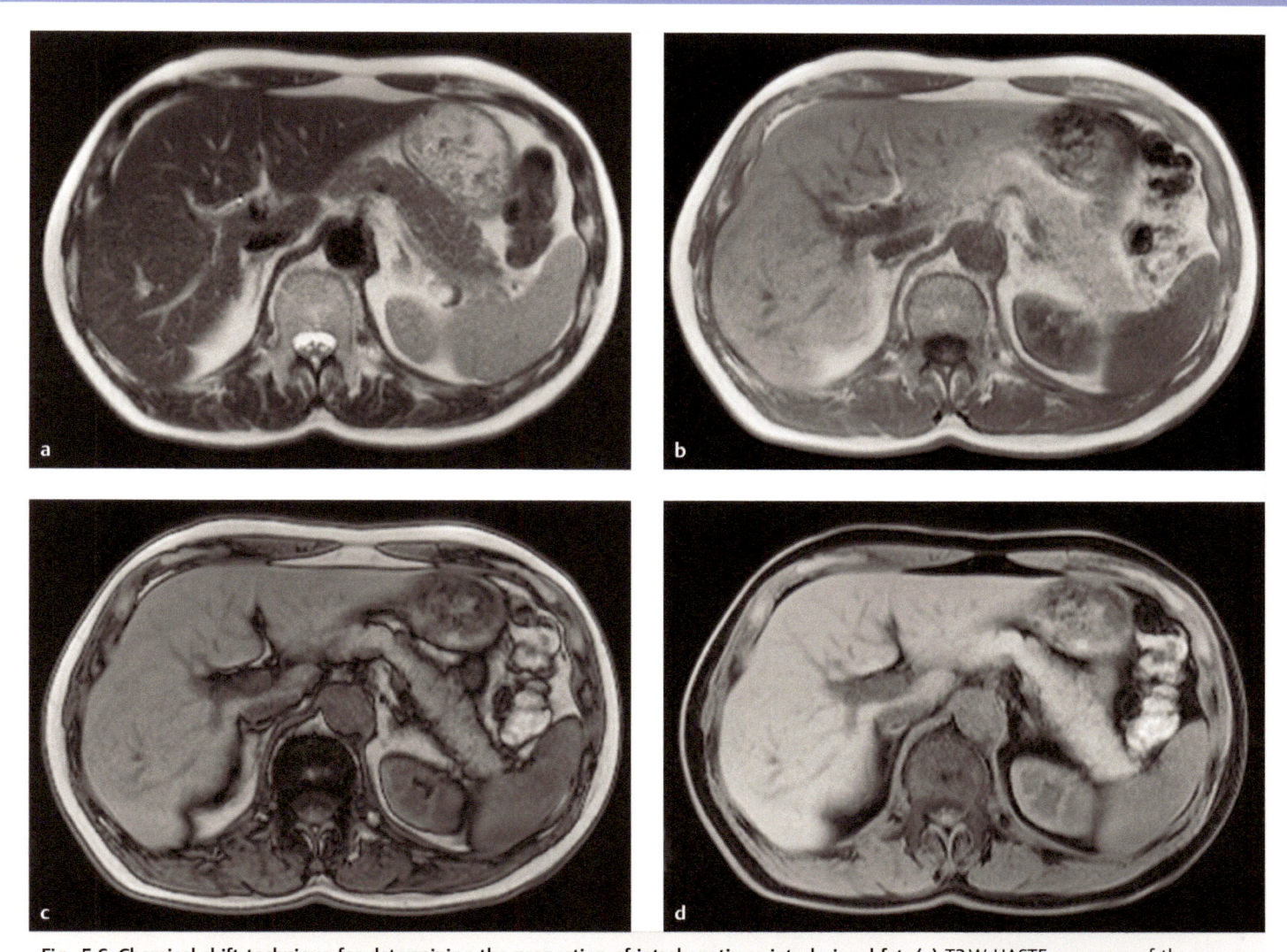

Fig. 5.6 Chemical shift technique for determining the proportion of intrahepatic or intralesional fat. **(a)** T2W HASTE sequence of the upper abdomen showing the liver, spleen, and pancreas. **(b)** T1W in-phase VIBE sequence. **(c)** T1W opposed-phase VIBE sequence. **(d)** Fat-suppressed T1W Dixon sequence. HASTE, half-Fourier acquisition single-shot turbo spin-echo. VIBE, volume-interpolated breath-hold examination.

the blood, and endothelial injury or dysfunction.[15] Typical Causative factors for portal vein thrombosis are:
- Slow blood flow in a setting of hepatic cirrhosis.
- Vascular stenosis due to pulmonary hilar lymphadenopathy.
- Invasion of the portal vein by a malignant tumor.
- Inflammatory changes relating to pancreatitis.
- Ascending and sclerosing cholangitis.
- Abdominal infections in general.
- Polycythemia vera.
- Obstruction by benign masses.

A typical cause of portal vein thrombosis in small children is the infection of an umbilical vein catheter. In cases of complete portal vein thrombosis, perfusion of the portal vein is maintained by periportal collateral veins. Extensive collaterals may develop in response to long-standing portal vein thrombosis, the most pronounced form being cavernous transformation of the portal vein, a spongelike plexus of many small, tortuous venous channels. Occasionally this condition may be mistaken for a patent portal vein on ultrasound examination.

▶ **Imaging signs.** Portal vein thrombosis is detectable sonographically by the absence of a Doppler signal and increased echogenicity in the vessel lumen. The thrombus can be directly visualized by CT, appearing as an intraluminal filling defect (▶ Fig. 5.10). Tumor thrombi may show enhancement in the portal venous phase. MRI is a noninvasive means of evaluating portal venous blood flow and the presence of partially occlusive intraluminal thrombi and collateral circulation.[16] Portal vein patency can be assessed even without contrast medium. Unlike ultrasound, MRI is not restricted by obesity, ascites or abdominal air, and therefore MRI supplies more diagnostic information than duplex ultrasound. Portal vein patency can be quickly evaluated in an SE sequence that demonstrates a flow void within the vessel. One potential pitfall is that turbulence at the confluence of the splenic vein and mesenteric veins may create an intraluminal signal. If portal vein thrombosis is present, the signal within the portal vein is typically isointense or slightly hyperintense to liver parenchyma in the T1W image and hyperintense in the T2W image (▶ Fig. 5.11). A diagnosis of portal vein thrombosis on unenhanced images is likely if a

Liver

| b = 50 | b = 400 | b = 800 | ADC |

a

| b = 50 | b = 400 | b = 800 | ADC |

b

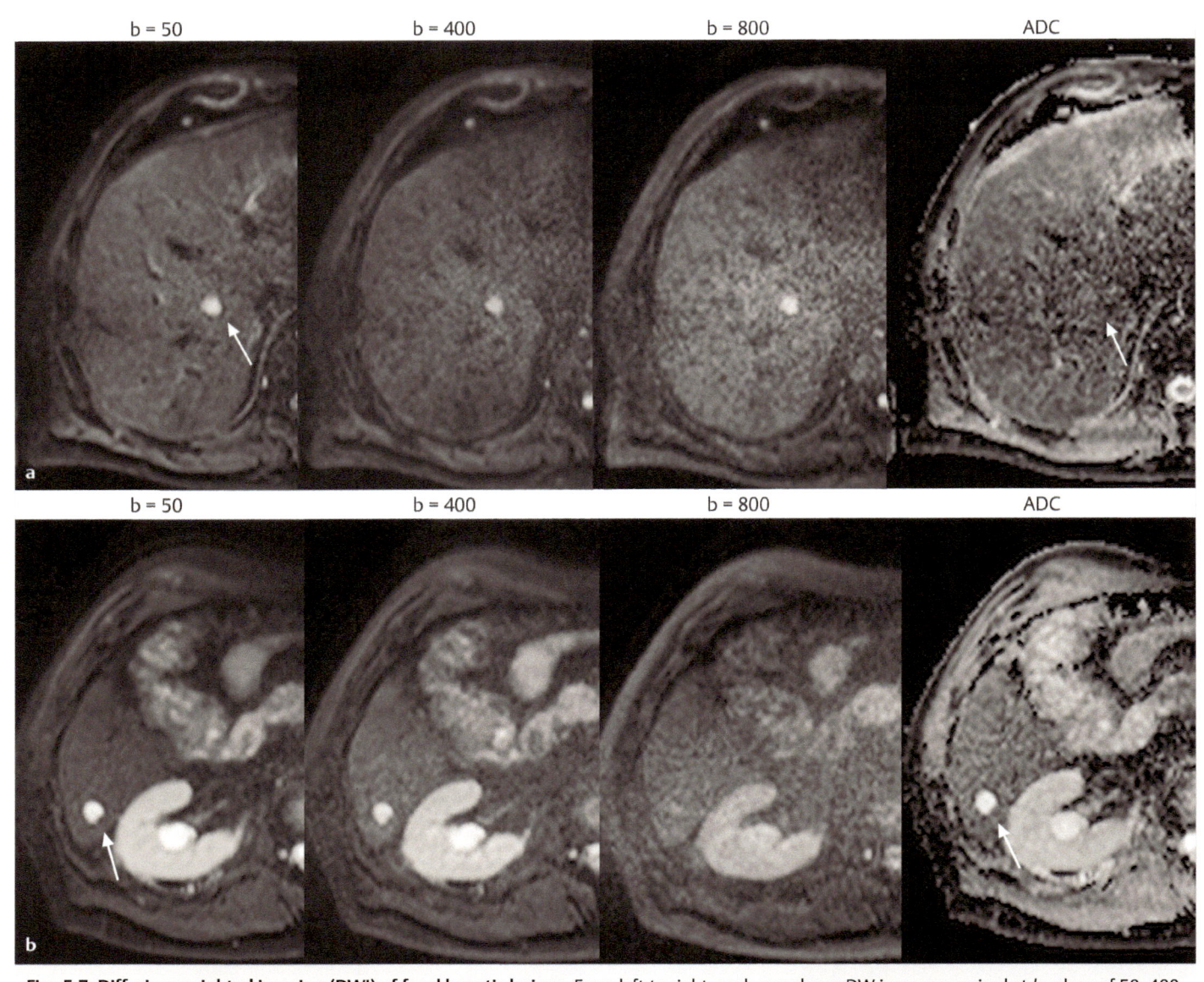

Fig. 5.7 **Diffusion-weighted imaging (DWI) of focal hepatic lesions.** From left to right, each row shows DW images acquired at *b* values of 50, 400, and 800 and the corresponding apparent diffusion coefficient (ADC) map at far right. While the metastasis shows definite hyperintensity even at high *b* values, the hepatic cyst is isointense to surrounding liver parenchyma at high *b* values. The metastasis is hypointense in the ADC map, while the cyst is hyperintense. **(a)** Hepatic metastasis (arrows) from a neuroendocrine tumor. **(b)** Hepatic cyst (arrows).

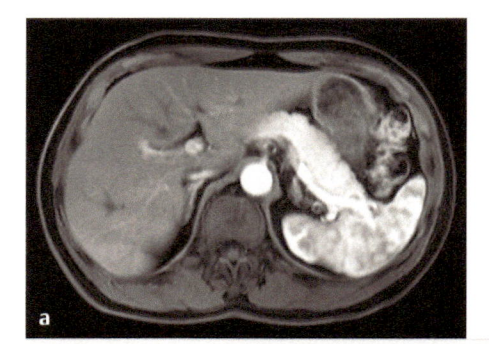

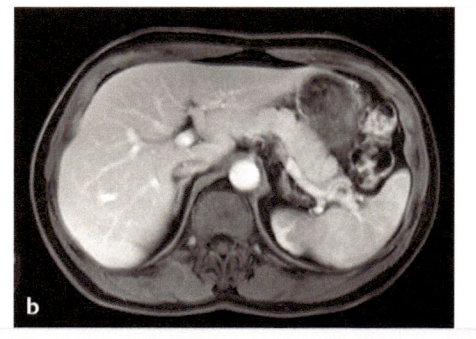

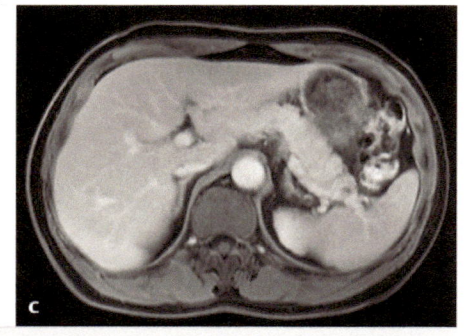

Fig. 5.8 **Dynamic contrast-enhanced imaging of the upper abdomen.** Dynamic fat-suppressed T1 W VIBE sequence after a bolus injection of Gd-BOPTA at 0.05 mmol/kg BW **(a)** Arterial phase. **(b)** Portal venous phase. **(c)** Equilibrium phase.

signal abnormality is found in the same area and has approximately the same size in all sequences. Suspected portal vein thrombosis can be confirmed or excluded by also acquiring flow-sensitive GRE images.[17] Administration of contrast medium can also be used to provide detailed views of small mural thrombi and of the collateral channels associated with cavernous transformation (▶ Fig. 5.12).

▶ **Clinical features.** Incomplete portal vein thrombosis often goes unnoticed. Complete portal vein thrombosis leads to prehepatic

5.4 Vascular Diseases

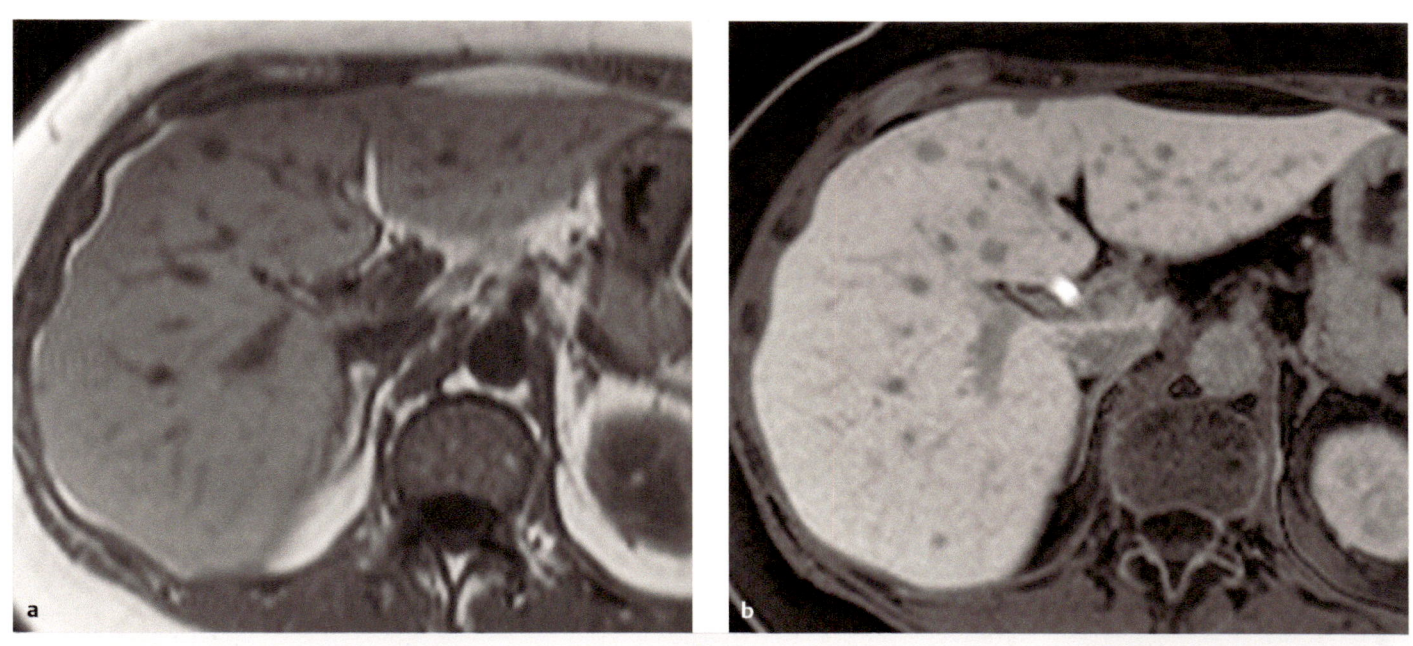

Fig. 5.9 **Liver imaging in the hepatobiliary phase of contrast excretion.** Dynamic fat-suppressed T1W VIBE sequence after bolus injection of 0.05 mmol/kg BW. Gd-BOPTA contrast medium. (a) T1W image of the upper abdomen before injection of contrast medium. (b) Fat-suppressed T1W image of the upper abdomen 45 minutes after the injection of 0.05 mmol/kg BW Gd-BOPTA. Although hepatic metastases are already visible in the precontrast image, they are more conspicuous in the contrast-enhanced image, which reveals multiple additional lesions.

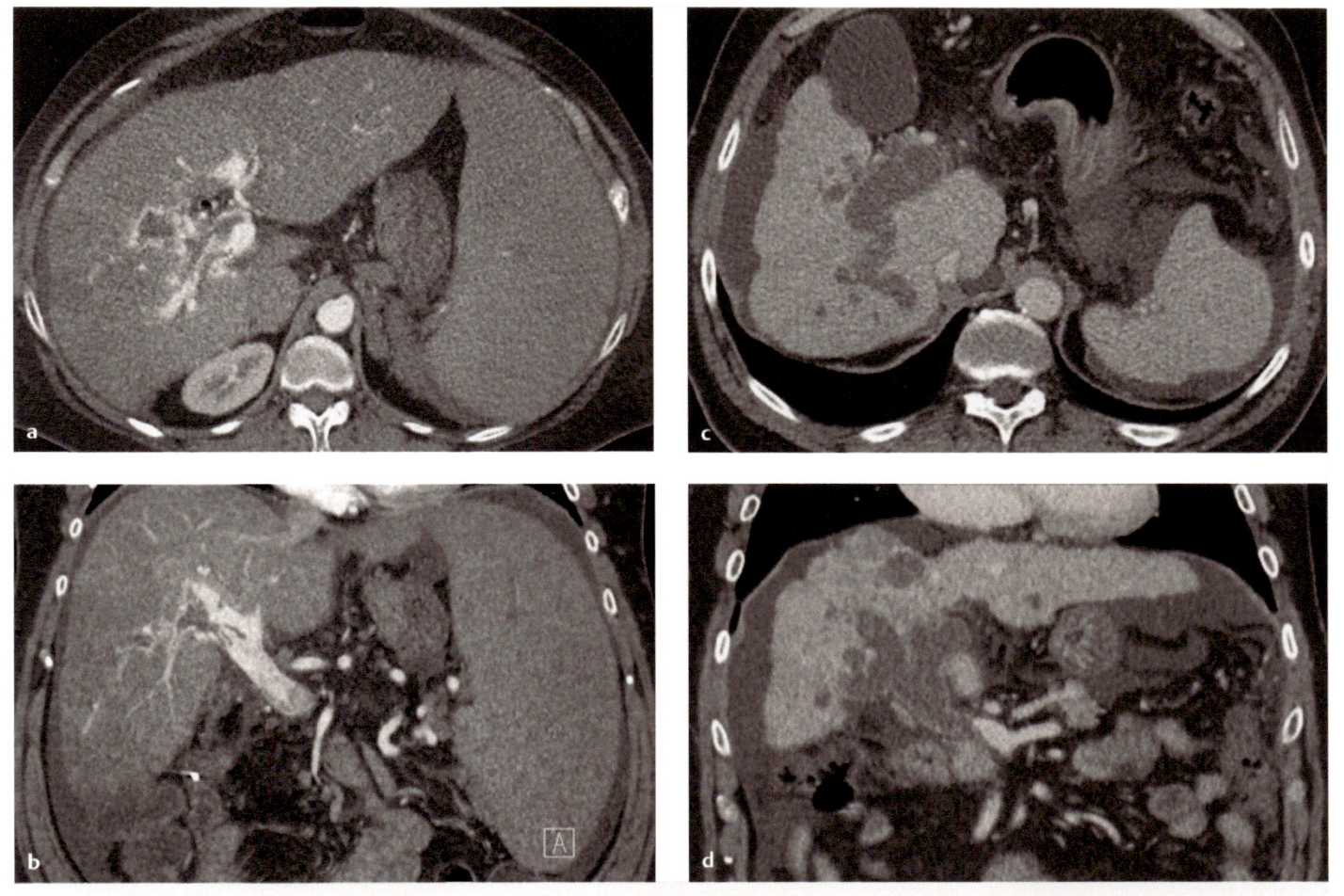

Fig. 5.10 **Portal vein thrombosis.** Postcontrast CT shows a thrombus outlined by contrast medium (a, b) and invasion of the portal vein by hepatocellular carcinoma with intravascular tumor growth (c, d). Portal vein enlargement extends to the periphery. (a) Axial image of the porta hepatis. (b) Coronal reformatted image of the portal vein. (c) Axial image of carcinoma invading the portal vein. (d) Coronal reformatted image of carcinoma invading the portal vein.

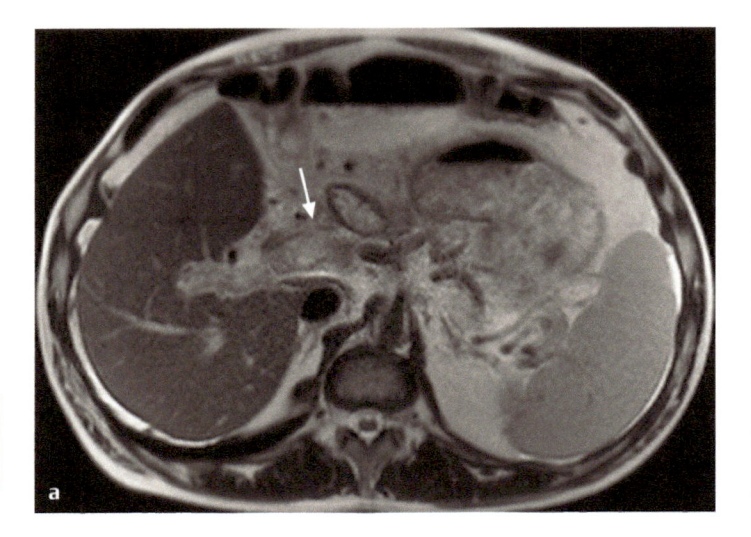

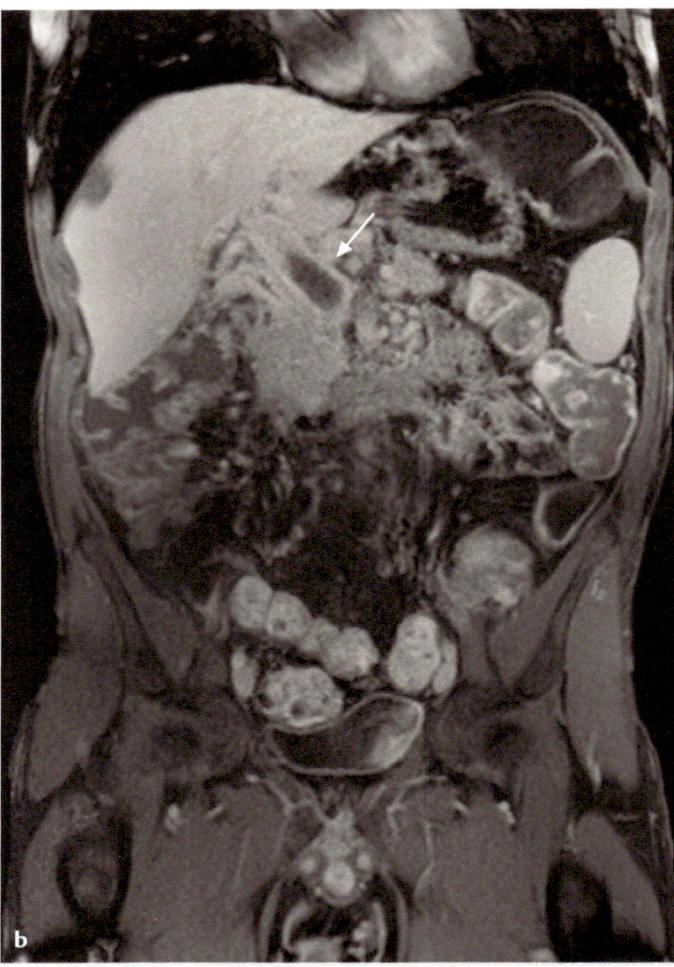

Fig. 5.11 Acute portal vein thrombosis. (a) Axial HASTE sequence shows markedly increased signal intensity in the portal vein (arrow; compare with flow void in the inferior vena cava). **(b)** Corresponding contrast-enhanced fat-suppressed T1W sequence shows the nonenhancing thrombus (arrow).

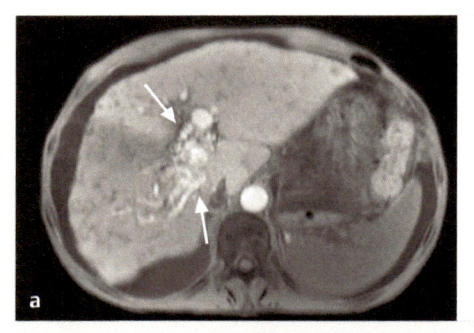

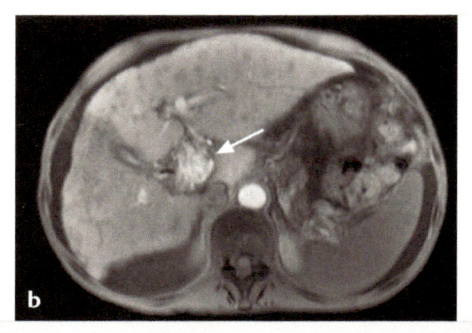

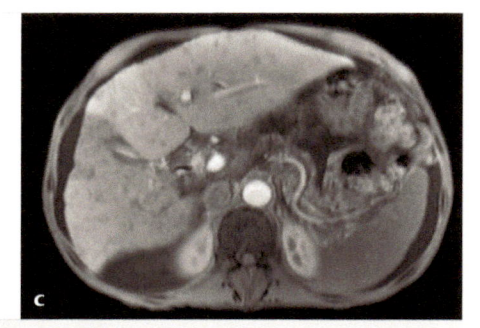

Fig. 5.12 Portal vein thrombosis. Cavernous transformation with multiple small collaterals detected about the porta hepatis (arrows). **(a)** Scan through the upper portion of the porta hepatis. **(b)** Midlevel scan through the porta hepatis. **(c)** Scan through the lower portion of the porta hepatis. The portal vein is occluded.

portal hypertension, and the associated collateral flood flow produces symptoms. Bleeding esophageal varices may occur, and ascites may develop.

▶ **Differential diagnosis.** It is important in portal vein thrombosis to differentiate a thrombus from invasion of the portal vein by a tumor, as hepatocellular carcinoma has a propensity for vascular invasion.

▶ **Key points.** Ultrasound, CT, and MRI are all suitable modalities for the diagnosis of portal vein thrombosis. Tumor thrombi enhance after IV administration of contrast medium.

5.4.2 Budd–Chiari Syndrome

▶ **Brief definition.** Budd–Chiari syndrome is caused by the obstruction of venous outflow from the sinusoidal bed of the liver. Both the large and small hepatic veins may be affected. The syndrome leads to portal hypertension, ascites, and progressive liver failure.[18,19] Budd–Chiari syndrome typically involves an obstruction of the large hepatic veins, usually at the confluence of the hepatic veins, with or without associated thrombosis of the intrahepatic segment of the inferior vena cava. This contrasts with veno-occlusive disease, which is characterized by

5.4 Vascular Diseases

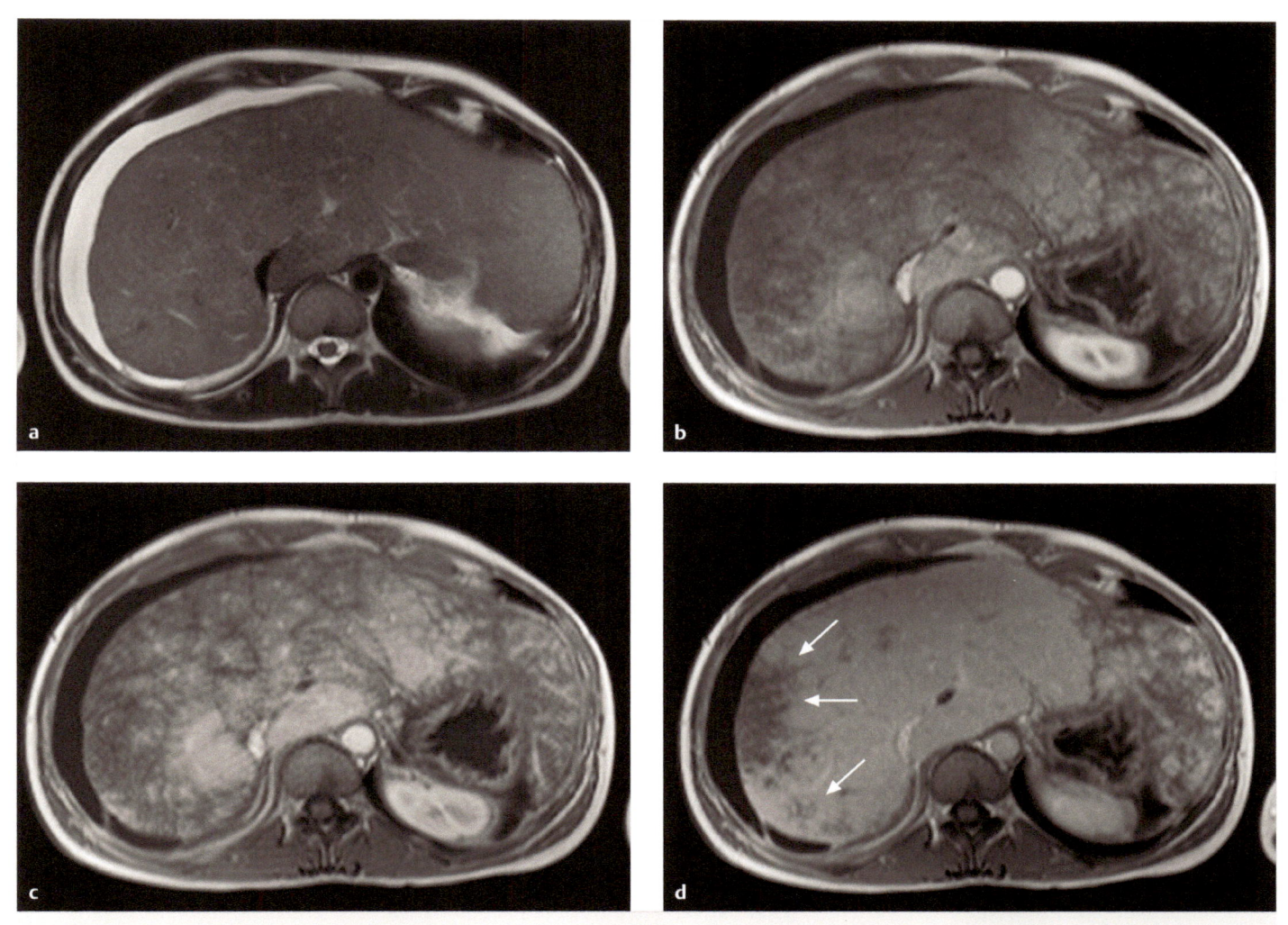

Fig. 5.13 **Budd–Chiari syndrome of the liver.** Marked ascites is present during the acute phase (a–c). (a) T2 W image shows marked swelling of the liver. The hepatic veins are not visualized. (b) T1 W image in the arterial phase after injection of contrast medium. The liver parenchyma shows only faint enhancement due to increased intrahepatic resistance. (c) T1 W image in the portal venous phase after injection of contrast medium. Arterial perfusion is noted, and the liver parenchyma shows marked peripheral hypoperfusion in segment VII. (d) T1 W image 15 minutes after injection of contrast medium still shows peripheral hypoperfusion in segment VII (arrows).

obstruction of the small intrahepatic veins, often with continued patency of the large hepatic veins.[20] When Budd–Chiari syndrome is suspected, therefore, it is important to evaluate for possible inferior vena cava thrombosis during imaging.

▶ **Imaging signs.** Typical morphological signs of Budd–Chiari syndrome are as follow (▶ Fig. 5.13):
- Marked swelling and rounding of the liver borders in the T2 W image, and increased signal intensity of the liver.
- Complete obstruction of the hepatic veins at the level of their confluence, with or without associated inferior vena cava thrombosis.
- Sparing of hepatic segment 1, which typically has its own venous drainage.
- Markedly delayed perfusion of the liver, typically affecting the peripheral portions of the liver parenchyma more than the center. Also, the arterial supply to the peripheral liver parenchyma is increased because the portal-vein perfusion pressure is no longer adequate to supply those regions.

Long-standing Budd–Chiari syndrome may give rise to intrahepatic venous collaterals in the upper part of the liver. Regenerating nodules are also found.[21]

▶ **Clinical features.** The obstruction of hepatic venous outflow leads to hepatomegaly. Liver failure may occur in the acute stage. Portal hypertension leads to ascites and collateralization. Chronic cases gradually progress to hepatic cirrhosis with associated symptoms.

▶ **Differential diagnosis.** Imaging features similar to those described above are seen in hepatic veno-occlusive disease, which is distinguished from Budd–Chiari syndrome by the occlusion of small postsinusoidal hepatic veins while the large hepatic veins remain patent. This disease is more commonly associated with chemotherapy, especially in patients who have undergone bone marrow transplantation. A pure radiological diagnosis is difficult, but a presumptive diagnosis can be made based on the similarity of parenchymal changes to those in Budd–Chiari syndrome. The diagnosis is confirmed by liver biopsy.

▶ **Key points.** Budd–Chiari syndrome is characterized by the obstruction of hepatic venous outflow, leading to posthepatic portal hypertension. Patients develop ascites and collaterals, and chronic cases gradually progress to cirrhosis.

5.4.3 Rendu–Osler–Weber Disease

▶ **Brief definition.** Rendu–Osler–Weber disease (synonym: hereditary hemorrhagic telangiectasia) is an autosomal dominant disorder characterized by a defect in transforming growth factor-beta (TGF-β). This leads to the development of arteriovenous malformations and telangiectasias. Four diagnostic criteria for Rendu–Osler–Weber disease have been described:
- Epistaxis.
- Multiple telangiectasias on the lips, tongue, fingers, or nose.
- Visceral arteriovenous malformations (in the lung, liver, brain, and spine).
- A first-degree relative with the disease.

The diagnosis is classed as likely if two of these criteria are present, and as definite if three or four criteria are present. Five different phenotypes are known, and the genetic mutation site has been identified for three of them. The phenotypes differ in the location of the arteriovenous fistulas (▶ Table 5.1). The HHT 1 and 2 phenotypes are characterized by the presence of hepatic arteriovenous malformations.

▶ **Imaging signs.** The hepatic veins are markedly dilated due to the arteriovenous shunting of blood. The liver may be enlarged. The arteriovenous malformations show intense contrast enhancement, similarly to the vessels, and appear as well-circumscribed round or tubular structures (▶ Fig. 5.14). The hepatic

Table 5.1 Phenotypes of Rendu–Osler–Weber disease

Phenotype	Mutation (gene)	Features
HHT1	ENG	Most common form; pulmonary arteriovenous malformation
HHT2	ALK1	Phenotype, pulmonary arteriovenous malformation rare
HHT3	Unknown	Hepatic arteriovenous malformation, pulmonary arteriovenous malformation
HHT4	Unknown	Arteriovenous malformation in lung/brain
JPHT	SMAD4	Arteriovenous malformation variable, juvenile polyposis

Abbreviations: HHT, hereditary hemorrhagic telangiectasia. JPHT, juvenile polyposis/hereditary hemorrhagic telangiectasia syndrome.

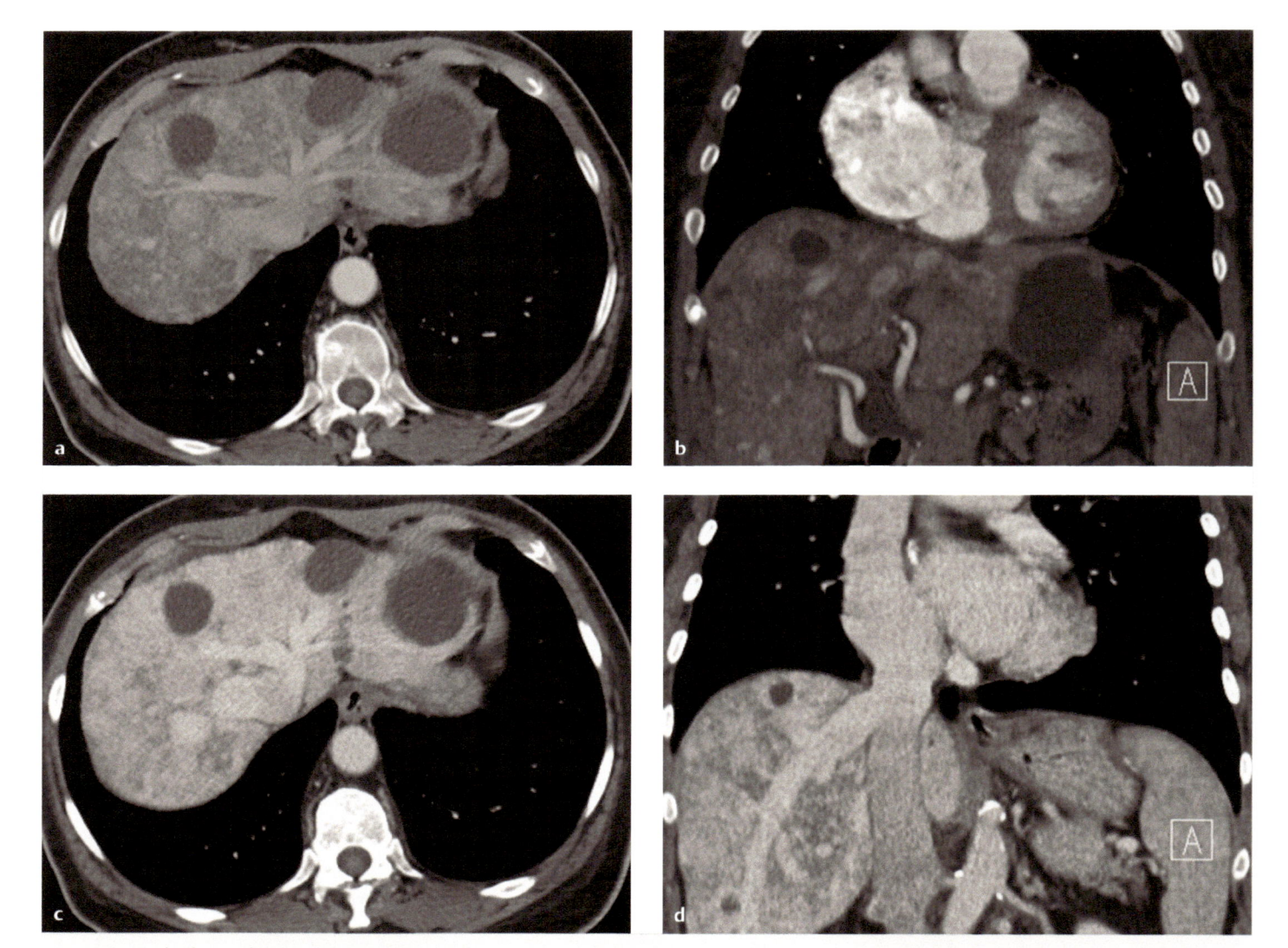

Fig. 5.14 Multiple intrahepatic arteriovenous malformations in Rendu–Osler–Weber disease. (a) Arterial phase. Early enhancement of the hepatic veins occurs due to multiple arteriovenous fistulas. (b) Coronal reformatted image shows the hypertrophic hepatic artery and its branches. (c) Portal venous phase. The liver parenchyma typically shows only faint enhancement. The multiple arteriovenous malformations appear as well-circumscribed round or tubular structures. (d) Coronal reformatted image shows dilatation of the hepatic veins.

artery is usually hypertrophic. Because of the arteriovenous shunt, the hepatic veins show very early enhancement during the arterial phase.

▶ **Clinical features.** Patients exhibit rapid fatigability due to the arteriovenous shunt. Heart failure may develop. From 30 to 50% of all patients suffer one or more transient ischemic attacks or stroke. An additional 10% of patients develop a brain abscess.

▶ **Key points.** Arteriovenous malformations may be present in Rendu–Osler–Weber disease, depending on the phenotype. They are detectable by ultrasonography, CT, and MRI. The hepatic veins show early enhancement after IV administration of contrast medium.

5.5 Focal Hepatic Lesions

Hepatic lesions are classified according to their histological origin. Three main categories are primary hepatic lesions, secondary hepatic lesions, and pseudolesions. Primary hepatic lesions can be subdivided further into mesenchymal, hepatocytic, and cholangiocytic lesions. Each of these subdivisions includes both benign and malignant lesions, and their imaging features may overlap. The accurate characterization of primary focal hepatic lesions requires a comprehensive review of all findings, including precontrast images, dynamic contrast-enhanced images, and hepatobiliary-phase images. The following techniques are utilized for these:
- Unenhanced T2 W sequences.
- Unenhanced T1 W sequences.
- Dynamic T1 W imaging with extracellular contrast agents.
- Hepatobiliary T1 W imaging with liver-specific contrast agents.

Initial lesion characterization is based upon findings detected on unenhanced MRI. The presence of intralesional fat, high T2 W or T1 W signal intensity, and other factors are useful for narrowing the differential diagnosis. The unenhanced MRI features of various focal hepatic lesions are reviewed in ▶ Fig. 5.15 and ▶ Fig. 5.16.

Dynamic images acquired in the arterial, portal venous, and equilibrium phases after injection of contrast medium are also useful for the classification of focal hepatic lesions. Arterial-phase imaging is particularly useful as it differentiates arterial hypervascular and hypovascular lesions and also identifies lesions that show delayed, persistent enhancement. The flowcharts in ▶ Fig. 5.17, ▶ Fig. 5.18, and ▶ Fig. 5.19 show how these features can be used for characterization of lesion.

Additionally, hepatobiliary contrast agents can be used to detect the presence of functional hepatocytes within a hepatic lesion. Lesions that do not contain functioning hepatocytes are not enhanced by these agents in the hepatocyte-specific biliary phase. ▶ Fig. 5.20 shows how these MRI criteria are applied in the differential diagnosis of focal hepatic lesions.

5.5.1 Primary Hepatic Lesions

Mesenchymal Lesions

Benign Mesenchymal Tumors

Hepatic Hemangioma

▶ **Brief definition.** The most common mesenchymal hepatic lesions, and the most common true focal hepatic lesions in general, are hemangiomas, which may occur in a cavernous or capillary form. The incidence of hepatic hemangioma is up to 20% in

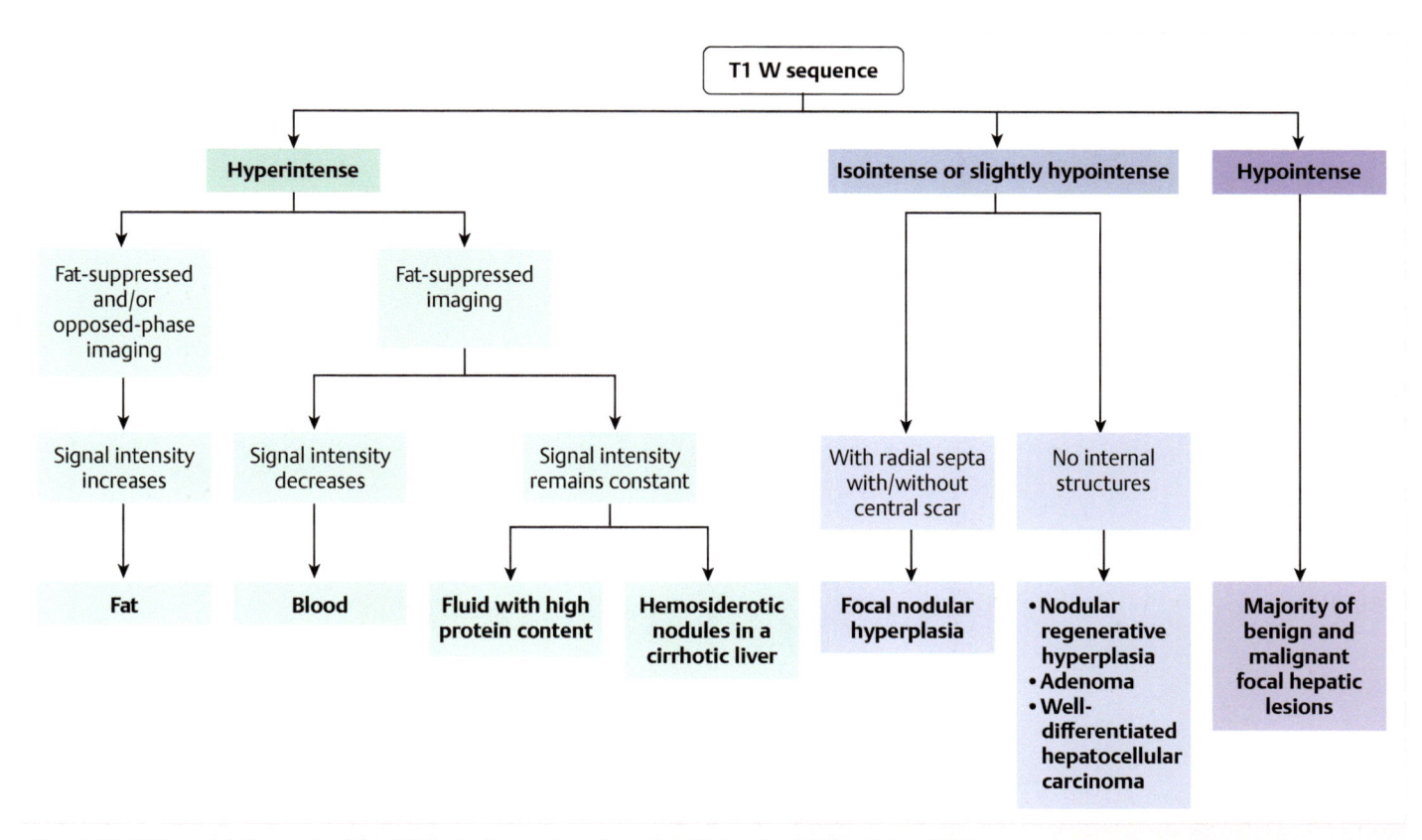

Fig. 5.15 Differential diagnosis of focal hepatic lesions based on signal intensity in T1-weighted MRI.

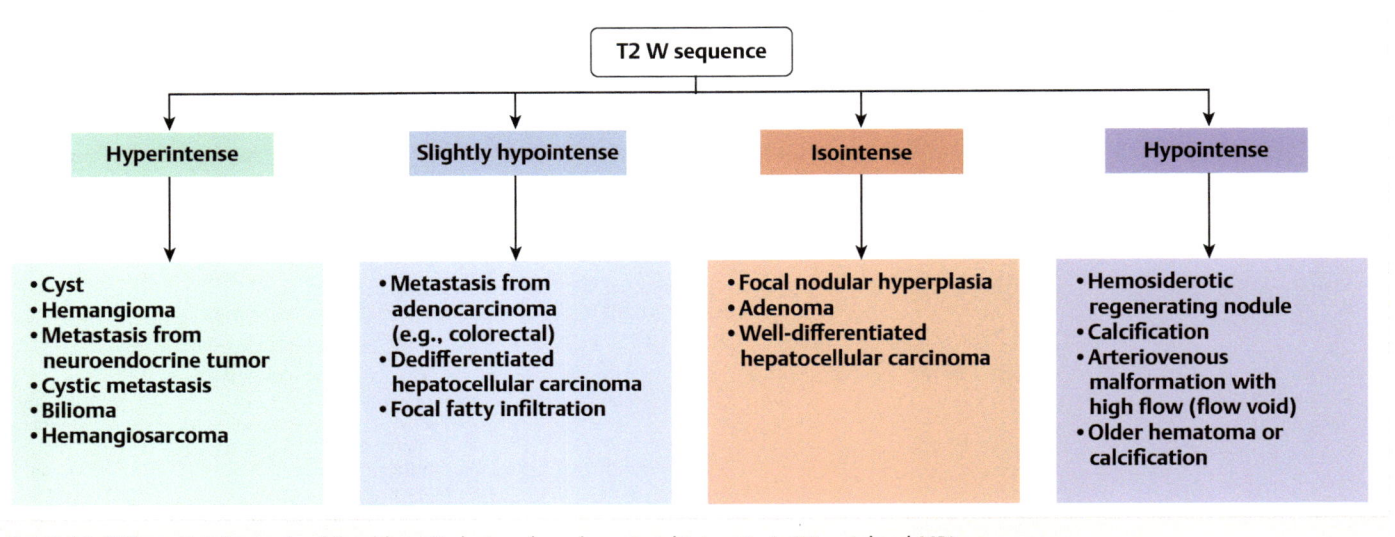

Fig. 5.16 Differential diagnosis of focal hepatic lesions based on signal intensity in T2-weighted MRI.

T2 W sequence

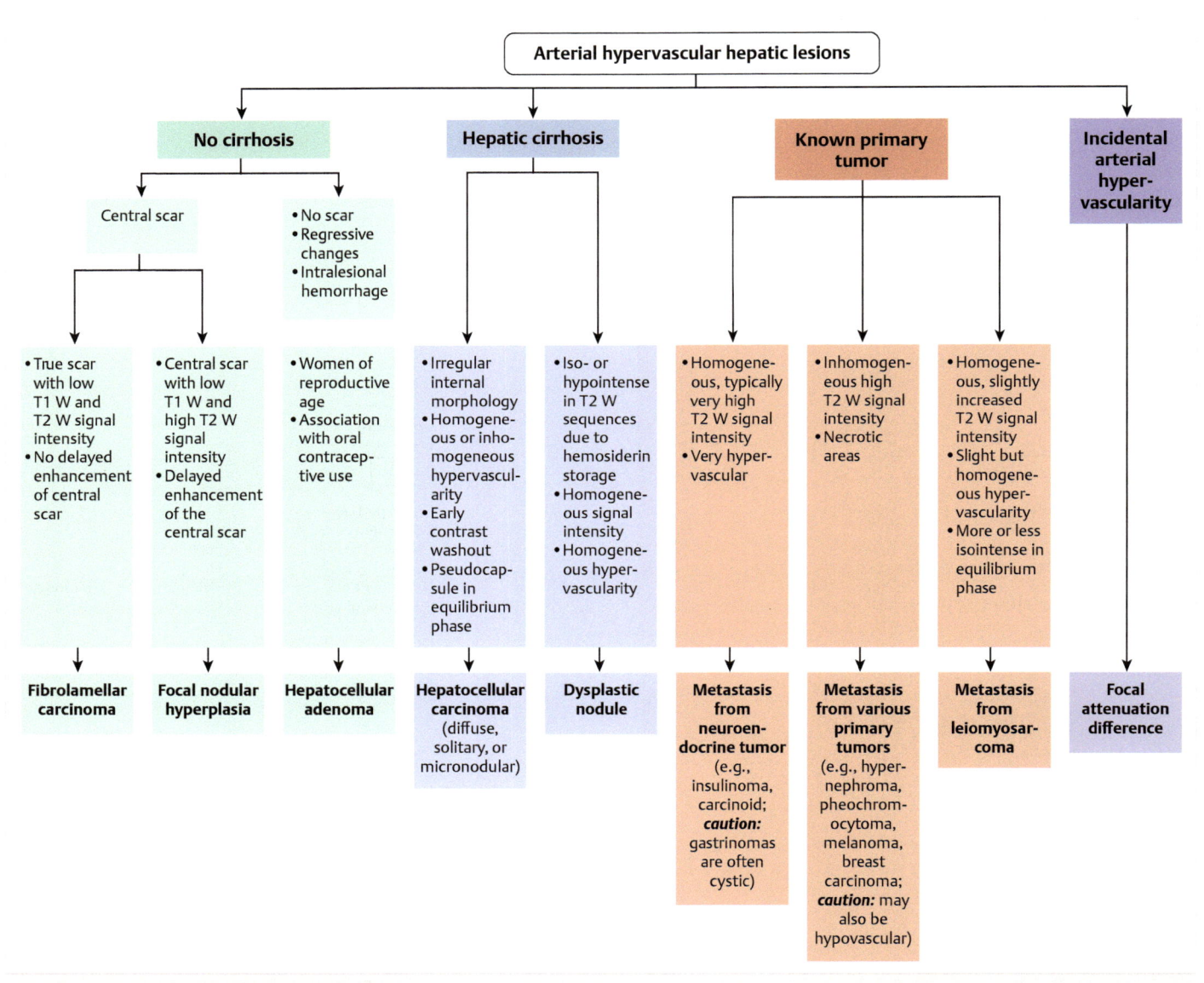

- **Hyperintense**
  - Cyst
  - Hemangioma
  - Metastasis from neuroendocrine tumor
  - Cystic metastasis
  - Bilioma
  - Hemangiosarcoma

- **Slightly hypointense**
  - Metastasis from adenocarcinoma (e.g., colorectal)
  - Dedifferentiated hepatocellular carcinoma
  - Focal fatty infiltration

- **Isointense**
  - Focal nodular hyperplasia
  - Adenoma
  - Well-differentiated hepatocellular carcinoma

- **Hypointense**
  - Hemosiderotic regenerating nodule
  - Calcification
  - Arteriovenous malformation with high flow (flow void)
  - Older hematoma or calcification

Fig. 5.17 Differential diagnosis of arterial hypervascular hepatic lesions.

Arterial hypervascular hepatic lesions

- **No cirrhosis**
  - Central scar
    - True scar with low T1 W and T2 W signal intensity; No delayed enhancement of central scar → **Fibrolamellar carcinoma**
    - Central scar with low T1 W and high T2 W signal intensity; Delayed enhancement of the central scar → **Focal nodular hyperplasia**
  - No scar / Regressive changes / Intralesional hemorrhage
    - Women of reproductive age; Association with oral contraceptive use → **Hepatocellular adenoma**

- **Hepatic cirrhosis**
  - Irregular internal morphology; Homogeneous or inhomogeneous hypervascularity; Early contrast washout; Pseudocapsule in equilibrium phase → **Hepatocellular carcinoma (diffuse, solitary, or micronodular)**
  - Iso- or hypointense in T2 W sequences due to hemosiderin storage; Homogeneous signal intensity; Homogeneous hypervascularity → **Dysplastic nodule**

- **Known primary tumor**
  - Homogeneous, typically very high T2 W signal intensity; Very hypervascular → **Metastasis from neuroendocrine tumor (e.g., insulinoma, carcinoid; caution: gastrinomas are often cystic)**
  - Inhomogeneous high T2 W signal intensity; Necrotic areas → **Metastasis from various primary tumors (e.g., hypernephroma, pheochromocytoma, melanoma, breast carcinoma; caution: may also be hypovascular)**
  - Homogeneous, slightly increased T2 W signal intensity; Slight but homogeneous hypervascularity; More or less isointense in equilibrium phase → **Metastasis from leiomyosarcoma**

- **Incidental arterial hypervascularity**
  - → **Focal attenuation difference**

5.5 Focal Hepatic Lesions

```
                            Arterial hypovascular hepatic lesions
        ┌──────────────────────┬──────────────────┬──────────────────────┐
   Cystic appearance    Arterial hypervascular                  History of abdominal
                                rim                              trauma or surgery
```

Cystic appearance:
- Sharply demarcated from surroundings
- No change in surrounding vascularity

→ Cyst (solitary or multiple)
- Caroli's disease
- Polycystic liver/kidney disease

- Hypointense rim
- Internal septa
- Daughter cysts

→ Echinococcal cyst

Arterial hypervascular rim:
- Peripheral washout 10–15 min after contrast injection
- Donut or halo sign in T2 W sequences

→ Metastasis from adenocarcinoma (pancreatic, colon, gastric carcinoma and other primaries)

- Cystic appearance
- Irregular cyst wall
- Enhancing internal septa
- Solid components

→ Cystic metastasis (e.g., ovarian carcinoma)

- Isointense in equilibrium phase
- Does not displace liver tissue

→ Non-Hodgkin's lymphoma
- Hodgkin's disease

- Arterial hypervascular rim with persistent enhancement
- No central enhancement
- High T2 W signal intensity (near-cystic appearance)
- Gas formation within the lesion

→ Hepatic abscess

History of abdominal trauma or surgery:
- Cystic
- Tendency to enlarge
- High T2 W signal intensity
- Displaces surrounding structures

→ Bilioma

- Irregular margins
- Inhomogeneous T1 W and T2 W signal intensity
- Hyperintense rim in T1 W sequences due to extracellular methemaglobin

→ Hepatic hematoma
- Hepatic rupture

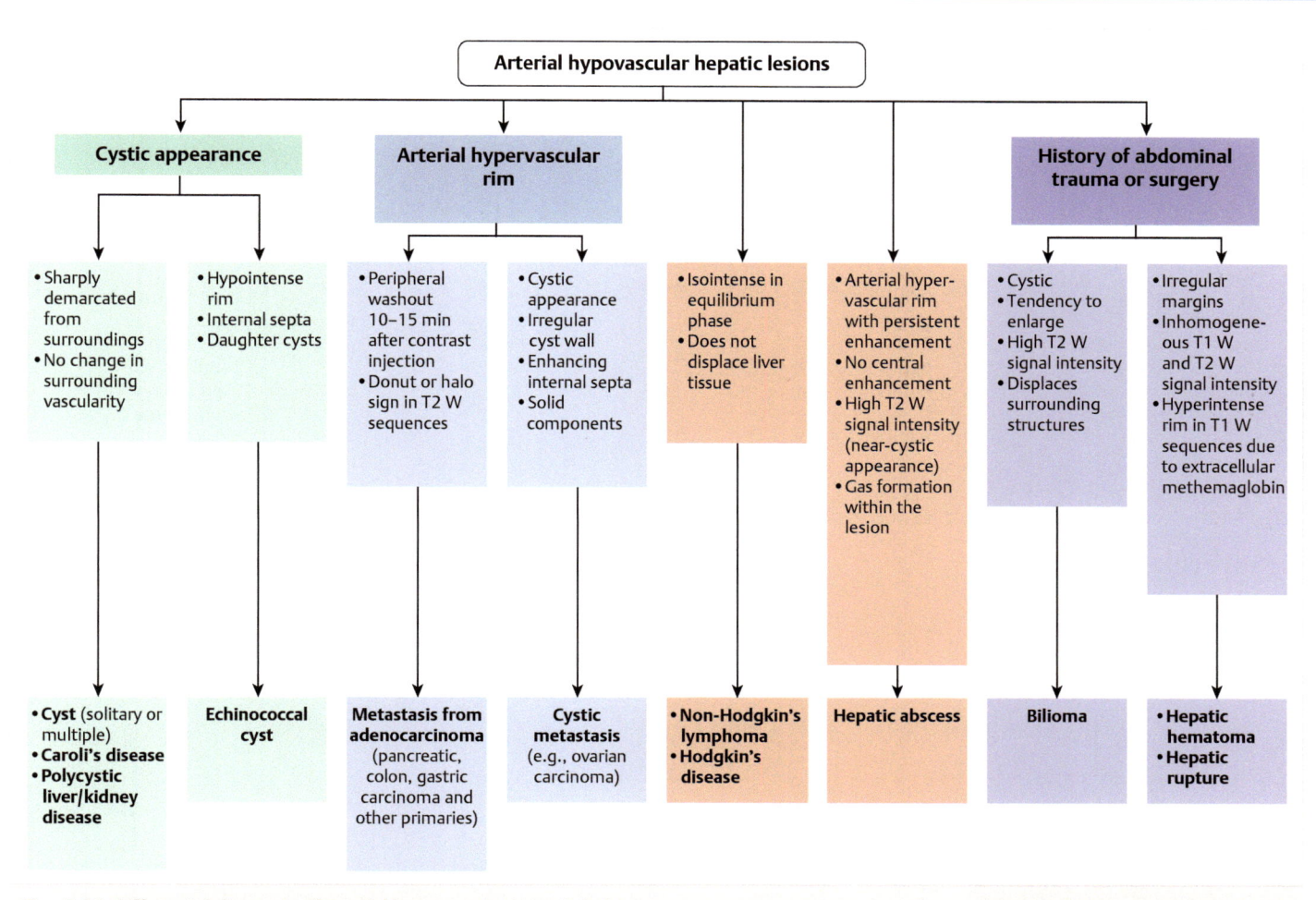

Fig. 5.18 Differential diagnosis of arterial hypovascular hepatic lesions.

Hepatic lesions showing persistent delayed enhancement

- Nodular peripheral enhancement in arterial phase
- Centripetal spread of enhancement
- High T2 W signal intensity

→ Hemangioma

- Infiltration along bile ducts
- Segmental biliary obstruction
- Hypovascular with irregular peripheral enhancement in arterial phase

→ Intrahepatic cholangiocellular carcinoma

- Known or unknown primary
- Hypervascular in arterial phase

→ Metastasis from leiomyosarcoma or gastrointestinal stromal tumor

- Irregular, partially nodular enhancement in arterial phase
- Centrifugal or irregular enhancement pattern
- Irregular margins

→ Hemangiosarcoma
- Hemangioendothelioma
- Hemangiopericytoma

- Homogeneous, sometimes early enhancement
- Irregular margins
- High T2 W signal intensity
- Iso- or hyperintense in equilibrium phase

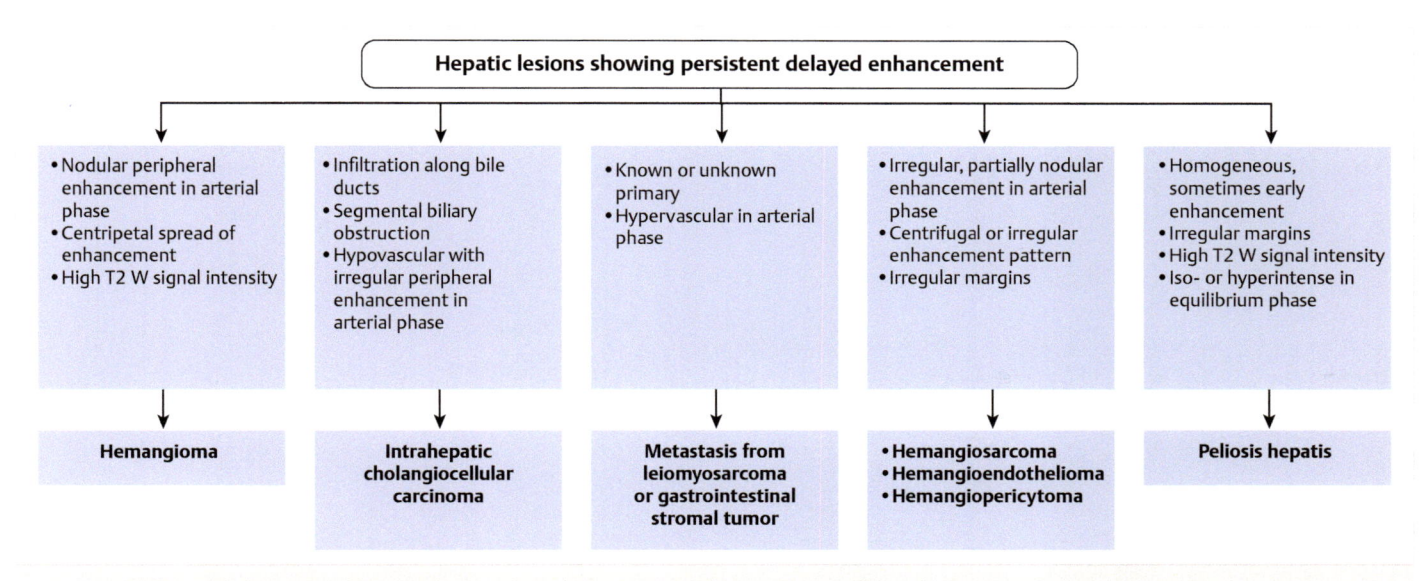

→ Peliosis hepatis

Fig. 5.19 Differential diagnosis of hepatic lesions showing persistent enhancement on delayed images.

---

the normal population, based on various sources in the literature. An association with focal nodular hyperplasia is observed in 15 to 20% of cases.[22] Two main types are distinguished:
- *Pediatric hepatic hemangioma*: Lesions of this type often undergo spontaneous regression. Solitary hepatic hemangioma is a somewhat unusual finding in the pediatric age group. It is more common to find multiple hemangiomas in association with viscerocutaneous hemangiomatosis. These cases may develop right heart failure due to the functional left-to-right shunt and will require chemotherapy for primary benign hemangiomatosis.

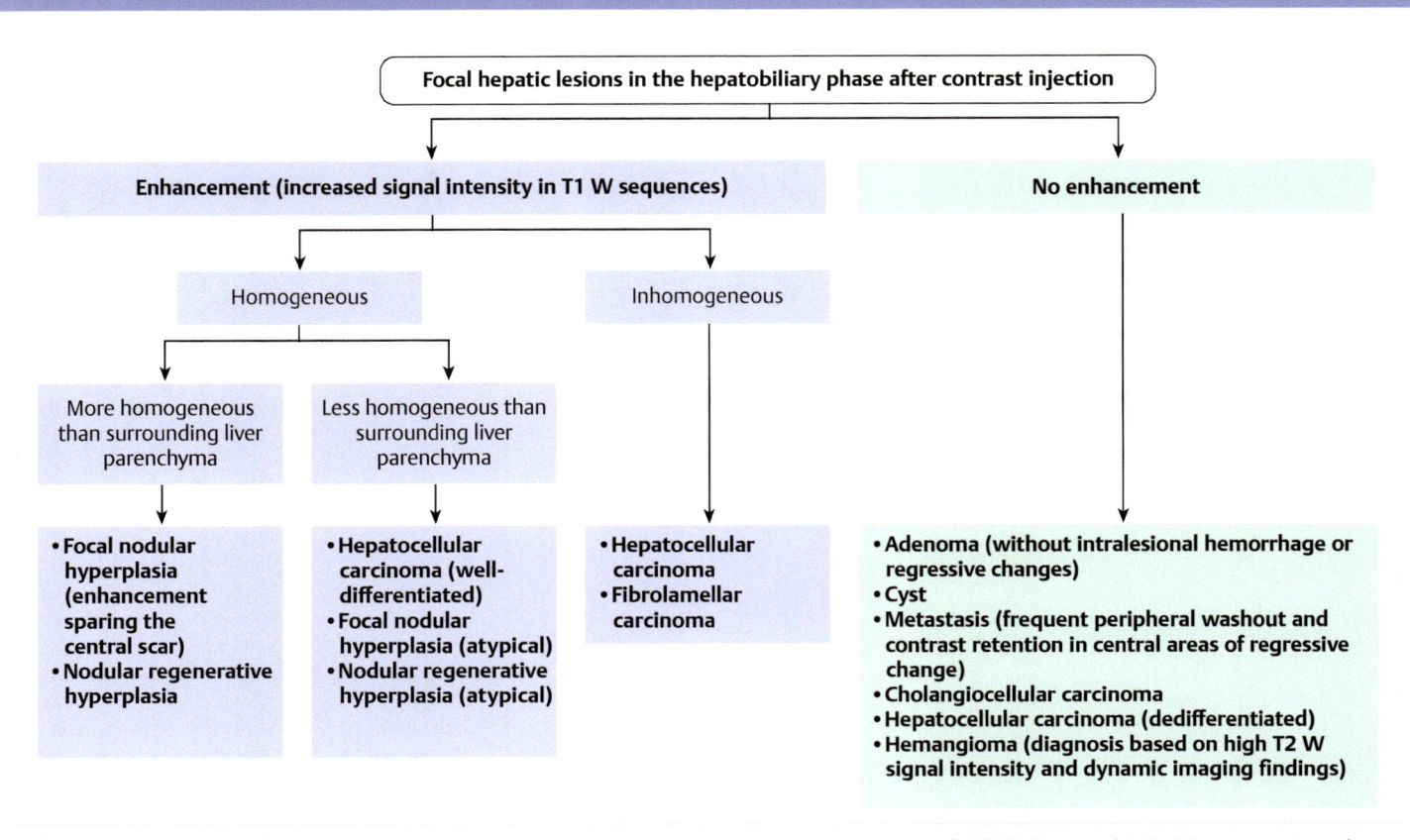

```
Focal hepatic lesions in the hepatobiliary phase after contrast injection
├── Enhancement (increased signal intensity in T1 W sequences)
│   ├── Homogeneous
│   │   ├── More homogeneous than surrounding liver parenchyma
│   │   │   • Focal nodular hyperplasia (enhancement sparing the central scar)
│   │   │   • Nodular regenerative hyperplasia
│   │   └── Less homogeneous than surrounding liver parenchyma
│   │       • Hepatocellular carcinoma (well-differentiated)
│   │       • Focal nodular hyperplasia (atypical)
│   │       • Nodular regenerative hyperplasia (atypical)
│   └── Inhomogeneous
│       • Hepatocellular carcinoma
│       • Fibrolamellar carcinoma
└── No enhancement
    • Adenoma (without intralesional hemorrhage or regressive changes)
    • Cyst
    • Metastasis (frequent peripheral washout and contrast retention in central areas of regressive change)
    • Cholangiocellular carcinoma
    • Hepatocellular carcinoma (dedifferentiated)
    • Hemangioma (diagnosis based on high T2 W signal intensity and dynamic imaging findings)
```

Fig. 5.20 Differential diagnosis of focal hepatic lesions in the hepatobiliary phase after injection of Gd-BOPTA or Gd-EOB-DTPA contrast media.

- **Adult hepatic hemangioma**: Lesions of this type may be solitary or multiple and are usually asymptomatic. Patients may occasionally become symptomatic due to thrombosis or hemorrhage, although hemorrhage is very rare.

Hemangiomas typically present as well-defined lesions ranging from a few millimeters to 20 or 30 cm in size.[23] Hemangiomas larger than 10 cm are called "giant hemangiomas." Microscopically, hemangiomas consist of multiple vascular channels with a single layer of endothelial cells. Larger lesions almost always have a heterogeneous tissue composition with areas of fibrosis, necrosis, cystic changes, and occasional coarse intratumoral calcifications.

▶ **Imaging signs.** Hemangiomas appear sonographically as hyperechoic lesions with well-defined margins (▶ Fig. 5.21). Cavernous hemangiomas show an almost pathognomonic enhancement pattern on CT: The enhancement is intense, comparable to that of major vessels. The enhancement pattern is called "lacunar" for its resemblance to tiny lakes. On delayed images the hemangioma shows progressive centripetal enhancement spreading from the periphery toward the center (▶ Fig. 5.22). On T1-weighted MRI, the lesions appear as hypointense masses with a round or lobulated shape that are sharply demarcated from surrounding liver tissue. T2 W sequences show very high signal intensity that is homogeneous in small hemangiomas and inhomogeneous in larger lesions.[24] Imaging with an extracellular gadolinium-based contrast agent demonstrates lacunar enhancement in the arterial phase. Later images show an iris diaphragm sign similar to that seen on CT (▶ Fig. 5.23).[25] Images in the equilibrium phase show more or less complete, homogeneous uptake in the lesion, depending on the size of the hemangioma and the presence or absence of central fibrotic changes (▶ Fig. 5.24).[26] Capillary hemangiomas show a different enhancement pattern on both CT and MRI: these lesions already show marked, homogeneous enhancement in the early arterial phase (▶ Fig. 5.25); but unlike lesions such as focal nodular hyperplasia and hepatocellular adenoma or carcinoma, which also show arterial hypervascul-arity, capillary hemangiomas show high T2 W signal intensity and a persistence of enhancement in the portal venous and equilibrium phases.

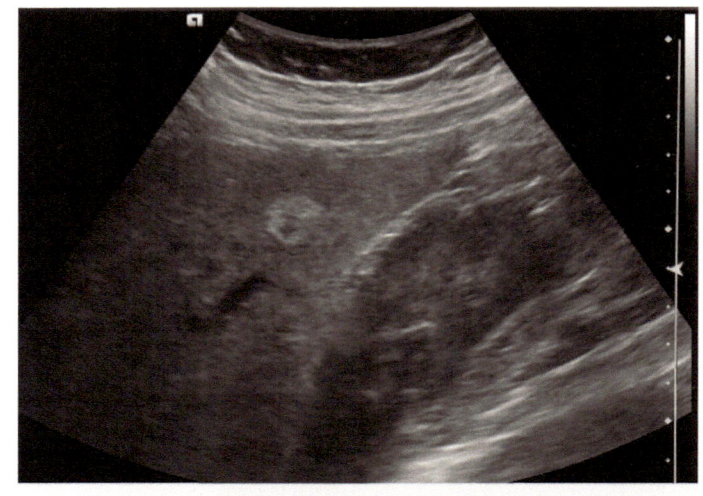

Fig. 5.21 **Hemangioma.** Ultrasound displays the hemangioma as a hyperechoic mass with well-defined margins.

5.5 Focal Hepatic Lesions

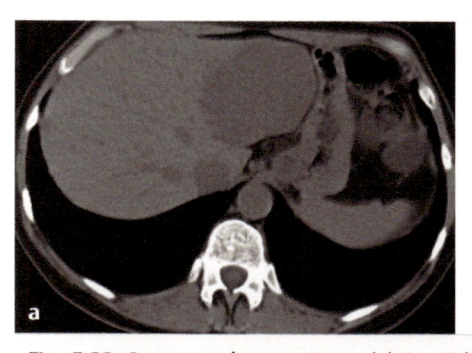

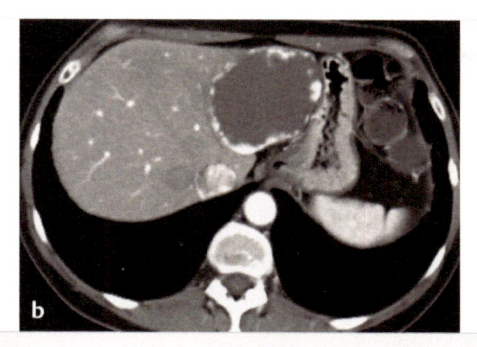

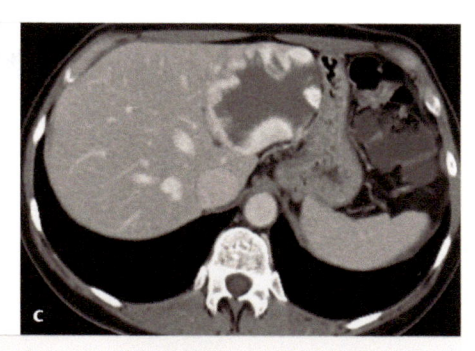

Fig. 5.22 Cavernous hemangioma. (a) On CT before injection of contrast medium, the hemangioma is isoattenuating to the vena cava. (b) Arterial phase. The hemangioma shows a lacunar enhancement pattern from the periphery to the center. (c) Centripetal spread of enhancement, called the iris diaphragm sign, continues in the portal venous phase.

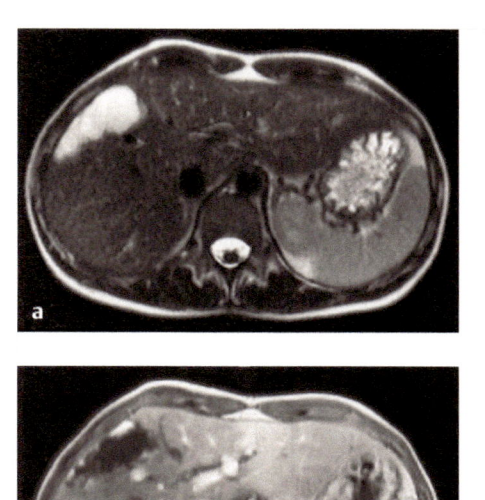

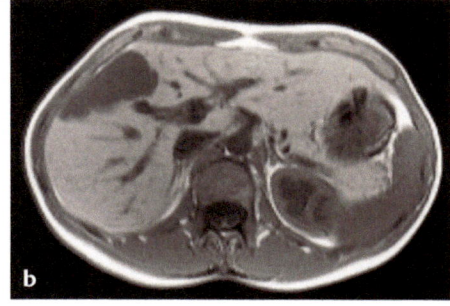

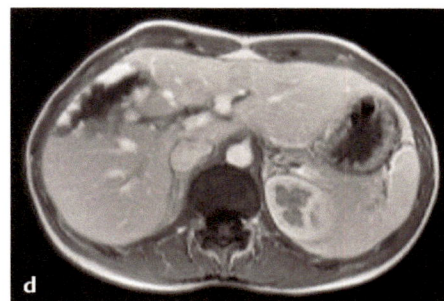

Fig. 5.23 Cavernous hemangioma in an asymptomatic patient. (a) T2 W image shows a hyperintense, sharply circumscribed lesion with homogeneous internal signal intensity. (b) T1 W image. The lesion appears uniformly hypointense. (c) T1 W image in the arterial phase after injection of contrast medium. The lesion shows nodular rim enhancement. (d) T1 W image in the portal venous phase after injection of contrast medium shows spreading enhancement. (e) T1 W image in the equilibrium phase after injection of contrast medium shows almost complete enhancement of the hemangioma (iris diaphragm sign).

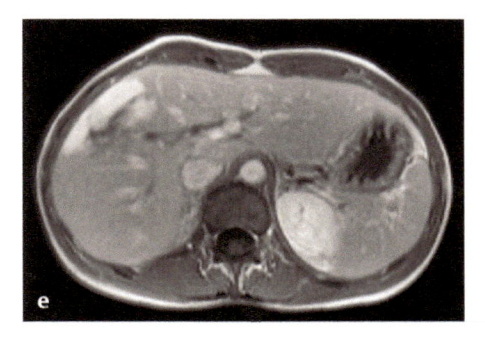

Note

Hemangiomas occasionally show a "shine through" effect on diffusion-weighted imaging. This means that the lesion, even when imaged at high b values, shows a high signal consistent with restricted diffusion. This effect is based on high T2 W signal intensity that "shines through" to the diffusion-weighted image. Viewed in isolation, this property is characteristic of a malignant hepatic lesion, but when combined with high signal intensity in the ADC map it is more suggestive of hemangioma than malignancy.[27]

▶ **Clinical features.** Hemangiomas are generally asymptomatic and are detected incidentally. Differentiation from other hepatic lesions is necessary.

▶ **Key points.** Cavernous hemangiomas have a pathognomonic enhancement pattern after IV injection of contrast medium. Capillary hemangiomas are difficult to distinguish from malignant hypervascular tumors and metastases on CT but are more accurately characterized by MRI.

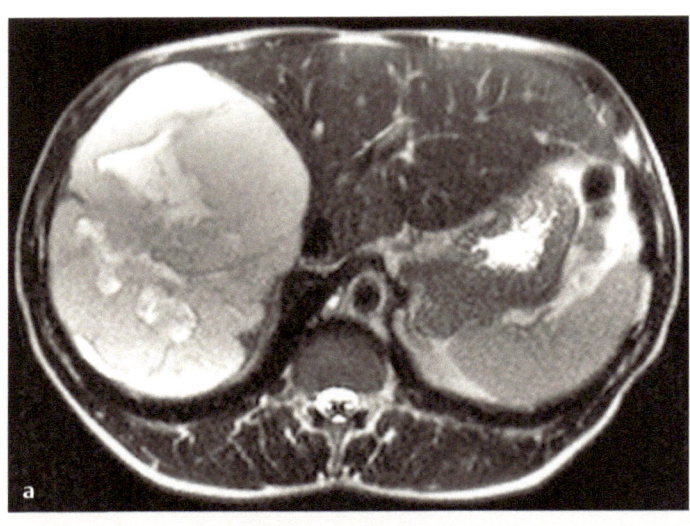

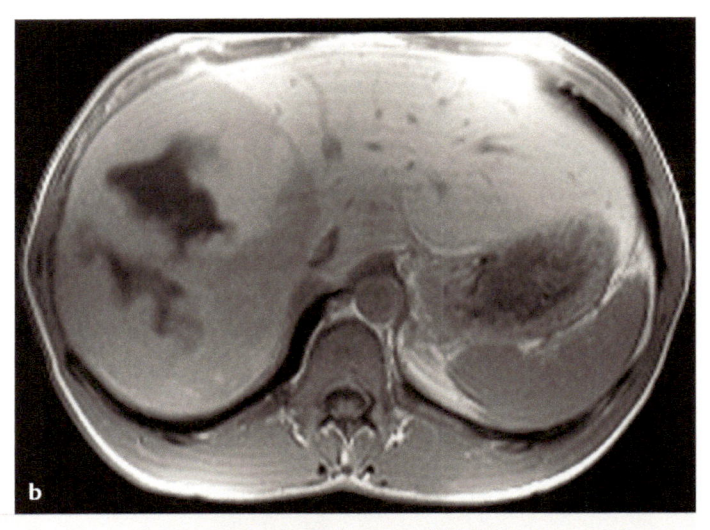

Fig. 5.24 "Giant hemangioma" in the right lobe of the liver. (a) T2 W image shows inhomogeneous hyperintensity. (b) T1 W image 15 minutes after injection of contrast medium. Enhancement is still inhomogeneous, consistent with the presence of central fibrotic components.

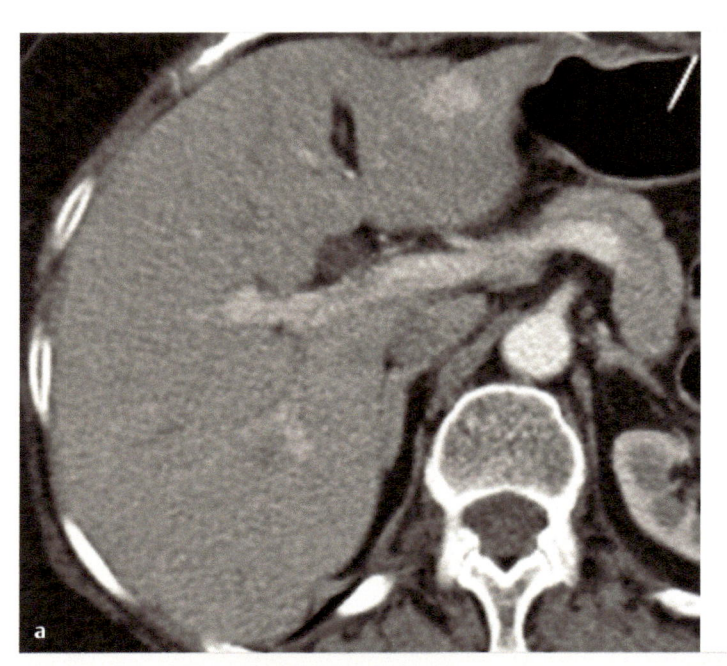

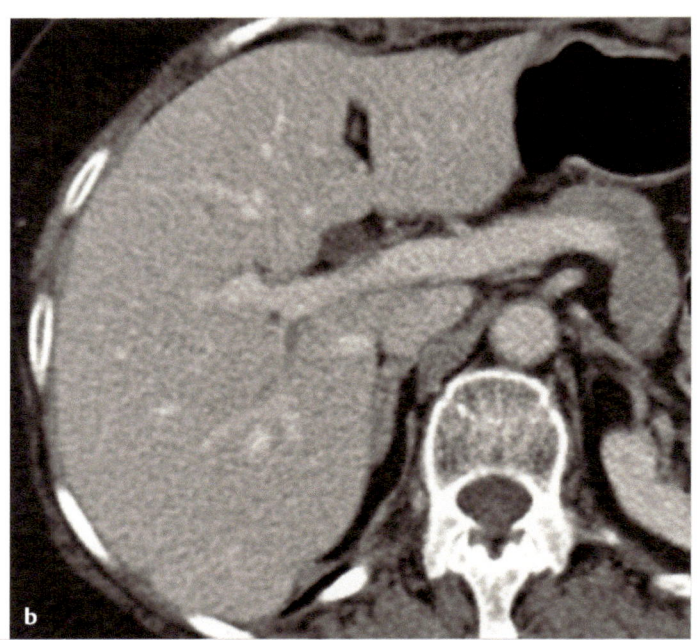

Fig. 5.25 Capillary hemangioma. (a) Arterial phase. The hemangioma shows intense enhancement. (b) Portal venous phase. The hemangioma has become isointense to surrounding parenchyma.

Lipomatous Masses

▶ **Brief definition.** Lipomatous masses constitute another group of benign mesenchymal liver tumors. Benign hepatic tumors that are composed partially or entirely of fat cells are lipomas, angiomyolipomas, myolipomas, and angiomyelolipomas.[28] Most lipomatous tumors are solitary, round, sharply circumscribed masses that occur in noncirrhotic livers. They contain variable proportions of fat, smooth muscle tissue, and thick-walled blood vessels. Hematopoietic components may also be present, in which case the term "myelolipoma" or "angiomyelolipoma" is used. Angiomyelolipomas are rare, usually asymptomatic solid tumors. Multiple angiomyelolipomas, which are sometimes symptomatic and show progressive growth, may be found in patients with Bourneville–Pringle syndrome.

▶ **Imaging signs.** On CT, angiomyolipomas show areas of fat attenuation along with intensely enhancing areas and areas of intermediate density (▶ Fig. 5.26). Their signal intensity on MRI reflects the tumor composition, and masses with predominantly lipomatous components have high signal intensity on both T1 W and T2 W images (▶ Fig. 5.27). By contrast, lipomatous masses with a dominant vascular or smooth muscle component will have low T1 W signal intensity and intermediate T2 W signal intensity. A presumptive diagnosis can be confirmed by fat-suppressed T1 W sequences and opposed-phase sequences to guide the detection of fat cells within the mass.[29,30]

▶ **Clinical features.** Patients are generally asymptomatic. Symptoms result from intratumoral hemorrhage, which may lead to

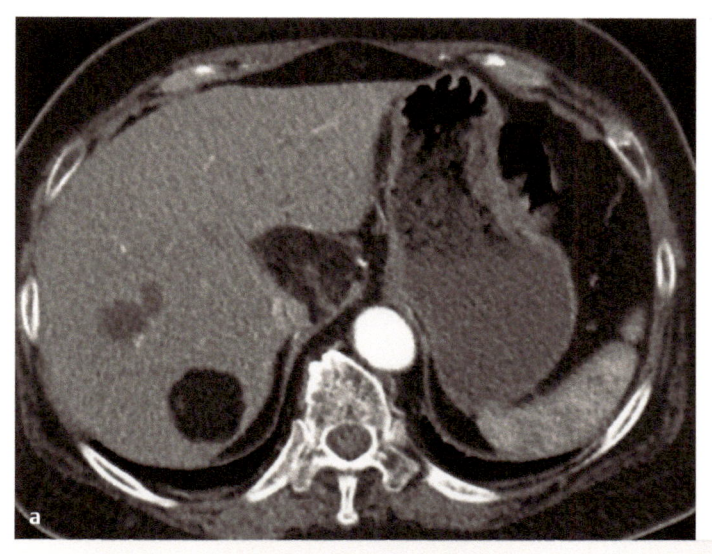

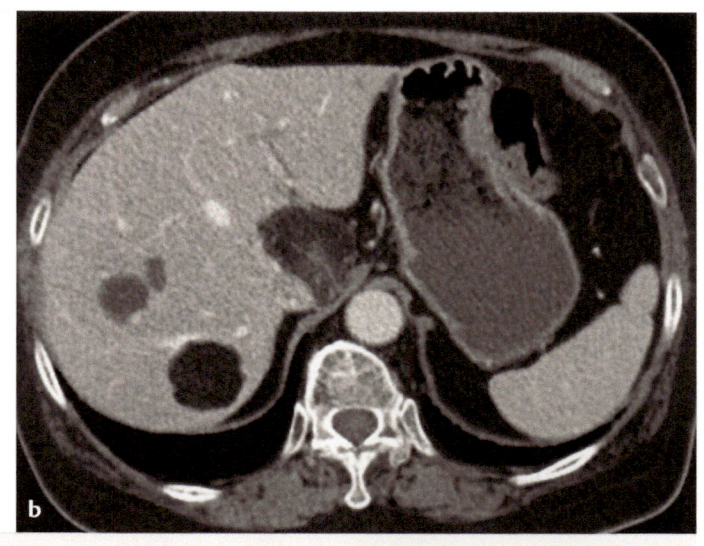

Fig. 5.26 Angiomyolipomas in segments I, VII, and VIII. (a) Arterial phase. (b) Portal venous phase. The angiomyolipomas show mixed density with large components of fat attenuation.

sudden pain or, in the case of capsular rupture, to hemoperitoneum and shock.

▶ **Key points.** Hepatic lipomas are rare tumors. As in the kidney, their imaging appearance is that of a mixed tumor with fatty components, vessels, and smooth muscle.

Hepatic Cysts

▶ **Brief definition.** Hepatic cysts are fluid-filled cavities lined with a single layer of epithelium. They are present in up to 10% of the population, so they are a common imaging finding. The etiology and pathogenesis of solitary hepatic cysts are not fully understood and it is also uncertain whether they are congenital lesions or true neoplasms.

▶ **Imaging signs.** When imaged with ultrasound, cysts are echo-free and have smooth margins (▶ Fig. 5.28). They are associated with posterior acoustic enhancement. Because ultrasound waves travel freely through the cyst and are not reflected as they are in the liver parenchyma, they are less attenuated at the far end of the liver than in the adjacent parenchyma. This causes the parenchyma behind the cyst to appear more echogenic, creating the impression of acoustic enhancement in that area. Cysts also have smooth margins on CT and do not enhance after IV injection of contrast medium. Simple cysts have an attenuation of approximately 10 HU (▶ Fig. 5.29). In rare cases, larger cysts may show intralesional hemorrhage producing an inhomogeneous signal pattern. Typically the lesions are hypointense with well-defined margins on T1 W images and are uniformly hyperintense on T2 W images. Postcontrast images show unchanged arterial vascularity around the cysts, and no enhancement occurs in the cyst wall or in the lesions themselves (▶ Fig. 5.30). This is an important aid to differential diagnosis as it excludes lesions such as hepatic abscess, parasitic cysts, and biliary hamartomas, which show peripheral rim enhancement.

▶ **Clinical features.** Cysts are asymptomatic. Very large cysts may cause a pressure sensation in the upper abdomen.

▶ **Differential diagnosis.** The differential diagnosis includes echinococcal cysts and cystic tumors.

▶ **Key points.** Hepatic cysts are present in approximately 10% of the population and are usually asymptomatic. On ultrasound, simple cysts are echo-free and show posterior acoustic enhancement. Cysts show smooth, nonenhancing walls on CT and have an attenuation of approximately 10 HU. On MRI, cysts are hyperintense in T2 W sequences and are hypointense and nonenhancing in T1 W sequences.

Benign Mesenchymal Tumors in Children

▶ **Brief definition.** Benign mesenchymal tumors that occur exclusively in children include infantile hemangioendothelioma and mesenchymal hamartoma:

- *Infantile hemangioendothelioma*: This is the most common benign liver tumor in the pediatric age group.[31] It is a vascular tumor derived from endothelial cells that proliferate in the form of vascular channels. Infantile hemangioendothelioma is responsible for approximately 10 to 15% of all liver tumors in children. Approximately 90% of infantile hemangioendotheliomas are detected during the first 6 months of life. They are usually multiple or diffuse; a solitary lesion is a somewhat unusual variant.
- *Mesenchymal hamartoma*: These entities comprise approximately 10% of all liver tumors in children. Mesenchymal hamartoma probably represents a localized abnormality of embryonic development that persists after birth. Histologically, mesenchymal hamartomas are composed of mesenchymal tissue and bile ducts, so that the tumors contain cystic components with internal septa. Accordingly, mesenchymal hamartoma is considered more a benign cystic malformation than a true neoplasm.[32] Mesenchymal hamartomas resolve spontaneously in most cases, although there have been sporadic reports of malignant transformation to sarcoma. Mesenchymal hamartomas occur exclusively in young children (average age 15 months). Progressive abdominal distention may occur, depending on tumor size. Because

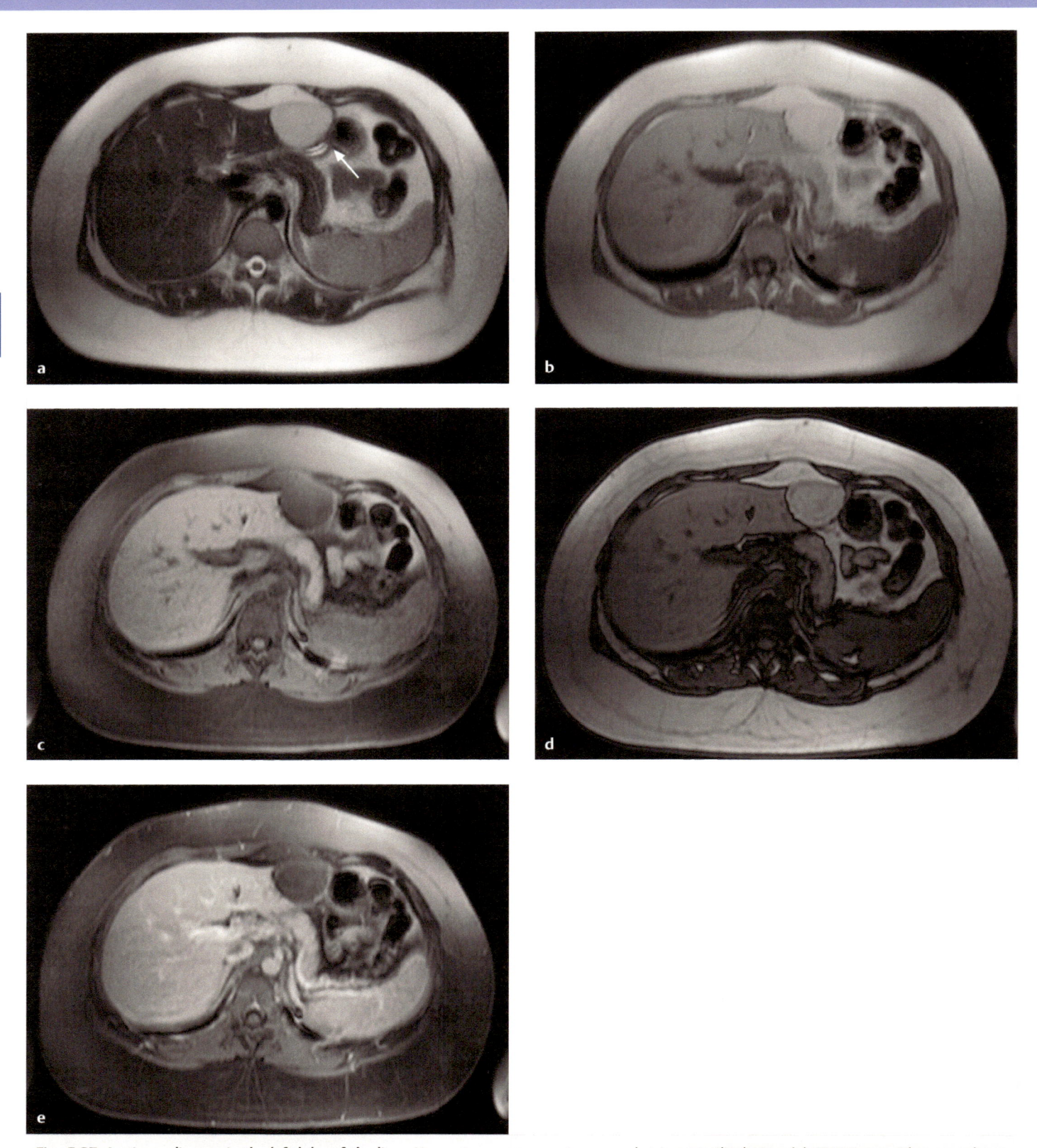

Fig. 5.27 Angiomyolipoma in the left lobe of the liver. Lipomatous components are predominant in this lesion. (a) T2W image. The mass shows high signal intensity (arrow). (b) T1W image. The mass also appears hyperintense in this sequence. (c) Fat-suppressed T1W image shows a marked loss of signal intensity. (d) Opposed-phase sequence does not show significant signal loss because the lesion consists mostly of fat cells. (e) Fat-suppressed T1W image after injection of contrast medium. The lesion shows virtually no enhancement.

imaging cannot positively differentiate mesenchymal hamartoma from other liver tumors (hepatoblastoma, embryonic sarcoma, hepatocellular carcinoma), histological confirmation is always required.

▶ **Imaging signs**
- *Infantile hemangioendothelioma*: Hemangioendotheliomas appear very echogenic on ultrasound (▶ Fig. 5.31). The presence of vascular channels and cystlike components with

5.5 Focal Hepatic Lesions

well-defined margins explains the hypointense pattern in T1 W images. The lesions usually show homogeneous hyperintensity in T2 W sequences, similarly to hemangiomas, although small areas of intralesional hemorrhage, thrombosis, fibrosis, or calcifications may create low T2 W signal intensity. Postcontrast images show an inhomogeneous pattern with mainly peripheral enhancement that fills in toward the center (▶ Fig. 5.32). Incomplete filling in the equilibrium phase indicates central regressive changes.

- *Mesenchymal hamartoma*: Mesenchymal hamartomas show mixed echogenicity at ultrasound. Cystic components are usually present, although the tumor may be completely solid. Ultrasound is the modality of choice for follow-ups. Most mesenchymal hamartomas will undergo spontaneous regression over time. They show mixed density on CT, with a combination of cystic and enhancing components. Prior intralesional hemorrhage may increase the density of the cyst contents. The MRI features of mesenchymal hamartoma are based on the dominant tissue structure, which may be stromal or cystic. Lesions with a dominant stromal component show low signal intensity in T1 W and T2 W images. Conversely, lesions that are predominantly cystic will show somewhat higher T1 W signal intensity and very high T2 W signal intensity, like other cystic tumors. Lesions typically have different signal intensities arising from multiple cystic components with intervening septa (▶ Fig. 5.33) due to differences in the concentration of protein-rich fluid.[32] The varying protein content identifies the lesions as mesenchymal hamartoma rather than simple cysts.

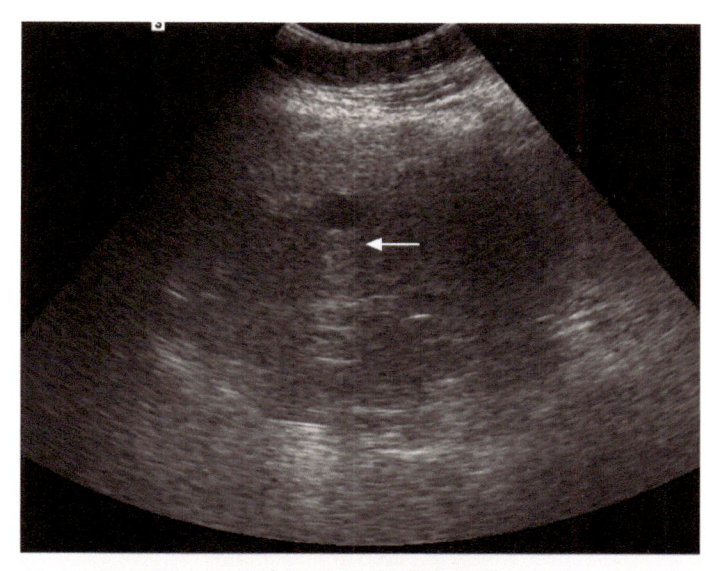

Fig. 5.28 Hepatic cyst. The cyst is echo-free and has smooth margins. Posterior acoustic enhancement occurs at the far side of the cyst (arrow) because the cyst causes less sound attenuation than the surrounding tissue.

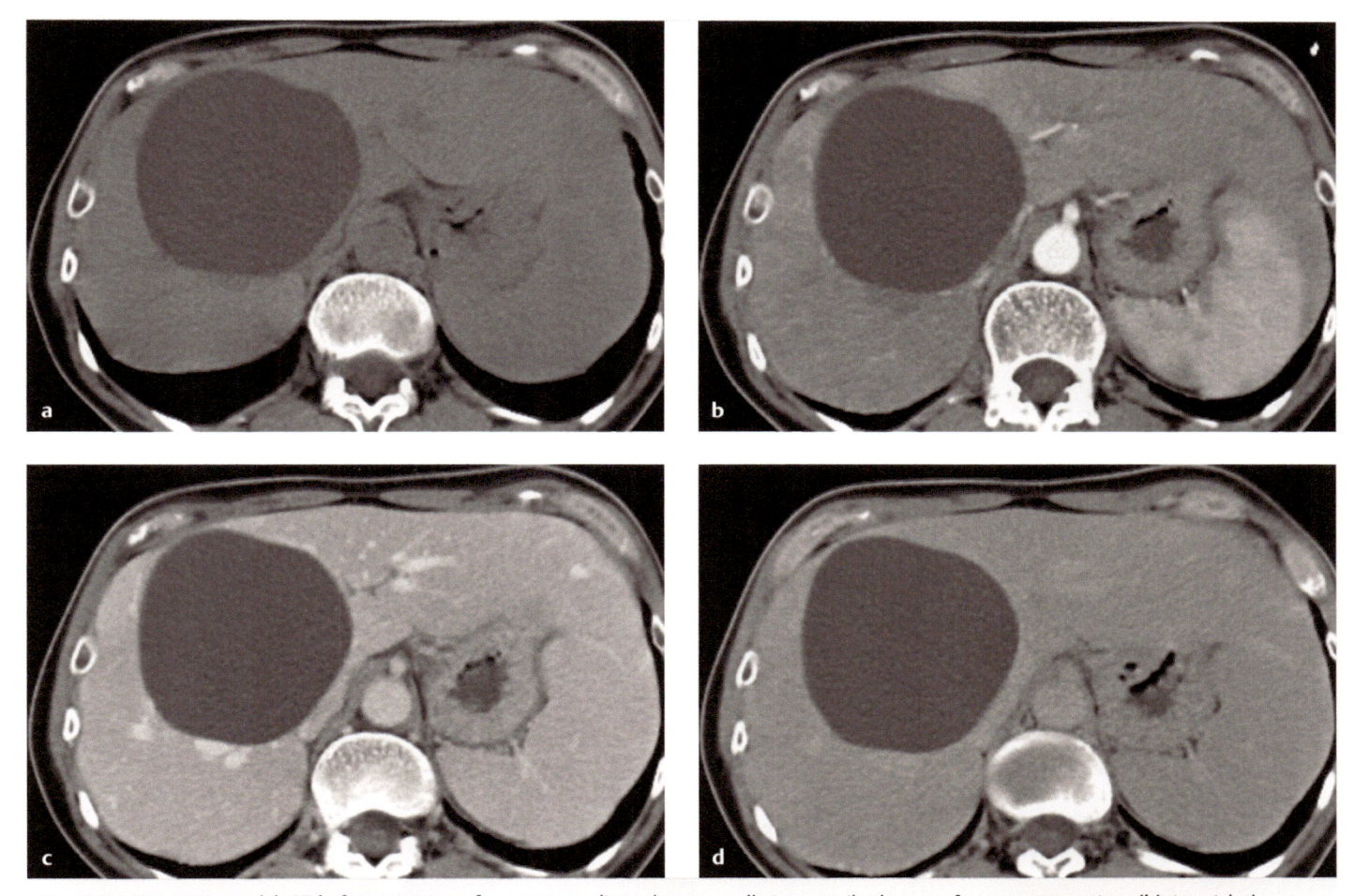

Fig. 5.29 Hepatic cyst. (a) CT before injection of contrast medium shows a well-circumscribed mass of water attenuation. (b) Arterial phase. (c) Portal venous phase. (d) Equilibrium phase. The cyst is nonenhancing in all phases.

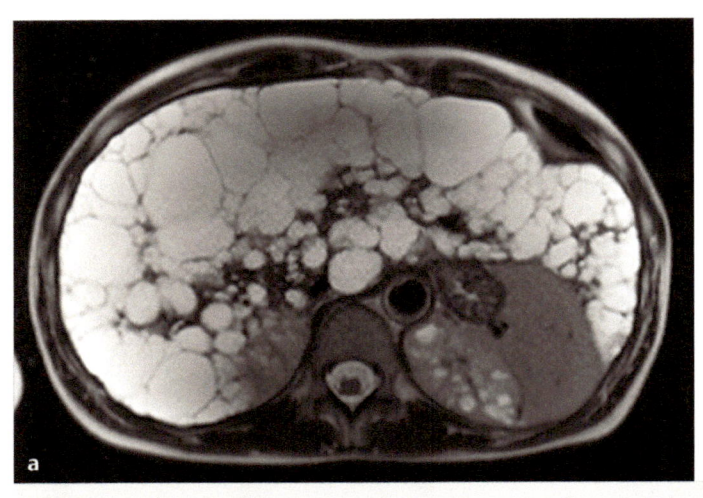

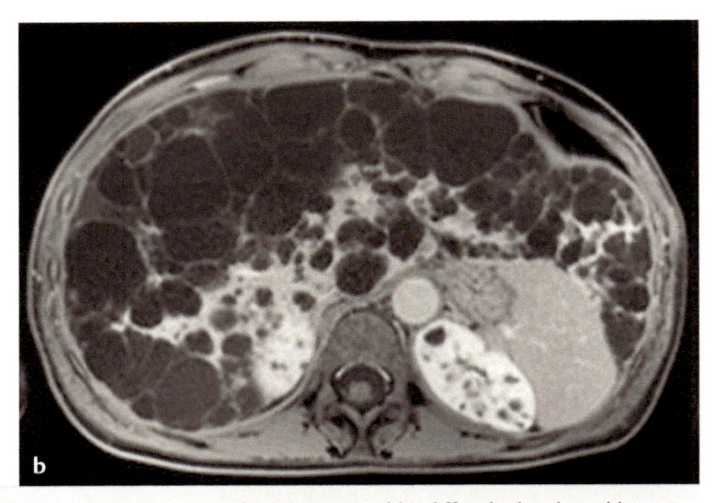

Fig. 5.30 **Multilocular hepatic cysts in a patient with polycystic kidney disease.** (a) T2 W image shows innumerable, diffusely distributed hepatic cysts with homogeneous high signal intensity. (b) Fat-suppressed T1 W image after injection of contrast medium. The liver parenchyma enhances without appreciable enhancement of the cyst walls or the cysts themselves.

▶ **Clinical features**
- *Infantile hemangioendothelioma*: The tumor must be relatively large to produce symptoms, which include hepatomegaly, right heart failure due to the left-to-right shunt,[33] and Kasalbach–Merritt syndrome due to thrombocytopenia. There have been rare cases of hemoperitoneum caused by the rupture of infantile hemangioendothelioma. The natural history of the tumor is benign, and lesions typically regress over a period of several months.[34] There are rare reports of infantile hemangioendothelioma undergoing malignant transformation to angiosarcoma.
- *Mesenchymal hamartoma*: This tumor may present initially as a palpable abdominal mass. Compression of the stomach or bowels may cause feeding difficulties in some infants. Mesenchymal hamartomas undergo spontaneous regression.

▶ **Differential diagnosis**
- *Infantile hemangioendothelioma*: The differential diagnosis includes angiosarcoma and cavernous hemangioma.
- *Mesenchymal hamartoma*: The differential diagnosis in this age group consists mainly of hepatoblastoma, embryonic sarcoma, and hepatocellular carcinoma. Differentiation cannot rely on imaging alone and requires histological confirmation.

▶ **Key points**
- *Infantile hemangioendothelioma*: This entity occurs as a benign tumor in children with a peak incidence in the first 6 months of life. It is distinct from the low-grade epithelioid hemangioendotheliomas that occur in adults.
- *Mesenchymal hamartoma*: The peak age of incidence of mesenchymal hamartoma is in infancy, and this entity is diagnosed almost exclusively before 1 year of age. Given its histology, the tumor presents a mixed appearance in all modalities. It cannot be positively differentiated from malignant liver tumors in the pediatric age group, so histological confirmation is always required. After initial detection by ultrasound, the next imaging

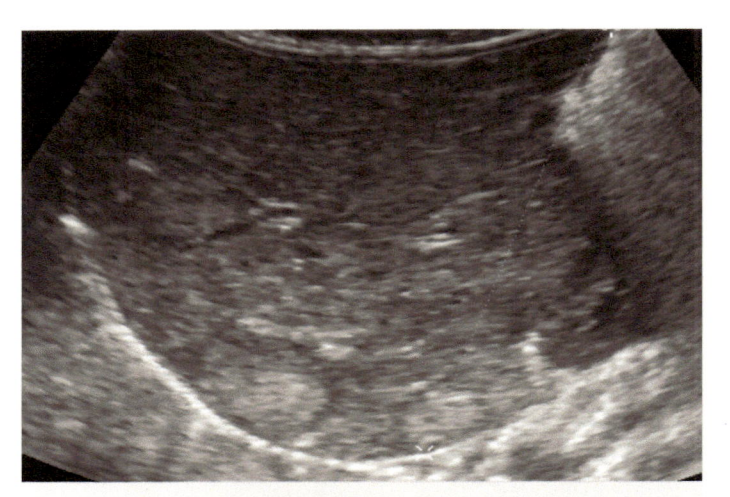

Fig. 5.31 **Hemangioendothelioma** in a 10-month-old child. Ultrasound findings are nonspecific, showing hyperechoic masses. But ultrasound is still a useful modality for follow-up.

study is usually MRI. Definitive lesion characterization requires biopsy. Since mesenchymal hamartomas generally resolve spontaneously, cases can be managed by sonographic follow-up.

Malignant Mesenchymal Tumors

Hepatic Angiosarcoma

▶ **Brief definition.** Hepatic angiosarcoma has a bimodal age distribution with one peak in early childhood and another in the sixth to seventh decade. Hepatic angiosarcoma in children is extremely rare and is viewed as a malignant form of infantile hemangioendothelioma.[35] Angiosarcoma in children may have an initial presentation similar to infantile hemangioendothelioma, but it does not regress over time. Instead it spreads diffusely into the surrounding tissue, identifying it as a malignant lesion. Hepatic angiosarcoma in adults is responsible for only about 1.8% of all primary hepatic neoplasms and is approximately 30 times rarer than hepatocellular carcinoma.[36] A predisposing factor is

5.5 Focal Hepatic Lesions

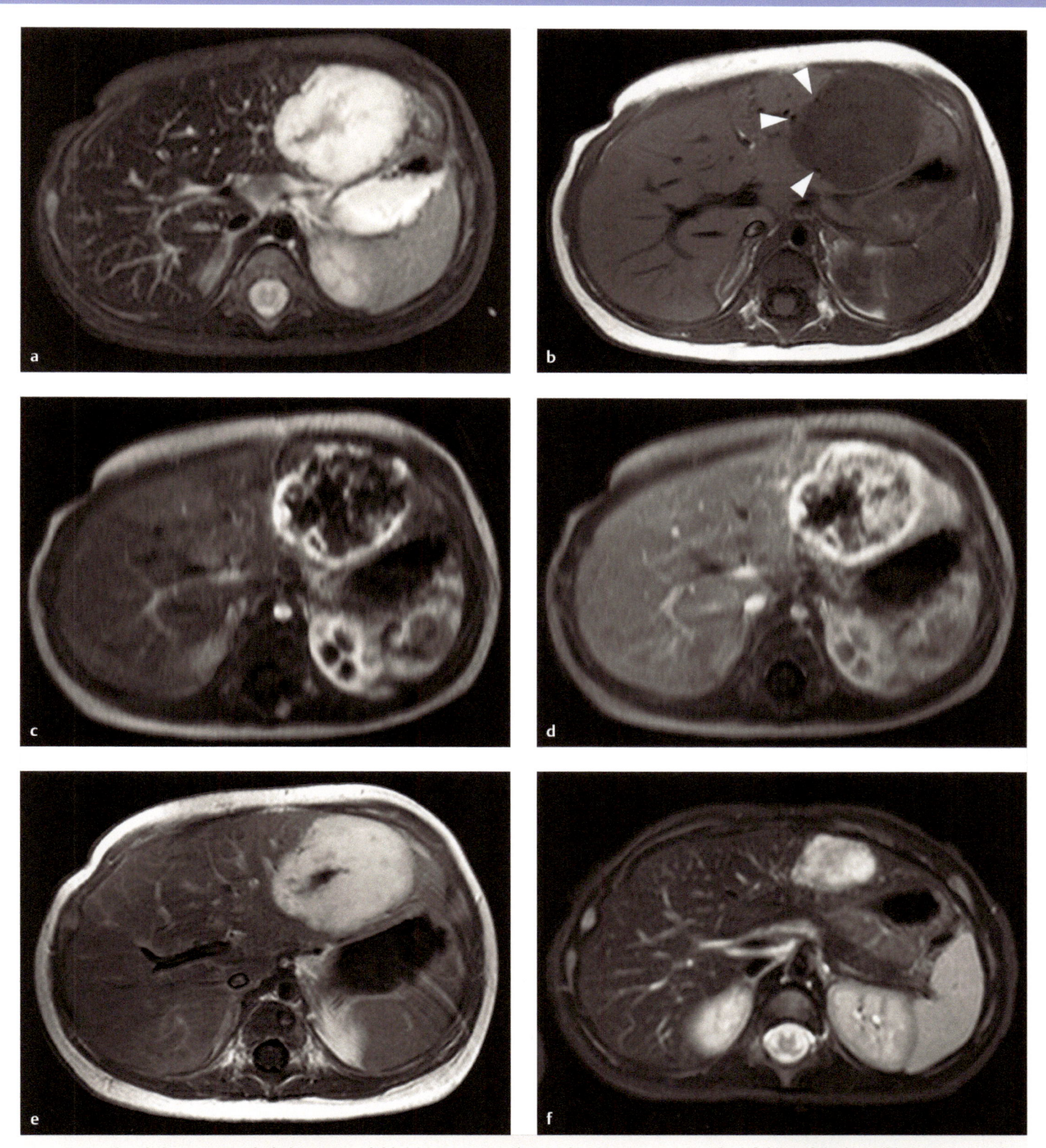

Fig. 5.32 **Infantile hemangioendothelioma in a child.** (a) T2W image shows a hyperintense mass in the left lobe of the liver. (b) T1W image. The mass shows low signal intensity. Vessels with flow voids (arrowheads) are visible at the periphery of the lesion. (c) T1W image after injection of contrast medium. Initial enhancement is mainly peripheral, though some central enhancement is also noted. (d) T1W image after injection of contrast medium, later phase. The lesion now shows inhomogeneous enhancement. (e) T1W image after injection of contrast medium, later phase than in (d). The lesion now shows inhomogeneous enhancement with sparing of central components, a signal pattern that is typical of infantile hemangioendothelioma. (f) T2W image 9 months later documents a significant, spontaneous decrease in lesion size.

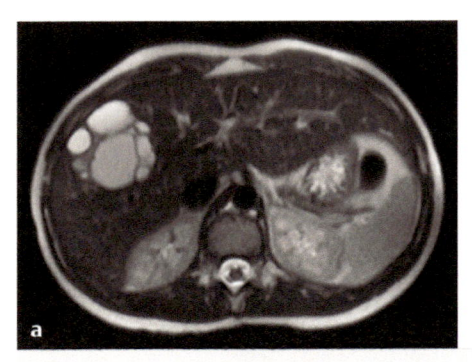

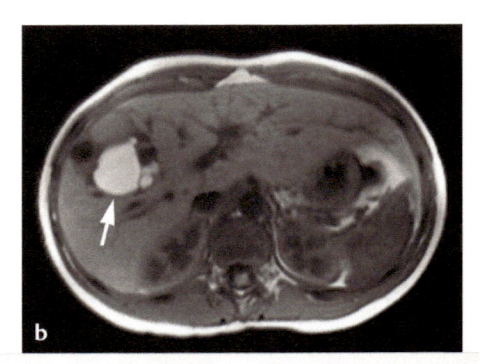

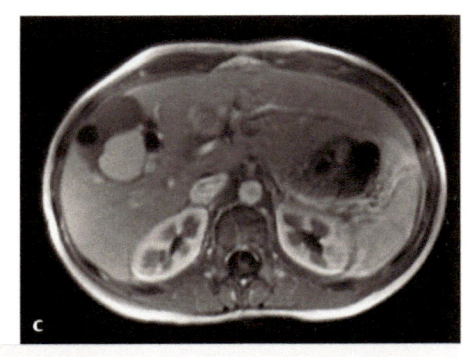

Fig. 5.33 Mesenchymal hamartoma of the liver in a child. (a) T2W image shows multiple contiguous cysts of varying signal intensity. (b) T1W image shows the contrasting signal intensities even more clearly. One large cyst has very high signal intensity (arrow) indicating the presence of protein-rich fluid. (c) T1W image after injection of contrast medium shows no enhancement of the cysts or cyst walls.

exposure to vinyl chlorides, arsenic, steroids, and radium. An increased incidence is also found in association with chronic idiopathic hemochromatosis and Recklinghausen's disease. Angiosarcomas arise from endothelial cells and do not have a capsule. The tumors consist of a disordered array of vessel-like clefts and structures and may show a nodular growth pattern or may aggressively infiltrate surrounding tissue in a very diffuse pattern.

▶ **Imaging signs.** Hepatic angiosarcomas have indistinct margins due to the absence of a capsule. They enhance intensely, and the enhancement persists into the equilibrium phase. Regressive changes are often visible within the lesion, and intratumoral cysts may form. Intratumoral hemorrhage is common with angiosarcomas, which may also bleed into their surroundings. As a result, large tumors may be accompanied by hemorrhagic ascites. Angiosarcomas may invade the hepatic vessels, leading to thrombosis. The combination of intratumoral cysts, regressive changes, and intratumoral hemorrhage give the tumor a heterogeneous imaging appearance in all modalities. Hepatic angiosarcoma in children may show early central enhancement and inhomogeneously enhancing areas (▶ Fig. 5.34), a pattern that differs from hemangioma but is similar to angiosarcoma in adults.

▶ **Clinical features.** Like other malignant tumors, hepatic angiosarcoma usually presents initially with B symptoms such as weakness and weight loss. Rapid growth may cause pain due to tension on the liver capsule. Biliary tract compression may cause jaundice. Tumor rupture with hemoperitoneum has been described. A large tumor volume may lead to consumption coagulopathy due to the large intravascular space as well as intratumoral thrombosis and hemorrhage. Many patients develop anemia. The mean survival time after diagnosis is 6 months.

▶ **Differential diagnosis.** Angiosarcomas require differentiation from metastases and vascular tumors such as epithelioid hemangioendothelioma, which occurs very rarely in adults (peak incidence: second to fourth decade with a female preponderance).

▶ **Key points.** Hepatic angiosarcomas are rare tumors that arise from endothelial cells and form disordered vascular spaces. This leads to intense enhancement on imaging. The tumors may develop regressive changes, creating a heterogeneous appearance.

Primary Hepatic Lymphoma

▶ **Brief definition.** Hodgkin's lymphoma and non-Hodgkin's lymphoma, like the leukemias, tend to affect the liver secondarily, but primary hepatic lymphomas have been reported increasingly. It is important to recognize these tumors because of the markedly better prognosis of primary hepatic lymphoma. The tumor may occur at any age from childhood to adulthood and shows a 4:1 predilection for males. It may be found in association with autoimmune diseases, chronic hepatitis, cirrhosis, and HIV infection. Most primary hepatic lymphomas present as solid masses, but diffuse infiltration occasionally occurs.[37]

▶ **Imaging signs.** At ultrasound the tumor usually has sharp margins and is hypoechoic to liver parenchyma. On CT, areas of intrahepatic lymphoma are hypodense following injection of contrast medium (▶ Fig. 5.35). On MRI the tumors often appear very similar to normal liver tissue in T1W and T2W images. After administration of contrast medium, however, the lesions appear hypovascular in the arterial and portal venous phases. They may return to isointensity in the equilibrium phase (▶ Fig. 5.36). The lesions are usually hypointense in the biliary phase while normal surrounding liver tissue shows a marked rise in signal intensity.

▶ **Clinical features.** The symptoms relating to secondary lymphomas are determined by the pattern of lymphoma spread. Primary hepatic lymphomas often cause a pressure sensation in the upper abdomen accompanied by B symptoms.

▶ **Differential diagnosis.** The most important differential diagnosis is hepatic metastasis. Diffuse involvement, like that found in secondary hepatic involvement by lymphoma, requires differentiation from hepatic steatosis (p. 232).

▶ **Key points.** Primary hepatic lymphoma is less common than secondary involvement of the liver by lymphoma. Primary lymphomas appear as circumscribed lesions and mainly require differentiation from hepatic metastases.

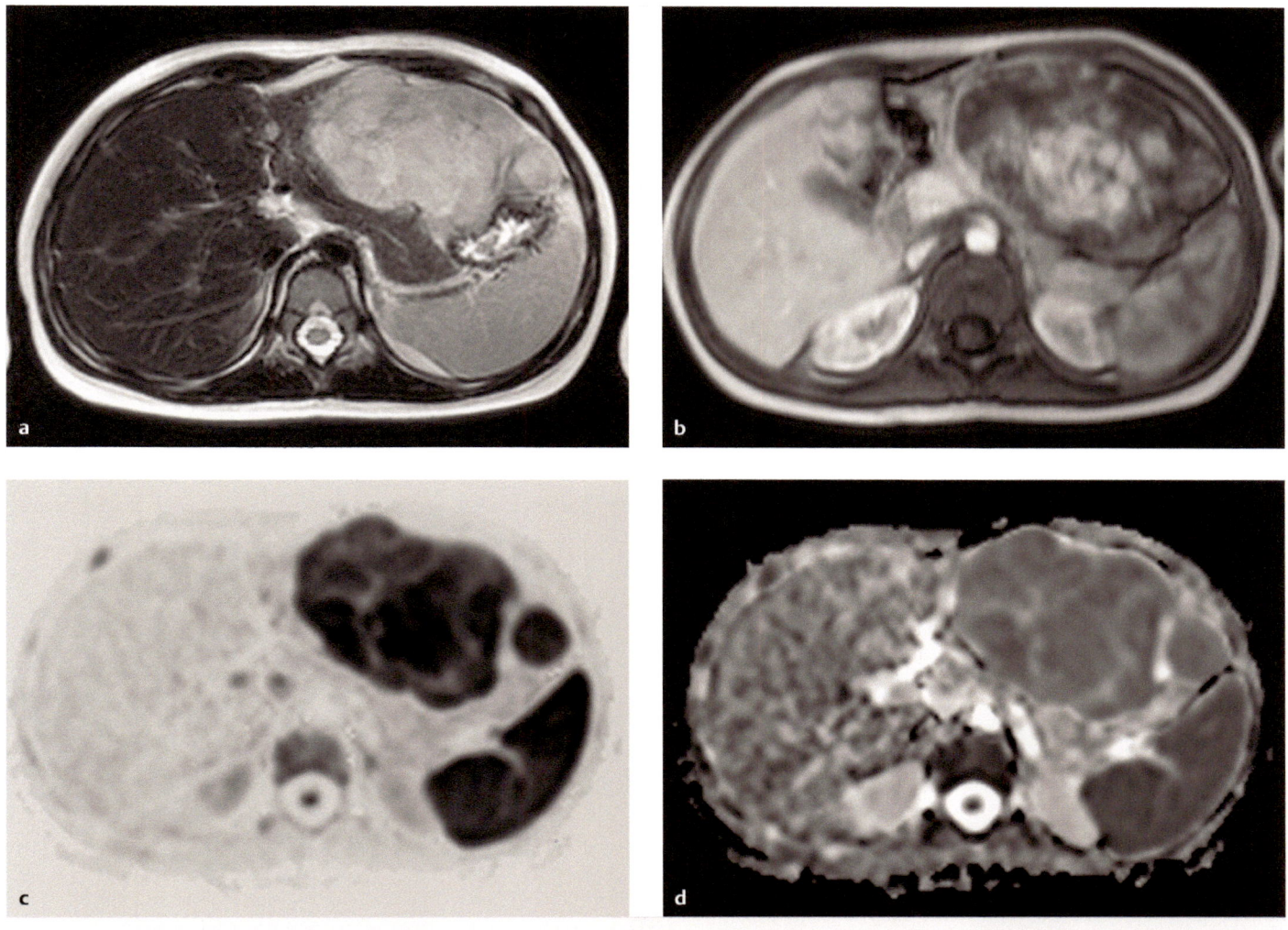

Fig. 5.34 Hepatic hemangiosarcoma in a child. (a) T2W image shows a large, relatively homogeneous, hyperintense tumor in the left lobe of the liver. (b) T1W image after injection of contrast medium shows inhomogeneous enhancement. (c) DWI with $b_0 = 1,400$. The lesion shows markedly restricted diffusion. (d) Hypointensity of the lesion in the ADC map is suspicious for malignancy.

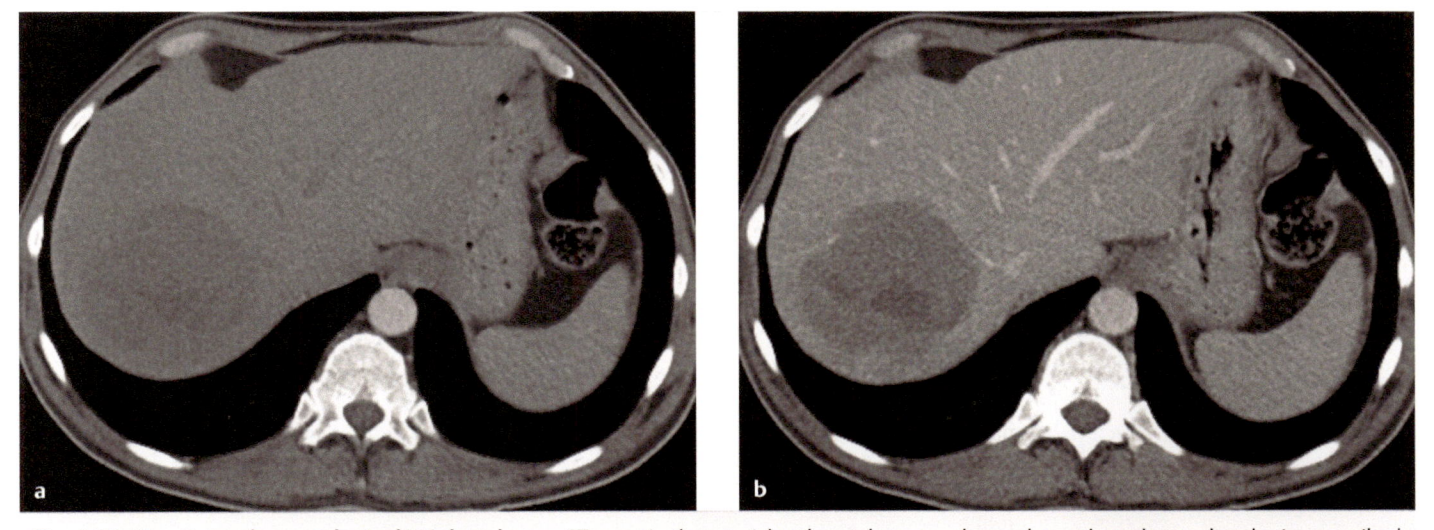

Fig. 5.35 Hepatic involvement by Burkitt's lymphoma. CT scans in the arterial and portal venous phases show a hypodense, sharply circumscribed mass with an inhomogeneous internal structure. (a) Arterial phase. (b) Portal venous phase.

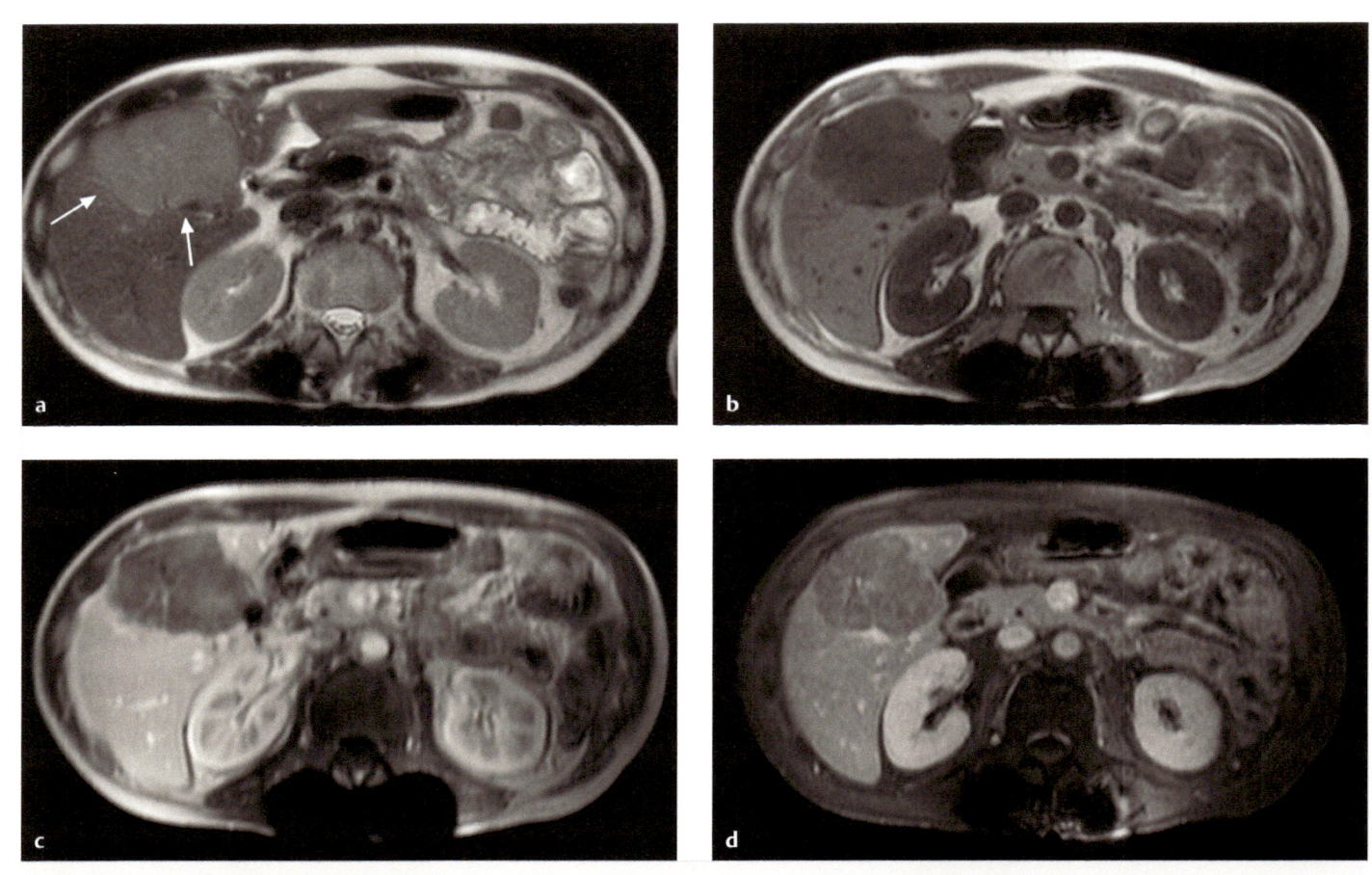

Fig. 5.36 Primary hepatic lymphoma. (a) T2 W image shows a homogeneous mass in the hepatic right lobe that is slightly hyperintense to the liver tissue (arrows). (b) T1 W image. The lesion shows homogeneous low signal intensity. (c) T1 W image in the portal venous phase after injection of contrast medium shows slight enhancement. Vessels pass undisplaced through the lesion. (d) Fat-suppressed T1 W image after injection of contrast medium. Image in the equilibrium phase shows homogeneous enhancement of the lesion, which is only slightly hypointense to normal liver tissue.

Primary Hepatocellular Lesions

Liver tumors of primary hepatocellular origin include both benign and malignant lesions. The most common benign lesions result from the nodular hyperplasia of liver tissue:
- Benign variants of hepatocellular lesions:
  - Focal nodular hyperplasia.
  - Regenerative nodular hyperplasia in association with Budd–Chiari syndrome.
  - Hepatocellular adenoma.
  - Regenerating nodules in response to parenchymal liver damage.
- Malignant variants of hepatocellular lesions:
  - Hepatocellular carcinoma.
  - Fibrolamellar carcinoma.
  - Hepatoblastoma in children.

Benign Primary Hepatocellular Lesions

▶ **Brief definition.** Focal nodular hyperplasia and adenoma occur predominantly in women 20 to 40 years of age. Regarding the etiology of focal nodular hyperplasia, the current prevailing theory is an underlying arteriovenous shunt leading to the focal hyperplasia of liver tissue.[38,39] These pathologic vessels occur at the center of the tumor, surrounded by connective tissue and appearing as a "central scar." Oral contraceptives may stimulate the growth of focal nodular hyperplasia but do not cause it. This differs from hepatocellular adenoma, which currently is believed to be caused by use of oral contraceptives.[40] Existing adenomas may regress following the cessation of contraceptive use. Similar considerations apply to regenerative nodular hyperplasia, in which concomitant underlying changes such as Budd–Chiari syndrome may be observed.[41,42,43] Adenomas may undergo malignant change.

▶ **Imaging signs.** Ultrasound imaging can rarely define the central scar of focal nodular hyperplasia. The tumors are smoothly marginated and may show varying echogenicity (▶ Fig. 5.37). Doppler ultrasound can detect the central vessels. On contrast-enhanced CT, focal nodular hyperplasia is hypervascular in the arterial phase of enhancement. The pathognomonic central scar can be clearly visualized in most patients. The tumors show rapid contrast washout and, by the portal venous phase, are usually isodense to the liver parenchyma (▶ Fig. 5.38). Adenomas have a nonspecific sonographic appearance. Central necrosis and prior intralesional hemorrhage create a heterogeneous pattern that may suggest a diagnosis of adenoma in the appropriate age group. Hepatic adenomas are usually hypodense on plain CT

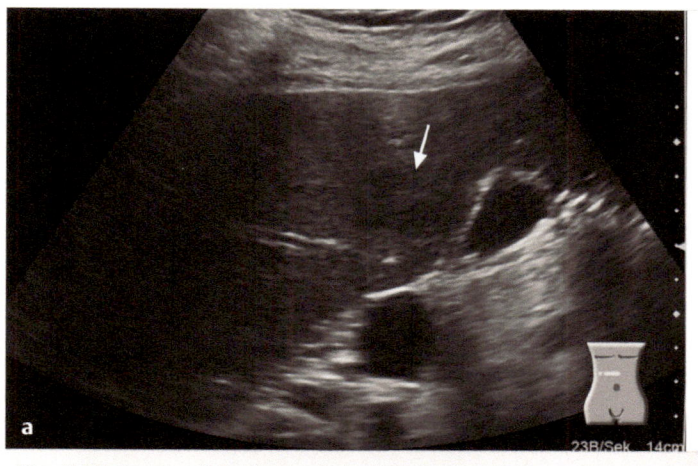

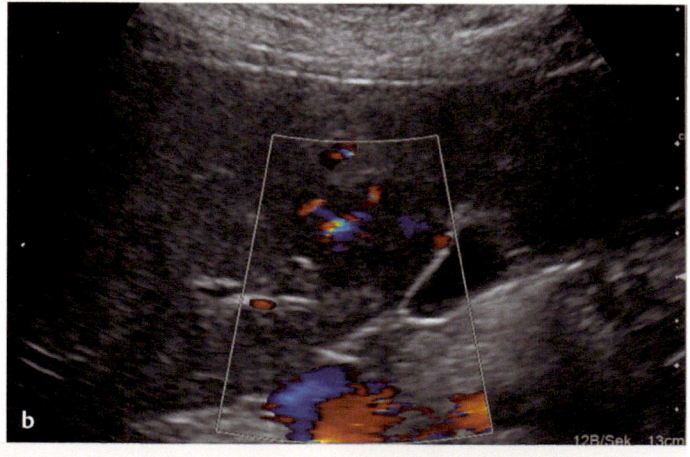

Fig. 5.37 Focal nodular hyperplasia. (a) Ultrasound demonstrates a hypoechoic mass with smooth margins (arrow). (b) Color Doppler scan shows typical convoluted vessels at the center of the mass.

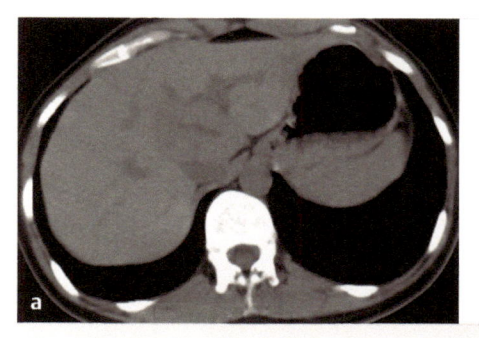

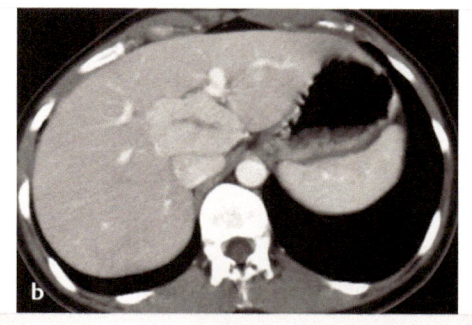

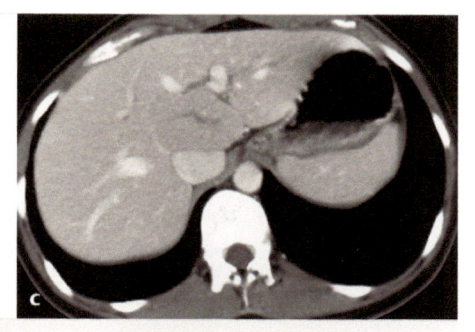

Fig. 5.38 Focal nodular hyperplasia in segment I of the liver. (a) Precontrast CT. A central scar is already visible without contrast medium. (b) Scan in the late arterial phase shows marked hypervascularity. (c) Portal venous phase. The area of focal nodular hyperplasia is isodense to the liver parenchyma.

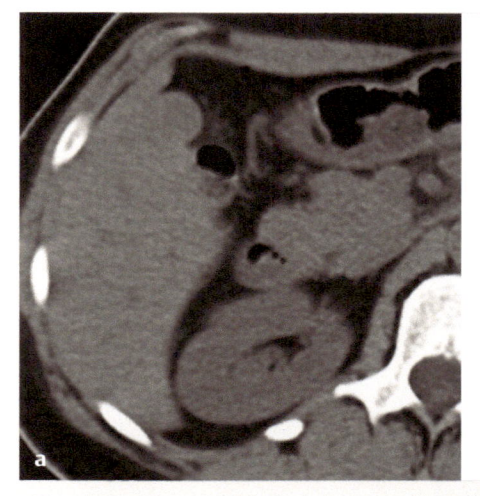

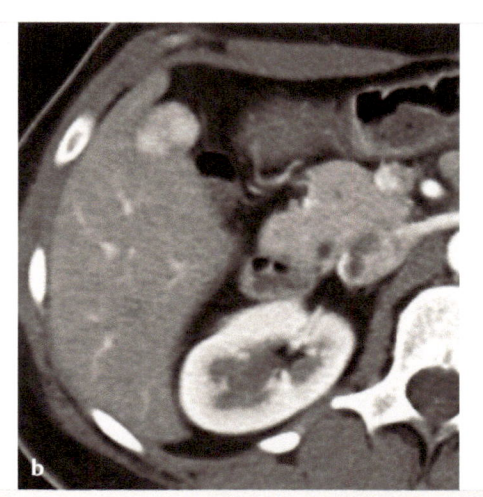

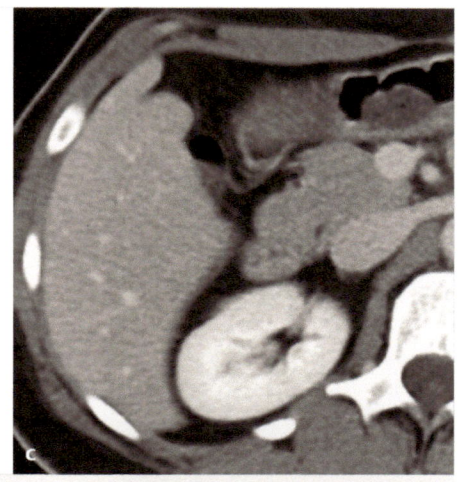

Fig. 5.39 Adenoma. (a) The adenoma is hypodense on precontrast CT. (b) Scan in the arterial phase shows intense enhancement. (c) Portal venous phase. The adenoma is isodense to surrounding parenchyma.

scans but may contain hyperdense areas due to prior intratumoral hemorrhage. Adenomas show homogeneous enhancement in the arterial phase, with possible heterogeneities due to necrosis and intralesional hemorrhage. Most adenomas are isodense to surrounding parenchyma in the portal venous phase (▶ Fig. 5.39, ▶ Fig. 5.40).

Note

Biliary contrast agents are very helpful in the differentiation of hepatocellular lesions on MRI, adding the characterization of lesion cellular structure to purely morphological distinctions (see ▶ Fig. 5.20).

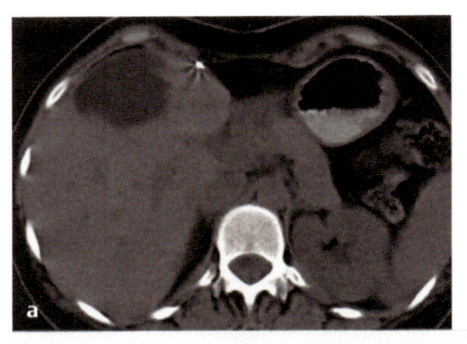

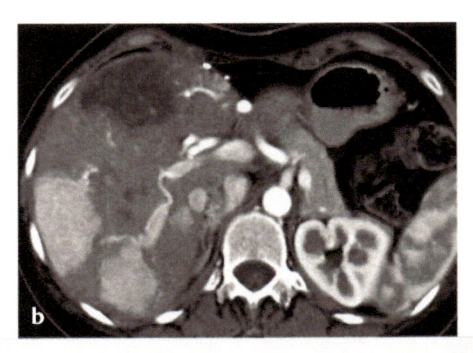

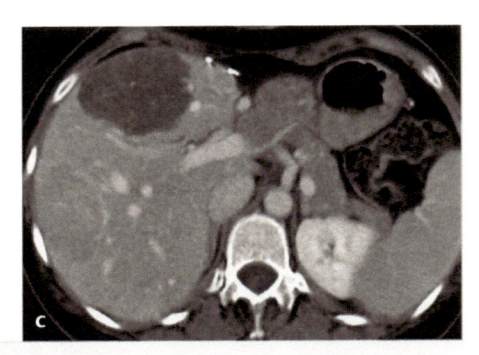

Fig. 5.40 Hepatic adenomas. (a) Precontrast CT. The adenoma in segment IV shows regressive changes and is already visible without contrast medium. **(b)** Scan in the arterial phase reveals two additional adenomas. **(c)** Portal venous phase. The other two adenomas are now isodense to surrounding liver parenchyma.

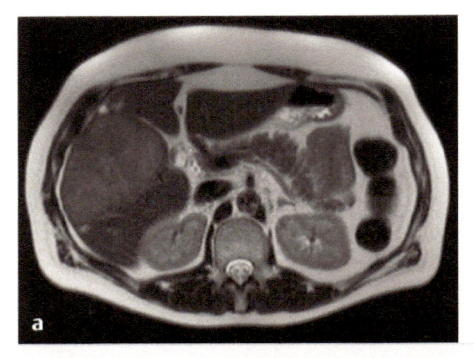

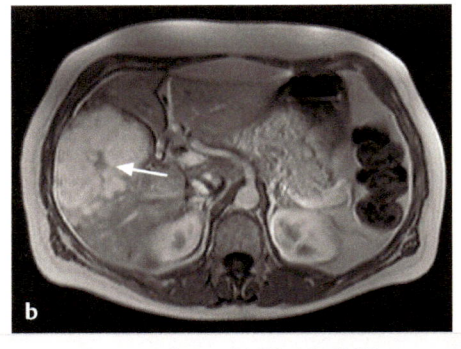

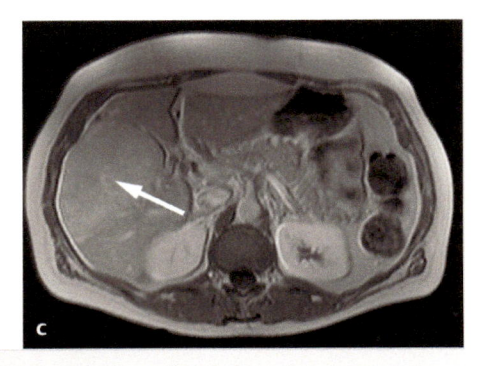

Fig. 5.41 Typical focal nodular hyperplasia. Dynamic contrast-enhanced MRI. **(a)** T2W sequence demonstrates a slightly hyperintense mass. **(b)** T1W sequence in the arterial phase of enhancement shows a very hypervascular mass with a central scar (arrow). **(c)** Equilibrium phase. The scar shows homogeneous uptake (arrow), identifying the mass as focal nodular hyperplasia.

Focal nodular hyperplasia and hepatocellular adenoma have similar features on unenhanced and contrast-enhanced MRI. Both show strong hypervascularity in the arterial phase, washout in the portal venous phase, and isointensity in the equilibrium phase (▶ Fig. 5.41). Although a central scar is found in typical focal nodular hyperplasia, this feature is absent in up to 30% of cases. This can make the lesion difficult to distinguish from hepatocellular adenoma, especially a small adenoma with no regressive changes or intralesional hemorrhage. However, focal nodular hyperplasia and hepatocellular adenoma do show histological differences, particularly regarding the presence of bile ducts: Focal nodular hyperplasia contains small biliary ducts that do not communicate with the larger bile ducts. This means that contrast agents that are excreted via the biliary system, such as Gd-BOPTA and Gd-EOB-DTPA, are taken up by the lesion. The lesion may even show greater uptake of contrast medium than normal liver tissue due to the absence of biliary drainage, causing it to appear isointense or hyperintense to liver tissue in the hepatobiliary phase (▶ Fig. 5.42). By contrast, biliary ducts are not present in hepatocellular adenoma, resulting in no uptake of contrast medium. Hepatocellular adenoma therefore appears hypointense to normal liver tissue in the biliary phase (▶ Fig. 5.43).[10,11] Both lesions are benign liver tumors that most commonly occur in young men and women of reproductive age who do not have hepatic cirrhosis. Resection is recommended for adenoma due to the risk of hemorrhage, while conservative management is preferred for focal nodular hyperplasia. Regenerating nodules[44] are typically found in cirrhotic livers; they may evolve in stages from a regenerating nodule to a hemosiderotic nodule, then to low- and high-grade dysplastic nodules, and finally hepatocellular carcinoma.[45,46] Hepatobiliary contrast agents cannot positively differentiate between hepatocellular carcinoma and benign precursor lesions. The literature contains numerous case reports of well-differentiated hepatocellular carcinomas that showed marked enhancement in the biliary phase.[47]

▶ **Clinical features.** Benign liver tumors are usually detected incidentally and remain asymptomatic. Adenomas are perfused at their margins and the tumor center may be hypoperfused, leading to necrosis. In turn this can lead to tumoral hemorrhage, which may become life-threatening if it breaks through the liver capsule. Given the risk of hemorrhage and malignant transformation in larger adenomas, tumors 5 cm or more in diameter should be resected.

▶ **Key points.** Benign liver tumors can often be differentiated from one another by their morphology and their enhancement characteristics on CT and MRI when liver-specific contrast agents are used. If this is unsuccessful, suspected hepatic adenomas should be biopsied because of the risk of malignant transformation and life-threatening hemorrhage with lesions larger than 5 cm. For these reasons, lesions 5 cm or more in diameter should be resected whenever possible. Focal nodular hyperplasia does not carry this risk, and so the differentiation of these entities has major therapeutic implications.

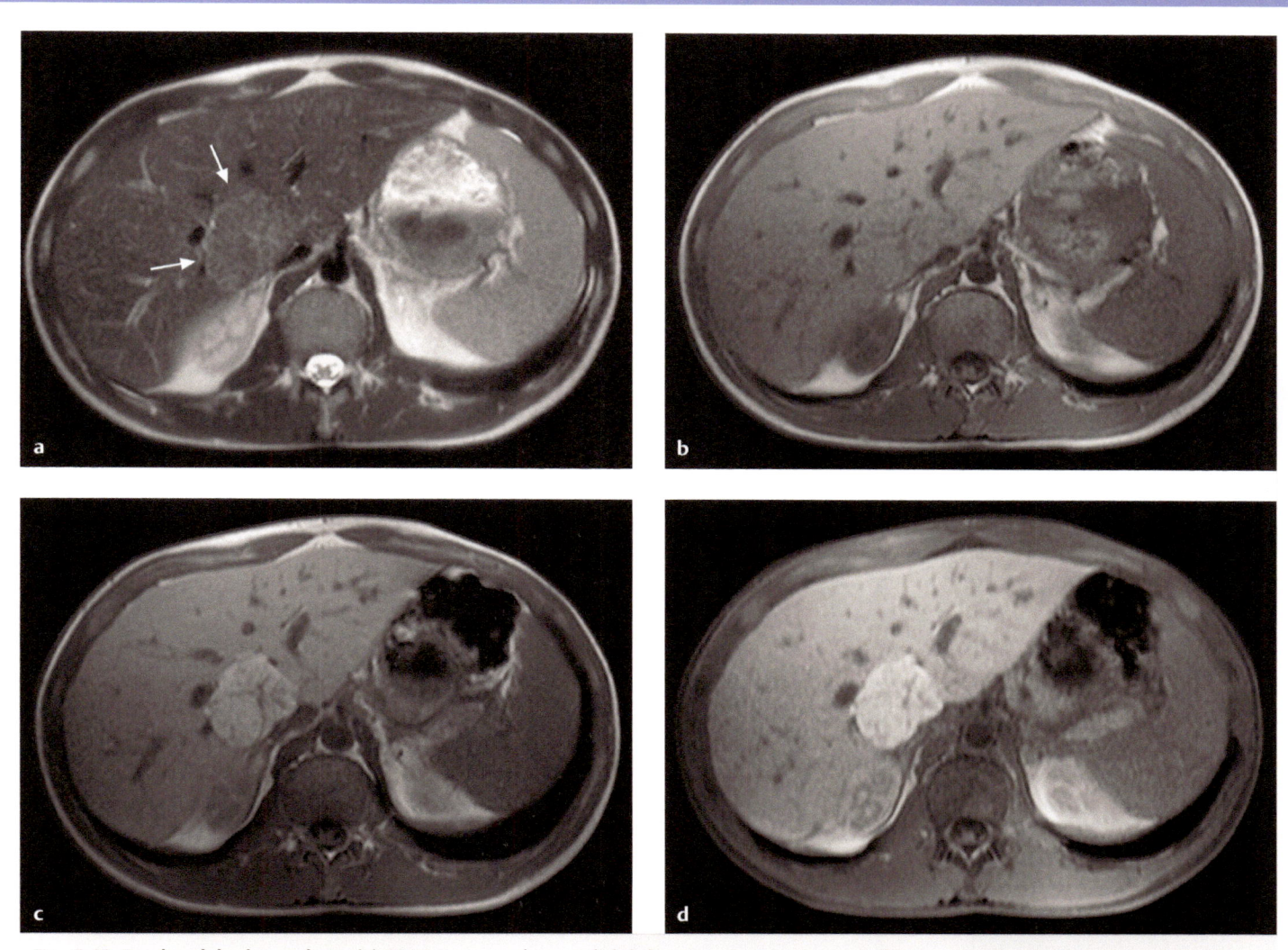

Fig. 5.42 Focal nodular hyperplasia. (a) T2W sequence shows a slightly hypointense mass (arrows). (b) Corresponding T1W sequence. The mass is isointense to liver tissue. (c) On dynamic contrast-enhanced imaging with a liver-specific contrast agent, the lesion was markedly hypervascular in the arterial phase (not shown). In the hepatobiliary phase 45 minutes after Gd-BOPTA injection at 0.05 mmol/kg BW, the T1W image shows markedly increased uptake relative to normal liver tissue, a pattern that is typical of focal nodular hyperplasia. (d) Corresponding fat-suppressed T1W sequence.

Malignant Primary Hepatocellular Lesions

Malignant primary hepatocellular lesions include hepatocellular carcinoma and fibrolamellar carcinoma in adolescents and young adults.

Fibrolamellar Carcinoma

▶ **Brief definition.** Fibrolamellar carcinoma is a rare tumor that occurs predominantly in children and young adults. Risk factors have not been identified and fibrolamellar carcinoma may occur in the absence of hepatic cirrhosis. Both sexes are affected equally. The prognosis is better than that of hepatocellular carcinoma because most fibrolamellar cancers are resectable and are not associated with other liver disease.

▶ **Imaging signs.** Fibrolamellar carcinoma may close resemble focal nodular hyperplasia in its imaging features (▶ Fig. 5.44).[48] However, 30% of fibrolamellar carcinomas are found to have central calcifications on CT,[49] a finding that is not observed in focal nodular hyperplasia. The presence of these calcifications makes a diagnosis of focal nodular hyperplasia unlikely. Moreover, fibrolamellar carcinoma does not show biliary enhancement on MRI, providing another useful differentiating criterion from focal nodular hyperplasia.[49] Fibrolamellar carcinoma is often similar to focal nodular hyperplasia in unenhanced T1W and T2W images, fat-suppressed sequences, and DWI (▶ Fig. 5.45). The tumor is definitely distinct from hepatocellular carcinoma and occurs in the absence of underlying cirrhosis.[50]

Hepatocellular Carcinoma

▶ **Brief definition.** Approximately 90% of all hepatocellular carcinomas occur in a cirrhotic liver. The tumor arises from initially benign regenerating nodules. The etiology has been linked to infection with the hepatitis B virus and exposure to exogenous agents such as aflatoxin. Hepatocellular carcinoma is more common in males than in females. Because patients with hepatic cirrhosis have a 4% annual risk of developing hepatocellular carcinoma, cirrhosis patients are screened by determination of their alpha-fetoprotein titer and by hepatic ultrasound.

▶ **Imaging signs.** In 2013, important recommendations on the radiology of hepatocellular carcinoma based on current study

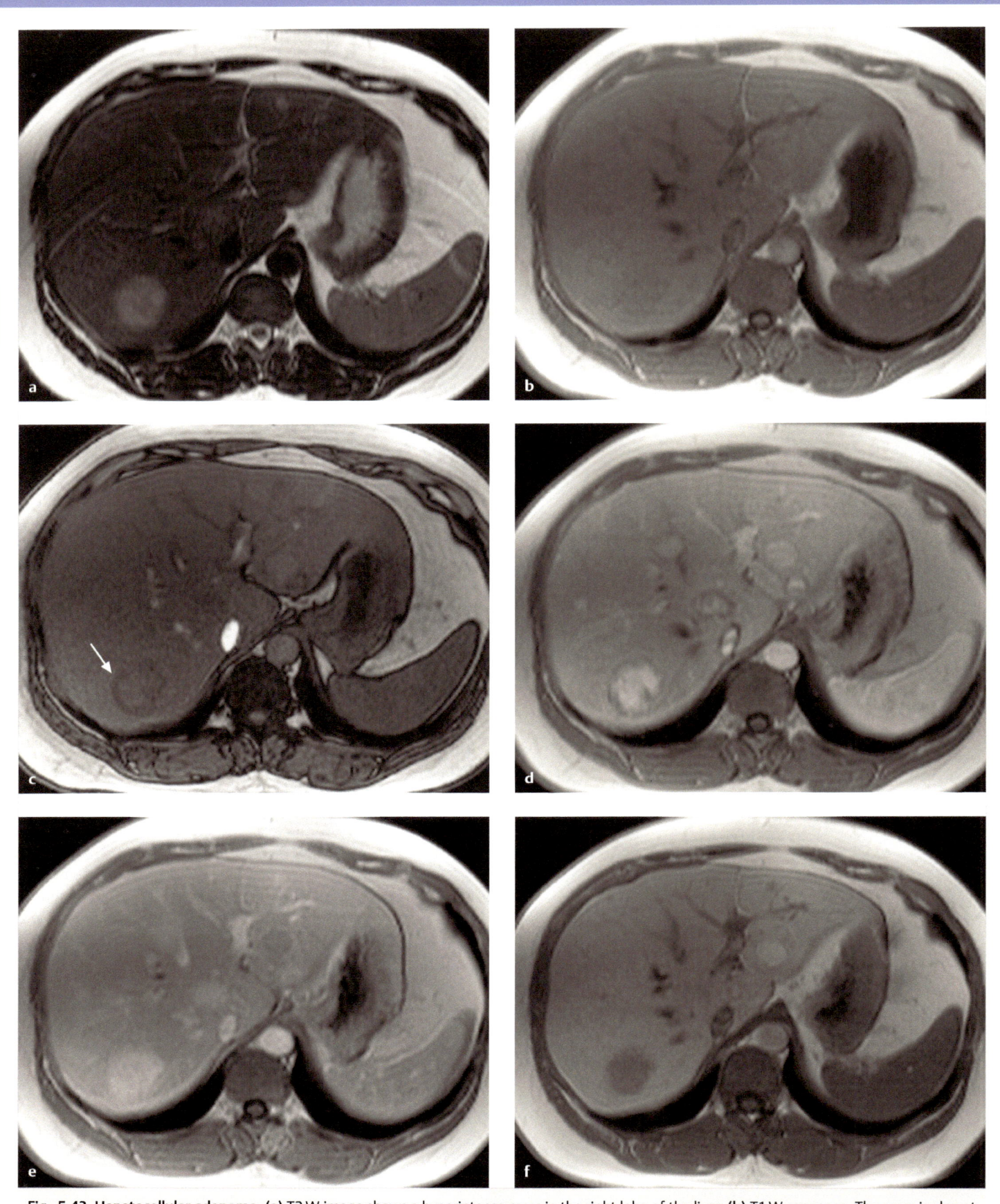

Fig. 5.43 **Hepatocellular adenoma.** (a) T2 W image shows a hyperintense mass in the right lobe of the liver. (b) T1 W sequence. The mass is almost isointense to liver tissue. (c) Opposed-phase sequence. Hypointense areas in the periphery of the mass suggest the presence of intralesional fat. This finding is not typical of focal nodular hyperplasia. (d) Arterial phase of dynamic contrast-enhanced imaging. The lesion shows marked hypervascularity. (e) Image in the portal venous phase shows persistent lesion enhancement. (f) T1 W image in the hepatobiliary phase of contrast excretion 45 minutes after Gd-BOPTA injection at 0.05 mmol/kg BW. Unlike focal nodular hyperplasia, the mass is hypointense to surrounding liver tissue, consistent with hepatocellular adenoma.

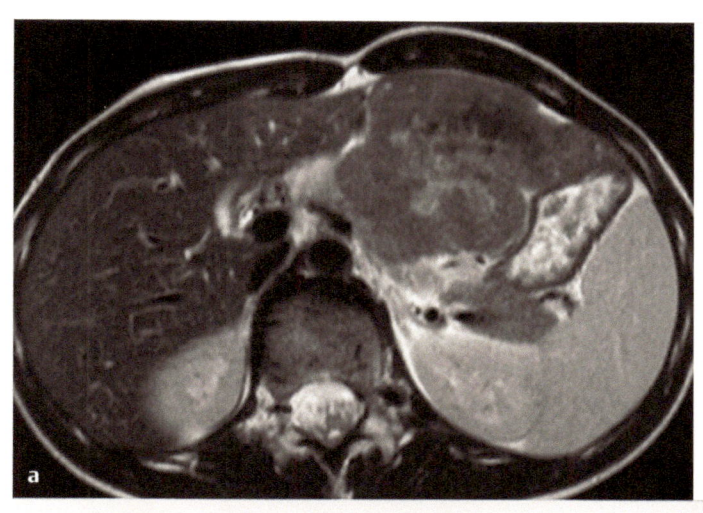

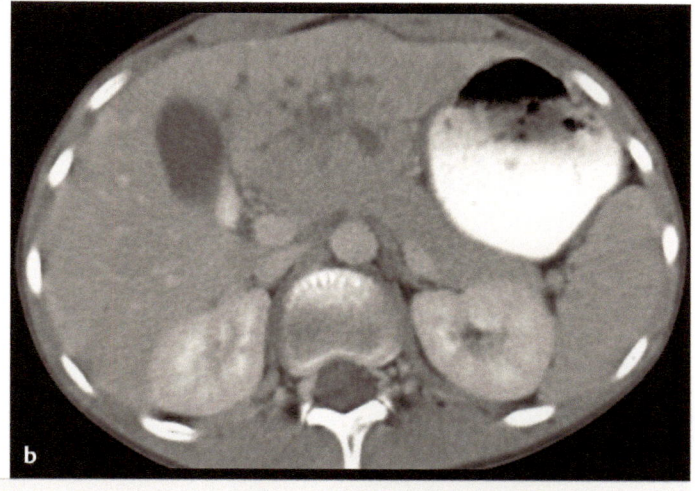

Fig. 5.44 Fibrolamellar carcinoma. (a) Axial T2 W TSE image. The carcinoma in the left lobe is hyperintense to liver parenchyma. (b) CT scan in the portal venous phase. The central scar is clearly visible.

data were published within the framework of S3 guidelines.[51] European guidelines recognize noninvasive imaging as the clinical standard for the diagnosis of hepatocellular carcinoma when lesions are more than 1 cm in diameter. Acceptable techniques are contrast-enhanced ultrasonography, CT, and MRI. For new lesions larger than 2 cm in a cirrhotic liver, diagnosis requires the detection of hyperperfusion in the arterial phase in two imaging techniques, or of arterial hyperperfusion combined with rapid washout in the portal venous phase in one imaging technique. For lesions larger than 1 cm but smaller than 2 cm, diagnosis requires the detection of arterial hyperperfusion and rapid washout.[52] A 2009 meta-analysis found that ultrasound had a sensitivity of 94% and specificity of 94% in the detection of hepatocellular carcinoma.[53] A comparative study also published in 2009 found that MRI had a sensitivity of 94% and specificity of 98%.[54] CT has a sensitivity of 67.5% and specificity of 92.5%.[55] The sensitivity of all modalities depends critically on the size of the hepatocellular carcinoma.

Note

With tumors smaller than 2 cm that are suspicious for hepatocellular carcinoma and do not show typical enhancement characteristics on initial imaging, biopsy provides the highest sensitivity. For lesions larger than 2 cm, histology and a second sectional imaging technique have equivalent sensitivity and specificity, so a second imaging technique should be used. If enhancement hallmarks of hepatocellular carcinoma are found in the second technique, a diagnosis of hepatocellular carcinoma can be made in a cirrhotic liver without further histological investigation, allowing treatment to be initiated. Biopsy is appropriate only if its result could have therapeutic implications.

The risk of seeding tumor cells into the needle track is negligibly small in image-guided percutaneous biopsy of hepatocellular carcinoma.[56] A major diagnostic criterion for hepatocellular carcinoma is the presence of a hypervascular lesion in the arterial phase in a cirrhotic liver.[57,58,59] Other criteria are early washout of the contrast material in the portal venous phase and lesion hypointensity in the equilibrium phase (▶ Fig. 5.46, ▶ Fig. 5.47).

Another enhancement characteristic of hepatocellular carcinoma is the detection of a pseudocapsule around the lesion (see ▶ Fig. 5.47f), which typically is observed in the equilibrium phase.[60] If the lesion does not enhance in the biliary phase, this would support a diagnosis of hepatocellular carcinoma (▶ Fig. 5.48).[61,62,63] If the lesion does enhance, hepatocellular carcinoma cannot be excluded, as noted above.[47] Hepatocellular carcinomas are often very inhomogeneous tumors, and this property is reflected in T1 W and T2 W images: Hepatocellular carcinoma may contain both fatty and cystic areas, causing the tumor to have a heterogeneous internal structure on images.

▶ **Clinical features.** Because hepatocellular carcinoma arises in a cirrhotic liver, the dominant symptoms are those of hepatic cirrhosis. The tumor itself may eventually become symptomatic as it enlarges. As with other malignant tumors, the cardinal symptoms are fatigue, night sweats, and undesired weight loss. Jaundice usually does not occur until the late stage. In rare cases, spontaneous rupture and intraperitoneal hemorrhage may occur. The new guideline has introduced a new treatment recommendation in patients with hepatic cirrhosis. Primary surgical treatment is indicated only for patients *without* hepatic cirrhosis who have a resectable hepatocellular carcinoma. Several radiological techniques are available for the treatment of hepatocellular carcinoma:

- *Radiofrequency ablation*: Radiofrequency ablation is a potentially curative procedure in which a percutaneous needle is inserted into the liver and delivers an alternating current to the targeted lesion. The alternating current excites increased molecular motion in the tissue, generating heat and inducing local necrosis through the denaturation of proteins. Lesions up to 5 cm in diameter can be ablated with this technique. In patients with 1 to 3 foci of hepatocellular carcinoma at child stage A or B and the largest lesion less than 3 cm in diameter, primary treatment should consist of radiofrequency ablation or surgical resection. Both procedures result in identical survival rates. In patients with 1 to 3 hepatocellular carcinomas larger than 3 cm but smaller than 5 cm, the decision between radiofrequency ablation and resection can be made on an individual basis by an interdisciplinary tumor board. If radiofrequency ablation is opted for, it should be preceded by

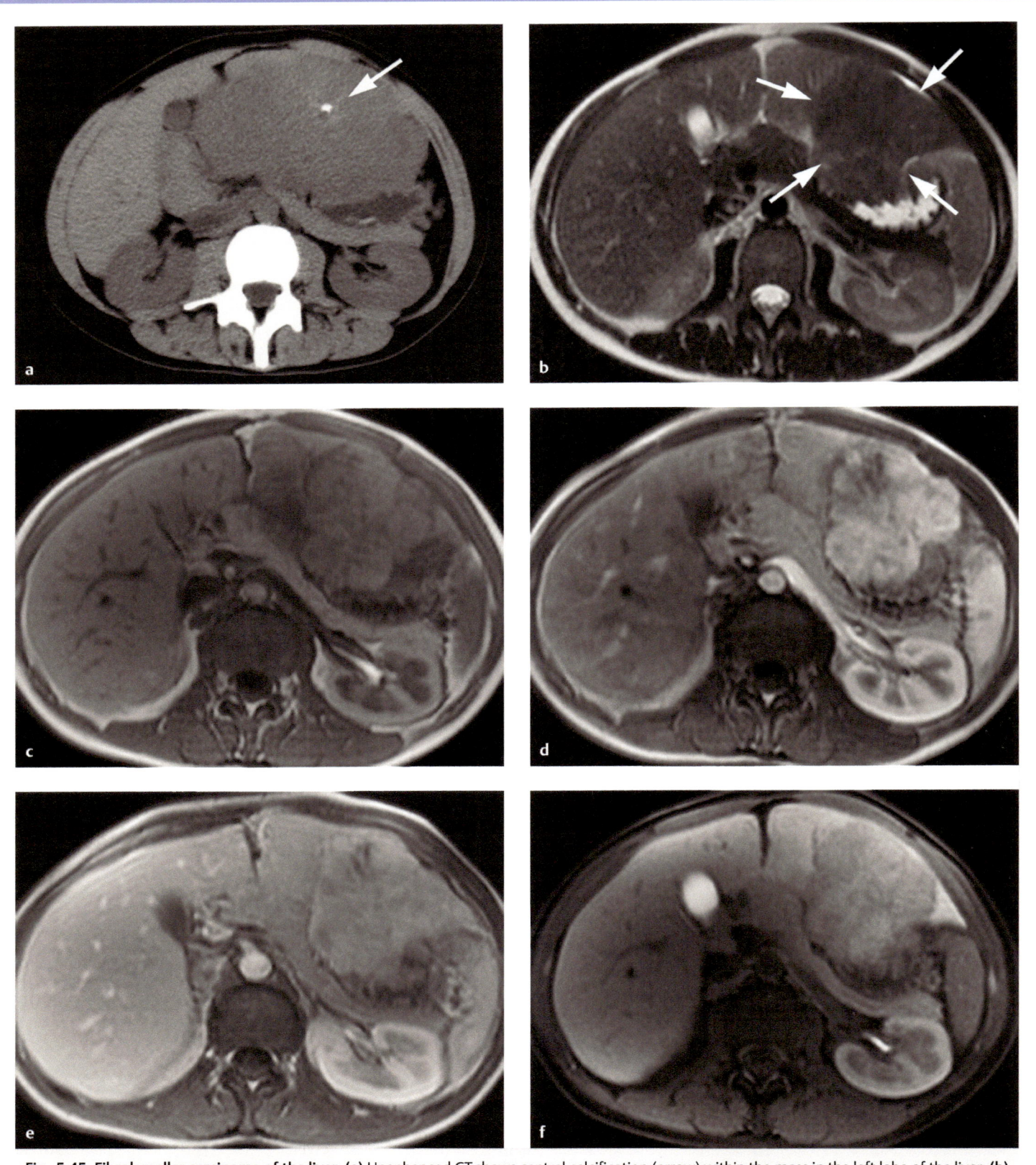

Fig. 5.45 Fibrolamellar carcinoma of the liver. (a) Unenhanced CT shows central calcification (arrow) within the mass in the left lobe of the liver. **(b)** T2W sequence. The mass appears hypointense (arrows). **(c)** T1W sequence. The mass appears almost isointense. **(d)** Dynamic T1W contrast-enhanced MRI. **(e)** Dynamic T1W contrast-enhanced image in a later phase. As in the unenhanced image, the lesion resembles focal nodular hyperplasia. **(f)** Hepatobiliary phase 45 minutes after Gd-BOPTA injection at 0.05 mmol/kg BW. The lesion is not enhanced in this phase. This indicates a lesion with nonfunctioning hepatocytes, in this case fibrolamellar carcinoma.

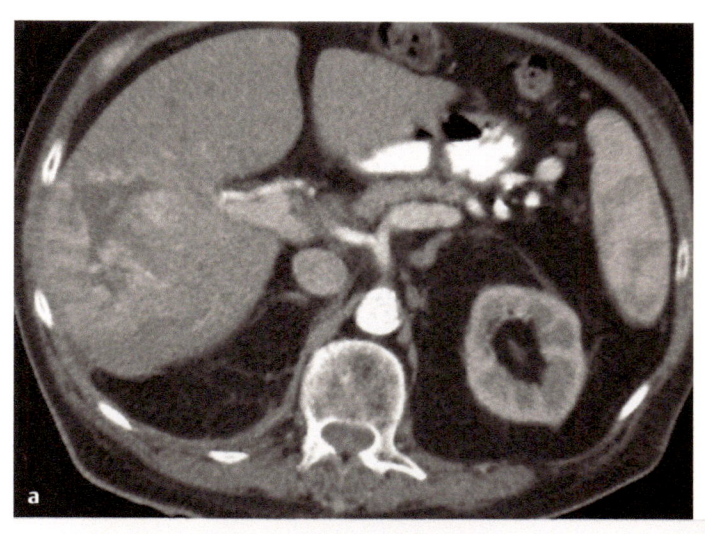

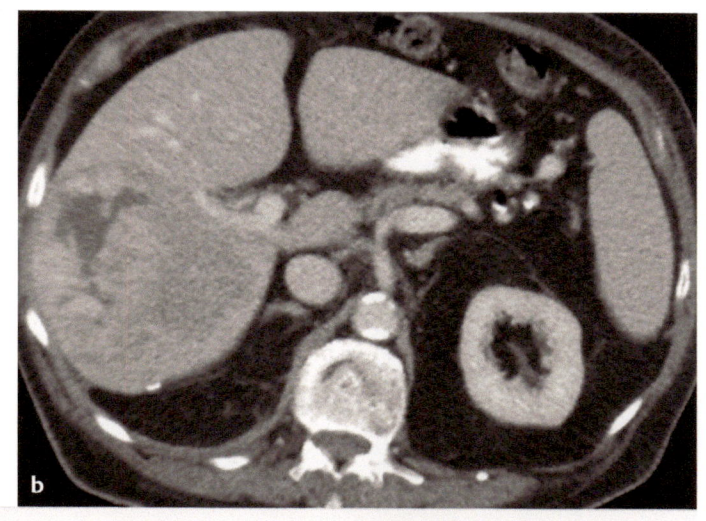

Fig. 5.46 **Hepatocellular carcinoma.** (a) Arterial phase. The hepatocellular carcinoma appears hypervascular. (b) Portal venous phase. The lesion is still enhanced and exhibits a necrotic center.

chemoembolization, which will significantly reduce the local recurrence rate. Radiofrequency ablation is recommended as the standard percutaneous ablation technique.
- *TACE (transarterial chemoembolization)*: Unlike radiofrequency ablation, TACE is a palliative therapy that can extend survival. While the liver receives approximately 75% of its blood supply from the portal vein and 25% from the hepatic artery, hepatocellular carcinoma derives almost 100% of its blood supply from the hepatic artery. This provides the rationale for TACE, in which embolization is performed through a catheter advanced into the segmental branches of the hepatic artery. TACE is recommended if curative procedures are no longer an option and there is no extrahepatic spread. In patients with systemic metastasis, TACE is reserved for selected cases in which extrahepatic spread is not the principal manifestation. The guideline for TACE expressly recommends simultaneous delivery of the embolic and chemotherapeutic agents. Embolization alone is appropriate if use of the chemotherapeutic agent is contraindicated. The intra-arterial administration of a chemotherapeutic agent without embolization is not advised, however. The guideline also states that the catheter should be selectively positioned as close to the tumor as possible. Tumor response is evaluated by contrast-enhanced CT or MRI performed at least 4 weeks after the TACE procedure. TACE may employ a mixture of lipiodol and the chemotherapeutic agent. Lipiodol is an oily contrast agent that produces capillary occlusion while also providing delayed release of the chemotherapeutic agent. Alternatively, TACE can be performed with microspheres containing the chemotherapeutic drug (▶ Fig. 5.49). The microspheres are composed of polyvinyl alcohol and are of uniform size. Because they induce occlusion of all tumor vessels, response is evaluated using the Modified Response Evaluation Criteria in Solid Tumors (mRECIST, ▶ Table 5.2, ▶ Fig. 5.50). Purely morphological measurements of tumor size based on RECIST criteria do not reflect response to treatment. But the mRECIST criteria are based on uptake of contrast medium, which is a better indicator of tumor response.
- *SIRT (selective internal radiation therapy)*: SIRT is also an available treatment option. Hepatocellular carcinoma requires a dose of 70 Gy, but healthy liver parenchyma can tolerate only 30 Gy; radiation above that dose will cause parenchymal damage. SIRT overcomes this limitation by the intra-arterial injection of particles loaded with yttrium 90. These beta-emitters have a penetration depth of just a few millimeters, so that liver damage is avoided. The activity lasts approximately 11 days. When SIRT is used, however, it must be determined whether significant shunts exist in the lung or gastrointestinal tract. This is done by injecting technetium Tc macroalbumin into the hepatic artery and determining the activity. Shunts via the gastroduodenal artery can be embolized. A pulmonary shunt volume greater than 13% is a contraindication to SIRT.

▶ **Key points.** Approximately 90% of hepatocellular carcinomas occur in cirrhotic livers. Patients with hepatic cirrhosis have a 4% annual risk of developing hepatocellular carcinoma, and therefore cirrhosis is considered a precancerous condition. Imaging in all contrast-enhanced modalities typically shows early uptake of contrast medium with washout in the portal venous phase and enhancement of the surrounding parenchyma. Based on current worldwide guidelines, these enhancement characteristics are considered proof of hepatocellular carcinoma in patients with hepatic cirrhosis, eliminating the need for histological confirmation in this group of patients. Radiological treatment options include the potentially curative procedure of radiofrequency ablation, which is equivalent to surgical excision in terms of survival benefit. TACE and SIRT are palliative options that can extend survival.

Hepatoblastoma

▶ **Brief definition.** Hepatoblastoma is the most common liver tumor in children, with a peak incidence before 4 years of age. There are about 100 newly diagnosed cases of hepatoblastoma per year in the US. The incidence is often considered as too low to be computed. It originates from fetal and embryonic hepatocytes. Like many pediatric tumors, hepatoblastoma may contain fatty components as well as calcifications and fibrotic areas. The alpha-fetoprotein level is elevated in up to 80% of affected children and can serve as a tumor marker in many patients.

▶ **Imaging signs.** The initial imaging study in most cases is ultrasound. If a liver tumor is detected, ultrasound scans should be followed by abdominal MRI or CT and thoracic CT. Ultrasound and

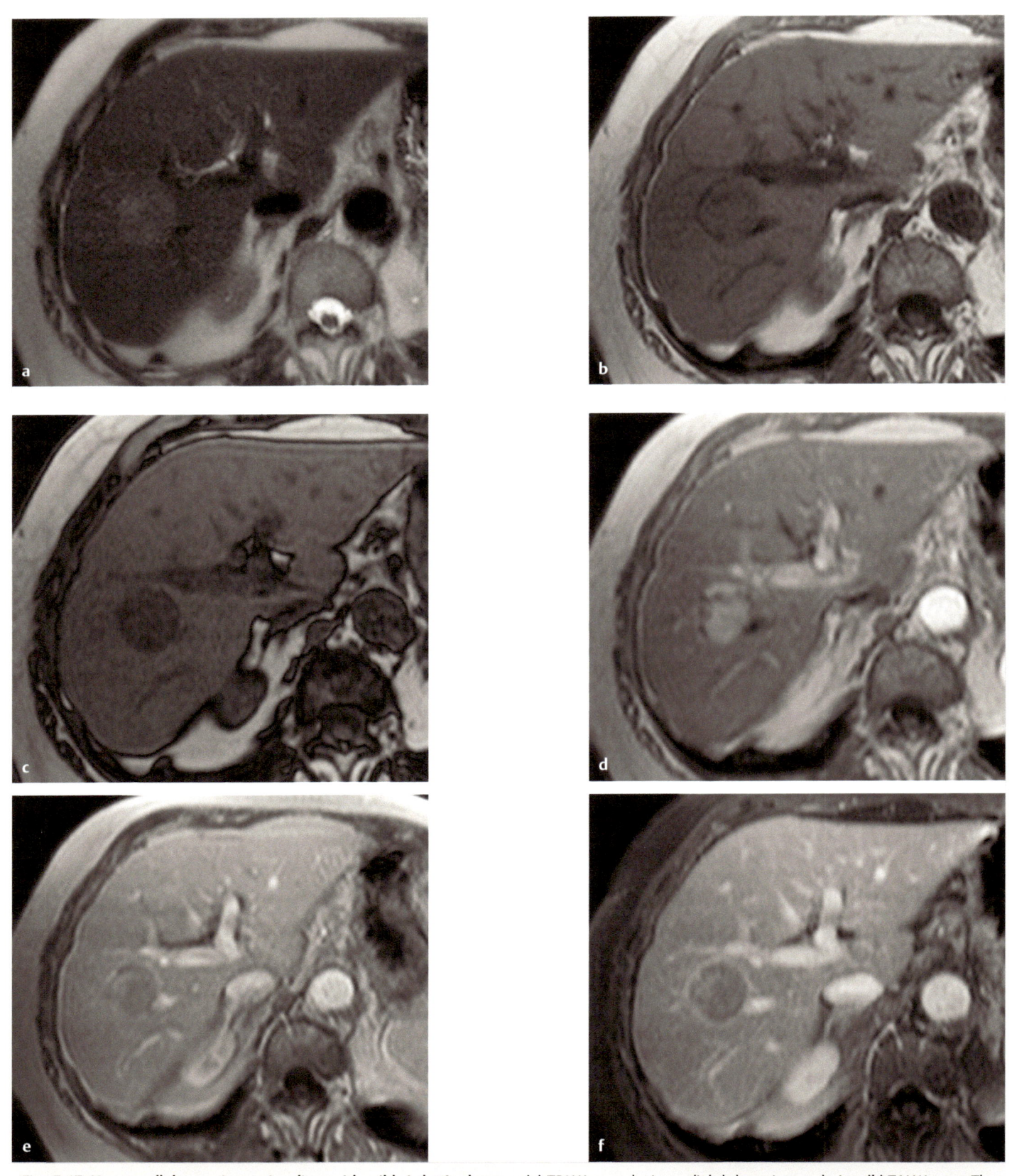

Fig. 5.47 Hepatocellular carcinoma in a liver with mild cirrhotic changes. (a) T2W image depicts a slightly hyperintense lesion. (b) T1W image. The mass is almost isointense to surrounding liver. (c) Opposed-phase sequence shows decreased signal intensity consistent with intralesional fat. (d) Arterial phase after injection of contrast medium. The lesion shows marked hypervascularity. (e) Image in the portal venous phase shows early washout of contrast material. (f) Fat-suppressed T1W image in the equilibrium phase. The lesion displays a pseudocapsule typical of hepatocellular carcinoma.

5.5 Focal Hepatic Lesions

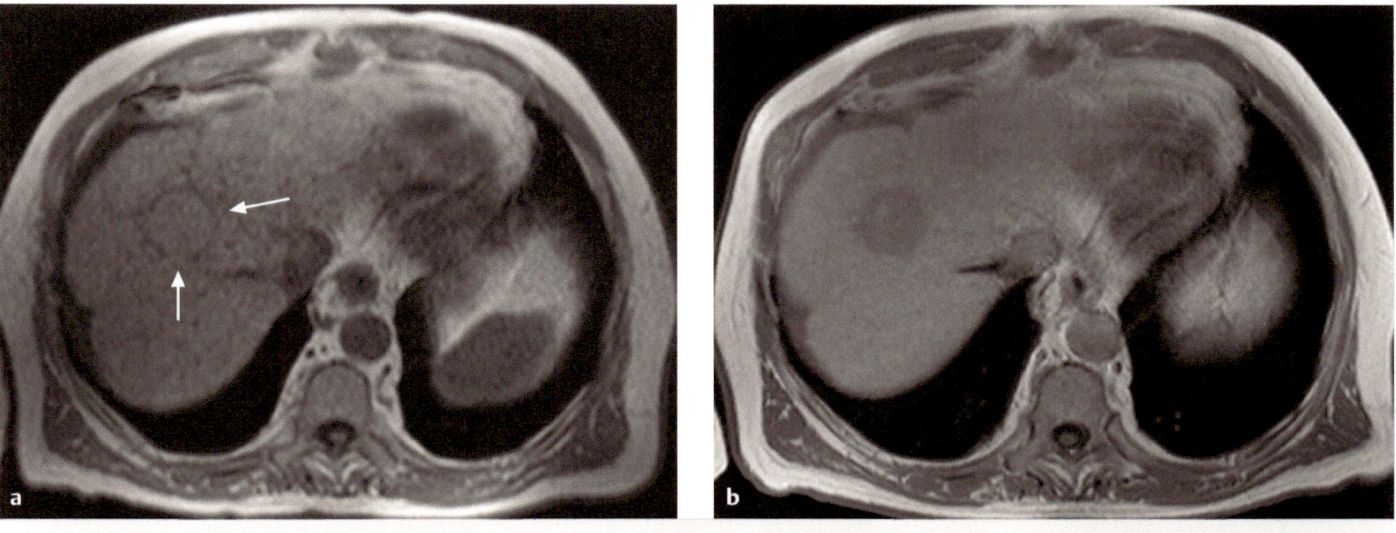

Fig. 5.48 Hepatocellular carcinoma in a cirrhotic liver. (a) Unenhanced T1 W sequence shows nodular transformation of the liver parenchyma with a detectable isointense mass (arrows). (b) Hepatobiliary phase image 45 minutes after Gd-BOPTA injection at 0.05 mmol/kg BW. The mass is not enhanced, indicating an absence of functioning hepatocytes in the lesion, in this case an hepatocellular carcinoma.

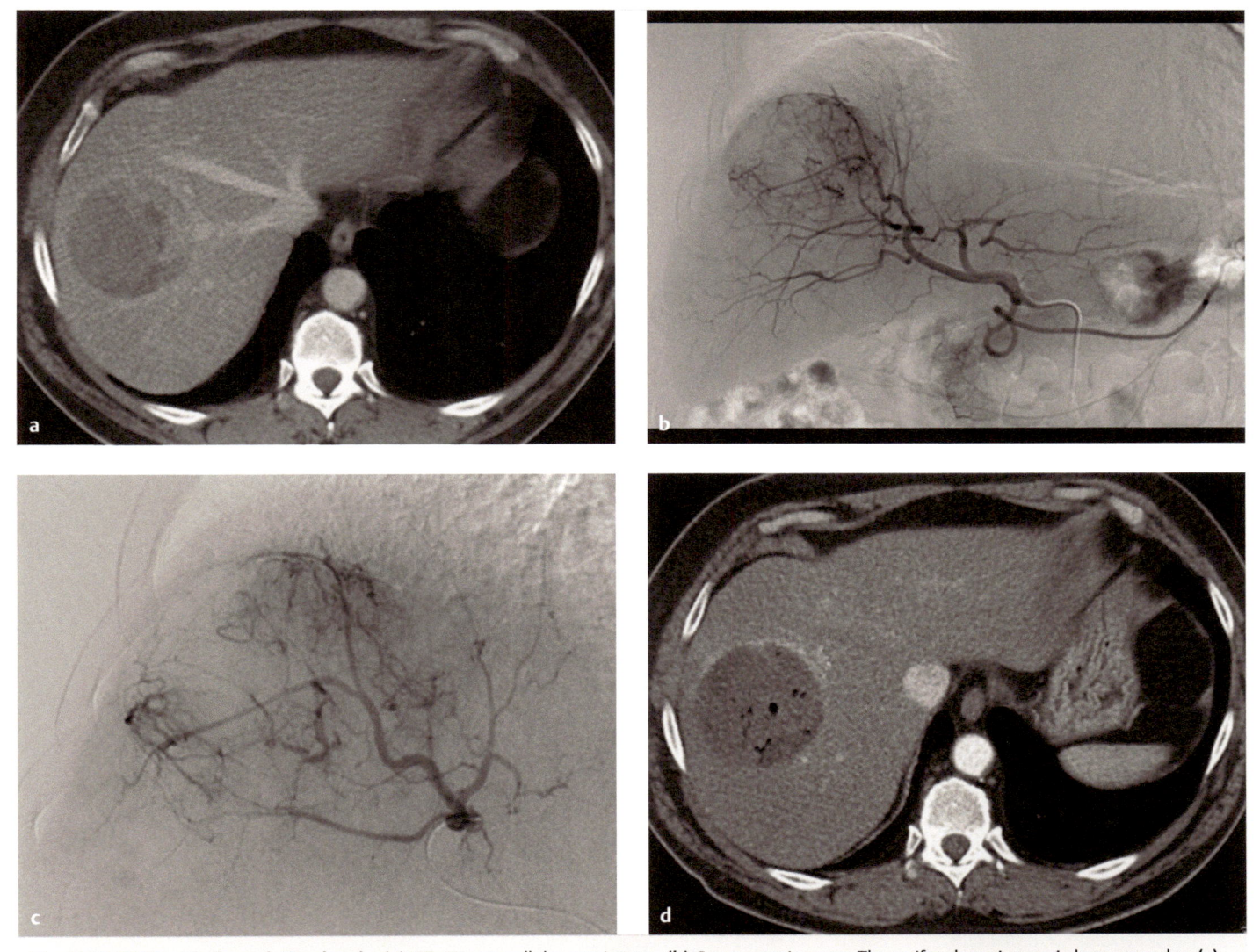

Fig. 5.49 TACE with drug-eluting beads. (a) CT. Hepatocellular carcinoma. (b) Survey angiogram. The unifocal carcinoma is hypervascular. (c) Selective catheter placement before embolization. (d) Postembolization CT shows that the tumor is no longer enhanced. Typical air inclusions within the tumor indicate necrosis.

Table 5.2 RECIST and mRECIST criteria[64]

Criteria	RECIST	mRECIST
Complete response	Disappearance of all lesions	Disappearance of any intratumoral arterial enhancement
Partial response	At least a 30% decrease in the diameters of the target lesions (reference: baseline diameters of the target lesions)	At least a 30% decrease in the diameters of lesions that enhance in the arterial phase (reference: baseline diameters of the target lesions)
Stable disease	Any cases that do not qualify for either partial response or progressive disease	Any cases that do not qualify for either partial response or progressive disease
Progressive disease	An increase of at least 20% in the diameters of the target lesions relative to the smallest diameters of the target lesions during treatment	An increase of at least 20% in the diameters of enhancing target lesions relative to the smallest diameters of enhancing target lesions during treatment

Abbreviation: (m)RECIST, modified response evaluation criteria in solid tumors.

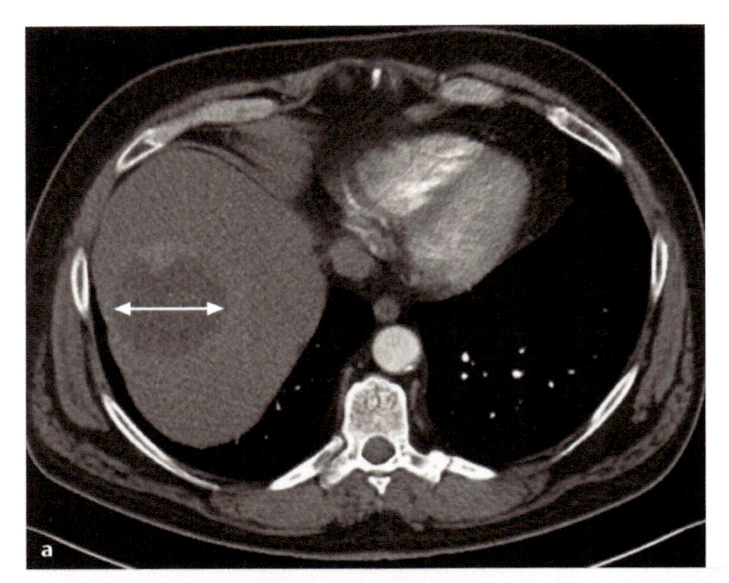

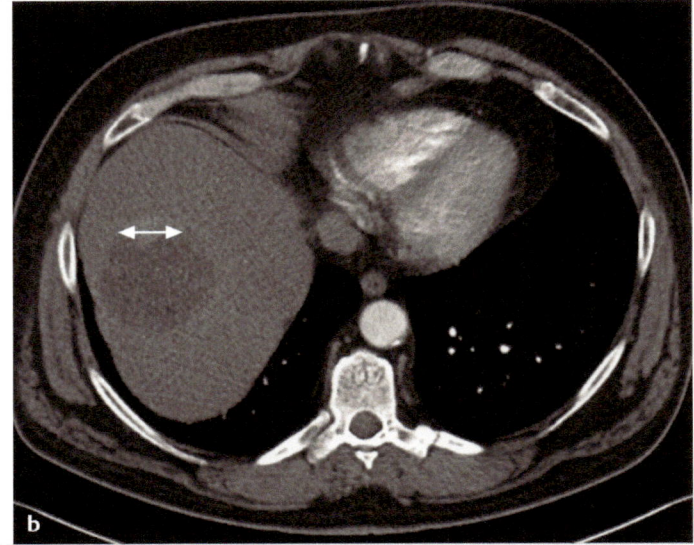

Fig. 5.50 Hepatocellular carcinoma after transarterial chemoembolization with drug-eluting beads. (a) Tumor measurement based on RECIST criteria. (b) Tumor measurement based on mRECIST criteria. The mRECIST assessment more accurately reflects tumor viability.

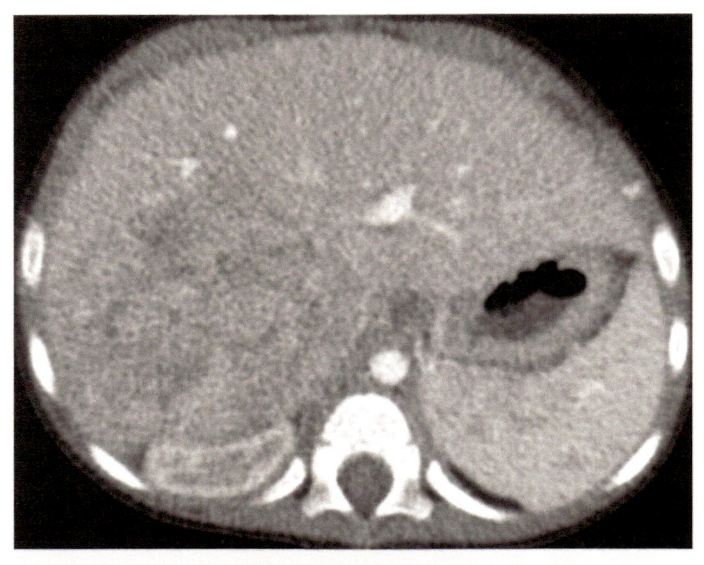

Fig. 5.51 Hepatoblastoma. Contrast-enhanced CT shows an inhomogeneous tumor in the late arterial phase.

CT are nonspecific due to the heterogeneous tumor appearance, but they can define the size and location of the hepatoblastoma (▶ Fig. 5.51). MRI typically shows inhomogeneous hypervascular tumors with inhomogeneous high T2W signal intensity and low T1W signal intensity (▶ Fig. 5.52). The tumors may cause significant hepatomegaly.[65] Often the tumors are quite large at diagnosis, already occupying more than 30% of the liver volume. The PRETEXT system is widely used for the staging, treatment planning and risk stratification of liver tumors.[66] This grouping system was designed by the International Childhood Liver Tumor Strategy Group (SIOPEL). It describes tumor extent prior to treatment as a basis for evaluating radiological findings. The Couinaud liver segments are grouped into four sections, with each section comprising two segments (▶ Fig. 5.53a). PRETEXT numbers are assigned according to the number of adjoining sections not involved by tumor, as shown in ▶ Fig. 5.53b and ▶ Table 5.3. "Additional criteria" are also evaluated in PRETEXT staging (▶ Table 5.4). The caudate lobe is not included among the four sections but is evaluated as part of the additional criteria. All of the PRETEXT criteria should be reassessed after chemotherapy and before surgical resection of the tumor and recorded as POSTEXT.

▶ **Clinical features.** Swelling of the upper abdomen is often the earliest symptom of hepatoblastoma. Other commonly observed symptoms are fever and decreased appetite. Precocious puberty is rarely observed.

5.5 Focal Hepatic Lesions

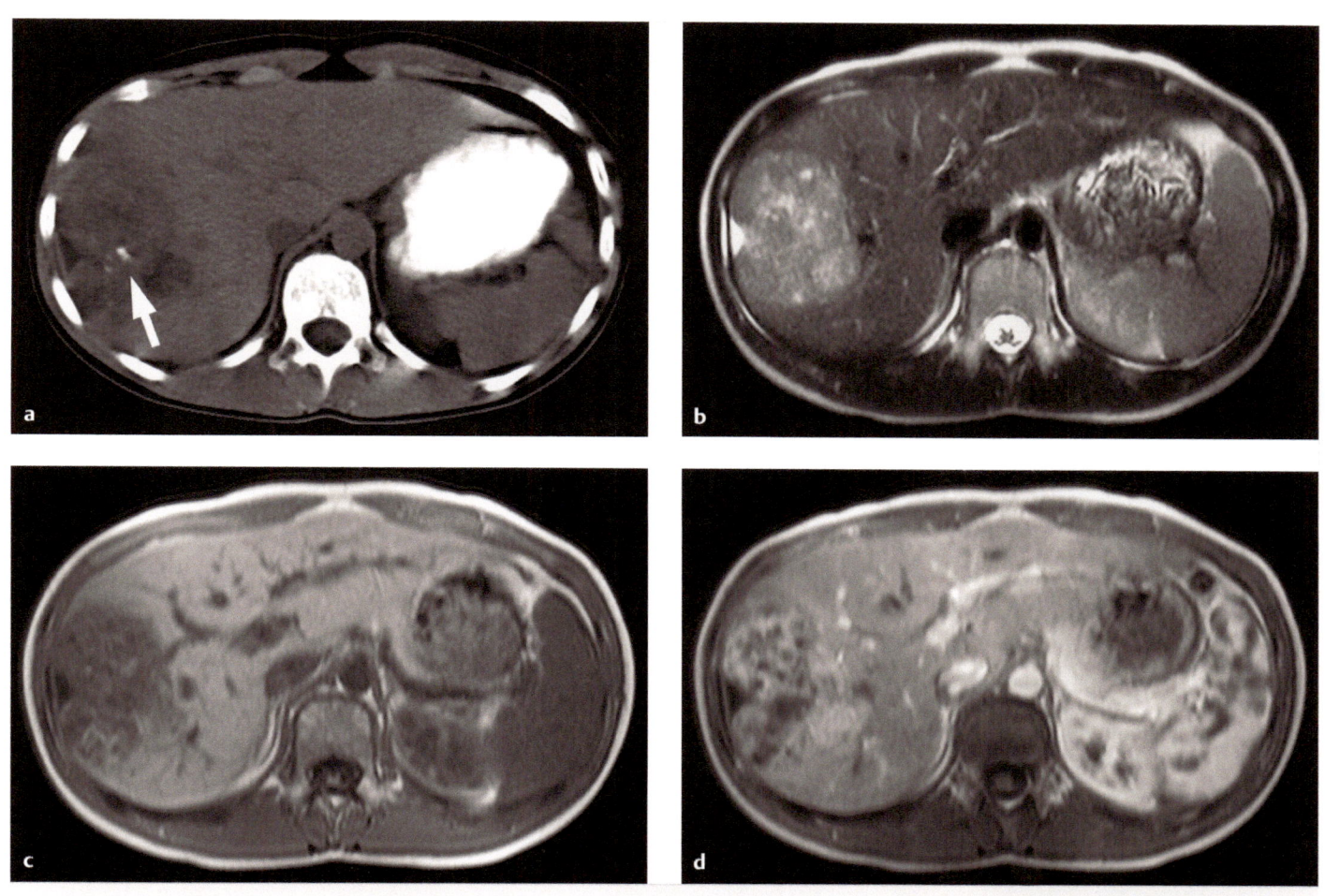

Fig. 5.52 Hepatoblastoma. (a) CT demonstrates calcifications within the lesion (arrow). (b) T2 W sequence. The lesion is inhomogeneous but markedly hyperintense. (c) T1 W sequence. The lesion is inhomogeneous and hypointense. (d) Contrast wash-in. Inhomogeneous hypervascularity.

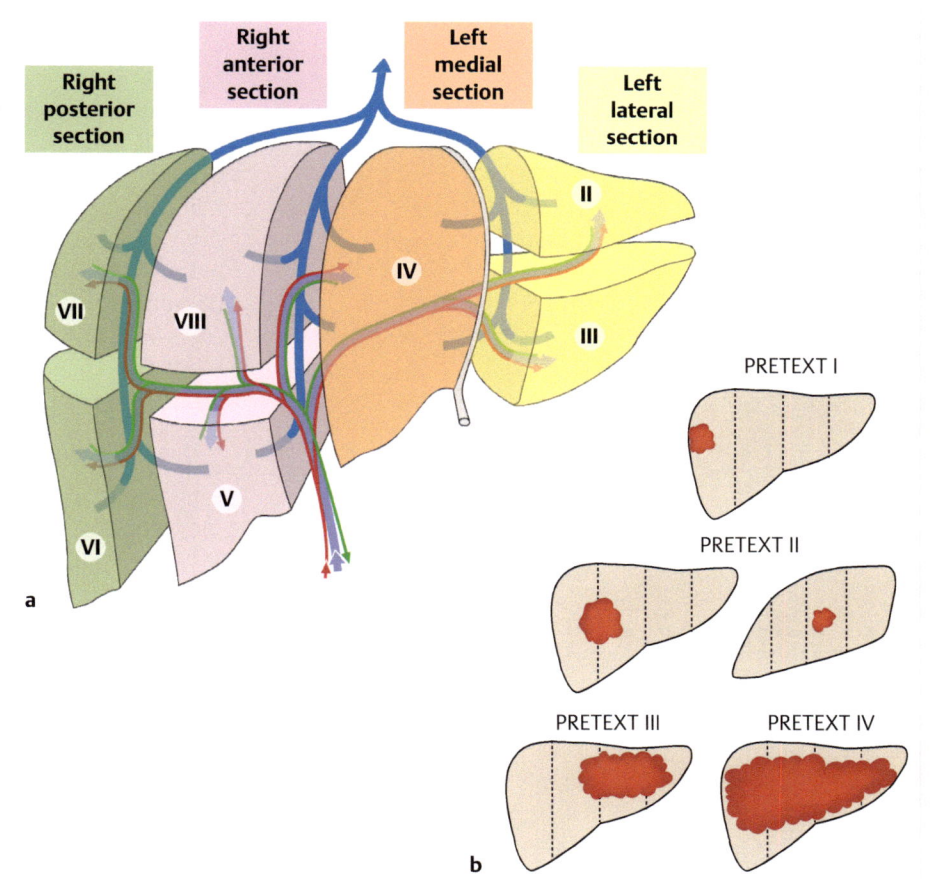

Fig. 5.53 PRETEXT system for staging hepatoblastoma and other liver tumors in children. (a) The segments of the liver are grouped into four *sections* that comprise segments II and III, IVa and IVb, V and VIII, and VI and VII. Segment I is considered separately and is evaluated within the framework of additional criteria (▶ Table 5.4). (b) PRETEXT grouping based on involved sections. (Reproduced from Schünke M, Schulte E, Schumacher U. Prometheus. LernAtlas der Anatomie: Innere Organe. Illustrated by M. Voll/K. Wesker. 2nd ed. Stuttgart: Thieme; 2009.)

217

▶ **Differential diagnosis.** Given the heterogeneous tumor appearance, other entities such as mesenchymal hamartoma and angiosarcoma should be considered. The differential diagnosis relies on laboratory values: In the age group from 6 months to 4 years, a rise in the α-fetoprotein level to more than 1000 ng/mL, or at least 3 times the age-normal value, is indicative of hepatoblastoma. Histological confirmation may be omitted in these cases in accordance with current guidelines.[67]

▶ **Key points.** Hepatoblastoma is the most common liver tumor in children. The PRETEXT grouping system is used for treatment planning and risk stratification.

5.5.2 Secondary Hepatic Lesions

Secondary hepatic lesions include:
- Metastases.
- Inflammatory changes.
- Parasitic liver diseases.

Hepatic Metastases

▶ **Brief definition.** The two main imaging presentations of hepatic metastases are hypervascular and hypovascular. Some lesions may also have a cystic appearance.

Table 5.3 PRETEXT numbers for staging hepatoblastoma and other liver tumors in children

PRETEXT number	Definition
I	One section is involved and three adjoining sections are free
II	One or two sections are involved, but two adjoining sections are free
III	Two or three sections are involved, and no two adjoining sections are free
IV	All four sections are involved

Abbreviation: PRETEXT, PRETreatment EXTent of disease.

Table 5.4 Additional criteria used in PRETEXT staging of hepatoblastoma and other liver tumors in children. All the criteria are individually evaluated and the corresponding suffix is added to the PRETEXT stage

Tumor manifestation	Criterion	Suffix
Caudate lobe involvement	Tumor involving the caudate lobe	C1
	All other patients	C0
Extrahepatic abdominal disease	No evidence of tumor spread in the abdomen (except M or N)	E0
	Direct extension of tumor into adjacent organs or diaphragm	E1
Tumor rupture or intraperitoneal hemorrhage	Imaging and clinical findings of intraperitoneal hemorrhage	H1
	All other patients	H0
Distant metastases	No metastases	M0
	Any metastasis (except E and N)	M1 (add one or more suffixes to indicate major sites of metastasis: p for pulmonary, s for skeletal, c for central nervous system, m for bone marrow, and x for other sites)
Lymph node metastases	No nodal metastases	N0
	Abdominal lymph node metastases only	N1
	Extra-abdominal lymph node metastases (with or without abdominal lymph node metastases)	N2
Portal vein involvement	No involvement of the portal vein or its left or right branches	P0
	Involvement of either the left or right branch of the portal vein	P1
	Involvement of the main portal vein	P2
Involvement of the inferior vena cava and/or hepatic veins	No involvement of the hepatic veins or inferior vena cava	N0
	Involvement of one hepatic vein but not the inferior vena cava	V1
	Involvement of two hepatic veins but not the inferior vena cava	V2
	Involvement of all three hepatic veins and/or the inferior vena cava	V3

Abbreviation: PRETEXT, PRETreatment EXTent of disease.

- *Hypervascular hepatic metastases*: The majority of hypervascular metastases are derived from very vascular primary tumors such as neuroendocrine tumors (e.g., carcinoids, islet cell tumors), renal cell carcinoma, thyroid carcinoma, pheochromocytoma, melanoma, and breast carcinoma.[68] Special considerations apply to malignant melanomas and metastases from ovarian cancer.
- *Hypovascular hepatic metastases*: These are the most common hepatic malignancies. Typically they are metastatic to adenocarcinomas such as colorectal carcinoma. Hypovascular metastases usually have a rounded shape and are often larger than 3 cm when diagnosed.

▶ Imaging signs

- *Hypervascular hepatic metastases*: On CT, hypervascular hepatic metastases show intense enhancement in the arterial phase. These tumors are typically hypointense in T1 W sequences but hyperintense in T2 W sequences. The occasionally very high signal intensity of metastases from neuroendocrine tumors is caused by hormones stored in fluid-filled vacuoles in the tumor cells, similarly to hemangiomas.[69] An exception to the typical unenhanced appearance of metastases on MRI is melanin-forming metastases from melanoma. The paramagnetic effect of the melanin in these lesions creates high signal intensity on unenhanced T1 W images (▶ Fig. 5.54). Metastases show restricted diffusion on DWI at high *b* values, and they are hypointense in the ADC map. On dynamic contrast-enhanced imaging, hypervascular metastases show increased, homogeneous enhancement relative to liver parenchyma in all modalities (▶ Fig. 5.55) and may be hyperintense or isointense in the portal venous phase. They show relatively rapid washout of enhancement (similar to hepatocellular carcinoma) and usually appear more hypointense in the equilibrium phase (▶ Fig. 5.56, ▶ Fig. 5.57). The lesions are not enhanced in the hepatobiliary phase and are hypointense when either Gd-BOPTA or Gd-EOB-DTPA is used.
- *Hypovascular hepatic metastases*: At ultrasound, these metastases may be less echogenic or more echogenic than the surrounding parenchyma. Larger lesions often show central necrosis due to rapid peripheral growth that outstrips the blood supply. This is why hypovascular metastases also have a relatively hypodense center on CT (▶ Fig. 5.58), creating a pattern called the "target sign." Accordingly, the lesions have a hyperintense rim on T2 W MRI with an even more hyperintense center (necrosis), similarly to cystic lesions. The lesions are hypointense to varying degrees in T1 W images. Postcontrast imaging shows increased peripheral vascularity in the growth zone; central areas are usually hypointense in the early arterial and portal venous phases. This is followed by increasing enhancement that encompasses the tumor center. Peripheral washout is often observed in the equilibrium phase (▶ Fig. 5.59). Peripheral washout is highly specific for the presence of malignant lesions, appearing as a hypointense ring around an enhancing center. The hypointense ring represents the growing portions of the tumor that are still perfused and therefore show contrast washout, while the central enhancement results from incipient necrosis with diffusion of contrast material into the necrotic

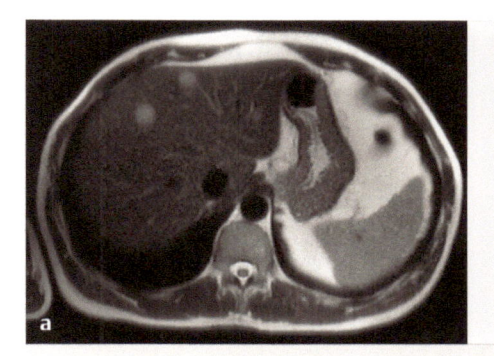

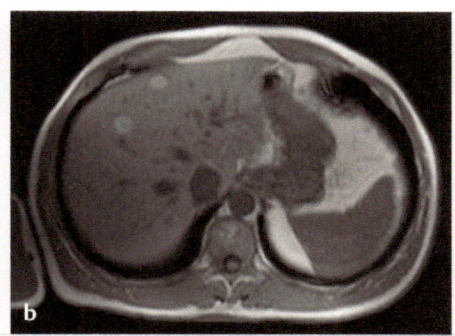

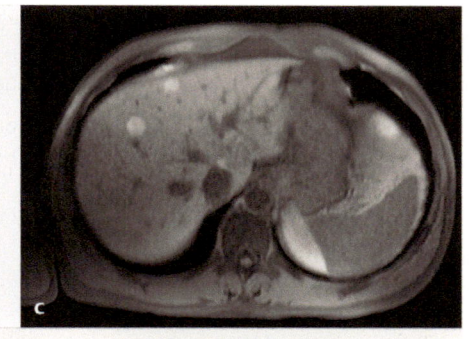

Fig. 5.54 Hepatic metastases from malignant melanoma. (a) T2 W image reveals multiple hyperintense masses (arrows). (b) The lesions are also hyperintense in the T1 W image due to their melanin content, which acts like a paramagnetic contrast agent. (c) The lesions are still hyperintense in the fat-suppressed sequence.

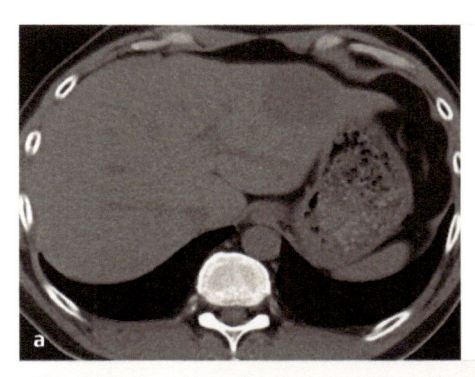

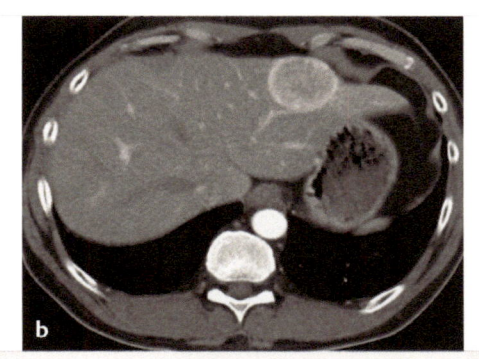

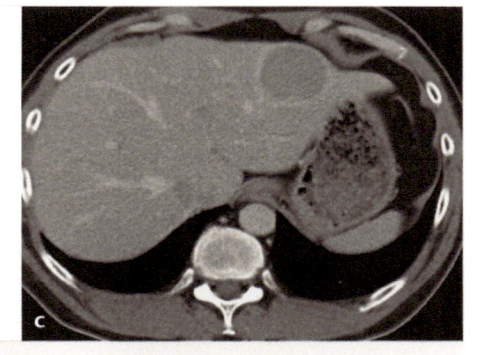

Fig. 5.55 Hypervascular metastasis from hemangiopericytoma. (a) Precontrast CT. The metastasis is hypodense. (b) Arterial phase image shows intense lesion enhancement. (c) Image in the portal venous phase shows an enhancing rim. The center of the metastasis is hypodense.

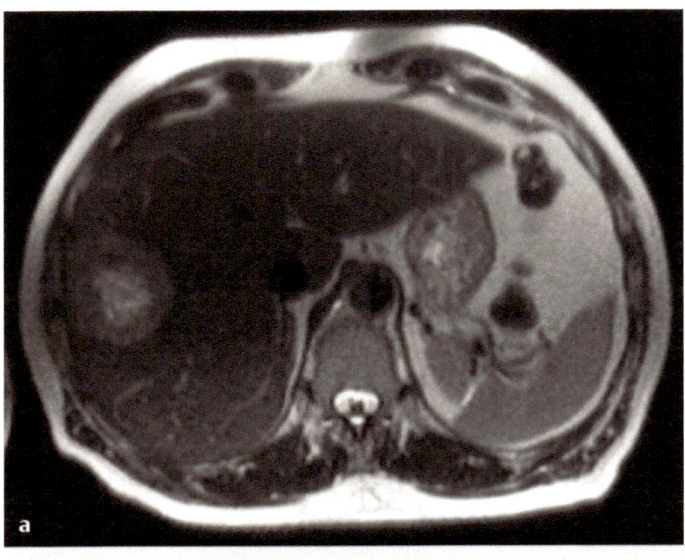

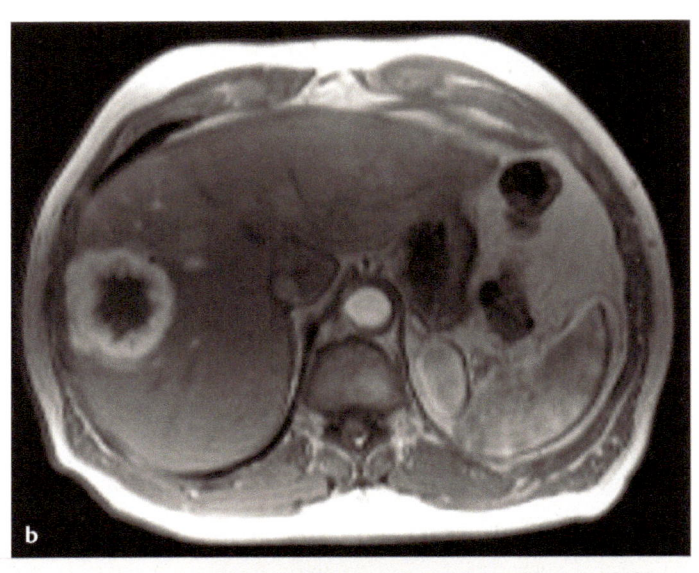

Fig. 5.56 Hypervascular metastasis from renal cell carcinoma. (a) Unenhanced T2 W sequence. The metastasis is hyperintense. **(b)** Arterial phase after injection of contrast medium. The metastasis is markedly hypervascular and shows extensive central necrosis.

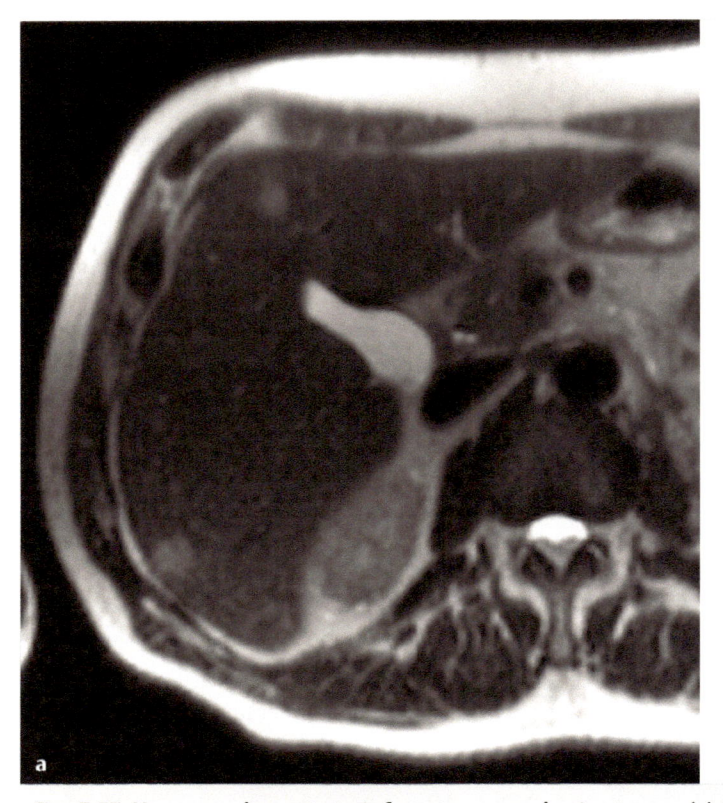

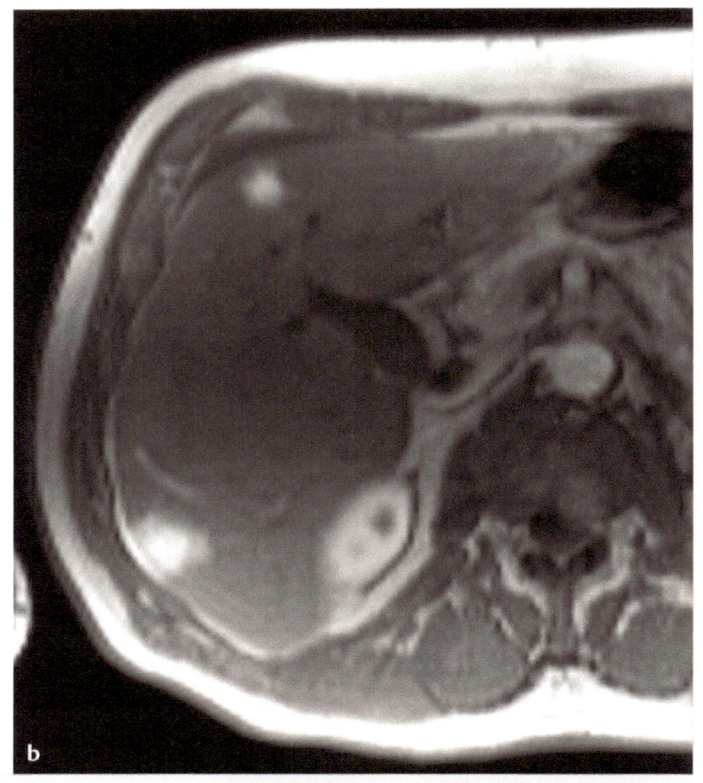

Fig. 5.57 Hypervascular metastasis from a neuroendocrine tumor. (a) Unenhanced T2 W sequence. The metastases appear hyperintense. **(b)** Arterial phase after injection of contrast medium. The metastases are markedly hypervascular.

areas.[69] These areas may still show enhancement in the hepatobiliary phase due to diffusion of contrast agent into the necrotic center. The peripheral hypointense ring often appears accentuated in this case. The overall detection rate of metastases in the hepatobiliary phase is significantly increased after the administration of a hepatobiliary contrast agent compared with unenhanced T1 W sequences.[70]

Note

Chloroma is a special type of secondary hepatic malignancy that occurs in patients with acute leukemia. The lesions are similar in behavior to hypovascular metastases of solid tumors but often show enhancement in the equilibrium phase. An example is shown in ▶ Fig. 5.60.

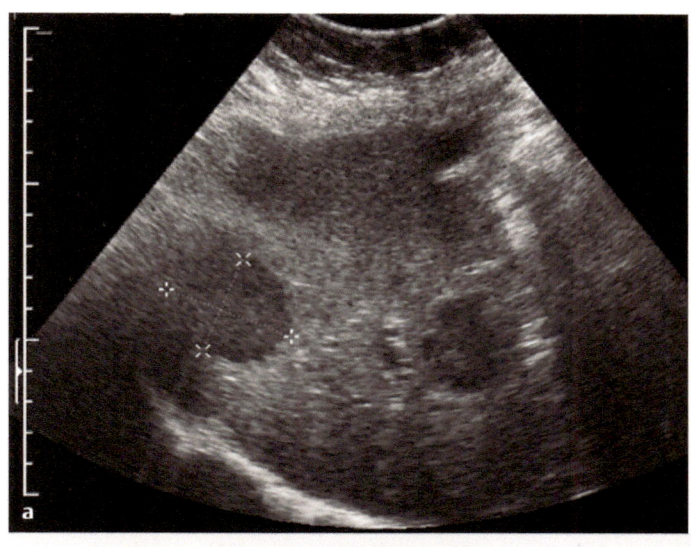

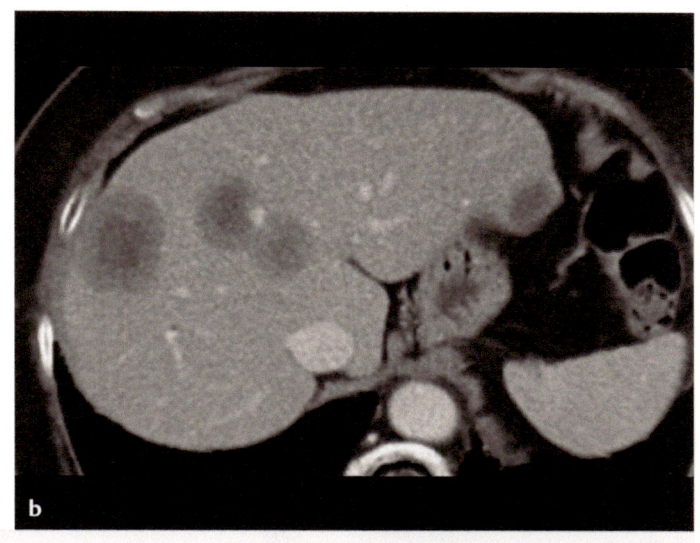

Fig. 5.58 Hypovascular metastases from colorectal carcinoma. (a) The metastases are hypoechoic at ultrasound. (b) Portal venous phase. The hypovascular metastases appear hypodense with a target pattern of rim enhancement.

▶ **Differential diagnosis.** Differentiation is required from metastases of benign primary liver tumors.

▶ **Key points.** Hepatic metastases are perfused by the hepatic artery, not by the portal vein. They may be hypovascular or hypervascular and are differentiated by this perfusion pattern on contrast-enhanced imaging.

Inflammatory Changes: Hepatic Abscess

▶ **Brief definition.** Hepatic abscess is a secondary benign lesion that may be caused by bacterial infection (*Escherichia coli*, *Enterococcus fecalis*, *Staphylococcus aureus*, *Klebsiella* species, or anaerobes) as well as amebic or fungal infection and is associated with a localized accumulation of inflammatory cells and parenchymal destruction.[71] Initial pathology is marked by inflammatory infiltration of the tissue without liquefaction. This is followed within a week by colliquation with central liquefaction, pus accumulation, and the formation of an abscess membrane composed of granulation tissue. Insertion of a drain and saline irrigation of the abscess may be curative at this stage. The formation of a liver abscess may occur through any of five main pathways[72]:
- *Biliary ducts*: in a setting of ascending cholangitis resulting from a benign or malignant biliary obstruction.
- *Portal vein*: due to pyophlebitis secondary to appendicitis, diverticulitis, proctitis, or other gastrointestinal tract infections.
- *Hepatic arteries*: typically in association with septicemia.
- *Direct extension to the liver from surrounding inflammatory processes.*
- *Trauma*: relating to blunt or penetrating injuries of the upper abdomen.

▶ **Imaging signs.** The initial imaging study is often by ultrasound, in which the still-immature abscess appears as a hypoechoic area. Following liquefaction, the abscess cavity is fluid-filled and hypoechoic, while the abscess membrane is echogenic. CT is usually used in seriously ill patients to define the overall extent of the abscess and, if necessary, for CT-guided percutaneous drainage. Abscesses are most conspicuous on CT during the portal venous phase (▶ Fig. 5.61, ▶ Fig. 5.62). The center of a mature abscess is hypodense while the rim shows contrast enhancement and may be very thin, especially in later stages. The initial presence of gas inclusions before percutaneous drainage suggests infection with gas-forming bacteria. MRI shows an area of low signal intensity on T1 W images and high signal intensity on T2 W images. The lesions are typically surrounded by hyperintense edematous liver tissue in T2 W sequences. A peripheral rim of granulation tissue is occasionally visible on T2 W images. The rim of granulation tissue around the central, nonenhancing liquefied area is usually depicted more clearly on contrast-enhanced T1 W images (▶ Fig. 5.63). The arterial phase image often shows peripheral hypervascularity around the abscess, reflecting inflammatory change with increased blood flow.[73]

▶ **Clinical features.** Clinical manifestations include fever, acute onset of right upper quadrant pain, nausea, and vomiting. Hepatic abscesses are usually associated with hepatomegaly and marked leukocytosis.

▶ **Differential diagnosis.** Tumors can be differentiated from abscesses by their typical clinical presentation and laboratory findings.

▶ **Key points.** Hepatic abscess appears in all modalities as a well-circumscribed mass with a nonenhancing center.

Parasitic Lesions

Parasitic lesions most commonly consist of amebic abscesses or hydatid cysts due to infestation with *Echinococcus granulosus* or *E. alveolaris* (*E. multilocularis*).

Amebic Abscess

▶ **Brief definition.** Amebic abscesses are caused by the parasite *Entamoeba histolytica*. Endemic regions are the tropics, Mexico,

Liver

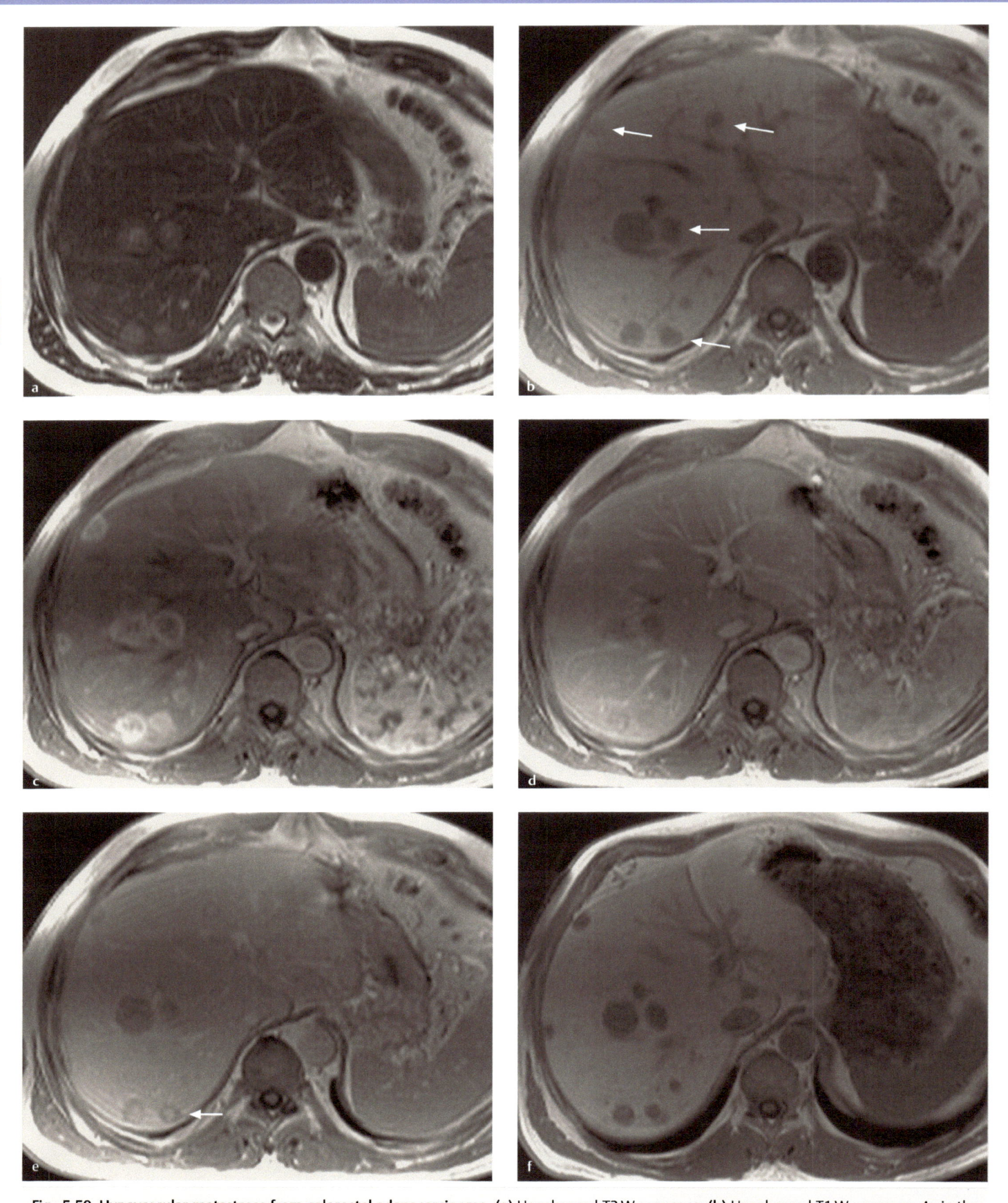

Fig. 5.59 Hypovascular metastases from colorectal adenocarcinoma. (a) Unenhanced T2W sequence. (b) Unenhanced T1W sequence. As in the unenhanced T2W sequence, multiple hepatic metastases are visualized (arrows). (c) Arterial phase. The lesions have hypervascular rims and hypointense centers. (d) Portal venous phase. The metastases appear hypointense. (e) Equilibrium phase. The lesions show peripheral washout (arrow), a feature that is highly specific for malignancy. (f) Hepatobiliary phase. The lesions are not enhanced and contrast more sharply with the enhancing liver tissue than in the unenhanced image.

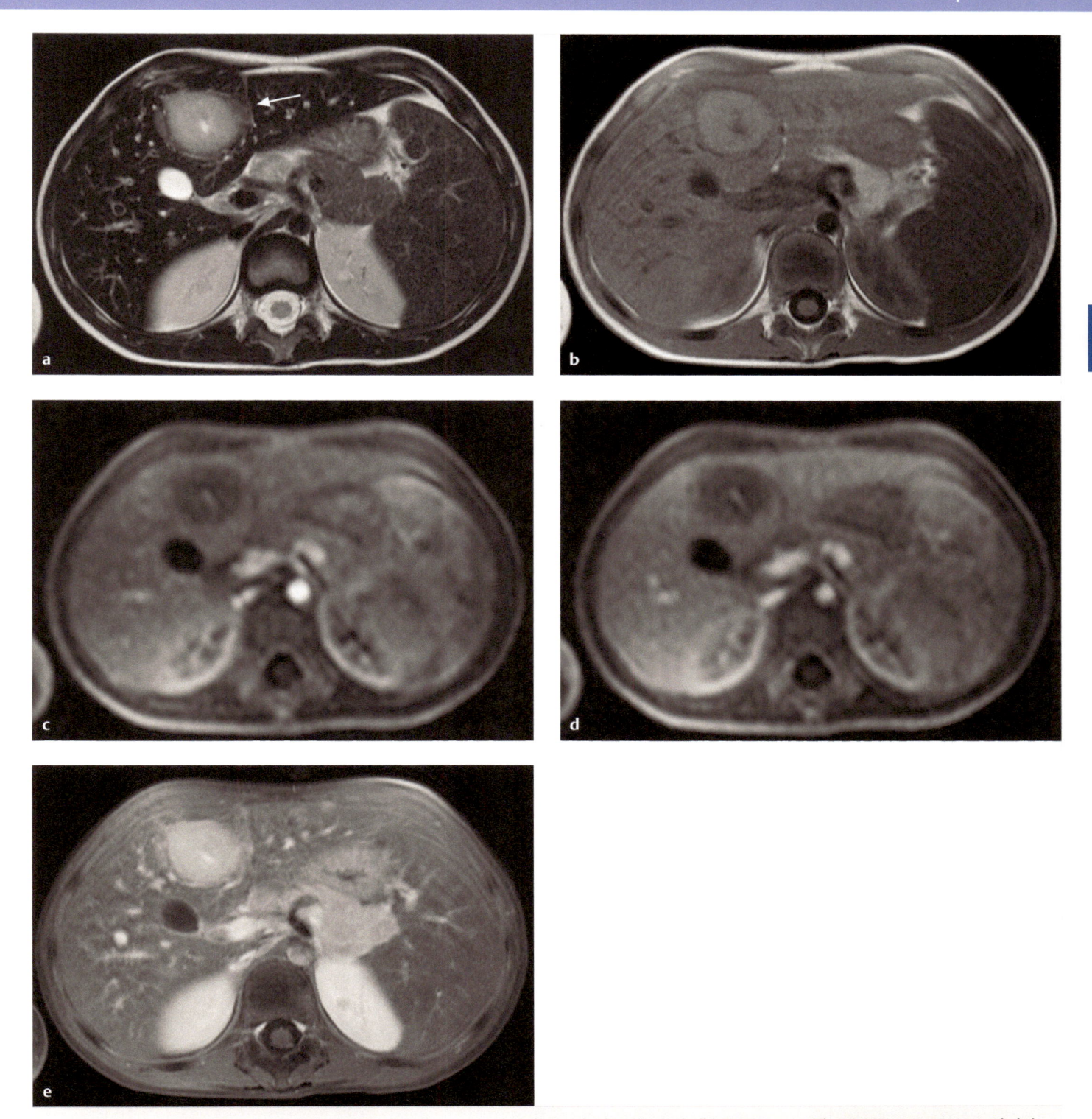

Fig. 5.60 Hepatic chloroma. (a) T2W image shows a hyperintense mass in the liver (arrow). (b) T1W image. The mass is isointense to slightly hyperintense. (c) Image after injection of contrast medium. The lesion is hypovascular. (d) Later phase after injection of contrast medium. The lesion still appears hypovascular. (e) Fat-suppressed T1W image in the equilibrium phase shows homogeneous lesion enhancement.

Central and South America, Africa, and West Asia. Following oral ingestion of the parasite, the liver may become infected by any of three pathways[74]:
- Portal venous system.
- Lymphatic vessels.
- Direct spread through the colon wall, through the peritoneum, and then through the hepatic capsule into the liver.

▶ **Imaging signs.** When imaged by CT and MRI, amebic abscesses usually have sharper margins than hepatic abscesses of pyogenic origin.[75] They are hypointense in T1W sequences and hyperintense in T2W sequences. The perifocal reaction is less pronounced than with pyogenic liver abscesses. Persistent enhancement may be observed in the area of the capsule. Otherwise their imaging features are similar to those of pyogenic abscesses.

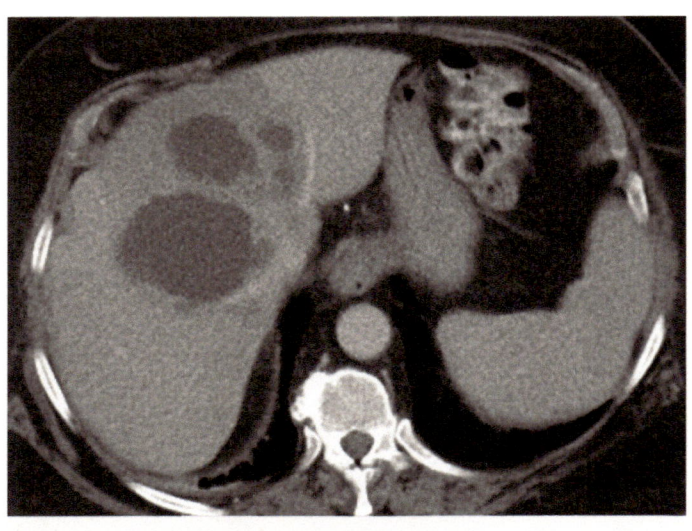

Fig. 5.61 Hepatic abscess. CT in the portal venous phase shows a hypodense lesion with absence of central enhancement.

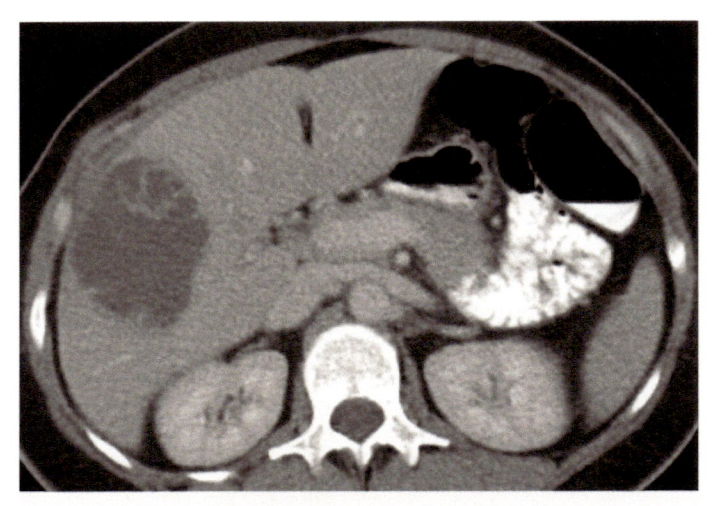

Fig. 5.62 Hepatic abscess. CT in the portal venous phase. Intralesional septa can be identified.

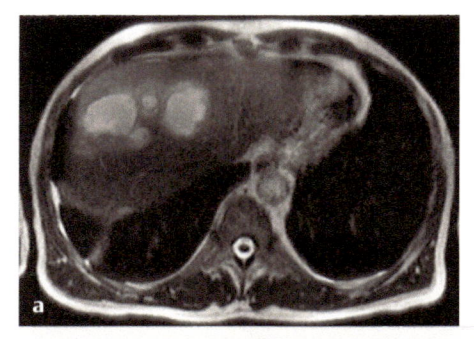

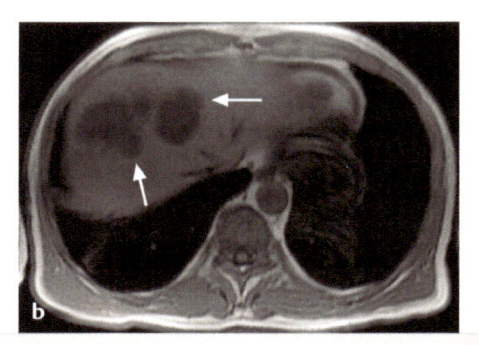

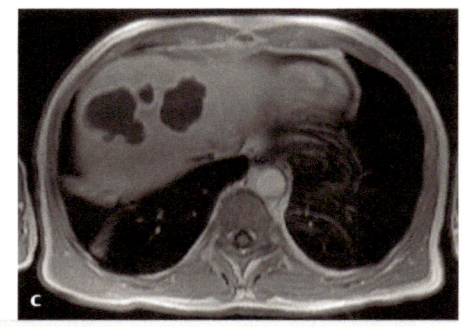

Fig. 5.63 Multiple abscesses in the superior part of the liver. (a) T2W image shows marked edema of the liver tissue with multiple liquefied areas of fluid signal intensity. **(b)** T1W image. The areas of liquefaction are hypointense with a hypointense rim composed of granulation tissue (arrows). **(c)** Equilibrium phase. The granulation tissue shows marked enhancement.

▶ **Clinical features.** In typical cases the liver feels firm and enlarged, and patients complain of right upper quadrant pain. Amebae can usually be identified in the stool. Serological tests are positive in approximately 90% of patients.

▶ **Differential diagnosis.** Differentiation is required mainly from abscesses caused by other organisms.

▶ **Key points.** Amebic abscess accounts for the largest proportion of hepatic abscesses worldwide. It is endemic in the tropics, Mexico, Central and South America, Africa, and Asia. Intralesional septa are found on imaging.

Hydatid Disease Caused by the Dog Tapeworm

▶ **Brief definition.** *Echinococcus granulosus* (dog tapeworm), the causative organism of unilocular hydatid disease, is found throughout Europe. Humans become infected mainly through contact with dogs. The tapeworm infects two species of mammal in its life cycle: The definitive host (dog or wolf) sheds tapeworm eggs in its feces, which are then ingested by an intermediate host, usually a grazing herbivore. The human is an accidental host that becomes infected orally through direct contact (e.g., by stroking contaminated fur). The tapeworm larvae penetrate the intestinal wall and, in 75% of cases, travel to the liver via the portal venous system. There they form cysts that grow slowly over a period of years and may compress the bile ducts or incite a bacterial infection. The lung is also involved in the approximately 15% of cases. Involvement of the kidneys, brain, heart, or other sites is rare. The cysts may measure up to 30 cm in size and are surrounded by a fibrous outer layer called the pericyst. Inside the cyst, daughter cysts may develop from the germinal layer.[76,77] Scolices form within the daughter cysts and, when the daughter cysts are ingested by carnivores (dog, wolf), may lodge in the small intestine and grow into adult tapeworms. The treatment of hydatid cysts is by surgical resection. Patients with multiple lesions or lesions at a nonresectable site can be treated medically with mebendazole or albendazole. Cysts of types I to III can be killed by the direct percutaneous injection of hypertonic saline solution.

▶ **Imaging signs.** Cysts are divided into five morphological types based on their imaging features at different stages of development (▶ Table 5.5). These types can be identified in all imaging modalities. The wall layers are often definable on CT (▶ Fig. 5.64). Additional cysts may be detected, or solid components may be found in the hydatids (▶ Fig. 5.65). Homogeneous calcification is the only imaging proof of a nonviable cyst (▶ Fig. 5.66). The cystic portion of an *E. granulosus* cyst has a similar MRI appearance as other liver cysts,[78] i.e., low signal intensity on T1W images and high signal intensity on T2W images. The fibrous capsule around the cyst is usually defined more clearly on T2W images. Membranes are often visible within the cyst (▶ Fig. 5.67), representing portions of the endocyst that have detached from the ectocyst.[79,80]

> **Note**
>
> The detachment of the germinal layer creates a floating membranelike structure, the "water lily sign," that is virtually pathognomonic for *Echinococcus granulosus*.

▶ **Clinical features.** The hydatid cysts develop very slowly. Complaints are often nonspecific and may include a pressure sensation in the upper abdomen. If a cyst ruptures, an anaphylactoid reaction may occur in response to dissemination of the daughter cysts.

▶ **Differential diagnosis.** Differentiation is mainly required from hepatic cysts and cystic liver tumors.

▶ **Key points.** Humans are an irregular intermediate host for *E. granulosus* infections. Hydatid cysts have a characteristics imaging appearance that correlates with their developmental stage.

Table 5.5 Imaging features of hydatid cysts

Type	Features
I	Echo-free (nonseptated) cyst
II	Septated cyst with strandlike septa
III	Daughter cysts (cysts within a cyst)
IV	Daughter cysts plus solid components
V	Peripheral calcifications

Hydatid Disease Caused by the Fox Tapeworm

▶ **Brief definition.** The fox tapeworm (*Echinococcus multilocularis*) occurs in Europe, Russia, and Japan. It may be transmitted by contact with infected foxes (hunters) or by ingestion of contaminated berries. The life cycle is the same as for *E. granulosus*, but unlike the hydatid cysts formed by the dog tapeworm, the larval stages of the fox tapeworm form an infiltrative, tumorlike mass with a liquid center that can spread to surrounding tissues. In contrast to involvement by *E. granulosus*, percutaneous treatment is unlikely to be effective. The locally aggressive growth results in a high mortality rate of up to 75%. The liver is most commonly affected.

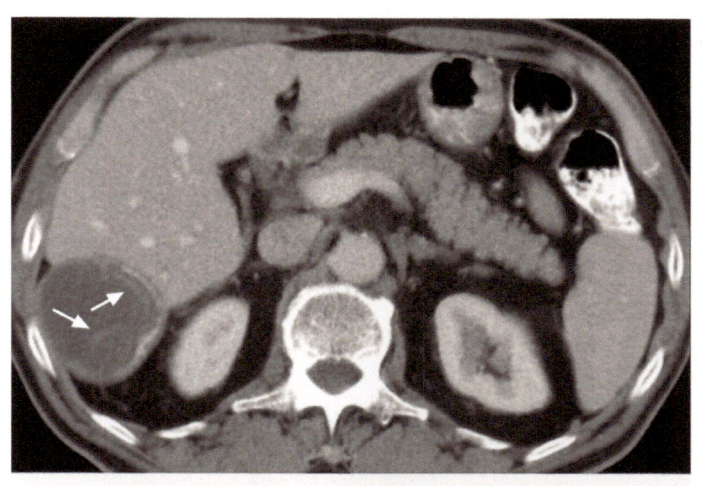

Fig. 5.64 *Echinococcus granulosus*. CT in the portal venous phase. The pericyst forms the outer layer. The germinal layer (upper arrow) is visible inside the cyst. Part of the germinal layer has detached to form a free-floating membrane within the cyst ("water lily sign," lower arrow).

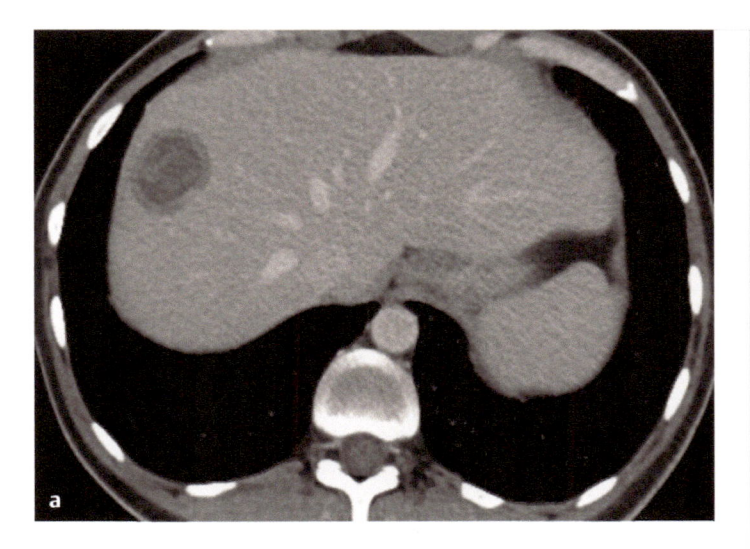

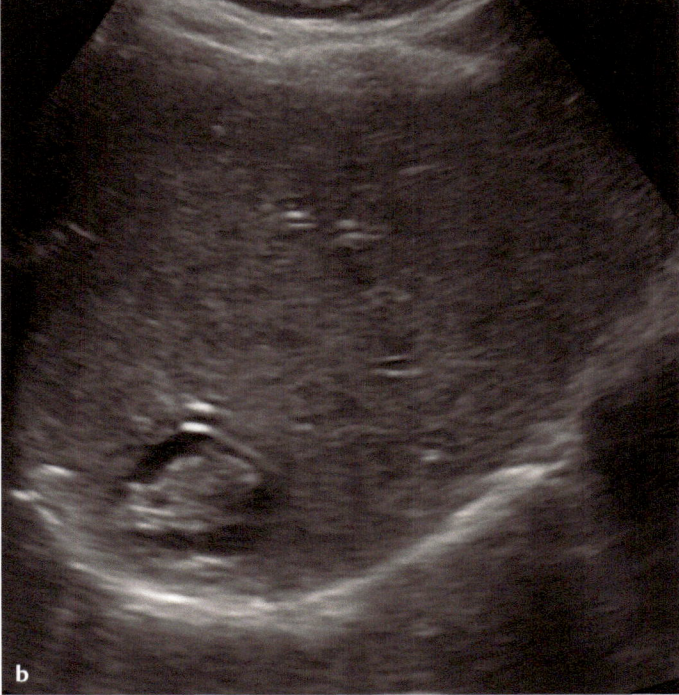

Fig. 5.65 *Echinococcus granulosus*. (a) Cysts within a cyst (type III). (b) Solid cyst contents 4 months after treatment (type IV).

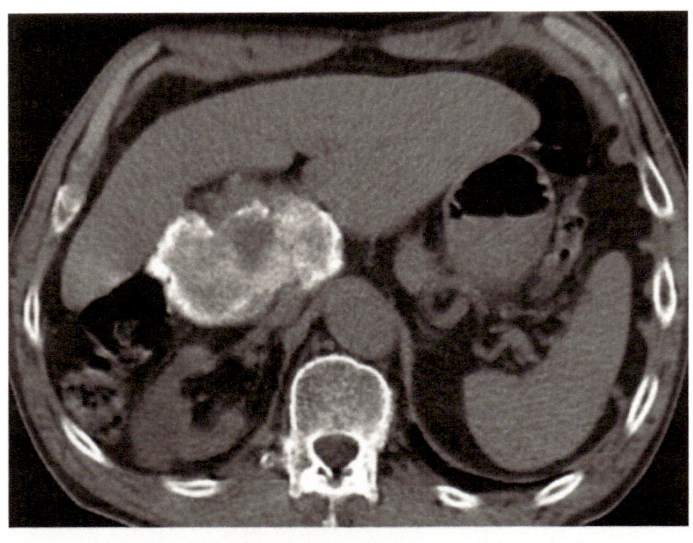

Fig. 5.66 **Echinococcus granulosus** after successful medical treatment. The cyst is calcified.

▶ **Imaging signs.** Involvement by *E. multilocularis* produces multiple cysts with irregular margins that invade the surrounding parenchyma like a malignant tumor. Central punctate calcifications (▶ Fig. 5.68) are a common finding even in untreated patients. The masses are poorly demarcated from surrounding tissue. When imaged by T1 W MRI, they show patchy low signal intensity with multiple small, hypointense cysts. On T2 W images the affected liver parenchyma is edematous and permeated by smaller cysts.[81] Postcontrast imaging shows inhomogeneous enhancement of the stroma between the cysts, with an overall infiltrative appearance (▶ Fig. 5.69).

▶ **Clinical features.** In contrast to *E. granulosus*, patients infected with *E. multilocularis* often have severe complaints such as hepatomegaly, jaundice, or ascites.

▶ **Differential diagnosis.** *E. multilocularis* cysts require differentiation mainly from hepatobiliary malignancies.

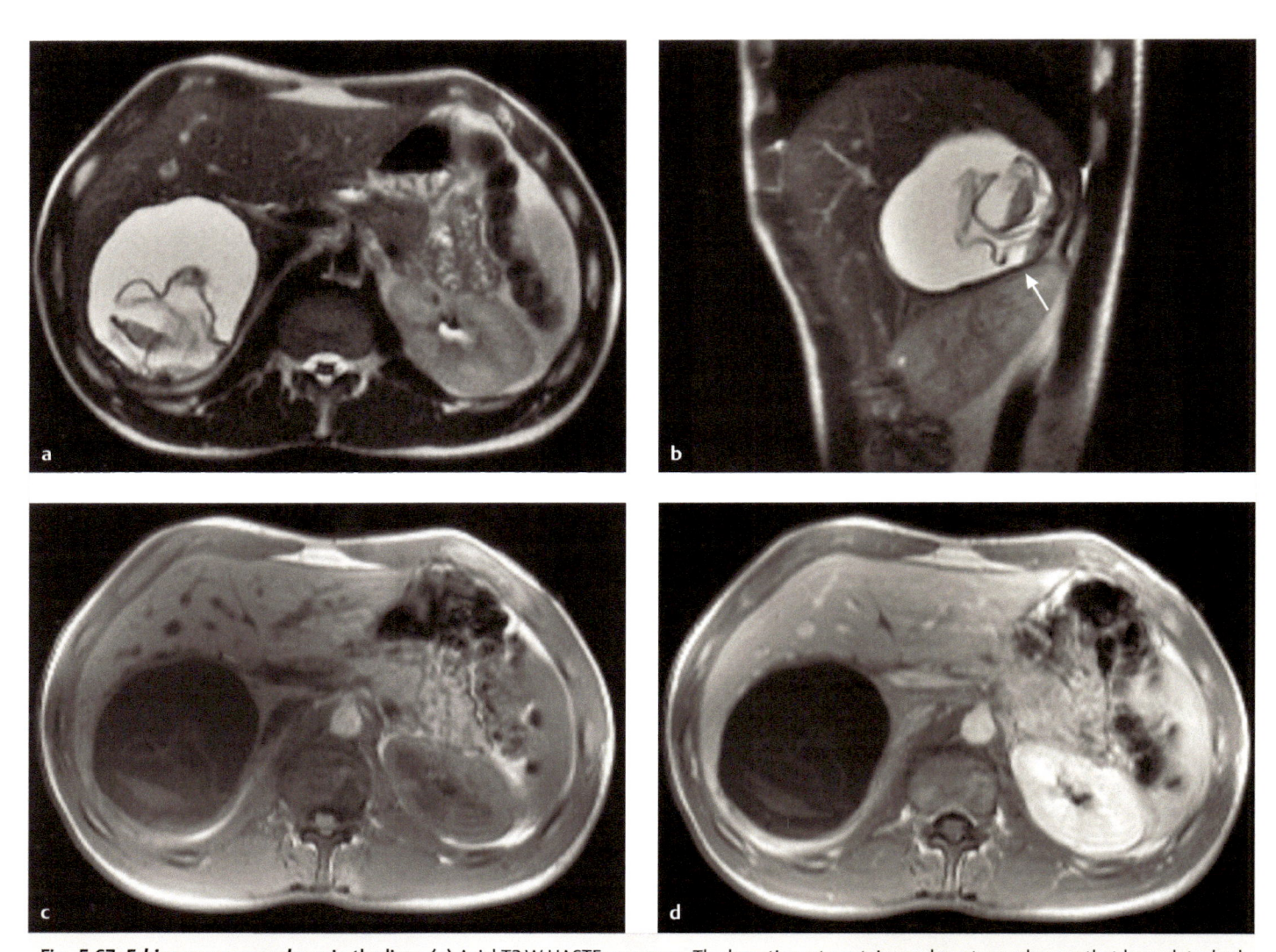

Fig. 5.67 **Echinococcus granulosus** in the liver. (a) Axial T2 W HASTE sequence. The hepatic cyst contains endocyst membranes that have detached from the ectocyst. (b) Corresponding sagittal T2 W HASTE sequence. (c) Unenhanced T1 W sequence. The cyst is hypointense. (d) Image in the equilibrium phase after injection of contrast medium. Enhancement is not observed in the cyst or its membranes.

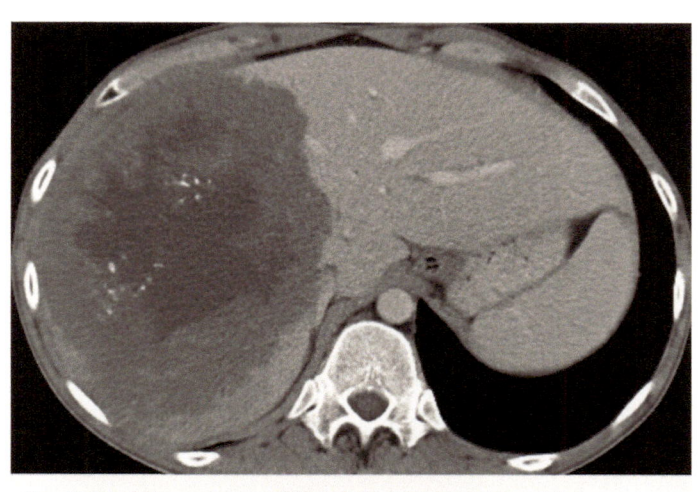

Fig. 5.68 *Echinococcus multilocularis*. The hydatid cyst has a hypodense center and contains calcifications.

▶ **Key points.** *E. multilocularis* has an external germinal layer, resulting in infiltrative growth of the hydatid cysts. At imaging, differentiation is mainly required from malignant tumors.

5.5.3 Pseudolesions of the Liver Parenchyma

The principal "pseudolesions" of the liver parenchyma are focal fatty infiltration, focal fatty sparing, and inflammatory pseudotumors.

Focal Fatty Infiltration and Fatty Sparing

▶ **Brief definition.** The accumulation of fat within hepatocytes is typically observed in diabetic and overweight patients, alcoholics, and patients exposed to other chemical toxins. Focal fatty infiltration may also result from the hepatotoxic effects of chemotherapy. Fatty infiltration may affect the entire liver homogeneously, or it may show a somewhat patchy, inhomogeneous distribution or may be confined to focal areas.[82] Focal fatty infiltration ultimately reflects differences in blood flow to different areas of the liver. Sites of predilection are the portal vein bifurcation and the area bordering the falciform ligament.[83]

▶ **Imaging signs**
- *Focal fatty infiltration*: Foci of fatty infiltration appear as areas of decreased attenuation on CT scans (▶ Fig. 5.70). These areas are hyperechoic on ultrasound. On MRI, focal fatty infiltration typically shows high signal intensity in both T1 W and T2 W sequences. The foci may also be isointense to surrounding liver on T1 W images, depending on their fat content. Opposed-phase and fat-suppressed sequences show a marked signal loss in areas affected by focal fatty infiltration. The areas do not enhance after IV injection of contrast medium (▶ Fig. 5.71). Vessels run undisplaced through the infiltrated liver parenchyma, although areas with mass effect will usually cause appreciable vascular displacement. It should be added that adenomas may also show a relatively homogeneous fat distribution. As a result, it is necessary in some cases to supplement unenhanced imaging with contrast-enhanced imaging to exclude focal fatty infiltration. The same considerations apply to the homogeneous fatty infiltration of hepatocellular carcinoma.
- *Focal fatty sparing*: Focal hepatic areas spared from fatty infiltration in diffuse steatosis often represent areas of regeneration in the liver parenchyma. Standard and fat-suppressed T1 W images and the opposed-phase sequence often display opposite signal patterns (▶ Fig. 5.72).

▶ **Differential diagnosis.** Focal fatty infiltration and fatty sparing require differentiation from true lesions such as hepatic metastases.

▶ **Key points.** Focal fatty infiltration and fatty sparing are based on blood flow differences and most commonly occur along the falciform ligament, in the gallbladder bed, and in the region of the porta hepatis. An awareness of these typical sites is important, as fatty infiltration and fatty sparing need to be differentiated from metastases.

5.6 Diffuse Liver Diseases

5.6.1 Cirrhosis

▶ **Brief definition.** Hepatic cirrhosis is a condition leading to irreversible fibrosis of the liver parenchyma. The changes are found in the space between the portal plates and destroy the normal hepatic architecture. As a general rule, hepatic cirrhosis is diagnosed by histological examination of a liver biopsy, while imaging is used to analyze the anatomical distribution of the disease.[84] As described earlier in connection with hepatocellular carcinoma, hepatic cirrhosis is considered a premalignant condition that is important in the early diagnosis of hepatocellular carcinoma. Portal hypertension with the development of collaterals is a common problem arising in approximately 30% of patients. Patients with refractory ascites or prior bleeding esophageal varices should be evaluated for the placement of a transjugular intrahepatic portosystemic shunt (TIPS). The device, consisting of a Gore-Tex-lined stent, creates an intrahepatic connection between the portal vein and hepatic vein (usually the right hepatic vein).

▶ **Imaging signs.** The earliest imaging sign is hepatomegaly. Typical imaging findings in advanced hepatic cirrhosis are a nodular surface contour of the liver and an enlarged caudate lobe combined with enlargement of the lateral segments of the left lobe and atrophy of the right lobe (▶ Fig. 5.73). Portal hypertension is manifested by collateral vessels and an enlarged spleen (▶ Fig. 5.74, ▶ Fig. 5.75). But since hepatic cirrhosis is often accompanied by hepatitis or inflammatory changes, it is not unusual to find prolonged T1 and/or T2 relaxation times. Accumulation of iron is also common in the cirrhotic liver and may cause decreased signal intensity. Associated changes in hepatic cirrhosis are ascites, signs of portal hypertension (▶ Fig. 5.76), and fluid in the gallbladder bed.[85,86]

▶ **Clinical features.** The dominant symptoms are those of impaired hepatic synthetic function. Disease is classified under the Child–Pugh system based on laboratory values (albumin, bilirubin, Quick value) and the presence of ascites.

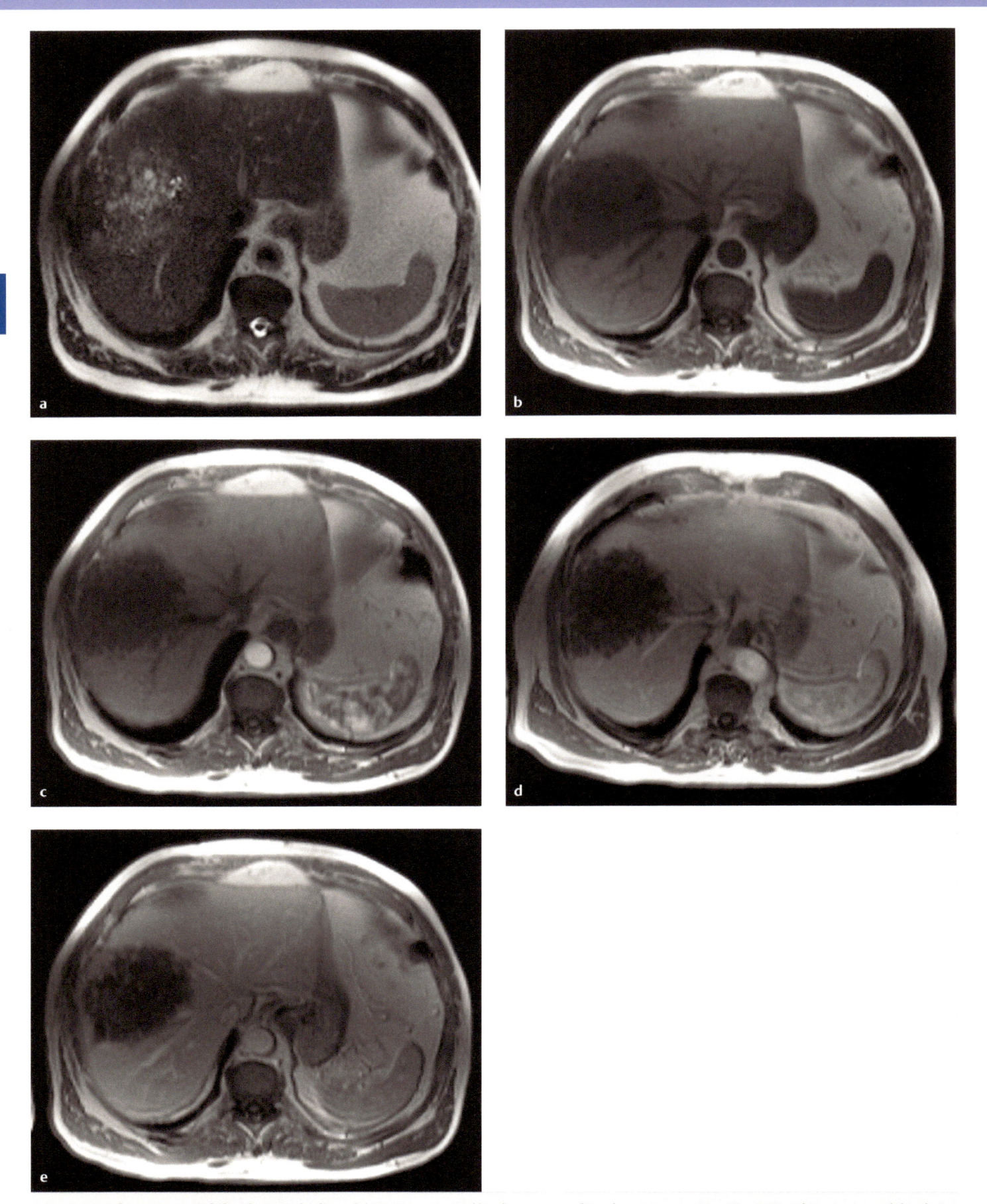

Fig. 5.69 *Echinococcus multilocularis* in the liver. (a) T2 W image. Unlike the pattern of involvement seen in ▶ Fig. 5.67, *Echinococcus multilocularis* produces multiple small cysts showing an almost infiltrative type of growth. **(b)** T1 W image. The cysts are hypodense. **(c)** Arterial phase image after injection of contrast medium shows enhancement of the tissue between the cysts, which are poorly demarcated from normal liver tissue. **(d)** Image in the portal venous phase shows increasing enhancement. **(e)** Equilibrium phase image shows a further increase of enhancement.

5.6 Diffuse Liver Diseases

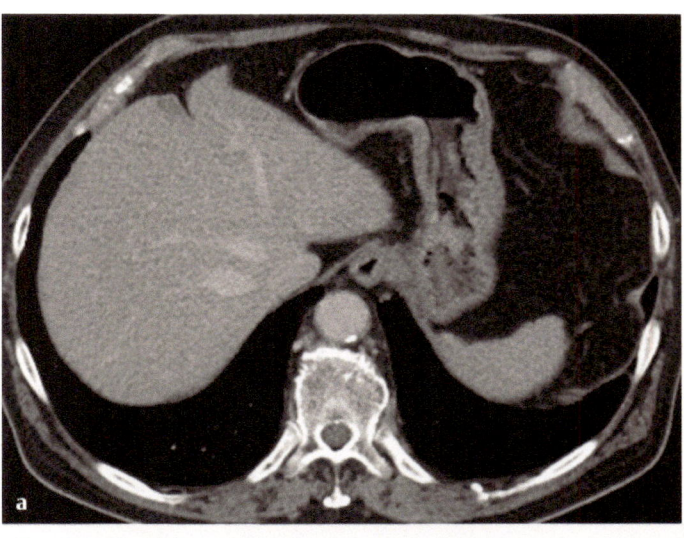

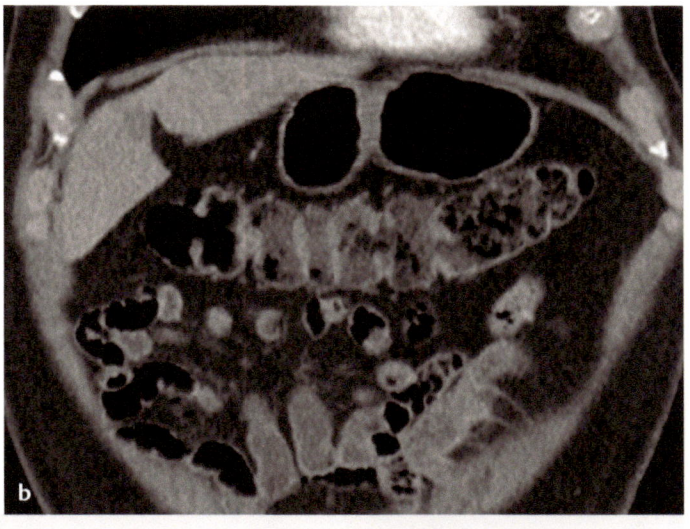

Fig. 5.70 Focal fatty infiltration at a typical site along the falciform ligament. (a) Portal venous phase. (b) Coronal reformatted image.

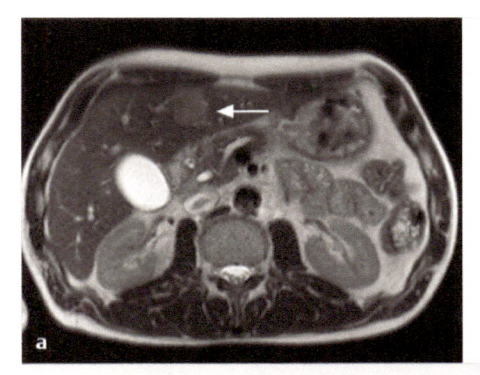

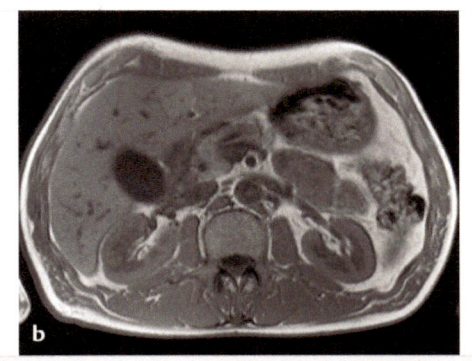

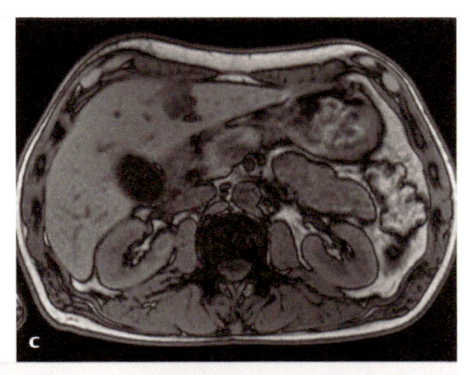

Fig. 5.71 Focal fatty infiltration at a typical site along the falciform ligament. (a) T2 W HASTE sequence shows a hyperintense mass in proximity to the falciform ligament (arrow). (b) Corresponding T1 W image. The mass is also hyperintense in this sequence. (c) Opposed-phase image shows a marked loss of signal intensity in the mass. This pattern is diagnostic of focal fatty infiltration.

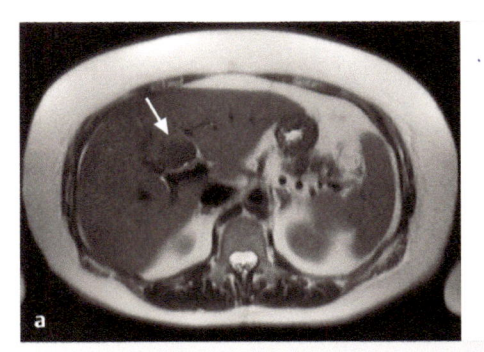

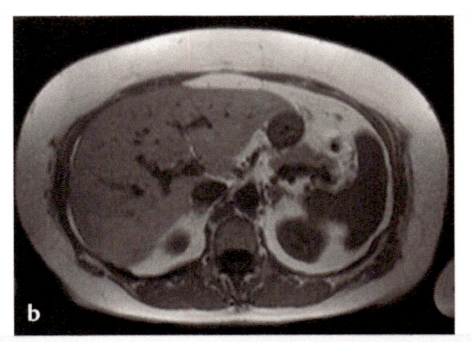

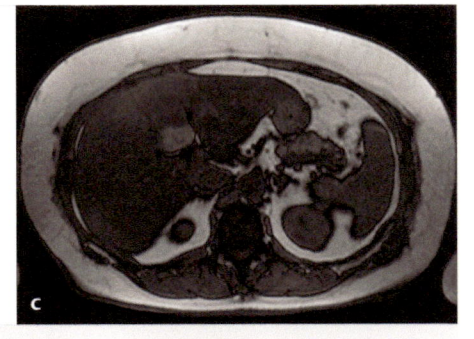

Fig. 5.72 Focal fatty sparing in the liver. (a) T2 W HASTE sequence shows generally increased signal intensity in the liver with a hypointense focus at the portal vein bifurcation (arrow). (b) Corresponding T1 W image. The lesion is isointense to surrounding liver tissue. (c) Opposed-phase sequence shows markedly decreased signal intensity in the liver consistent with hepatic steatosis. But the pseudolesion caused by focal fatty sparing shows no signal change and appears hyperintense, indicating an absence of fatty infiltration.

▶ **Differential diagnosis.** Hepatic cirrhosis can be differentiated from other diseases by typical imaging signs, laboratory values, and, if necessary, by histological findings. The etiology usually suggests the correct diagnosis: alcohol abuse is the leading cause of hepatic cirrhosis, present in 70% of cases, followed by hepatitis B. Systemic diseases such as cystic fibrosis, Wilson's disease, etc. are less common.

▶ **Key points.** Portal hypertension due to hepatic cirrhosis may lead to the development of collateral vessels bypassing the liver, with risk of bleeding esophageal varices. This condition and refractory ascites are indications for TIPS placement. Patients with hepatic cirrhosis should be followed for the possible development of hepatocellular carcinoma.

Liver

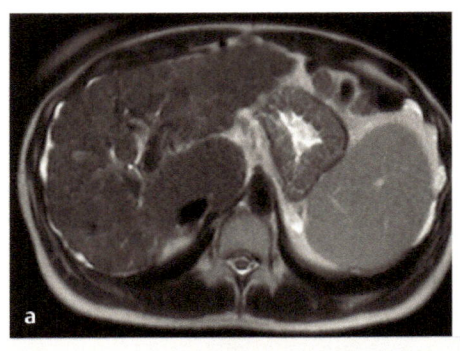

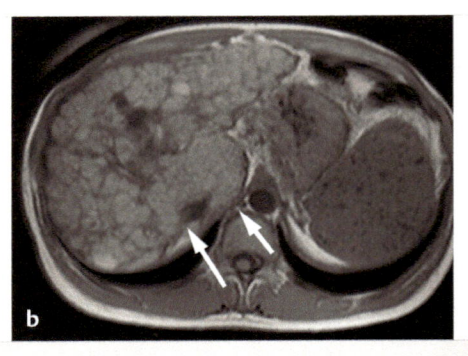

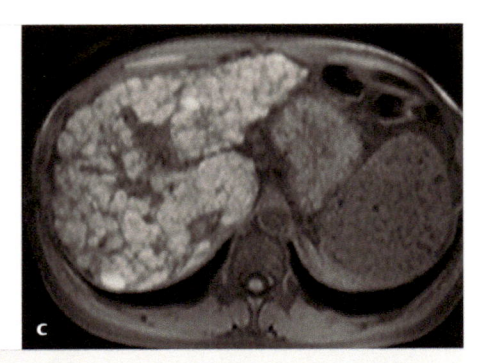

Fig. 5.73 Changes associated with advanced hepatic cirrhosis. All three sequences show multiple regenerating nodules in the liver, creating a nodular contour in the liver surface. Only the caudate lobe ([b], arrow) is less affected by the changes and still shows a relatively normal signal. **(a)** T2W sequence. **(b)** T1W sequence. **(c)** Fat-suppressed T1W sequence.

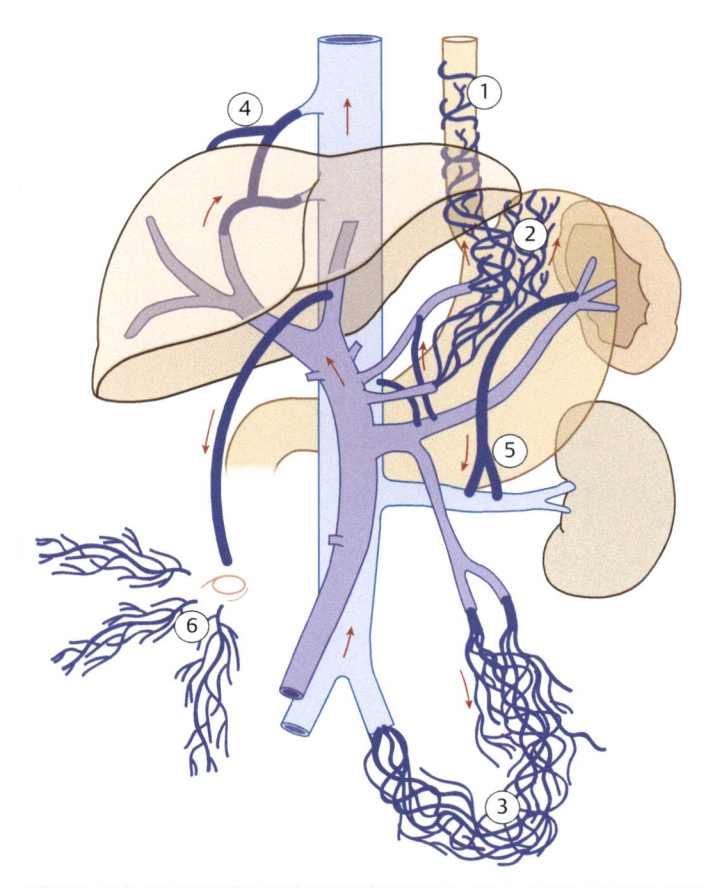

Fig. 5.74 Collateral pathways that may develop in portal hypertension: 1, through the esophageal veins; 2, through the short gastric veins; 3, through the middle and inferior rectal veins; 4, through veins in the anterior diaphragm; 5, through the splenic veins and renal vein (splenorenal shunt); 6, through the umbilical vein and inferior epigastric vein, and also through the thoracoepigastric and lateral thoracic veins.

5.6.2 Iron Storage Diseases

Hemochromatosis

▶ **Brief definition.** Hemochromatosis is an autosomal recessive disorder caused by an increase in intestinal iron absorption. The absorbed iron is stored as ferritin or hemosiderin, and there is an excessive accumulation of iron in the pancreas.[87] The disease becomes symptomatic in the fourth to fifth decades. The organs primarily affected by hemochromatosis are the liver, pancreas (approximately 50% of cases), and heart (approximately 15% of cases). Accordingly, hemochromatosis is associated with changes such as hepatic cirrhosis, diabetes mellitus, and cardiomyopathy in patients with cardiac involvement.

> **Note**
>
> Patients with a long history of hemochromatosis have a significantly increased risk of developing hepatocellular carcinoma.

Patients with hemochromatosis also show decreased reticuloendothelial function, and the iron deposition in hemochromatosis occurs principally in the liver cells,[88] where the iron has a cytotoxic effect. This explains the development of cirrhosis and the markedly increased risk of hepatocellular carcinoma.

▶ **Imaging signs.** Excessive iron accumulation in the liver and pancreas leads to decreased signal intensity in T1W and T2W sequences. This process spares the spleen (▶ Fig. 5.77).

▶ **Clinical features.** The most common symptoms are those of hepatic cirrhosis, diabetes mellitus, and eventual heart failure in patients with cardiac involvement. Other typical clinical manifestations are hyperpigmentation of the skin due to intracutaneous iron, decreased libido, and a slightly increased incidence of extrahepatic malignancies. Hemochromatosis is also referred to as "bronze diabetes" due to hyperpigmentation of the skin and diabetes mellitus.

▶ **Differential diagnosis.** Hemochromatosis secondary to multiple blood transfusions requires differentiation from the primary form. This is best accomplished by analysis of the affected organs. The primary form, hemochromatosis, spares the spleen.

▶ **Key points.** Hemochromatosis is an autosomal recessive disorder caused by increased intestinal iron absorption. The genetic defect also causes reticuloendothelial system dysfunction.

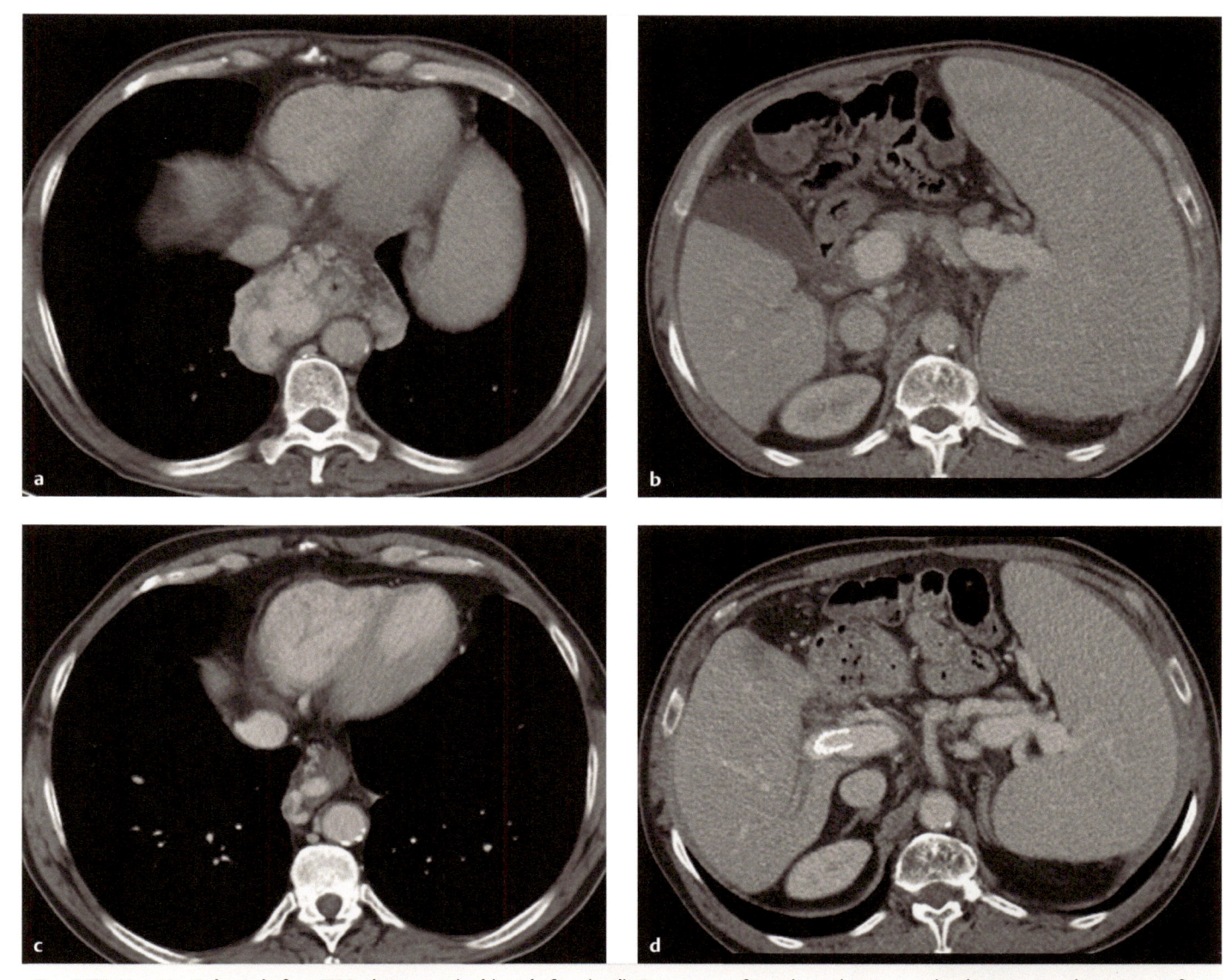

Fig. 5.75 Hepatic cirrhosis before TIPS placement (a, b) and after (c, d). Regression of esophageal varices and a decrease in spleen size confirm that portal pressure has been reduced following shunt placement. **(a)** Severe esophageal varices. **(b)** Marked splenomegaly. **(c)** Marked regression of esophageal varices after shunt placement. **(d)** Reduction in spleen size.

Excessive iron is stored in the cells of the liver, pancreas, skin, and heart. The cytotoxic effect of the iron leads to diabetes mellitus and hepatic cirrhosis with risk for development of hepatocellular carcinoma.

Hemosiderosis

▶ **Brief definition.** Hemochromatosis is distinguished from the secondary form of iron overload, hemosiderosis. This condition may result from parenteral iron administration, such as multiple blood transfusions with an associated hemolytic reaction. The iron accumulates in the cells of the reticuloendothelial system; hence the liver and spleen are affected by the changes (▶ Fig. 5.78), while the pancreas and other parenchymal organs are largely spared.[89] This is of key importance in differentiating hemosiderosis from the primary form—hemochromatosis—since an iron overload in parenchymal cells such as hepatocytes has a much more toxic effect.

Note

Hemosiderosis is characterized by iron accumulation in the liver and spleen. In hemochromatosis, iron is deposited in the liver, pancreas and heart, sparing the spleen.

▶ **Imaging signs.** The CT attenuation of the liver is more than 70 HU on unenhanced scans (▶ Fig. 5.79). The blood vessels are hypodense to the liver parenchyma. Because iron deposition shortens the T2 relaxation time on MRI, the liver shows decreased signal intensity in T2W or T2*W images. Greater degrees of iron overload also cause decreased signal intensity in T1W images. The distribution of the iron overload is important: If the changes spare the spleen, the most likely diagnosis is hemochromatosis. But if the signal intensity of the spleen, normally isointense to muscle, is found to be decreased, the most likely diagnosis is transfusion hemosiderosis or siderosis due to another cause.

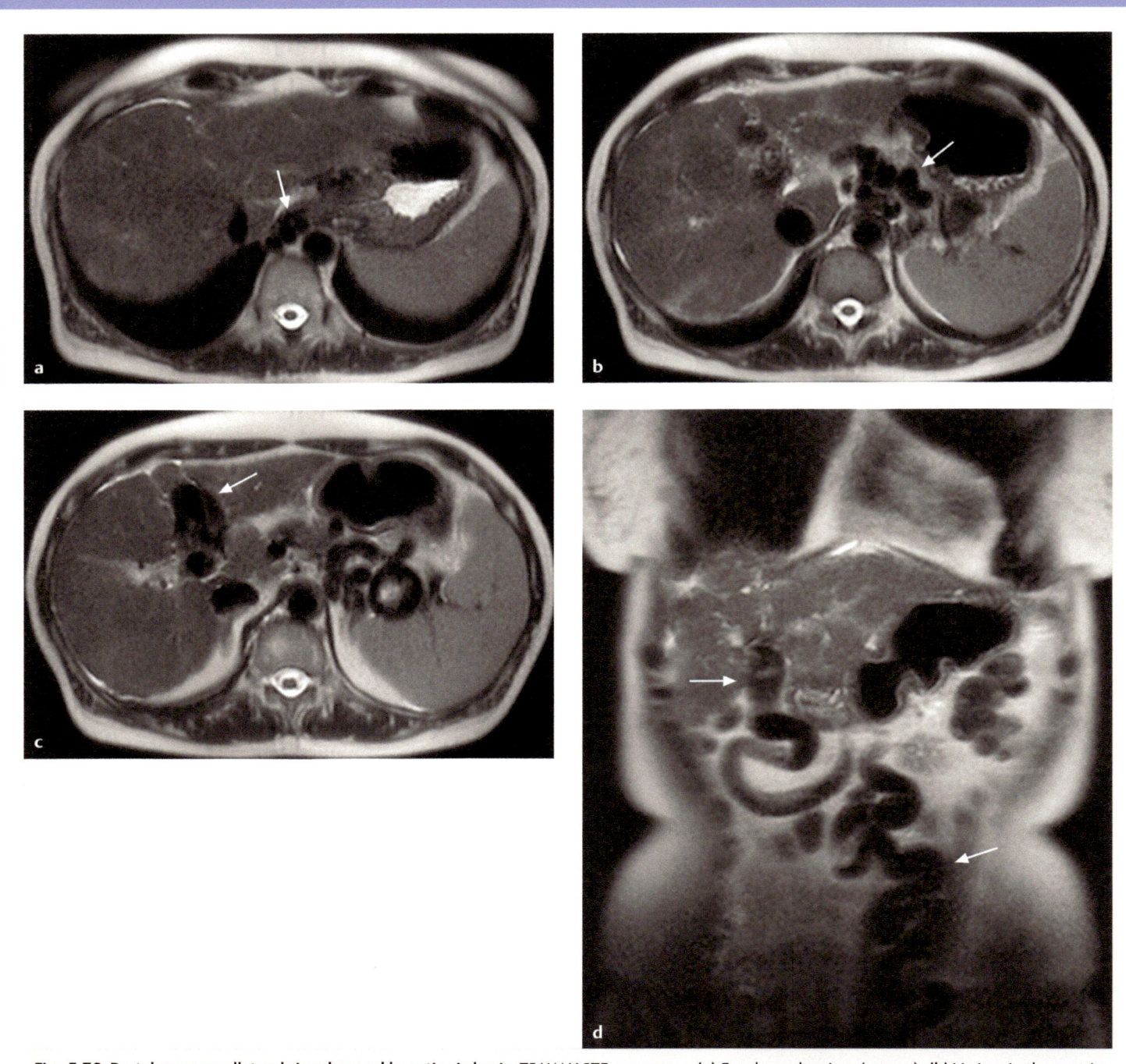

Fig. 5.76 Portal venous collaterals in advanced hepatic cirrhosis. T2 W HASTE sequences. (**a**) Esophageal varices (arrows). (**b**) Varices in the gastric region (arrow). (**c**) Recanalization of the umbilical vein in the falciform ligament (arrow). (**d**) Tortuous veins (arrows) run from the umbilical vein to the umbilicus and the epigastric vessels.

▶ **Differential diagnosis.** Hemochromatosis requires differentiation from secondary iron overload, hemosiderosis.

▶ **Key points.** Hemosiderosis results from secondary iron accumulation due to blood transfusion and hemolysis. The iron is stored in the reticuloendothelial system, explaining why the liver and spleen are most commonly affected. The pancreas is spared. The iron overload leads to increased density of the liver on unenhanced CT. Affected organs show decreased signal intensity on MRI.

Hepatic Steatosis

▶ **Brief definition.** Hepatic steatosis, or fatty liver disease, is an abnormal accumulation of fat within hepatocytes. As well as overeating, all potentially hepatotoxic agents may cause steatosis—most notably alcohol and chemotherapeutic drugs but also hepatitis. A subtype is nonalcoholic steatohepatitis (NASH), which is characterized histologically by fat accumulation with an inflammatory reaction and may progress to cirrhosis. Typical causes of NASH are obesity, gastrointestinal bypass, type II diabetes

5.6 Diffuse Liver Diseases

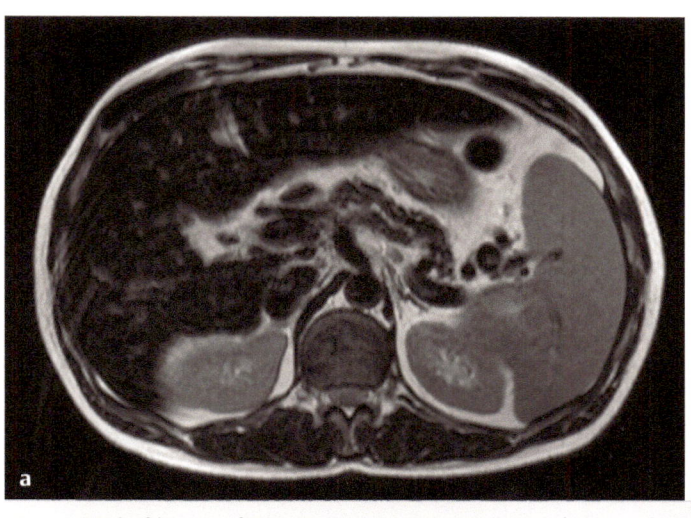

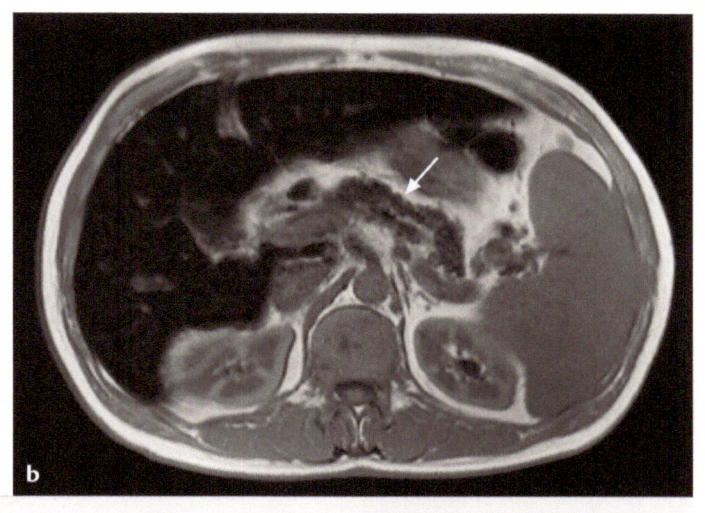

Fig. 5.77 (a, b) **Hemochromatosis.** Excessive iron accumulation in the liver and pancreas ([b], arrow) leads to a marked reduction of signal intensity in the T2W (a) and T1W (b) images. The spleen does not exhibit signal changes.

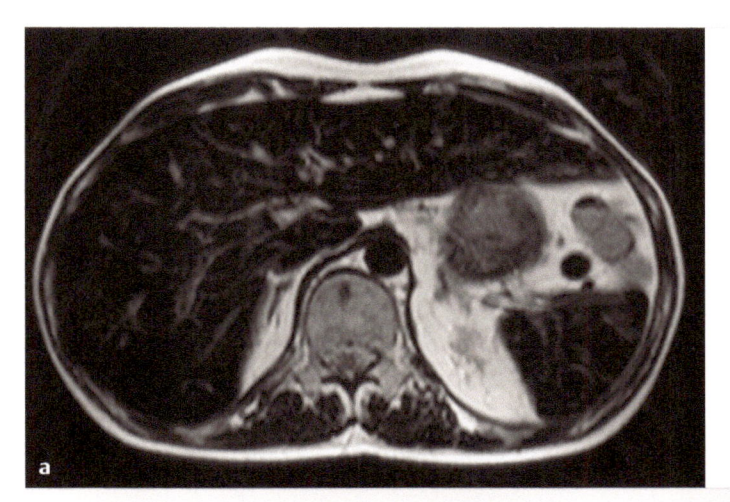

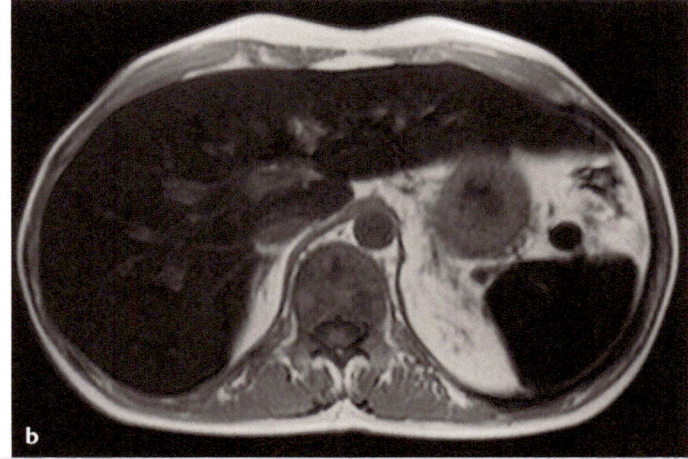

Fig. 5.78 (a, b) **Hemosiderosis.** Iron accumulation in the reticuloendothelial system in hemosiderosis, unlike in hemochromatosis, causes marked hypointensity of the liver and spleen in both T2W (a) and T1W (b) images while sparing the pancreas.

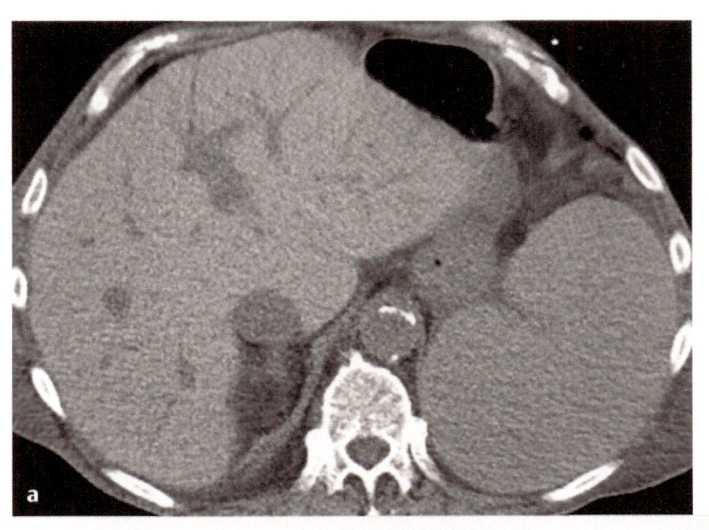

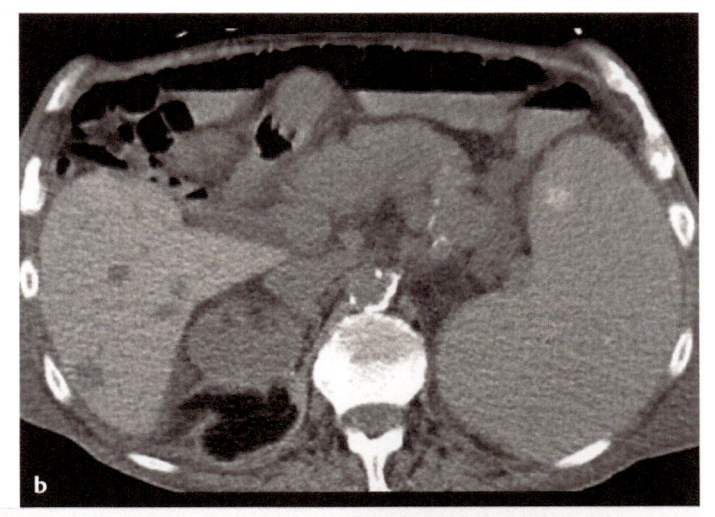

Fig. 5.79 **Hemosiderosis after multiple blood transfusions.** Unenhanced CT. (a) The density of the liver is significantly increased (to more than 70 HU). The spleen also shows increased density. (b) The pancreas appears normal. This distribution pattern is typical of hemosiderosis.

Liver

mellitus, and toxic liver damage due, for example, to parenteral nutrition or abetalipoproteinemia.[90]

▶ **Imaging signs.** As noted under pseudotumors of the liver (see Chapter 5.5.3), fatty infiltration of the parenchyma with liver damage may show a diffuse, patchy, or focal pattern of involvement (▶ Fig. 5.80, ▶ Fig. 5.81). Hepatic steatosis is diagnosed sonographically by comparing the echogenicity of the liver with that of the kidney. The echogenicity of the steatotic liver is greatly increased and far surpasses that of the kidney (▶ Fig. 5.82). While echogenicity is homogeneous, the sound is typically attenuated in liver areas farther from the probe (see ▶ Fig. 5.82). On CT, the liver shows markedly decreased density on unenhanced scans (▶ Fig. 5.83). Normal liver tissue has an unenhanced attenuation of 55 to 65 HU. The attenuation values decrease with increasing fat content, falling by approximately 15 HU per 10% increase. Normal contrast with intrahepatic vessels is reversed on unenhanced scans, as the vessels appear denser than the steatotic liver parenchyma.

Note

Hepatic steatosis alters the contrast between the liver parenchyma and hepatic tumors. Metastases are denser than the parenchyma on unenhanced scans.

With MRI, hepatic steatosis is difficult to diagnose on T2 W and T1 W images alone. But chemical shift imaging provides a simple

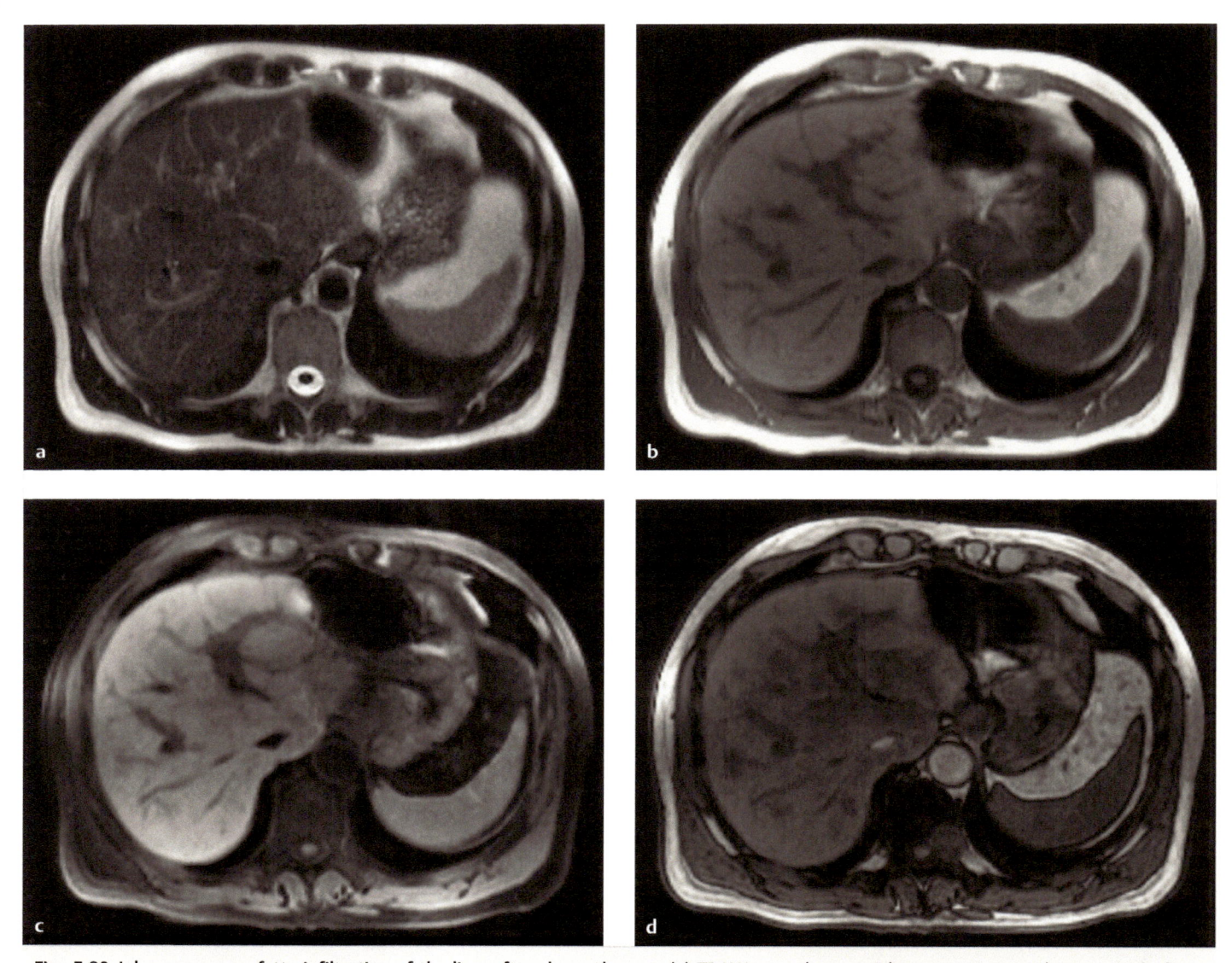

Fig. 5.80 Inhomogeneous fatty infiltration of the liver after chemotherapy. **(a)** T2 W image shows an inhomogeneous signal pattern in the liver. **(b)** Corresponding T1 W image. The inhomogeneous signal intensity of the liver is not apparent in this sequence. **(c)** Fat-suppressed T1 W image shows diffusely distributed areas of low signal intensity in the liver. **(d)** Opposed-phase sequence. The diffusely distributed areas of fatty infiltration are clearly depicted.

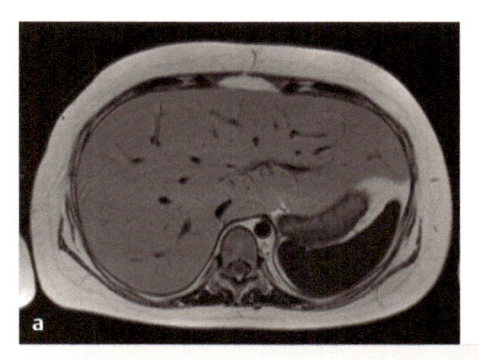

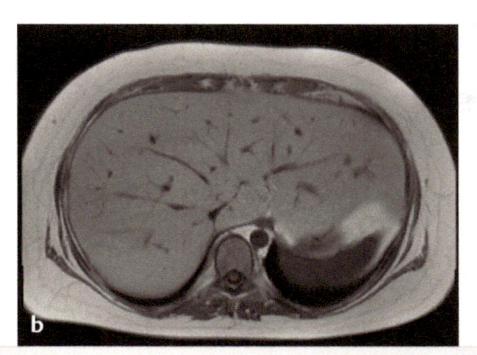

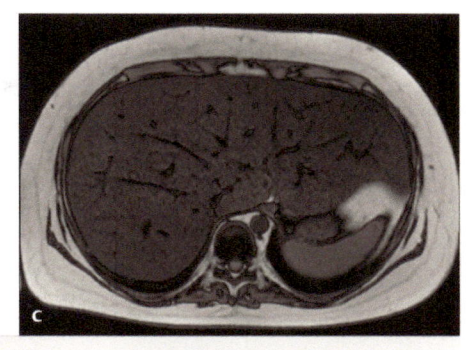

Fig. 5.81 NASH. All the sequences show massive fatty infiltration of the liver with hepatomegaly. **(a)** T2 W sequence. **(b)** T1 W sequence. **(c)** Opposed-phase sequence.

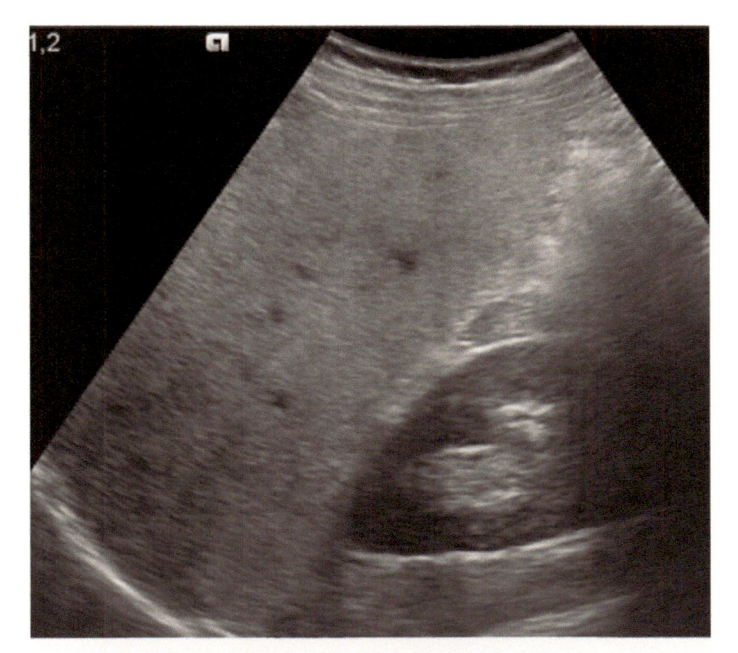

Fig. 5.82 Hepatic steatosis. The echogenicity of the liver is markedly increased relative to that of the kidney. Its echo pattern is homogeneous, but the far side of the liver shows acoustic shadowing due to the attenuating effect of the steatotic liver parenchyma.

and accurate way to differentiate steatosis from other parenchymal changes in the liver (see ▶ Fig. 5.6).[91] In chemical shift imaging, water and fat have different signal characteristics due to their different resonant frequencies. This permits an accurate diagnosis of focal or diffuse steatosis of the liver. Except for hepatic lipoma, opposed-phase and out-of-phase imaging are more sensitive than fat-suppressed imaging for detecting fatty infiltration of the liver parenchyma. The signal intensity in opposed-phase images is determined by the absolute value of water intensity minus fat intensity. For this reason, most tissues including fat have roughly the same appearance in in-phase and out-of-phase images, whereas fatty infiltration of the liver causes a marked loss of signal intensity. In the case of hepatic lipomas, which are composed almost entirely of fat, the signal intensity on opposed-phase imaging is not significantly altered (see ▶ Fig. 5.27). These lesions appear markedly hypointense in fat-suppressed images, however.

▶ **Differential diagnosis.** The cause of hepatic steatosis can be determined from the history.

▶ **Key points.** Hepatic steatosis is characterized by the intracellular accumulation of fat. Ultrasound shows increased echogenicity of the liver. The CT density of the liver declines in proportion to the degree of steatosis. Chemical shift imaging is the most effective MRI technique for diagnosing hepatic steatosis.

5.7 Liver Injuries

▶ **Brief definition.** Liver injuries are graded on a scale developed by the American Association for the Surgery of Trauma (AAST) (▶ Table 5.6).

▶ **Imaging signs.** CT is the modality of choice for imaging acutely symptomatic injuries such as liver rupture, laceration, subcapsular hematoma, or posttraumatic arteriovenous shunts because it can quickly survey the extent of changes and determine the possible need for surgery. At ultrasound, an acute intrahepatic hematoma may appear hyperechoic, hypoechoic, or isoechoic to the surrounding parenchyma. The hallmark of a liver injury is an inhomogeneous echo pattern in one area of the liver (▶ Fig. 5.84). The echogenicity of the injury tends to change over time. Subcapsular hematomas of the liver have a sharp boundary with the capsule but are poorly demarcated from the parenchyma.

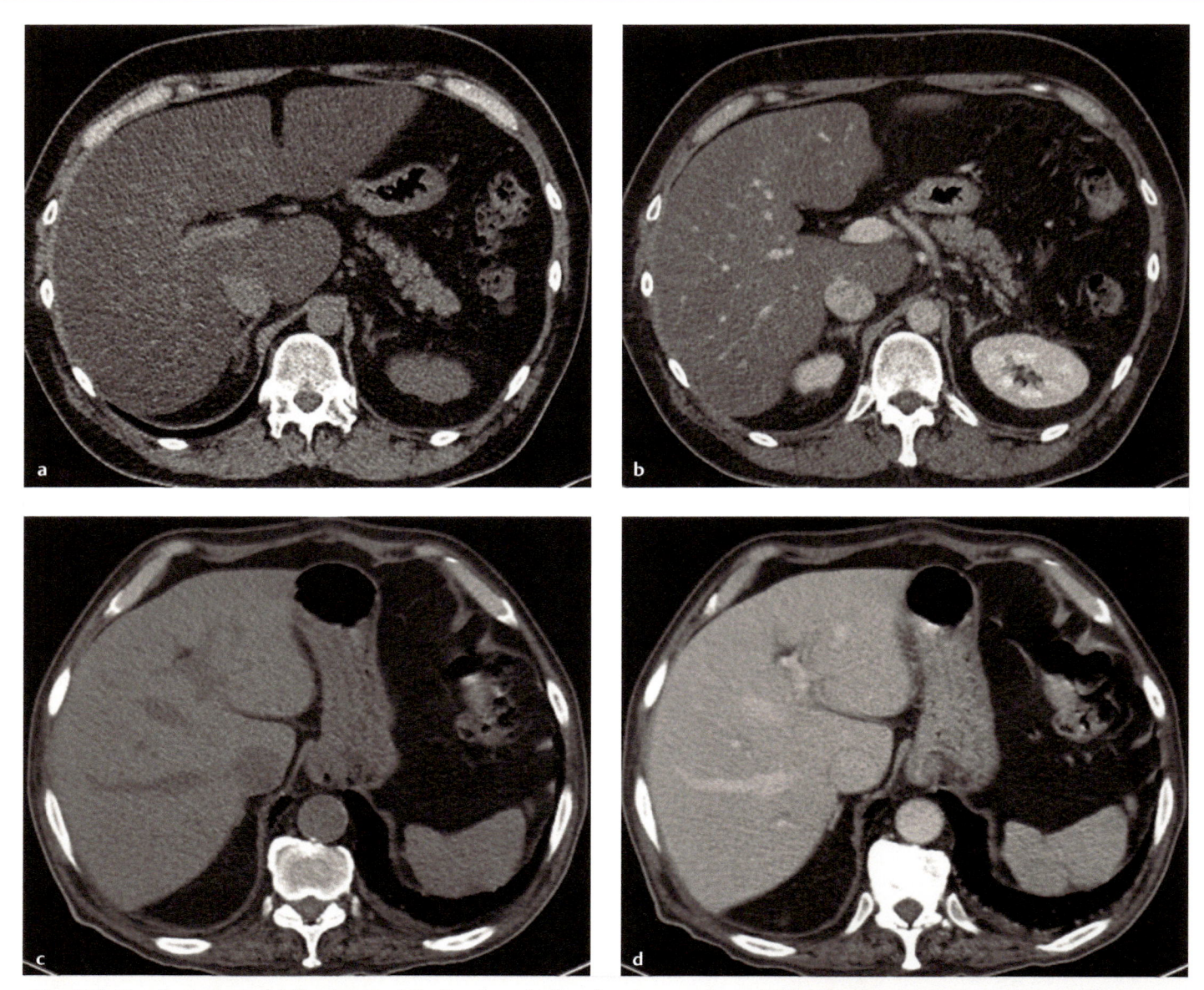

Fig. 5.83 Hepatic steatosis. (a) The density of the liver is markedly reduced on unenhanced CT, with a reversal of contrast between the liver parenchyma and vessels. **(b)** After injection of contrast medium, the liver parenchyma shows markedly less enhancement than a nonsteatotic liver. **(c)** Unenhanced CT scan of a healthy liver. **(d)** Healthy liver in the portal venous phase still shows greater density than the steatotic liver.

Table 5.6 Liver injury scale of the American Association for the Surgery of Trauma (AAST). The grade is advanced one number for multiple injuries up to grade III

Grade	Type of injury	Description
I	Hematoma/contusion	Subcapsular, <10% surface area
	Laceration	Capsular tear, <1 cm parenchymal depth
II	Hematoma/contusion	Subcapsular, 10–50% surface area Intraparenchymal <10 cm in diameter
	Laceration	Capsular tear 1–3 cm parenchyma depth, <10 cm in length
III	Hematoma/contusion	Subcapsular, >50% surface area of ruptured subcapsular or parenchymal hematoma; intraparenchymal hematoma >10 cm or expanding
	Laceration	>3 cm parenchymal depth
IV	Laceration	Parenchymal disruption involving 25–75% of hepatic lobe or 1–3 Couinaud segments
V	Laceration	Parenchymal disruption involving >75% of hepatic lobe or >3 Couinaud segments within a single lobe
	Vascular	Juxtahepatic venous injuries, i.e., retrohepatic vena cava/central major hepatic veins
VI	Vascular	Hepatic avulsion

5.7 Liver Injuries

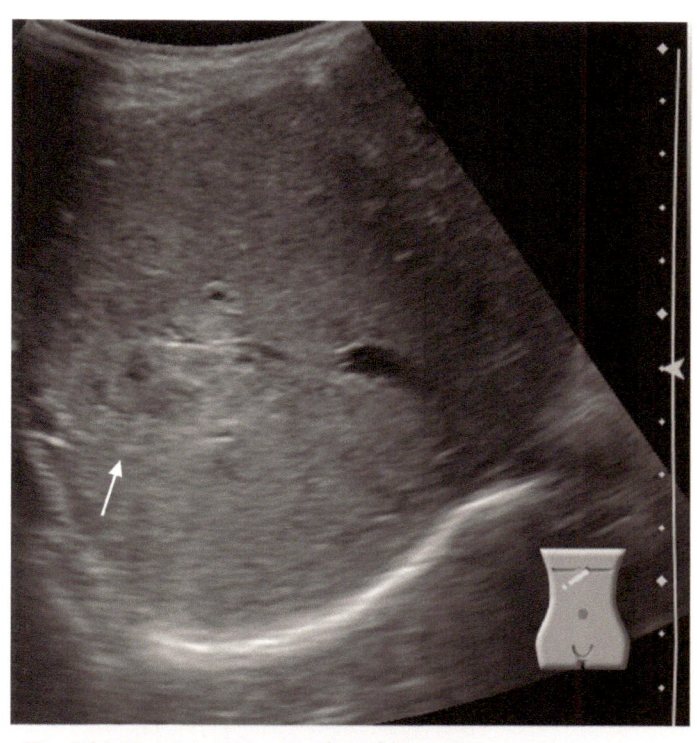

Fig. 5.84 Liver injury. A parenchymal laceration (arrow) appears hypoechoic in an ultrasound scan of the liver. The inhomogeneous echo pattern is characteristic of liver injury.

⚠ Caution
Ultrasound has low sensitivity for the direct detection of liver injuries following blunt abdominal trauma.[92]

Current guidelines for the examination and treatment of multiply injured patients approve ultrasound use for the detection of free intra-abdominal fluid, but diagnostic imaging should employ CT whenever possible.[93] Both lacerations and contusions of the liver are hypodense to surrounding parenchyma on CT (▶ Fig. 5.85, ▶ Fig. 5.86). A special form of posttraumatic or postoperative change is a bile leak following a cholecystectomy (stump leak) or anastomosis (anastomotic leak). In these cases it is difficult to distinguish a bile leak from a local postoperative fluid collection by unenhanced MRI or CT. This is an important application for biliary contrast agents.[94] When gadoxetalate is used, significant biliary excretion of the agent occurs within a short time after administration of contrast medium, and a bile leak is identified as an area of contrast extravasation. ▶ Fig. 5.87 illustrates the imaging appearance of a bile leak following cholecystectomy.

▶ **Key points.** CT is the imaging modality of choice in trauma patients with suspected liver injury. Liver injuries are graded by severity on the AAST scale.

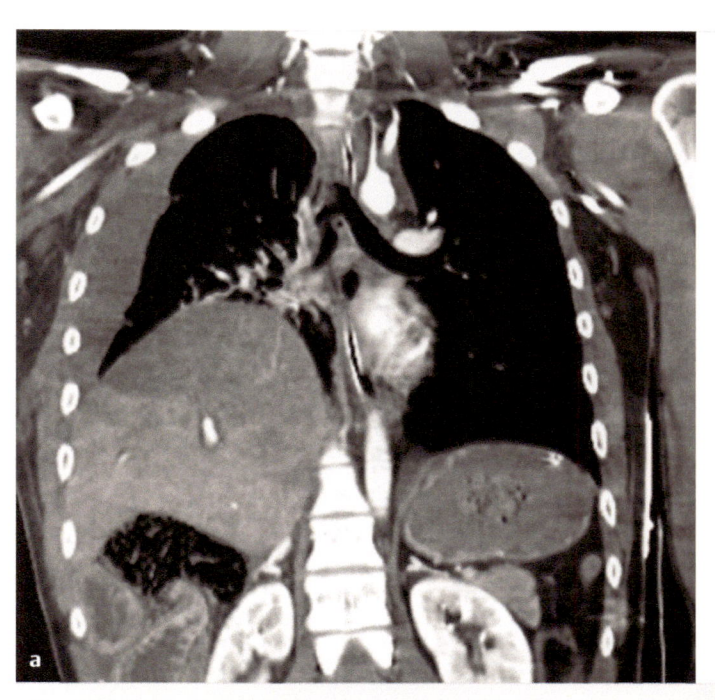

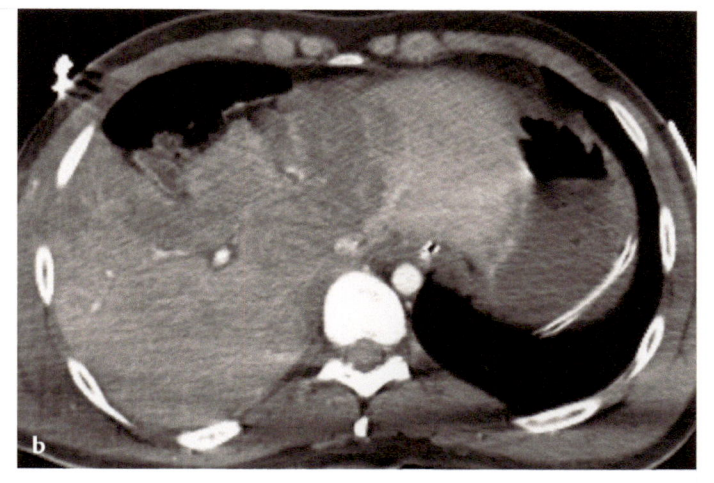

Fig. 5.85 Contusion of the liver and rupture of the diaphragm (AAST grade V injury). The injured parenchyma shows decreased density on CT. (a) Coronal image. (b) Axial image.

Liver

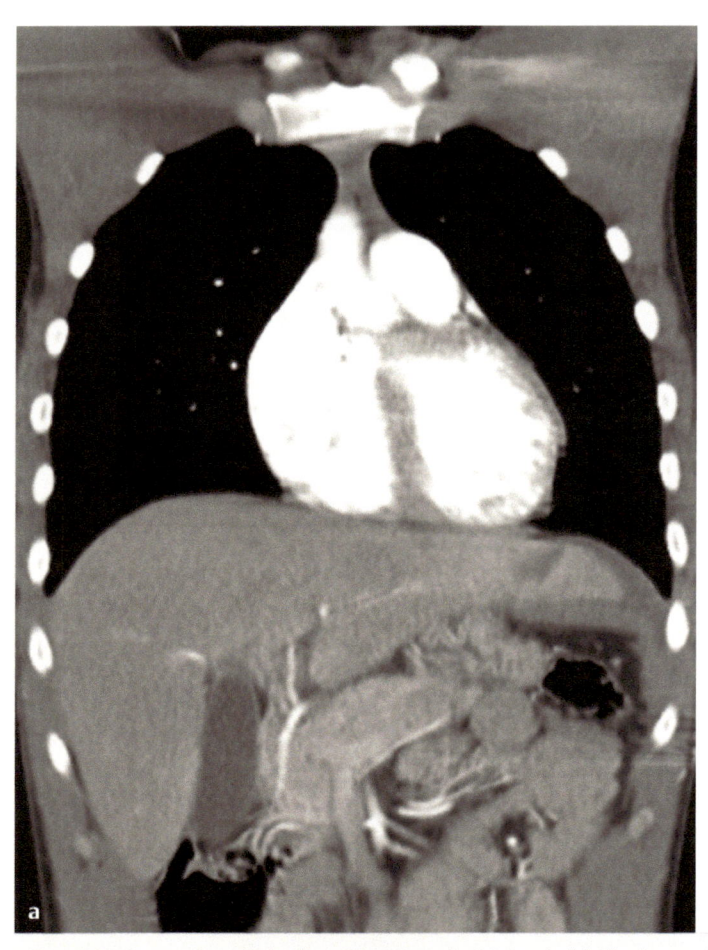

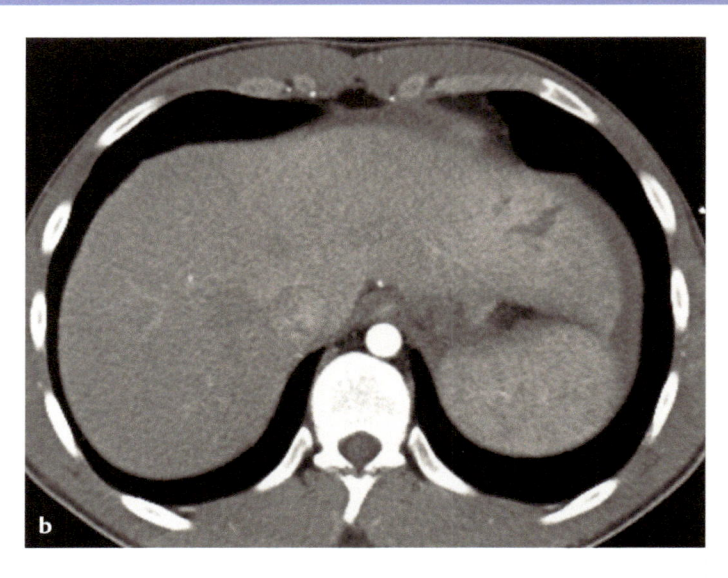

Fig. 5.86 Laceration of the liver (AAST grade II injury). (a) The laceration in segment II is less dense than its surroundings. **(b)** Capsular tear has resulted in a small hemoperitoneum.

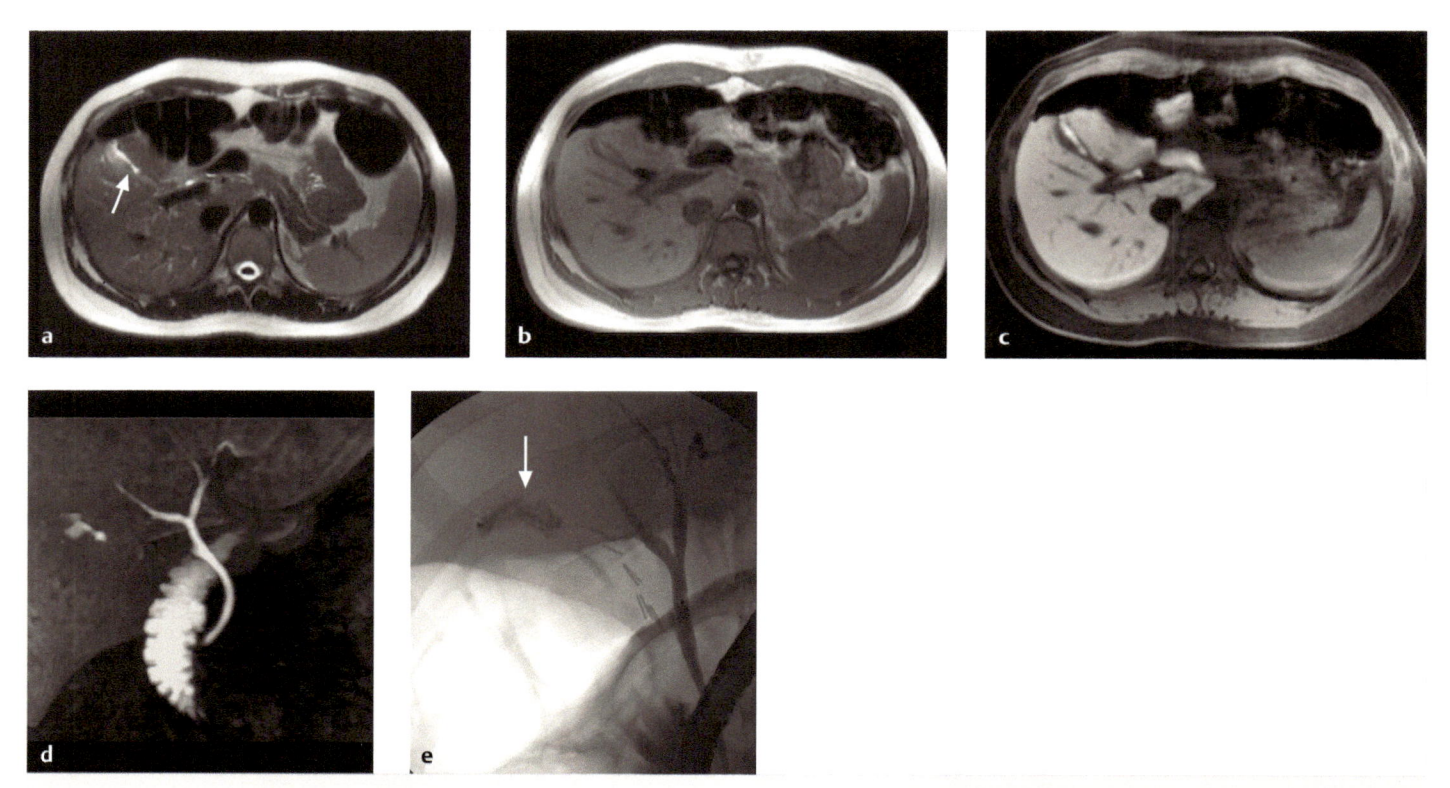

Fig. 5.87 Cystic duct stump leak following cholecystectomy. (a) T2 W image shows a small fluid collection in the former gallbladder bed (arrow). **(b)** The fluid appears hypointense in a T1 W image. **(c)** Fat-suppressed T1 W image 15 minutes after injection of Gd-EOB-DTPA at 0.025 mmol/kg BW. A bile leak in the former gallbladder bed is indicated by the presence of hyperintense contrast agent that is excreted through the biliary system. **(d)** Maximum intensity projection of a T1 W 3D data set provides an even clearer view of the bile leak. **(e)** Subsequent endoscopic retrograde cholangiopancreatography (ERCP) clearly demonstrates contrast extravasation from the cystic duct stump (arrow).

Bibliography

[1] Bismuth H. Surgical anatomy and anatomical surgery of the liver. World J Surg. 1982; 6(1):3–9

[2] Couinaud C. Le foie. Etudes anatomiques et chirurgicales. Paris: Masson & Cie; 1957

[3] Fasel JH, Gailloud P, Terrier F, Mentha G, Sprumont P. Segmental anatomy of the liver: a review and a proposal for an international working nomenclature. Eur Radiol. 1996; 6(6):834–837

[4] Reimer P, Schneider G, Schima W. Hepatobiliary contrast agents for contrast-enhanced MRI of the liver: properties, clinical development and applications. Eur Radiol. 2004; 14(4):559–578

[5] Galea N, Cantisani V, Taouli B. Liver lesion detection and characterization: role of diffusion-weighted imaging. J Magn Reson Imaging. 2013; 37(6):1260–1276

[6] Mitchell DG. Chemical shift magnetic resonance imaging: applications in the abdomen and pelvis. Top Magn Reson Imaging. 1992; 4(3):46–63

[7] Rofsky NM, Lee VS, Laub G, et al. Abdominal MR imaging with a volumetric interpolated breath-hold examination. Radiology. 1999; 212(3):876–884

[8] Hamm B, Staks T, Mühler A, et al. Phase I clinical evaluation of Gd-EOB-DTPA as a hepatobiliary MR contrast agent: safety, pharmacokinetics, and MR imaging. Radiology. 1995; 195(3):785–792

[9] Spinazzi A, Lorusso V, Pirovano G, Kirchin M. Safety, tolerance, biodistribution, and MR imaging enhancement of the liver with gadobenate dimeglumine: results of clinical pharmacologic and pilot imaging studies in nonpatient and patient volunteers. Acad Radiol. 1999; 6(5):282–291

[10] Grazioli L, Morana G, Kirchin MA, Schneider G. Accurate differentiation of focal nodular hyperplasia from hepatic adenoma at gadobenate dimeglumine-enhanced MR imaging: prospective study. Radiology. 2005; 236(1):166–177

[11] Grazioli L, Bondioni MP, Haradome H, et al. Hepatocellular adenoma and focal nodular hyperplasia: value of gadoxetic acid-enhanced MR imaging in differential diagnosis. Radiology. 2012; 262(2):520–529

[12] Low RN. Contrast agents for MR imaging of the liver. J Magn Reson Imaging. 1997; 7(1):56–67

[13] Schuhmann-Giampieri G, Mahler M, Röll G, Maibauer R, Schmitz S. Pharmacokinetics of the liver-specific contrast agent Gd-EOB-DTPA in relation to contrast-enhanced liver imaging in humans. J Clin Pharmacol. 1997; 37(7):587–596

[14] Tweedle MF. Physicochemical properties of gadoteridol and other magnetic resonance contrast agents. Invest Radiol. 1992; 27 Suppl 1:S2–S6

[15] Patriquin H, Lafortune M, Burns PN, Dauzat M. Duplex Doppler examination in portal hypertension: technique and anatomy. AJR Am J Roentgenol. 1987; 149(1):71–76

[16] Levy HM, Newhouse JH. MR imaging of portal vein thrombosis. AJR Am J Roentgenol. 1988; 151(2):283–286

[17] Silverman PM, Patt RH, Garra BS, et al. MR imaging of the portal venous system: value of gradient-echo imaging as an adjunct to spin-echo imaging. AJR Am J Roentgenol. 1991; 157(2):297–302

[18] Murphy FB, Steinberg HV, Shires GT, III, Martin LG, Bernardino ME. The Budd–Chiari syndrome: a review. AJR Am J Roentgenol. 1986; 147(1):9–15

[19] Stanley P. Budd–Chiari syndrome. Radiology. 1989; 170(3 Pt 1):625–627

[20] Spritzer CE. Vascular diseases and MR angiography of the liver. Magn Reson Imaging Clin N Am. 1997; 5(2):377–396

[21] Kane R, Eustace S. Diagnosis of Budd–Chiari syndrome: comparison between sonography and MR angiography. Radiology. 1995; 195(1):117–121

[22] Buetow PC, Pantongrag-Brown L, Buck JL, Ros PR, Goodman ZD. Focal nodular hyperplasia of the liver: radiologic-pathologic correlation. Radiographics. 1996; 16(2):369–388

[23] Popescu I, Ciurea S, Brasoveanu V, et al. Liver hemangioma revisited: current surgical indications, technical aspects, results. Hepatogastroenterology. 2001; 48(39):770–776

[24] Schima W, Saini S, Echeverri JA, Hahn PF, Harisinghani M, Mueller PR. Focal liver lesions: characterization with conventional spin-echo versus fast spin-echo T2-weighted MR imaging. Radiology. 1997; 202(2):389–393

[25] Leslie DF, Johnson CD, Johnson CM, Ilstrup DM, Harmsen WS. Distinction between cavernous hemangiomas of the liver and hepatic metastases on CT: value of contrast enhancement patterns. AJR Am J Roentgenol. 1995; 164(3):625–629

[26] Schimke M, Schulte E, Schumacher U. Prometheus. LernAtlas der Anatomie: Innere Organe. 2nd ed. Stuttgart: Thieme; 2009. Illustrated by M. Voll/K. Wesker

[27] Duran R, Ronot M, Kerbaol A, Van Beers B, Vilgrain V. Hepatic hemangiomas: factors associated with T2 shine-through effect on diffusion-weighted MR sequences. Eur J Radiol. 2014; 83(3):468–478

[28] Goodman ZD, Ishak KG. Angiomyolipomas of the liver. Am J Surg Pathol. 1984; 8(10):745–750

[29] Hooper LD, Mergo PJ, Ros PR. Multiple hepatorenal angiomyolipomas: diagnosis with fat suppression, gadolinium-enhanced MRI. Abdom Imaging. 1994; 19(6):549–551

[30] Murakami T, Nakamura H, Hori S, et al. Angiomyolipoma of the liver. Ultrasound, CT, MR imaging and angiography. Acta Radiol. 1993; 34(4):392–394

[31] Dachman AH, Lichtenstein JE, Friedman AC, Hartman DS. Infantile hemangioendothelioma of the liver: a radiologic-pathologic-clinical correlation. AJR Am J Roentgenol. 1983; 140(6):1091–1096

[32] Ros PR, Goodman ZD, Ishak KG, et al. Mesenchymal hamartoma of the liver: radiologic–pathologic correlation. Radiology. 1986; 158(3):619–624

[33] Levick CB, Rubie J. Haemangioendothelioma of the liver simulating congenital heart disease in an infant. Arch Dis Child. 1953; 28(137):49–51

[34] Pardes JG, Bryan PJ, Gauderer MW. Spontaneous regression of infantile hemangioendotheliomatosis of the liver. J Ultrasound Med. 1982; 1:349–353

[35] Alt B, Hafez GR, Trigg M, Shahidi NT, Gilbert EF. Angiosarcoma of the liver and spleen in an infant. Pediatr Pathol. 1985; 4(3–4):331–339

[36] Buetow PC, Buck JL, Ros PR, Goodman ZD. Malignant vascular tumors of the liver: radiologic–pathologic correlation. Radiographics. 1994; 14(1):153–166, quiz 167–168

[37] Gazelle GS, Lee MJ, Hahn PF, Goldberg MA, Rafaat N, Mueller PR. US, CT, and MRI of primary and secondary liver lymphoma. J Comput Assist Tomogr. 1994; 18(3):412–415

[38] Wanless IR, Mawdsley C, Adams R. On the pathogenesis of focal nodular hyperplasia of the liver. Hepatology. 1985; 5(6):1194–1200

[39] Wanless IR, Albrecht S, Bilbao J, et al. Multiple focal nodular hyperplasia of the liver associated with vascular malformations of various organs and neoplasia of the brain: a new syndrome. Mod Pathol. 1989; 2(5):456–462

[40] Wanless IR, Medlin A. Role of estrogens as promoters of hepatic neoplasia. Lab Invest. 1982; 46(3):313–320

[41] Brancatelli G, Federle MP, Grazioli L, Golfieri R, Lencioni R. Benign regenerative nodules in Budd–Chiari syndrome and other vascular disorders of the liver: radiologic–pathologic and clinical correlation. Radiographics. 2002; 22(4):847–862

[42] Dachman AH, Ros PR, Goodman ZD, Olmsted WW, Ishak KG. Nodular regenerative hyperplasia of the liver: clinical and radiologic observations. AJR Am J Roentgenol. 1987; 148(4):717–722

[43] Wanless IR, Solt LC, Kortan P, Deck JH, Gardiner GW, Prokipchuk EJ. Nodular regenerative hyperplasia of the liver associated with macroglobulinemia. Am J Med. 1981; 70:1203–1209

[44] Wada K, Kondo F, Kondo Y. Large regenerative nodules and dysplastic nodules in cirrhotic livers: a histopathologic study. Hepatology. 1988; 8(6):1684–1688

[45] Choi BI, Takayasu K, Han MC. Small hepatocellular carcinomas and associated nodular lesions of the liver: pathology, pathogenesis, and imaging findings. AJR Am J Roentgenol. 1993; 160(6):1177–1187

[46] Sakamoto M, Hirohashi S, Shimosato Y. Early stages of multistep hepatocarcinogenesis: adenomatous hyperplasia and early hepatocellular carcinoma. Hum Pathol. 1991; 22(2):172–178

[47] Choi YS, Rhee H, Choi JY, et al. Histological characteristics of small hepatocellular carcinomas showing atypical enhancement patterns on gadoxetic acid-enhanced MR imaging. J Magn Reson Imaging. 2013; 37(6):1384–1391

[48] Corrigan K, Semelka RC. Dynamic contrast-enhanced MR imaging of fibrolamellar hepatocellular carcinoma. Abdom Imaging. 1995; 20(2):122–125

[49] Ichikawa T, Federle MP, Grazioli L, Madariaga J, Nalesnik M, Marsh W. Fibrolamellar hepatocellular carcinoma: imaging and pathologic findings in 31 recent cases. Radiology. 1999; 213(2):352–361

[50] Craig JR, Peters RL, Edmondson HA, Omata M. Fibrolamellar carcinoma of the liver: a tumor of adolescents and young adults with distinctive clinico-pathologic features. Cancer. 1980; 46(2):372–379

[51] Leitlinienprogramm Onkologie der AWMF, Deutsche Krebsgesellschaft e.V., Deutsche Krebshilfe e.V. Diagnostik und Therapie des hepatozellulären Karzinoms. AWMF Register-Nr. 032–053OL; 2013

[52] European Association for the Study of the Liver, European Organisation for Research and Treatment of Cancer. EASL-EORTC clinical practice guidelines: management of hepatocellular carcinoma. J Hepatol. 2012; 56(4):908–943

[53] Singal A, Volk ML, Waljee A, et al. Meta-analysis: surveillance with ultrasound for early-stage hepatocellular carcinoma in patients with cirrhosis. Aliment Pharmacol Ther. 2009; 30(1):37–47

[54] Kim SH, Kim SH, Lee J, et al. Gadoxetic acid-enhanced MRI versus triple-phase MDCT for the preoperative detection of hepatocellular carcinoma. AJR Am J Roentgenol. 2009; 192(6):1675–1681

[55] Colli A, Fraquelli M, Casazza G, et al. Accuracy of ultrasonography, spiral CT, magnetic resonance, and alpha-fetoprotein in diagnosing hepatocellular carcinoma: a systematic review. Am J Gastroenterol. 2006; 101(3):513–523

[56] Caturelli E, Solmi L, Anti M, et al. Ultrasound guided fine needle biopsy of early hepatocellular carcinoma complicating liver cirrhosis: a multicentre study. Gut. 2004; 53(9):1356–1362

[57] Murakami T, Kim T, Takamura M, et al. Hypervascular hepatocellular carcinoma: detection with double arterial phase multi-detector row helical CT. Radiology. 2001; 218(3):763–767

[58] Yamashita Y, Fan ZM, Yamamoto H, et al. Spin-echo and dynamic gadolinium-enhanced FLASH MR imaging of hepatocellular carcinoma: correlation with histopathologic findings. J Magn Reson Imaging. 1994; 4(1):83–90

[59] Yu JS, Kim KW, Kim EK, Lee JT, Yoo HS. Contrast enhancement of small hepatocellular carcinoma: usefulness of three successive early image acquisitions during multiphase dynamic MR imaging. AJR Am J Roentgenol. 1999; 173 (3):597–604

[60] Grazioli L, Olivetti L, Fugazzola C, et al. The pseudocapsule in hepatocellular carcinoma: correlation between dynamic MR imaging and pathology. Eur Radiol. 1999; 9(1):62–67

[61] Choi JW, Lee JM, Kim SJ, et al. Hepatocellular carcinoma: imaging patterns on gadoxetic acid-enhanced MR Images and their value as an imaging biomarker. Radiology. 2013; 267(3):776–786

[62] Grazioli L, Morana G, Caudana R, et al. Hepatocellular carcinoma: correlation between gadobenate dimeglumine-enhanced MRI and pathologic findings. Invest Radiol. 2000; 35(1):25–34

[63] Manfredi R, Maresca G, Baron RL, et al. Delayed MR imaging of hepatocellular carcinoma enhanced by gadobenate dimeglumine (Gd-BOPTA). J Magn Reson Imaging. 1999; 9(5):704–710

[64] Lencioni R, Llovet JM. Modified RECIST (mRECIST) assessment for hepatocellular carcinoma. Semin Liver Dis. 2010; 30(1):52–60

[65] Helmberger TK, Ros PR, Mergo PJ, Tomczak R, Reiser MF. Pediatric liver neoplasms: a radiologic–pathologic correlation. Eur Radiol. 1999; 9(7):1339–1347

[66] Roebuck DJ, Aronson D, Clapuyt P, et al. International Childhood Liver Tumor Strategy Group. 2005 PRETEXT: a revised staging system for primary malignant liver tumours of childhood developed by the SIOPEL group. Pediatr Radiol. 2007; 37(2):123–132; quiz 249–250

[67] Czauderna P, Otte JB, Aronson DC, et al. Childhood Liver Tumour Strategy Group of the International Society of Paediatric Oncology (SIOPEL). Guidelines for surgical treatment of hepatoblastoma in the modern era—recommendations from the Childhood Liver Tumour Strategy Group of the International Society of Paediatric Oncology (SIOPEL). Eur J Cancer. 2005; 41(7):1031–1036

[68] Goodman ZD. Nonparenchymal and metastatic malignant tumors of the liver. In: Haubrich WS, Schaffner F, Berk JE, eds. Bockus Gastroenterology. Philadelphia: WB Saunders; 1995:2488–2500

[69] Lewis KH, Chezmar JL. Hepatic metastases. Magn Reson Imaging Clin N Am. 1997; 5(2):319–330

[70] Runge VM, Lee C, Williams NM. Detectability of small liver metastases with gadolinium BOPTA. Invest Radiol. 1997; 32(9):557–565

[71] Ralls PW. Focal inflammatory disease of the liver. Radiol Clin North Am. 1998; 36(2):377–389

[72] Goldman IS, Farber BF, Brandborg LL. Bacterial and miscellaneous infections of the liver. In: Zakim D, Boyer TD, eds. Hepatology. 3rd ed. Philadelphia: WB Sauders; 1996:1232–1242

[73] Balci NC, Semelka RC, Noone TC, et al. Pyogenic hepatic abscesses: MRI findings on T1- and T2-weighted and serial gadolinium-enhanced gradient-echo images. J Magn Reson Imaging. 1999; 9(2):285–290

[74] Lee KC, Yamazaki O, Hamba H, et al. Analysis of 69 patients with amebic liver abscess. J Gastroenterol. 1996; 31(1):40–45

[75] Veranghen F, Poey C, Lebras Y, et al. X-ray computed tomographic tests in the diagnosis and treatment of amebic liver abscesses [in French]. J Radiol. 1996; 77:23–28

[76] Caremani M, Benci A, Maestrini R, Rossi G, Menchetti D. Abdominal cystic hydatid disease (CHD): classification of sonographic appearance and response to treatment. J Clin Ultrasound. 1996; 24(9):491–500

[77] Lewall DB. Hydatid disease: biology, pathology, imaging and classification. Clin Radiol. 1998; 53(12):863–874

[78] Murphy BJ, Casillas J, Ros PR, Morillo G, Albores-Saavedra J, Rolfes DB. The CT appearance of cystic masses of the liver. Radiographics. 1989; 9(2):307–322

[79] Kalovidouris A, Gouliamos A, Vlachos L, et al. MRI of abdominal hydatid disease. Abdom Imaging. 1994; 19(6):489–494

[80] Polat P, Kantarci M, Alper F, Suma S, Koruyucu MB, Okur A. Hydatid disease from head to toe. Radiographics. 2003; 23(2):475–494, quiz 536–537

[81] Kantarci M, Bayraktutan U, Karabulut N, et al. Alveolar echinococcosis: spectrum of findings at cross-sectional imaging. Radiographics. 2012; 32(7):2053–2070

[82] Kammen BF, Pacharn P, Thoeni RF, et al. Focal fatty infiltration of the liver: analysis of prevalence and CT findings in children and young adults. AJR Am J Roentgenol. 2001; 177(5):1035–1039

[83] Brawer MK, Austin GE, Lewin KJ. Focal fatty change of the liver, a hitherto poorly recognized entity. Gastroenterology. 1980; 78(2):247–252

[84] The Clinical NMR Group. Magnetic resonance imaging of parenchymal liver disease: a comparison with ultrasound, radionuclide scintigraphy and X-ray computed tomography. Clin Radiol. 1987; 38(5):495–502

[85] Mitchell DG. MR imaging of cirrhosis and its complications. Abdom Imaging. 2000; 25(5):455

[86] Stark DD, Goldberg HI, Moss AA, Bass NM. Chronic liver disease: evaluation by magnetic resonance. Radiology. 1984; 150(1):149–151

[87] Holland HK, Spivak JL. Hemochromatosis. Med Clin North Am. 1989; 73 (4):831–845

[88] McLaren GD, Muir WA, Kellermeyer RW. Iron overload disorders: natural history, pathogenesis, diagnosis, and therapy. Crit Rev Clin Lab Sci. 1983; 19 (3):205–266

[89] Siegelman ES, Mitchell DG, Rubin R, et al. Parenchymal versus reticuloendothelial iron overload in the liver: distinction with MR imaging. Radiology. 1991; 179(2):361–366

[90] Permutt Z, Le TA, Peterson MR, et al. Correlation between liver histology and novel magnetic resonance imaging in adult patients with non-alcoholic fatty liver disease - MRI accurately quantifies hepatic steatosis in NAFLD. Aliment Pharmacol Ther. 2012; 36(1):22–29

[91] Wenker JC, Baker MK, Ellis JH, Glant MD. Focal fatty infiltration of the liver: demonstration by magnetic resonance imaging. AJR Am J Roentgenol. 1984; 143(3):573–574

[92] Kendall JL, Faragher J, Hewitt GJ, Burcham G, Haukoos JS. Emergency department ultrasound is not a sensitive detector of solid organ injury. West J Emerg Med. 2009; 10(1):1–5

[93] Deutsche Gesellschaft für Unfallchirurgie. S3-Leitlinie Polytrauma/Schwerverletzten-Behandlung. AWMF Register-Nr. 012/019; 2011

[94] Kantarcı M, Pirimoglu B, Karabulut N, et al. Non-invasive detection of biliary leaks using Gd-EOB-DTPA-enhanced MR cholangiography: comparison with T2-weighted MR cholangiography. Eur Radiol. 2013; 23(10):2713–2722

[95] Agildere AM, Haliloglu M, Akhan O. Biliary cystadenoma and cystadenocarcinoma. AJR Am J Roentgenol. 1991; 156(5):1113

[96] Bilgin M, Shaikh F, Semelka RC, Bilgin SS, Balci NC, Erdogan A. Magnetic resonance imaging of gallbladder and biliary system. Top Magn Reson Imaging. 2009; 20(1):31–42

[97] Buetow PC, Buck JL, Pantongrag-Brown L, et al. Biliary cystadenoma and cystadenocarcinoma: clinical–imaging–pathologic correlations with emphasis on the importance of ovarian stroma. Radiology. 1995; 196(3):805–810

[98] Caldwell SH, Hespenheide EE, Harris D, de Lange EE. Imaging and clinical characteristics of focal atrophy of segments 2 and 3 in primary sclerosing cholangitis. J Gastroenterol Hepatol. 2001; 16(2):220–224

[99] Chapman RW, Arborgh BA, Rhodes JM, et al. Primary sclerosing cholangitis: a review of its clinical features, cholangiography, and hepatic histology. Gut. 1980; 21(10):870–877

[100] Coffey RJ, Wiesner RH, Beaver SJ, et al. Bile duct carcinoma: a late complication of end-stage primary sclerosing cholangitis s [Abstract]. Hepatology. 1984; 4:1056–1059

[101] Devaney K, Goodman ZD, Ishak KG. Hepatobiliary cystadenoma and cystadenocarcinoma. A light microscopic and immunohistochemical study of 70 patients. Am J Surg Pathol. 1994; 18(11):1078–1091

[102] Flisak ME, Budris DM, Olson MC, Zarling EJ. Inflammatory pseudotumor of the liver: appearance on MRI. Clin Imaging. 1994; 18(1):1–3

[103] Hadjis NS, Adam A, Blenkharn I, Hatzis G, Benjamin IS, Blumgart LH. Primary sclerosing cholangitis associated with liver atrophy. Am J Surg. 1989; 158(1):43–47

[104] Helmberger H, Kammer B. Inflammatory diseases of the gall bladder and biliary system. II. Acute and chronic inflammation of the biliary system–primary biliary cirrhosis [in German]. Radiologe. 2005; 45(6):569–578, quiz 579

[105] Horiuchi R, Uchida T, Kojima T, Shikata T. Inflammatory pseudotumor of the liver. Clinicopathologic study and review of the literature. Cancer. 1990; 65(7):1583–1590

[106] Kim K, Choi J, Park Y, Lee W, Kim B. Biliary cystadenoma of the liver. J Hepatobiliary Pancreat Surg. 1998; 5(3):348–352

[107] Klatskin G. Adenocarcinoma of the hepatic duct at its bifurcation within the porta hepatis: an unusual tumor with distinctive clinical and pathological features. Am J Med. 1965; 38:241–256

[108] Krausé D, Cercueil JP, Dranssart M, Cognet F, Piard F, Hillon P. MRI for evaluating congenital bile duct abnormalities. J Comput Assist Tomogr. 2002; 26(4):541–552

[109] Krech RH, Erhardt-Domagalski M, Neumann H. Inflammatory pseudotumor of the liver: morphologic and cytophotometry studies and differential diagnosis [in German]. Pathologe. 1995; 16(6):415–420

[110] Lee JH, Yang HM, Bak UB, Rim HJ. Promoting role of Clonorchis sinensis infection on induction of cholangiocarcinoma during two-step carcinogenesis. Korean J Parasitol. 1994; 32(1):13–18

[111] Levy AD, Rohrmann CA, Jr, Murakata LA, Lonergan GJ. Caroli's disease: radiologic spectrum with pathologic correlation. AJR Am J Roentgenol. 2002; 179(4):1053–1057

[112] Marcos-Alvarez A, Jenkins RL. Cholangiocarcinoma. Surg Oncol Clin N Am. 1996; 5(2):301–316

[113] Miller WJ, Sechtin AG, Campbell WL, Pieters PC. Imaging findings in Caroli's disease. AJR Am J Roentgenol. 1995; 165(2):333–337

[114] Nakajima T, Sugano I, Matsuzaki O, et al. Biliary cystadenocarcinoma of the liver. A clinicopathologic and histochemical evaluation of nine cases. Cancer. 1992; 69(10):2426–2432

[115] Reiner CS, Merkle EM, Bashir MR, Walle NL, Nazeer HK, Gupta RT. MRI assessment of biliary ductal obstruction: is there added value of T1-weighted gadolinium-ethoxybenzyl-diethylenetriamine pentaacetic acid-enhanced MR cholangiography? AJR Am J Roentgenol. 2013; 201(1):W49–56

[116] Semelka RC, Sofka CM. Hepatic hemangiomas. Magn Reson Imaging Clin N Am. 1997; 5(2):241–253

[117] Tajima T, Honda H, Kuroiwa T, et al. Radiologic features of intrahepatic bile duct adenoma: a look at the surface of the liver. J Comput Assist Tomogr. 1999; 23(5):690–695

[118] Vitellas KM, Keogan MT, Freed KS, et al. Radiologic manifestations of sclerosing cholangitis with emphasis on MR cholangiopancreatography. Radiographics. 2000; 20(4):959–975; quiz 1108–1109, 1112

[119] Wiesner RH, LaRusso NF. Clinicopathologic features of the syndrome of primary sclerosing cholangitis. Gastroenterology. 1980; 79(2):200–206

[120] Worawattanakul S, Semelka RC, Noone TC, Calvo BF, Kelekis NL, Woosley JT. Cholangiocarcinoma: spectrum of appearances on MR images using current techniques. Magn Reson Imaging. 1998; 16(9):993–1003

[121] Yoshida Y, Imai Y, Murakami T, et al. Intrahepatic cholangiocarcinoma with marked hypervascularity. Abdom Imaging. 1999; 24(1):66–68

6 Gallbladder and Biliary Tract

Horst D. Litzlbauer

6.1 Anatomy

6.1.1 Biliary Fluid

Biliary fluid is composed of 85% water, 10% bile salts, 3% glycoproteins, 1% fat, and 0.7% inorganic salts. A total volume of approximately 1 liter of this "liver bile" is produced daily.[1] When the papilla is closed, the initially low-viscosity liver bile is stored in the gallbladder where water is absorbed from the fluid, raising its viscosity and concentrating it to approximately 10% of its initial volume (100 to 150 mL).

When lipids enter the small intestine, they stimulate production of the hormone cholecystokinin in the intestinal mucosa. Cholecystokinin stimulates the smooth muscle of the gallbladder wall, causing it to contract and release stored bile into the duodenum. Increased vagus nerve activity has the same effect.

The bile enables fat digestion by emulsifying ingested lipids, making them accessible to attack by lipases. Moreover, water-insoluble substances and toxins are excreted in the bile. Another important function is neutralization of the acidic gastric juice by the alkaline bile.

Bile derives its characteristic color from the bile pigments bilirubin and biliverdin, which are formed from the breakdown of porphyrins and hemoglobin in the hepatocytes. Bile acids, bilirubin, and cholesterol participate in the enterohepatic circulation; 90% of these substances are absorbed in the terminal ileum and transported back to the liver through the portal vein. This recirculation process maintains a total bile salt pool of 2 to 4 g in the body, which is sufficient to meet the fat absorption requirement of 20 to 30 g/day.

6.1.2 Biliary Capillaries and Bile Ducts

The functional units of the liver, the lobules, are approximately 2 mm high and 1 to 1.5 mm in diameter and are arranged in a honeycomb pattern. Branches of the portal vein and hepatic artery are found at the corners of each lobule. Both vessels supply a three-dimensional space composed of specialized capillaries, called sinusoids, which are permeated by cords of hepatocytes. The sinusoids drain into the central vein located at the center of each lobule, so that the blood flow is directed from the periphery of the lobule toward its center.[2]

The system of bile ducts begins between the walls of adjacent lobules in the form of bile canaliculi 0.1 to 1 mm in diameter. The canaliculi between two hepatocytes are arranged in such a way that part of the hepatocyte is interposed between the biliary network and sinusoids. This creates a physical separation between the biliary network and vascular system at the cellular level.

The flow of biliary fluid is directed oppositely to the blood flow, i.e., from the center of the lobule toward its periphery (▶ Fig. 6.1a). Special short connecting channels at the edge of each lobule, called the canals of Hering (30 μm in diameter), interconnect the bile capillary network with the interlobular bile ducts.

The interlobular bile ducts accompany the intrahepatic branches of the portal vein and hepatic vein. Together these vessels form the "portal triad" (Glisson's triad), which is embedded in periportal connective tissue (▶ Fig. 6.1b). Following the branching pattern of the portal vein, they merge to form increasingly larger ducts that finally become the ducts of the hepatic segments. The segmental ducts of the hepatic right lobe unite to form the right main trunk, while those of the left lobe join to form the left main trunk: the right and left hepatic ducts (▶ Fig. 6.1c). The common hepatic duct is formed by the junction of the right and left ducts, which may unite within the liver parenchyma or just after emerging from the liver. The common hepatic duct is 3 to 4 cm long and 6 mm in diameter.

The extrahepatic duct formed by the union of the common hepatic duct and cystic duct is called the common bile duct (ductus choledochus). Measuring approximately 4 to 8 cm long and 6 mm in diameter, the common bile duct is divided into a supraduodenal segment and a retroduodenal (or pancreatic) segment (▶ Fig. 6.2a).

The common bile duct terminates at the papilla of the duodenum. The papilla is a muscular valve that controls the passage of bile and pancreatic secretions into the small intestine. Its closure mechanism consists of three sphincters, one each for the bile duct and pancreatic duct plus a common sphincter in the duodenal wall called the sphincter of Oddi (▶ Fig. 6.2b). The oblique course of the ducts through the intestinal wall helps to prevent the reflux of small bowel secretions into the biliary tree. In 70% of cases the terminal segments of the common bile duct and main pancreatic duct unite at a common junction, the ampulla of Vater. In 10% of cases the common bile duct and main pancreatic duct enter the duodenum at separate sites. In the remaining 20% the ducts unite to form a common long terminal segment (▶ Fig. 6.2c).[3]

6.1.3 Gallbladder

The gallbladder is connected to the common hepatic duct by the cystic duct. It occupies a small fossa on the undersurface of the liver at the junction of the right and left lobes and is fused to the liver at that location. The gallbladder's surface facing the abdominal cavity is covered by peritoneum. The gallbladder extends from the porta hepatis to the anterior border of the liver. It consists of a blind pouch (the fundus), a body, and a neck (see ▶ Fig. 6.2a). The fundus extends down past the inferior border of the liver in many cases. The body of the gallbladder is in contact with the duodenum and right colic flexure. The gallbladder neck, from which the cystic duct arises, is adjacent to the porta hepatis.

> **Note**
>
> A spiral arrangement of mucosal folds in the initial part of the cystic duct prevents the passive drainage of bile from the gallbladder but does allow bile to enter from the common hepatic duct when the papilla is closed.[1]

The gallbladder has a total capacity of 40 to 50 mL. Its volume is variable owing to the specialized structure of the gallbladder wall.

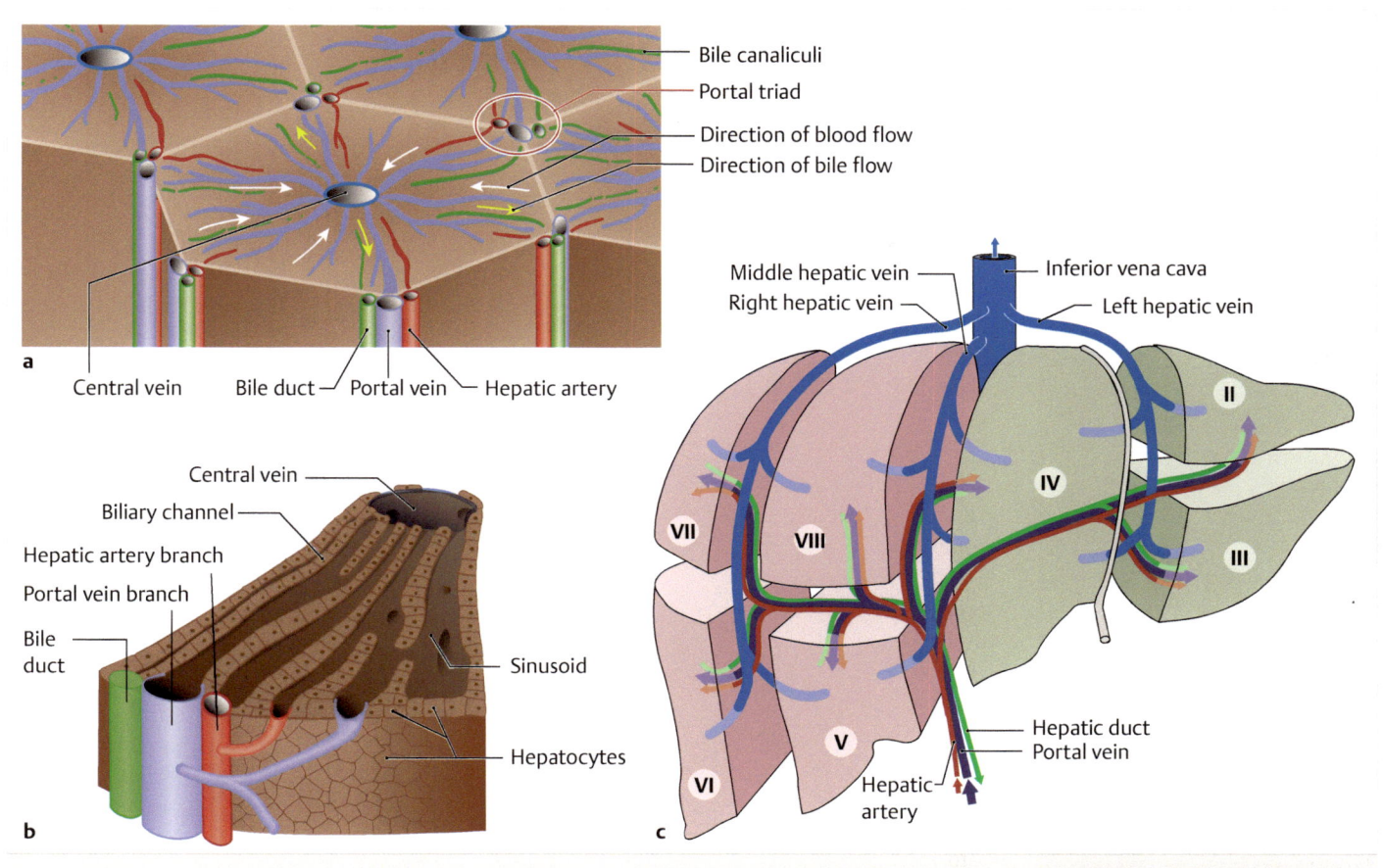

Fig. 6.1 Flow of bile and blood in the liver. Schematic representation. (a) Bile flows from the center to the periphery of the hepatic lobules, opposite to the direction of blood flow. (b) The small ducts merge at the portal triad, following the distribution of the portal vein, and unite to form increasingly larger ducts. (c) The segmental ducts unite to form the right and left hepatic ducts and finally the common hepatic duct. Roman numerals indicate the Couinaud segments of the liver. (Reproduced from Schünke M, Schulte E, Schumacher U. Prometheus. LernAtlas der Anatomie: Innere Organe. Illustrated by M. Voll/K. Wesker. 2nd ed. Stuttgart: Thieme; 2009.)

6.1.4 Blood Vessels, Lymphatics, and Nerves

The gallbladder receives its blood supply (▶ Fig. 6.3) from the cystic artery, which generally arises from the right hepatic artery (see ▶ Fig. 6.3a). Possible variations are shown in ▶ Fig. 6.4. A normal variant in which the right hepatic artery arises from the superior mesenteric artery is clearly demonstrable by CT. Normal variants in the origin of the cystic artery itself can be demonstrated only by conventional angiography. Venous blood is drained by the cystic vein to the portal vein or directly to the intrahepatic portal vein (see ▶ Fig. 6.3c). The portal vein occupies a far posterior position in the hepatoduodenal ligament, just behind the hepatic artery. The bile ducts are anterior (see ▶ Fig. 6.4a). The intrahepatic bile ducts are supplied by accompanying branches of the hepatic artery and portal vein.

The lymphatic vessels of the gallbladder communicate with those of the liver. The regional lymph nodes are located at the porta hepatis in the hepatoduodenal ligament.

The gallbladder and bile ducts derive their autonomic nerve supply from sympathetic and parasympathetic fibers of the hepatic plexus.

6.2 Physiology and Pathophysiology

6.2.1 Cholestasis (Obstructive Jaundice)

Cholestasis results from a disturbance of bile secretion leading to the retention of substances such as bilirubin and bile acids. The clinical hallmark of cholestasis is jaundice accompanied by generalized pruritus; the itchiness is caused by the deposition of bile acids in the skin. Pruritus may be absent in some forms of intrahepatic cholestasis. Obstructive jaundice is characterized by beer-brown urine and pale (acholic) stools. Laboratory tests show hyperbilirubinemia and elevated alkaline phosphatase activity.

Note

Except for rare hereditary forms (Alagille's syndrome and various forms of progressive familial intrahepatic cholestasis), cholestatic jaundice is always acquired.

Gallbladder and Biliary Tract

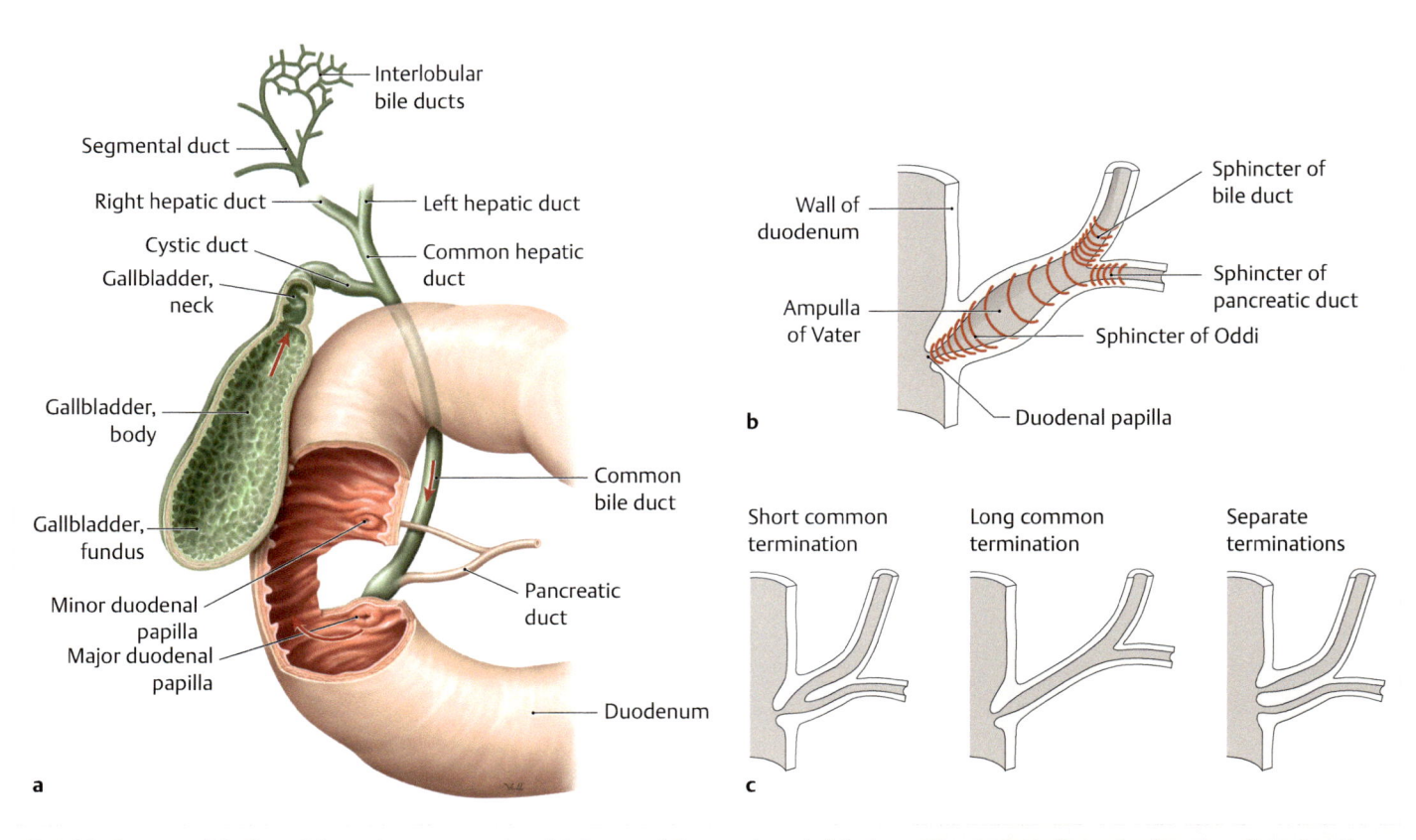

Fig. 6.2 Common bile duct. Schematic representation. **(a)** Course of the extrahepatic bile ducts. The arrows indicate the direction of bile flow from the gallbladder. **(b)** Duodenal papilla. **(c)** Variations of the duodenal papilla. (Reproduced from Schünke M, Schulte E, Schumacher U. Prometheus. LernAtlas der Anatomie: Innere Organe. Illustrated by M. Voll/K. Wesker. 2nd ed. Stuttgart: Thieme; 2009.)

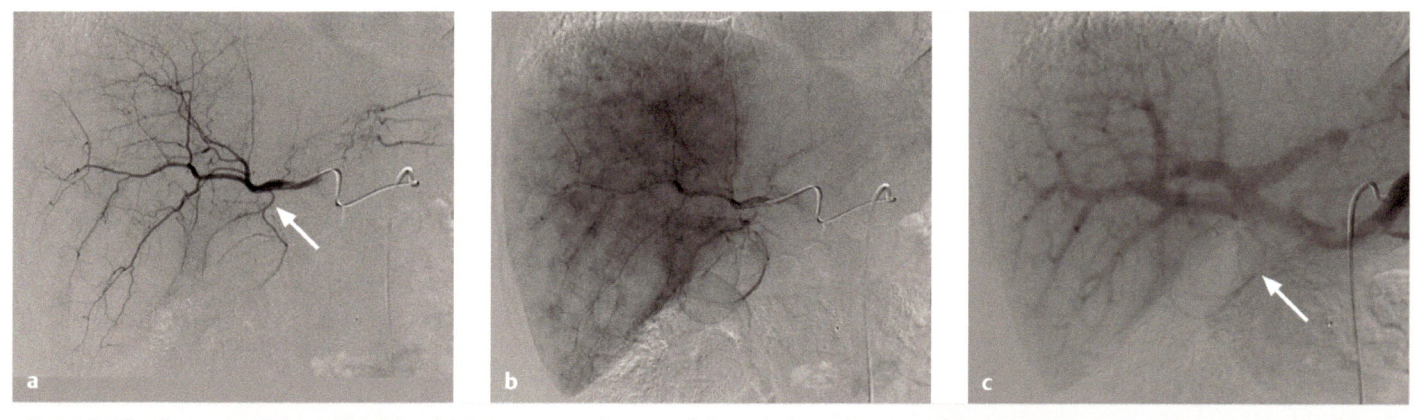

Fig. 6.3 Blood vessels of the gallbladder. **(a)** Selective visualization of the right hepatic artery and cystic artery (arrow). **(b)** Opacification of the hepatic right lobe and gallbladder wall in the parenchymal phase. **(c)** Indirect portography via the celiac trunk defines the veins of the gallbladder (arrow), which drain into the right main branch of the portal vein.

Cholestatic jaundice can have two main causes[4] (▶ Table 6.1):
- *Nonobstructive cholestasis*: caused by a primary disturbance of bile secretion in the hepatocytes themselves.
- *Obstructive cholestasis*: caused by a mechanical outflow obstruction in the common hepatic duct or common bile duct.

The unilateral obstruction of a hepatic duct usually does not cause jaundice, as the unaffected half of the liver can still maintain an almost normal level of bilirubin excretion.

Intrahepatic nonobstructive cholestasis is most commonly caused by impaired secretion from hepatocytes and occurs in the following entities, among others:
- All forms of cirrhosis.
- Cholestatic viral hepatitis.
- Drug-induced cholestatic jaundice.
- Cholestatic steatohepatitis.

The bile ducts are not dilated in any of these conditions. On the other hand, jaundice caused by a mechanical outflow obstruction

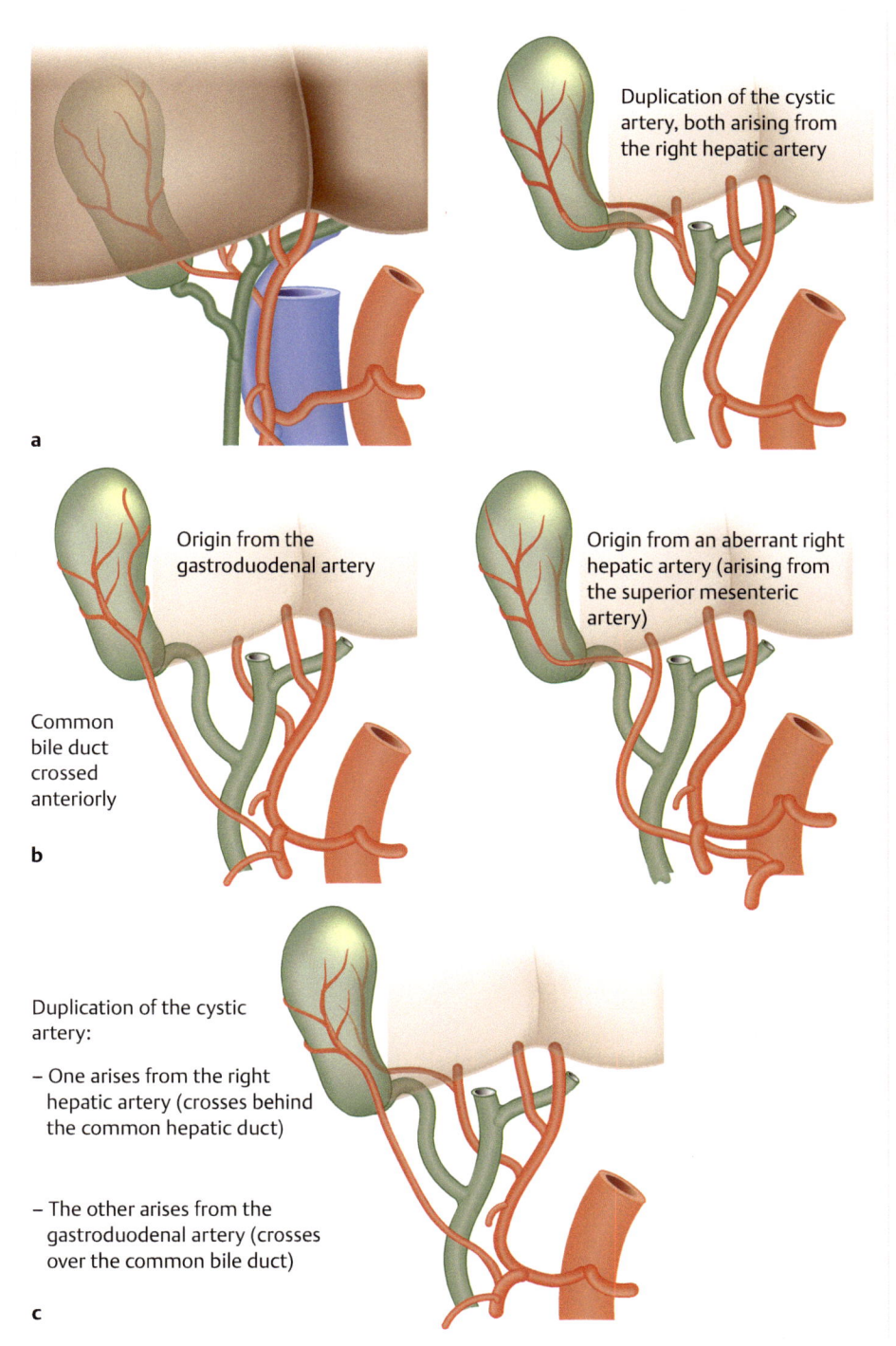

Fig. 6.4 Variants in the arterial blood supply of the gallbladder. (a) Normal origin of the cystic artery from the right hepatic artery. The vessel may be single (left) or duplicated (right). (b) Normal variant in which the cystic artery arises from the gastroduodenal artery (left) or from an aberrant right hepatic artery (right). (c) Dual blood supply from the right hepatic artery and gastroduodenal artery.

Duplication of the cystic artery, both arising from the right hepatic artery

a

Origin from the gastroduodenal artery

Origin from an aberrant right hepatic artery (arising from the superior mesenteric artery)

Common bile duct crossed anteriorly

b

Duplication of the cystic artery:

– One arises from the right hepatic artery (crosses behind the common hepatic duct)

– The other arises from the gastroduodenal artery (crosses over the common bile duct)

c

is almost always associated with increasing dilatation of the bile ducts (▶ Fig. 6.5).

6.3 Imaging
6.3.1 Conventional Radiography

The abdominal plain film is not suitable for evaluating diseases of the biliary system. However, calcified gallstones, calcifications of the gallbladder wall (porcelain gallbladder), and air in the bile ducts (▶ Fig. 6.6), gallbladder, or gallbladder wall may be visible on radiographs obtained for a different indication.

6.3.2 Ultrasonography
Initial Ultrasound Examination

Ultrasound and MRI are the principal modalities for biliary tract imaging, providing an almost 100% detection rate for gallstones and acute cholecystitis.

The diameter of the common bile duct does not exceed 6 to 7 mm in a healthy individual. The normal intrahepatic bile ducts are always smaller than the accompanying portal vein branches. The right and left hepatic ducts can be defined with ultrasound and are approximately 2 mm in diameter. Dilatation of the intrahepatic bile ducts is characterized initially by a unilateral thickening of the periportal connective tissue.

Table 6.1 Acquired cholestatic jaundice

Pathophysiology	Examples
Intrahepatic cholestasis	
Caused by impaired bile secretion from hepatocytes without dilatation of the bile ducts	• All forms of cirrhosis • All cholestatic hepatitis • Drug-induced jaundice • Sepsis
Caused by diffuse impairment of drainage in the liver with dilatation of the intrahepatic bile ducts only	• Primary biliary cirrhosis
Caused by proximal intrahepatic obstructions with dilatation of the intrahepatic bile ducts only	• Metastases and liver tumors • Cholangiocellular carcinoma (Klatskin's tumor) • Cholangitis, especially oriental cholangiohepatitis • Inflammatory or infiltrative diseases of the periportal fields • Hepatolithiasis secondary to hepatic cirrhosis
Extrahepatic cholestasis	
Caused by distal extrahepatic obstructions with dilatation of the extrahepatic and intrahepatic bile ducts	• Choledocholithiasis • Biliary sludge • Mirizzi's syndrome • Biliary stricture • Common bile duct carcinoma • Gallbladder carcinoma • Common bile duct metastasis • Choledochal cyst • Papillary carcinoma • Pancreatic carcinoma • Pancreatitis (chronic, acute) • Duodenal diverticulum • Biliary atresia • Extrinsic compression by masses in the hepatoduodenal ligament

Note

With increasing dilatation, the intrahepatic bile ducts can be identified as a second linear duct system accompanying the portal vein branches in the periportal connective tissue. This phenomenon is called the "double-barrel shotgun sign" and is also known as the "parallel channel sign" (see ▶ Fig. 6.5a).

Ultrasound Evaluation of Gallbladder Function

Ultrasound can be used to evaluate gallbladder emptying (▶ Fig. 6.7) after a cholecystokinin injection or the ingestion of a provocative meal (with chocolate). Gallbladder volume is measured sonographically in the fasting state and again after stimulation. Volume determination is based on the assumption of a rotational ellipsoid using a simplified geometric formula:

$$\text{Volume} = \frac{1}{2} \times \text{Length} \times \text{Width} \times \text{Height}$$

Gallbladder volume should decrease by at least 50% in response to the provocative meal.

6.3.3 Computed Tomography

Computed tomography (CT) is less sensitive than ultrasound in the detection of gallstones. The density of gallstones may vary with their composition and ranges from fat attenuation to dense calcification. Approximately 20% of gallstones are isodense to biliary fluid and therefore are not visualized on CT scans. The detection rate for gallbladder sludge is even lower.

The strength of CT lies in its ability to define the tissues around the gallbladder. CT is also better than ultrasound for detecting masses of the bile ducts, gallbladder, and pancreas and for identifying secondary tumor signs. CT is the imaging modality of choice for the evaluation and staging of pancreaticobiliary masses.

6.3.4 Magnetic Resonance Imaging and Magnetic Resonance Cholangiopancreatography

Heavily T2-weighted sequences can be used to visualize the fluid-filled bile ducts (and the pancreatic duct) with magnetic resonance imaging (MRI). In contrast to direct visualization of the ducts with contrast material, conventional MRI can simultaneously demonstrate the parenchyma and vasculature along with the bile ducts. MRI is somewhat better than CT for imaging tumors of the biliary tract.

The spatial resolution of magnetic resonance cholangiopancreatography (MRCP) is less than that of direct visualization with contrast material in endoscopic retrograde cholangiopancreatography (ERCP). One limitation of MRI is its susceptibility to artifacts from indwelling biliary drains or stents.

6.3 Imaging

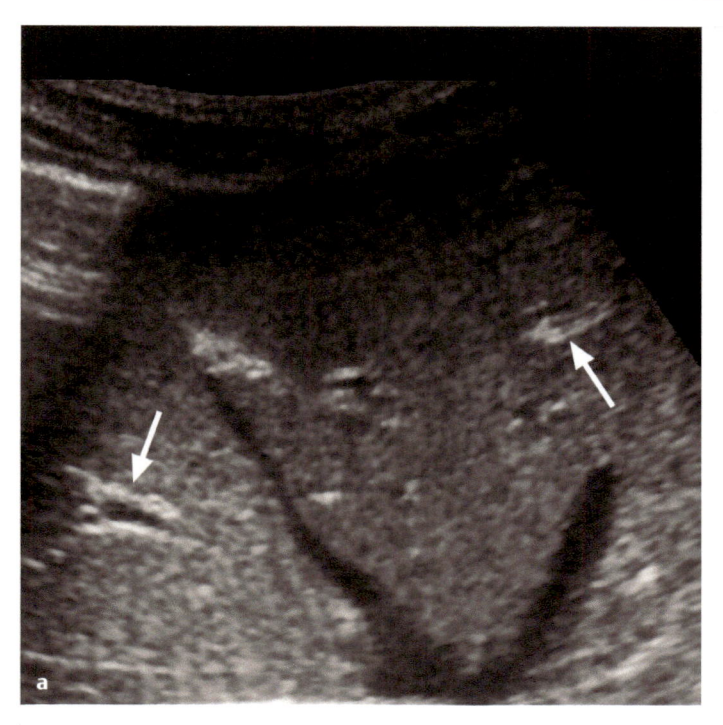

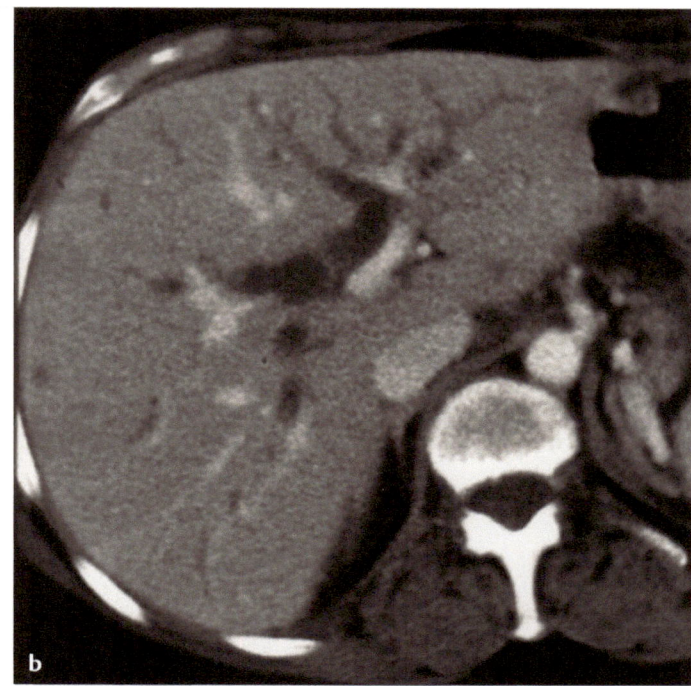

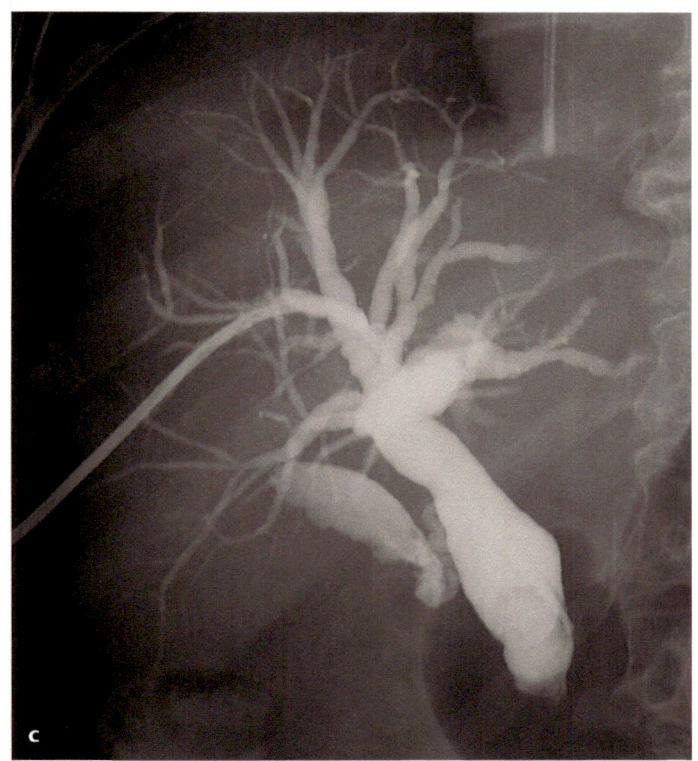

Fig. 6.5 Dilatation of the bile ducts. (a) Ultrasound shows initial intrahepatic biliary obstruction with unilateral thickening of periportal fields (arrows). **(b)** Symmetrical intrahepatic biliary obstruction on axial CT. **(c)** Obstructive jaundice due to pancreatic head carcinoma. Contrast medium was instilled through an external biliary drain.

Note
Imaging of the biliary tree with MRI is significantly improved by administering secretin, which stimulates distension of the ducts.

The level of detail can be improved by the administration of liver-specific contrast agents that are excreted in the bile.

6.3.5 Percutaneous Transhepatic Cholangiodrainage

Percutaneous transhepatic cholangiodrainage (PTCD) is important in the treatment of biliary obstruction. It is used in cases where the bile ducts are not accessible endoscopically (e.g., after a Whipple operation) or if an obstruction cannot be crossed from the duodenal side.

Gallbladder and Biliary Tract

In these cases the obstruction is reached and crossed percutaneously via the intrahepatic bile ducts. This provides access for the implantation of a suitable biliary stent, allowing the temporary drain to be removed ("internalized" drainage by stent placement).

6.4 Normal Variants, Developmental Anomalies, and Congenital Disorders

Various disorders, known collectively as *fibropolycystic liver disease*, may develop depending on the location of the developmental abnormality in the biliary tract (▶ Fig. 6.8):

- *Congenital hepatic fibrosis*: abnormal development of bile ducts in the hepatic lobules.
- *Biliary hamartomas of interlobular ducts*: microhamartomas, von Meyenburg's complex.
- *Autosomal dominant polycystic liver disease*: small ducts that are separate from the actual duct system (▶ Fig. 6.9).
- *Caroli's syndrome*: cystic dilatation of large (segmental) ducts with hepatic fibrosis.

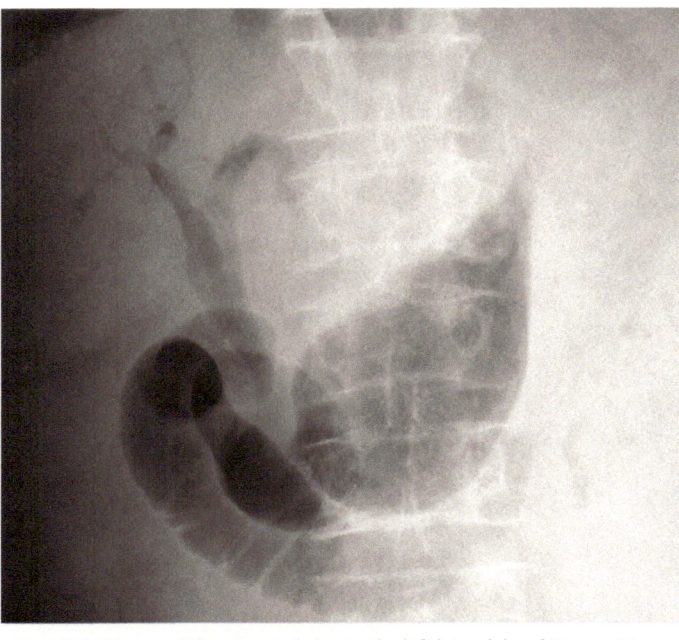

Fig. 6.6 Pneumobilia. Rotated view in the left lateral decubitus position.

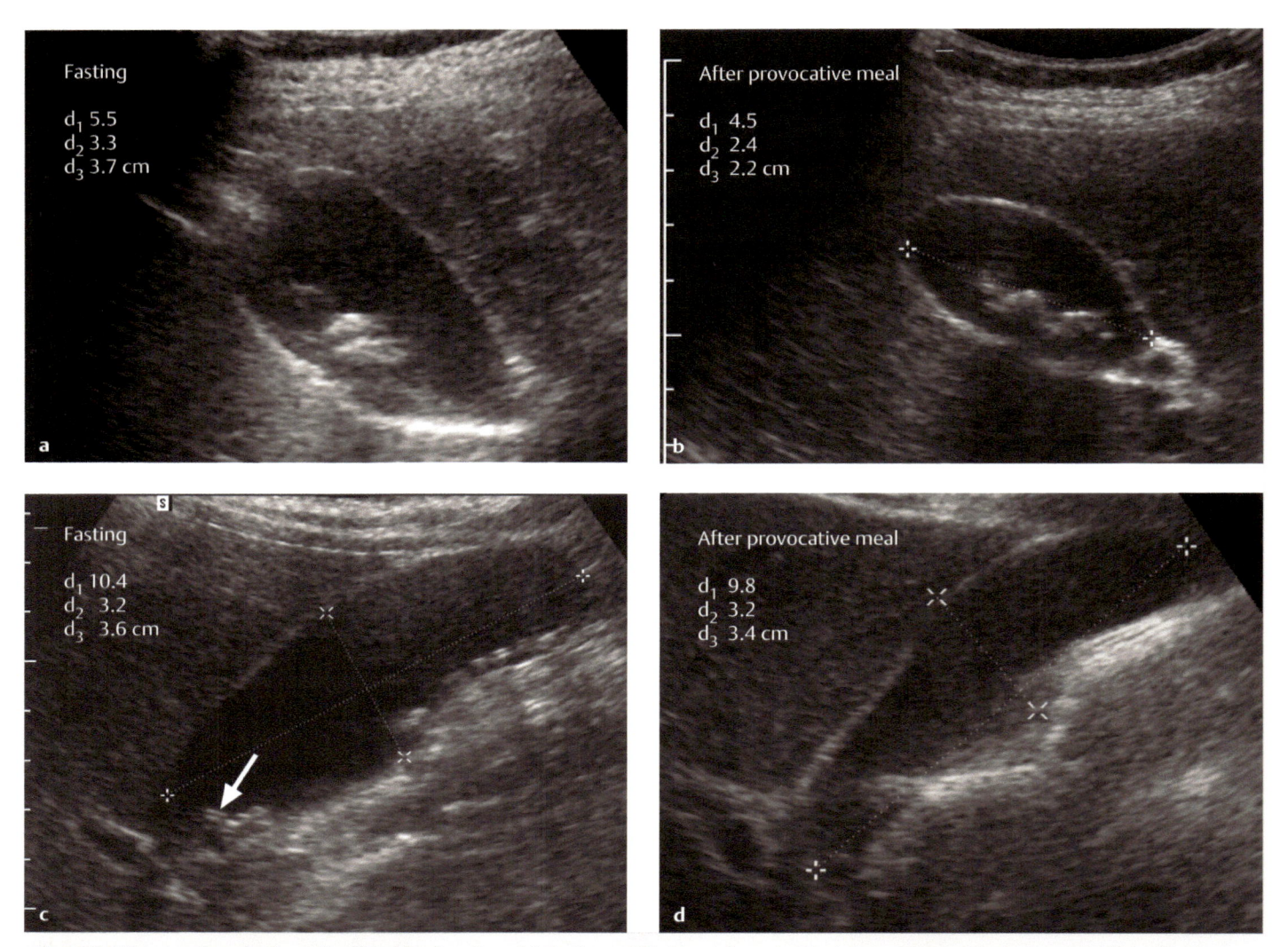

Fig. 6.7 Ultrasound evaluation of gallbladder function. (a) Fasting gallbladder volume is 35 mL in a patient with cholecystolithiasis. (b) The gallbladder shows normal volume reduction (12 mL) after a provocative meal. (c) Fasting gallbladder volume is 63 mL in a patient with sludge in the infundibulum (arrow). (d) Emptying does not occur (56 mL) in response to a provocative meal.

6.4 Normal Variants, Developmental Anomalies, and Congenital Disorders

The cystic duct is also variable in its course and termination. For example, the cystic duct may run parallel to the common hepatic duct for some distance before joining it at the level of the pancreas just above the papilla (▶ Fig. 6.12). In other cases the cystic duct may open immediately into the right hepatic duct. Rarely, accessory bile ducts may arise from the liver and enter the gallbladder.

Variants of the Bile Ducts and Biliary Vessels

Note

Anatomical variants of the biliary system have no pathologic significance. Their danger lies in their possible misinterpretation at imaging. Unless normal duct variants are identified and described, there is a potential for duct injury or ligation of the wrong duct during laparoscopic cholecystectomy. Duct anomalies may also be significant if liver transplantation is planned.

▶ **Brief definition.** The posterior duct of the hepatic right lobe that drains segments VI and VII shows the most variable termination (15% incidence of variants in the general population). It may open into the left main duct ("crossed anomaly," ▶ Fig. 6.13a), into the confluence of the right and left main ducts ("triple confluence," ▶ Fig. 6.13b), or less commonly into the cystic duct, the common bile duct, the gallbladder, or even the pancreatic duct (▶ Fig. 6.14). A frequent anomaly of the cystic duct is a "long cystic duct" that joins the common hepatic duct at a low level close to the papilla. In other cases the cystic duct may open into the right or left hepatic duct (▶ Fig. 6.12a).[7] Variations in the arterial supply to the gallbladder may have surgical implications. For example, the cystic artery may arise from the left hepatic artery or from the proper hepatic artery. The biliary artery may have multiple trunks. The right hepatic artery may be misidentified as the cystic artery (see ▶ Fig. 6.4).[3]

▶ **Imaging signs**
- *Normal variants of intra- and extrahepatic bile ducts*: Normal variants of these ducts can be recognized during magnetic resonance cholangiopancreatography (volume-rendered MRCP images, maximum intensity projection, respiratory-triggered 3D TSE sequence) or during endoscopic retrograde cholangiopancreatography(ERCP). CT cholangiography provides the highest spatial resolution and can be used for special investigations (e.g., before liver transplantation) in cases where MRCP findings are equivocal or MRI is contraindicated.
- *Normal variants of extrahepatic bile ducts*: These ducts can also be identified in a detailed analysis of axial MR images (heavily T2-weighted sequences, T2 W or T1 W TrueFISP sequences) or thin-slice CT scans.
- *Normal variants of blood vessels*: Besides conventional angiography, thin-slice arterial CT angiography (CTA) images are best for demonstrating normal variants of vascular anatomy.

▶ **Key points.** It is common to find normal variants in the bile duct and vascular anatomy. Generally they have no pathologic significance but may become important during laparoscopic gallbladder procedures or transplantation surgery.

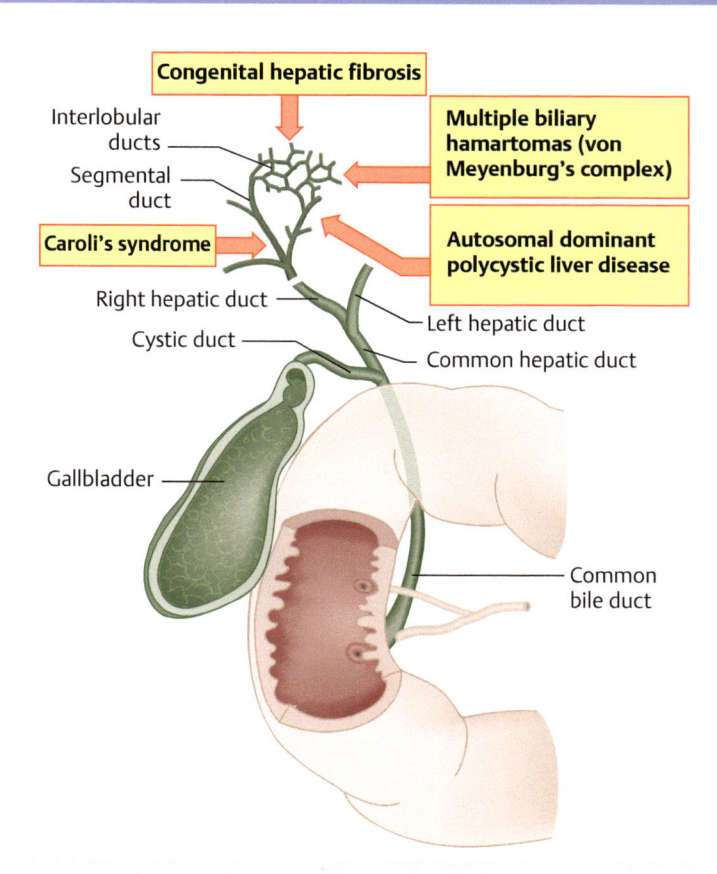

Fig. 6.8 Fibropolycystic liver disease. The specific disease depends on the anatomical location of the affected bile ducts. In autosomal dominant polycystic liver disease, the cysts form in small ducts that are separate from the actual duct system.[5]

The Todani system is used to classify malformations involving cystic dilatation of the common bile duct and/or the intrahepatic ducts (▶ Fig. 6.10)[6]:
- *Todani type I*: dilatation of the common bile duct (which may extend into the common hepatic duct and main ducts).
- *Todani type II*: diverticulum of the common bile duct.
- *Todani type III*: choledochocele (dilatation of the intramural small-bowel segment with herniation in the papillary region).
- *Todani type IV*: dilatation of intra- and extrahepatic bile ducts.
- *Todani type V*: cystic dilatation of intrahepatic bile ducts (synonym: Caroli disease or Caroli syndrome when hepatic fibrosis is also present).

6.4.1 Anatomical Variants
Variants of the Gallbladder

▶ **Brief definition.** Variants of gallbladder morphology are congenital and may involve the presence of internal septa (▶ Fig. 6.11a) or angulations. The most familiar congenital morphological variant of the gallbladder is the Phrygian cap, in which the fundus is elongated and folded over (▶ Fig. 6.11b). Morphological variants are incidental imaging findings that do not have pathologic significance.

Note

Circumscribed constrictions or diverticula of the gallbladder are predisposing factors for gallstone formation.

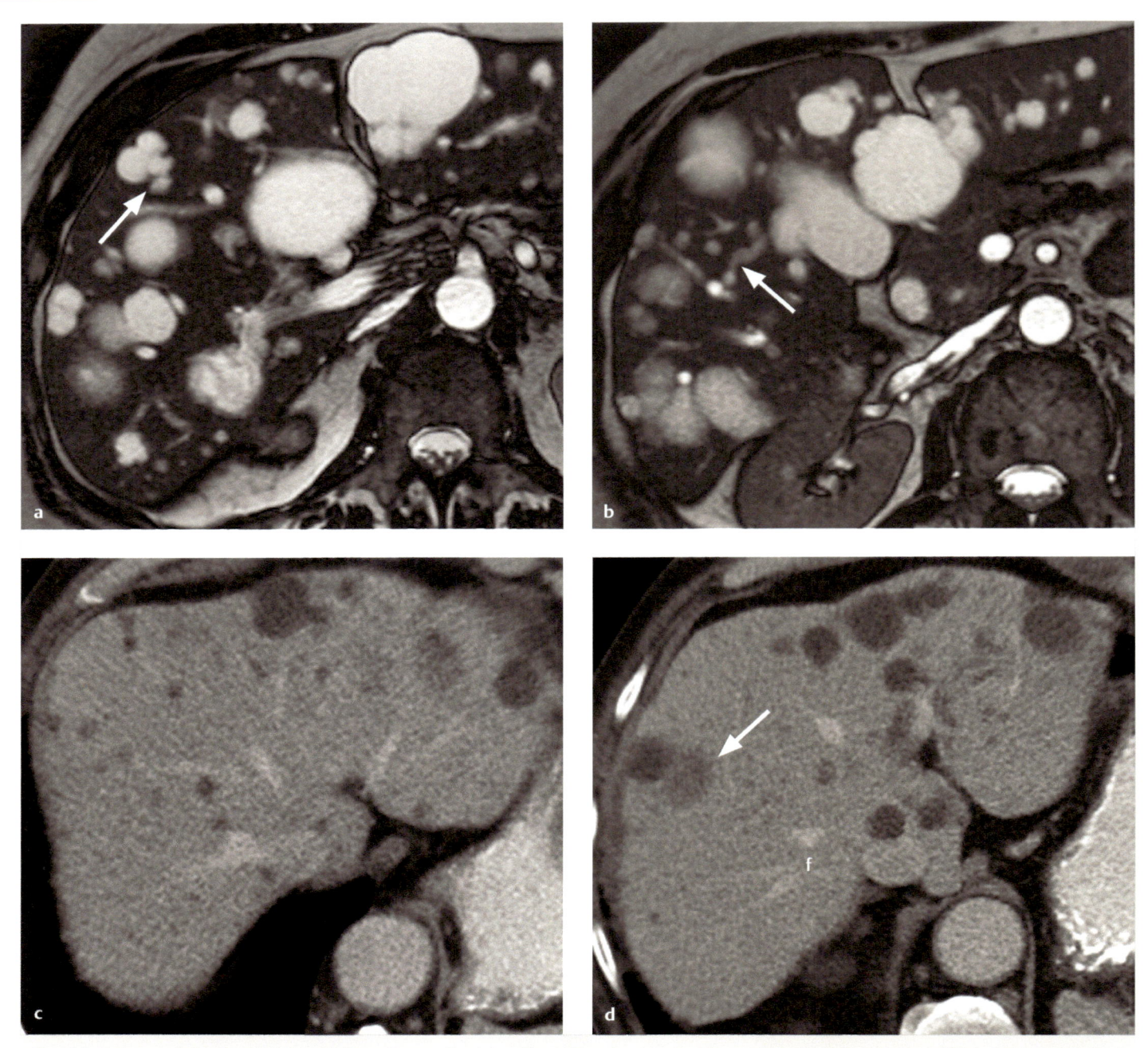

Fig. 6.9 **Autosomal dominant polycystic liver disease.** Ductal malformation characterized by small, isolated ducts in two different patients. Patient 1 has adult polycystic liver change with branching cysts, some with a ductal appearance ([a] and [b], arrows). Patient 2 has a milder case with an associated anomaly (solitary biliary hamartoma; [d], arrow). (a) Patient 1. (b) Patient 1 (adjacent slice). (c) Patient 2. (d) Patient 2 (adjacent slice).

6.4.2 Biliary Atresia

▶ **Brief definition.** The prevalence of biliary atresia is approximately 1 in 10,000 to 13,000 live births. Intrahepatic ductal atresia (either syndromic or nonsyndromic) is much less common than atresia of extrahepatic bile ducts. Extrahepatic atresia may be confined to the common bile duct or may additionally affect the common hepatic duct. Atresia of both ducts is very rare. The gallbladder is present in one-fourth of cases. The cause of biliary atresia is not fully understood but presumably relates to a prenatal viral infection of the biliary tract leading to destructive inflammatory obliteration of the bile ducts. Thus, the disease is not a congenital absence of duct systems but a gradually progressive process that develops in postnatal life.[8] Approximately one-fourth of patients have associated congenital disorders (polysplenia syndrome, cardiac anomalies, portal vein anomalies).

▶ **Imaging signs.** The initial imaging study in newborns is ultrasound. The echogenicity of the liver is initially normal. The liver may already be enlarged at birth but will definitely enlarge during postnatal development. The common bile duct is invariably absent. In rare cases imaging may demonstrate the right and left hepatic ducts, the common hepatic duct, or dilated intrahepatic segments of the largely obliterated duct system ("bile lakes"). The common duct is replaced in the porta hepatis by an echogenic band. A gallbladder is demonstrable in 25% of cases. When present, it has an unusual shape and shows irregular wall thickening (▶ Fig. 6.15). Functional ultrasonography (initial scan after

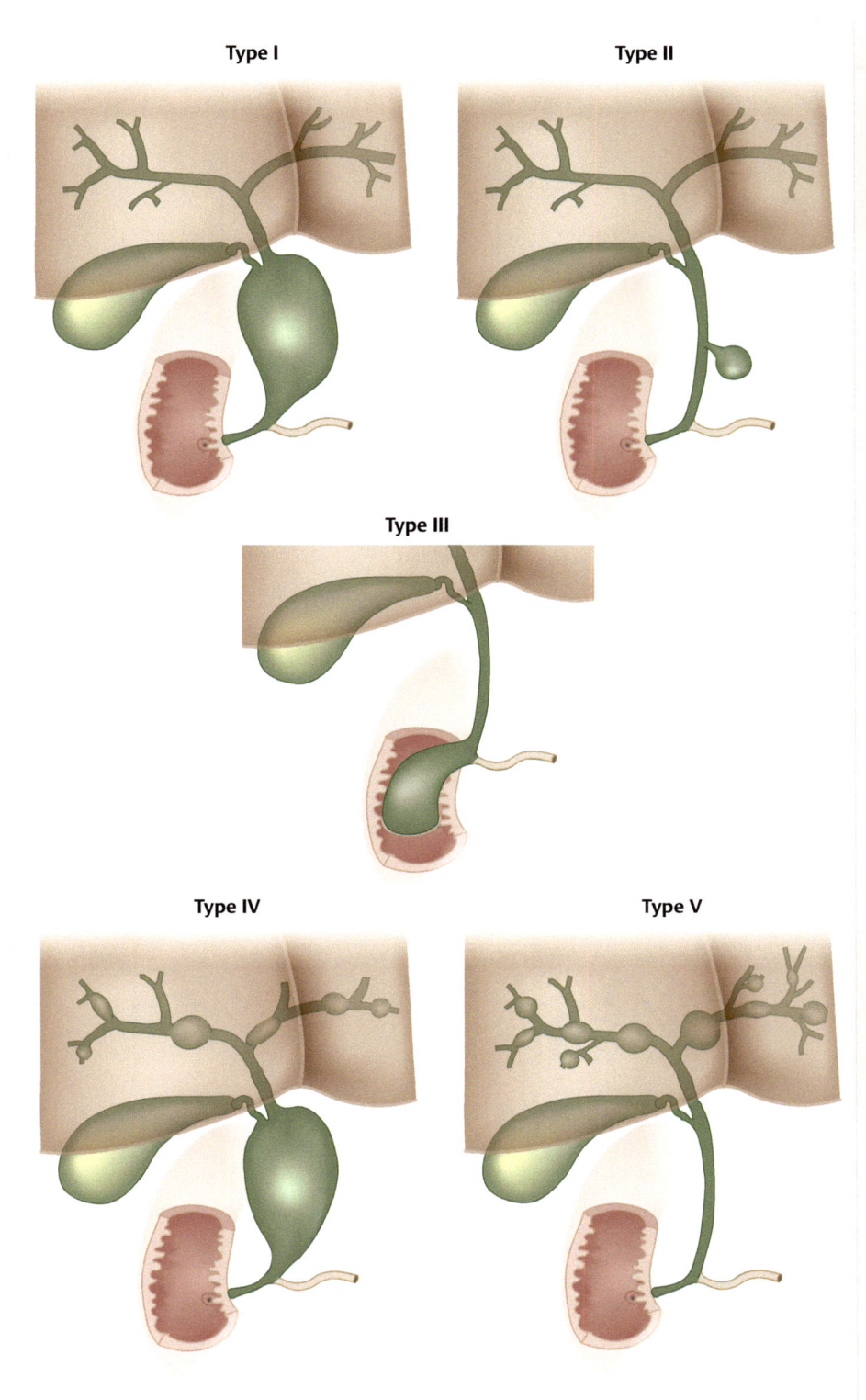

Fig. 6.10 Todani classification of choledochal cysts. Type I, cystic dilatation of the common bile duct, with possible extension into the cystic duct and right or left hepatic duct. Type II, diverticulum of the common duct. Type III, choledochocele. Type IV, dilatation of intra- and extrahepatic bile ducts. Type V, cystic dilatation of intrahepatic bile ducts.

a 4-hour fast; rescan after nursing) shows there to be no gallbladder contraction. Untreated patients will develop hepatic cirrhosis and portal hypertension. Both of these conditions are also diagnosed sonographically. Hepatobiliary scintigraphy (technetium Tc 99 m HIDA sequential scintigraphy) requires 5 days' preparation with phenobarbital (oral) to stimulate bile secretion from hepatocytes. Entry of the tracer into the small intestine excludes biliary atresia. Absence of detectable tracer in the small intestine by 24 hours confirms obstructive jaundice, which may be caused by biliary atresia (see ▶ Fig. 6.15b) or extrinsic compression of the common duct. The presence of inspissated bile should also be considered, especially in premature infants. CT is contraindicated in this age group due to radiation exposure concerns and the need for sedation.

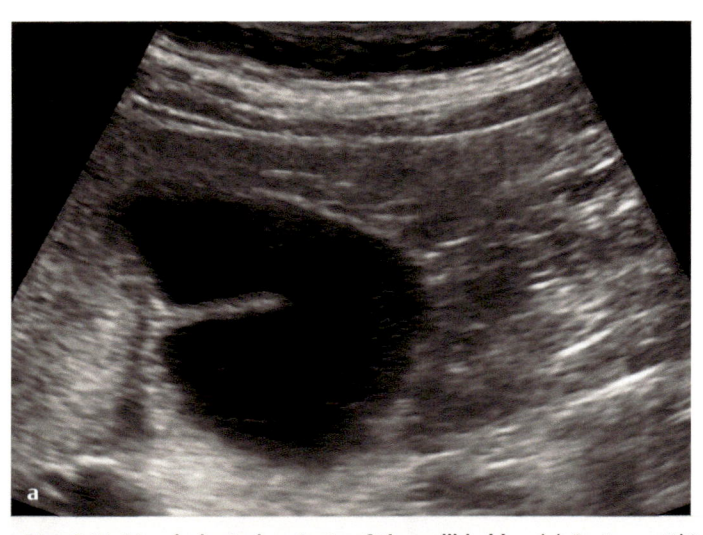

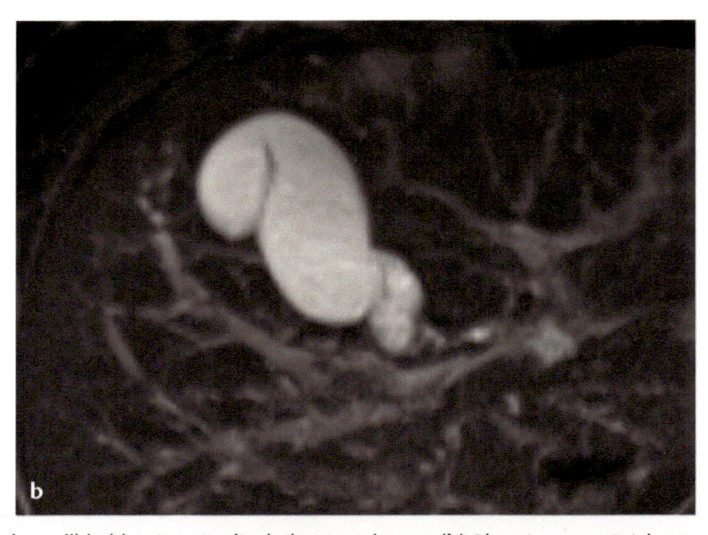

Fig. 6.11 Morphological variants of the gallbladder. (a) Septum within the gallbladder. Longitudinal ultrasound scan. (b) Phrygian cap. Axial fat-suppressed T2W MRI, maximum intensity projection (slice thickness 4 cm).

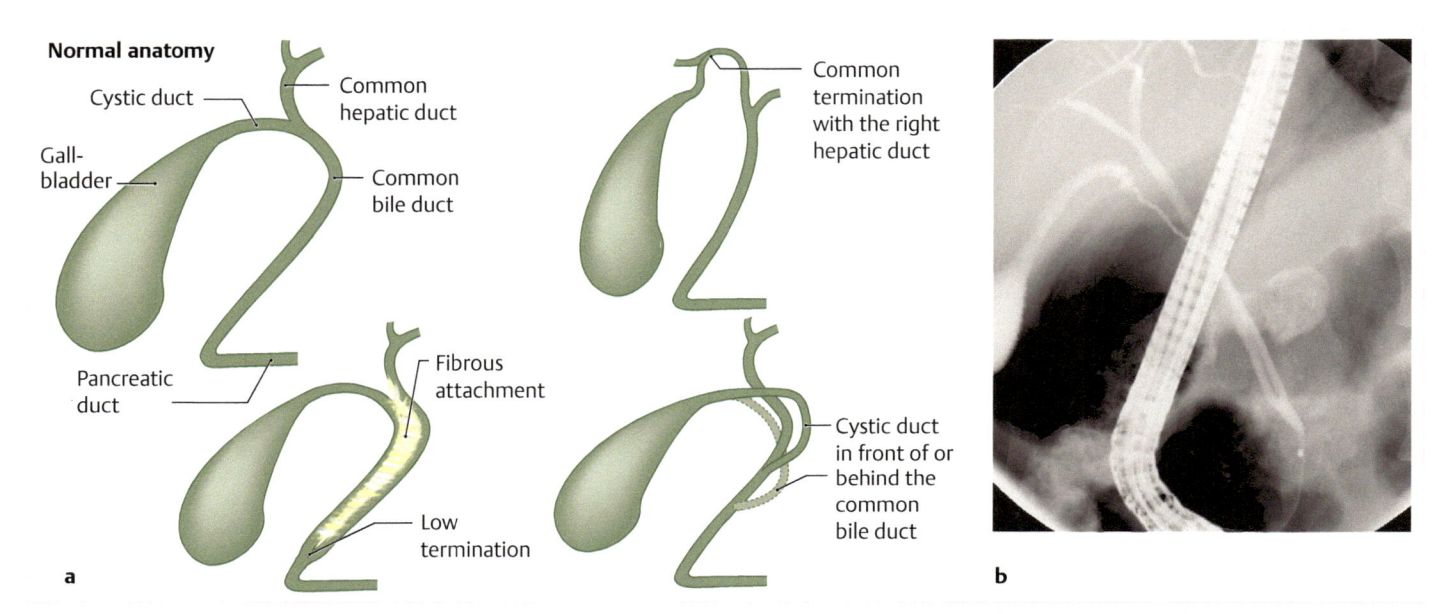

Fig. 6.12 Variants of the cystic duct. (a) Schematic diagrams showing possible variations in the course and termination of the cystic duct. (b) Endoscopic view. Low termination of the cystic duct.

> **Caution**
>
> Because the absence of extrahepatic bile ducts is the hallmark of biliary atresia, MRCP is of very limited value. Even normal bile ducts may be difficult to detect in infancy.

Both CT and MRCP can aid in the differentiation of extrinsic common bile duct compression, however. Nonvisualization of the common bile duct with a visible pancreatic duct on ERCP provides high diagnostic accuracy (see ▶ Fig. 6.15c). If the common bile duct can be visualized, there is no atresia.

▶ **Clinical features.** Affected children are born with normal body weight at term or occasionally before term. Approximately one-third of newborns are already jaundiced at birth, and jaundice will gradually develop in the rest. Because the jaundice has a mechanical causation, acholic stools and dark-brown urine are present. A progressive rise of conjugated bilirubin is found. The liver enlarges over time, with rapid development of hepatic cirrhosis. It takes just 2 months for irreversible liver damage to occur. Untreated children will die from biliary hepatic cirrhosis within 12 to 15 months. The only treatment option is a biliary–enteric anastomosis. In 10% of children the atresia affects only the common bile duct, allowing the hepatic duct to be used for a biliary–enteric reconstruction. The remaining 90% of atresias can be treated with a Kasai's hepatic portoenterostomy.[9] This procedure is 90% successful when performed during the first 2 months of life. When done after 3 months, its success rate falls to less than 50%. Even patients who have the Kasai's operation will eventually require liver transplantation.

▶ **Differential diagnosis**
- *Neonatal hepatitis*: This is the most frequent cause of neonatal jaundice besides physiologic jaundice (possible causes are hepatitis A and B, cytomegalovirus infection, rubella, or toxoplasmosis).

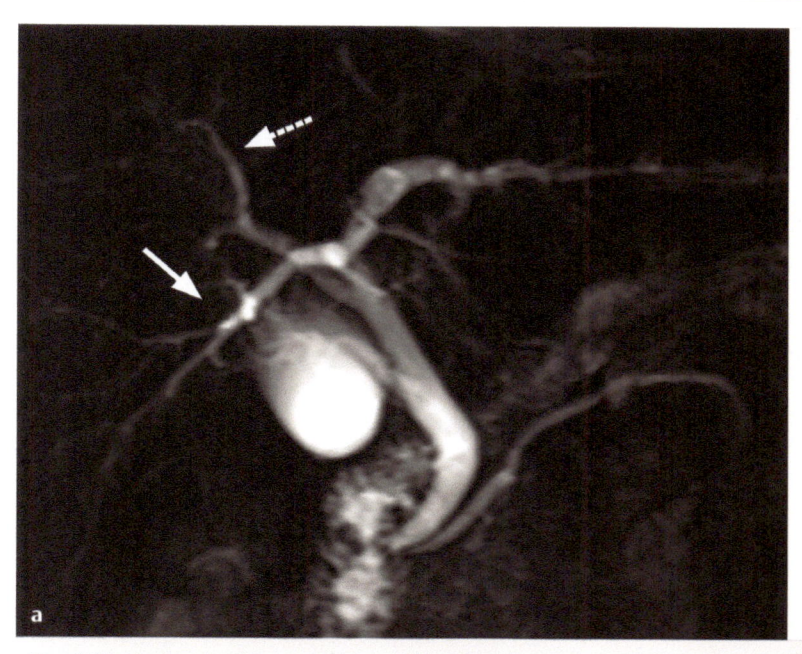

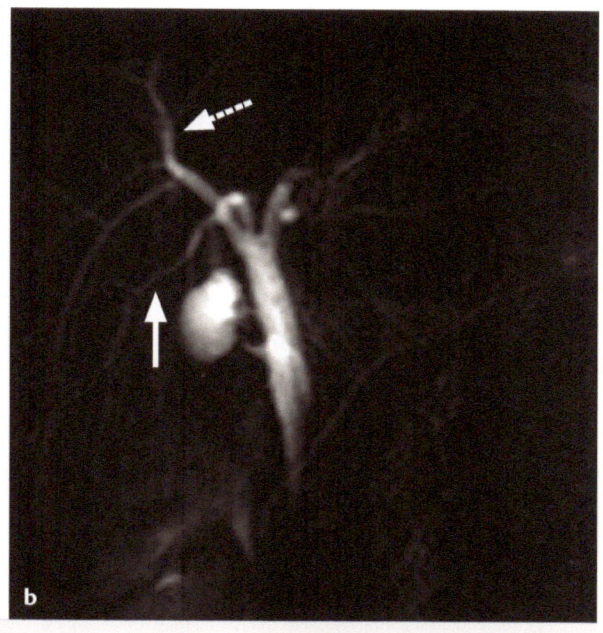

Fig. 6.13 Variants in the termination of the right posterior duct. The solid arrows indicate the right posterior duct; the dashed arrows indicate the anterior duct. **(a)** The right posterior duct opens into the left hepatic duct: crossed anomaly. **(b)** The duct opens into the confluence of the left and right anterior ducts: triple confluence.

- *Bile plug syndrome*: This may occur in cystic fibrosis, sepsis, or total parenteral nutrition.
- *Atresia of intrahepatic bile ducts*: Alagille's syndrome, common duct malformation, and obstructive jaundice due to extrinsic compression of the common duct (hydronephrosis, duodenal atresia, etc.).

▶ **Key points.** Biliary atresia is a rare but important differential diagnosis in newborns with persistent obstructive jaundice and in infants with progressive obstructive jaundice. It is not a primary congenital anomaly but results from inflammatory destruction of the bile ducts. The key to diagnosis is nonvisualization of the common bile duct on ultrasound. Visualization of the gallbladder does not exclude biliary atresia. The diagnosis is confirmed by hepatobiliary scintigraphy and endoscopy. The only effective treatment option is hepatic portoenterostomy (Kasai's operation) before 2 months of age. Ten percent of cases can be treated with a simple biliary–enteric anastomosis.

6.4.3 Choledochal Cysts

▶ **Brief definition.** Five types of choledochal cyst are distinguished by their site of occurrence in the Todani classification (see ▶ Fig. 6.10). Cyst size varies from 1 cm to more than 15 cm. The prevalence of choledochal cysts is approximately 1:100,000 live births in the United states and 1:1,000 live births in Japan. Approximately one-third of all documented cases originate in Japan. Girls are affected more frequently than boys. Three causal factors are considered:
- Failure of recanalization.[10]
- Pancreaticobiliary reflux due to a long, common terminal segment.[11]
- Distal obstruction.[10]

Approximately one-half of infants become symptomatic before 1 year of age, but complaints may not appear until much later in life.[12]

▶ **Imaging signs.** Ultrasound is ideal for revealing dilatation of the extra- and intrahepatic bile ducts. If the diameter of the common bile duct is greater than 10 mm in childhood, the most likely cause is a choledochal anomaly (▶ Fig. 6.16). MRCP is the technique of choice for noninvasive ductal imaging. Hepatobiliary scintigraphy can be used for functional evaluation.

▶ **Clinical features.** Infants younger than 12 months show intermittent obstructive jaundice combined with hepatomegaly and vomiting. Sixty percent of older children and adults manifest the classic triad of upper abdominal pain, jaundice, and a right-upper-quadrant mass. The remaining 40% have nonspecific upper abdominal complaints that may be accompanied by fever, intermittent jaundice, nausea, and vomiting. Stones are found in 30% of adult patients.[13] Pancreatitis may also occur. Biliary cirrhosis may be present as an initial diagnosis. Patients with a choledochal cyst are at increased risk for the development of bile duct cancer (cholangiocarcinoma).

Treatment decisions are based on the Todani classification:
- *Type I*: complete surgical resection with biliary–enteric reconstruction (typically in the form of a Roux-en-Y choledochojejunostomy).
- *Type II*: resection of the diverticulum, preserving the biliary tree.
- *Type III*: endoscopic papillotomy, or open transduodenal removal for larger cysts.
- *Type IV*: resection tailored to the location and extent of the dilatations.
- *Type V*: options ranging from segmental resection to hemihepatectomy; the diffuse type requires liver transplantation.

▶ **Differential diagnosis**
- Chronic cholangitis with stricture and secondary cystic ductal dilatation.
- Obstructive cholelithiasis.

Gallbladder and Biliary Tract

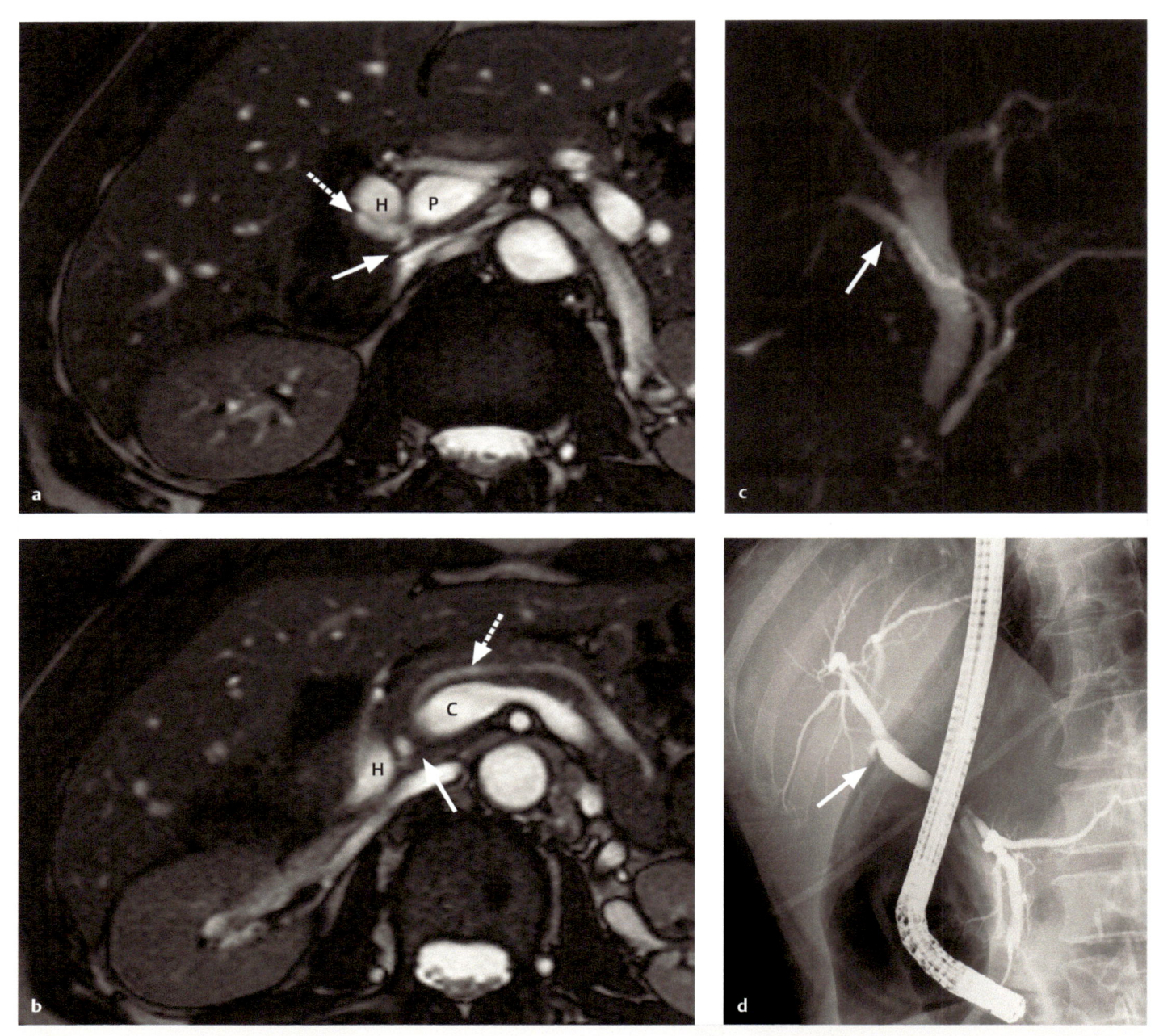

Fig. 6.14 **Aberrant bile duct opening into the pancreatic duct** in a woman who underwent cholecystectomy for recurrent attacks of biliary pancreatitis. (**a**) Aberrant duct (solid arrow) and cystic duct stump (dashed arrow) behind the dilated common hepatic duct. (**b**) Aberrant duct (arrow), dilated major pancreatic duct (dashed arrow). (**c**) MRCP shows the posterior right duct inserting into the pancreatic duct (arrow). The rest of the biliary tree is dilated. (**d**) Pancreatogram shows opacification of the right posterior duct and cystic duct stump (arrow). Note the associated anatomical variant of the pancreas. C, venous confluence; H, common hepatic duct; P, portal vein.

- Pancreatic pseudocysts.
- Echinococcal cysts.

▶ **Key points.** Choledochal anomalies in children are easily detected sonographically and are diagnosed when the diameter of the common bile duct is 10 mm or more. Choledochal cysts may be as large as 15 cm. In one-half of children the anomaly becomes symptomatic during the first year of life, but many cases are not diagnosed until adulthood. Symptoms are obstructive jaundice, an abdominal mass, and recurrent episodes of cholangitis. Possible complications are lithiasis or even biliary pancreatitis. Patients with choledochal cysts are at increased risk for developing cholangiocarcinoma.

6.4.4 Caroli's Disease and Caroli's Syndrome

▶ **Brief definition.** Since intrahepatic segmental bile duct cysts were first described by Caroli in 1958, two main types of disease have been distinguished[1]:
- *Caroli's disease*: a simple but very rare type without associated hepatic fibrosis.
- *Caroli's syndrome*: a congenital type of fibrosis.

The simple form results from anomalous development of the large, central bile ducts. Its cause is not known. Caroli's disease, unlike Caroli's syndrome, occurs sporadically. It consists of nonobstructive,

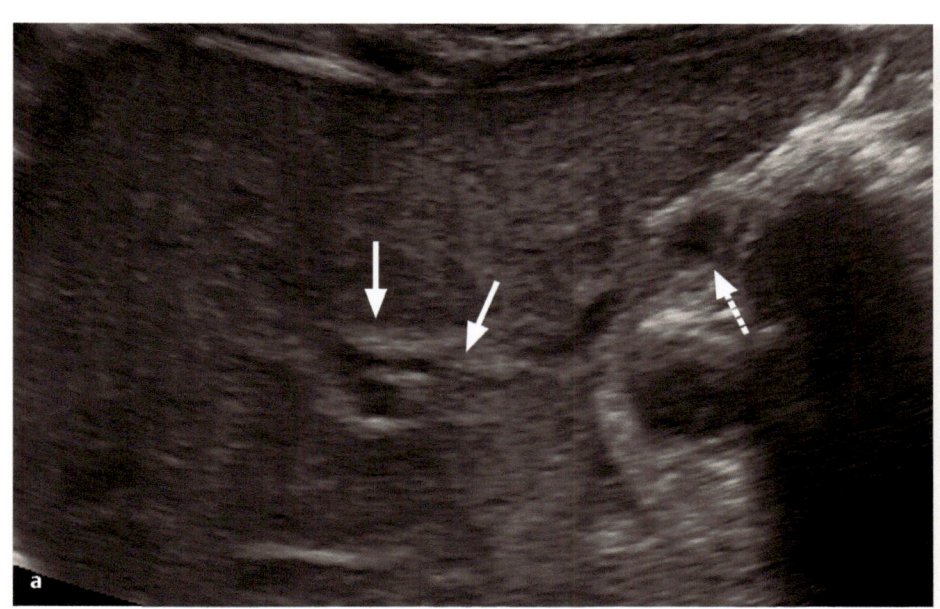

Fig. 6.15 Biliary atresia in a 1-month-old boy. (a) Bandlike widening of the periportal field at the site of the common hepatic duct (arrows). The gallbladder (dashed arrow) is small and shows irregular wall thickening. (Image [a] with kind permission of Professor Berthold, Hannover Medical School, Germany.) (b) Hepatobiliary scintigraphy. Image at 6 hours shows hepatic tracer uptake with no excretion into the bowel. Tracer in the bladder (arrow) results from ectopic excretion. (Image [b] with kind permission of Dr. Steiner, Nuclear Medicine, University Hospital Giessen, Germany.) (c) Only the pancreatic duct is visualized on ERCP. (Image [c] with kind permission of Dr. Collet, University Hospital Giessen, Germany.)

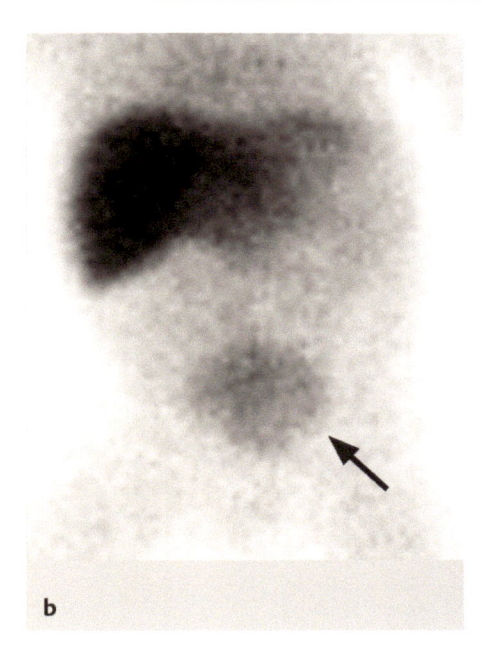

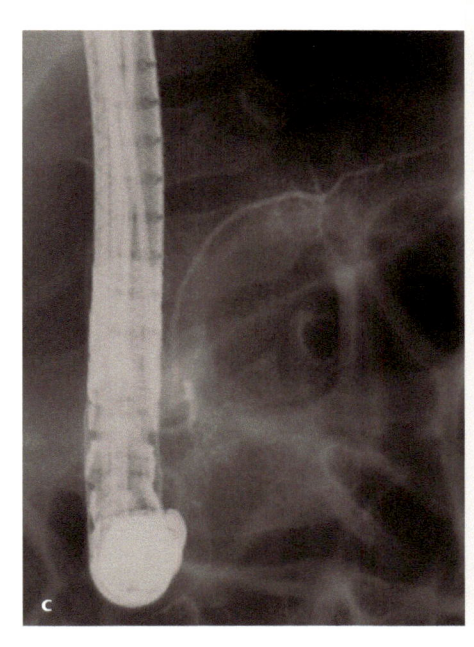

cavernous dilatations of intrahepatic bile ducts (diffuse, lobar, or segmental). If all portions of the intrahepatic biliary system are affected and cystic dilatation of the ducts is accompanied by congenital fibrosis, the condition is Caroli's syndrome. Caroli's syndrome has an autosomal recessive mode of inheritance and is associated in 60% of cases with autosomal recessive polycystic kidney disease.[14]

▶ **Imaging signs.** The principal imaging sign is intrahepatic biliary obstruction with the cystic dilatation of bile ducts, which is clearly demonstrable by ultrasound. Intraductal sludge or gallstones may be found within the intrahepatic ducts. The portal vein branches may pass through areas of cystic duct dilatation[15]; this finding can be confirmed by duplex ultrasound scanning. Caroli's syndrome may also be associated with signs of hepatic cirrhosis and portal hypertension.

Contrast-enhanced CT defines the extent and distribution of the ductal dilatation. The presence of opacified portal vein branches within the dilated intrahepatic ducts ("central dot sign") is considered pathognomonic.[16] CT is less effective than ultrasound or MRI in the detection of intrahepatic gallstones. Cyst contents of high attenuation should suggest hepatic abscess. CT can also diagnose hepatic cirrhosis and its sequelae, splenomegaly with portomesenteric varices. MRI (using T2 W sequences and contrast-enhanced T1 W sequences) can detect cystic dilatation of the intrahepatic ducts in addition to the presence of portal vein branches within the dilatations (▶ Fig. 6.17). MRCP has the ability to detect intrahepatic gallstones and biliary strictures due to scarring.[17]

▶ **Clinical features.** The simple type, Caroli's disease, is much rarer than the fibrosing type, Caroli's syndrome. Both types may become clinically apparent at any age, but most patients become symptomatic in the second decade of life. The most common presenting symptom is right upper quadrant pain. Simple Caroli's disease presents with recurrent episodes of cholangitis with fever and jaundice. Patients develop intrahepatic duct stones and hepatic abscesses. The clinical manifestations of Caroli's syndrome

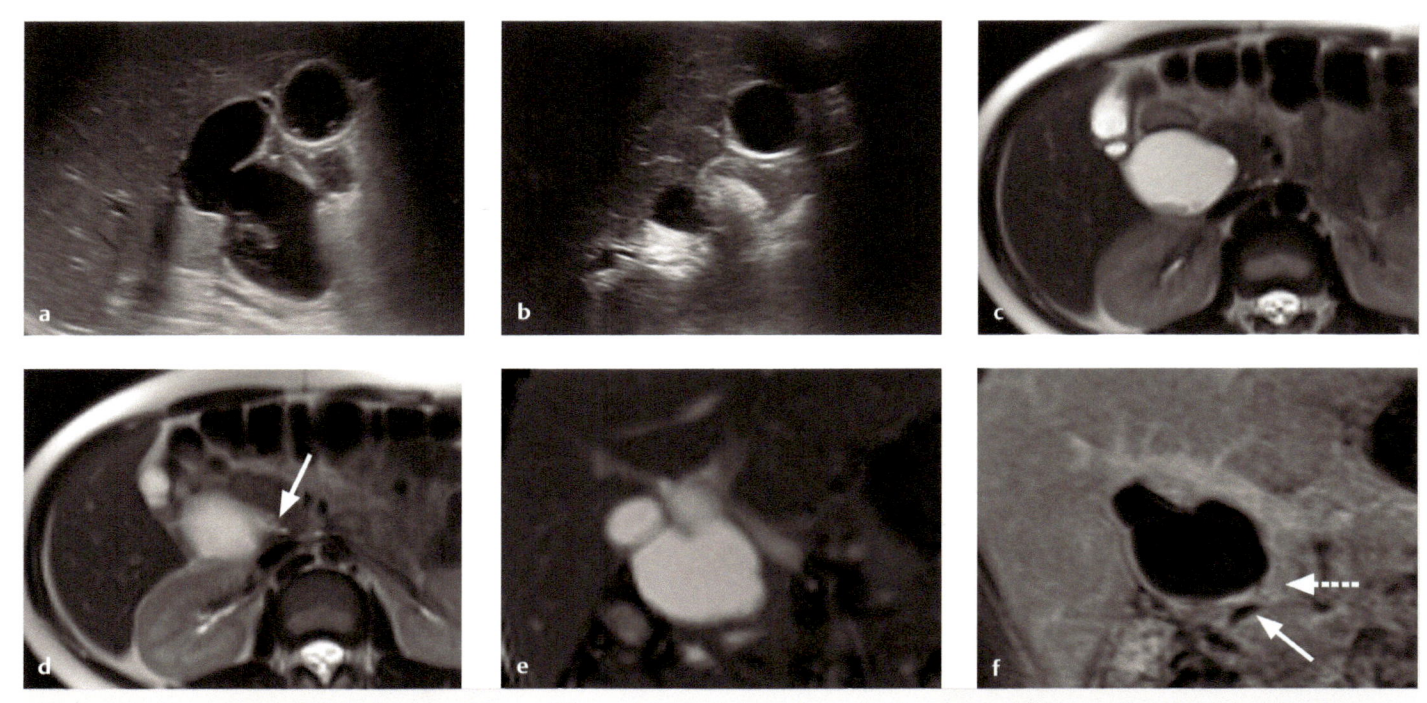

Fig. 6.16 Todani type I choledochal cyst in a 10-year-old boy with upper abdominal pain. **(a)** The common bile duct is dilated to 4 cm. **(b)** Sludge in the common bile duct. **(c)** Maximum transverse diameter of the common bile duct. **(d)** Major pancreatic duct is dilated and opens into a long, common terminal segment (arrow). **(e)** Dilatation of the common bile duct extends into the cystic duct. **(f)** Fat-suppressed T1 W MRI after administration of contrast medium shows a filiform choledochal stenosis (dashed arrow) just proximal to its junction with the pancreatic duct (solid arrow).

are determined by hepatic cirrhosis and portal hypertension. Cholangitis is less common and usually occurs only after portal hypertension has developed.[1] The risk of cholangiocarcinoma is increased by a factor of 100 (ca. 7% of patients develop bile duct cancer). Intrahepatic cholelithiasis can be treated conservatively with ursodeoxycholic acid.[18] The first-line treatment option for cholangitis is antibiotic therapy. Localized forms should be treated surgically (by lobectomy or segmentectomy). Drainage may be necessary for biliary decompression. Liver transplantation is indicated for patients with refractory cholangitis or biliary cirrhosis.

▶ **Differential diagnosis**
- Polycystic kidney disease.
- Primary sclerosing cholangitis.
- Recurrent suppurative cholangitis and hepatic abscess.
- Biliary hamartomas.

▶ **Key points.** Simple, nonobstructive dilatation of the large intrahepatic ducts (Caroli's disease) is distinguished from a congenital fibrosing type that additionally involves the small ducts (Caroli's syndrome). There is also a pure congenital fibrosing type in which only the small ducts are affected. Presentation in early adulthood is common. The cardinal symptom is intrahepatic biliary obstruction with cystic dilatation of the ducts. Caroli's disease is manifested by recurrent attacks of cholangitis, intrahepatic gallstones, and hepatic abscesses. Caroli's syndrome rarely presents with cholangitis; its manifestations are determined by hepatic cirrhosis and portal hypertension. The risk of cholangiocarcinoma is increased 100-fold.

6.5 Acquired Diseases
6.5.1 Gallstones and Their Sequelae

Note

Gallstones are the leading cause of biliary tract disease. Frequently they are asymptomatic ("silent cholelithiasis").

The spectrum of symptomatic cholelithiasis ranges from nonspecific upper abdominal pain and colic to life-threatening conditions such as biliary pancreatitis, gallbladder perforation, or gallstone ileus. Gallbladder carcinoma may develop as a potential late complication of chronic mechanical stone irritation.

Gallstones are caused by an imbalance in the soluble substances contained in bile. They almost always form in the gallbladder. About 15% of patients with gallbladder stones (cholecystolithiasis) also have stones in the common bile duct (choledocholithiasis).

Gallstones are classified by their chemical composition as follows:
- *Pure gallstones* (5–10%): composed chiefly of one component of bile.
- *Mixed gallstones* (80–90%): faceted stones made up of various components.
- *Combination stones* (5–10%): different compositions of core and shell.

A statistical analysis of autopsy study in Leipzig from 1980 to 1989 documented the following frequency distribution: 10% pure

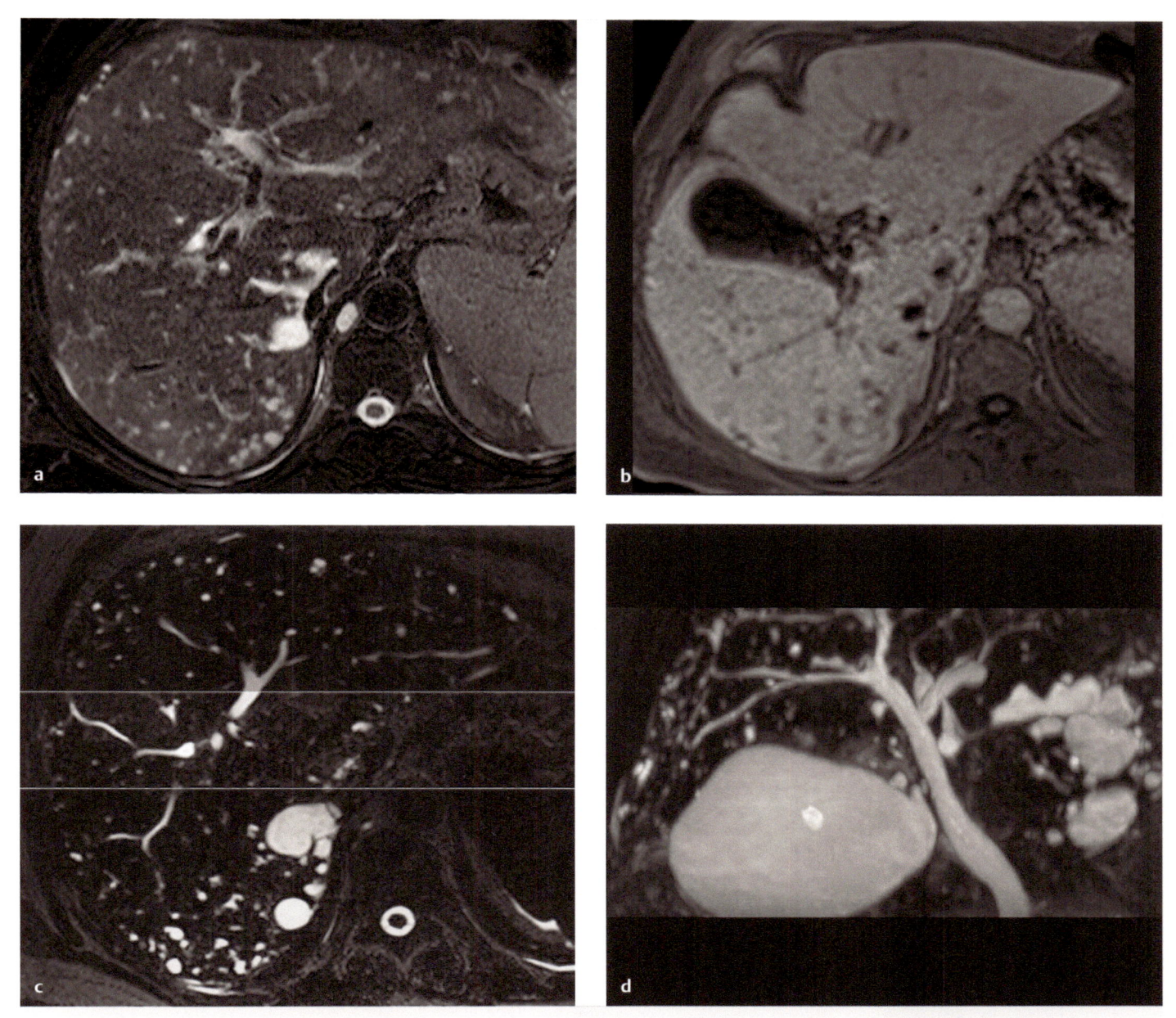

Fig. 6.17 Caroli's syndrome. (a) T2W image shows multiple hyperintense, oval, saccular dilatations of small intrahepatic bile ducts. (b) The intrahepatic ducts are only slightly dilated. (c) Axial maximum intensity projection. (d) Coronal maximum intensity projection. (Images with kind permission of Prof. Berthold, Hannover Medical School, Germany)

cholesterol stones, 85% cholesterol-pigment-calcium stones, 1% pigment stones, and 3% sludge (sand).[19] For simplicity, two main types of gallstone are distinguished:
- *Cholesterol stones*: stones composed mainly of cholesterol (75% of all gallstones).
- *Pigment stones*: stones composed mainly of calcium bicarbonate (25% of all gallstones).

The two subtypes of pigment stones are termed brown and black stones. Cholesterol stones consist of at least 70% hardened cholesterol. They have an oval shape, while small stones are spherical. They are faceted, have a small cholesterol-pigment core, and may calcify. The formation of cholesterol stones is influenced by three factors:
- *Cholesterol oversaturation of bile*: This results from increased hepatic cholesterol secretion (or decreased hepatic secretion of bile acids). Genetic factors play a role and involve the increased transport of cholesterol from the hepatocyte into the biliary tree (ABCG8 mutation of sterolin).[20] Other risk factors are age, obesity, rapid weight loss, female sex, pregnancy, a high-fat diet, intestinal disorders, and lipid-lowering drugs (clofibrate, etc.).
- *Nucleation-promoting factors*: These factors include gallbladder mucus and calcium.
- *Impaired gallbladder emptying*: This is caused by reduced gallbladder motility. Risk factors are pregnancy, rapid weight loss, and medications (contraceptives, octreotide [a somatostatin analogue]).

Pigment stones form under two conditions: Black pigment stones are associated with hemolysis or hepatic cirrhosis and are most commonly found in the gallbladder. They may also form in the intrahepatic bile ducts of a cirrhotic liver. Brown pigment stones form in association with biliary tract infections and therefore occur in the biliary tree. Pigment stones are small (1–10 mm) and

Gallbladder and Biliary Tract

usually multiple. Their color is derived from the presence of iron and copper.

Gallbladder sludge consists of small particles that precipitate from the biliary fluid. It most commonly forms in response to conditions such as rapid weight loss, consumptive illness, pregnancy, medication use (lipid-lowering drugs), and organ or bone marrow transplantation. It consistently forms in patients on prolonged parenteral nutrition (e.g., ICU patients); this underscores the importance of gallbladder emptying in the pathogenesis of lithiasis. Biliary sludge is asymptomatic in most patients. If the cause is eliminated, it may resolve. When symptoms occur, they result from duct obstruction and present as biliary colic. Like gallstones, gallbladder sludge may also cause acute cholecystitis or even biliary pancreatitis.

Silent Cholelithiasis

▶ **Brief definition.** Gallstones are a common occurrence, affecting approximately 10% of adults and 2% of children. Females are affected 2 to 3 times more frequently than males. There is also a familial disposition. Hepatic cirrhosis, biliary tract diseases, and infections predispose to gallstone formation. Other factors play a role in children: congenital bile duct anomalies, short bowel syndrome with impaired enterohepatic circulation, prolonged parenteral nutrition, hemolytic anemia, and cystic fibrosis. Asymptomatic stones are found almost exclusively in the gallbladder. Stones in the common bile duct will generally produce symptoms.

▶ **Imaging signs.** Only 20% of cholesterol stones are calcified and radiopaque (▶ Fig. 6.18).

Diagnosis of gallstones is the domain of ultrasound (▶ Fig. 6.19). A normal gallbladder is echo-free. A stone presents the following triad of sonographic features:
- Curved, high-level echo with a posterior acoustic shadow.
- Visualizability in two planes.
- Mobility with changes in patient position.

Small stones may not cast an acoustic shadow (see ▶ Fig. 6.18c).

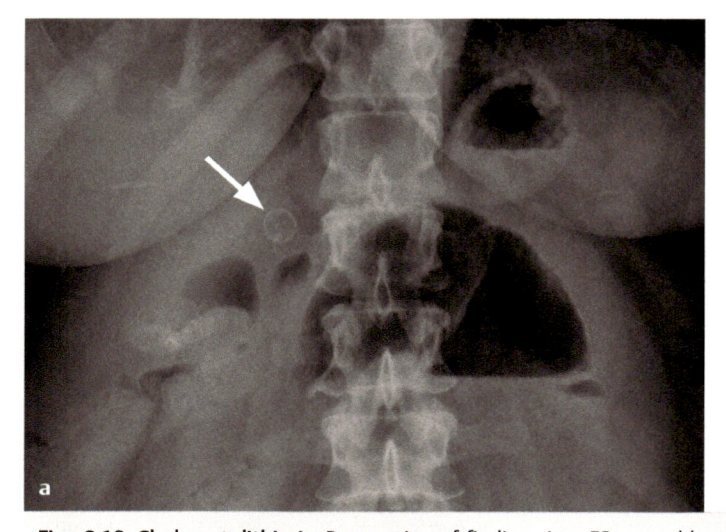

Note
The size, number, and location of the stones should be noted in the radiology report.

Small stones (4–6 mm) are potentially passable. They may occlude the infundibulum or incite a choledocholithiasis leading to biliary tract obstruction or even biliary pancreatitis. A large gallstone may completely occupy the gallbladder lumen ("giant gallstone," ▶ Fig. 6.20). Small cholesterol stones may float within the gallbladder lumen. Often they do not cast an acoustic shadow and are visible as round or polygonal bodies (see ▶ Fig. 6.19c). Gallbladder sludge appears as a mobile sediment that may be hyperechoic or isoechoic to the liver. If the gallbladder is completely filled with sludge, it may be difficult to delineate from the adjacent liver (▶ Fig. 6.21). Gallbladder sludge can mask the presence of actual stones (see ▶ Fig. 6.21d). Ultrasound is a reliable modality for detecting stones in the common bile duct, thickening of the duct wall, and intrahepatic biliary obstruction (see ▶ Fig. 6.5). Stone detection by CT is limited by the variable density of gallstones. Hyperdense calcified stones, mixed stones with a calcium component, and hypodense fatty cholesterol stones are distinguishable from biliary fluid. Approximately 20% of gallstones are isodense to the surrounding fluid and are therefore not detectable by CT; gallbladder sludge is often undetectable as well. CT is less accurate than ultrasound for evaluating the gallbladder wall (▶ Fig. 6.22). Bile is hyperintense in T2W sequences on MRI, and these sequences provide the highest sensitivity for stone detection (▶ Fig. 6.23). Fat-suppressed T1W sequences after administration of contrast medium have special importance as they can distinguish stones from gallbladder polyps based on enhancement characteristics (see ▶ Fig. 6.23d, f). MRCP is available as an adjunct to sectional imaging. MRI can detect stones as small as 2 mm in the gallbladder and biliary tree.

▶ **Clinical features.** Silent cholecystolithiasis remains asymptomatic in two-thirds of cases; generally it is detected incidentally

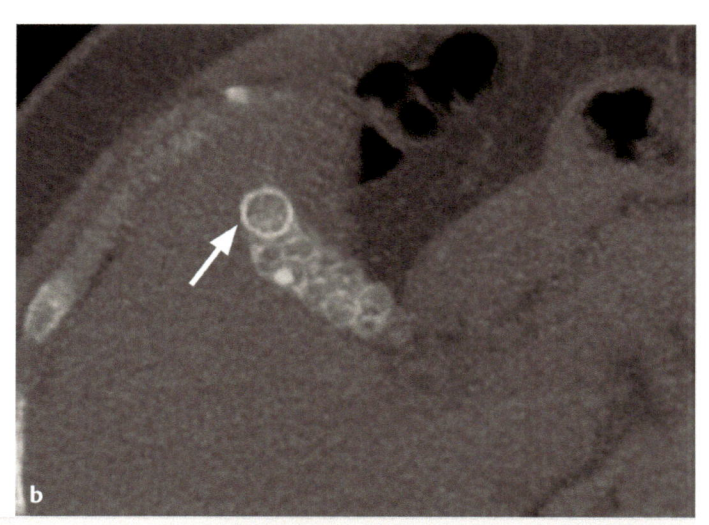

Fig. 6.18 Cholecystolithiasis. Progression of findings in a 52-year-old man with sarcoidosis and nonspecific upper abdominal complaints without local tenderness. Antral gastritis was diagnosed by endoscopy (not shown). **(a)** Radiograph shows a cholesterol stone with a calcified rim in the gallbladder infundibulum (arrow). Additional small stones are present in the fundus. **(b)** CT scan for sarcoidosis 6 months before image [a] shows a small, stone-filled gallbladder. Here the infundibulum stone is located in the fundus (arrow).

6.5 Acquired Diseases

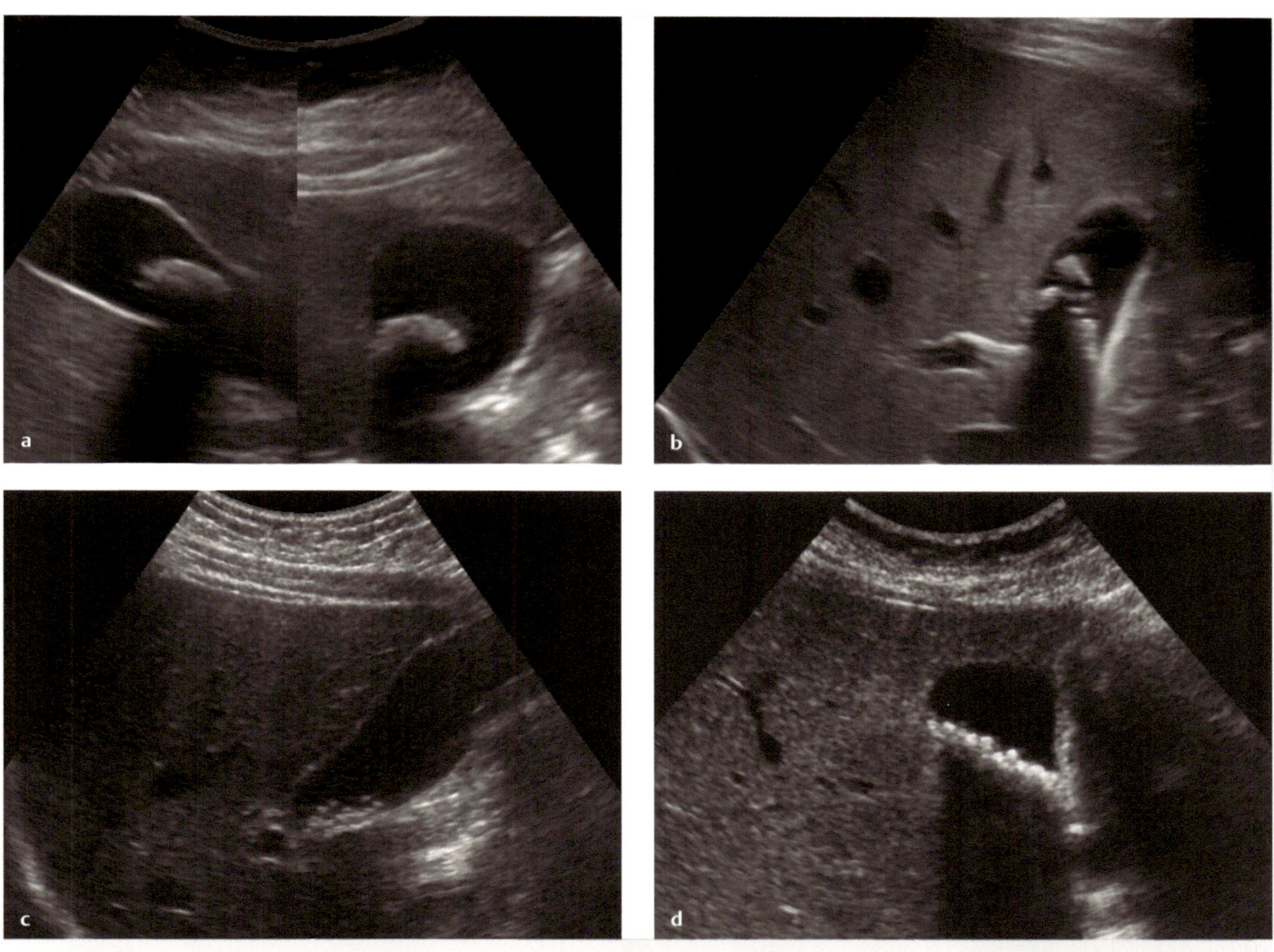

Fig. 6.19 **Gallbladder stones.** Ultrasound features. (a) Large, solitary, shadowing cholesterol stone imaged in two planes (longitudinal and transverse). (b) Medium-sized stones. (c) Small, nonshadowing cholesterol stones. (d) Multiple small stones with dense acoustic shadows. Pigment stones in spherocytosis.

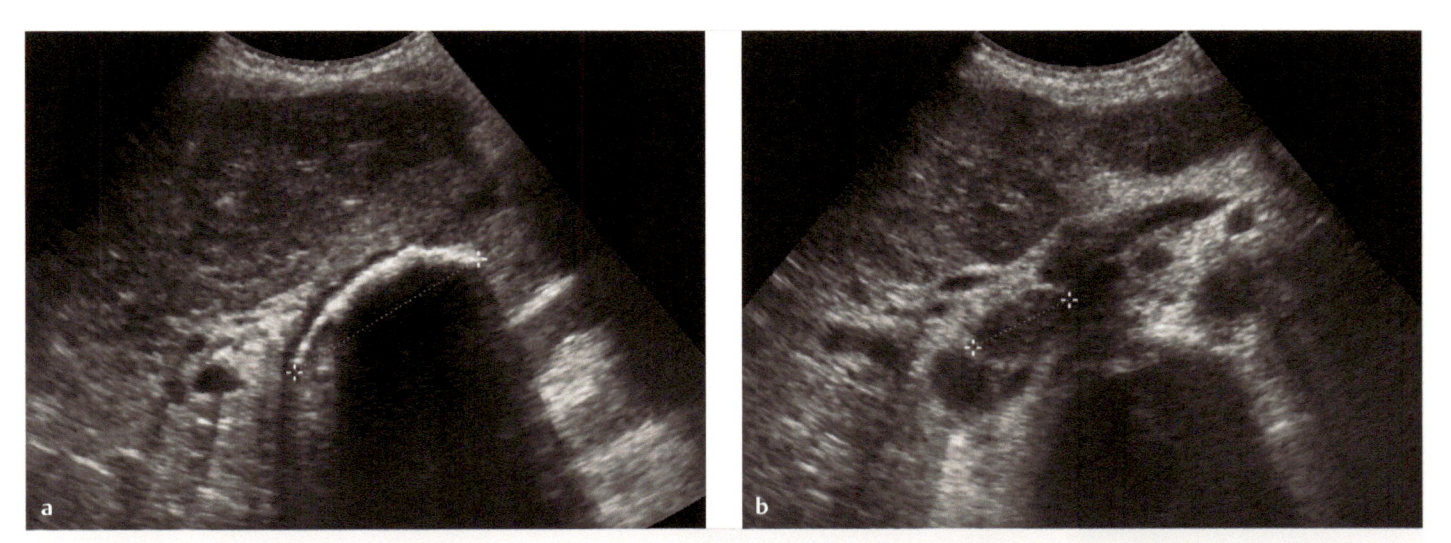

Fig. 6.20 **Giant gallstone** in an 84-year-old woman with weight loss. At surgery: chronic atrophic cholecystitis with gallbladder carcinoma and nodal metastases. (a) Giant gallstone casts a large acoustic shadow that obscures the porta hepatis and posterior gallbladder wall. (b) Scan at a more caudal level shows enlarged lymph nodes in the hepatoduodenal ligament.

Gallbladder and Biliary Tract

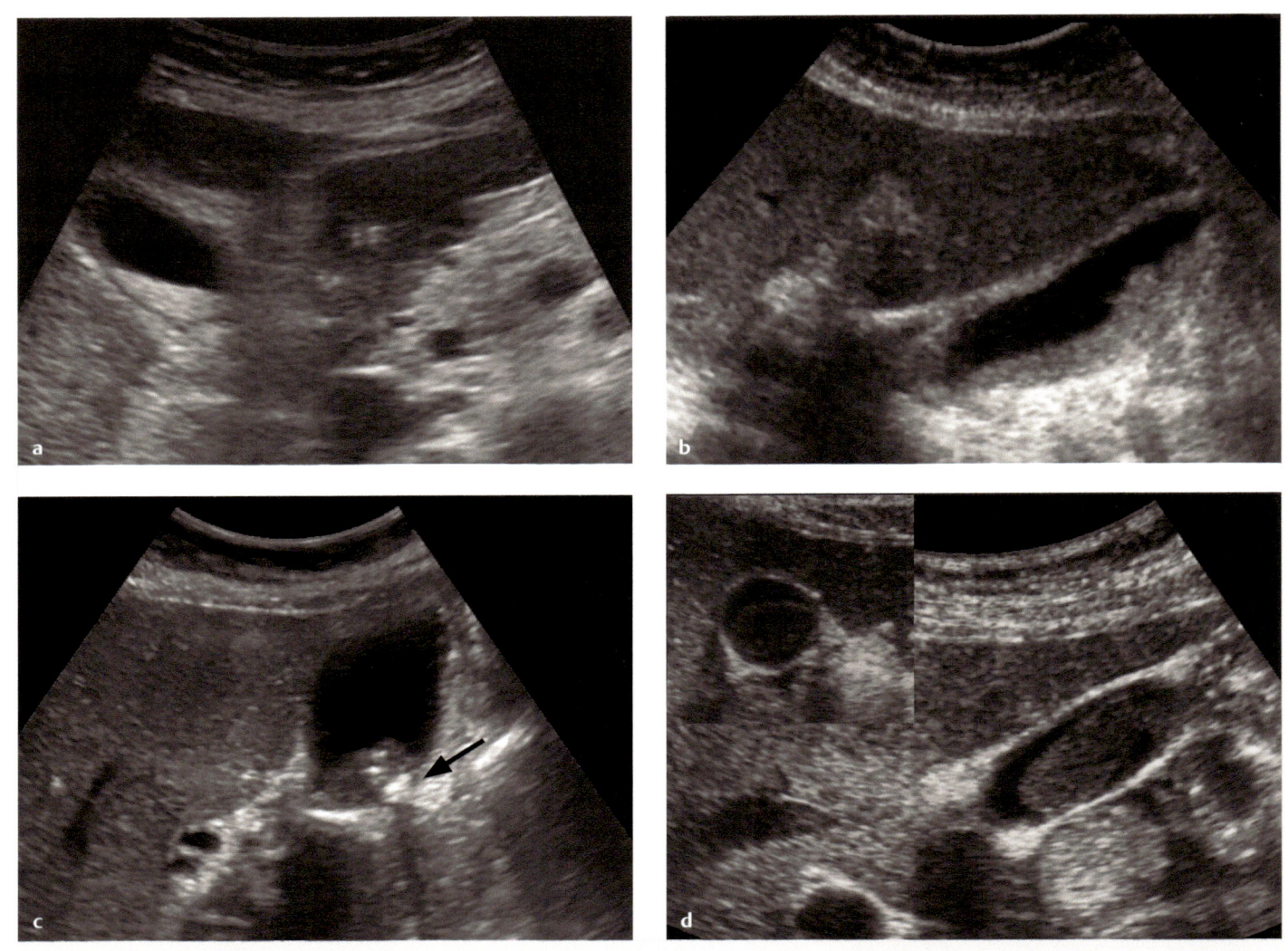

Fig. 6.21 Gallbladder sludge. (a) Dependent layering of echogenic sediment. (b) Sediment layer shows a partially lobulated surface. (c) Rounded sludge mass isoechoic to liver includes small stones and a larger stone with an acoustic shadow (arrow). (d) Sludge forming an ellipsoidal cast of the gallbladder lumen (inset: transverse scan).

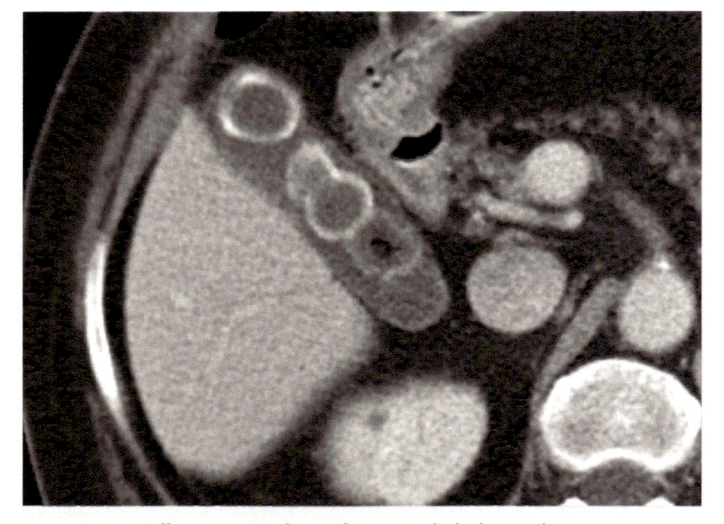

Fig. 6.22 Gallstones. CT shows five mixed cholesterol stones (cholesterol, pigment and calcium stones) with surface calcifications diminishing posteriorly. The interior of the stones is isodense to biliary fluid. The posterior stone is barely identifiable.

at ultrasound. On the other hand, gallstones are the most frequent cause of upper abdominal pain. Patients often present with nonspecific complaints such as nausea and occasional vomiting, especially after heavy, fat-rich meals. A history of aversion to fatty, spicy foods is another classic sign.

> **Note**
>
> An important indicator of whether acute upper abdominal pain is due to acute cholecystitis is the tenderness of the gallbladder to pressure (Murphy's sign). If the gallbladder is not tender, it is probably not the source of the acute upper abdominal pain.

Asymptomatic stones in an otherwise normal gallbladder do not require treatment.

▶ **Differential diagnosis**
- *Gallbladder polyps*: Polyps are not mobile in response to position changes; they are fixed to the gallbladder wall. They do not

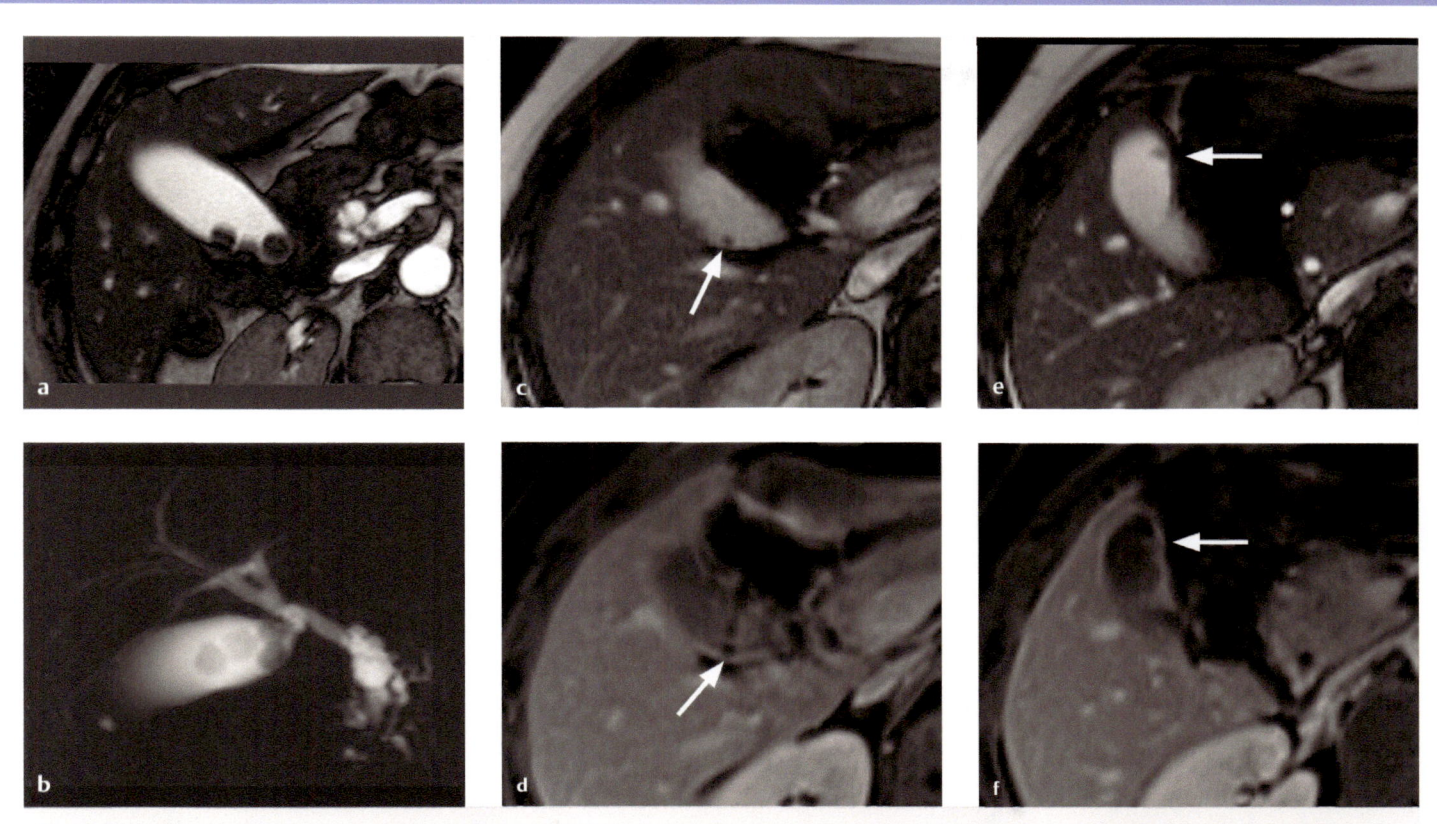

Fig. 6.23 **Gallstones.** MRI features. (a) Venography. (b) MR cholangiopancreatography. (c) T2 W image shows a small stone in the gallbladder fundus (arrow). (d) Coronal fat-suppressed T1 W image shows absence of enhancement (arrow), consistent with a stone. (e) T2 W image of a small stone in the infundibulum (arrow). (f) Coronal fat-suppressed T1 W image shows enhancement (arrow) consistent with a gallbladder polyp.

cast an acoustic shadow, and they enhance on T1-weighted MRI after IV administration of contrast medium.
- *Adenomyomatosis*: This condition involves a segmental or diffuse wall thickening that enhances after IV administration of contrast medium.
- *Gallbladder tumor*: Generally it is not difficult to distinguish between a stone and gallbladder tumor at ultrasound owing to the immobility of the tumor. The main criterion on CT and MRI is the occurrence of tumor enhancement. If CT or MRI findings are equivocal, the gallbladder should also be examined by ultrasound.

▶ **Key points.** Silent gallbladder stones can be found in 10% of adults and 2% of children. They are detected incidentally during an ultrasound examination. Approximately one-third of patients with silent stones will go on to develop symptomatic cholecystolithiasis or choledocholithiasis. The risk of symptomatic cholelithiasis depends on stone size and is greater with small, potentially passable stones. The finding of gallbladder wall changes in an asymptomatic patient is sufficient to exclude silent cholecystolithiasis. These patients should be evaluated for possible gallbladder carcinoma.

Symptomatic Cholecystolithiasis

▶ **Brief definition.** When gallstones migrate, they may become impacted at any level of the biliary tree and cause an obstruction. The consequent rise in pressure leads to biliary colic. Impaired bile drainage may lead to obstructive jaundice and is a risk factor for biliary tract infection. Over time the infection may ascend and reach the gallbladder. Colic may also be caused by an infundibular stone that prevents the contracting gallbladder from emptying. Stone-associated symptoms may resolve spontaneously in one-half of cases. But they may also cause potentially life-threatening complications.

▶ **Imaging signs.** The gallbladder is always found to be tender on initial ultrasound scanning. Ultrasound can detect the stones and determine their size and location. Dilatation of the bile ducts may be noted depending on the site and duration of the obstruction. The normal diameter of the common bile duct is 6 mm. A value of 10 mm or more in a patient not previously operated on indicates dilatation. Stones in the gallbladder infundibulum are easily detected, whereas common duct stones are not, especially if the duct is not dilated (▶ Fig. 6.24, ▶ Fig. 6.25). If the gallbladder wall is thickened, there is cholecystitis.

The advantage of CT is that it permits a rapid, noninvasive evaluation. It should be performed as a multiphase contrast-enhanced study. The arterial phase defines the vascular status in the hepatoduodenal ligament and gallbladder region. The parenchymal phase (portal venous phase) defines local findings. It is superior to ultrasound for imaging common duct stones and the area around the gallbladder (▶ Fig. 6.26). CT is the modality of choice for the diagnosis of biliary pancreatitis.

MRI can also define even small common duct stones. As well as axial images, coronal T2 W images are recommended (▶ Fig. 6.27). Biliary obstruction is best demonstrated by MRCP. Fat-suppressed T1 W images after administration of contrast medium are useful for detecting wall changes in the common bile duct and gallbladder. MRI is more time-consuming, however, and therefore less suitable for emergency diagnosis.

Gallbladder and Biliary Tract

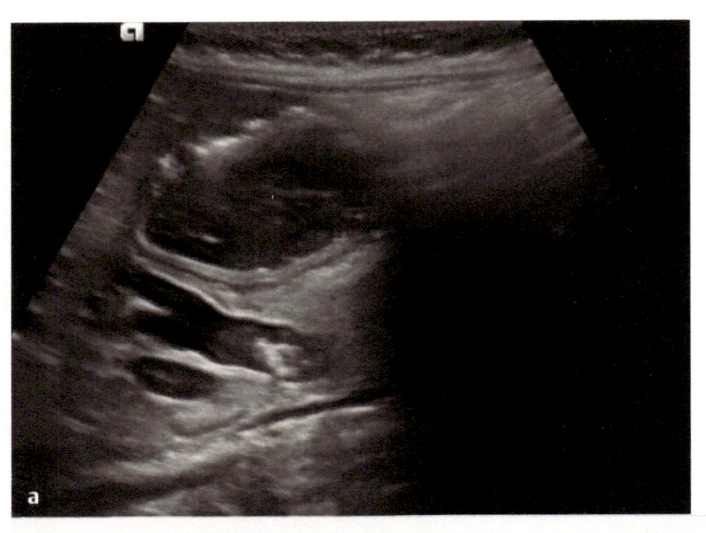

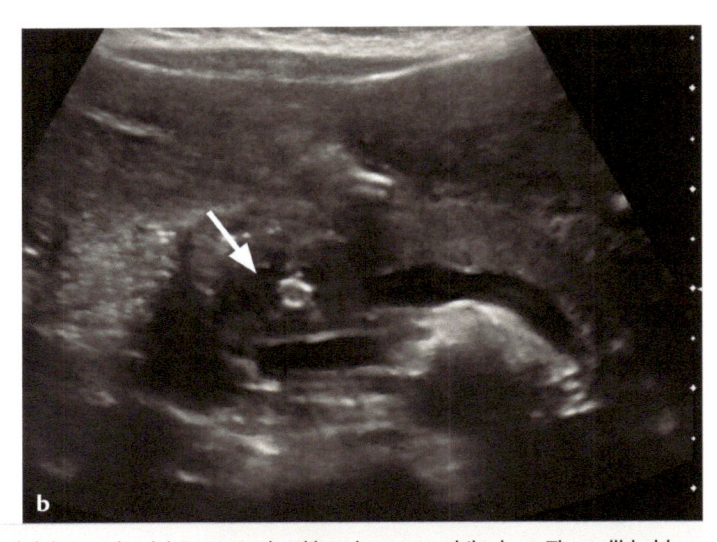

Fig. 6.24 Choledocholithiasis. Ultrasound findings in an 8-year-old boy with biliary colic. **(a)** Stone in the dilated common bile duct. The gallbladder wall is thickened, and sludge is present in the gallbladder lumen. **(b)** Hypoechoic swelling (arrow) surrounds the pancreatic segment of the common bile duct in biliary head pancreatitis.

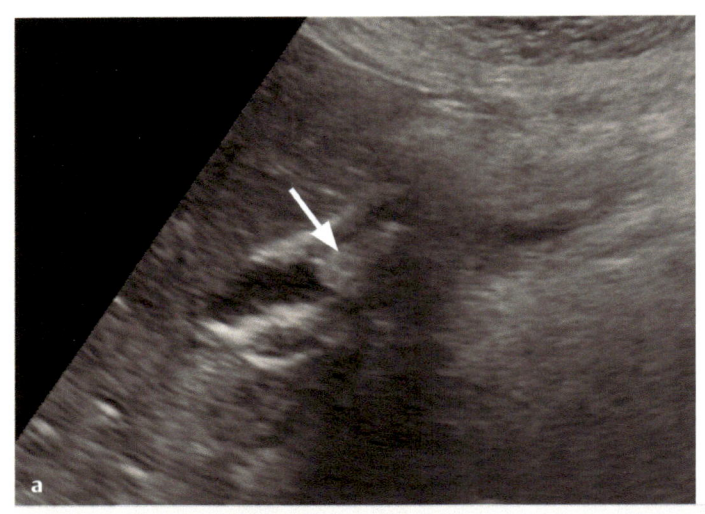

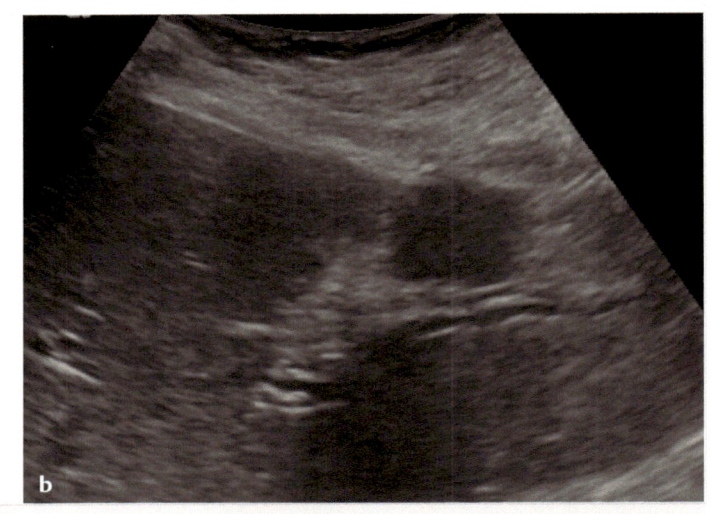

Fig. 6.25 Choledocholithiasis. Ultrasound findings in an 82-year-old woman with biliary colic. **(a)** Dilated common bile duct with a large stone. **(b)** Intrahepatic biliary obstruction with associated jaundice.

Note

An impacted papillary stone is an indication for emergency endoscopic retrograde cholangiopancreatography with a papillotomy.

▶ **Clinical features.** Classic biliary colic consists of severe right upper quadrant pain that comes in waves and may radiate to the right flank, back, or shoulder. In contrast to renal colic, the patient here assumes an antalgic posture. Biliary colic is often accompanied by nausea and vomiting. If the stone is obstructing only the gallbladder infundibulum and not the bile ducts, the colic is not accompanied by jaundice. The isolated gallbladder may become infected over time, and gallbladder empyema may develop. If the stone migrates to the common bile duct, the patient may have obstructive jaundice with acholic stools and beer-brown urine, depending on the degree of obstruction. Obstruction at the papillary level leads to biliary pancreatitis, which may be life-threatening depending on its severity. Biliary pancreatitis is responsible for one-third of all cases of acute pancreatitis. Treatment depends on various factors:

- *Treatment in the acute phase*: The cornerstones of acute therapy are withholding solid foods while giving analgesics and spasmolytics (hyoscine butylbromide, no morphine preparations). Any infection is treated with antibiotics.
- *Therapy in symptom-free periods*: Symptomatic cholecystolithiasis should be treated surgically whenever possible. Choledocholithiasis should be excluded prior to laparoscopic cholecystectomy. Open cholecystectomy can be combined with exploration of the common bile duct.
- *Treatment for common duct stones after cholecystectomy*: ERCP with papillotomy and stone extraction may be tried in cases of this kind.
- *Pharmacologic stone dissolution*: Reportedly, oral treatment with ursodeoxycholic acid can dissolve all stones in up to 70% of patients within 1 to 2 years. The recurrence rate is up to 50% within 5 years. Stones reduced in size by drug therapy may migrate, with an associated risk of biliary pancreatitis. Other prerequisites for medical therapy are a maximum stone size of

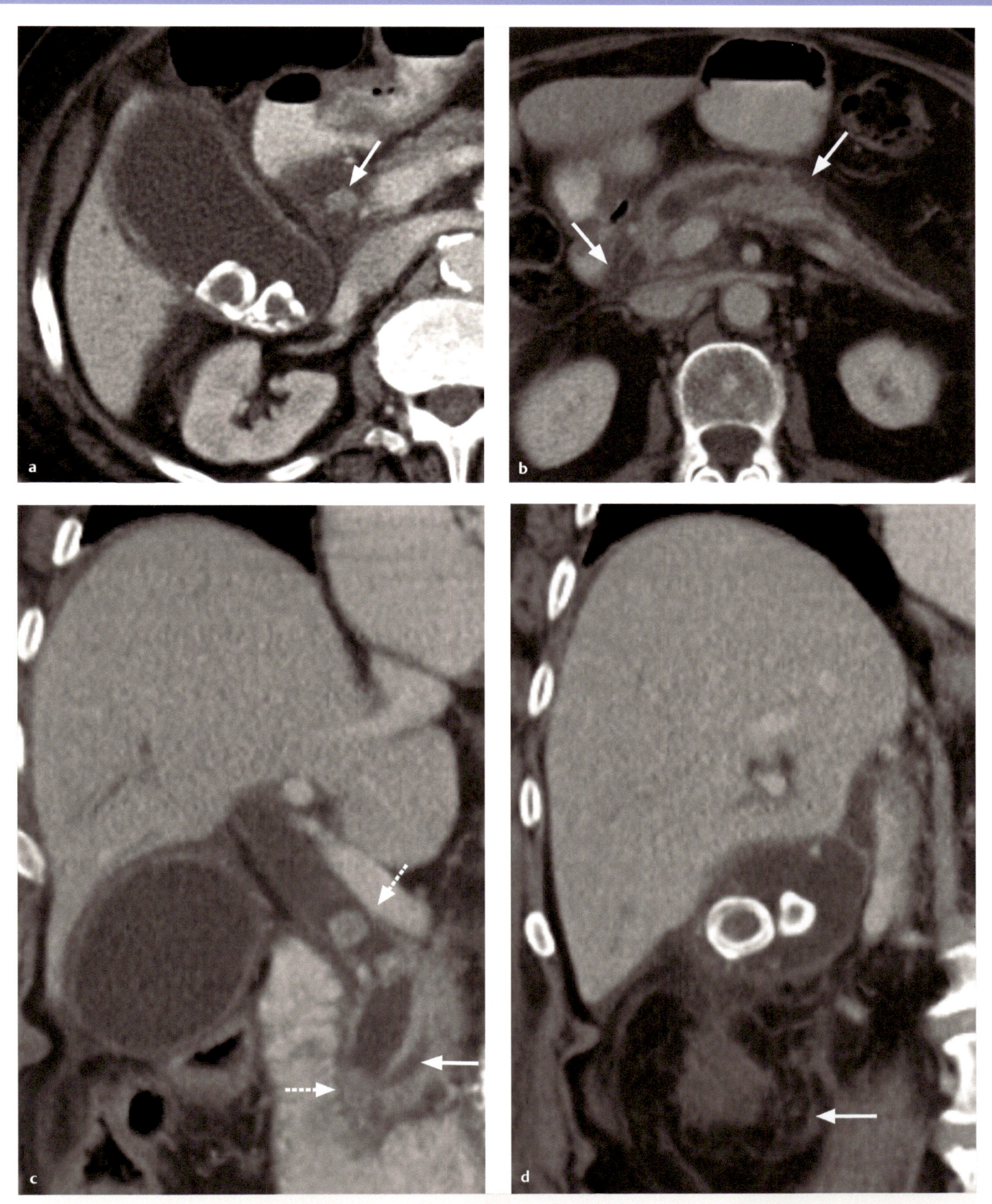

Fig. 6.26 Cholecystolithiasis and choledocholithiasis with obstructive jaundice, acute cholecystitis, and biliary pancreatitis in a 90-year-old woman with upper abdominal pain, jaundice, and fever. (a) Enlarged gallbladder with a thickened wall. Calcified gallbladder stones and a common duct stone (arrow). (b) Biliary pancreatitis with duct dilatation and peripancreatic exudates (arrows). (c) Papillary stone and common duct stone (dashed arrows). Dilatation of the common bile duct and pancreatic duct (arrow). (d) Increased retroperitoneal density (arrow) in pericholecystitis.

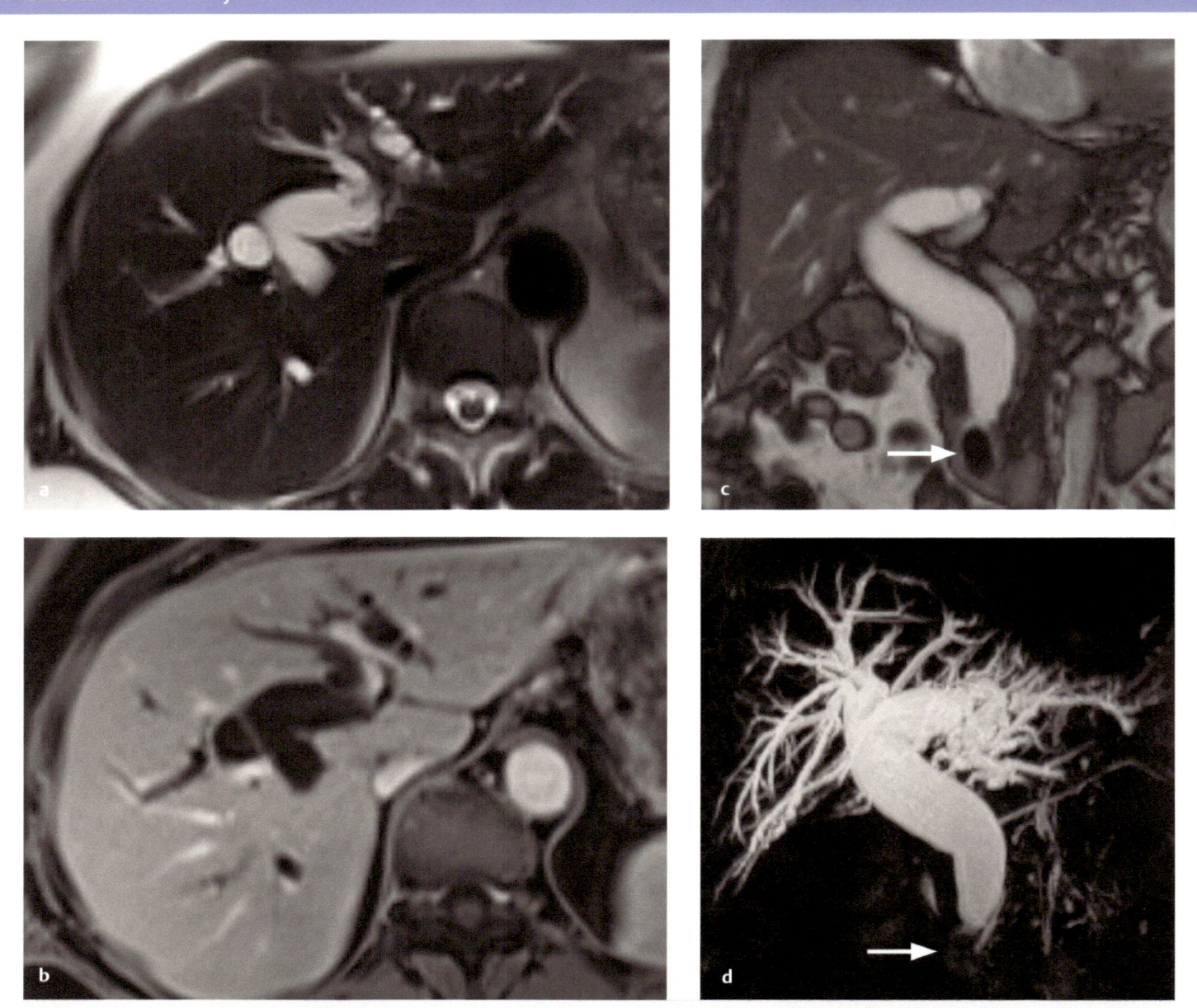

Fig. 6.27 **Obstructive jaundice secondary to a papillary stone.** MRI findings in a 75-year-old woman 35 years after cholecystectomy. The patient had a long history of recurrent bouts of colic; she presented now with jaundice. (a) T2 W image. Biliary obstruction. (b) Fat-suppressed T1 W image after administration of contrast medium. Biliary obstruction. (c) T2 W image. Papillary stone (arrow). (d) MR cholangiopancreatography. Biliary obstruction with a normal-appearing pancreatic duct. The stone appears as a filling defect (arrow).

5 mm, and that stones should occupy no more than half the gallbladder volume. Normal gallbladder function (at least 50% emptying after a "provocative meal") is another essential prerequisite.

▶ **Differential diagnosis.** Classic biliary colic is easily distinguished from right-sided renal colic by antalgic posturing, which is not observed with kidney stones. Acute mesenteric ischemia should be considered as a possible cause. The differential diagnosis of jaundice includes other causes of biliary tract obstruction. Painful jaundice may be due to chronic pancreatitis or pancreatic carcinoma. Cholangitis should be considered if fever is present.

▶ **Key points.** Biliary colic is caused by migration of a stone into the common bile duct and less commonly by a stone in the gallbladder infundibulum. Both conditions are easily diagnosed by ultrasound. Biliary colic may be complicated by obstructive jaundice or biliary tract infection.

Gallbladder Hydrops and Empyema

▶ **Brief definition.** The gallbladder is enlarged in both conditions. As in acute cholecystitis, the cause is an obstruction of the infundibulum. With gallbladder hydrops, the biliary fluid is not infected. The gallbladder is filled with sterile, clear mucinous fluid ("white bile"). The cause is passive back-diffusion of bile pigments from the bile into the gallbladder wall and from there into the vessels.

- *Gallbladder hydrops*: This condition is more common in children than adults, and pediatric cases are rarely caused by stones. The hydrops is often preceded by an infectious disease such as gastroenteritis, otitis media, or a respiratory tract infection.[1] Many cases resolve spontaneously. If the hydrops persists and an infection ensues, the result is acute cholecystitis or empyema. Gallbladder hydrops in adults is caused by an infundibulum stone or rarely by an obstructing tumor. In contrast to pediatric cases, the collection seldom resolves spontaneously in adults.

- *Gallbladder empyema*: This is a bacterial cholecystitis, usually caused by *Escherichia coli*, enterococci, or *Klebsiella* species, in which the gallbladder lumen is filled and distended by pus. Gallbladder empyema is often preceded by gallbladder hydrops caused by an obstructing stone in the infundibulum. Less commonly the obstruction is caused by a tumor. Empyema may also develop as a result of acute or chronic cholecystitis.

▶ **Imaging signs.** Enlargement of the gallbladder is easily detectable with ultrasound. Hydrops is associated with little or no thickening of the gallbladder wall (▶ Fig. 6.28, ▶ Fig. 6.29). If an infundibular stone is not detectable in an adult, a malignant stricture should be sought. Mild tenderness may be noted over the gallbladder. With empyema, the gallbladder wall is markedly thickened, usually with stratification, and the gallbladder is tender to probe pressure. Pus in the gallbladder lumen shows complex echogenicity, often with sedimentation (▶ Fig. 6.30), making it difficult to detect the presence of stones. With gallbladder hydrops, CT will also show an enlarged gallbladder with only slight wall thickening. Little or no change is noted in adjacent fatty tissue. Gallbladder empyema features a thickened, strongly enhancing wall with increased density of adjacent fat (see ▶ Fig. 6.30). Air is sometimes detectable within the gallbladder. MRI in hydrops shows an enlarged gallbladder that otherwise appears relatively normal (see ▶ Fig. 6.28, ▶ Fig. 6.29). Empyema features an enlarged gallbladder with stratified contents. T2W sequences depict pericholecystitis as hyperintense edema. T1W sequences after administration of contrast medium show a thickened, intensely enhancing gallbladder wall with associated enhancement of surrounding tissues.

▶ **Clinical features**
- *Gallbladder hydrops*: Gallbladder hydrops may be an asymptomatic incidental finding at ultrasound or may cause a pressure sensation in the right upper quadrant. Severe gallbladder distention may incite autonomic symptoms such as nausea and vomiting.
- *Gallbladder empyema*: This is an acute, severe, febrile disease. Patients are in a debilitated condition marked by extreme local tenderness and rigidity in the right upper quadrant.

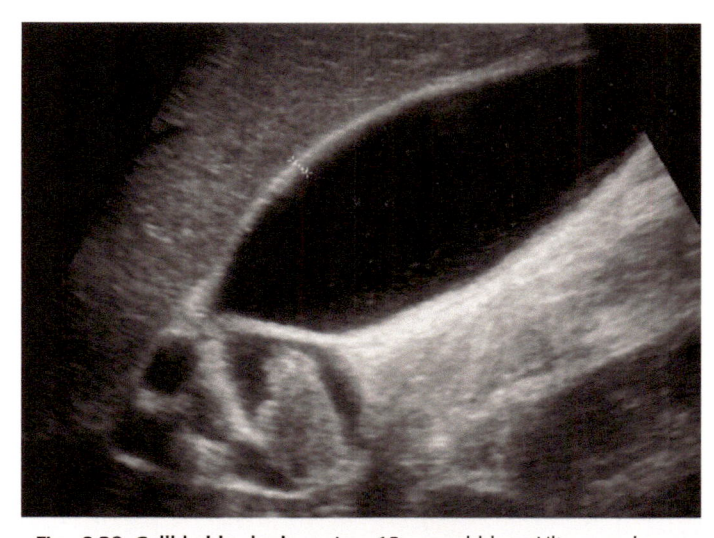

Fig. 6.28 Gallbladder hydrops in a 12-year-old boy. Ultrasound scan shows sludge in the gallbladder infundibulum and slight wall thickening (4 mm).

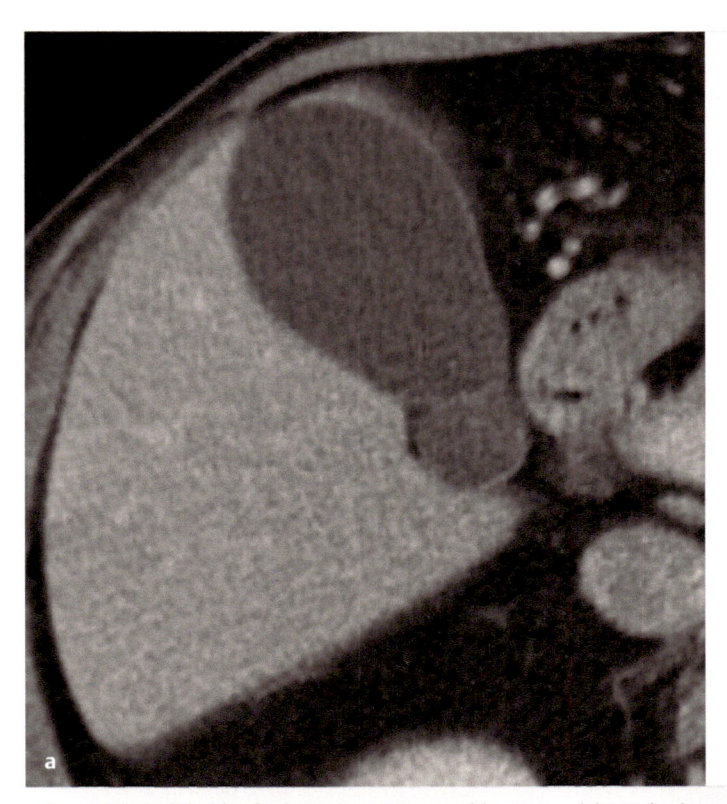

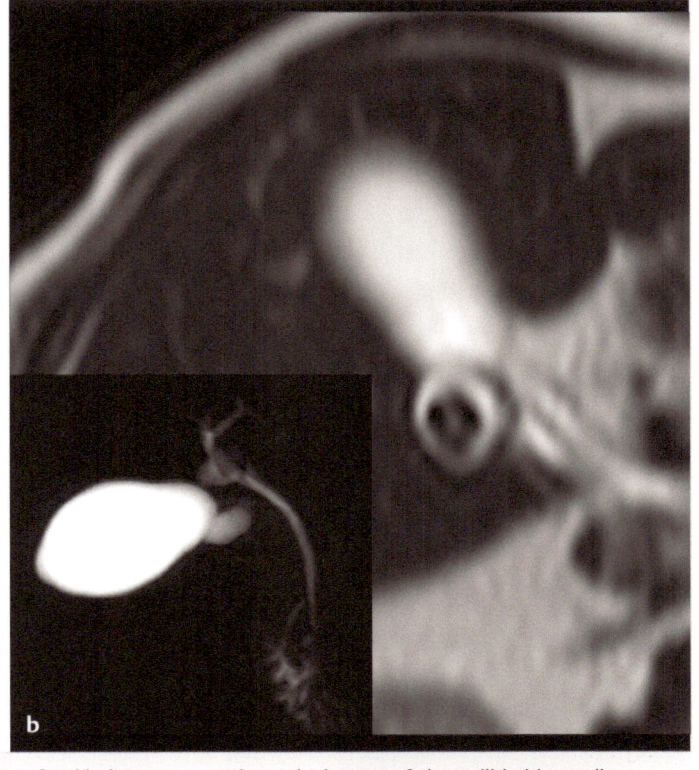

Fig. 6.29 Gallbladder hydrops in a 45-year-old woman. (a) CT displays an infundibulum stone with no thickening of the gallbladder wall. (b) Correlative MRI. The inset shows the MRCP image.

Gallbladder and Biliary Tract

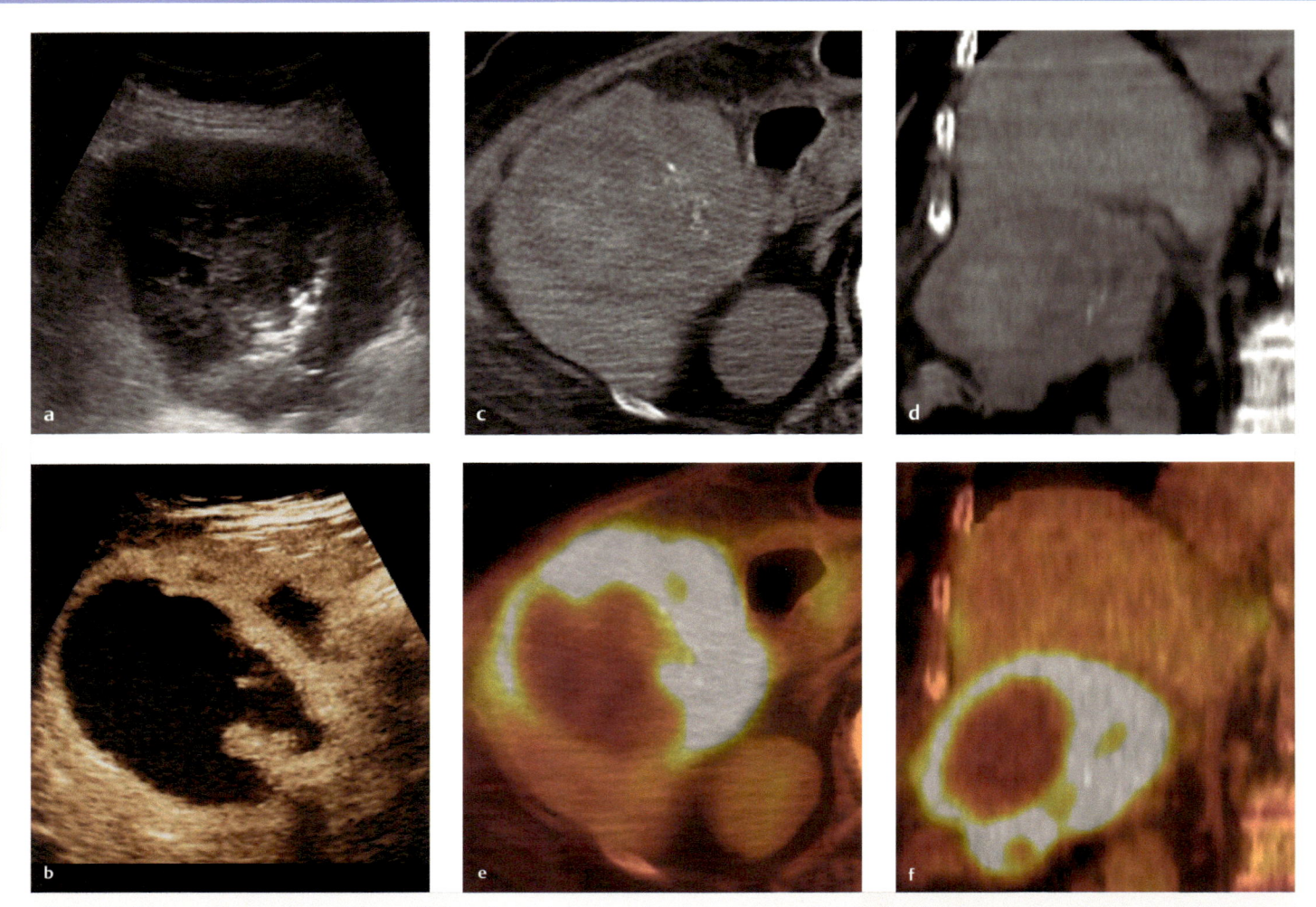

Fig. 6.30 **Empyema in a patient with renal failure.** Surgical specimen histology (not shown) indicated florid granulating cholecystitis with abscess formation in gallbladder empyema. (a) Ultrasound shows a complex mass at the site of the gallbladder with small, echogenic calculi. (b) Contrast-enhanced ultrasound shows central liquefaction plus additional liquefaction in a large adjacent mass. (c) CT shows a hypodense mass at the site of the gallbladder with hyperdense components and calcifications. (d) Coronal reformatted image with a discernible gallbladder and a large mass on the peritoneal side. (e) FDG scan shows sharp delineation from the liver. (f) Corresponding coronal FDG PET-CT scan.

Caution

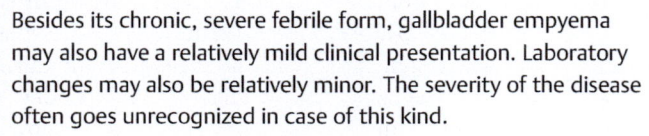

Besides its chronic, severe febrile form, gallbladder empyema may also have a relatively mild clinical presentation. Laboratory changes may also be relatively minor. The severity of the disease often goes unrecognized in case of this kind.

Gallbladder hydrops is treated conservatively or by cholecystectomy, depending on clinical findings. Gallbladder empyema is treated by cholecystectomy. Inoperable cases can be managed by CT-guided percutaneous decompression of the gallbladder or pericholecystic drainage of abscesses.

▶ **Differential diagnosis**
- *Gallbladder hydrops*: Symptomatic hydrops in children requires differentiation from appendicitis and small intestinal volvulus. This is easily accomplished with ultrasound.
- *Gallbladder empyema*: This condition requires differentiation from chronic cholecystitis and gallbladder carcinoma. Both are difficult to discriminate by imaging. Definitive diagnosis in some cases must wait until a surgical specimen is available.

▶ **Key points**
- *Gallbladder hydrops*: The gallbladder is distended by sterile fluid. Its wall is not thickened. Hydrops may be asymptomatic, or a markedly enlarged gallbladder may cause a pressure sensation and autonomic symptoms. Gallbladder hydrops is more common in children; it is not caused by an obstructing stone and may resolve without treatment.
- *Gallbladder empyema*: Empyema is a collection of pus in the gallbladder lumen, usually caused by a stone obstructing the infundibulum. It is more common in adults. Gallbladder empyema may present as an acute, severe septic illness or may take a relatively mild, chronic course. Differentiation is mainly required from chronic cholecystitis and gallbladder carcinoma.

Chronic Cholecystitis and Porcelain Gallbladder

▶ **Brief definition.** Chronic cholecystitis is approximately five times more common than acute inflammation of the gallbladder. Women are affected five times more frequently than men. Chronic cholecystitis may develop as a sequel to acute cholecystitis ("secondary chronic cholecystitis") or may occur as a

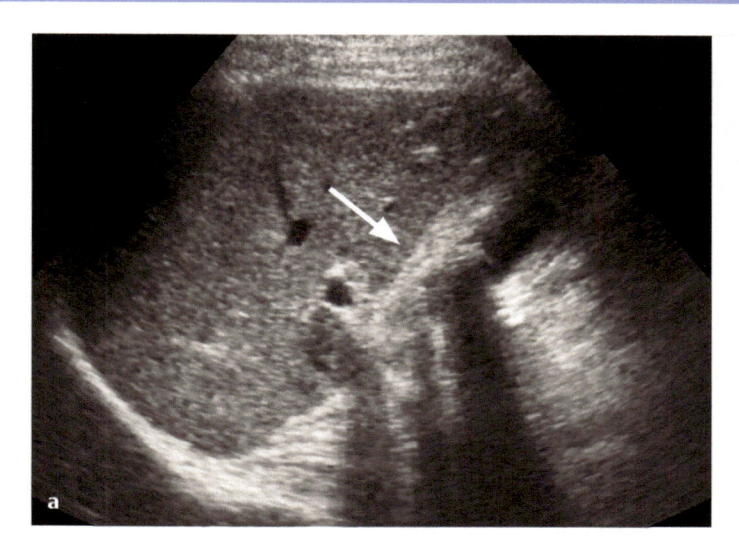

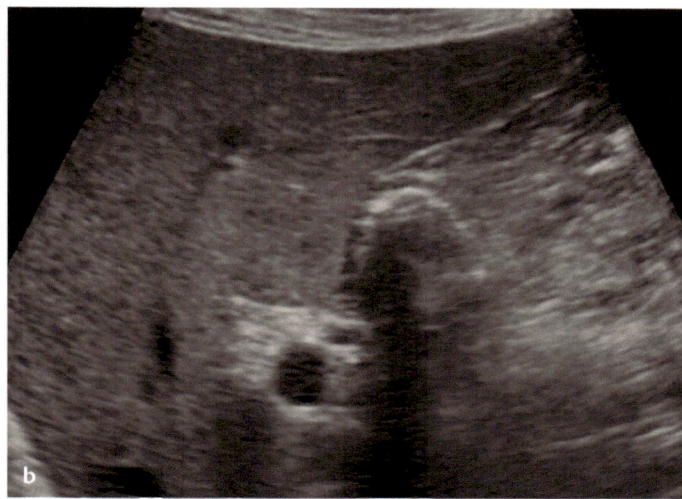

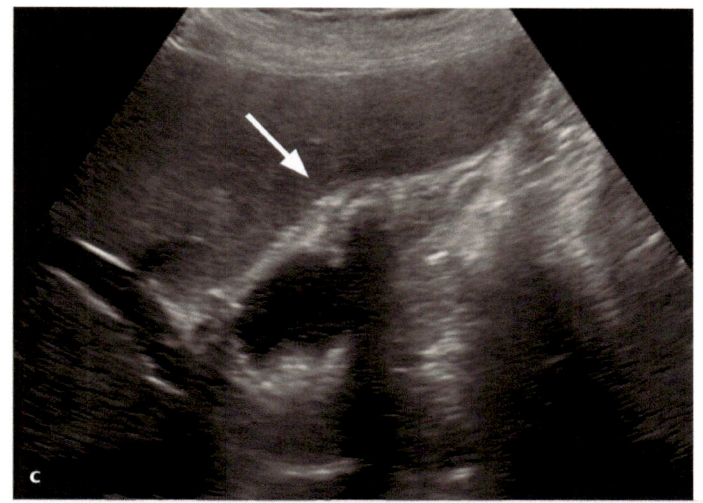

Fig. 6.31 **Chronic cholecystitis.** Ultrasound features. **(a)** Thickened gallbladder wall. Stones in gallbladder sludge (arrow) are identified only by their acoustic shadows. **(b)** Curved acoustic shadow in a porcelain gallbladder (differential diagnosis: giant gallstone). **(c)** Intramural stone (arrow).

primary chronic process without acute exacerbations. In 5% of cases the inflammation occurs in the absence of detectable gallbladder stones. Imaging features may include a chronic hypertrophic inflammation with wall thickening (▶ Fig. 6.31a). There is also a chronic atrophic form characterized by fibrotic scarring and thinning of the gallbladder wall. The disease may culminate in a shrunken gallbladder with a hyalinized wall or a porcelain gallbladder with a calcified wall (▶ Fig. 6.31b). Chronic cholecystitis is associated with an increased risk of gallbladder carcinoma. With a porcelain gallbladder, the risk of malignant transformation was originally estimated at 20%,[21] but more recent studies indicate a risk of only 0.5%.[22] Nearly all cases show associated pericholecystitis, and adhesions with an adjacent organ are common. If a gallstone or granulation tissue is incorporated into the gallbladder wall (▶ Fig. 6.31c), the stone may penetrate or perforate the wall. This may lead to a confined perforation into the liver, a free perforation into the abdominal cavity, or formation of a fistula. Fistulas may form a tract to the skin (biliocutaneous fistula), or bile may leak into surrounding areas. Gallstone ileus develops in 0.1% of gallstone patients.

▶ **Imaging signs.** Calcifications in the gallbladder wall and porcelain gallbladder are easily recognized on the abdomen plain film (▶ Fig. 6.32a). Generally they are noted incidentally on images obtained for a different indication. The main sonographic features of chronic cholecystitis are thickening of the wall (to more than 5 mm) and detection of stones (see ▶ Fig. 6.31). If these signs are found incidentally (not during an acute attack), the gallbladder will not be tender to pressure. Ultrasound during an acute attack will show a hypoechoic border signifying pericholecystitis. This sign is difficult to identify in the presence of a shrunken gallbladder. In addition to wall thickening, the gallbladder contents are hyperechoic.

> **Note**
>
> If the gallbladder is not visualized at ultrasound, there are three possible explanations:
> - Prior cholecystectomy.
> - Postprandial gallbladder contraction.
> - Chronic cholecystitis.
>
> Agenesis of the gallbladder is not a consideration in everyday practice.

Porcelain gallbladder cannot be evaluated sonographically because of its thickened, shadowing wall. Ultrasound cannot

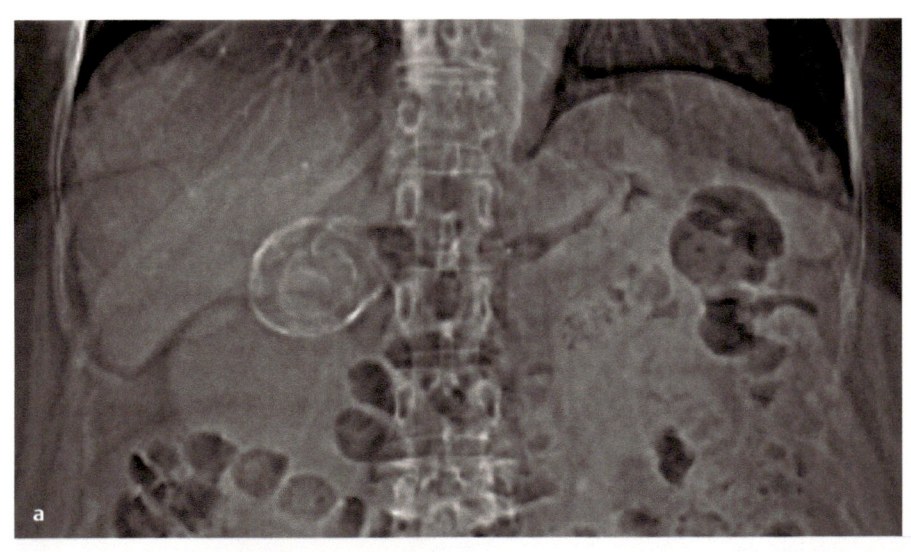

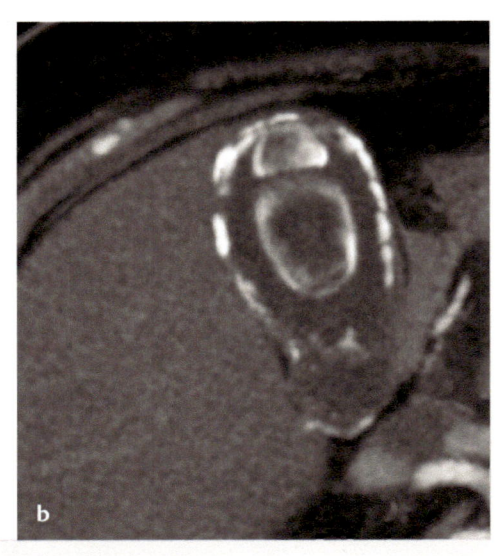

Fig. 6.32 Porcelain gallbladder with large calcified stones. (a) Scout image. (b) Thick-slice multiplanar reconstruction.

easily distinguish a porcelain gallbladder from a giant stone completely filling the gallbladder with a noncalcified wall (see ▶ Fig. 6.31b). Contrast-enhanced CT shows a small gallbladder with a thickened, strongly enhancing wall and pericholecystitic changes. Porcelain gallbladder is easy to diagnose (▶ Fig. 6.32b). Pericholecystitis appears as an enhancing soft tissue mass surrounding the gallbladder. On MRI, the wall of the small gallbladder appears hyperintense in T2W sequences and hypointense in unenhanced T1W sequences. The gallbladder wall enhances markedly after IV administration of contrast medium. Pericholecystitis is also detectable. Wall calcifications do not produce an MR signal. Fistulas are best appreciated in heavily T2-weighted sequences combined with fat-suppressed T1W sequences after contrast injection.

Note

No imaging modality can positively diagnose gallbladder carcinoma in chronic cholecystitis. This requires pathological examination after cholecystectomy. Finding nodal or hepatic metastases in a patient with chronic cholecystitis is strongly suggestive of gallbladder carcinoma (see ▶ Fig. 6.20).

▶ **Clinical features.** Patients with secondary chronic cholecystitis present with recurrent attacks of acute cholecystitis. Primary chronic forms often present with mild, nonspecific symptoms. In both cases the development of gallbladder carcinoma almost always goes unnoticed, as symptoms appear only at an advanced stage. A stone perforating into the free abdominal cavity will incite a local or diffuse biliary peritonitis, which presents as an acute abdomen. Fistulas to adjacent organs produce specific symptoms. Cholecystectomy is indicated even in asymptomatic patients to prevent complications and because of the potential for malignant change.

▶ **Differential diagnosis.** With chronic cholecystitis that is secondary to recurrent acute cholecystitis, the differential diagnosis is the same as for acute cholecystitis: hepatic abscess, pancreatitis, right-sided diverticulitis of the colon, and ulcer disease. The most important differential diagnosis is gallbladder carcinoma, which cannot be excluded by imaging alone in the absence of secondary tumor signs.

▶ **Key points.** Chronic cholecystitis as a complication of cholecystolithiasis may take a primary chronic course (with absent or nonspecific symptoms) or it may result from recurrent acute inflammations of the gallbladder. It often leads to a shrunken gallbladder with thickened walls. In the chronic atrophic form, the gallbladder wall is thinned. Perifocal inflammation (pericholecystitis) is consistently found. Incorporation of a stone in the gallbladder wall creates a nidus for fistula formation. The most feared complication of chronic cholecystitis is gallbladder carcinoma, which is almost always silent and is not diagnosed until an advanced stage. Early carcinoma confined to the gallbladder wall is not detectable by imaging, and this provides a rationale for cholecystectomy whenever chronic cholecystitis is diagnosed.

Mirizzi's Syndrome

▶ **Brief definition.** Mirizzi's syndrome is a rare complication of chronic cholecystitis that is characterized by obstructive jaundice due to benign stenosis of the common hepatic duct. Only 1 in 1,000 patients with symptomatic cholecystolithiasis develops Mirizzi's syndrome. It is observed in approximately 1% of all patients who have undergone biliary surgery.[23] Partial duct obstruction by an impacted stone with associated inflammation was first described by Kehr in 1905.[24] Mirizzi did not describe the condition until 1948.[25] Obstruction of the common hepatic duct is caused by pressure from a stone in the cystic duct or gallbladder infundibulum. The main cause of the obstruction is not mechanical compression, however, but the associated inflammatory change in the affected duct.[26] A long, common course of the common hepatic duct and cystic duct due to a low insertion of the cystic duct predisposes to the disorder.[27] Chronic inflammation of an infundibulum stone leads to formation of adhesions with the common hepatic duct. Eventually the stone may cause pressure necrosis. A biliobiliary or cholecystobiliary fistula may develop, with perforation of the incrusted stone into the common hepatic duct. At this stage the common hepatic duct may show a variable degree of wall destruction.[28]

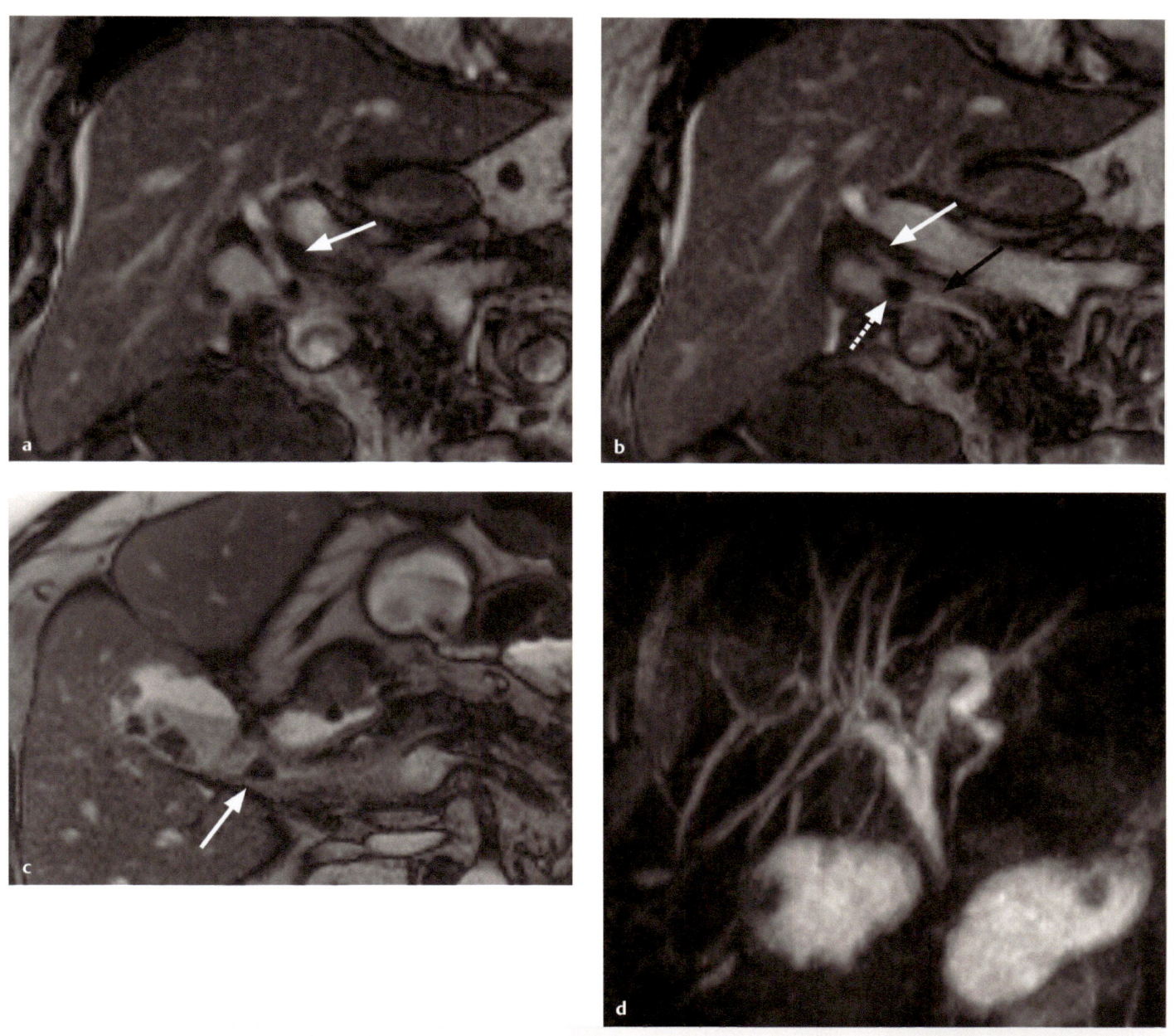

Fig. 6.33 Gallbladder empyema in Mirizzi's syndrome in a 64-year-old man with jaundice, cholangiogenic sepsis, and acute renal failure. (a) Common hepatic duct (arrow). (b) Stone in the cystic duct (white dashed arrow). Narrow common bile duct (black arrow). Common hepatic duct (white arrow). (c) Cholecystolithiasis with bile sediment. Cystic duct stone with wall thickening (arrow). (d) MR cholangiopancreatography shows intrahepatic bile stasis with obstruction of the common hepatic duct.

▶ **Imaging signs.** Ultrasound shows symmetrical intrahepatic biliary obstruction with an impacted gallstone in the gallbladder infundibulum. The common bile duct is not dilated. The gallbladder itself is usually shrunken.[29] CT reveals intrahepatic biliary obstruction and shows an infundibular stone with an absence of extrinsic compression.[30] Coronal reconstructions of the CT data set are better than ultrasound for defining the level of the obstruction, hepatoduodenal ligament anatomy, and the relationship of the obstruction to the portal vein and hepatic artery. MRCP is the best technique for demonstrating the biliary tract stenosis and intrahepatic biliary obstruction (▶ Fig. 6.33). Postcontrast imaging shows focal periductal enhancement due to periductal inflammatory and fibrotic changes.[31] Direct visualization of the ducts by ERCP gives the most detailed view of the stenosis (▶ Fig. 6.34). Stone compression, perforation, or fistulation can be detected. Differentiation from a malignant stricture may be difficult; in particular, direct ductal visualization cannot detect a mass in the porta hepatis. Today both techniques (MRCP and ERCP) are used only as part of temporizing interventional treatment prior to definitive surgery.

▶ **Clinical features.** The cardinal symptom is obstructive jaundice with a prior history of recurrent attacks of acute cholecystitis. Most patients present with right upper quadrant pain and a febrile infection. Other patients may have a painless obstructive jaundice. Treatment consists of cholecystectomy with dissection of the biliary tree and, if necessary, a biliary–enteric reconstruction.

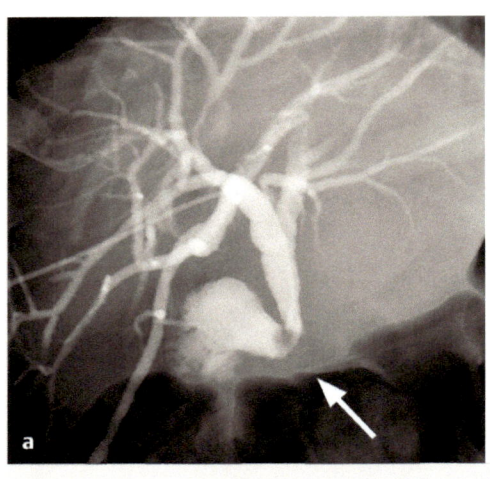

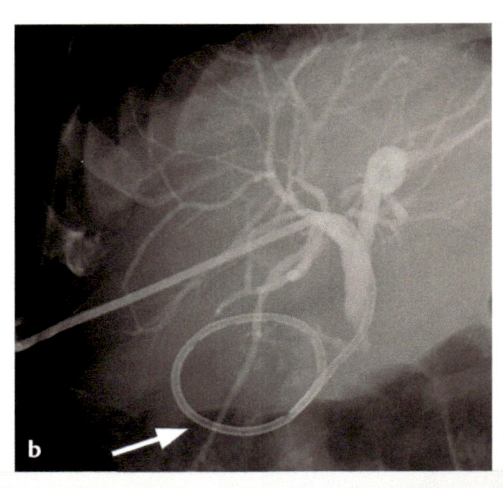

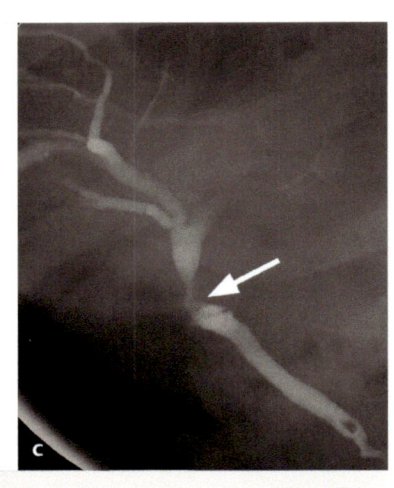

Fig. 6.34 Percutaneous transhepatic cholangiodrainage of suppurative cholangitis and gallbladder empyema. Same patient as in ▶ Fig. 6.33. (a) Stone compression of the common hepatic duct (arrow). (b) Drain insertion into the bile ducts and gallbladder (arrow). (c) Endoscopic retrograde cholangiopancreatography after cholecystectomy shows stenosis of the common hepatic duct (arrow).

▶ **Differential diagnosis.** Differentiation is required mainly from a malignant stricture caused by gallbladder cancer or cholangiocellular carcinoma. A lymph node metastasis in the hepatoduodenal ligament may cause extrinsic compression of the biliary tree.

▶ **Key points.** Mirizzi's syndrome is an obstructive jaundice resulting from benign stenosis of the common hepatic duct. It occurs as a complication of chronic cholecystitis and is caused by a stone in the gallbladder infundibulum with associated inflammation. It may involve uncomplicated compression alone, or a biliobiliary fistula may develop. When a fistula exists, the common hepatic duct shows a variable degree of wall destruction. Preoperative imaging is essential to avoid bile duct injuries. Imaging often consists of CT and MRI combined with MRCP.

6.5.2 Inflammatory and Infectious Biliary Tract Diseases

Inflammations of the biliary tract may be caused by infectious organisms or sterile inflammatory processes. Infections of the bile ducts result from an impairment or obstruction of bile flow.

Ascending Cholangitis

▶ **Brief definition.** Acute ascending cholangitis is caused by a bacterial infection secondary to impaired biliary drainage and stasis following an acute obstruction. Obstruction of the extrahepatic bile ducts is most commonly caused by a stone.[32] It may also result from the decompensation of a preexisting stenosis or invasion of the biliary tree by tumors in adjacent organs. The main causative organisms are *Escherichia coli*, enterococci, *Klebsiella* spp., and *Pseudomonas* spp. Ascending cholangitis most commonly affects younger patients 20 to 50 years of age. Cancer patients who develop cholangitis tend to be older. Both sexes are affected equally.

▶ **Imaging signs.** Stones in the gallbladder or bile ducts are detectable on initial ultrasound scans. A typical finding is dilatation of the extrahepatic and central intrahepatic bile ducts, which is accompanied by wall thickening. If the obstruction is in the common bile duct, the gallbladder will be large and filled with echogenic material. The gallbladder wall is also thickened. The inflamed bile ducts are hyperdense on unenhanced CT scans due to inflammatory exudate. Arterial-phase images show periportal hyperperfusion. Thin slices after injection of contrast medium can demonstrate the thickened, enhancing walls of the extrahepatic and large central intrahepatic bile ducts. Intrahepatic biliary obstruction is best appreciated in the portal venous phase. Diagnosis is aided by multiplanar reconstructions of the liver and extrahepatic bile ducts. FDG PET-CT can detect inflammation with high sensitivity based on FDG uptake in the portal fields. On MRI, duct dilatation and intraductal stones are best demonstrated in heavily T2-weighted images. Contrast-enhanced T1W images are also good for defining dilated ducts and adjacent periportal inflammatory changes. MRCP displays the dilated ducts along with filling defects (▶ Fig. 6.35). ERCP is used therapeutically to relieve biliary obstruction by drain implantation. Another option is percutaneous transhepatic cholangiodrainage (PTCD).

▶ **Clinical features.** The classic Charcot triad consists of right upper quadrant pain, fever, and jaundice. The disease may present with the features of cholangiogenic sepsis: severe debilitation, chills, and fever. Laboratory tests show definite signs of inflammation. Hepatic abscesses may form as a complication of ascending cholangitis. Untreated, the disease has a 100% mortality rate.

Treatment options:
- Antibiotic therapy.
- Surgical or interventional decompression of the obstruction by endoscopic or percutaneous drain insertion (PTCD).
- Endoscopic or percutaneous stone extraction if required.

> **Caution**
>
> A feared complication of endoscopic retrograde cholangiopancreaticography, especially when combined with papillotomy, is iatrogenic biliary pancreatitis.

▶ **Differential diagnosis**
- *Primary sclerosing cholangitis*: often differentiated by the clinical presentation. The disease also features characteristic

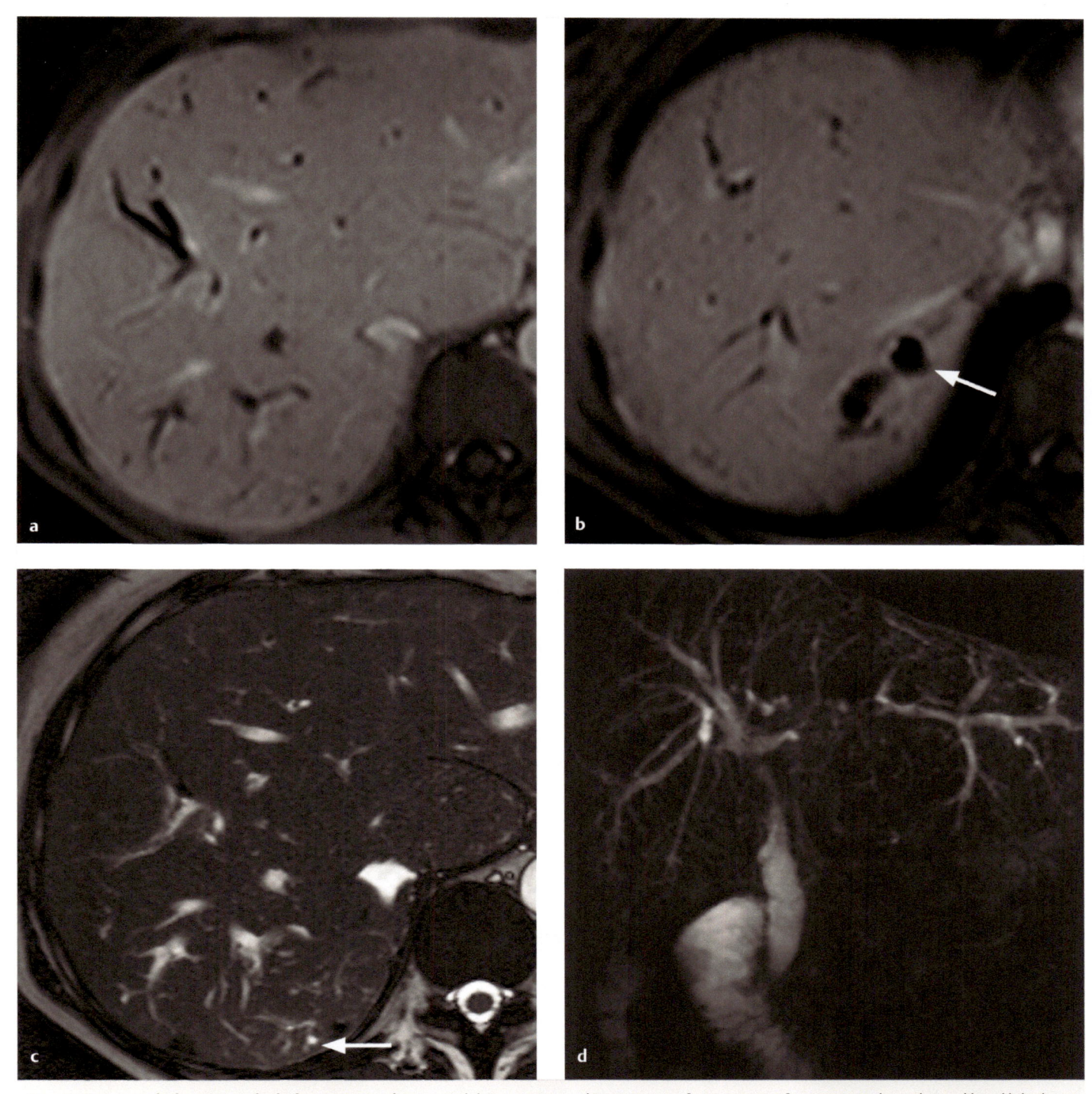

Fig. 6.35 **Acute cholangitis with cholangiogenic abscesses. (a)** Fat-suppressed T1 W image after injection of contrast medium shows dilated bile ducts with enhancement. **(b)** Duct-associated cystic dilatations. Cholangiogenic abscesses (arrow). **(c)** Bud-shaped outpouchings are also detectable at the level of the smallest ducts (arrow). **(d)** MR cholangiopancreatography demonstrates stenosis of the common hepatic duct and left hepatic duct.

deformities of the biliary tree with strictures and diverticulum-like dilatations.
- *Secondary sclerosing cholangitis*: AIDS-related cholangiopathy, ischemic cholangiopathy, eosinophilic cholangitis, and other secondary forms should also be considered.

Note
While some hepatic abscesses are cholangiogenic, others may result from the hematogenous spread of infectious organisms to the liver from a primary focus of sigmoid diverticulitis or chronic inflammatory bowel disease.

▶ **Key points.** Bacterial ascending cholangitis results from impaired biliary flow due to choledocholithiasis or biliary tract stenosis. It is difficult to distinguish noninflammatory bile stasis from cholangitis with imaging studies. The most useful study is PET-CT, which detects FDG uptake in the portal fields.

Primary Sclerosing Cholangitis

▶ **Brief definition.** Primary sclerosing cholangitis is a distinct entity—a progressive fibrosing biliary tract inflammation that probably has an autoimmune basis. The initiating event appears to be the release of antigens from damaged ductal epithelium. The antigens are absorbed by macrophages in the periportal connective tissue. Their interaction with T lymphocytes incites a self-perpetuating inflammation with connective tissue proliferation followed by sclerosis and obliterative duct destruction.[33] This process causes characteristic deformities of the biliary tree characterized by strictures and varicose dilatations. The disease affects intrahepatic and extrahepatic bile ducts. Simultaneous involvement of small and large ducts occurs in 75% of cases, isolated large duct involvement in 10%, and isolated small duct involvement in 15%.[34] The disease is typically manifested in the fourth decade, and 70% of patients are under 45 years of age. There is a slight male predilection. Approximately one-fourth of cases are idiopathic, lacking a definable cause. Three-fourths of cases occur in association with chronic inflammatory bowel disease (ulcerative colitis, Crohn's disease), autoimmune pancreatitis, or retroperitoneal fibrosis. The association with ulcerative colitis is highest, as approximately 70% of patients suffer from that disease. Primary sclerosing cholangitis takes a chronic progressive course that culminates in biliary cirrhosis with portal hypertension and liver failure. The chronic inflammation predisposes to cholangiocellular carcinoma, which is found in approximately 10% of patients. Cholangiocarcinoma occurs approximately 2 to 3 decades earlier than in patients without primary sclerosing cholangitis.[35] The 5-year survival rate of primary sclerosing cholangitis is 88%, with a mean survival of 12 years after diagnosis.

▶ **Imaging signs.** Imaging typically shows a string-of-beads configuration of the affected ducts with strictures and segmental dilatations. Prestenotic dilatations are mild or absent. Ultrasound demonstrates the intrahepatic duct dilatation along with thickening of the duct walls. Irregular widening of the periportal fields is found even in the absence of cirrhosis and is best demonstrated by ultrasound. Stones may be detectable in the intrahepatic ducts. If biliary cirrhosis has developed, ultrasound will display the features of hepatic cirrhosis. One-half of cases show gallbladder changes characterized by stones and wall thickening (▶ Fig. 6.36a).

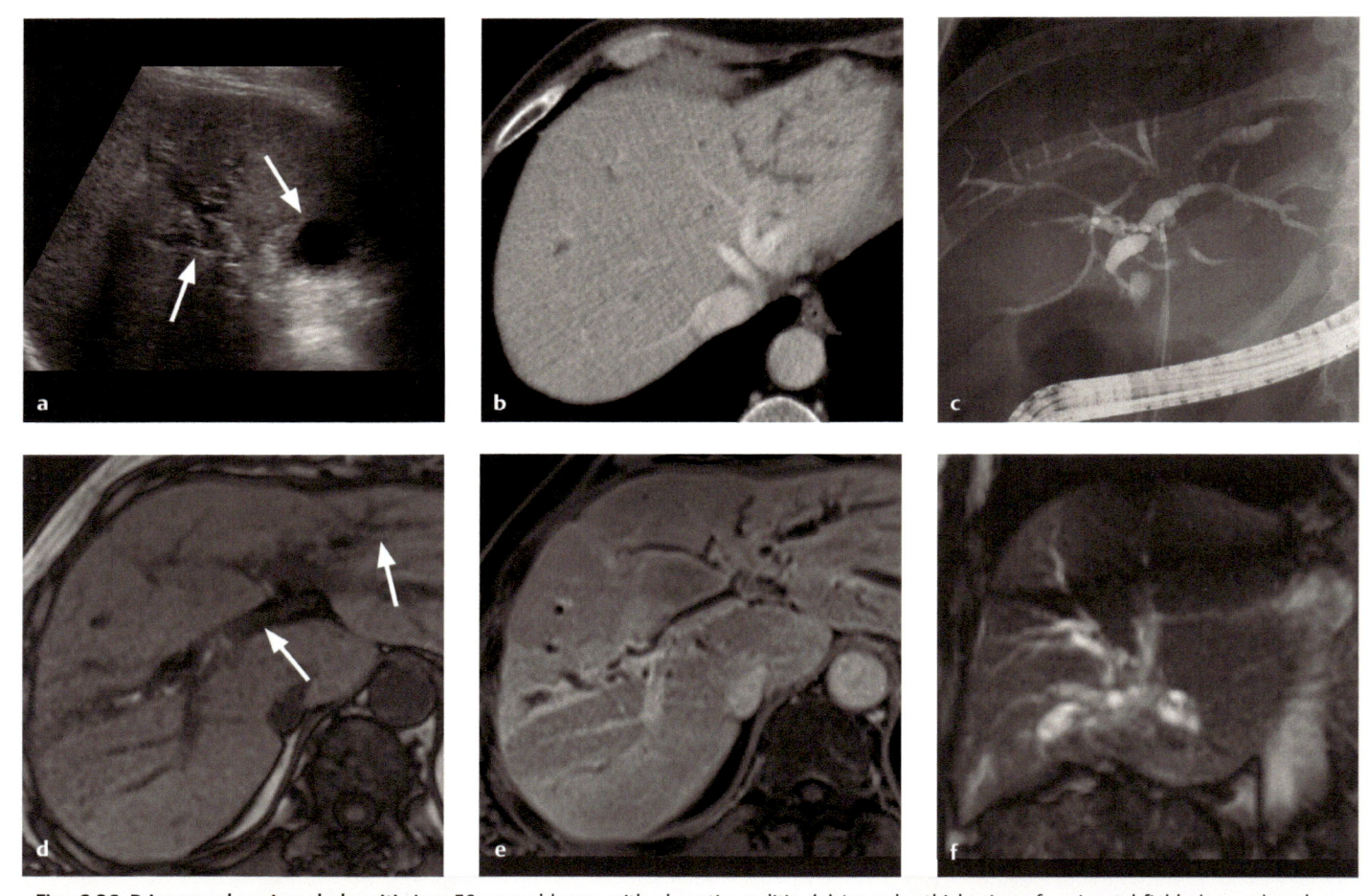

Fig. 6.36 Primary sclerosing cholangitis in a 50-year-old man with ulcerative colitis. (a) Irregular thickening of periportal fields (arrows) and dilatation of the bile ducts. Thickened gallbladder wall. (b) CT shows irregular obstruction with periportal enhancement. (c) Endoscopic retrograde cholangiopancreatography (ERCP) shows strictures with segmental dilatations and irregular margins. (Image [c] with kind permission of Professor Hardt, University Hospital of Giessen and Marburg, Germany.) (d) T1 W MRI shows irregular thickening of the hypointense periportal fields (arrows). (e) Postcontrast image shows marked enhancement and irregular biliary obstruction. (f) T2 W image shows irregular duct dilatation corresponding to ERCP.

Contrast-enhanced CT shows irregular biliary obstruction. In contrast to ordinary ductal dilatation, the ducts cannot be traced through successive axial scans. Thin-slice reconstructions may show thickening and enhancement of the duct walls. Associated periportal fibrosis is hypodense before administration of contrast medium and shows delayed enhancement (▶ Fig. 6.36b). The end stage is marked by hepatic cirrhosis with peripheral atrophy and central hypertrophy. This differs from the left-lobe hypertrophy found in classic hepatic cirrhosis (see Chapter 5.6).

> **Note**
>
> A pseudotumor of the caudate lobe is a relatively specific sign of primary sclerosing cholangitis, which precedes the onset of cirrhosis.

As well as showing enlargement, the caudate lobe appears hyperdense on unenhanced CT scans. Cholangiocellular carcinoma is difficult to diagnose. The presence of a mass, wall thickening to more than 4 mm, and increasing ductal dilatation over time are suggestive signs.[36,37] On MRI, the periportal fibrosis appears hypointense with irregular margins on unenhanced T1 W images (▶ Fig. 6.36d). Images after administration of contrast medium show periportal enhancement. The fibrosis is hyperintense in T2 W sequences (▶ Fig. 6.36e). T2 W images (▶ Fig. 6.36f) and MRCP show irregular ductal dilatations with strictures and segmental dilatation. MRI is equivalent to CT in its ability to detect morphological liver changes. Direct visualization of the ducts by ERCP is the diagnostic procedure of choice, providing the highest level of detail. It can detect multifocal strictures, irregular margins, segmental dilatations, and diverticula (▶ Fig. 6.36c) of the intrahepatic bile ducts.

▶ **Clinical features.** Primary sclerosing cholangitis presents with chronic intermittent episodes of jaundice with pruritus. The liver is enlarged, and right upper quadrant pain is present. The disease is unresponsive to drug therapy. The only curative treatment option is liver transplantation.

▶ **Differential diagnosis**
- *Secondary sclerosing cholangitis*: Differentiation from secondary forms of sclerosing cholangitis is most easily accomplished by noting the association of primary sclerosing cholangitis with ulcerative colitis. If the patient has no history of secondary sclerosing cholangitis, idiopathic primary sclerosing cholangitis can be differentiated only by its course (apart from histological examination).
- *Cholangiocellular carcinoma*: It is difficult to diagnosis this disease in the setting of primary sclerosing cholangitis.
- *Hepatic cirrhosis*: Differentiation from classic hepatic cirrhosis is based on the characteristic change in liver shape.

▶ **Key points.** Primary sclerosing cholangitis is a progressive biliary tract inflammation, probably autoimmune, that is characterized by extensive periportal fibrosis. Concomitant involvement of large and small bile ducts is detectable in 75% of cases. Isolated involvement of extrahepatic ducts may occur. Characteristic duct changes consist of strictures and varicose dilatations. The disease takes a progressive course and is unresponsive to therapy. It leads to a characteristic biliary cirrhosis with peripheral atrophy and central hypertrophy of the liver. Approximately one-fourth of cases do not have an identifiable cause. In three-fourths of cases the disease develops separately in a setting of chronic inflammatory bowel disease. The strongest association is with ulcerative colitis. Approximately 10% of patients develop cholangiocellular carcinoma, which occurs 2 to 3 decades earlier than in the general population.

6.5.3 Benign Tumors and Hyperplastic Changes

Benign lesions of the gallbladder and bile ducts consist mainly of epithelial tumors (polyps, adenomas) and benign, diffuse tumor-like wall thickening such as adenomyomatosis. Mesenchymal tumors are very rare.

Gallbladder Polyps

▶ **Brief definition.** Polyps are defined as grossly visible outgrowths of the mucosal wall; they may be sessile or pedunculated. Gallbladder polyps are relatively common (present in approximately 5% of the population) but rarely cause clinical symptoms, so they are usually detected incidentally during an ultrasound scan.[1] Histological studies have shown that cholesterol polyps are the most common type, accounting for approximately 50% of cases. Their occurrence correlates with obesity. Cholesterol polyps are followed by other hyperplastic-inflammatory processes. Adenomas are in third place, comprising about 20% of cases. Approximately 85% of polyps are smaller than 5 mm. Large studies found that all polyps smaller than 1 cm were benign while all polyps larger than 1.5 cm were malignant.[38,39] Sessile adenomas and multiple adenomas are also associated with an increased cancer risk.

▶ **Imaging signs.** Polyps appear sonographically as well-circumscribed echogenic masses that protrude from the gallbladder wall into the lumen. They do not cast an acoustic shadow. The most reliable differentiating criterion from small cholesterol stones (also nonshadowing) is their immobility within the gallbladder. An important consideration besides size is number—solitary or multiple (▶ Fig. 6.37). Polyps are inherently less visible on CT than on ultrasound because their density is similar to that of biliary fluid, but postcontrast CT can demonstrate them as enhancing masses. As a result, CT provides a higher detection rate for gallbladder polyps than for stones. On MRI, the bile in the gallbladder is hyperintense in T2 W sequences while stones or polyps are hypointense. Even small foci can be recognized owing to the high contrast with their surroundings. Differentiation from stones relies on contrast enhancement. If a polyp is isointense to the gallbladder wall in both T1 W and T2 W sequences, it is an adenoma (▶ Fig. 6.38).

▶ **Clinical features.** Polyps are generally asymptomatic. Large polyps in the gallbladder neck may cause biliary colic by obstructing the infundibulum. Treatment depends on the size of the polyps:
- *Asymptomatic polyps smaller than 10 mm*: Polyps of this size are left untreated. Ultrasound follow-ups should be scheduled at 6 months to avoid missing a fast-growing tumor.

Gallbladder and Biliary Tract

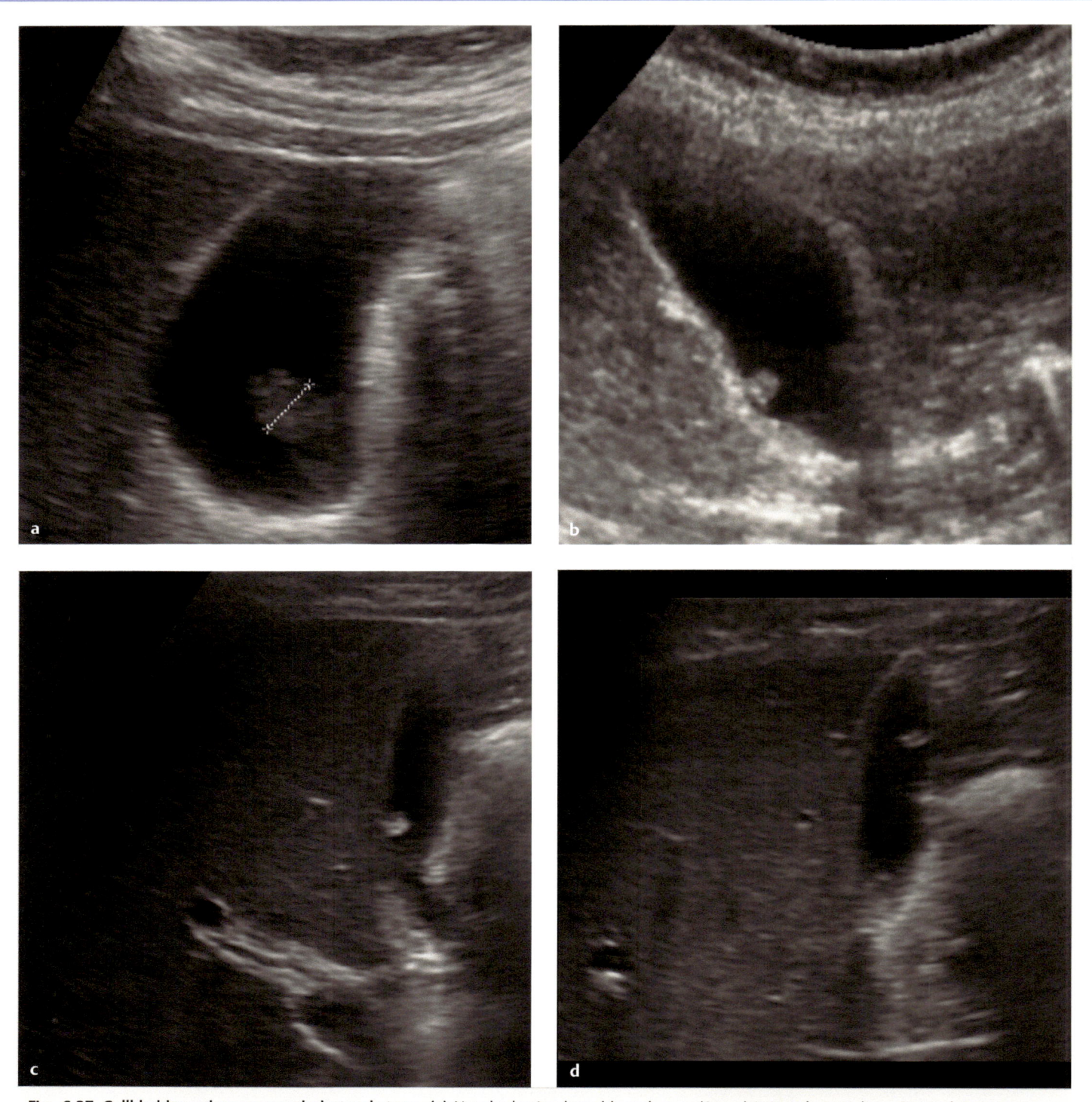

Fig. 6.37 Gallbladder polyps versus cholesterol stone. (a) Nonshadowing broad-based mass (8 mm) is isoechoic to liver. Surgical specimen: adenomatous polyp. (b) Slightly hyperechoic mass (5 mm) is nonshadowing and immobile on position changes: cholesterol polyp. (c) Hyperechoic mass with similar ultrasound features as [b]. Patient is supine. (d) Scan with the patient sitting upright: cholesterol stone.

- *Polyps larger than 10 mm*: Polyps of this size should be removed.
- *Polyps larger than 15 mm*: These lesions should be classified as suspicious for adenocarcinoma.

▶ **Differential diagnosis**
- *Focal sludge*: This material may resemble a polyp at ultrasound. Differentiation relies on mobility or absence of enhancement.
- *Gallstones*: These are distinguished by their acoustic shadow. Small, nonshadowing cholesterol stones are identified by their mobility.
- *Metastases*: Metastases appearing as focal polypous masses may occur rarely in the gallbladder. Unlike a polyp, a metastasis is associated with local change in the gallbladder wall.

▶ **Key points.** Polyps of the gallbladder wall are common and usually detected incidentally at ultrasound. Cholesterol polyps are the most common, followed by inflammatory-hyperplastic polyps and adenomas. Polyps are differentiated from stones by their immobility and enhancement. Only MRI can provide a specific diagnosis. If a polyp is isointense to the gallbladder wall in all sequences, it is an adenoma. Polyps smaller than 10 mm are

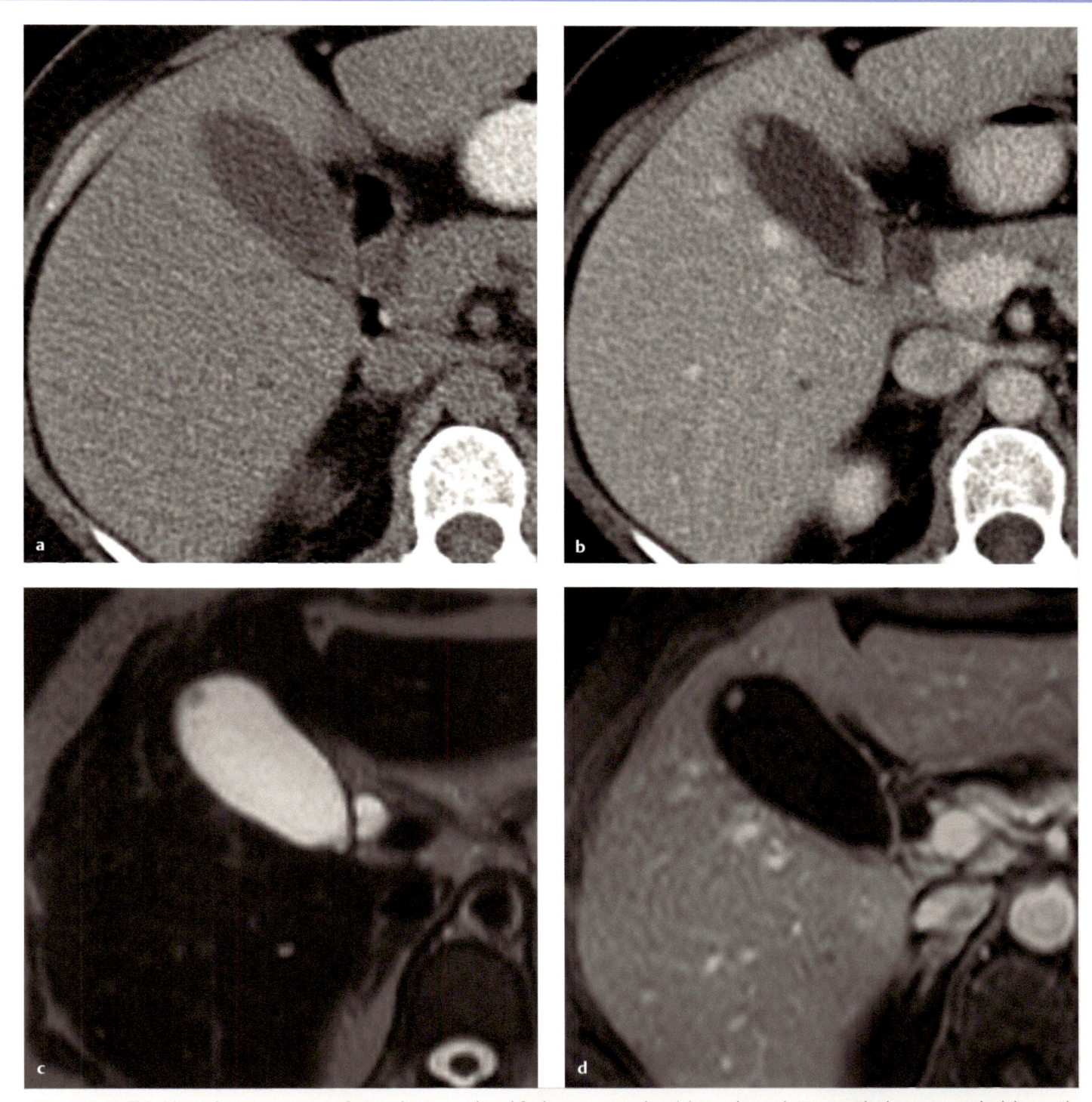

Fig. 6.38 **Gallbladder polyp.** Comparison of CT and MRI. Incidental finding: 4-mm polyp. (a) Unenhanced CT scan. The lesion is poorly delineated because it is almost isodense to biliary fluid. (b) The polyp is sharply delineated after administration of contrast medium. (c) T2 W image demonstrates a hypointense mass in the hyperintense biliary fluid. (d) Fat-suppressed T1 W sequence. The mass is isointense to the gallbladder wall.

followed sonographically. Polyps larger than 10 mm are removed by cholecystectomy. Polyps 15 mm or larger are highly suspicious for malignant transformation.

Benign Hyperplasia of the Gallbladder Wall (Adenomyomatosis and Cholesterolosis)

▶ **Brief definition**

- *Adenomyomatosis*: Adenomyomatosis is characterized by a diffuse or focal thickening of the gallbladder wall. There is hyperplasia of the mucosa (mucosal folds) and smooth muscle with the formation of characteristic intramural diverticula called Rokitansky–Aschoff sinuses.[40] Signs of adenomyomatosis or cholesterolosis are found in approximately 5 to 25% of cholecystectomy specimens. The etiology of the change is unknown. Gallstones are detectable in approximately 50% of cases.
- *Cholesterolosis*: Cholesterolosis refers to a change in the gallbladder wall due to excess fat absorption. It may result from an increased cholesterol content in the bile or impaired lymphatic drainage. It is marked by the subepithelial deposition of cholesterol esters in the gallbladder wall and the presence of cholesterol-laden foam cells. Like adenomyomatosis,

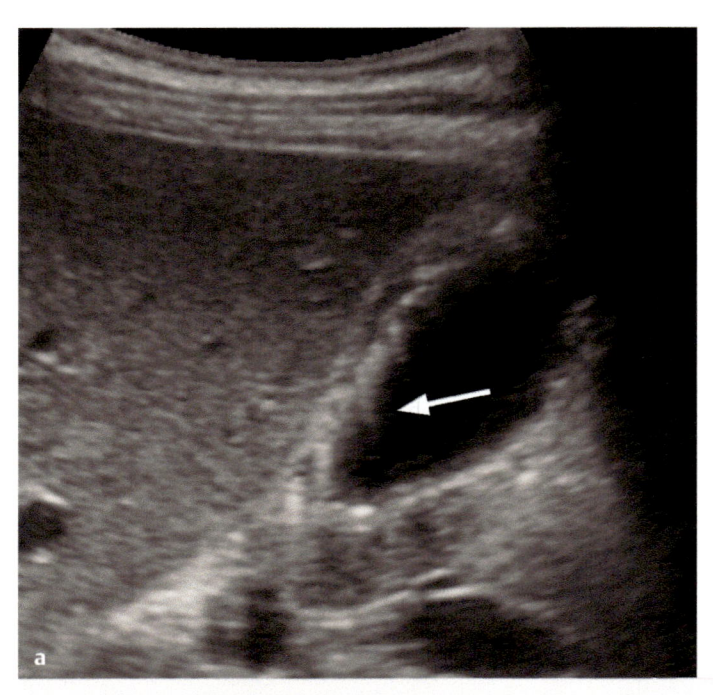

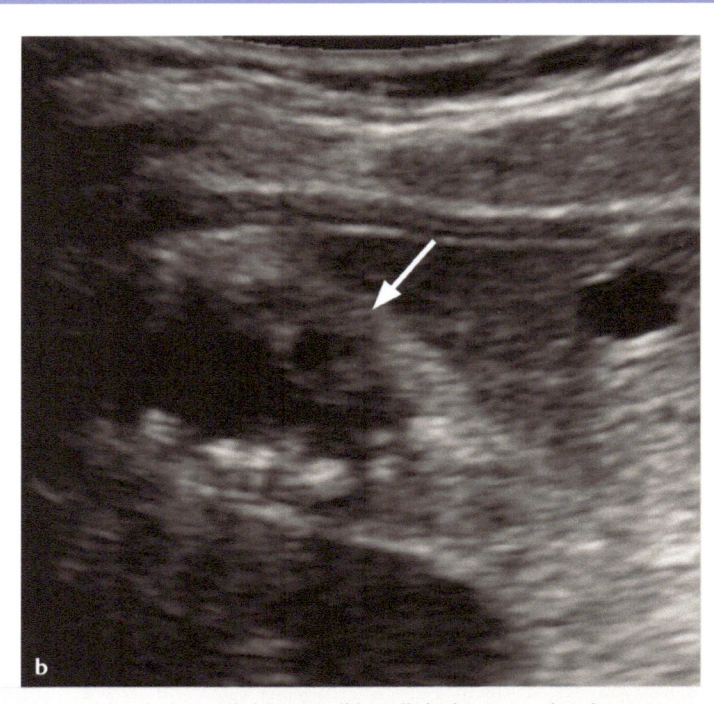

Fig. 6.39 **Adenomyomatosis.** (a) Comet-tail reverberation artifacts (arrow) caused by cholesterol deposits. (b) Wall thickening with echogenic deposits and intramural diverticula (arrow).

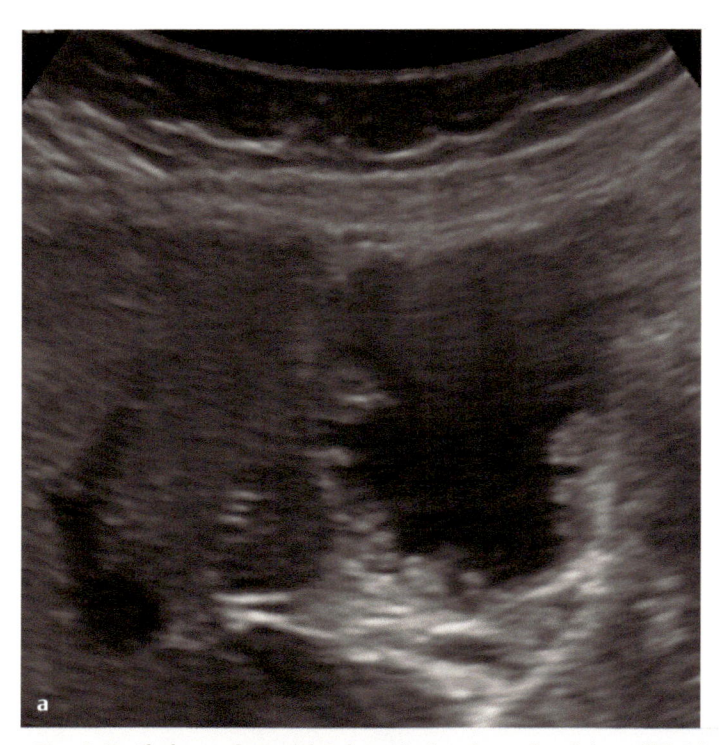

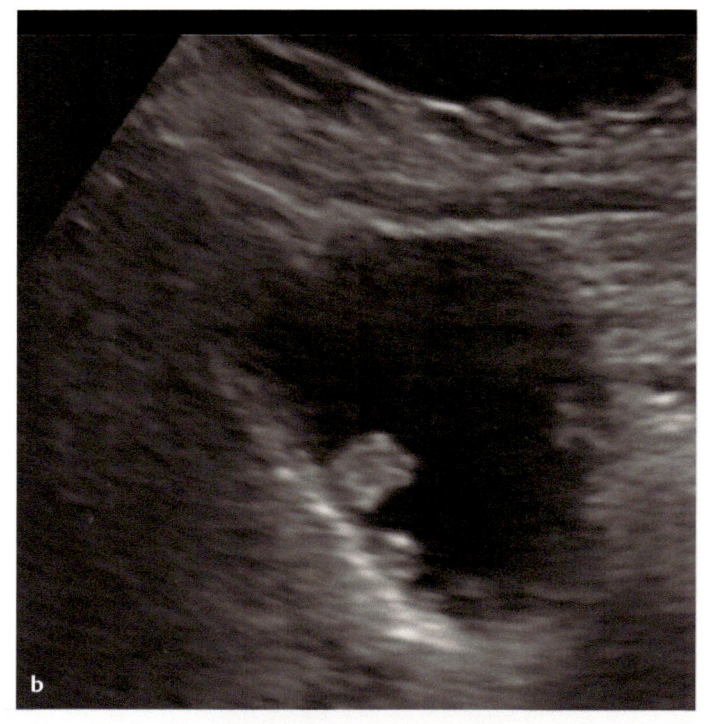

Fig. 6.40 **Cholesterolosis.** (a) Polyps blanket the walls of the gallbladder neck and body. (b) Small degree of echogenic wall thickening.

cholesterolosis has both a diffuse and localized form. Diffuse involvement is called a "strawberry gallbladder." The localized form is characterized by polyps.

▶ **Imaging signs.** Ultrasound in adenomyomatosis shows diffuse or local thickening of the gallbladder wall. Intramural diverticula (Rokitansky–Aschoff sinuses) appear as hypoechoic cystic inclusions. A typical finding is echogenic inclusions with comet-tail reverberation artifacts caused by intramural deposits of cholesterol crystals (▶ Fig. 6.39). Scans in cholesterolosis show numerous polyps (smaller than 10 mm), which may cover portions of the wall like a lawn (▶ Fig. 6.40). CT also demonstrates diffuse or localized wall thickening, and intense enhancement occurs after administration of contrast medium. Intramural diverticula are rarely visualized. Multiple polyps are present in cholesterolosis. In both adenomyomatosis and cholesterolosis, CT gives a less detailed view than ultrasound. MRI shows a thickened, enhancing gallbladder wall. Intramural diverticula are directly visualized in T2 W sequences.

▶ **Clinical features.** Both conditions are usually detected incidentally at ultrasound. Right upper quadrant pain may be present in rare cases. Clinical symptoms may stem from associated diseases of the gallbladder. No treatment options are available.

▶ **Differential diagnosis**
- *Adenomyomatosis*: The differential diagnosis of adenomyomatosis includes chronic cholecystitis, gallbladder carcinoma, and xanthogranulomatous cholecystitis. The sonographic features of adenomyomatosis are characteristic enough to exclude other possible diagnoses. Any unexplained thickening of the gallbladder wall detected by CT should be investigated further by ultrasound.
- *Cholesterolosis*: Differentiation is required from multiple polyps of the gallbladder wall.

▶ **Key points.** Cholesterol deposits are detectable in the gallbladder wall in both adenomyomatosis and cholesterolosis. Adenomyomatosis causes definite wall thickening with characteristic intramural diverticula (Rokitansky–Aschoff sinuses). Comet-tail reverberation artifacts caused by cholesterol deposits are another typical ultrasound finding. Numerous cholesterol polyps are found in cholesterolosis. CT diagnosis is difficult, so the use of ultrasound is recommended as an adjunct.

Intraductal Papillary Mucinous Neoplasm

▶ **Brief definition.** As its name suggests, this is a mucin-producing neoplasm (adenoma) of the bile ducts. Mucin consists of 95% water and 5% glycoproteins. Because of its high water content, mucin has imaging features equivalent to water or bile, making it difficult to discern. The inspissation of mucin alters its imaging appearance. The neoplasm develops in the mucosa. Besides a nodular form, the tumor may also spread longitudinally in the ductal mucosa. Much time is needed for the tumor to infiltrate the bile ducts and cause luminal obstruction leading to dilatation of dependent ducts. The site of occurrence determines the degree of ductal dilatation. Associated filling defects may resemble stones. The neoplasm may also occur in the gallbladder.[41] Extensive involvement—papillomatosis—is marked by a combination of adenomas, dysplastic adenomas, and adenocarcinomas of the bile ducts.

▶ **Imaging signs.** The most obvious sign is intrahepatic biliary obstruction. Mucus retention leads to aneurysmal dilatation of the intrahepatic bile ducts, which is often difficult to discern on ultrasound scans. Depending on the composition of the mucus, the bile may be echo-free, contain fine echoes, or show complex echogenicity. It is rarely possible to detect an intraductal mass. Aneurysmal dilatation of the ducts is clearly demonstrated by contrast-enhanced CT. The dilated ducts coalesce to form one duct with enhancing intraductal tumor tissue. In CT as in ultrasound, the composition of the secretion determines the density range from water-equivalent to hyperdense.[42] The dilated ducts are also depicted by T2 W MRI and MRCP (▶ Fig. 6.41). The signal intensity ranges from water-equivalent (T2 hyperintense, T1 hypointense) to proteinaceous (T2 hypointense, T1 hyperintense), depending on the composition of the bile and mucus. Fat-suppressed T1 W sequences after injection of contrast medium can demonstrate intraductal tissue.

Note
Transpapillary mucus detection on ERCP is pathognomonic.

▶ **Clinical features.** The dilated, mucus-filled bile ducts predispose to cholangitis, which determines the clinical picture (intermittent upper abdominal pain with fever and chills). Central duct involvement may lead to obstructive jaundice. Treatment consists of surgical resection of the affected liver segments.

▶ **Differential diagnosis.** Differentiation is mainly required from cholangiocarcinoma, recurrent pyogenic cholangitis, and pyogenic liver abscess. The degree of bile duct dilatation is greatest with intraductal papillary mucinous neoplasm.

▶ **Key points.** Intraductal papillary mucinous neoplasm of the bile ducts causes stenosis and mucus production leading to aneurysmal dilatation of the dependent biliary tree. Depending on its composition, the mucus may have the imaging appearance (in all modalities) of bile or proteinaceous fluid. Tumor growth characteristics are also variable, ranging from a nodular mass to longitudinal intraductal spread. A typical finding is marked, variable ductal dilatation, which may be focal and aneurysmal or may diffusely involve all of the bile ducts. Transpapillary mucus detection on ERCP is pathognomonic. Duct infiltration may occur in advanced stages.

6.5.4 Malignant Tumors

Malignant tumors of the gallbladder and biliary tree are mainly of epithelial origin. Over 80% of all gallbladder carcinomas and almost all bile duct carcinomas are adenocarcinomas. Ten percent are squamous cell carcinoma or anaplastic carcinoma.[43] Cystadenocarcinoma and mucinous carcinoma make up 5% of cases. Neuroendocrine carcinomas and malignant mesenchymal tumors (leiomyosarcoma, fibrosarcoma) are rare. Kaposi's sarcomas (in HIV infection) and lymphomas may also occur. Metastases to the gallbladder originate chiefly from melanoma. Colon carcinoma may metastasize to the bile ducts. Other tumors that metastasize to the bile ducts are lung cancer, breast cancer, pancreatic cancer, and prostate cancer.[44]

Gallbladder Carcinoma

▶ **Brief definition.** Gallbladder carcinoma is a rare malignancy (0.6–3.0% of all carcinomas). The incidence of gallbladder carcinoma in autopsy series is 0.24–0.50%.[45] Females predominate 3:1 over males. Because the tumor tends to grow slowly and silently, it remains undetected until it has reached an advanced stage. The peak age of incidence is in the seventh to eighth decades. The prognosis is poor. Approximately 75% of cases have metastasized by the time of diagnosis. The 5-year survival rate is less than 5%. Two macroscopic patterns of gallbladder carcinoma are distinguished:
- *Diffuse infiltrative carcinoma*: This pattern is more common. It is characterized by diffuse thickening of the gallbladder wall, while the gallbladder itself is shrunken (as in chronic cholecystitis).

Gallbladder and Biliary Tract

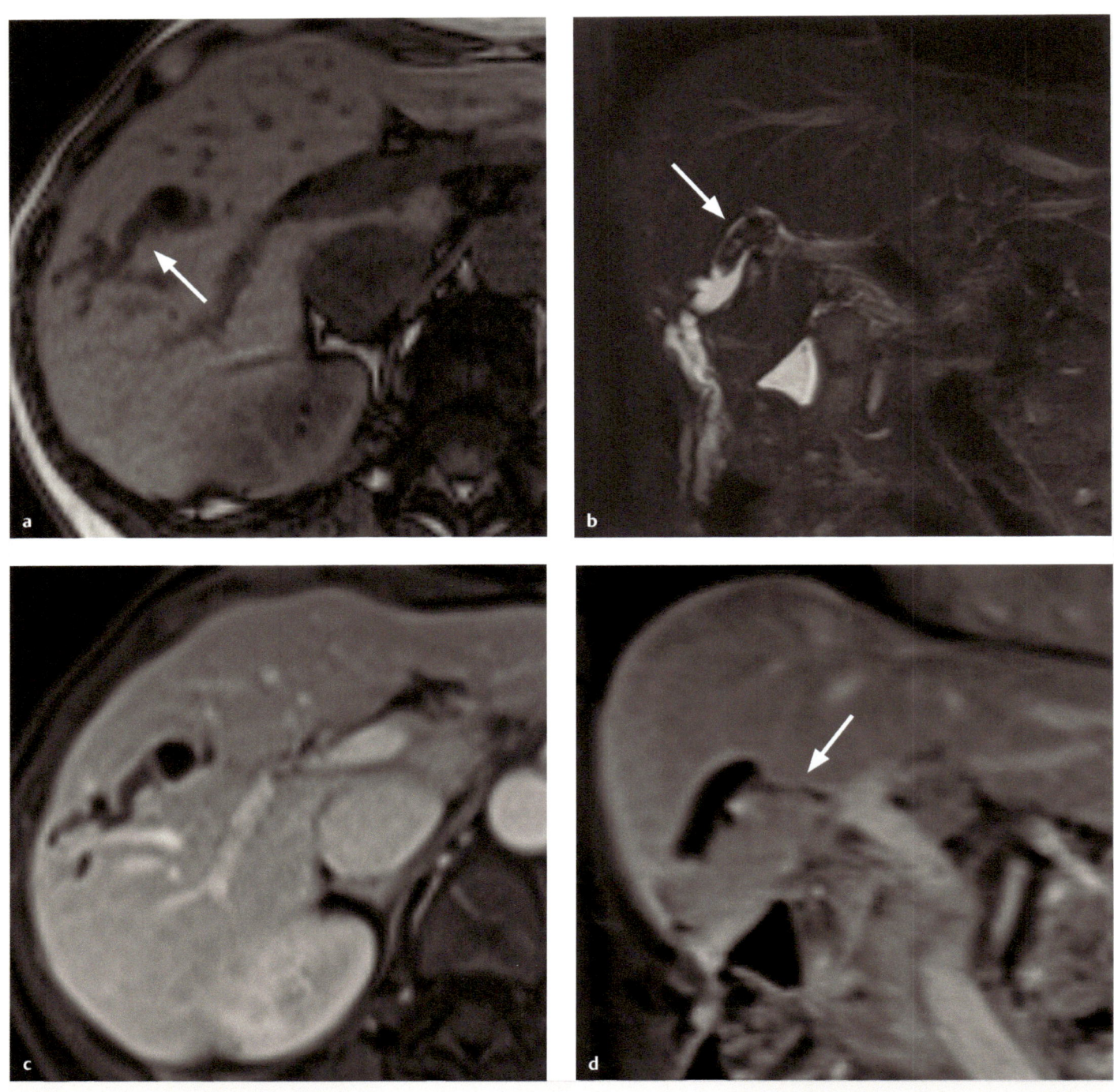

Fig. 6.41 **Intraductal papillary mucinous tumor of a bile duct.** (a) Aneurysmal dilatation of a bile duct (arrow). (b) Intraductal hypointense filling defect (arrow). Inspissated mucin. (c) Periductal enhancement. (d) Long-segment stenosis with an enhancing wall (arrow).

- *Nodular, polypoid mass*: This pattern is less common. The tumor forms a nodular, polypoid mass that completely occupies the gallbladder lumen. Empyema may develop if the gallbladder neck becomes obstructed.

In advanced stages the two patterns become indistinguishable. Typically the tumor spreads by direct invasion into the liver, bile ducts, and less commonly the pancreas, duodenum, and colon. Direct invasion of the liver will occur at some point during the disease. Spread along lymphatics is typical, resulting in characteristic intrahepatic satellite lesions around the liver area contiguous with the primary tumor. Peritoneal carcinomatosis develops in 25% of patients. Lymphogenous spread occurs to the lymph nodes in the hepatoduodenal ligament and to the lymph nodes of the stomach, pancreas, and retroperitoneum. Hematogenous spread occurs chiefly to the liver, lung, and skeleton.

Note

Approximately 75–90% of patients with gallbladder carcinoma also have stones in the gallbladder, but only about 2% of patients with gallbladder stones develop gallbladder carcinoma.

Stones can traumatize the epithelium and cause chronic inflammation. The inflammation may give rise to dysplasia, from which

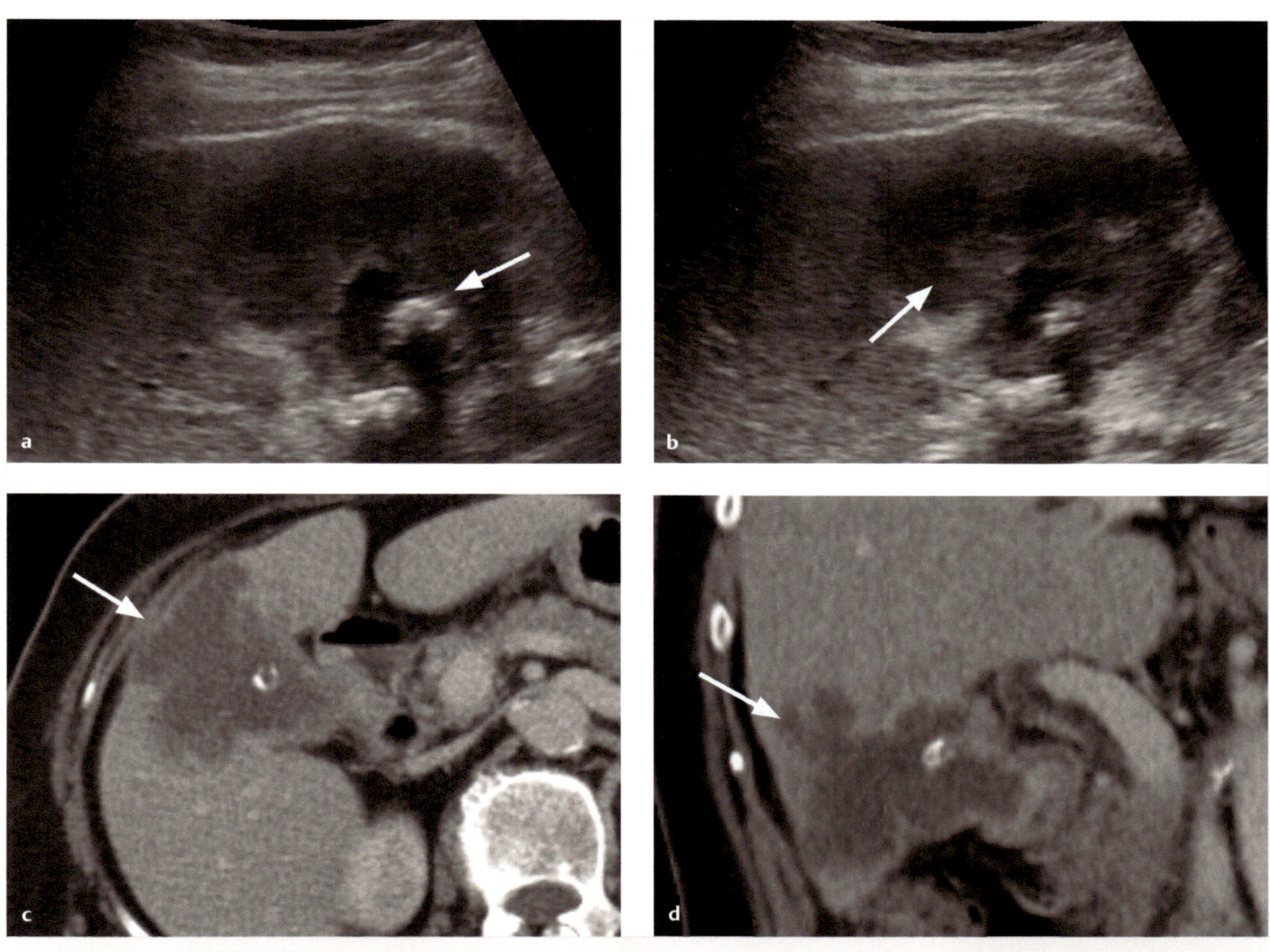

Fig. 6.42 Carcinoma of the gallbladder. (a) Irregular hypoechoic wall thickening. The arrow indicates a stone. Margins are indistinct due to invasion of the liver. (b) Hypodense adjacent liver parenchyma (arrow) due to tumor invasion. (c) Axial CT scan more clearly defines the extent of liver infiltration (arrow). (d) Coronal CT scan.

gallbladder carcinoma may gradually develop. The period from onset of dysplasia to detectable gallbladder carcinoma is estimated to be 15 years.[46]

A mechanical etiology is also supported by the fact that tumors most commonly originate in the gallbladder fundus (followed by the gallbladder neck and body). Other risk factors are adenomas and cystic anomalies of the biliary tree. Chronic salmonella excretors are also at increased risk.

Primary sclerosing cholangitis coexists with ulcerative colitis in 70% of cases and with Crohn's disease in 10%. It is characterized by a chronic biliary obstruction that progresses to biliary cirrhosis. The end stage is marked by the development of cholangiocarcinoma and gallbladder carcinoma.[47] Sites of epithelial dysplasia in the gallbladder are detectable in up to 40% of patients with familial polyposis coli.[48]

▶ **Imaging signs.** Besides supplying a diagnosis, imaging studies should determine local tumor extent. Tumor staging should include the identification of nodal and distant metastases. Ultrasound is the best initial imaging study for the detection of cholecystolithiasis and for evaluating the gallbladder wall. Early gallbladder carcinoma is an incidental finding at ultrasound. Its presence is suggested by focal, asymmetrical wall thickening. An advanced tumor shows infiltrative growth with an irregular nodular, hypoechoic mass. The mass extends through the gallbladder wall and into the lumen (▶ Fig. 6.42). This pattern is difficult to distinguish from chronic cholecystitis. Duplex ultrasound may be helpful in this regard. With a carcinoma larger than 2 cm, duplex scans will demonstrate hypervascular areas. Growth through the wall and into the liver suggests gallbladder carcinoma. Secondary tumor signs such as nodal and hepatic metastases and ascites are detectable by ultrasound. CT is the modality of choice for preoperative tumor staging and for defining local tumor extent (▶ Table 6.2). It should employ a multiphase protocol that includes arterial and portal enhancement phases. Thin-slice multiplanar reconstructions should also be obtained. The carcinoma appears as a hypodense mass. On MRI, gallbladder carcinoma appears on plain T1 W images as an infiltrative mass that is slightly hypointense to liver. After injection of contrast medium, the tissue is hypointense and is often more clearly delineated from the well-enhanced liver parenchyma. The mass is slightly hyperintense to liver in T2 W sequences. MRCP is helpful for evaluating the status of the intrahepatic and extrahepatic bile ducts.

▶ **Clinical features.** The symptoms are often nonspecific. The cardinal symptom is right upper quadrant pain; there may be nausea

with vomiting and weight loss. The symptoms are often attributed clinically to gallstones. Jaundice is an unfavorable prognostic sign. One in 5 patients has ascites at the time of diagnosis, and 1 in 10 already has a duodenal obstruction. Approximately 20% of gallbladder carcinomas are discovered incidentally at surgery (or on pathology) during a cholecystectomy performed for symptomatic cholecystolithiasis. Treatment depends on the tumor stage:
- *Stages I and II*: surgical resection (stage IIa includes partial hepatectomy, stage IIb includes lymph node dissection).
- *Stage III*: tumor spread not treatable by local resection.
- *Stage IV*: systemic disease with distant metastasis.

▶ **Differential diagnosis**
- *Chronic cholecystitis*: If secondary tumor signs are absent, the two entities cannot be differentiated from each other by their imaging features. Consequently, all chronic gallbladder inflammations are an indication for cholecystectomy and histological examination.
- *Gallbladder polyps larger than 1 cm*: The same rule applies for these lesions as for chronic cholecystitis.
- *Adenomyomatosis*: This is a benign wall thickening that requires differentiation. It does not invade the liver, and the cholesterol deposits produce characteristic reverberation echoes.
- *Metastases*: Hepatic metastases in the gallbladder fossa and metastases in the gallbladder wall should also be considered in the differential diagnosis.

▶ **Key points.** Gallbladder carcinoma often grows silently and is diagnosed at a late stage. Three-fourths of cases have metastasized by the time of diagnosis, and one-fourth of patients already have peritoneal carcinomatosis. The tumor pattern may be polypoid or nodular, but diffuse infiltrative growth is more common. The principal imaging sign is thickening of the gallbladder wall. Typically there is direct invasion of contiguous liver with associated satellite lesions. Risk factors are gallstones, chronic cholecystitis, porcelain gallbladder, polyps, primary sclerosing cholangitis, and familial polyposis coli. A diagnosis of chronic cholecystitis is an indication for cholecystectomy. Only histological examination can exclude carcinoma.

Biliary Cystadenocarcinoma

▶ **Brief definition.** Biliary cystadenocarcinoma is a rare, low-grade cystic tumor that occurs predominantly in the intrahepatic bile ducts (85% of cases). The extrahepatic bile ducts are less common sites of occurrence (15%), and gallbladder involvement is very rare (0.02%). The tumor develops from a benign biliary cystadenoma, which probably arises from ectopic primitive bile ducts.[50] Biliary cystadenocarcinomas are large cystic masses up to 20 cm in diameter with internal septations. They occur predominantly in middle-aged women; occurrence in males is extremely rare.

▶ **Imaging signs.** Ultrasound shows a large, multilocular cystic mass with internal septa. The cyst contents are usually complex with internal echoes. Fluid levels are noted where intralesional hemorrhage has occurred. CT shows a multilocular cystic mass (▶ Fig. 6.43), appearing in rare cases as a solitary cyst. The septa

Table 6.2 Staging of gallbladder carcinoma[49]

Stage	Characteristics	Stage groupings
I	Tumor confined to the mucosa (Ia) or gallbladder wall (Ib)	T1, 2 N0 M0
IIa	T3: tumor has penetrated the serosa or invades an adjacent organ	T3 N0 M0
IIb	N1: lymph node metastasis in the hepatoduodenal ligament	T1, 2, 3 N1 M0
III	T4: tumor invades the portal vein, hepatic artery, or at least two adjacent organs	T4 Any N M0
IV	Distant metastasis	Any T Any N M1

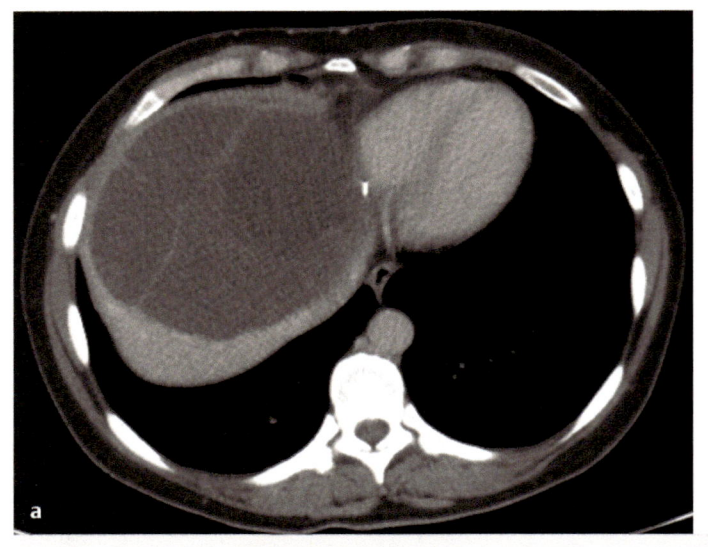

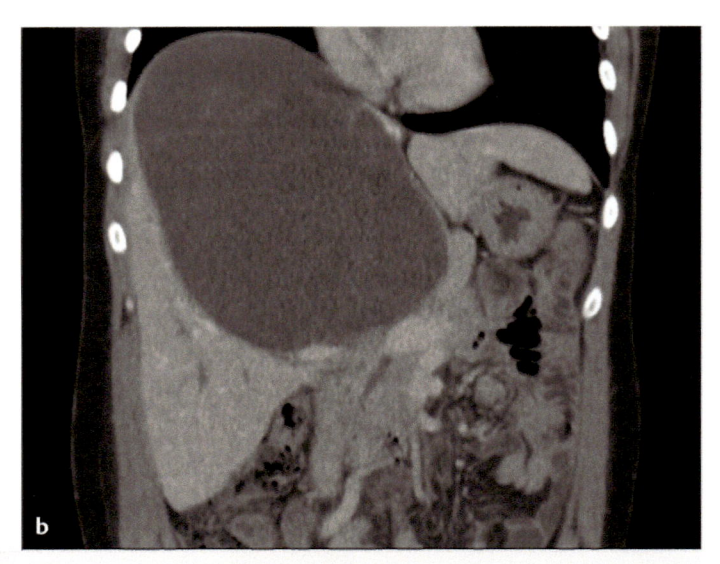

Fig. 6.43 Histologically confirmed cystadenocarcinoma. (a) Axial CT scan in the portal venous phase shows a large, well-circumscribed tumor with internal septa. (b) Coronal reformatted image defines the craniocaudal extent of the tumor. The bile ducts are slightly dilated.

may calcify or exhibit mural nodules. In the microcystic variant, the tumor has a spongy structure with a larger tissue component. The tumor capsule has lobulated margins and is thicker than the internal septa.[51] MRI can discriminate the cyst contents as serous, water-equivalent, or proteinaceous according to signal intensity. Septal calcifications are depicted less clearly. Enhancing mural nodules are suspicious for malignancy.

▶ **Clinical features.** Because of tumor size, the main presenting symptoms are abdominal pain and a palpable mass. Obstructive jaundice or pyloric stenosis may develop due to extrinsic compression. Possible complications include cyst rupture into the abdomen or retroperitoneum. Treatment consists of surgical resection.

▶ **Differential diagnosis.** Differentiation is required mainly from hepatic abscess and hemorrhagic liver cyst. The differential diagnosis should also include cystic metastases and echinococcal cyst involvement of the liver.

▶ **Key points.** Biliary cystadenocarcinoma is a rare tumor that most commonly arises from the intrahepatic bile ducts and less commonly from the extrahepatic ducts. It occurs almost exclusively in women. It presents as a large, encapsulated, multilocular cystic mass with internal septa. Development from cystadenoma may occur even after years of stability. The cyst contents are variable. The detection of enhancing mural nodules suggests malignant transformation. Cysts may rupture.

Cholangiocarcinoma

▶ **Brief definition.** Cholangiocarcinoma (cholangiocellular carcinoma) is a biliary tract carcinoma that develops from the epithelium of bile ducts. Histologically, 95% of these tumors are adenocarcinomas. Most patients are diagnosed in the sixth or seventh decade of life. In contrast to gallbladder carcinoma, males predominate by a 3:2 ratio. Cholangiocarcinoma develops in the setting of preexisting biliary tract disease. Liver fluke infection (caused by *Clonorchis sinensis* in Southeast Asia and Japan) with the formation of bile duct stones is the most frequent cause of cholangiocarcinoma throughout the world. Primary sclerosing cholangitis (ulcerative colitis, Crohn's disease, retroperitoneal fibrosis) and suppurative cholangitis predispose to the development of carcinoma in the small bile ducts. As noted earlier, cholangiocarcinoma occurs approximately two decades earlier in patients with primary sclerosing cholangitis.

Gallstones are detectable in approximately one-half of cholangiocarcinoma patients, usually in the form of gallbladder stones. Other risk factors are congenital disorders. The incidence of biliary tract carcinoma in patients with choledochal cysts is 5 to 35 times higher than in the general population.[52] The incidence of cholangiocarcinoma is also increased in patients with Caroli's disease (7% cancer risk).[1] Cholangiocarcinoma can occur at various locations:

- *Intrahepatic (peripheral) carcinoma of the small ducts*: These tumors are very rare (less than 10% of cases) and usually develop in a setting of sclerosing cholangitis. Nevertheless, intrahepatic cholangiocellular carcinoma is the second most common primary liver tumor after hepatocellular carcinoma.
- *Carcinoma at the hepatic duct bifurcation*: The most common site of occurrence is the hepatic duct bifurcation (junction of the right and left hepatic ducts with the common hepatic duct), accounting for approximately 50% of cases. A cholangiocarcinoma at this location is called a Klatskin tumor.
- *Common bile duct carcinoma*: Approximately one-third of all cholangiocarcinomas occur at this level.
- *Cystic duct carcinoma*: This site accounts for approximately 5% of cases. Cholangiocellular carcinomas in the papillary region are a special subtype.
- *Multifocal carcinomas*: Ten percent of cholangiocarcinomas develop at multiple sites.

Growth characteristics are also variable (▶ Fig. 6.44). Three main patterns have been identified: an exophytic mass-forming type, a periductal infiltrating type, and an intraductal growth type.[53] Initial spread is intraductal, followed by extension to the liver and pancreas. Over half of cholangiocarcinomas have already metastasized when diagnosed. Lymphogenous metastasis first occurs to lymph nodes along the bile ducts (in the hepatoduodenal ligament, liver, or pancreas) and later along the vessels. Peritoneal carcinomatosis can also occur. The prognosis varies with tumor location but is generally poor. Intrahepatic tumors have a 5-year survival rate of 30%. With carcinomas of the extrahepatic bile

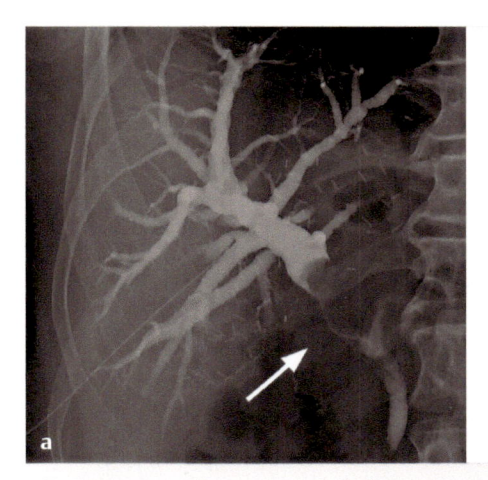

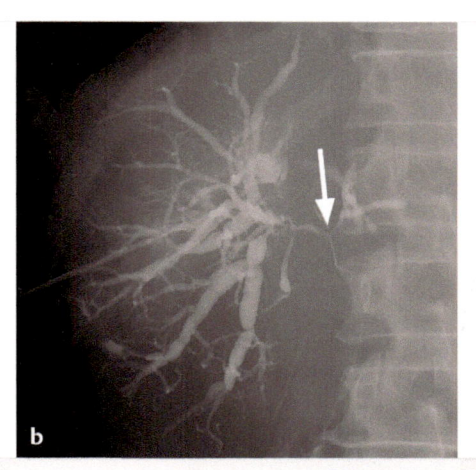

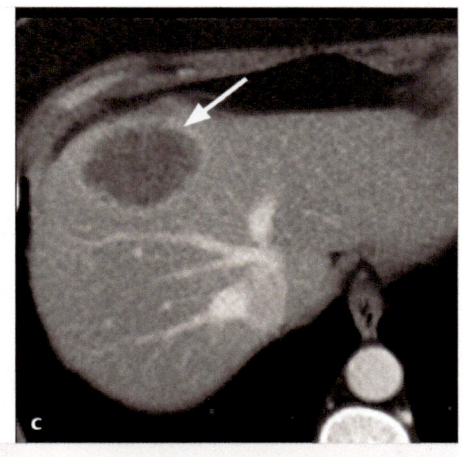

Fig. 6.44 Growth patterns of cholangiocarcinoma. (a) Polypoid intraductal recurrence after left hemihepatectomy. A long-segment stenosis (arrow) is associated with marked dilatation of intrahepatic bile ducts. (b) Infiltrative Klatskin's tumor with spread to the segmental ducts (arrow: hepatic duct bifurcation). (c) Exophytic tumor typically appears as a hypodense mass with an enhancing rim (arrow).

Gallbladder and Biliary Tract

ducts, the success rate for complete surgical resection dwindles in the proximal-to-distal direction, so that Klatskin tumors have the poorest prognosis. Tumors of the suprapancreatic and pancreatic segments of the common bile duct have a somewhat better prognosis. The median survival time for all extrahepatic biliary tract carcinomas is 5 months. Unfavorable factors besides an advanced tumor stage are advanced age, a high tumor site, and noncurative surgery. The most frequent causes of death are tumor progression, cholangitis with cholangiogenic sepsis, and hemorrhage.

▶ **Imaging signs.** Ultrasound is the most sensitive modality for detecting intrahepatic biliary obstruction in the investigation of jaundice (▶ Fig. 6.45). The level of occurrence determines whether scans show segmental intrahepatic dilatation or, with an extrahepatic tumor, generalized dilatation. The appearance of the gallbladder is also helpful in assessing tumor location. With a Klatskin's tumor, the intrahepatic bile ducts are greatly dilated while the gallbladder is small. With a carcinoma of the common bile duct, on the other hand, the gallbladder is enlarged. The level of an intrahepatic biliary obstruction can be determined in almost 100% of patients with ductal dilatation, while a tumor mass is detectable in only about one-third of cases.[54] The tumor itself appears as a hypoechoic mass that may be intraductal or may diffusely infiltrate the periductal tissue. A Klatskins' tumor is usually small and cannot be directly visualized with ultrasound. Mass-forming cholangiocarcinomas appear as hypoechoic focal hepatic lesions. Ultrasound is of limited value in the assessment of tumor spread and tumor staging. CT is the modality of choice for the diagnosis and preoperative staging of cholangiocarcinoma (▶ Table 6.3).[3] It should be performed as a multiphase study using thin-slice technique.

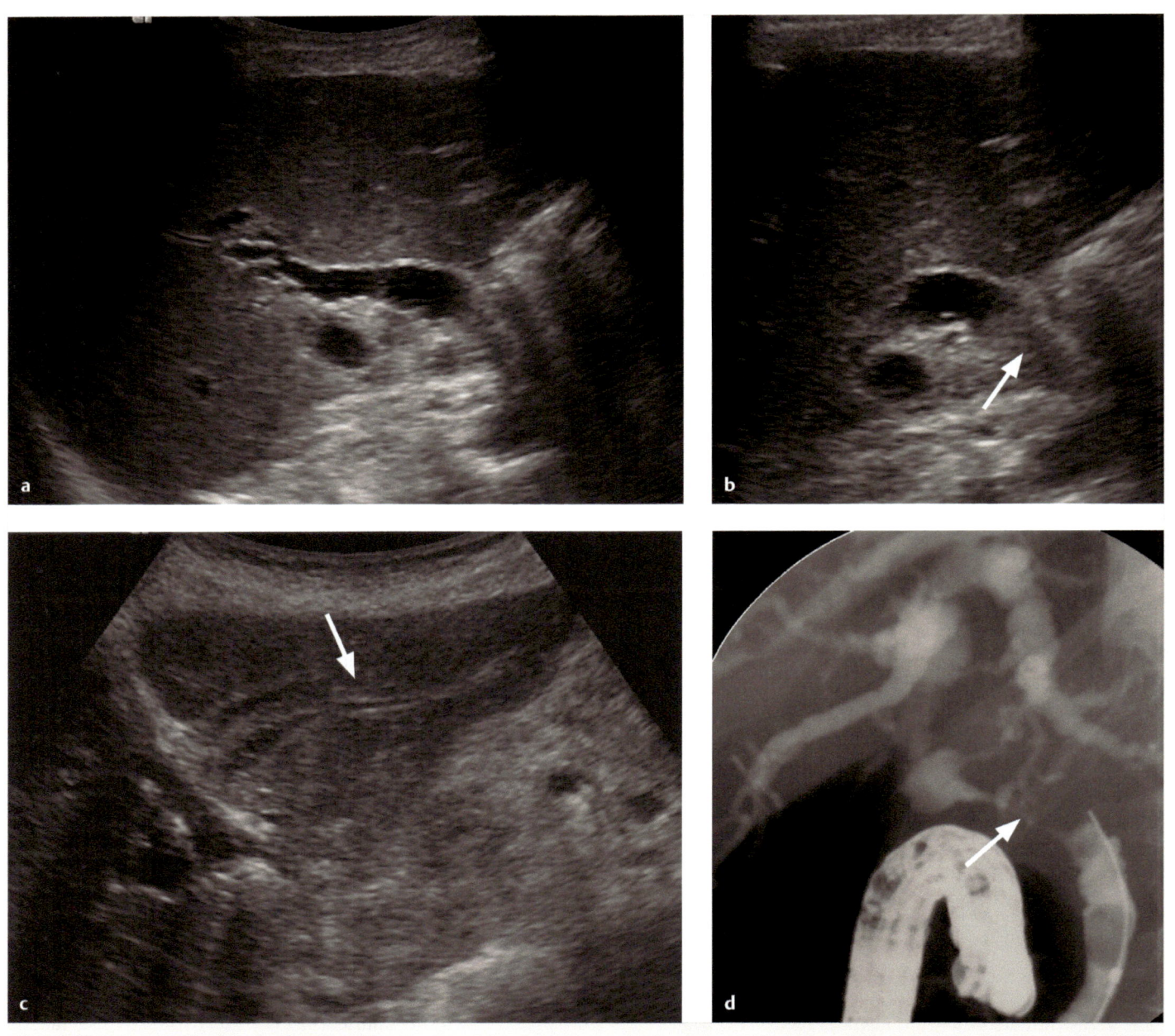

Fig. 6.45 Common bile duct carcinoma. (a) Long-segment intraluminal mass in the common bile duct with central ductal dilatation. (b) The inlet of the stenosis can be identified (arrow). (c) Symmetrical intrahepatic biliary obstruction (arrow). (d) Endoscopic retrograde cholangiopancreatography shows a malignant stricture (arrow) with marked dilatation of the intrahepatic ducts.

Table 6.3 Staging of cholangiocarcinoma[49]

Stage	Characteristics	Stage groupings
I	Tumor confined to the bile duct (Ia) or invades adjacent connective tissue (Ib)	T1, 2 N0 M0
IIa	T3: tumor invades the liver or gallbladder or unilateral portal vein branches or hepatic artery branches	T3 N0 M0
IIb	N1: lymph node metastasis in the hepatoduodenal ligament	T1, 2, 3 N1 M0
III	T4: tumor invades the portal vein or both branches, the hepatic artery, or adjacent organs	T4 Any N M0
IV	Distant metastasis	Any T Any N M1

Note: Lymph node metastasis in the hepatoduodenal ligament is classified as N1, lymph node metastasis beyond the hepatoduodenal ligament as M1.

Note

A CT examination for cholangiocarcinoma should include arterial and portal venous phase imaging in addition to delayed scans (3–5 minutes after injection of contrast medium).

The CT morphology of cholangiocarcinoma depends on its site of occurrence and growth pattern. Due to its hypovascular desmoplastic structure, the tumor is hypodense to liver parenchyma in the arterial and parenchymal phases and shows delayed enhancement.[55] CTA and multiplanar reconstructions permit vascular imaging, which is important for surgical planning. Contrast-enhanced CT can detect sites of abrupt biliary obstruction. Tumor spread and tumor stage can also be assessed. CT has some limitations in the detection of lymph node metastasis.[56] On MRI with dynamic MRA, mass-forming cholangiocarcinoma is hypointense to isointense in T1 W images and shows variable hyperintensity in T2 W sequences depending on tumor composition. Fat-suppressed T1 W images after administration of contrast medium show minimal peripheral enhancement with increasing enhancement in delayed images. Small tumors may show early, prominent enhancement (▶ Fig. 6.46). Intraductal tumors are more clearly depicted by MRI than by CT. MRCP demonstrates the biliary obstruction, and thin-slice T2 W images may even depict small intraluminal masses. Their appearance in T1 W and T2 W images is similar to that of mass-forming tumors. They usually show marked enhancement on T1 W images after administration of contrast medium. The site of the duct obstruction can be localized in nearly all cases. Reliable differentiation of a malignant from a benign stricture is not always possible with MRI.[3] These rare cases may require direct visualization of the duct by percutaneous transhepatic cholangiography (PTC) or ERCP. Both techniques allow for tissue sampling from intraductal tumors.

▶ **Clinical features.** The clinical presentation varies with site of occurrence. Klatskin's tumors and distal carcinomas of the extrahepatic bile ducts cause painless jaundice, but painful liver swelling is not uncommon. Because obstructive jaundice is present, patients suffer from pruritus. Obstruction of the common bile duct leads to gallbladder hydrops. Tumors of the intrahepatic bile ducts lead to variable intrahepatic biliary obstruction, depending on the tumor site. Jaundice (see Chapter 6.2.1) is a late feature in these cases. Tumors of the intrahepatic ducts are manifested by pain, palpable masses, and weight loss. Another potential complication of cholangiocarcinoma is bleeding, which presents as hemobilia. Complete surgical resection has the greatest prognostic benefit, but only about 20% of cases are resectable. Histologically clear margins (R0 resection) do not exclude a recurrence[57] but will significantly improve survival time.[35] A palliative treatment option for obstructive jaundice is the placement of a stent or drain via PTCD or endoscopy (see ▶ Fig. 6.48).

▶ **Differential diagnosis**
- *Pancreatic carcinoma*: The possibility of pancreatic cancer should always be considered in patients with obstructive jaundice. Cholangiocarcinoma of the extrahepatic bile ducts is often smaller and does not cause dilatation of the pancreatic duct.
- *Chronic pancreatitis*: This condition is easily diagnosed by CT. Pancreatic carcinoma is more difficult to diagnose in patients with chronic pancreatitis.
- *Choledocholithiasis*: This disease can be differentiated by MRCP, CT, and ultrasound.

Caution

Cholangiocarcinoma is difficult to distinguish in a setting of primary sclerosing cholangitis (p. 272).

▶ **Key points.** Cholangiocarcinoma is almost always an adenocarcinoma. It has various sites of occurrence (intrahepatic, hilar, extrahepatic) and various growth patterns (mass-forming, periductal infiltrating, and intraductal). Both factors determine the clinical and radiological features. The principal imaging sign is biliary obstruction; the tumor itself is often more difficult to define. Occurrence at the hepatic duct bifurcation (Klatskin's tumor) is the most common. Even small Klatskin's tumors cause obstructive jaundice. Common bile duct carcinomas cause obstructive jaundice with gallbladder hydrops. Intrahepatic cholangiocarcinomas often present as focal, mass-forming hepatic lesions. They may cause segmental biliary obstruction, but jaundice is a late occurrence. Only 20% of cholangiocarcinomas are resectable. Palliative options are drain insertion or stent implantation via PTCD or ERCP.

6.5.5 Injuries and Posttherapeutic Changes

Injuries of the Gallbladder and Biliary Tree

▶ **Brief definition.** Injuries to the biliary tree or gallbladder may occur in patients who have sustained blunt abdominal trauma. Penetrating injuries of the liver and biliary system are rare. The most common biliary injuries are iatrogenic and

Gallbladder and Biliary Tract

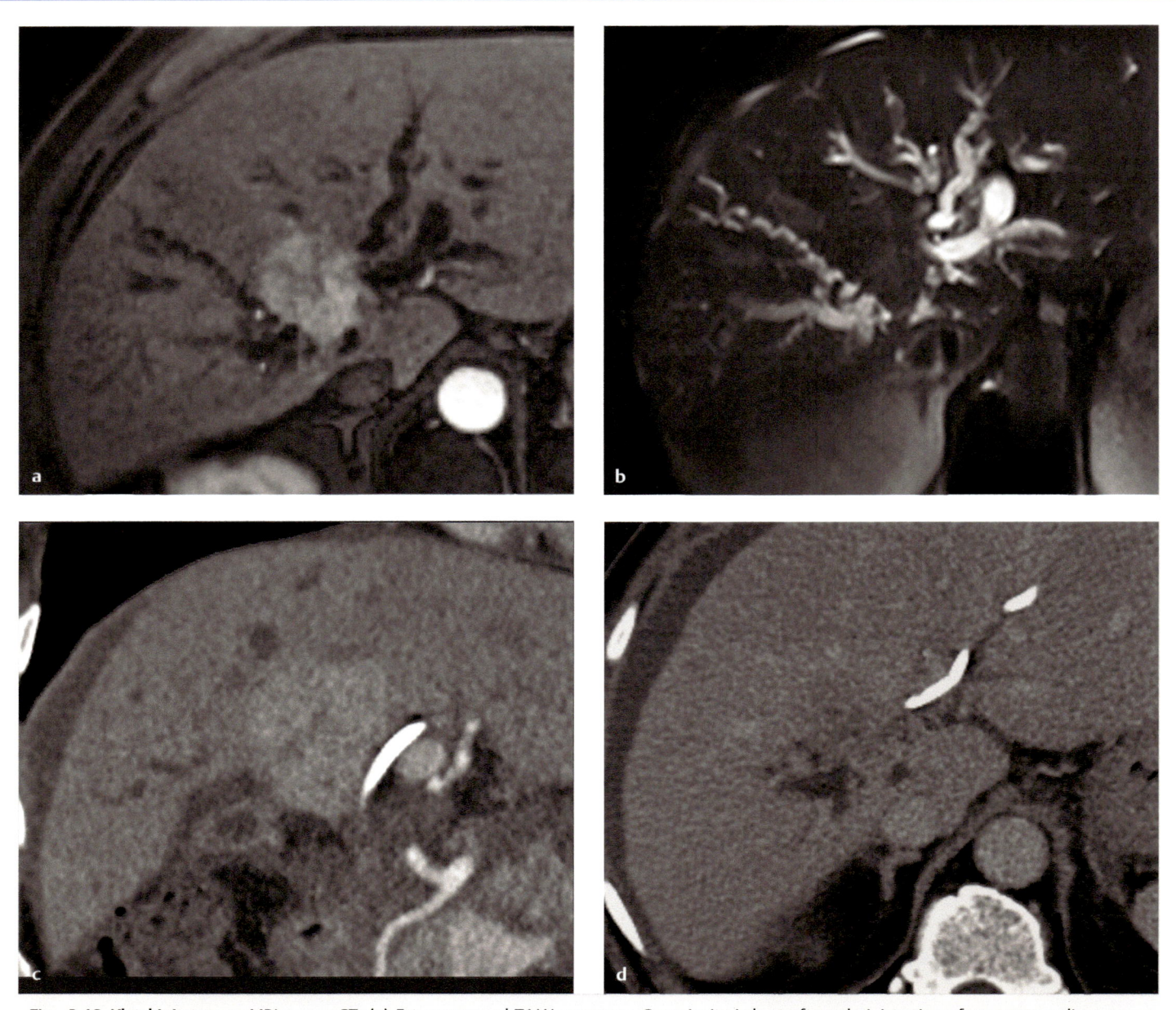

Fig. 6.46 Klatskin's tumor. MRI versus CT. **(a)** Fat-suppressed T1 W sequence. Conspicuity is best after administration of contrast medium. **(b)** Heavily T2-weighted sequence. Axial view of biliary obstruction. The tumor is not defined. **(c)** CT in the arterial phase. The tumor is hyperdense and well defined. **(d)** CT after drain insertion into the left biliary system. The tumor is poorly visualized in the parenchymal phase.

result from endoscopy, liver biopsy and catheterization, or surgery. When biliary injury occurs in the setting of blunt abdominal trauma, it is always combined with a liver injury and the clinical picture is dominated by that injury. An associated injury to the gallbladder or biliary tree is often undetected initially and is diagnosed later due to bilioma formation (▶ Fig. 6.47). Injuries of the gallbladder are subdivided into contusions and lacerations of the gallbladder wall. Very rarely, the gallbladder may be avulsed from the gallbladder bed. A laceration of the liver is associated with tearing of intrahepatic bile ducts and hematoma formation. The bile leak leads to biliary extravasation from the dependent region. A bilioma, or local bile collection, may develop over time. It may have either an intrahepatic or extrahepatic location. Biliomas may also result from injury to the gallbladder wall (see ▶ Fig. 6.47).[58] If the biliary tree is injured endoscopically, the pancreatic segment of the common bile duct is usually affected. Concomitant injury of the pancreas can be very problematic in cases of this kind (▶ Fig. 6.48). Frequently the course is aggravated by post-ERCP pancreatitis. The inadvertent division or ligation of an extrahepatic bile duct during surgery can cause a bile leak or biliary obstruction. There may occur biliary fistulas to adjacent organs, called internal fistulas (▶ Fig. 6.49). External fistulas with bile drainage to the skin along indwelling drains are rare (▶ Fig. 6.50). A particularly feared late complication of biliary tract injury is a biliary stricture due to scarring. The resulting biliary obstruction may progress to cirrhosis. Less commonly, the dependent liver parenchyma may atrophy.

▶ **Imaging signs.** Ultrasound in the acute phase shows only indirect signs such as perihepatic free fluid or hemoperitoneum from a lacerated liver (see ▶ Fig. 6.47d). The gallbladder wall may be thickened. Its lumen may appear echogenic due to intraluminal

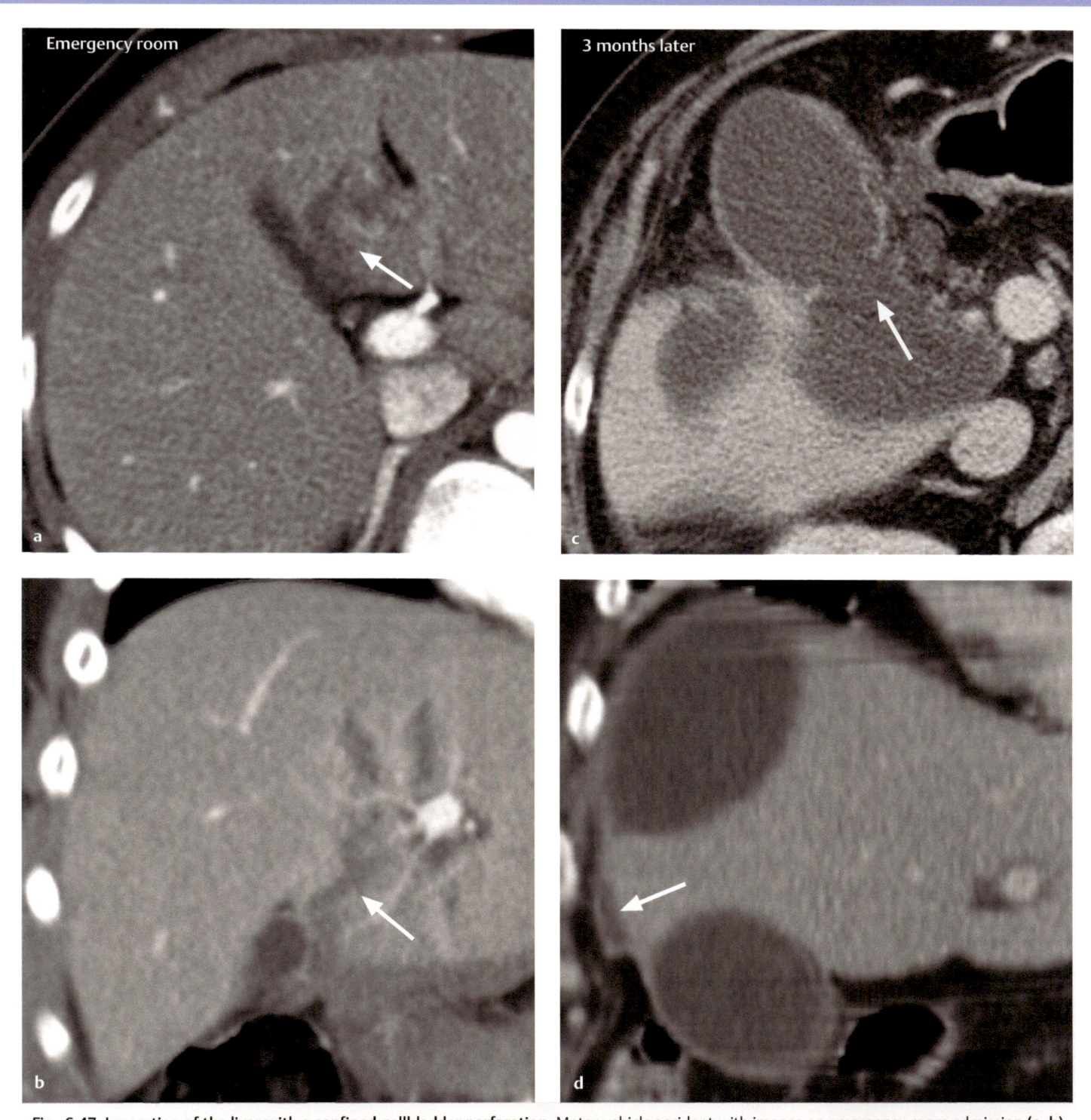

Fig. 6.47 Laceration of the liver with a confined gallbladder perforation. Motor vehicle accident with images on emergency room admission (a, b) and CT scans 3 months later (c, d). (a) Axial scan shows a liver laceration with an opposing gallbladder impression (arrow). (b) Coronal scan. (c) Perforation of the gallbladder wall (arrow). (d) Subcapsular bilioma in the gallbladder bed and the superior part of the liver (arrow: connection between both parts).

hemorrhage. A perforated gallbladder will be in a collapsed state. A bile leak is characterized by free fluid. Subsequent biliomas appear sonographically as cystic, echo-free masses located within the liver or closely adjacent to the liver capsule. They can be percutaneously aspirated and drained. If a biliary stricture develops over time, an intrahepatic biliary obstruction can be detected. CT is the modality of choice in patients with blunt abdominal trauma. CT at initial work-up shows a contusion or laceration of the liver (see ▶ Fig. 6.47a, b). With isolated iatrogenic injuries of the biliary tree, scans may show retroperitoneal air or free intraperitoneal air in addition to the normal pneumobilia that follows a papillotomy. The duodenal wall is thickened and there is increased density of adjacent fat often accompanied by pancreatitis of the pancreatic head (see ▶ Fig. 6.48a, b). MRI does not have a role in the acute setting but when used with MRCP it is the most effective modality for investigating complications, especially biliary strictures.[59] Hepatobiliary scintigraphy aids in the detection of bile leak, as tracer uptake at an extrahepatic site will confirm the leak. With direct

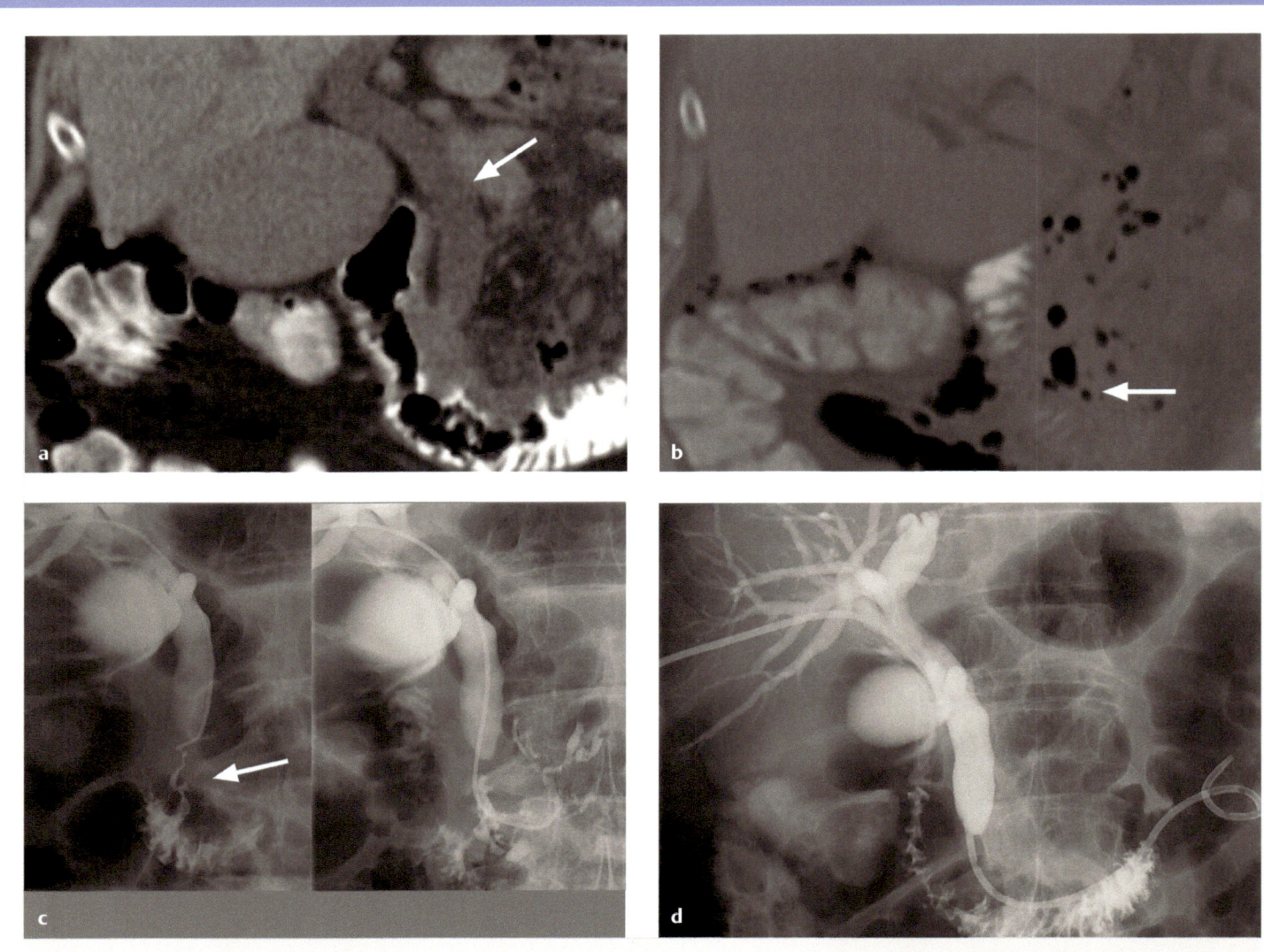

Fig. 6.48 Obstructive jaundice: retroperitoneal perforation. (a) Unenhanced CT 2 hours after endoscopic retrograde cholangiopancreatography shows dilated extrahepatic bile ducts (arrow). (b) Retroperitoneal air along the duodenum (arrow) and below the liver. (c) Percutaneous transhepatic cholangiodrainage to occlude the leak. The stenosis is visualized. The arrow indicates the perforation. The perforation was inadvertently catheterized, with retroperitoneal contrast extravasation. (d) PTCD. Transpapillary catheter placement toward the duodenum.

visualization of the ducts by ERCP, it is often possible to demonstrate a leak in the extrahepatic bile ducts. Injuries to intrahepatic ducts cannot be visualized in most cases.

▶ **Clinical features.** The symptoms arising from blunt abdominal trauma are determined by the liver injury. If there is a tear in the gallbladder wall with bile spillage into the free abdominal cavity, the patient will develop biliary peritonitis that presents as an acute abdomen. Right upper quadrant pain and rigidity are accompanied by nausea and vomiting. If the perforation is confined, a bilioma will form. Biliomas generally remain asymptomatic for some time. Large biliomas cause a pressure sensation and upper abdominal pain. If an injury leads to biliary obstruction, the clinical presentation is determined by jaundice. Endoscopic injury to the biliary tree is manifested clinically by post-ERCP pancreatitis. A retroperitoneal perforation leads to pain and fever. Biliary strictures may cause obstructive jaundice, depending on the extent of the dependent region. Treatment in the acute setting is geared toward the liver injury: A gallbladder perforation or avulsion requires surgical treatment. The procedure of choice for injuries of the extrahepatic bile ducts and strictures with biliary obstruction is interventional treatment (PTCD or ERCP) with drain insertion or stent implantation.[60] If a biliary stricture is not correctible, a biliary–enteric anastomosis may be required. A bile leak can be repaired only if unrestricted biliary drainage to the bowel can be established. Treatment in these cases centers on eliminating any outflow obstruction. A leak or fistula cannot close spontaneously in an obstructed biliary tract.

▶ **Differential diagnosis**
- *Bilioma*: A bilioma requires differentiation from a liver cyst, liquefied hematoma, or encapsulated abscess. This is most easily done by needle aspiration.
- *Endoscopic injuries*: These require differentiation from pancreatitis.
- *Biliary stricture*: The differential diagnosis includes pancreatic carcinoma, cholangiocarcinoma, or primary sclerosing cholangitis depending on the site of occurrence. The history and imaging findings will suggest the correct diagnosis.

▶ **Key points.** When biliary injury occurs in the setting of blunt abdominal trauma, the initial clinical presentation and imaging

6.5 Acquired Diseases

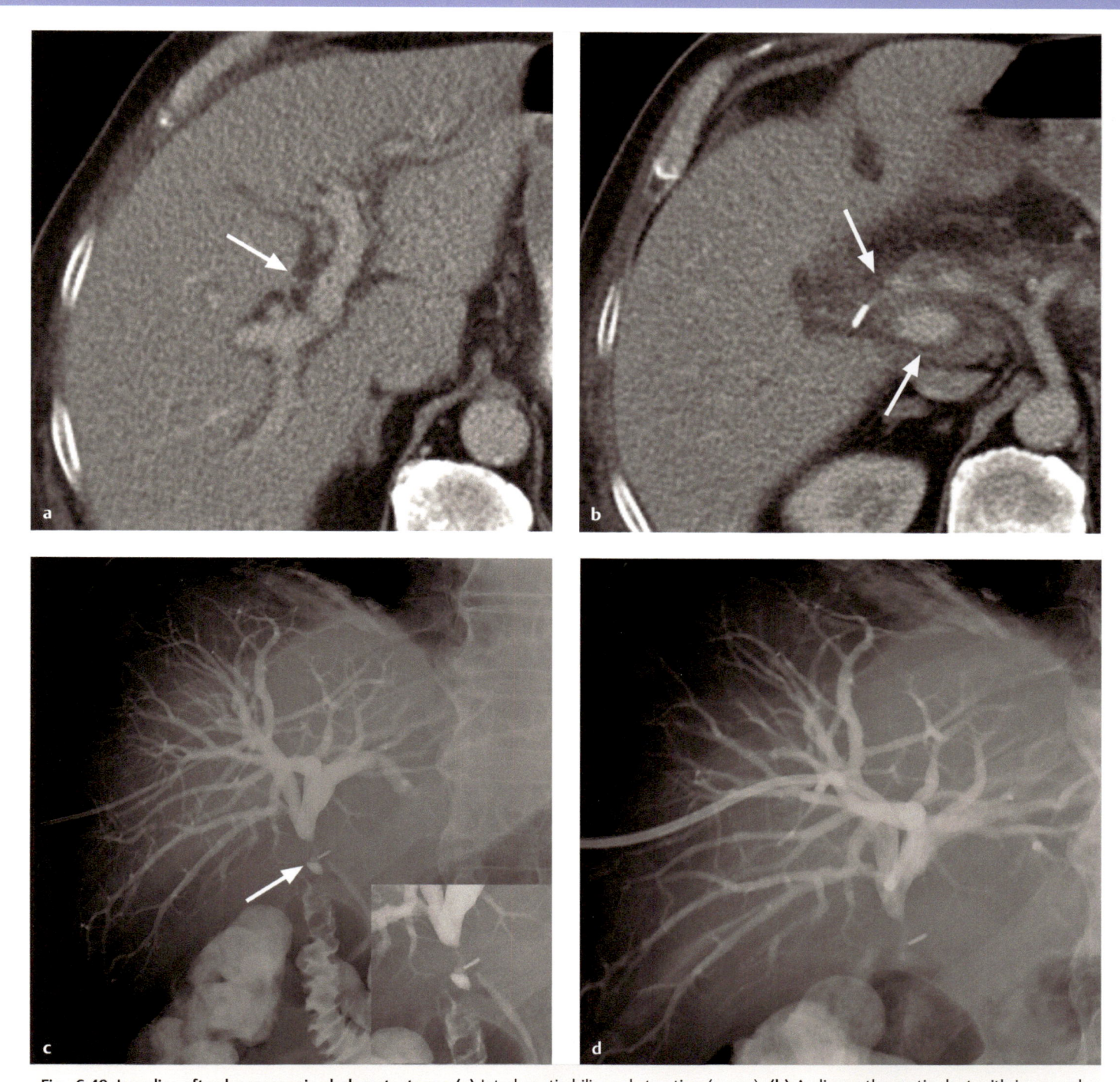

Fig. 6.49 Jaundice after laparoscopic cholecystectomy. (a) Intrahepatic biliary obstruction (arrow). (b) A clip on the cystic duct with increased density in the hepatoduodenal ligament (arrows). (c) Leakage next to the clip with a fistula to the duodenum (arrow). Inset: detail view. (d) Placement of an external drain before biliary–enteric anastomosis.

findings are dominated by the liver injury. Biliomas and bile leaks are generally diagnosed at a later time. Iatrogenic injuries of the biliary tree during endoscopy or liver biopsy/catheterization should pose no diagnostic difficulties. CT is the modality of choice in the acute phase. MRCP is best for demonstrating a posttraumatic biliary stricture. ERCP and PTCD have therapeutic applications.

Changes after Cholecystectomy

▶ **Brief definition.** After the gallbladder has been removed, some dilatation of the extrahepatic bile ducts will occur over time.

Note

Dilatation of the common bile duct to 10 mm is not abnormal after cholecystectomy.

Greater dilatation as well as dilatation of the intrahepatic bile ducts, especially segmental dilatation in the right lobe, may signify inadvertent ligation of the duct (see ▶ Fig. 6.49). Other possible causes are ischemic biliary stenosis or a thermally induced stricture. Bile leak from the cystic duct stump is manifested by a fluid collection found at the surgical site in the postoperative period (▶ Fig. 6.51). A dislodged clip is detectable in some cases.⁶¹ Strictures may be secondary to scarring or inflammation. Malignant strictures may be caused by recurrent tumor, peritoneal carcinomatosis, lymph node metastasis, or de novo cholangiocellular carcinoma originating at a scar. Biliary–enteric reconstructions predispose to ascending cholangitis.

▶ **Imaging signs.** Ultrasound is a good initial study for detecting biliary obstruction. A bilioma can be identified as a subhepatic collection. Surgical anastomoses cannot be evaluated with ultrasound in most cases. CT is the imaging modality of choice, as it gives an excellent view of postsurgical changes and can define the relationship of any collections to an anastomosis. MRI with MRCP is the principal modality for the investigation of biliary strictures.⁵⁹ Direct visualization of the ducts by ERCP or PTCD can often demonstrate a leak in the extrahepatic biliary tract. Injuries to intrahepatic bile ducts are not visualized as a rule. Hepatobiliary scintigraphy (with technetium Tc 99 m HIDA) is recommended for the investigation of an equivocal bile leak.

▶ **Clinical features.** Bile leakage from the cystic duct stump causes right upper quadrant pain. Biliary peritonitis presents clinically as an acute abdomen. A biliary stricture may be clinically silent or may lead to obstructive jaundice. The first step in treating a bile leak from the cystic duct stump is to improve biliary drainage with a papillotomy. This is followed by endoscopic stenting to occlude the leak.⁶⁰ Biliary tract strictures are treated initially by endoscopic stenting or the interventional placement of a drain or stent. Balloon dilatation may also be tried. If attempts to bypass or correct a scar stricture are unsuccessful, a biliary–enteric anastomosis may be required.

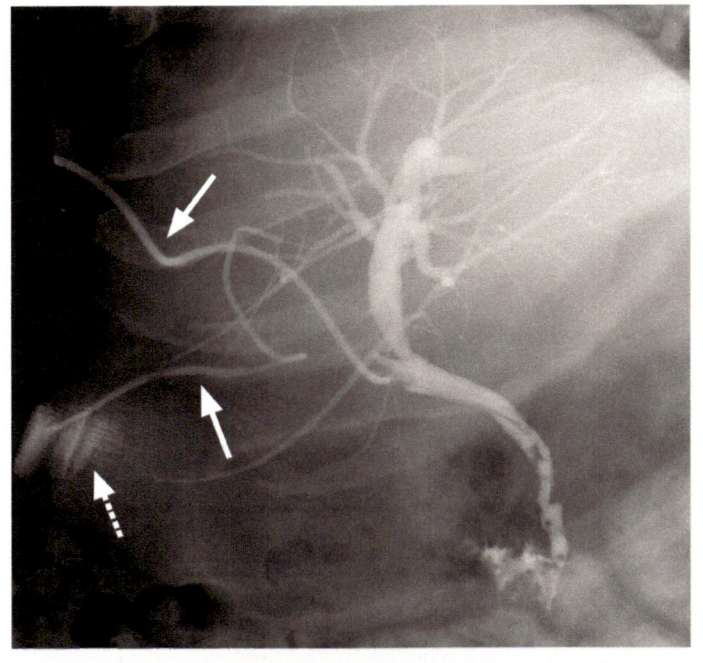

Fig. 6.50 Biliary-cutaneous fistula after removal of an intrahepatic biliary drain. View of the T-drain (middle arrow) with opacification of the left biliary tree. The image demonstrates a curved fistulous tract (top arrow) with contrast medium staining a gauze pad on the skin (dashed white arrow).

▶ **Differential diagnosis**
- *Bilioma from a leaking cystic duct stump*: This requires differentiation from a hematoma or seroma at the surgical site.

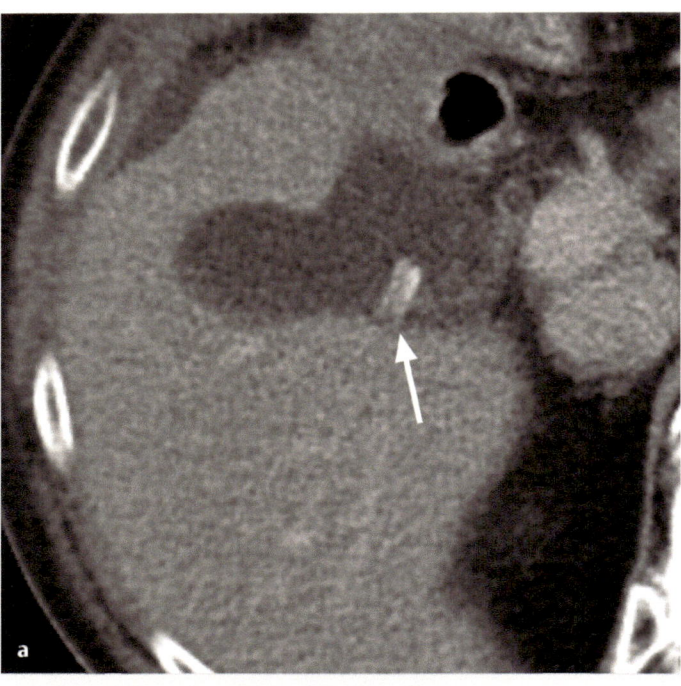

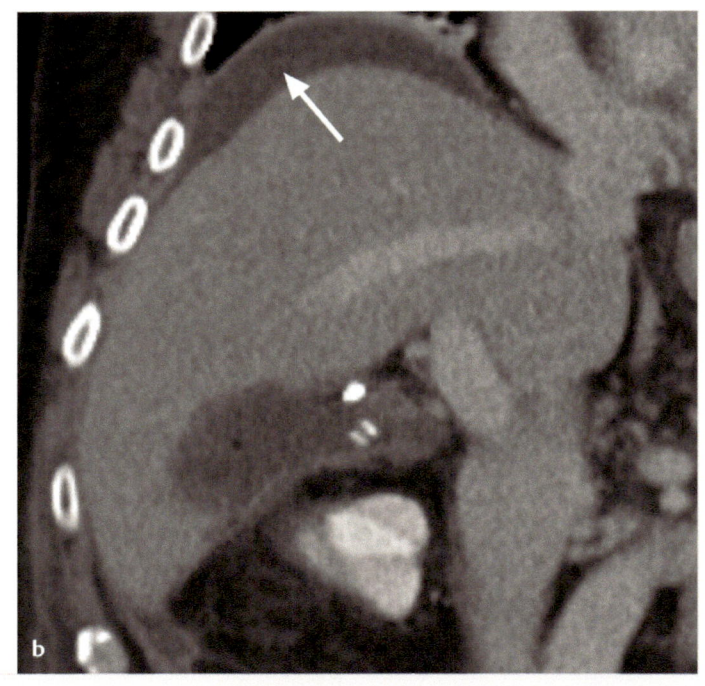

Fig. 6.51 Bile leak from the cystic duct stump. (a) Bilioma in the former gallbladder bed. Dislodged clip (arrow). **(b)** Perihepatic subphrenic bilioma (arrow).

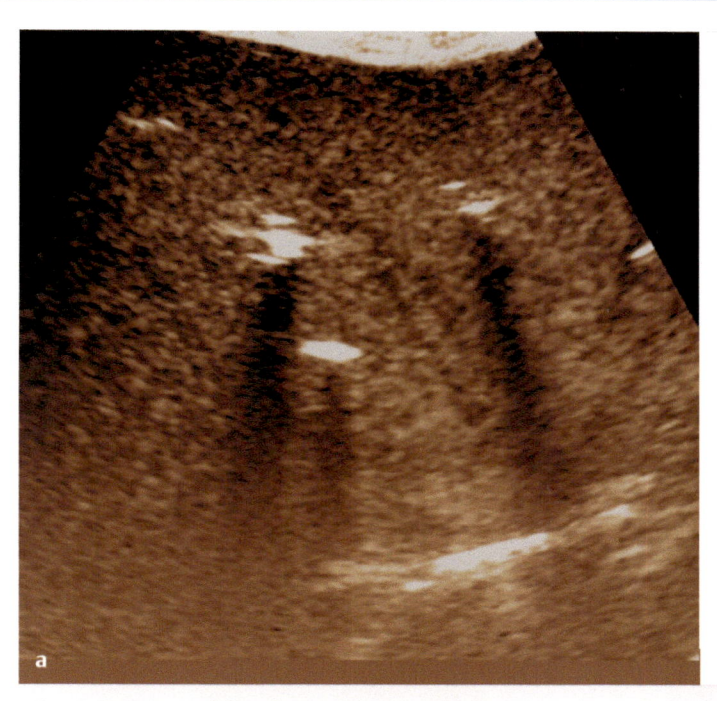

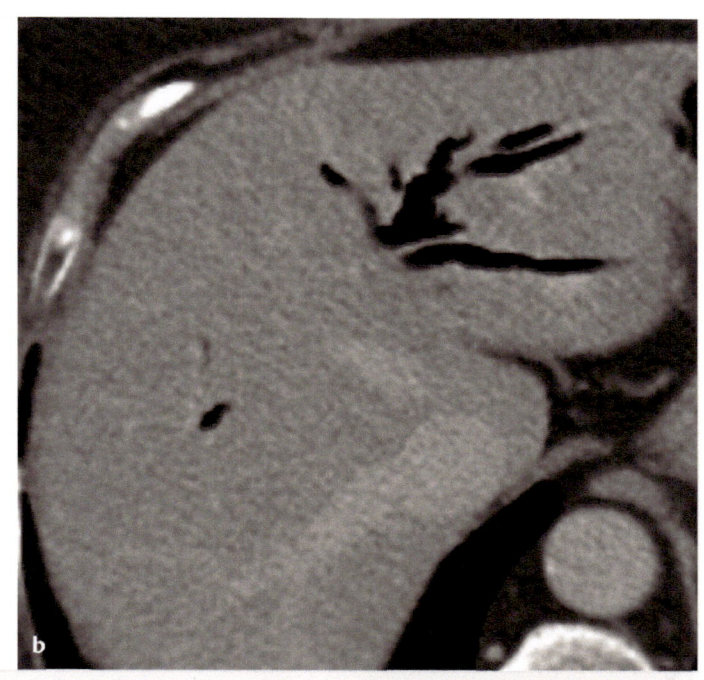

Fig. 6.52 Pneumobilia after papillotomy. (a) Contrast-enhanced ultrasound scan with conspicuous reverberation echoes. **(b)** Pneumobilia with dilated intrahepatic bile ducts and a congested liver.

- *Biliary stricture*: This may result from ischemia, thermal injury, or ligation. If the surgery was done some time ago, the possibility of a malignant stricture should be considered.

▶ **Key points.** Cholecystectomy is followed by dilatation of the extrahepatic bile ducts. The common bile duct may enlarge to 10 mm. Dilatation of the intrahepatic bile ducts is suggestive of a stricture. Ligation, thermal injury, or ischemic stenosis or scarring may be present, depending on the length of time after surgery. A bile leak is manifested by bilioma formation. The primary treatment goal for all these changes is to reestablish unobstructed bile flow.

Changes after Endoscopic Retrograde Cholangiopancreatography and Percutaneous Transhepatic Cholangiodrainage

▶ **Brief definition**
- *After ERCP*: Papillotomy is consistently followed by pneumobilia (▶ Fig. 6.52). The main complications of ERCP and papillotomy are pancreatitis, duodenal perforation, and biliary tract injury. Arteries of the pancreaticoduodenal arcade may be injured during papillotomy. Papillotomy also predisposes to ascending cholangitis. The nonfunctioning gallbladder after ERCP should be removed.
- *After PTCD*: If an artery is injured as a catheter is passed through the liver for transhepatic biliary drainage, a hepatic subcapsular hematoma will usually form. If an adjacent branch of the hepatic artery is injured during puncture of a bile duct, a biliary–vascular fistula may develop, leading to hemobilia (▶ Fig. 6.53). Biliary–vascular fistulas may develop as a late complication of biliary stenting if the stent perforates the bile duct and damages the wall of the adjacent artery (▶ Fig. 6.54). Another possible complication is bacterial contamination through a drain, leading to cholangitis and cholangiogenic hepatic abscess (▶ Fig. 6.55).

▶ **Imaging signs.** Ultrasound can demonstrate the hepatic subcapsular hematoma and its relation to the drain. Pneumobilia is easily recognized. Cholangitis cannot be diagnosed directly with ultrasound, but biliary obstruction is a suggestive sign. CT is the modality of choice as it can display the relationship of a hematoma or pseudoaneurysm to a drain without superimposed structures. When hemobilia is present, a pseudoaneurysm is detectable in the liver. Depending on the extent of the hemobiliary fistula, the blood-filled bile ducts may appear as hyperdense tubular structures on unenhanced CT. Inflammatory changes are also clearly depicted (see ▶ Fig. 6.55). The diagnosis of pancreatitis is the domain of CT. MRI is the best modality for imaging iatrogenic cholangitis and hepatic abscess. MRCP is of limited use when there is pneumobilia. CT is superior for the emergency diagnosis of a hematoma.

▶ **Clinical features.** A hematoma following insertion of a biliary drain causes right upper quadrant pain. Biliary–vascular fistulas are manifested by hemobilia with colicky upper abdominal pain. A significant fistula may lead to upper gastrointestinal bleeding or even circulatory collapse. Jaundice is a rare manifestation of a biliary–vascular fistula. Infection presents with right upper quadrant pain and fever. Obstructed bile flow leads relatively quickly to cholangiogenic sepsis and hepatic abscess formation. Hepatic subcapsular hematoma is usually managed conservatively. If extravasation of contrast medium is noted on CT or a pseudoaneurysm or biliary-vascular fistula is detected, angiography

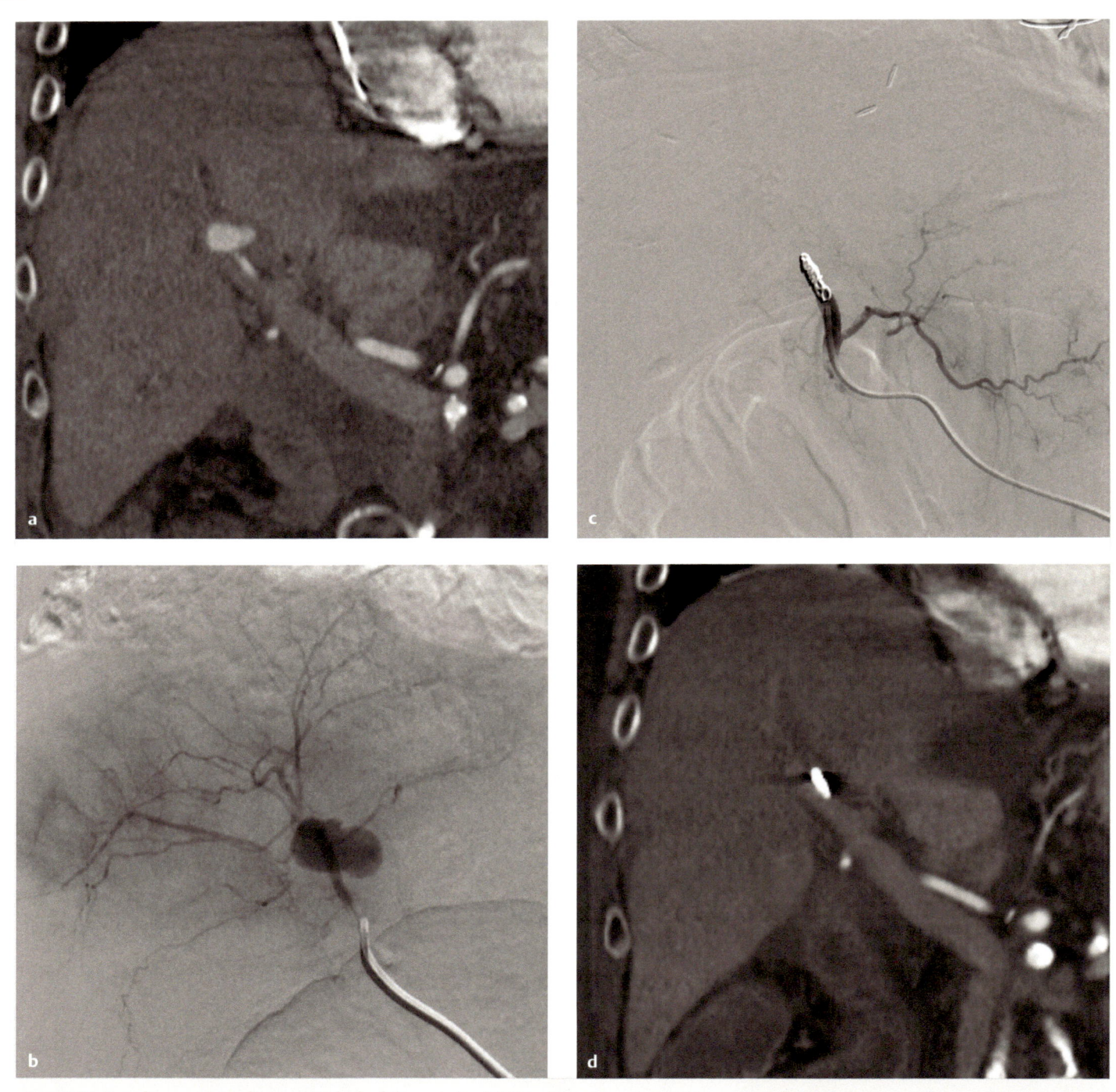

Fig. 6.53 Pseudoaneurysm after removal of a biliary drain. (**a**) Pseudoaneurysm arising from the right hepatic artery. (**b**) Angiographic view. (**c**) Endovascular occlusion with coils. (**d**) After embolization.

should be undertaken. The procedure of choice for establishing hemostasis is endovascular occlusion (usually by coil embolization, see ▶ Fig. 6.53). This also applies to bleeding from the pancreaticoduodenal arcade after papillotomy. It is difficult to treat drain- or stent-induced cholangitis; removal of the foreign material is unavoidable but is not always sufficient. The goal of treatment must be to improve biliary flow in the affected area. This may require a combined endoscopic–radiological approach.

▶ **Differential diagnosis.** Right upper quadrant pain after an interventional procedure (ERCP or PTCD) may be caused by a hematoma, bleeding, or pancreatitis. A hematoma or gastrointestinal hemorrhage after an interventional procedure should pose no problems of differential diagnosis. The possibility of biliary peritonitis due to retrograde bile leakage from the drainage channel should be considered. Fever and elevated bilirubin levels or jaundice always signify cholangitis or a cholangiogenic liver abscess.

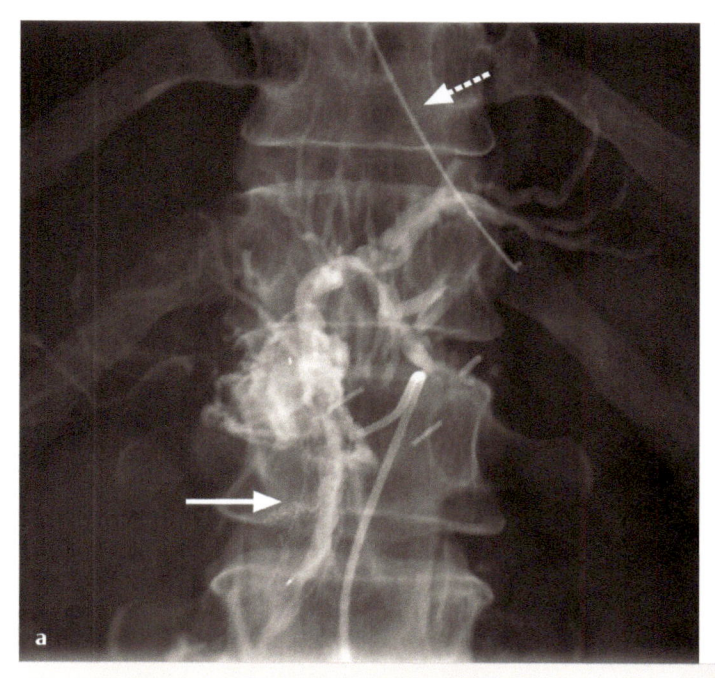

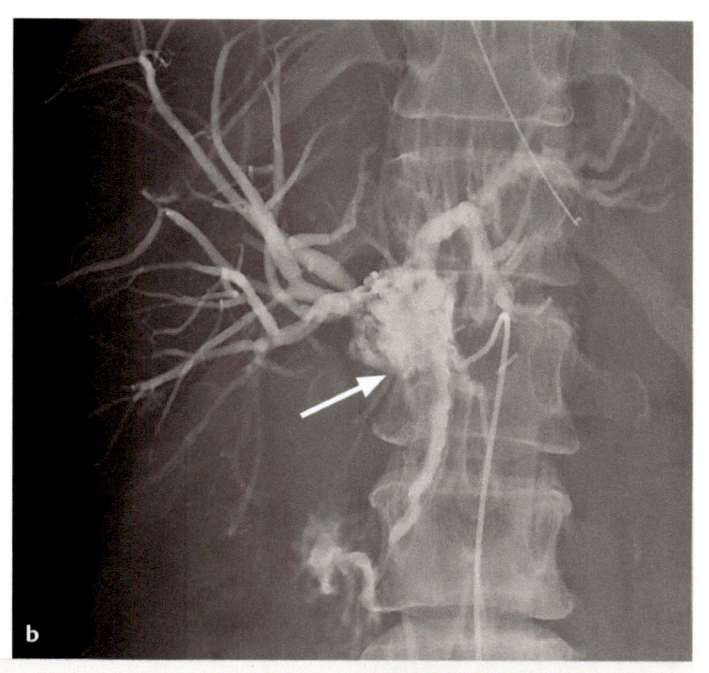

Fig. 6.54 **Biliary-vascular fistula after stenting.** Angiography of the celiac trunk. **(a)** Catheter in the ostium of the celiac trunk. A stent (arrow) was placed across a stenotic biliary–enteric anastomosis. A gastric tube was placed for bleeding in the upper gastrointestinal tract (dashed arrow). **(b)** Opacification of the intrahepatic bile ducts with contrast extravasation through the biliary stent into the small intestine. A degenerative cavity (arrow) is also opacified.

▶ **Key points.** Specific complications may arise, depending on the approach:
- *ERCP*: In ERCP, especially when ductal access is established by papillotomy, the papilla and pancreatic segment of the common bile duct are affected. The problem in that segment is pancreatitis. Duodenal injury and retroperitoneal perforation may also occur. Vascular injuries in the pancreaticoduodenal arcade are a particularly serious complication.
- *PTCD*: The transhepatic approach for biliary drainage may cause vascular injury with a hepatic subcapsular hematoma or, very rarely, a biliary–vascular fistula.

Another potential complication in both procedures is cholangitis. It should be noted that bacterial inoculation through the skin with sterile technique is less likely to occur than in an endoscopic procedure.

Chemotherapy-induced Cholangitis and Cholecystitis

▶ **Brief definition.** These conditions involve a drug-induced, fibrosing inflammation of the biliary tree, or less commonly an inflammation of the gallbladder, that may occur in response to intra-arterial chemotherapy for primary or secondary liver tumors. The fibrosis is caused by the interaction of a toxic insult and vasculitis leading to ischemia.[62] The concurrent administration of dexamethasone during chemotherapy infusion can significantly reduce the incidence of these inflammatory complications (from 20% to 3%).[63] The distal common bile duct is typically unaffected. One complication is ischemic cholecystitis, which can potentially lead to biliary peritonitis with a high mortality rate. The most serious complication is acute liver failure. Most patients do not survive the development of biliary cirrhosis because of the poor prognosis of their underlying disease.

During selective internal radiation therapy (SIRT) of the liver, particles may embolize to the cystic artery, provoking a radiogenic cholecystitis. This risk can be reduced by prior prophylactic embolization. Ischemic cholecystitis may develop in isolated cases.[64]

▶ **Imaging signs.** Ultrasound can demonstrate intrahepatic biliary obstruction. Thickening of the bile duct walls is sometimes found. Concomitant gallbladder involvement presents as cholecystitis with thickening of the gallbladder wall (▶ Fig. 6.56). CT can exclude biliary obstruction due to extrinsic duct compression by a nodal or hepatic metastasis. An enhancing area of wall thickening can be seen in thin-slice reconstructions. Associated periportal fibrosis is hypodense on precontrast scans and shows delayed enhancement. On unenhanced T1W MRI, the fibrosis along the periportal fields appears hypointense with irregular borders. The fibrosis is hyperintense in T2W sequences. A mixed T2W/T1W TrueFISP sequence is useful for luminal evaluation of the bile ducts. MRCP shows irregular ducts with segmental strictures. Direct visualization of the ducts by ERCP or PTCD is performed for therapeutic reasons. Biliary obstruction can be treated by drain insertion or stenting.

▶ **Clinical features.** Acute cases present with upper abdominal pain, fever, and jaundice. Laboratory tests show cholestasis with elevated titers of bilirubin and alkaline phosphatase. If liver

Gallbladder and Biliary Tract

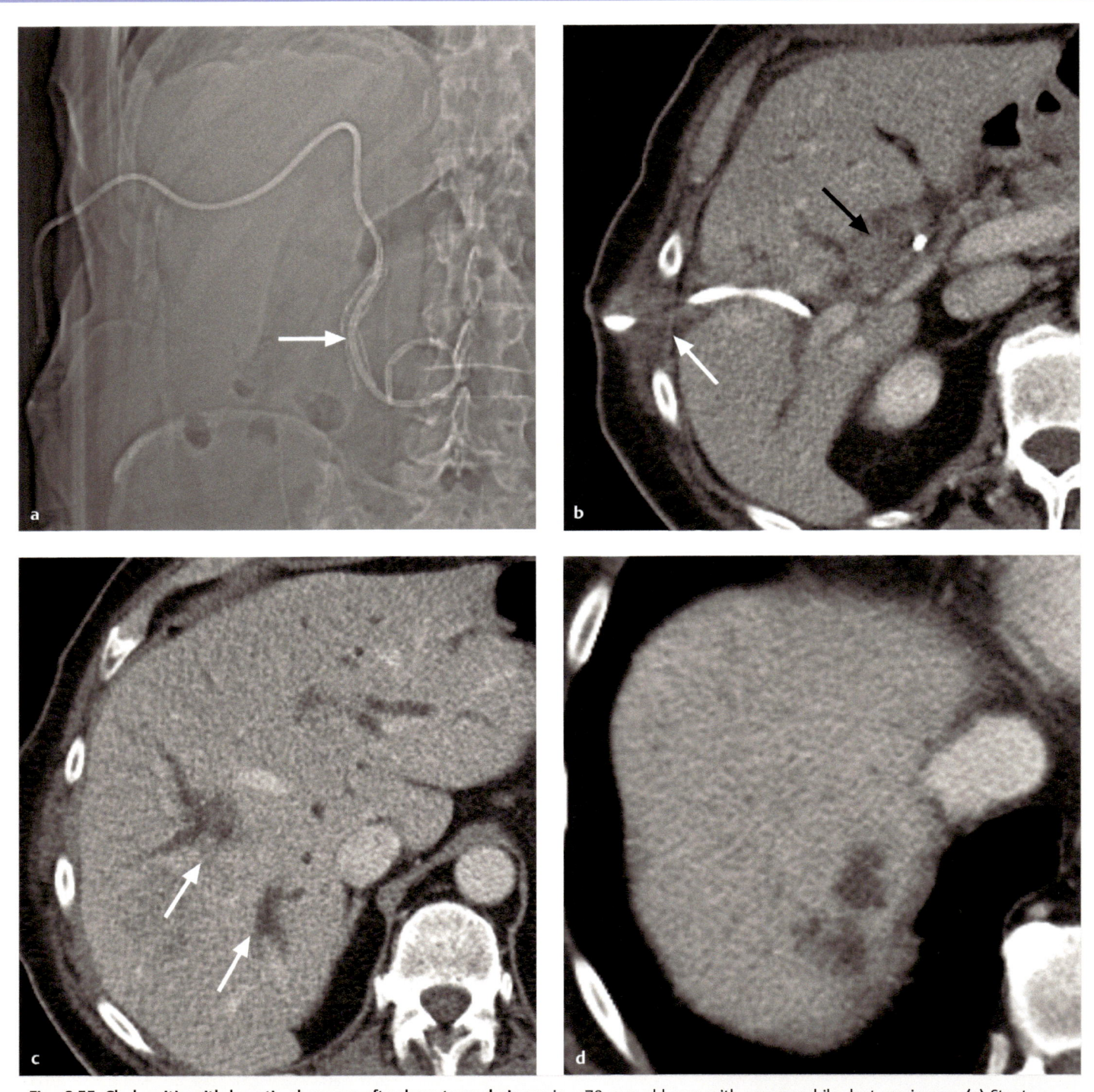

Fig. 6.55 Cholangitis with hepatic abscesses after long-term drainage in a 70-year-old man with common bile duct carcinoma. (a) Stent implanted initially (arrow). A drain was inserted after stent occlusion. (b) Infection along the drain (white arrow). Common bile duct carcinoma (black arrow). (c) Dilated bile ducts with cholangitis (arrows). (d) Abscesses in the superior part of the liver (segment VII).

function deteriorates in the absence of tumor progression, it is important to consider sclerosing cholangitis in addition to direct drug-induced liver damage. Treatment consists of discontinuing intra-arterial chemotherapy. Dilatation of biliary strictures may be performed if required.

▶ **Differential diagnosis**
- Primary sclerosing cholangitis and other forms of secondary sclerosing cholangitis: These conditions require differentiation from chemotherapy-induced cholangitis.
- Extrinsic biliary tract compression by metastasis: This should be excluded as a potential cause of jaundice.
- Chemotherapy-induced liver failure: Hepatic jaundice due to chemotherapy-induced liver failure is distinguished by an absence of biliary obstruction.

▶ **Key points.** Local chemotherapy can induce a vasculitis that may lead to ischemic fibrosing cholangitis or cholecystitis. These conditions may present clinically as cholecystitis. Cholangitis may be associated with obstructive jaundice, which requires differentiation from extrinsic tumor compression and from toxic liver damage induced by chemotherapy.

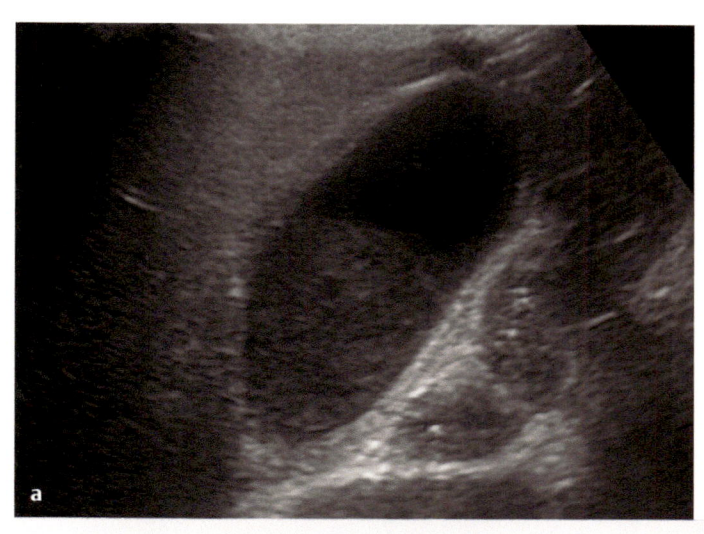

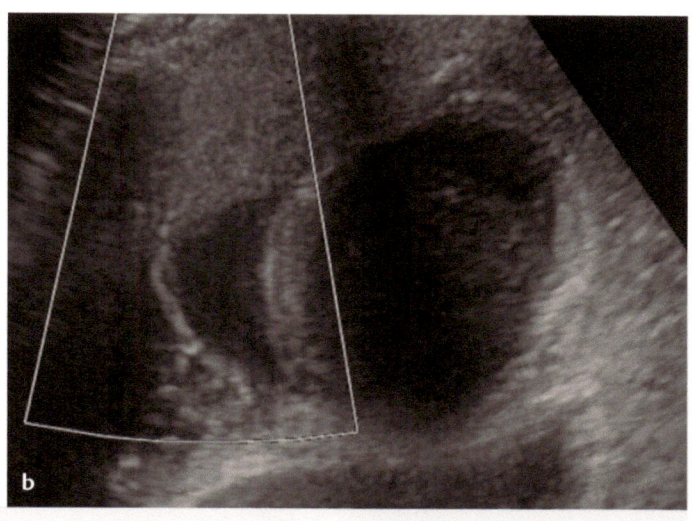

Fig. 6.56 **Acute cholecystitis in response to chemotherapy.** The patient underwent chemotherapy for leukemia. (a) The gallbladder wall is thickened, and its lumen is filled with sludge. (b) Pericholecystitis on the hepatic side.

Bibliography

[1] Remmele W. Gallenblase und extrahepatische Gallengänge, Vater-Papille. In: Remmele W, ed. Pathologie. Vol 3. 2nd ed. Berlin: Springer; 1999:219–331

[2] Drenckhahn D, Fahimi HD. Gallenwege, Gallenblase. In: Benninghoff A, Drenckhahn D, eds. Anatomie. Makroskopische Anatomie, Histologie, Embryologie, Zellbiologie. Vol 1. 17th ed. München: Urban & Fischer; 2008:715–720

[3] Sainani NI, Catalano OA, Holalkere NS, Zhu AX, Hahn PF, Sahani DV. Cholangiocarcinoma: current and novel imaging techniques. Radiographics. 2008; 28 (5):1263–1287

[4] Moradpour D. Leber. In: Siegenthaler W, Blum HE, eds. Klinische Pathophysiologie. 9th ed. Stuttgart: Thieme; 2006: 860–888

[5] Schünke M, Schulte E, Schumacher U. Prometheus. LernAtlas der Anatomie: Innere Organe. 2nd ed. Stuttgart: Thieme; 2009. Illustrated by M. Voll/K. Wesker

[6] Todani T, Watanabe Y, Narusue M, Tabuchi K, Okajima K. Congenital bile duct cysts: classification, operative procedures, and review of thirty-seven cases including cancer arising from choledochal cyst. Am J Surg. 1977; 134(2):263–269

[7] Mortelé KJ, Rocha TC, Streeter JL, Taylor AJ. Multimodality imaging of pancreatic and biliary congenital anomalies. Radiographics. 2006; 26(3):715–731

[8] Hartley JL, Davenport M, Kelly DA. Biliary atresia. Lancet. 2009; 374 (9702):1704–1713

[9] Kasai M, Suzuki H, Ohashi E, Ohi R, Chiba T, Okamoto A. Technique and results of operative management of biliary atresia. World J Surg. 1978; 2(5):571–579

[10] Tsang TM, Tam PKH, Chamberlain P. Obliteration of the distal bile duct in the development of congenital choledochal cyst. J Pediatr Surg. 1994; 29 (12):1582–1583

[11] Moss RL, Traverso LW. Biliary atresia and cysts. Curr Opin Gastroenterol. 1992; 8:791–895

[12] Wiseman K, Buczkowski AK, Chung SW, Francoeur J, Schaeffer D, Scudamore CH. Epidemiology, presentation, diagnosis, and outcomes of choledochal cysts in adults in an urban environment. Am J Surg. 2005; 189(5):527–531, discussion 531

[13] Cheney M, Rustad DG, Lilly JR. Choledochal cyst. World J Surg. 1985; 9(2): 244–249

[14] Sato Y, Ren XS, Nakanuma Y. Caroli's disease: current knowledge of its biliary pathogenesis obtained from an orthologous rat model. Int J Hepatol. 2012; 2012:107945

[15] Tomà P, Lucigrai G, Pelizza A. Sonographic patterns of Caroli's disease: report of 5 new cases. J Clin Ultrasound. 1991; 19(3):155–161

[16] Choi BI, Yeon KM, Kim SH, Han MC. Caroli disease: central dot sign in CT. Radiology. 1990; 174(1):161–163

[17] Asselah T, Ernst O, Sergent G, L'herminé C, Paris JC. Caroli's disease: a magnetic resonance cholangiopancreatography diagnosis. Am J Gastroenterol. 1998; 93(1):109–110

[18] Ros E, Navarro S, Bru C, Gilabert R, Bianchi L, Bruguera M. Ursodeoxycholic acid treatment of primary hepatolithiasis in Caroli's syndrome. Lancet. 1993; 342(8868):404–406

[19] Rodewohl E. Ausgewählte Erkrankungen der Gallenblase und extrahepatischen Gallengänge—einschließlich der Papilla Vateri—im Sektionsgut des Pathologisch-Bakteriologischen Instituts des Städtischen Klinikums "St. Georg" Leipzig—eine Analyse der Jahre 1980–1989 unter Berücksichtigung des Zusammenhangs von biliärem System und Pankreas [dissertation]. Leipzig: Universität Leipzig; 1996

[20] Buch S, Schafmayer C, Völzke H, et al. A genome-wide association scan identifies the hepatic cholesterol transporter ABCG8 as a susceptibility factor for human gallstone disease. Nat Genet. 2007; 39(8):995–999

[21] Ashur H, Siegal B, Oland Y, Adam YG. Calcified gallbladder (porcelain gallbladder). Arch Surg. 1978; 113(5):594–596

[22] Stephen AE, Berger DL. Carcinoma in the porcelain gallbladder: a relationship revisited. Surgery. 2001; 129(6):699–703

[23] Yonetci N, Kutluana U, Yilmaz M, Sungurtekin U, Tekin K. The incidence of Mirizzi syndrome in patients undergoing endoscopic retrograde cholangiopancreatography. Hepatobiliary Pancreat Dis Int. 2008; 7(5):520–524

[24] Kehr H. Die in meiner Klinik geübte Technik der Gallenstein Operationen, mit einen Hinweis auf die Indikationen und die Dauererfolge. München: JF Lehmann; 1905

[25] Mirizzi PL. Sindrome del conducto hepatico. J Int Chir. 1948; 8:731–777

[26] Lai EC, Lau WY. Mirizzi syndrome: history, present and future development. ANZ J Surg. 2006; 76(4):251–257

[27] Pedrosa CS, Casanova R, de la Torre S, Villacorta J. CT findings in Mirizzi syndrome. J Comput Assist Tomogr. 1983; 7(3):419–425

[28] Tanaka N, Nobori M, Furuya T, et al. Evolution of Mirizzi syndrome with biliobiliary fistula. J Gastroenterol. 1995; 30(1):117–121

[29] Strunk H, Teifke A, Menke H. [Typical radiologic findings in Mirizzi syndrome]. Rontgenblatter. 1988; 41(8):345–347

[30] Yun EJ, Choi CS, Yoon DY, et al. Combination of magnetic resonance cholangiopancreatography and computed tomography for preoperative diagnosis of the Mirizzi syndrome. J Comput Assist Tomogr. 2009; 33(4):636–640

[31] Choi BW, Kim MJ, Chung JJ, Chung JB, Yoo HS, Lee JT. Radiologic findings of Mirizzi syndrome with emphasis on MRI. Yonsei Med J. 2000; 41(1):144–146

[32] Attasaranya S, Fogel EL, Lehman GA. Choledocholithiasis, ascending cholangitis, and gallstone pancreatitis. Med Clin North Am. 2008; 92(4): 925–960, x

[33] Vierling JM. Immune disorders of the liver and bile duct. Gastroenterol Clin North Am. 1992; 21(2):427–449

[34] LaRusso NF, Shneider BL, Black D, et al. Primary sclerosing cholangitis: summary of a workshop. Hepatology. 2006; 44(3):746–764

[35] Burak K, Angulo P, Pasha TM, Egan K, Petz J, Lindor KD. Incidence and risk factors for cholangiocarcinoma in primary sclerosing cholangitis. Am J Gastroenterol. 2004; 99(3):523–526

[36] Campbell WL, Ferris JV, Holbert BL, Thaete FL, Baron RL. Biliary tract carcinoma complicating primary sclerosing cholangitis: evaluation with CT, cholangiography, US, and MR imaging. Radiology. 1998; 207(1):41–50

[37] Campbell WL, Peterson MS, Federle MP, et al. Using CT and cholangiography to diagnose biliary tract carcinoma complicating primary sclerosing cholangitis. AJR Am J Roentgenol. 2001; 177(5):1095–1100

[38] Colecchia A, Larocca A, Scaioli E, et al. Natural history of small gallbladder polyps is benign: evidence from a clinical and pathogenetic study. Am J Gastroenterol. 2009; 104(3):624–629

[39] Ozmen MM, Patankar RV, Hengirmen S, Terzi MC. Epidemiology of gallbladder polyps. Scand J Gastroenterol. 1994; 29(5):480

[40] Yoshimitsu K, Honda H, Jimi M, et al. MR diagnosis of adenomyomatosis of the gallbladder and differentiation from gallbladder carcinoma: importance of showing Rokitansky–Aschoff sinuses. AJR Am J Roentgenol. 1999; 172(6):1535–1540

[41] Lee NK, Kim S, Kim HS, et al. Spectrum of mucin-producing neoplastic conditions of the abdomen and pelvis: cross-sectional imaging evaluation. World J Gastroenterol. 2011; 17(43):4757–4771

[42] Lim JH, Jang KT, Rhim H, Kim YS, Lee KT, Choi SH. Biliary cystic intraductal papillary mucinous tumor and cystadenoma/cystadenocarcinoma: differentiation by CT. Abdom Imaging. 2007; 32(5):644–651

[43] Rashid A. Cellular and molecular biology of biliary tract cancers. Surg Oncol Clin N Am. 2002; 11(4):995–1009

[44] Menias CO, Surabhi VR, Prasad SR, Wang HL, Narra VR, Chintapalli KN. Mimics of cholangiocarcinoma: spectrum of disease. Radiographics. 2008; 28(4):1115–1129

[45] Albores-Saavedra J, Henson DE. Tumors of gallbladder and extrahepatic bile ducts. USAF Atlas of Tumor Pathology. 2nd series. Fasc 22. Washington, DC: Armed Forces Institute of Pathology under the auspices of Universities Associated for Research and Education in Pathology; 1986. For sale by the Armed Forces Institute of Pathology

[46] Strasberg SM, Drebin JA. Tumors of the biliary tree. In: Yamada T, Alpers DH, Kaplowitz N, et al, eds. Textbook of Gastroenterology. Vol 1. 4th ed. Philadelphia: Lippincott Williams & Wilkins; 2003:2234–2251

[47] Yamamoto T, Uki K, Takeuchi K, et al. Early gallbladder carcinoma associated with primary sclerosing cholangitis and ulcerative colitis. J Gastroenterol. 2003; 38(7):704–706

[48] Nugent KP, Spigelman AD, Talbot IC, Phillips RK. Gallbladder dysplasia in patients with familial adenomatous polyposis. Br J Surg. 1994; 81(2):291–292

[49] Rubin P, Hansen JT, eds. TNM Staging Atlas. Philadelphia: Lippincott Williams &Wilkins; 2008

[50] Devaney K, Goodman ZD, Ishak KG. Hepatobiliary cystadenoma and cystadenocarcinoma. A light microscopic and immunohistochemical study of 70 patients. Am J Surg Pathol. 1994; 18(11):1078–1091

[51] Mortelé KJ, Ros PR. Cystic focal liver lesions in the adult: differential CT and MR imaging features. Radiographics. 2001; 21(4):895–910

[52] Reveille RM, Van Stiegmann G, Everson GT. Increased secondary bile acids in a choledochal cyst. Possible role in biliary metaplasia and carcinoma. Gastroenterology. 1990; 99(2):525–527

[53] Yamasaki S. Intrahepatic cholangiocarcinoma: macroscopic type and stage classification. J Hepatobiliary Pancreat Surg. 2003; 10(4):288–291

[54] Neumaier CE, Bertolotto M, Perrone R, Martinoli C, Loria F, Silvestri E. Staging of hilar cholangiocarcinoma with ultrasound. J Clin Ultrasound. 1995; 23(3):173–178

[55] Slattery JM, Sahani DV. What is the current state-of-the-art imaging for detection and staging of cholangiocarcinoma? Oncologist. 2006; 11(8):913–922

[56] Lee HY, Kim SH, Lee JM, et al. Preoperative assessment of resectability of hepatic hilar cholangiocarcinoma: combined CT and cholangiography with revised criteria. Radiology. 2006; 239(1):113–121

[57] Cameron JL. Proximal cholangiocarcinomas. Br J Surg. 1988; 75(12):1155–1156

[58] Howard R, Bansal S, Munshi IA. Biloma: a delayed complication of blunt hepatic injury. J Emerg Med. 2008; 34(1):33–35

[59] Hoeffel C, Azizi L, Lewin M, et al. Normal and pathologic features of the postoperative biliary tract at 3D MR cholangiopancreatography and MR imaging. Radiographics. 2006; 26(6):1603–1620

[60] Pawa S, Al-Kawas FH. ERCP in the management of biliary complications after cholecystectomy. Curr Gastroenterol Rep. 2009; 11(2):160–166

[61] Kapoor V, Baron RL, Peterson MS. Bile leaks after surgery. AJR Am J Roentgenol. 2004; 182(2):451–458

[62] Fukuzumi S, Moriya Y, Makuuchi M, Terui S. Serious chemical sclerosing cholangitis associated with hepatic arterial 5FU and MMC chemotherapy. Eur J Surg Oncol. 1990; 16(3):251–255

[63] Kemeny N, Conti JA, Cohen A, et al. Phase II study of hepatic arterial floxuridine, leucovorin, and dexamethasone for unresectable liver metastases from colorectal carcinoma. J Clin Oncol. 1994; 12(11):2288–2295

[64] McWilliams JP, Kee ST, Loh CT, Lee EW, Liu DM. Prophylactic embolization of the cystic artery before radioembolization: feasibility, safety, and outcomes. Cardiovasc Intervent Radiol. 2011; 34(4):786–792

[65] Bergman KS, Harris BH. Oriental cholangitis. J Pediatr Surg. 1986; 21(7):573–575

[66] Bismuth H, Nakache R, Diamond T. Management strategies in resection for hilar cholangiocarcinoma. Ann Surg. 1992; 215(1):31–38

[67] Leung JWC, Venezuela RR. Cholangiosepsis: endoscopic drainage and antibiotic therapy. Endoscopy. 1991; 23(4):220–223

[68] Lim JH. Oriental cholangiohepatitis: pathologic, clinical, and radiologic features. AJR Am J Roentgenol. 1991; 157(1):1–8

[69] Mahajani RV, Uzer MF. Cholangiopathy in HIV-infected patients. Clin Liver Dis. 1999; 3(3):669–684, x

[70] Martel JP, McLean CA, Rankin RN. Melanoma of the gallbladder. Radiographics. 2009; 29(1):291–296

[71] Schwemmle K. Gallenwege. In: Koslowski L, Bushe KA, Junginger T, Schwemmle K, eds. Die Chirugie. 4th ed. Stuttgart: Schattauer; 1999:659–669

[72] Shuto R, Kiyosue H, Komatsu E, et al. CT and MR imaging findings of xanthogranulomatous cholecystitis: correlation with pathologic findings. Eur Radiol. 2004; 14(3):440–446

[73] Whitesell FB, Jr. Gallstone ileus. Am Surg. 1970; 36(5):317–322

7 Pancreas

Lars Grenacher and Franziska L. Fritz

7.1 Anatomy

7.1.1 Position

The pancreas is a secondarily retroperitoneal, intra-abdominal gland that is covered anteriorly by peritoneum.[1] The abdominal aorta and inferior vena cava run posterior to the pancreas. The pancreas is directed transversely with its right extremity, the head, nestled in the C-loop of the duodenum. It borders anteriorly on the posterior gastric wall and extends to the left toward the spleen. It forms the posterior boundary of the omental bursa, an intra-abdominal space that communicates with the rest of the abdominal cavity through a small lateral passage, the omental foramen.

The pancreas is approximately 15 cm long, 5 cm wide, and 2 to 3 cm thick and weighs 80 to 120 g.[2] It is a yellowish, lobulated gland whose exocrine tissues produce the pancreatic enzymes (including amylase and lipase) and whose endocrine tissues secrete the hormones insulin and glucagon, which are important in glucose metabolism.[2]

The pancreas is divided into three main parts:
- *Head*: The head of the pancreas rests within the curve of the duodenum and borders on the right side of the superior mesenteric artery and vein. The part of the pancreatic head that is posterior to the two mesenteric vessels is called the uncinate process. A short segment of the common bile duct passes through the pancreatic head. Normally it joins with the pancreatic duct and opens into the duodenum at the major duodenal papilla (of Vater).
- *Body*: The body of the pancreas borders the pancreatic head and is formed by the portions that are anterior to the mesenteric vessels.
- *Tail*: The pancreatic tail is located to the left of the portal vein and closely approaches the spleen.

Histology

The *acinus* is the smallest unit of the pancreas. This terminal glandular element is connected to a side branch, or ductule, into which it secretes its enzymes. Multiple acini combine to form a lobule, hence the description of the pancreas as a "lobulated organ." This lobulation is variable in degree and may be lost as a result of disease.

7.1.2 Blood Supply

The pancreas receives its blood supply from branches of the celiac trunk and the superior mesenteric artery:
- Celiac trunk:
  - The celiac trunk gives rise to the common hepatic artery, from which arises the gastroduodenal artery. The latter vessel, in turn, carries blood to the superior pancreaticoduodenal artery (anterior and posterior branches), which supplies the pancreatic head.[2]
  - The celiac trunk also gives rise to the splenic artery, which gives off branches that supply the tail of the pancreas—the greater pancreatic artery, the artery to the pancreatic tail, and the dorsal pancreatic artery.[2]
- *Superior mesenteric artery*: The head of the pancreas is additionally supplied by the inferior pancreaticoduodenal artery, which arises from the superior mesenteric artery.[1]

The pancreatic head is circled by a vascular anastomosis formed by the superior pancreaticoduodenal artery (from the common hepatic artery) and posterior branches of the inferior pancreaticoduodenal artery (from the superior mesenteric artery).[2]

The pancreatic head is drained by the pancreaticoduodenal veins, which empty into the superior mesenteric vein or open directly into the portal vein. The pancreatic veins drain from the body and tail of the pancreatic into the splenic vein (see ▶ Fig. 7.1).[1]

7.1.3 Development

The pancreas develops from one ventral bud and one dorsal bud, which fuse during embryonic development to form one organ (▶ Fig. 7.2).[1] Each of the buds has one duct, and he two ducts normally unite during development to form the main pancreatic duct.[1] Failure of the two ducts to unite may result in two ducts running the length of the pancreas. With incomplete union of the ducts in the pancreatic head, a remnant of the duct of the dorsal bud may remain as the accessory pancreatic duct (of Santorini).

Exocrine secretions are channeled by the side branches into the pancreatic duct (of Wirsung) and are discharged into the duodenum through the major duodenal papilla (of Vater). The normal diameter of the pancreatic duct is 3 to 5 mm. If an accessory pancreatic duct is present, it may have its own papilla, the minor duodenal papilla, which opens into the duodenum at a more proximal level than the greater duodenal papilla.[2] As a variant, the pancreatic duct may fail to fuse with the common bile duct, so that the latter opens into the duodenum through a separate papilla. Thus, there may be up to three papillae.

Note
The diameter of the pancreatic duct is less than 5 mm.

7.1.4 Imaging Landmarks

▶ **Landmarks in CT and MRI**
- The superior mesenteric artery and vein run at right angles to the pancreas.
- The splenic vein runs along the pancreatic tail from the spleen toward its confluence with the superior mesenteric vein; their union forms the hepatic portal vein. Viewed in coronal section, the splenic vein runs a slightly oblique course and usually descends slightly from the splenic hilum to the splenic–mesenteric confluence.

Pancreas

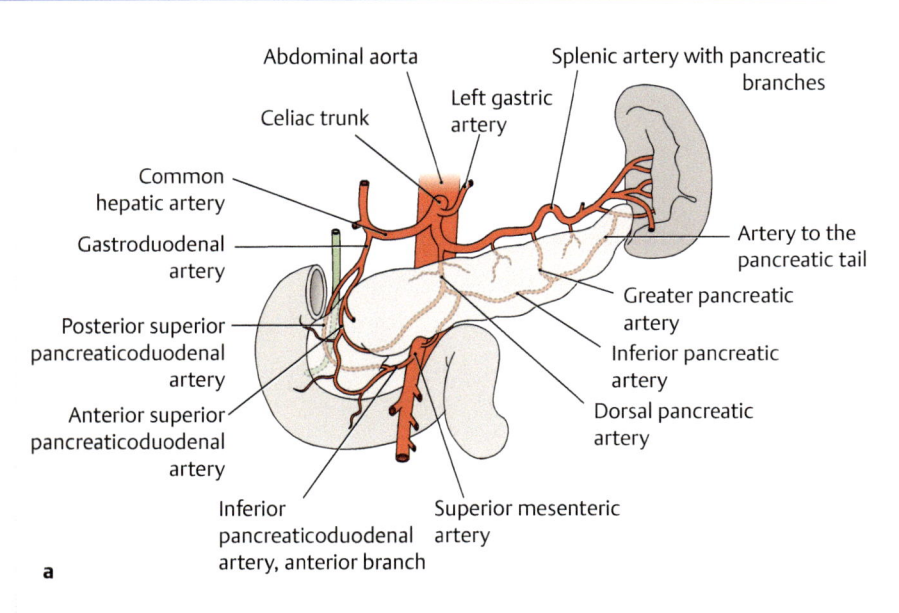

Fig. 7.1 Blood supply of the pancreas and duodenum. Anterior view. (a) Arterial supply. (b) Venous drainage. (Reproduced from Schünke M, Schulte E, Schumacher U. Prometheus. Lern-Atlas der Anatomie: Innere Organe. Illustrated by M. Voll/K. Wesker. 2nd ed. Stuttgart: Thieme; 2009.)

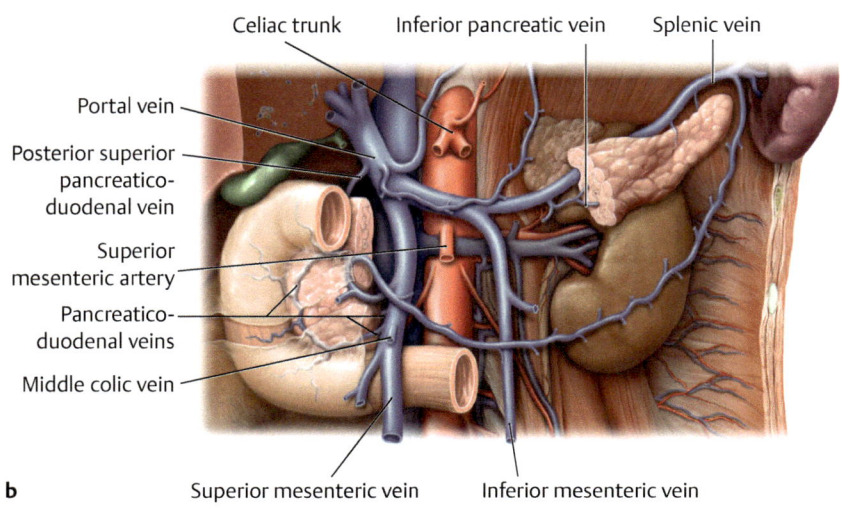

- The head of the pancreas is situated within the duodenal C loop. The uncinate process of the pancreatic head is posterior to the superior mesenteric vein and artery. The "hydro CT" technique (administering IV hyoscine butylbromide to immobilize the bowel, giving 0.5 to 1.5 L of water orally within 30 minutes of imaging, and positioning the patient in 45° left lateral decubitus)[3] can be used to improve contrast between the pancreatic head and surrounding bowel.
- The pancreatic tail is located to the left of the portal vein.

▶ **Sonographic Landmarks**
- Blood vessels are useful landmarks for ultrasound scanning of the pancreas. Orientation can be established by locating the portal vein at the porta hepatis and tracing the vein upward to the portal vein junction, around which lies the pancreatic head.
- Another localizing technique is to image the inferior vena cava and aorta in a transverse scan and follow them to the mesenteric vessels, which are bordered anteriorly by the body of the pancreas.
- The splenic vein is posterior to the pancreas (▶ Fig. 7.1) and provides a landmark for imaging the pancreatic tail.

Note
Because the pancreatic tail is angled slightly upward relative to the pancreatic head, the ultrasound probe should be angled somewhat when positioned below the left costal arch and should be aimed slightly cephalad relative to the left side of the patient.

▶ **Selection of Imaging Modalities.** The initial imaging study in most patients with clinical suspicion of pancreatic disease is upper abdominal ultrasound, as it is widely available and can provide an effective survey centered on the pancreas. Ultrasound can establish a pancreatic cause for the patient's complaints when correlated with other findings. If the cause is still unclear, further investigation by CT or MRI is definitely indicated to exclude a malignant process or detect complications. The preferred imaging modality is decided on an individual basis according to availability and the patient's clinical status. The appropriate application of a given technique for specific entities is described in the sections below. Note that patient-specific parameters such as pain and contraindications to CT or MRI may require some deviation from the gold standard.

7.2 Nonneoplastic Diseases

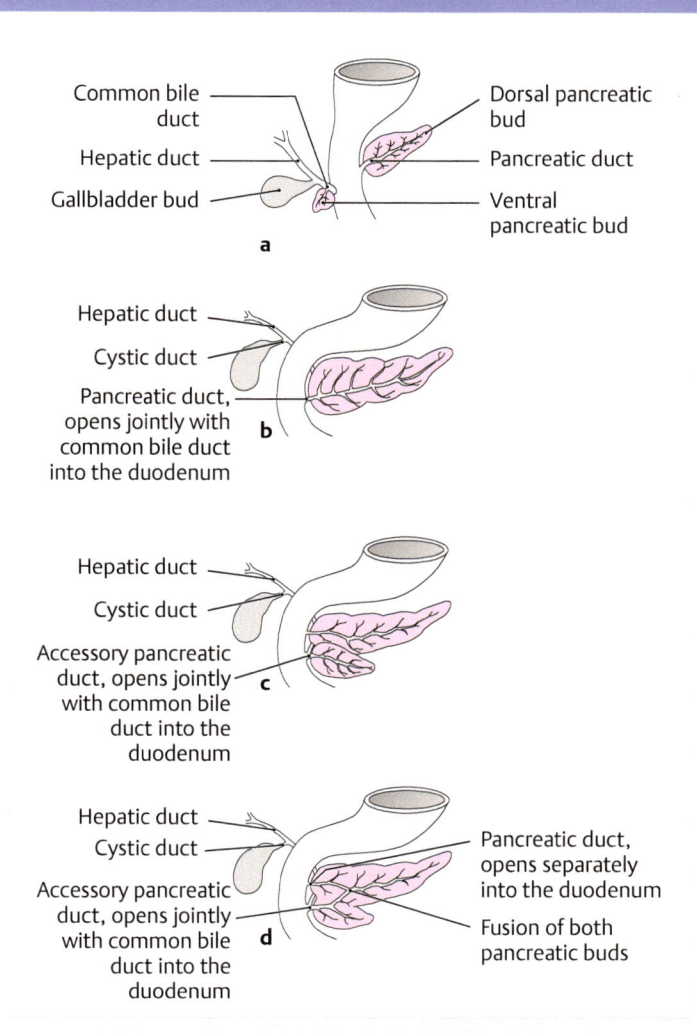

Fig. 7.2 Embryonic development of the pancreas. (a) Dorsal and ventral pancreatic buds. (b) Fusion of the two buds. (c) Failure of fusion of the two ducts of the dorsal and ventral buds. (d) Incomplete fusion of the dorsal and ventral ducts. (Reproduced from Schünke M, Schulte E, Schumacher U. Prometheus. LernAtlas der Anatomie: Innere Organe. Illustrated by M. Voll/K. Wesker. 2nd ed. Stuttgart: Thieme; 2009.)

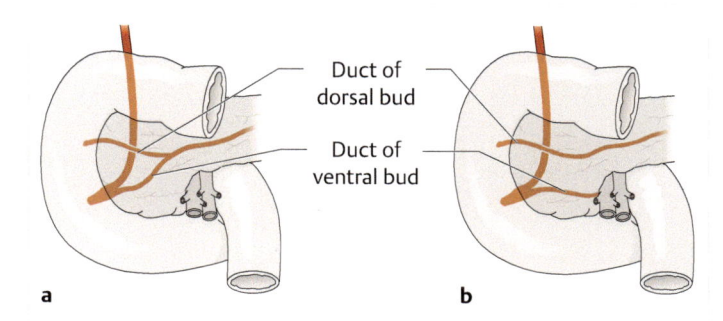

Fig. 7.3 Pancreas divisum. Schematic representation. (a) Incomplete pancreas divisum. (b) Complete pancreas divisum. (Reproduced from Schünke M, Schulte E, Schumacher U. Prometheus. LernAtlas der Anatomie: Innere Organe. Illustrated by M. Voll/K. Wesker. 2nd ed. Stuttgart: Thieme; 2009.)

7.1.5 Normal Variants and Congenital Anomalies

Pancreas Divisum

▶ **Brief definition.** Pancreas divisum is one of the most common congenital malformations of the pancreas.[4] It may be complete or incomplete and results from absent or incomplete fusion of the dorsal and ventral pancreatic buds during embryonic development.[5] Each of the buds has its own duct, and the two ducts normally fuse and drain into the duodenum at the major papilla. In the complete form of pancreas divisum, the ducts fail to unite due to absent or incomplete fusion of the buds, with the result that the pancreatic duct has a separate opening at the minor duodenal papilla (▶ Fig. 7.3a).[5] Secretions from the larger dorsal bud (pancreatic duct) drain through the lesser papilla while the smaller ventral bud drains through an accessory pancreatic duct to the major papilla.[5] With incomplete pancreas divisum, the main pancreatic duct and accessory duct are interconnected by a small channel (▶ Fig. 7.3b, ▶ Fig. 7.4).

▶ **Imaging signs.** Besides the main pancreatic duct, an additional duct is found within the parenchyma of the pancreatic head when pancreas divisum is present. In the complete form of the anomaly, the main pancreatic duct opens at the minor papilla as described above while the accessory pancreatic duct opens jointly with the common bile duct at the major papilla. MRCP is the imaging study of first choice, as it is superior to CT for ductal imaging (see Chapter 6.3.4). A relatively narrow accessory pancreatic duct leads to a rise of intraductal pressure.[6] There is disagreement whether the elevated pressure predisposes to chronic pancreatitis.

Annular Pancreas

▶ **Brief definition.** Annular pancreas is an embryonic malformation of the pancreas that occurs during the fourth week of gestation.[7] It is the second most common congenital anomaly of the pancreas, with a prevalence of 0.05%.[7] Like pancreas divisum, it involves a developmental abnormality of the two pancreatic buds. The ventral bud consists of right and left parts; the left part generally regresses, while the right part migrates around the back of the duodenum and fuses with the dorsal bud.[1] If the left part does not regress but migrates around the front of the duodenum and fuses with the right part, a ring of pancreatic tissue is formed around the C loop of the duodenum (▶ Fig. 7.5). This ring may cause constriction of the duodenum in adults.[1]

▶ **Imaging signs.** CT displays the duodenum surrounded by a continuous ring of uniformly enhancing pancreatic tissue. This tissue is continuous with the pancreatic body and forms the ring from which the condition derives its name (see ▶ Fig. 7.5a). On MRI the tissue is isointense to pancreas in all sequences and encircles the descending part of the duodenum as described above.

▶ **Pitfalls.** An inexperienced examiner may misinterpret the ring of the pancreatic tissue around the duodenum as a complex "cyst" located at the center of the pancreatic head (see ▶ Fig. 7.5a).

7.2 Nonneoplastic Diseases

7.2.1 Acute Pancreatitis

▶ **Brief definition.** Acute pancreatitis is an acute inflammation of the pancreas that runs a mild, self-limiting course in the great

297

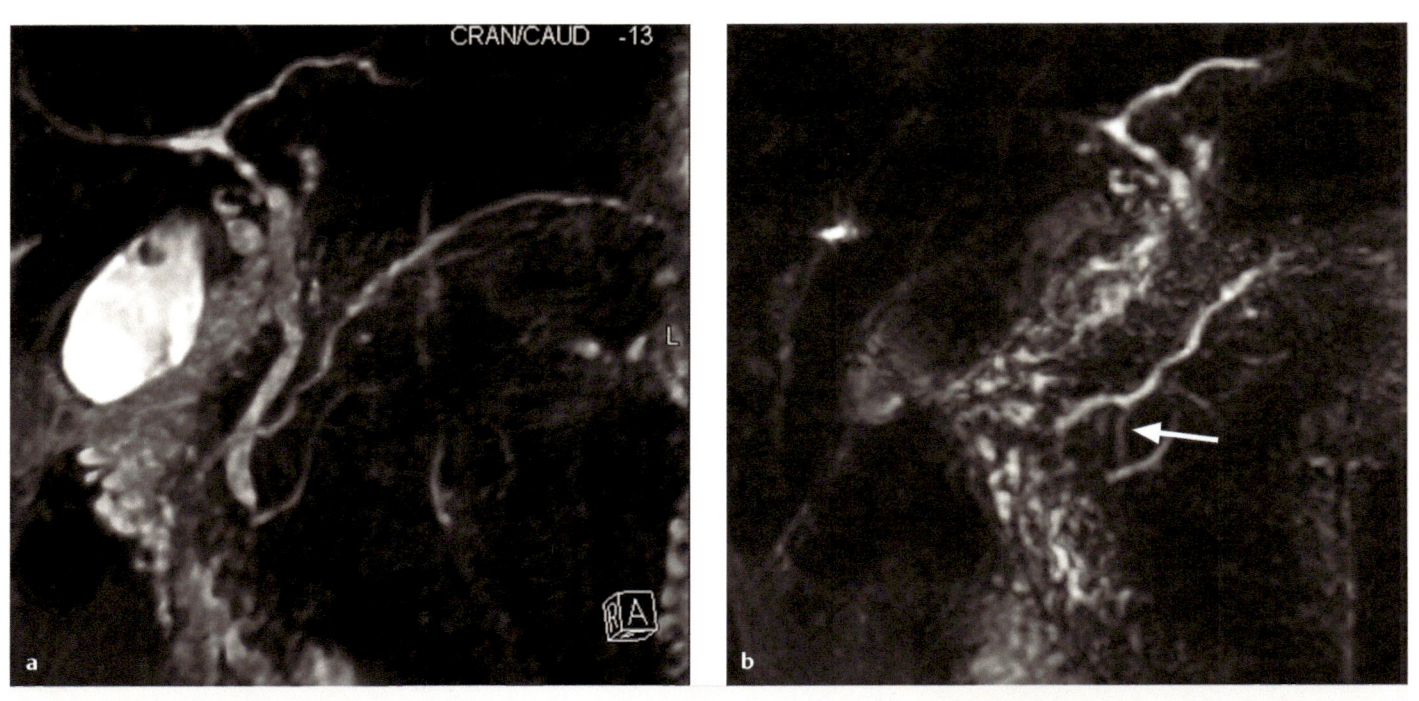

Fig. 7.4 Incomplete pancreas divisum. MRCP. **(a)** The pancreatic ducts open separately into the duodenum. **(b)** The pancreatic ducts are interconnected by a small channel (arrow).

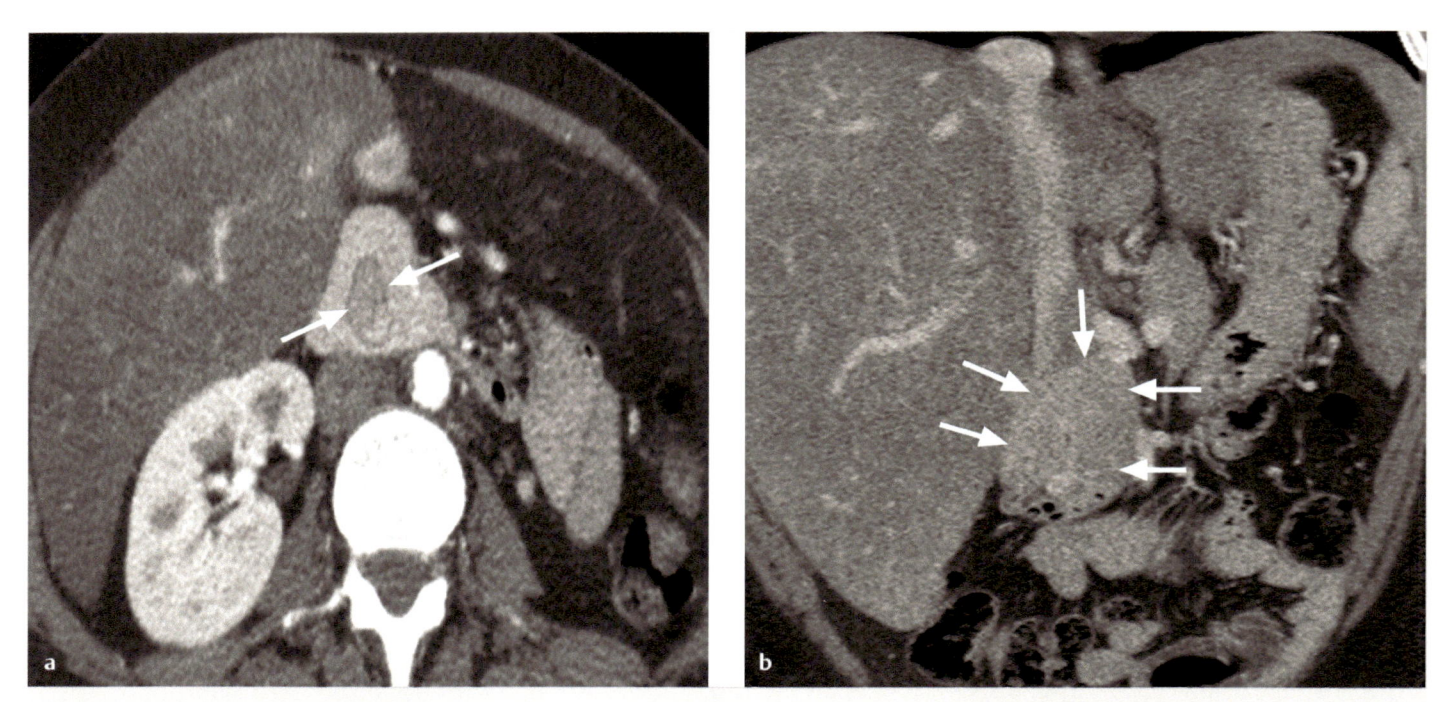

Fig. 7.5 Annular pancreas. Incomplete fusion of the dorsal and ventral pancreatic buds (fourth week of gestation). Pancreatic tissue encircles the duodenum (arrows). **(a)** Axial CT. **(b)** Coronal CT.

majority of cases. In approximately 20% of cases, however, the disease takes a severe course that leads to various complications as well as life-threatening conditions and permanent organ dysfunction.[8] The pathophysiology is believed to involve an uncontrolled activation of the enzyme trypsin in the acinar cells, leading to autodigestion of the pancreas with resulting inflammation and necrosis.[8] A cause cannot be identified in 15 to 20% of adult patients, who are said to have "idiopathic pancreatitis."[8]

An etiology can be established in the remaining 80 to 85% and most commonly involves a biliary cause. The second most frequent cause is alcohol abuse, followed by drug toxicity (corticosteroids, diuretics, etc.), trauma, iatrogenic causes (post-ERCP), infection (mumps, cytomegalovirus, coxsackievirus, etc.), and elevated serum calcium levels as in primary hyperparathyroidism.[8] Acute pancreatitis may lead to many pathologic changes in the organ itself and in regional tissues.[9]

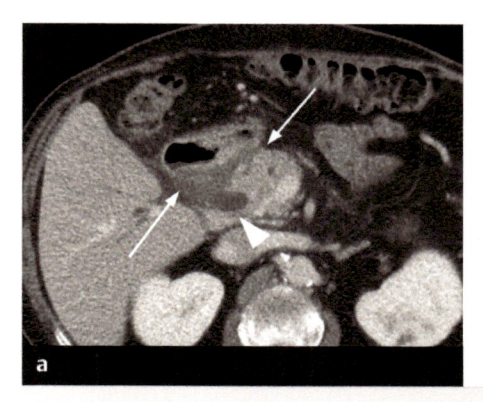

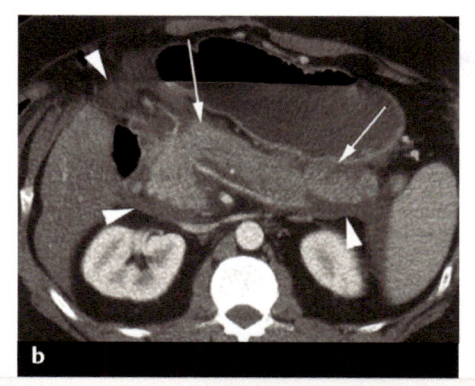

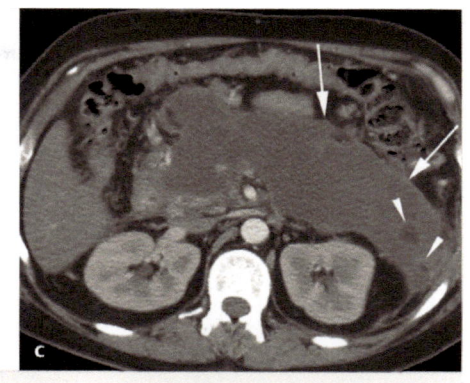

Fig. 7.6 Acute pancreatitis. CT. **(a)** Paraduodenal pancreatitis. Axial CT shows a faintly enhancing fluid collection between the pancreatic head and thickened duodenal wall (arrows) with a typical intramural cyst (arrowhead). **(b)** Edematous interstitial pancreatitis. Enlargement of the pancreas (arrows) and peripancreatic exudates (arrowheads) are typical findings. **(c)** Encapsulated colliquative necrosis (arrows) in necrotizing pancreatitis with fat inclusions (arrowheads) and loss of the normal lobulated structure.

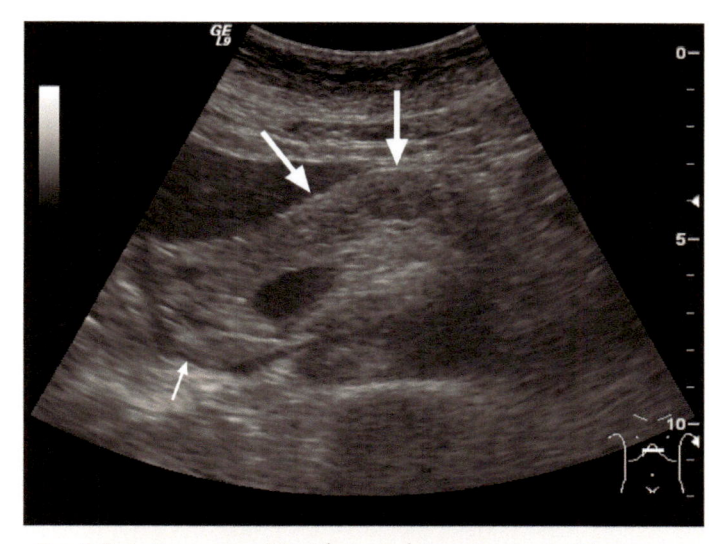

Fig. 7.7 Acute pancreatitis. Ultrasound in acute pancreatitis shows edematous swelling of the pancreatic head and body–tail junction (large arrows) with fluid tracking around the pancreatic head (small arrow).

Caution

Pancreatic necrosis is one of the most serious complications involving the pancreas and should be diagnosed or excluded as early as possible.[8]

Besides complications involving the organ itself, various types of intra-abdominal fluid collections and fat necrosis may occur.[9] Several scoring systems have been developed for assessing severity, including the APACHE II (Acute Physiology and Chronic Health Evaluation), SOFA (Sequential Organ Failure Assessment), and Ranson scores.[10,11,12,13] They all employ a point system for scoring various organ systems. The higher the total score, the more complicated the course.[10] Organs that are affected and scored include the kidney, central nervous system, cardiovascular system, respiratory tract, and hematologic system. Most complications are diagnosed from the clinical examination and laboratory tests.

▶ **Special form: paraduodenal pancreatitis.** Paraduodenal pancreatitis, also called groove pancreatitis, is a type of focal pancreatitis in which the inflammatory process affects the groove between the pancreatic head, the duodenum, and the common bile duct (▶ Fig. 7.6a). If scarring occurs in that area, sectional images may show apparent thickening of the duodenal wall at the level of the papilla or a tumorlike lesion of the pancreatic head, leading to errors in diagnosis.[5] Paraduodenal pancreatitis may also occur in association with a duodenal tumor: The thickened duodenal wall obstructs the papilla and blocks the drainage of biliary and pancreatic secretions, resulting in autolysis of the pancreas.

Note

The findings of paraduodenal pancreatitis include edematous swelling of the pancreatic head and typical fluid collections in the groove between the pancreatic head and the duodenum. The inflammation usually spares the rest of the pancreas. Whenever imaging reveals the typical fluid track, paraduodenal pancreatitis should be suspected and the duodenum evaluated further by endoscopy and biopsy to exclude a malignant process.

▶ **Imaging signs.** The main role of imaging in acute pancreatitis is follow-up and the (prompt) detection of complications. Pancreatitis can be diagnosed from clinical and laboratory findings. Transabdominal ultrasound can be added when scanning conditions are good and will show a hypoechoic, edematous pancreas with fluid collections and possible cholestasis (▶ Fig. 7.7). CT and MRI are unnecessary for making a diagnosis. Both modalities are used if complications arise.

Caution

The radiological exclusion of pancreatic necrosis should be delayed at least 72 hours after onset of symptoms to avoid false-negative results, as some time is needed for the visible demarcation of necrosis. MRI and CT are equivalent in their ability to detect necrosis, but contrast-enhanced CT is preferred from the standpoint of examination time and patient tolerance, as patients with acute pancreatitis are seriously ill and a shorter scan time may be beneficial.

CT demonstrates fluid collections around the pancreas (▶ Fig. 7.6b). Necrosis appears as an ill-defined hypodense area in the pancreas with loss of normal lobular architecture and loss of definition of normal organ boundaries (▶ Fig. 7.6c). Infection of the necrotic area by ascending intestinal organisms leads to abscess formation, with such typical imaging as air inclusions and an enhancing abscess wall. Intra- and/or extrahepatic cholestasis may be noted, depending on location and etiology. Portal vein thrombosis with ascites may develop. Pleural effusion and other pulmonary complications such as infiltrates may also be found. A unilateral pleural effusion (usually on the left side) in pancreatitis is called a "sympathetic" pleural effusion. Opacity of both lungs is suspicious for ARDS as a complication of pancreatitis. Some patients develop a reactive paralytic ileus in response to retroperitoneal irritation, characterized by distended bowel loops and air–fluid levels. Coagulation defects in a setting of severe acute pancreatitis may lead to spontaneous intra-abdominal hemorrhage, and CT may show diffuse stranding of the intra-abdominal fat. CT is also used to direct the percutaneous drainage of necrotic areas and abscesses.

▶ Clinical features. The main clinical findings are acute upper abdominal pain combined with at least a 3-fold elevation of amylase and lipase activity and increased C-reactive protein activity. The upper abdominal pain may be a girdling pain that radiates to the back. Nausea and vomiting may also be present.[14] Other possible symptoms are jaundice due to obstruction of the common bile duct, ascites, and pleural effusion, which indicate a severe course. On physical examination, the Grey–Turner sign may be noted in the flank region and Cullen's sign around the umbilicus.[8] Bruising in the flank and periumbilical regions is considered pathognomonic for severe acute pancreatitis (▶ Fig. 7.8). It occurs when the autodigestive process spreads from sites of pancreatic necrosis into adjacent abdominal compartments and causes disruption of cutaneous vessels with formation of hematoma.[8] The central question to be addressed in acute pancreatitis is whether it is a mild or severe form:
- *Mild form*: In the Atlanta Classification, the mild form of acute pancreatitis is associated with minimal organ dysfunction and a self-limiting course. It requires fluid replacement along with antiemetic and analgesic therapy.[15]
- *Severe form*: Severe cases require patient surveillance in ICU due to the potential for systemic complications with sepsis, hypovolemic shock, and multisystem organ failure.[15]

The Atlanta Classification of acute pancreatitis has been revised since its inception. In addition to mild and severe forms, the latest revision distinguishes between an early phase (within the first week of onset) and a late phase (after the first week of onset).[16] In the early phase of acute pancreatitis, a severe form is defined as organ failure of more than 48 hours' duration; in the late phase it is defined as permanent organ failure, death, or complications.[16] In the revised Atlanta Classification, the Marshall score is used to evaluate organ failure based on scores for the respiratory, cardiovascular, and renal systems.[16]

Note
A daily clinical examination that includes the above scores is important, as it is the only way to ensure the prompt detection of complications and the institution of appropriate treatment and surveillance.

Serum amylase and serum lipase are the two pancreatic enzymes that are determined in patients with acute pancreatitis. At least a 3-fold increase in amylase activity combined with increased lipase activity support the diagnosis when correlated with clinical findings. The enzyme activities remain elevated for approximately 3 to 5 days.[8] Enzyme elevation in the absence of clinical findings, or the presence of atypical clinical findings, is insufficient for a diagnosis of pancreatitis, and a differential diagnosis is required. Pancreatic enzymes are not useful parameters for follow-up.

▶ Differential diagnosis
- Acute exacerbation of chronic pancreatitis.
- A malignant process in the pancreatic head or adjacent duodenum that has caused pancreatitis due to compression of the common bile duct.

▶ Pitfalls. The premature use of CT to exclude necrosis may yield false-negative findings. On the whole, sectional imaging should be used sparingly in acute pancreatitis because mild cases do not require it.

▶ Key points. In 80% of cases acute pancreatitis is a mild, self-limiting disease that does not require sectional imaging. In the 20% of patients with severe disease, sectional imaging should be used for the exclusion of necrosis and other complications. It should not be scheduled earlier than 72 hours after symptom onset.

7.2.2 Chronic Pancreatitis
▶ Brief definition. Chronic pancreatitis is a chronic inflammation of the pancreas that leads to fibrotic changes in the organ

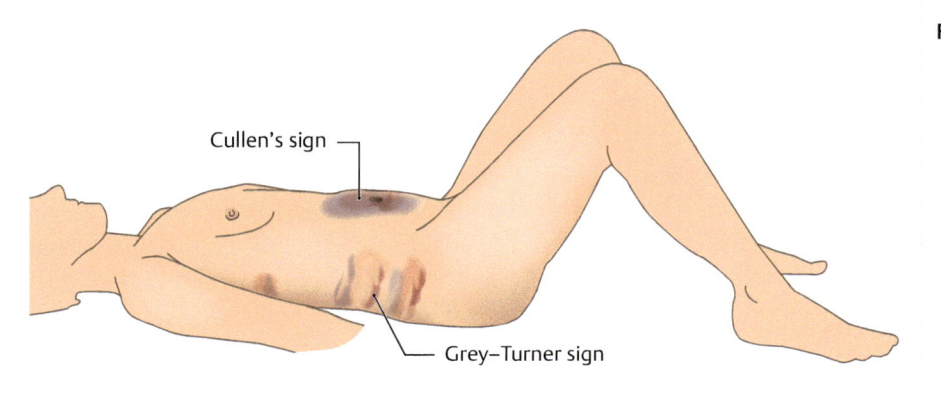

Fig. 7.8 Cullen's sign and Grey–Turner sign.

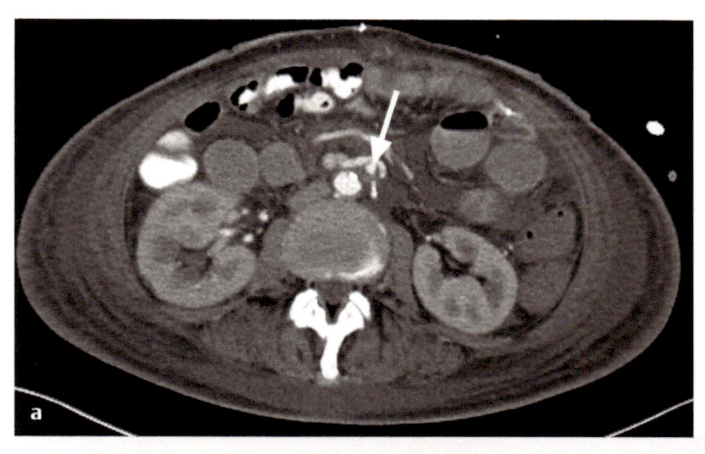

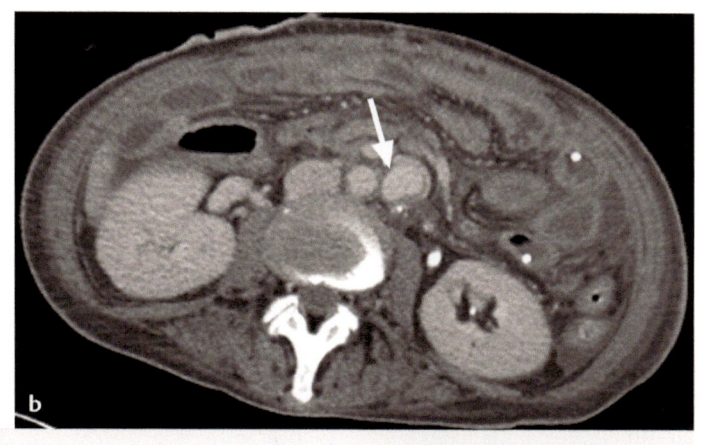

Fig. 7.9 Superior mesenteric artery pseudoaneurysm in pancreatitis. CT. **(a)** Scan in the arterial phase shows a small pseudoaneurysm of the superior mesenteric artery (arrow) following a pylorus-preserving pancreatic head resection. **(b)** Scan in the venous phase 3 weeks later shows marked enlargement of the pseudoaneurysm (arrow).

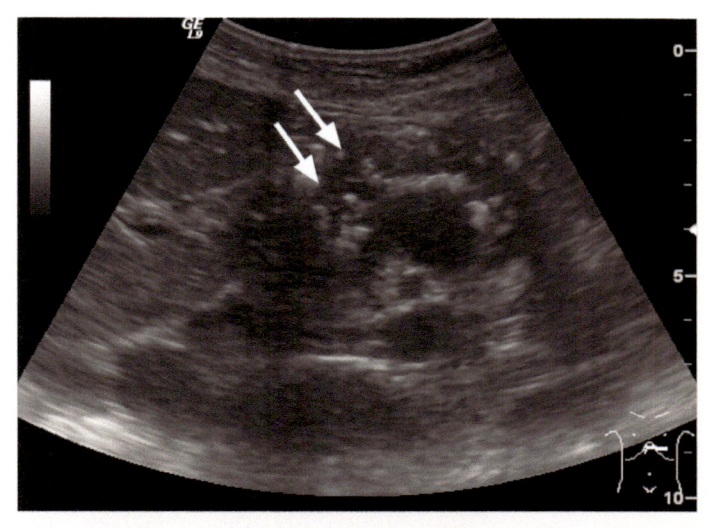

Fig. 7.10 Chronic pancreatitis. Ultrasound. The pancreatic parenchyma has a very inhomogeneous overall texture. It is permeated by acoustic shadows (echo-free areas, arrows) arising from stippled intrapancreatic calcifications.

and destruction of the duct system with consequent long-term exocrine and endocrine pancreatic insufficiency.[17] The disease leads to functional and morphological organ damage. Chronic pancreatitis has a worldwide incidence of 1.6 to 2.3/100,000 population per year, with a rising prevalence.[18] The leading cause of chronic pancreatitis in adults is alcohol abuse, which underlies 50 to 84% of cases.[17,19] Daily alcohol consumption of 80 g or more for a period of 6 to 12 years is considered a risk factor for the development of chronic pancreatitis.[20] Idiopathic chronic pancreatitis ranks second, accounting for 28% of cases.[17] Approximately 45% of these cases are referable to genetic factors.[17] Researchers have identified several gene mutations that predispose to chronic pancreatitis, such as the cationic trypsinogen gene (*PRSSI*). Mutations of this gene lead to chronic pancreatitis with a penetrance of up to 80%.[21] Another, less common cause is hyperparathyroidism. Pancreas divisum is suspected of increasing the risk of chronic pancreatitis, but this link has not been proven.[17] Besides long-term exocrine and endocrine pancreatic insufficiency, other typical complications have been identified: Pseudocyst formation may be clinically silent or may lead to infection and intralesional hemorrhage. Moreover, the infection of necrotic tissue may have severe and potentially fatal consequences. Pseudoaneurysms of the splenic artery or superior mesenteric artery may form in the chronically inflamed pancreas. There may also be biliary tract obstruction with impaired biliary drainage, pyloric and duodenal stenosis, and fistulation to the skin, adjacent hollow organs, or the (retro)peritoneum (▶ Fig. 7.9). Imaging cannot always positively distinguish between inflammation and neoplasia, and equivocal findings always require histological investigation. Patients with chronic pancreatitis are at increased risk for developing pancreatic cancer.[22]

> **Note**
>
> Chronic pancreatitis is a chronic inflammation of the pancreas leading to fibrotic organ changes and duct destruction with consequent long-term exocrine and endocrine insufficiency. The leading cause is alcohol abuse. Complications include pseudocysts, necrosis, pseudoaneurysms, strictures, fistulas, and malignant transformation.

▶ **Imaging signs.** Imaging in chronic pancreatitis is the third diagnostic pillar along with clinical examination and function tests. Imaging is also used for follow-up, for the investigation of complications, and if necessary to direct preoperative planning. The initial imaging study of choice is transabdominal ultrasound (▶ Fig. 7.10). This is useful for initial diagnosis and for detecting complications such as pseudocysts (echo-free with posterior acoustic enhancement) and biliary tract obstruction with cholestasis (diameter of the common bile duct up to 7 mm in patients with a gallbladder, up to 10 mm after cholecystectomy). Other imaging modalities are contrast-enhanced ultrasound for detection of necrosis (preferred over CT with iodinated contrast in patients with impaired renal function)[17]; endoscopic ultrasound, which can detect early parenchymal changes owing to its higher spatial resolution[17]; and CT and MRI, which have an adjunctive role. CT and MRI are particularly useful for differentiating chronic pancreatitis from tumor, the follow-up of complications, and preoperative planning. Sectional imaging can also be important in determining etiology, as it can detect congenital anomalies such as pancreas divisum as well as autoimmune pancreatitis. Signs of

Pancreas

chronic pancreatitis are parenchymal calcifications (▶ Fig. 7.11), parenchymal atrophy, and, in an acute flare, edematous enlargement of the pancreas with peripancreatic fluid collections. Pseudocysts are sharply circumscribed lesions of fluid density or fluid signal intensity that do not communicate with the duct system and usually originate from necrotic areas. Pseudoaneurysms can be detected in the arterial phase of enhancement. Necrotic areas appear hypodense on CT scans. Air inclusions signify the infection of a necrotic area (▶ Fig. 7.12).

Note

The addition of MRCP to the MRI protocol has replaced ERCP in recent years because it eliminates the risk of post-ERCP pancreatitis.

MRCP uses a T2 W sequence that depicts fluid-filled structures in the upper abdomen with high signal intensity. Thus, MRCP can provide ERCP-like visualization of the gallbladder and secretion-filled ductal structures, but with noninvasive technique. The progression of chronic pancreatitis can be described in terms of the changes found in the side branches of the main pancreatic duct. The changes begin at the periphery of the side branches, causing distal expansion and obstruction, and then advance toward the main duct, which shows progressive dilatation and irregularities. The diagnostic use of ERCP is still recommended in selected cases, as in patients with suspected autoimmune pancreatitis. Researchers have identified four ERCP criteria that are diagnostic of autoimmune pancreatitis with high sensitivity and specificity[17]:

- Stenosis of the pancreatic duct involving more than one-third of the duct length.
- No distal dilatation of the pancreatic duct.
- Dilatation of the side branches.
- Multifocal strictures along the full length of the pancreatic duct ("sausage-shaped pancreas").

ERCP is also used as a minimally invasive therapeutic procedure.

▶ **Clinical features.** Possible symptoms of chronic pancreatitis are recurrent abdominal pain (usually a girdling pain of the upper abdomen), vomiting, jaundice, weight loss, and laboratory tests showing increased activity of serum amylase and serum lipase to more than three times normal values. There may as

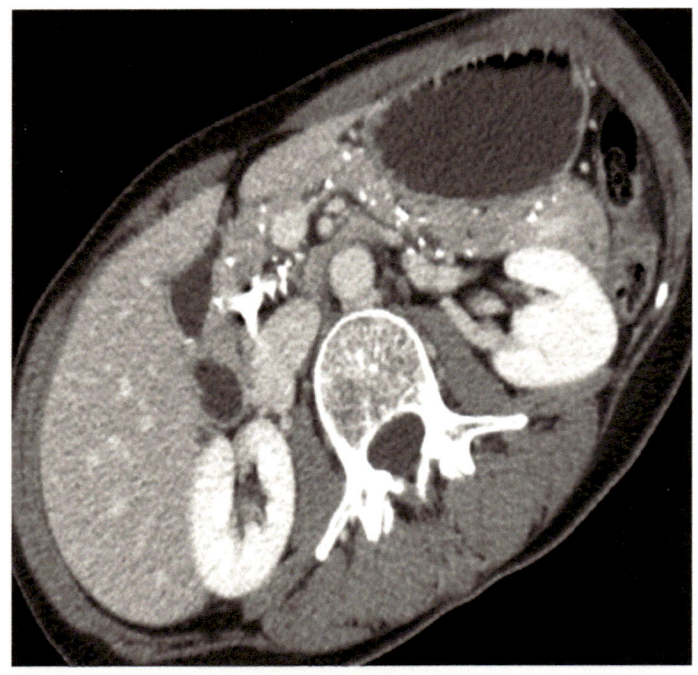

Fig. 7.11 **Chronic pancreatitis.** CT shows atrophy of the pancreas (here, in the body) accompanied by stippled and/or flocculent peri- or intraductal calcifications.

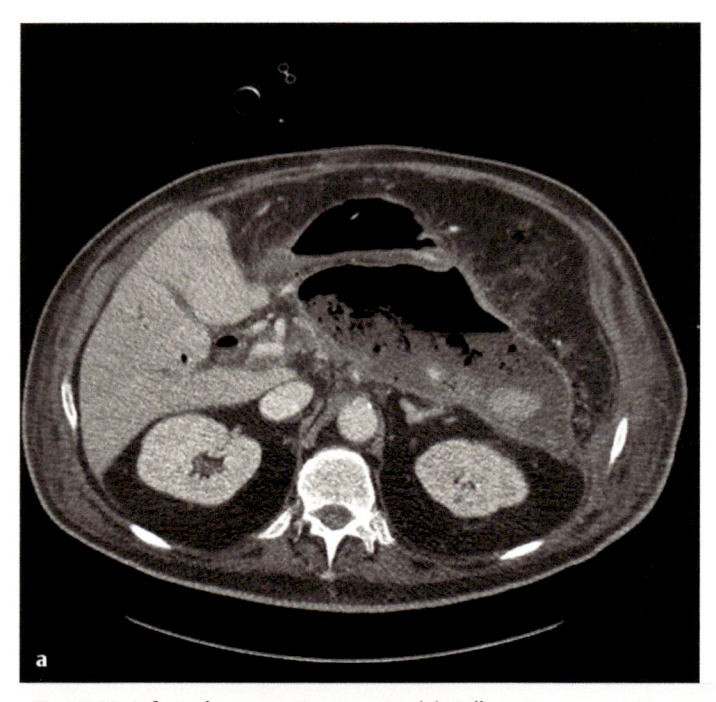

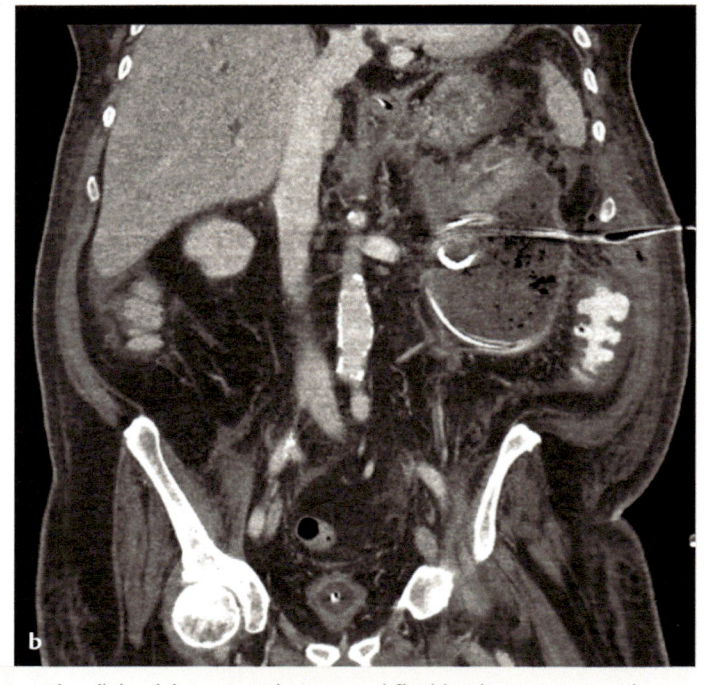

Fig. 7.12 **Infected pancreatic necrosis.** (a) Colliquative pancreatic necrosis with cellular debris, air inclusions, and fluid levels consistent with infected pancreatic necrosis. (b) Interventional placement of a 16F drain into the infection cavity, with drainage of putrid fluid.

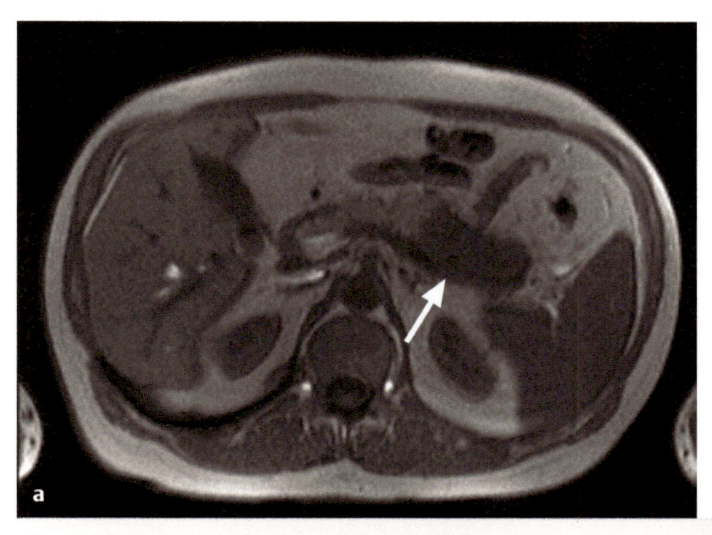

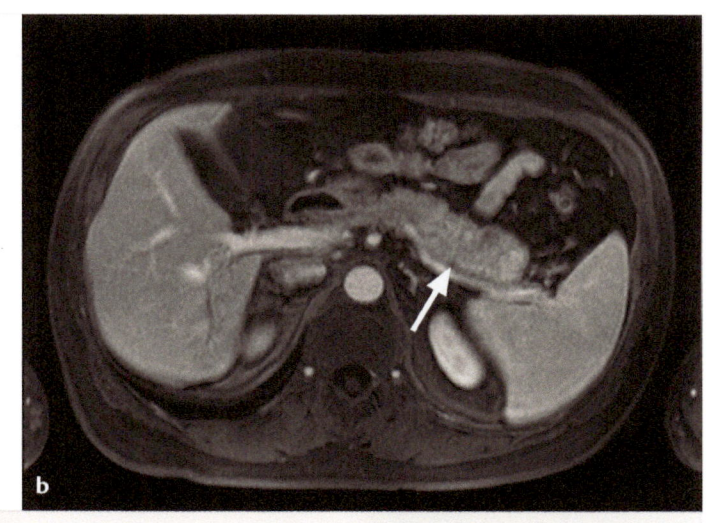

Fig. 7.13 Autoimmune pancreatitis. MRI. (a) T1W image shows a tumorlike lesion that is markedly hypointense to the rest of the pancreas (arrow). (b) Image in the late venous phase shows typical delayed enhancement (arrow).

associated symptoms relating to complications of chronic pancreatitis, such as sepsis, respiratory insufficiency, renal failure, and exocrine and endocrine pancreatic insufficiency due to tissue necrosis.[17]

▶ **Differential diagnosis.** Differentiation is mainly required from pancreatic cancer; this cannot always be positively accomplished by imaging. Etiology should also be considered in the differential diagnosis.

▶ **Pitfalls.** Undertaking CT imaging less than 72 hours after onset of symptoms may cause necrosis to be missed. On the other hand, hypoperfusion of the inflamed pancreas at the start of an acute flare may be misinterpreted as necrosis. The most serious error is a delay in diagnosing pancreatic cancer, so that histological confirmation should be obtained whenever uncertainty exists. Pseudoaneurysms that are not diagnosed may become a source of active bleeding.

▶ **Key points.** Abdominal ultrasound is the initial imaging study of choice in chronic pancreatitis. ERCP, MRI/MRCP, and CT can be used to investigate etiology and complications and for follow-up. Chronic pancreatitis always requires differentiation from pancreatic cancer, and equivocal imaging findings require histological confirmation.

Subtype: Autoimmune Pancreatitis

▶ **Brief definition.** Autoimmune pancreatitis is a rare cause of chronic pancreatitis and has been recognized as a separate entity only since 1995.[23] The process involves an elevation of serum immunoglobulins leading systemically to inflammatory fibrosis in multiple organs, including the pancreas. Autoimmune pancreatitis has a nonspecific clinical presentation marked by upper abdominal pain, weight loss, and jaundice.[17,19,24] The disease shows excellent response to steroid therapy.[17] Four main histological criteria have been identified[17,24]:
- Interstitial fibrosis.
- Lymphoplasmacytic infiltration.
- Predominantly periductal infiltration.
- Periphlebitis.

▶ **Imaging signs.** ERCP and ultrasound can demonstrate segmental or diffuse narrowing of the pancreatic duct along with nonspecific signs such as pancreatic edema. Sectional imaging aids differentiation from pancreatic cancer. Unenhanced MRI in autoimmune pancreatitis shows an area of decreased T1W signal intensity and increased T2W signal intensity in approximately one-half of cases. The area is hypointense in the arterial phase after IV injection of contrast medium, hyperintense in the venous phase in approximately 65% of cases, and hyperintense in the late venous phase (delayed enhancement) in 74% of cases. This hyperintensity in the venous and late venous phases is strongly suggestive of autoimmune pancreatitis.[24] CT does not show corresponding high attenuation in the venous phase, and MRI is therefore superior to CT for this application[24] (▶ Fig. 7.13).

▶ **Differential diagnosis.** As in other types of chronic pancreatitis, differentiation is mainly required from pancreatic cancer.

7.3 Neoplastic Diseases

The most important pancreatic tumors are reviewed in ▶ Table 7.1.

7.3.1 Ductal Adenocarcinoma

▶ **Brief definition.** Ductal adenocarcinoma of the pancreas, commonly known as "pancreatic cancer" or "pancreatic carcinoma," is by far the most common pancreatic tumor, accounting for 75 to 90% of cases.[2] Approximately 53,070 new cases of pancreatic cancer are expected each year in the United States[25] according to the American Cancer Society. It has the poorest prognosis of all malignancies, with a relative 5-year survival rate of approximately 5%.[26] The etiology of pancreatic cancer is not fully understood. There are risk factors that increase the likelihood that individuals will develop pancreatic cancer at some point during their lifetime; these include nicotine abuse, alcohol abuse, obesity, and chronic pancreatitis.[22,27,28] Ductal adenocarcinoma arises from the exocrine pancreas. It invades surrounding structures at an early stage and undergoes early metastasis.[2] Only about 15 to 20% of

Table 7.1 Principal tumors of the pancreas[2]

Exocrine/endocrine	Malignancy	Entities	Frequency (%)
Exocrine (epithelial) tumors	Malignant	• Ductal adenocarcinoma	75–90
		• Adenosquamous carcinoma	4
		• Intraductal papillary mucinous carcinoma	3
		• Mucinous cystadenocarcinoma	1
		• Acinar cell adenocarcinoma	1
		• Serous cystadenocarcinoma	<1
		• Pancreatoblastoma (in children)	<1
	Borderline	• Mucinous cystic neoplasm with dysplasia	
		• Intraductal papillary mucinous neoplasm with dysplasia	
		• Solid pseudopapillary tumor	
	Benign	• Serous cystadenoma	
		• Mucinous cystadenoma	
		• Intraductal papillary mucinous adenoma	
		• Mature teratoma	
Neuro endocrine tumors		• Insulinoma	
		• Gastrinoma	
		• VIPoma	
		• Glucagonoma	
		• Somatostatinoma	
		• Non–hormone-secreting tumors	

pancreatic cancers are resectable at the time of diagnosis. A complete R0 resection plus adjuvant chemotherapy is the only treatment strategy that significantly prolongs survival time, achieving 5-year survival rates of 24%.[2,29,30,31] It is essential, therefore, to determine tumor resectability so that patients can be triaged to appropriate therapies. This ensures the best possible prognosis while also sparing patients the risks and morbidity of surgery for unresectable disease. All diagnostic modalities can be used for diagnostic confirmation, TNM staging, and assessment of resectability. ▶ Table 7.2 shows the TNM classification system for pancreatic cancer recommended by the Union for International Cancer Control (UICC). The corresponding stage groupings are shown in ▶ Table 7.3.

Note

Invasion of the peripancreatic arteries is a key factor in determining local resectability. The relevant vessels are the superior mesenteric artery, celiac trunk, common hepatic artery, portal vein, and superior mesenteric vein.[2] If the vessels are free of tumor tissue, the tumor is considered resectable. If tumor tissue extends to the vessels, however, it becomes difficult to evaluate vascular invasion.[2]

There are several approaches for determining resectability. In some, contact of the tumor with the vessel is expressed as percentage or degrees of encasement (where 90–180° of encasement indicates invasion), while other methods use caliber reduction or occlusion to indicate vascular invasion (see ▶ Fig. 7.9b).[2,33,34,35,36] Newer versions of these classifications differentiate between arterial and venous invasion.[39] Frequently, venous invasion is not a criterion for nonresectability at pancreatic surgery centers where involved veins are resected.[2] Distant metastasis is generally considered to indicate nonresectability, but again there are centers where case-by-case decisions are made. For example, a single hepatic metastasis may be present and could be resected along with a locally resectable pancreatic cancer.[2]

▶ **Imaging signs.** Transabdominal ultrasound has only a limited role in the diagnosis of pancreatic cancer. Adenocarcinoma is hypoechoic or isoechoic to normal pancreatic tissue on ultrasound scans, which may also show dilatation of the pancreatic duct and atrophy of the pancreas. Adenocarcinoma can be diagnosed with an accuracy of 87.8% when ultrasound contrast agents are used.[40] The first attempts to quantify transabdominal ultrasound with contrast agents showed an information gain for discriminating between pancreatitis and pancreatic cancer, although the sensitivity and specificity of this method have not yet been fully investigated. Endoscopic ultrasound scanning through the duodenum or posterior gastric wall can detect pancreatic tumors smaller than 1 cm in diameter.[41,42] Endoscopic ultrasound-guided fine needle aspiration can be used for preoperative histological differentiation of solid pancreatic tumors.

It has been shown, however, that 31% of patients with negative fine needle histology were subsequently found to have pancreatic cancer.[43]

Table 7.2 TNM classification of exocrine pancreatic carcinoma[32]

Designation	Description
Primary tumor	
Tis	Carcinoma in situ
T1	Tumor limited to the pancreas, 2 cm or less in greatest dimension
T2	Tumor limited to the pancreas, more than 2 cm in greatest dimension
T3	Tumor extends past the pancreas but does not invade the celiac trunk or superior mesenteric artery
T4	Tumor invades the celiac trunk or superior mesenteric artery
Lymph nodes	
N0	No regional lymph node metastasis
N1	Regional lymph node metastasis (peripancreatic, pancreaticoduodenal, pyloric, splenic hilum, proximal mesenteric and celiac nodes)
Distant metastasis	
M0	No distant metastasis
M1	Distant metastasis (liver, lung, skeleton, brain)

Table 7.3 Staging of pancreatic carcinoma[32]

Stage	Groupings
0	Tis N0 M0
I	T1 N0 M0 to T2 N0 M0
• IA	T1 N0 M0
• IB	T2 N0 M0
II	T3 N0 M0 to T1–T3 N1 M0
• IIA	T3 N0 M0
• IIB	T1–T3 N1 M0
III	T4 Any N M0
IV	Any T Any N M1

Note

CT is the most widely used diagnostic modality for suspected pancreatic cancer because of its high spatial resolution. The examination should employ a multidetector-row scanner, a biphasic contrast protocol with a pancreatic parenchymal phase and portal venous phase, and a maximum slice thickness of 3 mm. Use of the hydro-CT technique is also recommended.

Hypovascular pancreatic cancer generally appears on CT as an ill-defined lesion that is hypodense to surrounding tissue (▶ Fig. 7.14a, b). Approximately 11% of pancreatic cancers are isodense to surrounding tissue, however, and must be diagnosed indirectly from secondary signs such as cholestasis, interruption of the pancreatic duct with prestenotic ductal dilatation, and atrophy of the remaining pancreas.[44] Contiguous obstruction of the pancreatic and common bile ducts is called the "double duct sign" and indicates a mass in the pancreatic head (▶ Fig. 7.14c). MRI should employ at least a 1.5 T field strength and standard pulse sequences with a slice thickness of 5 to 7 mm. As well as unenhanced T1 W and T2 W sequences, a contrast-enhanced T1 W sequence should also be obtained to exclude hemangiomas, for example, in patients with equivocal hepatic lesions. Diagnostic ERCP can be performed in palliative settings where biopsy confirmation is needed prior to palliative chemotherapy or radiation.[45] There is no significant difference between CT and MRI in the detection of pancreatic cancer, and both modalities yield almost identical results in the assessment of resectability.[46]

Note

The questions that the radiologist should answer for the surgeon pertain to local tumor extent (location? contiguity to surrounding structures?), the presence or absence of distant metastasis, and the invasion of peripancreatic arteries. The lymph nodes should be described, especially when lymphadenopathy is found. A nonpathologic lymph node status does not exclude nodal metastasis, however.

▶ **Clinical features.** Pancreatic cancer usually goes undetected in its early stages because it produces no symptoms.[47] Clinical manifestations occur only at advanced stages when the tumor has invaded surrounding tissue or metastasized to other organs. The three most common symptoms of pancreatic cancer are:
- Epigastric pain (pancreatic head carcinoma) or back pain (carcinoma of the pancreatic body or tail).
- Painless obstructive jaundice due to pancreatic head carcinoma.
- B symptoms including more than 10% undesired weight loss during the previous 6 months.

Other symptoms are recurrent pancreatitis due to obstruction of the pancreatic duct by pancreatic head carcinoma and venous thrombosis caused, for example, by tumor-induced secretion of procoagulant mediators or activation of the coagulation system.[48] Approximately 25% of patients have diabetes mellitus when their pancreatic cancer is initially diagnosed, and approximately 40% have reduced glucose tolerance.[47]

Note

Pancreatitis of unknown cause after 50 years of age is always suspicious for carcinoma and requires appropriate evaluation.[45]

If ascites is already present at the time of diagnosis, this suggests that hepatic metastasis or peritoneal seeding has already occurred.

▶ **Differential diagnosis.** Rare pancreatic tumors such as aggressive anaplastic carcinoma or acinar–endocrine carcinoma

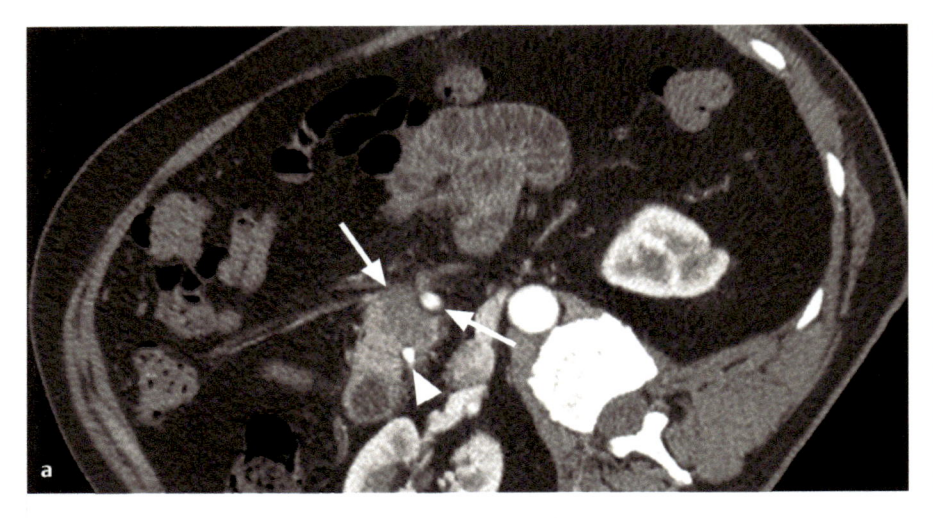

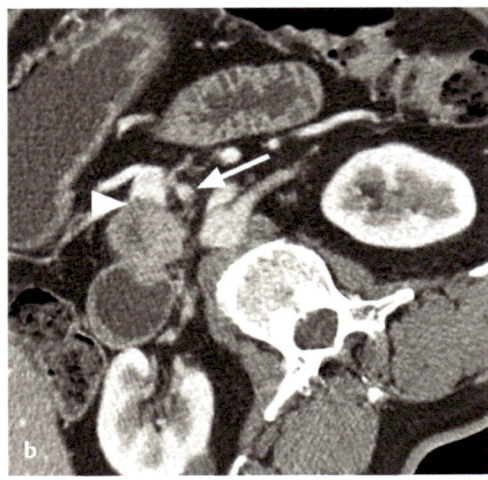

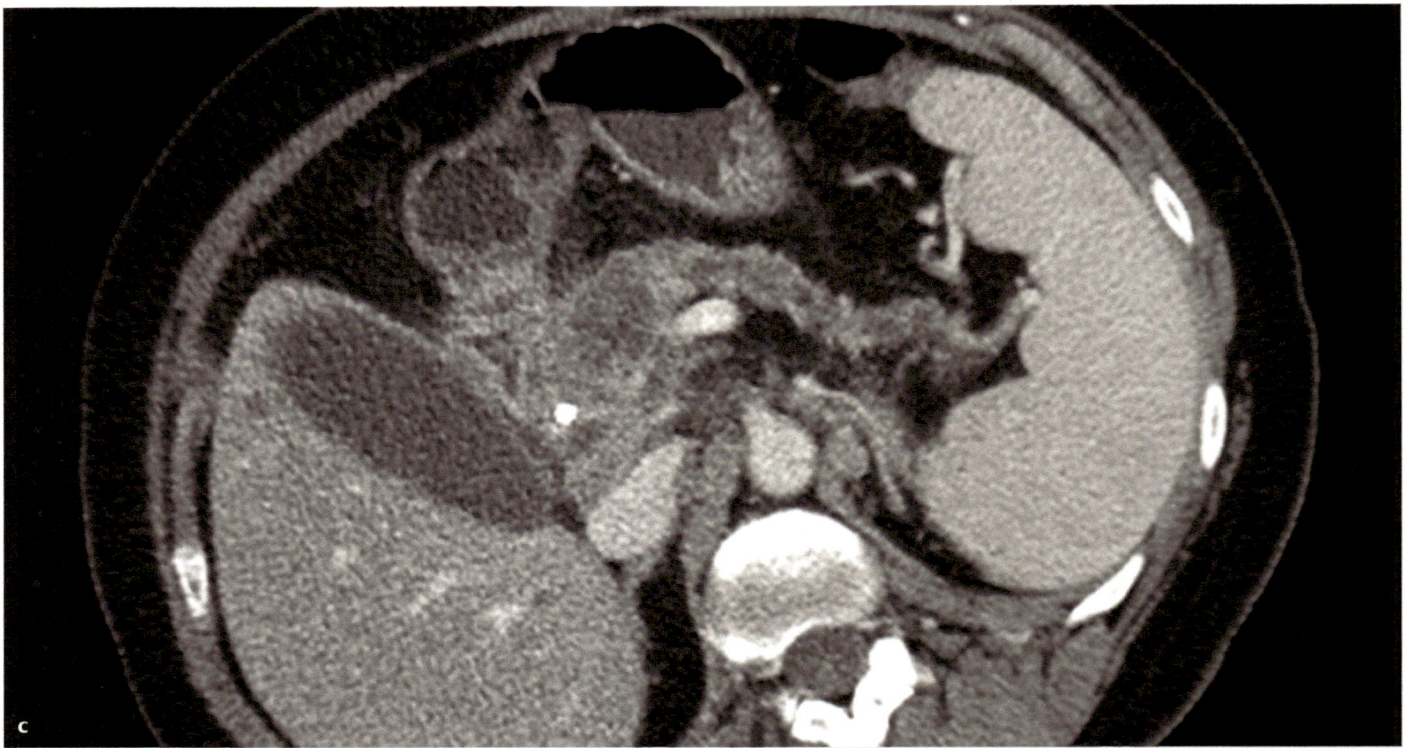

Fig. 7.14 Pancreatic carcinoma. (a) CT in the arterial phase. Despite the presence of an endoprosthesis (arrowhead), the hypodense tumor (arrow) is clearly defined at a spatial resolution of 0.33 mm. Its relationship to nearby vessels (upward-pointing arrow) is also well defined. **(b)** CT in the venous phase. The pancreatic head carcinoma is hypodense in the venous phase, showing 90–180° invasion of the superior mesenteric vein (arrowhead) and 90° invasion of the superior mesenteric vein (arrow). **(c)** CT in the venous phase. Advanced pancreatic carcinoma is hypodense to surrounding parenchyma, with an interrupted duct sign and dilatation of the pancreatic duct distal to the tumor. The rest of the pancreas is atrophic. The tumor has invaded the peripancreatic tissue and peripancreatic vessels.

may present the same CT features. Differentiation in this case must rely on histology.

Pancreatitis is the most important differential diagnosis for pancreatic cancer and is a frequent cause of misdiagnosis.[46]

▶ **Key points.** The only treatment for pancreatic cancer that can significantly improve prognosis is an R0 resection followed by adjuvant chemotherapy. Thus, an accurate preoperative assessment of resectability by sectional imaging is of prime importance for the patient. CT is the most widely used modality for the detection of pancreatic cancer, although MRI and CT are comparable in their ability to detect the disease and determine its resectability.

7.3.2 Neuroendocrine Tumors

▶ **Brief definition.** Neuroendocrine tumors are rare, slow-growing tumors of the pancreas that originate from the islets of Langerhans.[2,49,50] They are classified as hormone-producing or non-hormone-producing tumors. The latter are also called "nonfunctioning islet cell tumors."[50,51] Patients with hormone-producing neuroendocrine tumors develop typical hormone-associated symptoms. Over time, tumor-related symptoms such as pain and jaundice also occur. The non-hormone-producing tumors do not cause such specific symptoms. Hormone-producing tumors are named for the principal hormone that they produce, such as "insulinoma," "gastrinoma," and "glucagonoma":[2]

- *Insulinoma*: Insulinoma is the most common neuroendocrine tumor and the most frequent cause of endogenous hypoglycemia.[52] In 90% of cases insulinoma is a benign, solitary tumor less than 2 cm in diameter.[2]
- *Gastrinoma*: Gastrinoma is the second most common neuroendocrine tumor (synonym: Zollinger–Ellison syndrome). The overproduction of gastrin gives rise to multiple gastrointestinal ulcers.[53] Approximately 60% of gastrinomas are malignant, and 30 to 50% of these have metastasized at the time of diagnosis.[2] Some 80 to 90% of all gastrinomas occur in the "gastrinoma triangle," an area bounded by the inferior duodenal flexure, the pancreatic head, and the hepatoduodenal ligament (▶ Fig. 7.15).[2] Gastrinomas are slightly larger than insulinomas, with an average diameter of 3.5 cm.[2]
- *Islet cell tumor*: This is the third most common neuroendocrine tumor. It may reach 5 to 10 cm in size, so it is common to find areas of central necrosis and intralesional hemorrhage.[2]

▶ **Imaging signs.** Neuroendocrine tumors are usually diagnosed from the clinical presentation and laboratory findings. Imaging is used for localization of the tumor(s). The standard technique used in the diagnosis of neuroendocrine tumors is multidetector-row CT. MRI provides high sensitivity in the detection of these lesions. Neuroendocrine tumors are hypervascular masses and are portrayed as such in the arterial phase of contrast-enhanced CT. From the standpoint of surgical planning, it is important to establish the location of the tumors, determine their number, and evaluate for possible metastasis (▶ Fig. 7.16).[2] On MRI, neuroendocrine tumors are hyperintense to the pancreas in T2W sequences and hypointense in unenhanced T1W sequences. After IV injection of contrast medium, they show intense enhancement in the arterial phase followed by early washout of enhancement (▶ Fig. 7.17). If the neuroendocrine tumor is small, superficial or not contiguous with the pancreatic duct, tumor enucleation is sufficient. Partial pancreatectomy is indicated for tumors that are contiguous with the pancreatic duct and cause a reduction in its caliber.[2]

Note

Imaging is of key importance for the localization and quantification of neuroendocrine tumors.

▶ **Clinical features.** Neuroendocrine tumors are distinguished clinically by their hormone production[2,50]:
- *Insulinoma*: Excessive insulin production by this tumor leads to hypoglycemia, with associated neurologic symptoms such as fatigue, weakness, syncope, seizures, and possible related falls and injuries.[52]
- *Gastrinoma*: Increased gastrin secretion by these tumors induces excessive hydrochloric acid production in the gastrointestinal tract, leading to gastric and duodenal ulcers that may become complicated by perforation or bleeding.[53]

Non-hormone-producing tumors do not produce such typical symptoms but may eventually become symptomatic due to their mass effect. Neuroendocrine tumors of the pancreas may be evidence of multiple endocrine neoplasia (MEN) syndrome type I, in

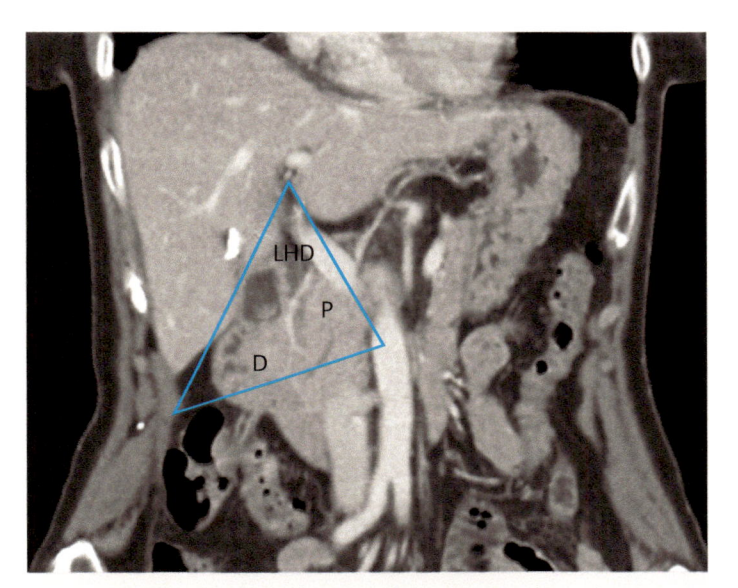

Fig. 7.15 Normal pancreas. The "gastrinoma triangle" is the area in which 80–90% of gastrinomas occur. D, duodenum with inferior duodenal flexure; LHD, hepatoduodenal ligament; P, pancreatic head.

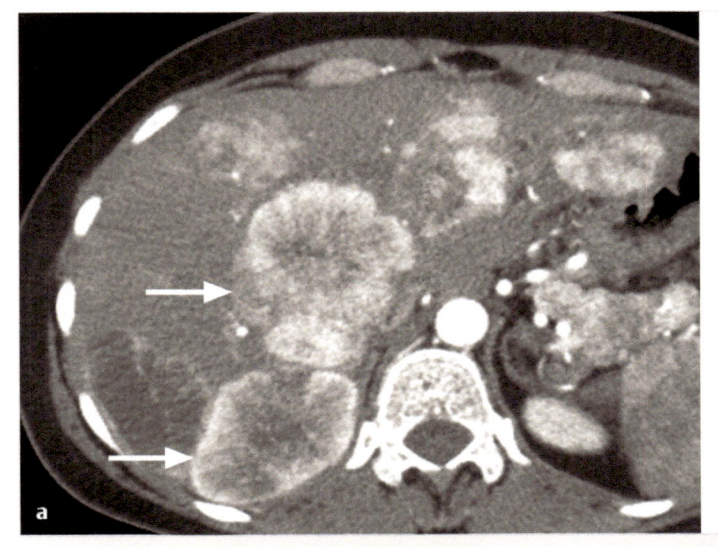

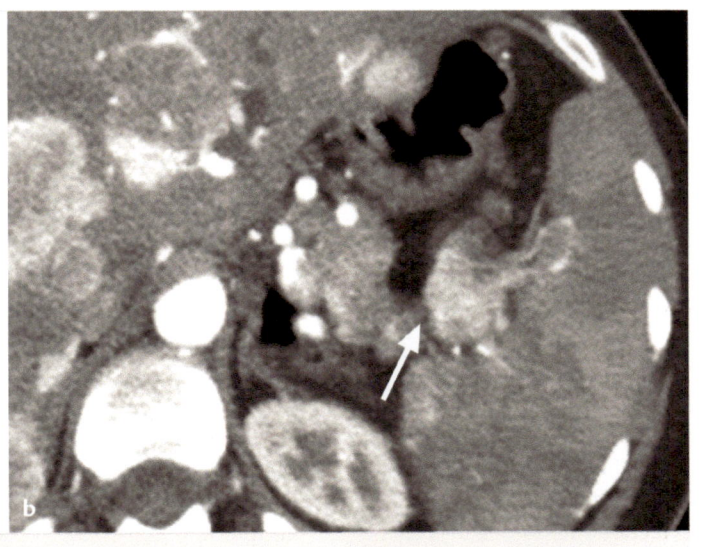

Fig. 7.16 Hypervascular masses. (a) Hypervascular hepatic metastases (arrows) and a neuroendocrine tumor with a target sign. **(b)** Typical hypervascular primary tumor (neuroendocrine tumor) of the pancreatic tail (arrow).

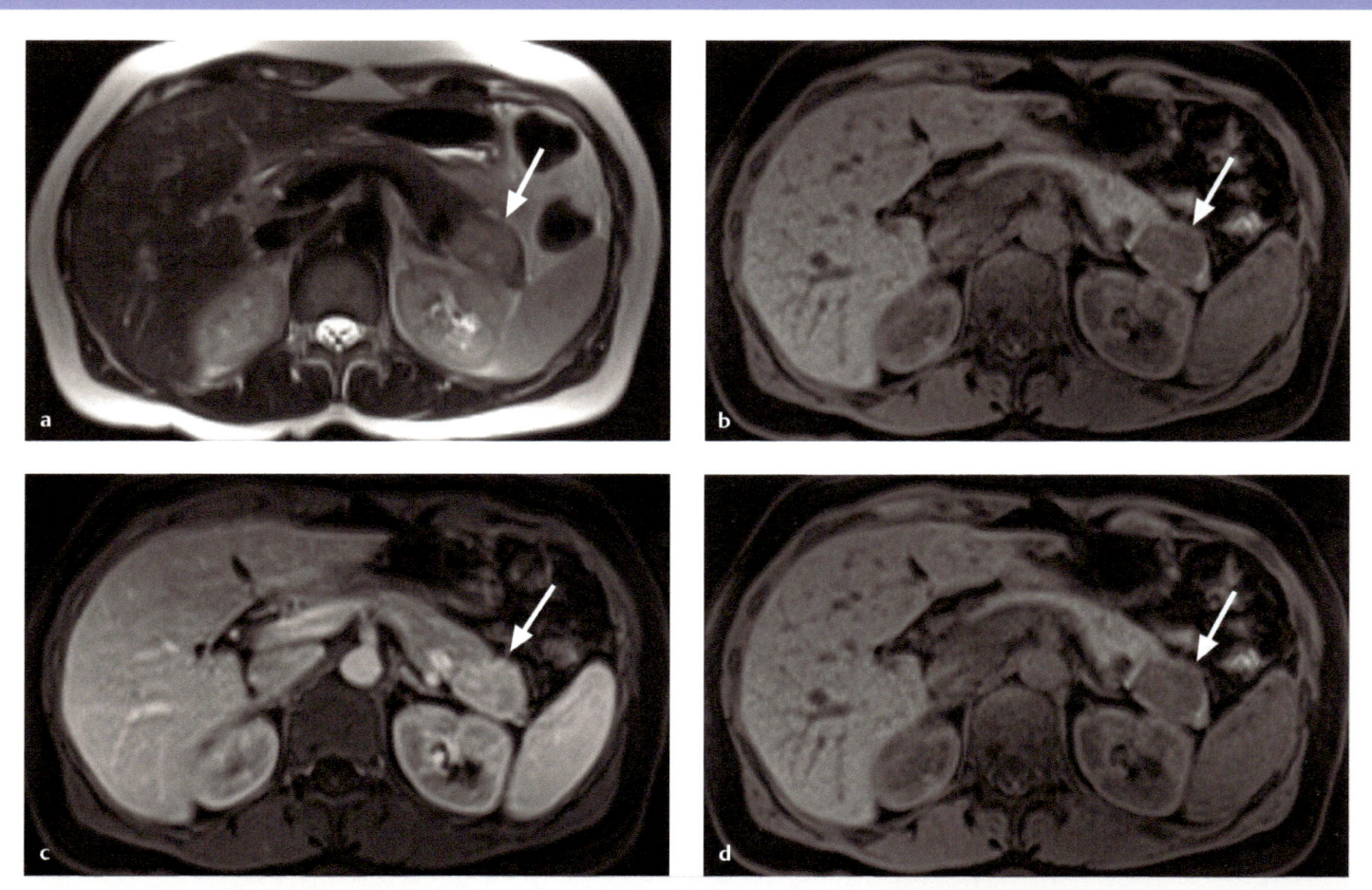

Fig. 7.17 Insulinoma of the pancreas. Arrows indicate the insulinoma. (a) T2 W sequence. The tumor appears hyperintense. (b) Unenhanced T1 W GRE sequence. The tumor is hypointense. (c) After IV injection of contrast medium the tumor shows intense enhancement in the arterial phase. (d) The tumor shows early washout of enhancement.

which neuroendocrine tumors are present not just in the pancreas but also in the pituitary and parathyroid glands.[53]

▶ **Differential diagnosis**
- *Intrapancreatic accessory spleen (IPAS)*: IPAS is a hypervascular nodule that may occur in the pancreas. It has the same enhancement characteristics as the spleen on CT scans, and this can be objectively confirmed by determining the HU values (▶ Fig. 7.18). When imaged by MRI, IPAS is hypointense to surrounding pancreatic tissue in the unenhanced T1 W sequence and hyperintense in the T2 W sequence. The main criterion for diagnosing IPAS is that the signal intensities of the lesions are identical to those of the spleen in all phases.[54] Superparamagnetic iron oxide (SPIO)-enhanced MRI uses a special contrast agent (nano-sized iron oxide crystals coated with dextran or carboxydextran) that is retained mainly in the cells of the reticuloendothelial system, and thus in splenic tissue. Because of the iron in the particles, the spleen is hypointense on SPIO-enhanced MRI, and IPAS is hypointense as well.[55] Unfortunately, iron oxide-based contrast agents are not commercially available at present.
- *Metastases*: Hypervascular metastases in the pancreas are another possible differential diagnosis. The primary tumors that most commonly metastasize to the pancreas are malignant melanoma and renal cell carcinoma ▶ Fig. 7.19).[5]

▶ **Key points.** Neuroendocrine tumors are slow-growing tumors named for the principal hormone that they produce. Non-hormone-producing lesions are called "nonfunctioning islet cell tumors." They can be differentiated clinically by their hormone production and are detectable by CT as hypervascular tumors.

7.3.3 Cystic Lesions

Approximately 90% of all primary cystic neoplasms of the pancreas are serous cystadenomas, intraductal papillary mucinous neoplasms (IPMNs), and mucinous cystic neoplasms (▶ Table 7.4).[56] Cystic pancreatic lesions, like other masses, require a very precise and uniform morphological description. This led to the development of a classification system based on the Bosniak classification for renal cysts.[2,57,58] In this system, pancreatic cysts are classified into four subtypes[58]:
- Unilocular cysts without a solid component, internal septa, or calcifications.
- Microcystic lesions.
- Macrocystic lesions.
- Cysts with a solid component.

This classification has significant implications for further management. Another morphological criterion is the relationship of the cystic lesion to the main pancreatic duct or a side branch.

Unilocular Cysts: Pseudocysts

▶ **Brief definition.** Unilocular cysts are most commonly pseudocysts but may also be IPMNs or unilocular serous cystadenomas,

7.3 Neoplastic Diseases

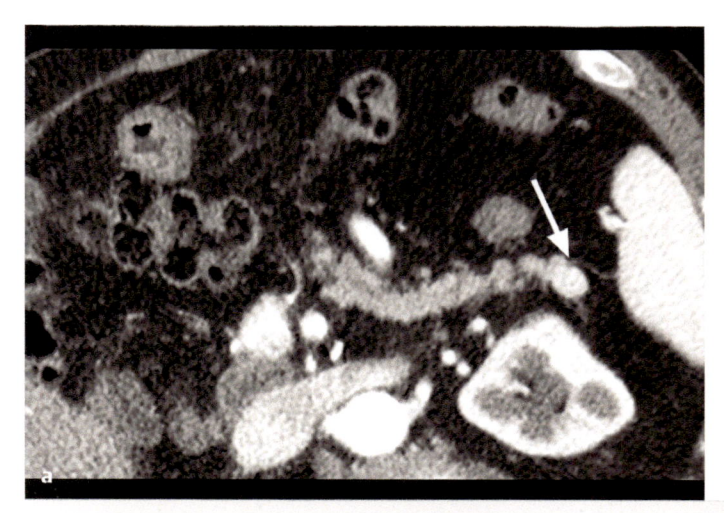

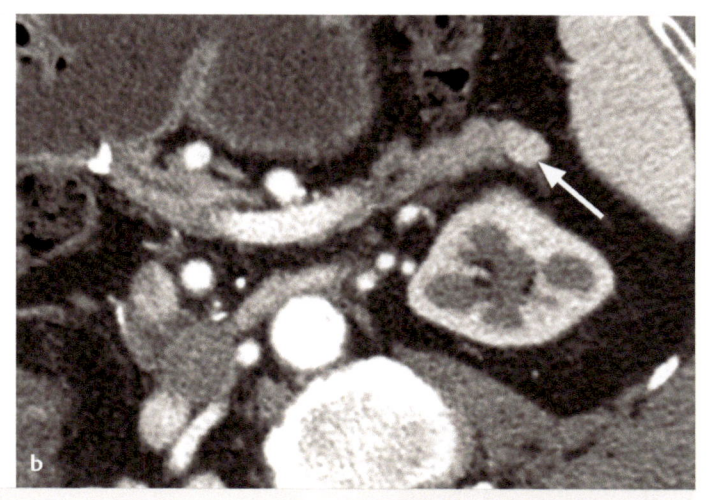

Fig. 7.18 Intrapancreatic accessory spleen (IPAS). The IPAS (arrows) always shows the same imaging characteristics as the splenic parenchyma. (a) CT, arterial phase. (b) CT, venous phase.

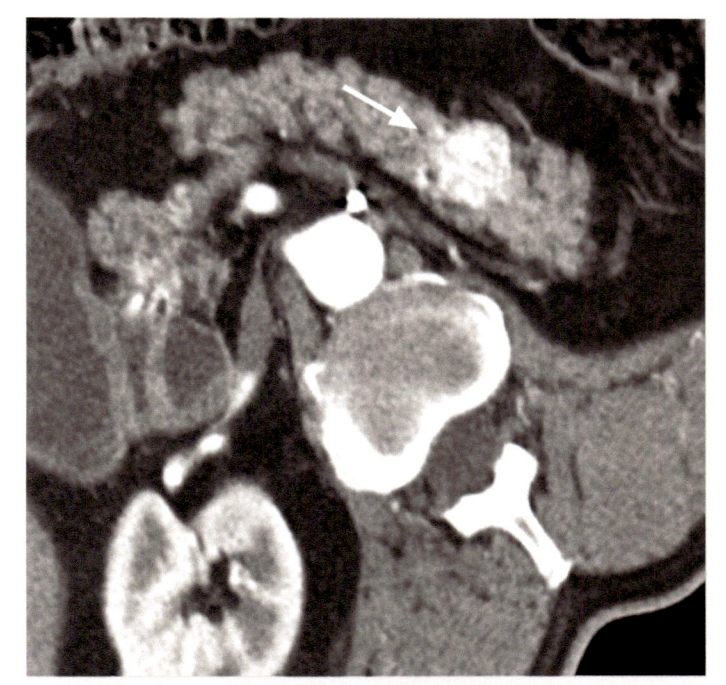

Fig. 7.19 Metastasis of renal cell carcinoma. CT, arterial phase. The metastasis (arrow) appears hypervascular.

Table 7.4 Classification of cystic pancreatic lesions.[56]

Groups	Lesions
Pseudocyst	
Common cystic pancreatic neoplasms	• Serous cystadenoma • Mucinous cystic neoplasm • IPMN
Rare cystic pancreatic neoplasms	• Solid pseudopapillary tumor (Franz's tumor) • Acinar cell cystadenocarcinoma • Lymphangioma • Hemangioma • Paraganglioma
Solid pancreatic lesions with cystic degeneration	• Adenocarcinoma of the pancreas • Cystic islet cell tumor • Metastasis • Cystic teratoma • Sarcoma
True epithelial cyst	Associated with von Hippel–Lindau disease, autosomal dominant polycystic kidney disease, and cystic fibrosis

Abbreviation: IPMN, intraductal papillary mucinous neoplasm.

the latter being much less common.[2] The lesions are almost always pseudocysts in patients with a known history of pancreatitis. The same applies to multiple unilocular pancreatic cysts less than 3 cm in diameter.[2] Pseudocysts may also form after abdominal trauma and may be distributed beyond the pancreas to other intra-abdominal sites.[59] If the cyst communicates with the pancreatic duct, a diagnosis of IPMN (p. 311) should be considered. A unilocular cyst with lobulated margins located in the pancreatic head may be a macrocystic serous cystadenoma (p. 311). The presence of irregular wall thickening is suggestive of aggressive growth.[58]

▶ **Imaging signs.** A pseudocyst is usually evaluated by CT, as this modality can simultaneously detect calcifications (chronic pancreatitis) and allows for a possible interventional procedure in the same session. CT can also detect pancreatic atrophy as a sign of chronic inflammation, which can help confirm a diagnosis of pseudocyst. T2W MRI demonstrates a fluid-filled cyst of high signal intensity. Pseudocysts may be permeated by very fine internal septa (▶ Fig. 7.20). The pseudocyst also has a thin wall; the cystic lesion should have no nodular components or wall irregularities, as these would be considered suspicious features.[59]

▶ **Clinical features.** Asymptomatic patients with small unilocular cysts can be followed with CT or MRI. Symptomatic patients should be managed by decompression or resection of the cysts.[2]

Microcystic Lesions: Serous Cystadenoma

▶ **Brief definition.** Serous cystadenoma accounts for all microcystic lesions of the pancreas.[2] It is a benign pancreatic lesion composed of multiple cysts with an epithelioid lining.[60] Serous cystadenoma constitutes 10 to 29% of cystic pancreatic neoplasms.⁶¹ Differentiation is required from serous cystadenocarcinoma, which was found to have a prevalence of 3% among serous cystic neoplasms.⁶²

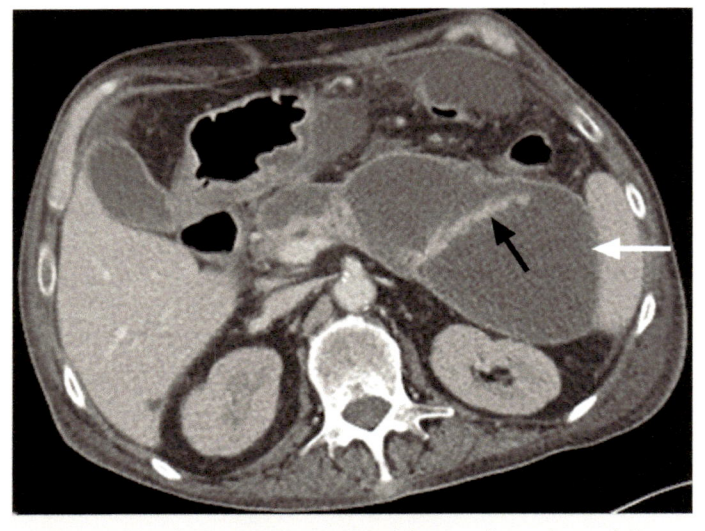

Fig. 7.20 Pseudocyst. CT appearance of a pseudocyst in exudative pancreatitis (white arrow) with an internal septum (black arrow).

▶ **Imaging signs.** Imaging typically reveals a polycystic or microcystic mass composed of at least six cysts, each ranging from a few millimeters to 2 cm in size. The lesions has a median overall size of 2.5 to 3.0 cm and is usually smaller than 5 cm.² Common findings are fine outer lobulation and contrast enhancement of the septa and cyst wall. A central scar with or without stellate calcification (30% of cases) surrounded by cuboid epithelial cells is pathognomonic for serous cystadenoma.[59,60,63] Histology may reveal a honeycomb pattern of equal-sized cysts or a spongelike pattern with larger cysts at the lesion's periphery. On CT the lesions usually show soft tissue attenuation values with good delineation from vessels. On MRI, the cystic character of the lesion is most clearly depicted in T2 W sequences (▶ Fig. 7.21).[2,59]

▶ **Clinical features.** Obstructive jaundice and obstruction of the pancreatic duct are rare. In most cases the duct is displaced, and this finding aids differentiation from ductal adenocarcinoma in equivocal cases.[59,60] Women are affected approximately three times more often than men, with a peak age of incidence of 65 years.[2,59,60] Serous cystadenomas are benign tumors. Resection is unnecessary in asymptomatic patients unless there is a high index of suspicion for malignancy due to uncertain differentiation from mucinous cystic neoplasms or rapid growth.

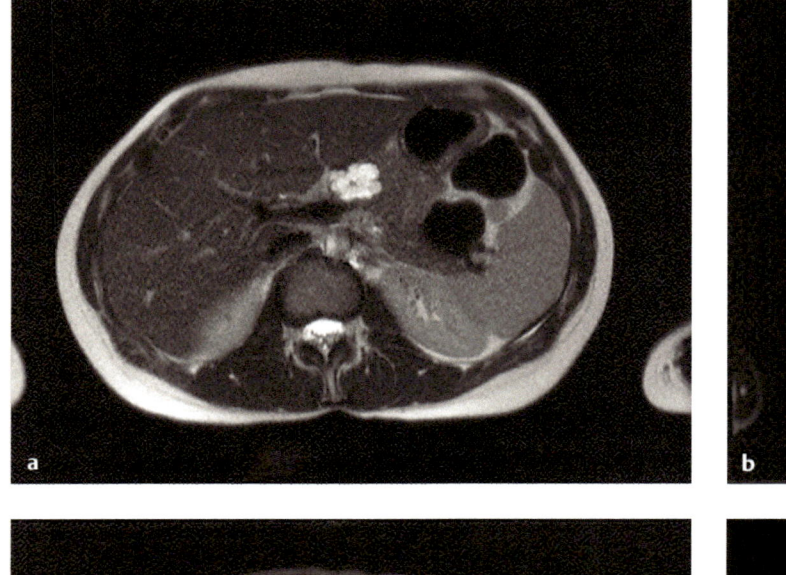

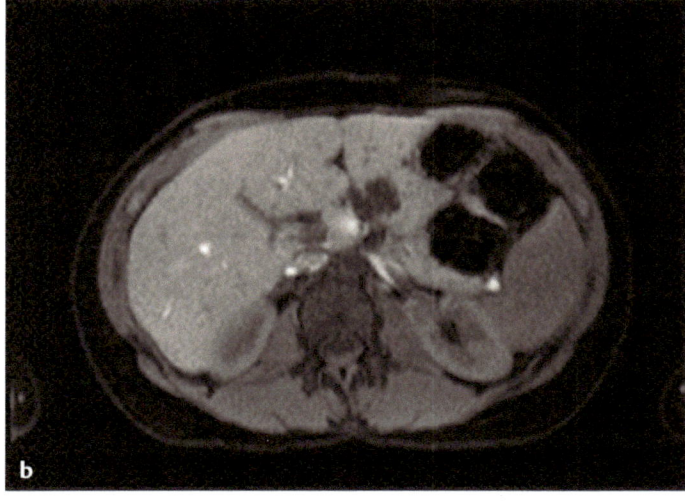

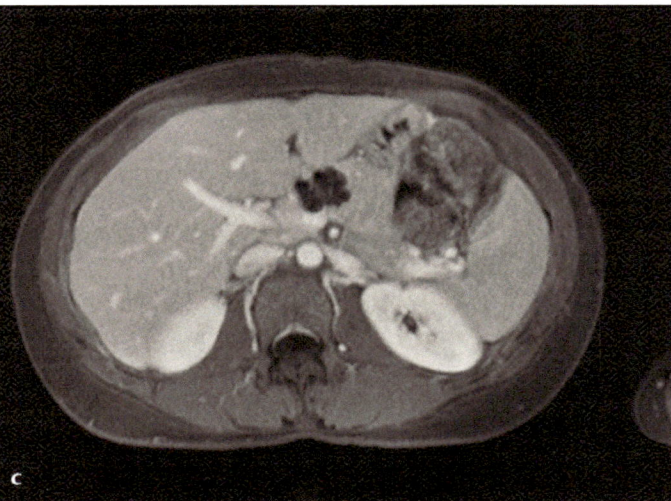

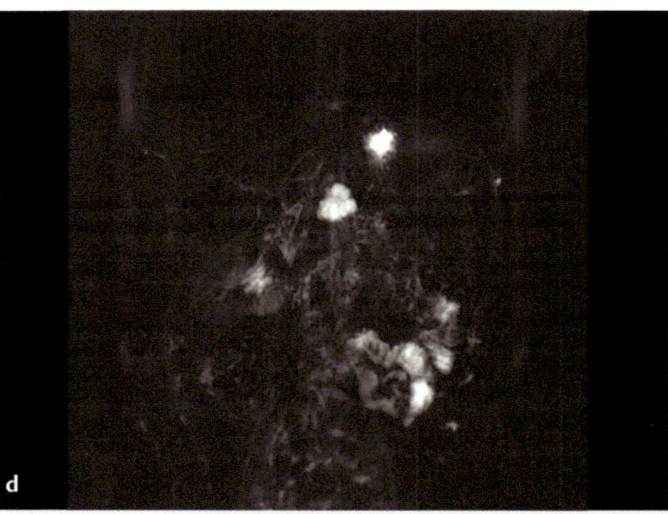

Fig. 7.21 Microcystic cystadenoma. MRI. (a) T2 W sequence shows a "cluster of grapes" arrangement of small cysts around a central scar. (b) Unenhanced T1 W sequence. The small cysts appear hypointense. (c) T1 W sequence after administration of contrast medium. The small cysts still appear hypointense. (d) MRCP demonstrates the microcystic appearance of the lesion.

Macrocystic Lesions

Macrocystic lesions of the pancreas include mucinous cystic neoplasms and IPMNs. Macrocystic neoplasms are distinguished by the presence of multilocular cysts with individual compartments more than 2 cm in diameter.[2]

Intraductal Papillary Mucinous Neoplasm

▶ **Brief definition.** IPMN has a predilection for the pancreatic head. It predominantly affects older men in the sixth or seventh decade.[2,59] IPMNs originate from the epithelium of the pancreatic duct (main-duct IPMN), its side branches (branch-duct IPMN), or both (mixed-type IPMN) (▶ Fig. 7.22).[59] They account for 30% of cystic neoplasms of the pancreas and 0.5 to 1.0% of all pancreatic neoplasms.[61,63] They are classified by their degree of cellular atypia as adenoma, moderate dysplasia, carcinoma in situ, or invasive carcinoma. IPMNs are believed to follow a pattern similar to the adenoma–carcinoma sequence for colorectal cancer, with an eventual transition from adenoma to invasive carcinoma.

Invasive carcinoma is detectable in 25 to 48% of resected IPMNs.[63,64,65] IPMNs do not metastasize to lymph nodes as frequently as adenocarcinomas and have a better overall prognosis.[2] The 5-year survival rate is 77 to 100% for noninvasive stages and 24 to 65% for invasive lesions.[66,67] Main-duct and mixed-type IPMNs are more likely to have malignant components or undergo malignant transformation than branch-duct IPMNs, so this distinction has clinical relevance for therapeutic decision making.[2] There is a risk of recurrence after the resection of an IPMN, but these cases can be successfully managed by reexcision.[63,64,65] Adequate follow-up is essential, therefore, and can be done with MRI.

Absence of the relationship of a cyst to the duct does not definitely exclude IPMN. Differentiation from mucinous cystic lesions can be difficult. A narrow cyst neck at the cyst–ductal junction is suggestive of IPMN.

▶ **Imaging signs.** Currently there is no clear consensus on the preferred imaging modality. CT has advantages owing to its high resolution and variable reconstruction options. MRI with MRCP permits visualization of the pancreaticobiliary system, provides better delineation of the lesion from the main duct, and thus improves the differentiation of main-duct and branch-duct IPMN.[2] Isolated dilatation of the main pancreatic duct to 10 mm or more is defined as main-duct IPMN (▶ Fig. 7.23). If the pancreatic duct measures less than 6 mm in diameter and a cystic lesion larger than 15 cm communicates with the main duct, the lesion is classified as branch-duct IPMN (▶ Fig. 7.24). If the side branch diameters are less than 15 mm, the term "branch-duct IPMN" should be avoided and the finding should be described simply as "branch-duct dilatation." If the main and branch ducts are dilated in a "fishbone" pattern, a mixed type of IPMN is present (▶ Fig. 7.25). The following morphological imaging signs are suggestive of malignancy[42]:

- Cyst larger than 3 cm.
- Mural nodule larger than 8 mm (almost never definable).
- Dilatation of the main pancreatic duct.
- Irregular thickness of septa.
- Accompanying soft-tissue mass.

Mucinous Cystic Neoplasm

▶ **Brief definition.** Most mucinous cystic neoplasms are solitary masses composed of multiple, thick-walled cysts.[68] Mucinous cystic neoplasms range from 6 to 35 cm in size.[2] They occur almost exclusively in premenopausal women around 40 years of age.[69] This is reflected histologically in the presence of ovarian stroma underlying the cyst epithelium.[59,70] The body or tail of the pancreas are sites of predilection.[2,59] The neoplasm does not communicate with the pancreatic duct but may produce a mass effect causing ductal obstruction. Mucinous cystic neoplasms are precursors of malignant tumors and therefore should be resected if there are no contraindications to surgery.[2,59] A mucinous cystic neoplasm that undergoes malignant transformation is called a "mucinous cystadenocarcinoma."

▶ **Imaging signs.** The cysts in a mucinous cystic neoplasm have variable contents (hemorrhagic, inspissated, watery), so the cysts do not necessarily show central isodensity to fluid. The thickened cyst wall is definable on CT scans, and MRCP can show absence of communication with the pancreatic duct. As noted above, this finding does not exclude IPMN as a differential diagnosis.[2] Solid components in the cyst, irregularities in the cyst wall, peripheral calcifications, and hypervascularity may be evidence of a malignant process.[2,57,59] Peripheral eggshell calcifications, while rare, are pathognomonic for mucinous cystic neoplasm. When they are present, the likelihood of malignant transformation is high.[2] MRI (▶ Fig. 7.26) and endoscopic ultrasound are the best tools for differentiating mucinous cystic neoplasm from serous cystadenoma.[2,57,70]

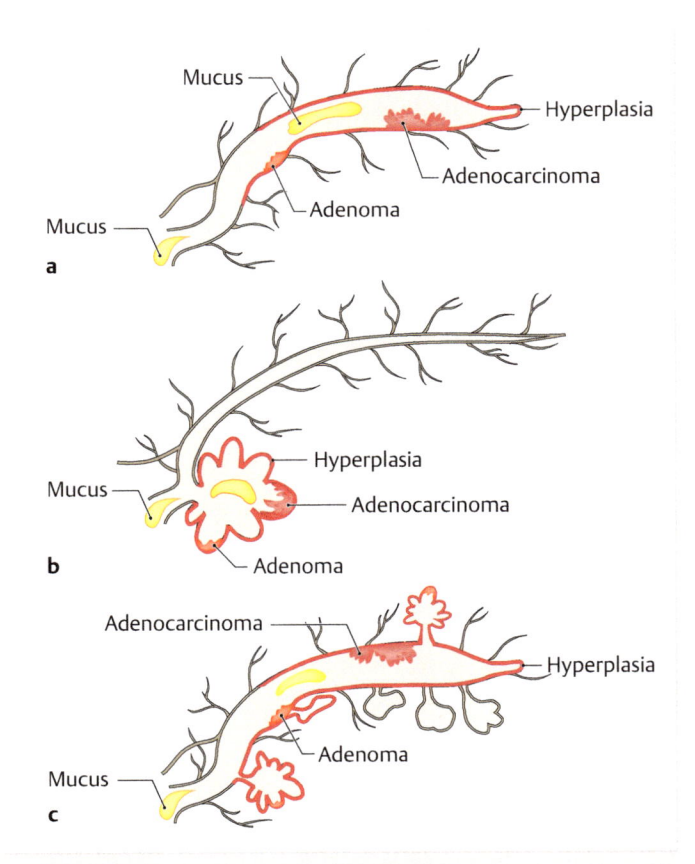

Fig. 7.22 IPMN. (a) Main-duct type. (b) Branch-duct type. (c) Mixed type.

Pancreas

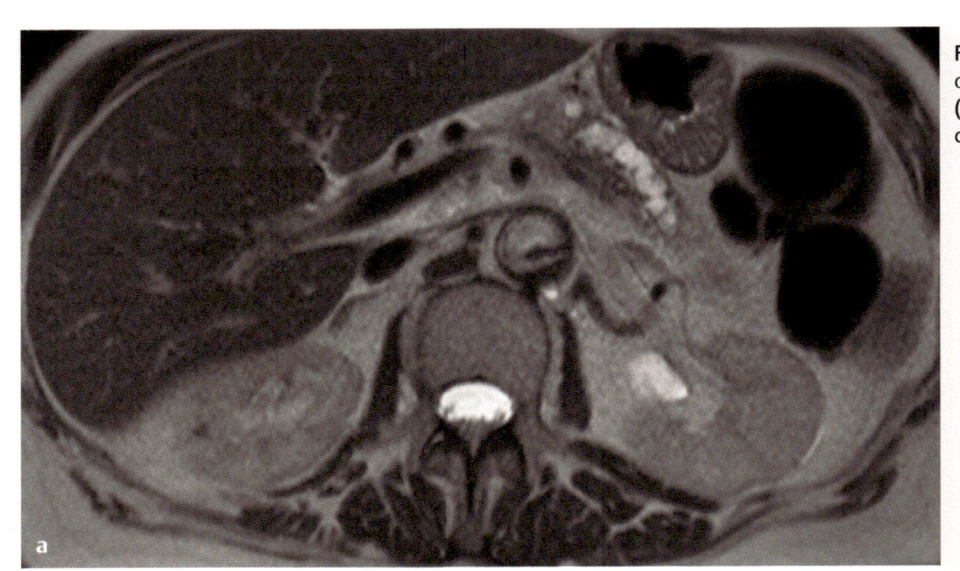

Fig. 7.23 Main-duct IPMN. Isolated dilatation of the main duct on MRI. **(a)** T2W sequence. **(b)** T1W sequence after administration of contrast medium.

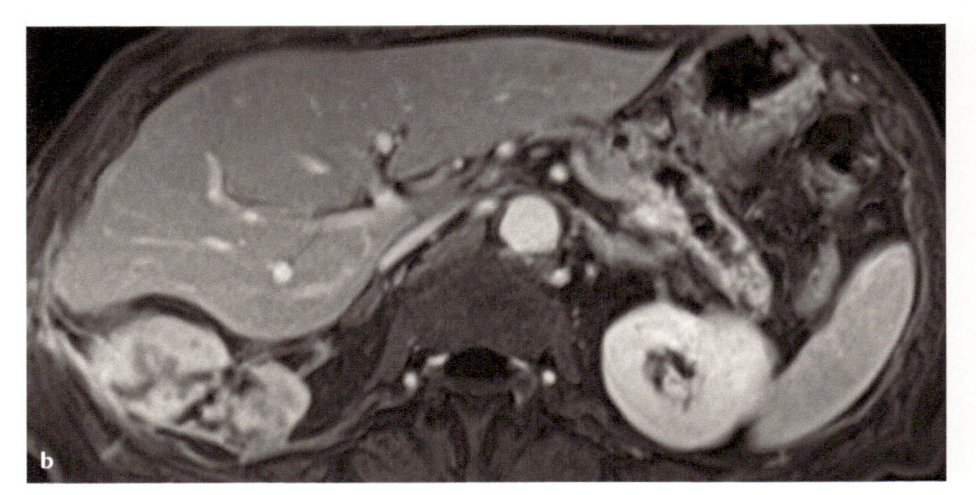

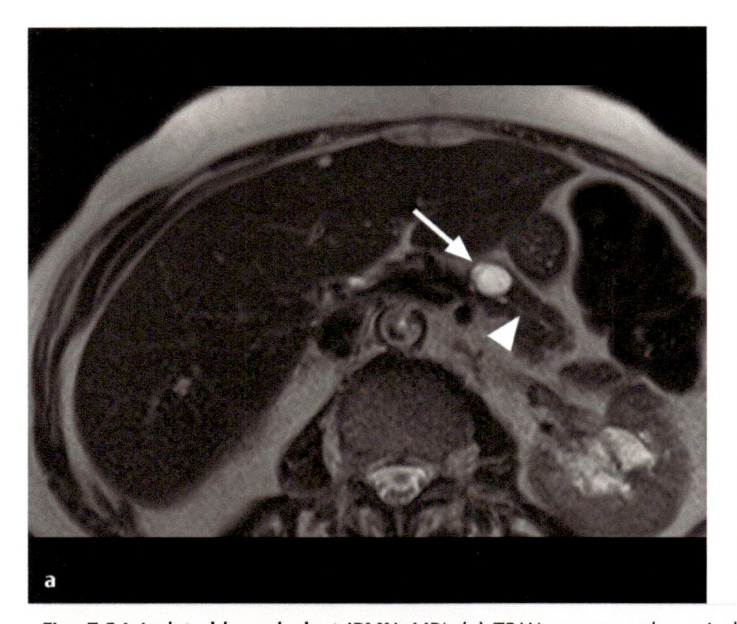

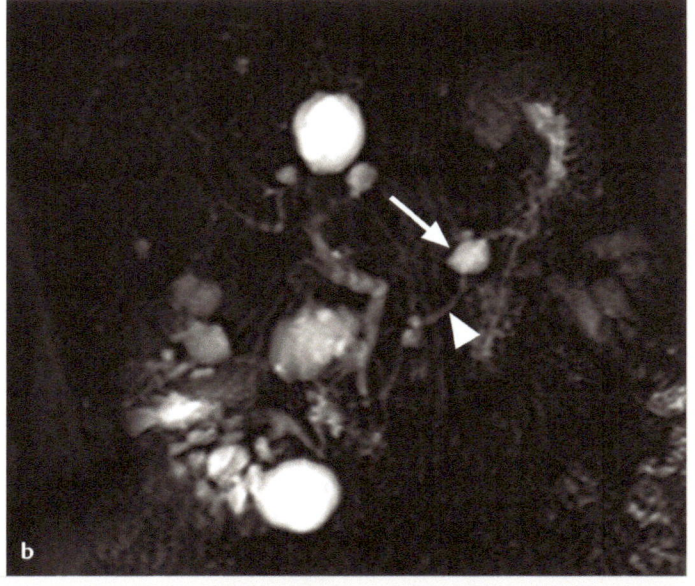

Fig. 7.24 Isolated branch-duct IPMN. MRI. **(a)** T2W sequence shows isolated cystic dilatation of a branch duct to 18 mm (arrow) and a narrow main duct (arrowhead). **(b)** MRCP shows a narrow main duct running the length of the pancreas. The branch-duct IPMN (arrow) is projected over the main duct (arrowhead).

tumor with solid components or a solid tumor with cystic components. Both forms are at least potentially malignant and are therefore are managed by surgical resection.[2] In the case of cystic tumors with a solid component, the solid component is called a "mural nodule" if it is hypointense on T2W images and enhances after IV administration of contrast medium.[2] Solid pseudopapillary tumors are initially solid tumors that have undergone massive degeneration with necrosis and cyst formation. Their malignant potential is low.[59,71] They occur exclusively in women around 30 years of age, are usually larger than 10 cm,[66] and are most commonly located in the pancreatic tail (▶ Fig. 7.27). The cysts are filled with debris and foam cells (macrophages).[2] Resection with clear margins is necessary to prevent metastasis. A complete resection is curative in 80% of cases.[71]

▶ **Imaging signs.** Imaging shows a well-circumscribed mass with a cystic center and an irregular, solid peripheral capsule. Central calcifications may be present in 30% of cases.[2,59] The capsule shows enhancement after IV administration of contrast medium.[59]

▶ **Clinical features.** Unexplained abdominal pain and a palpable abdominal mass bring most patients to medical attention. Weight loss may also occur.

Differential Diagnosis of Cystic Tumors

Adenocarcinoma may contain cystic components due to necrosis. Neuroendocrine tumors also develop cystic areas, not as a result of necrosis but due to their rich blood supply.[2]

Pancreatic cysts may also occur in patients suffering from von Hippel–Lindau syndrome, and so the imaging study should cover the suprarenal glands and any masses in that region should be described. In this case as well, MRI may be helpful in evaluating both the cyst and possible suprarenal masses.

Another differential diagnosis is acinar cell carcinoma, which also forms cysts. Typical imaging findings in this case include a well-defined lesion that shows central necrosis when larger than 5 cm. The prognosis is better than with ductal adenocarcinoma, but the tumor is still an aggressive malignancy (▶ Fig. 7.28).[2]

Summary

The main role of imaging studies in patients with pancreatic cystic lesions is to provide a detailed, comprehensive morphological description so that the malignant potential of the lesion can be predicted as accurately as possible and an accurate risk–benefit assessment can be made with regard to surgical treatment. The most important cystic lesions of the pancreas are reviewed in ▶ Table 7.5.

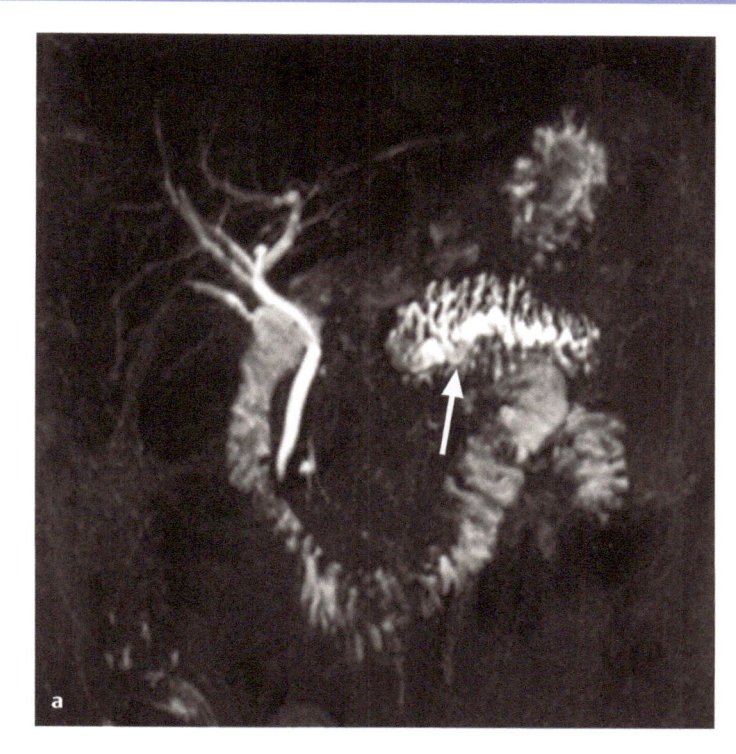

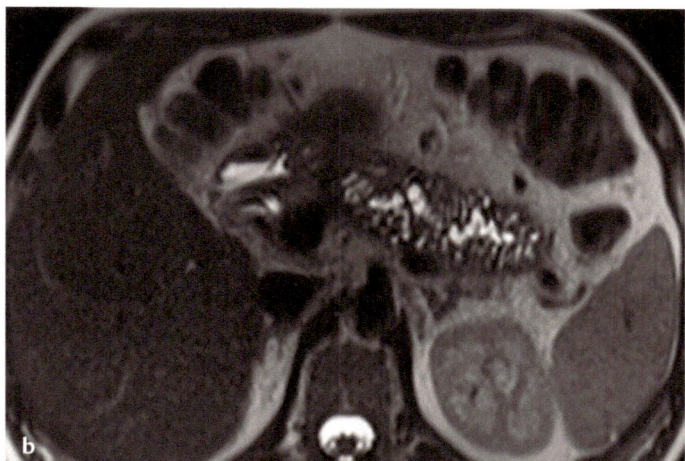

Fig. 7.25 Mixed-type IPMN. Dilatation of the main and branch ducts on MRI. **(a)** Oblique coronal MRCP image. The arrow indicates massive dilatation of the pancreatic duct and side branches. **(b)** Axial T2W image shows a dilated main duct and side branches in the pancreatic tail and body.

▶ **Clinical features.** Like IPMN and other pancreatic neoplasms, mucinous cystic neoplasm may be manifested by upper abdominal pain radiating to the back, jaundice, new-onset diabetes mellitus, or recurrent episodes of pancreatitis, depending on its site of occurrence. There are no typical clinical features that could distinguish mucinous cystic neoplasm from other tumors.

Cysts with Solid Components: Solid Pseudopapillary Tumor

▶ **Brief definition.** Cysts with solid components (also called solid pseudopapillary epithelial neoplasms, Hamoudi's tumors, Franz's tumors) include all neoplasms that are either a cystic

7.4 Generalized Pancreatic Changes

7.4.1 Pancreatic Lipoma

▶ **Brief definition.** Lipomas are benign fatty tumors that may occur anywhere in the body, including the pancreatic tissue.

Pancreas

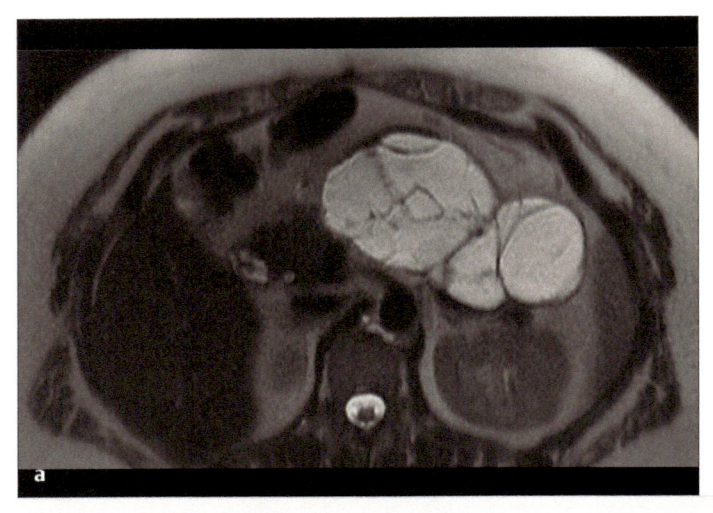

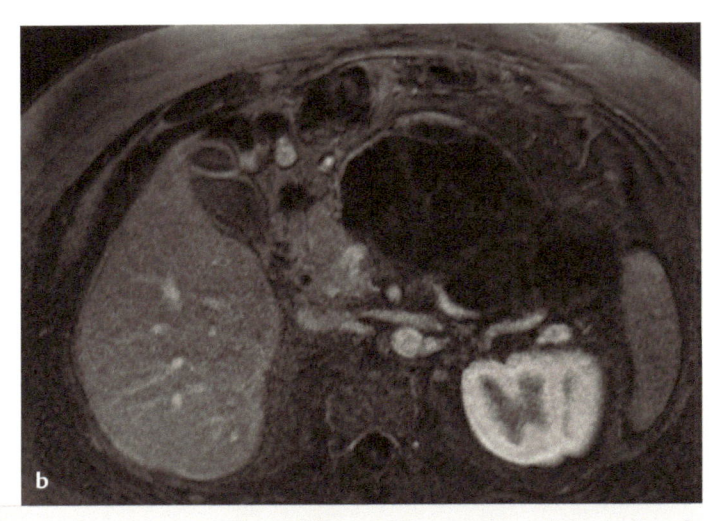

Fig. 7.26 Mucinous cystic neoplasm with multiple hyperintense macrocysts. MRI. (a) T2 W sequence. (b) T1 W sequence after administration of contrast medium shows enhancement of the cyst wall and septa.

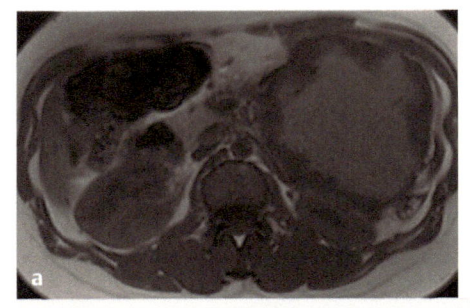

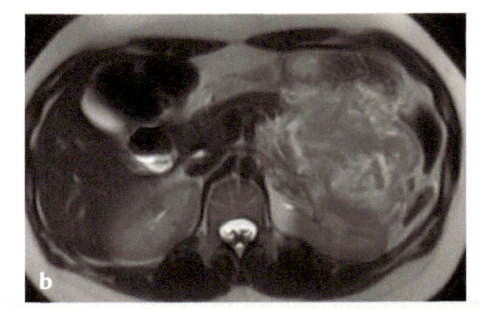

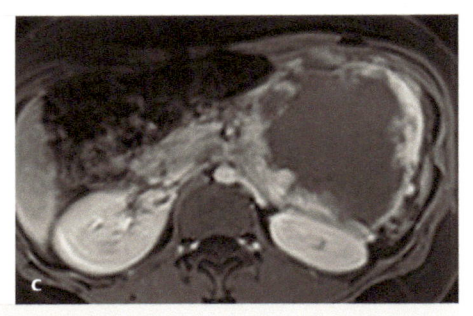

Fig. 7.27 Solid pseudopapillary tumor (Franz's tumor). MRI. (a) Unenhanced T1 W sequence shows a tumor with central necrosis. Tumor diameter is greater than 10 cm. (b) T2 W sequence clearly demonstrates the inhomogeneous "contents" with cellular debris. (c) T1 W sequence after administration of contrast medium shows central necrosis and an active peripheral tumor rim.

▶ **Imaging signs.** Pancreatic lipoma is isodense to fat on CT, showing negative attenuation values. MRI is superior to CT for this application. Pancreatic lipoma is isointense to fat in T1 W and T2 W sequences (▶ Fig. 7.29). Mesenteric fat can be used as an internal reference standard. A homogeneous reduction of signal intensity is noted in the fat-suppressed T2 W sequence.

▶ **Clinical features.** Most pancreatic lipomas are clinically silent. Lipoma is a likely diagnosis if the lesion is homogeneously isodense or isointense to fat, has no solid components, and is smaller than 3 cm.[72] If there is any doubt as to whether the lesion is benign or malignant, resection should be considered.

▶ **Differential diagnosis.** The differential diagnosis of pancreatic lipoma includes teratoma and liposarcoma.[72] Small lipomas may be misidentified as a malignant mass on CT.

▶ **Key points.** The diagnosis of lipoma should be considered for a pancreatic lesion having the same density or signal intensity as the surrounding mesenteric fat.

7.4.2 Cystic Fibrosis

▶ **Brief definition.** In cystic fibrosis, a defect in the chloride channels of epithelial cells, inherited as an autosomal recessive trait, leads to the formation of very viscous mucus in the exocrine glands (sweat glands, bronchi, pancreas, bile ducts, small intestine, and gonads). Damage to the pancreas can occur quite early as a result of the obstructed drainage of secretions. This damage may take the form of pancreatic atrophy, cyst formation, or diffuse fatty replacement of the organ. All of these changes are associated with exocrine and endocrine pancreatic insufficiency.

7.4 Generalized Pancreatic Changes

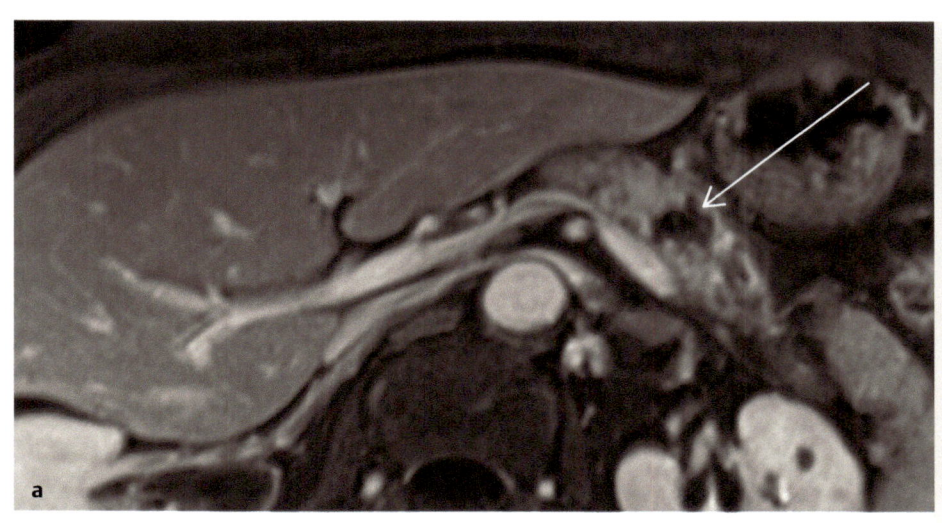

Fig. 7.28 **Acinar cell carcinoma.** MRI. Arrows indicate the carcinoma. **(a)** Venous-phase image shows a cystic-appearing mass approximately 5 cm in diameter with central necrosis. **(b)** Expansile morphology with an irregularly enhancing wall.

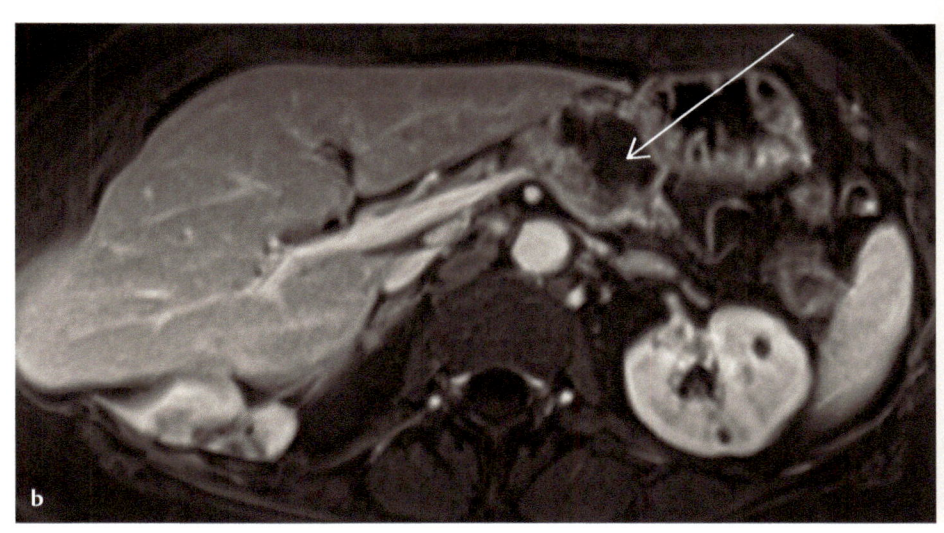

Table 7.5 Major cystic tumors of the pancreas and their characteristics

Tumor	Size	Patient characteristics	Sites of predilection	Distinctive features
Pseudocyst	Variable	History of pancreatitis	Ubiquitous	May be distributed throughout the abdomen
Serous cystadenoma	2.5–3.0 cm	3:1 female predominance, average age 65 years	None	Pathognomonic feature: central scar with or without central stellate calcification
IPMN	Variable	Most common in older males (sixth to seventh decade)	Pancreatic head	Adenoma-carcinoma sequence
Mucinous cystic neoplasm	6–35 cm	Occurs almost exclusively in women around age 40 years	Pancreatic head and tail	Pathognomonic feature: peripheral eggshell calcifications
Franz's tumor	>10 cm	Occurs exclusively in women around age 30 years	None	Occasionally forms a palpable mass

Abbreviation: IPMN, intraductal papillary mucinous neoplasm.

Pancreas

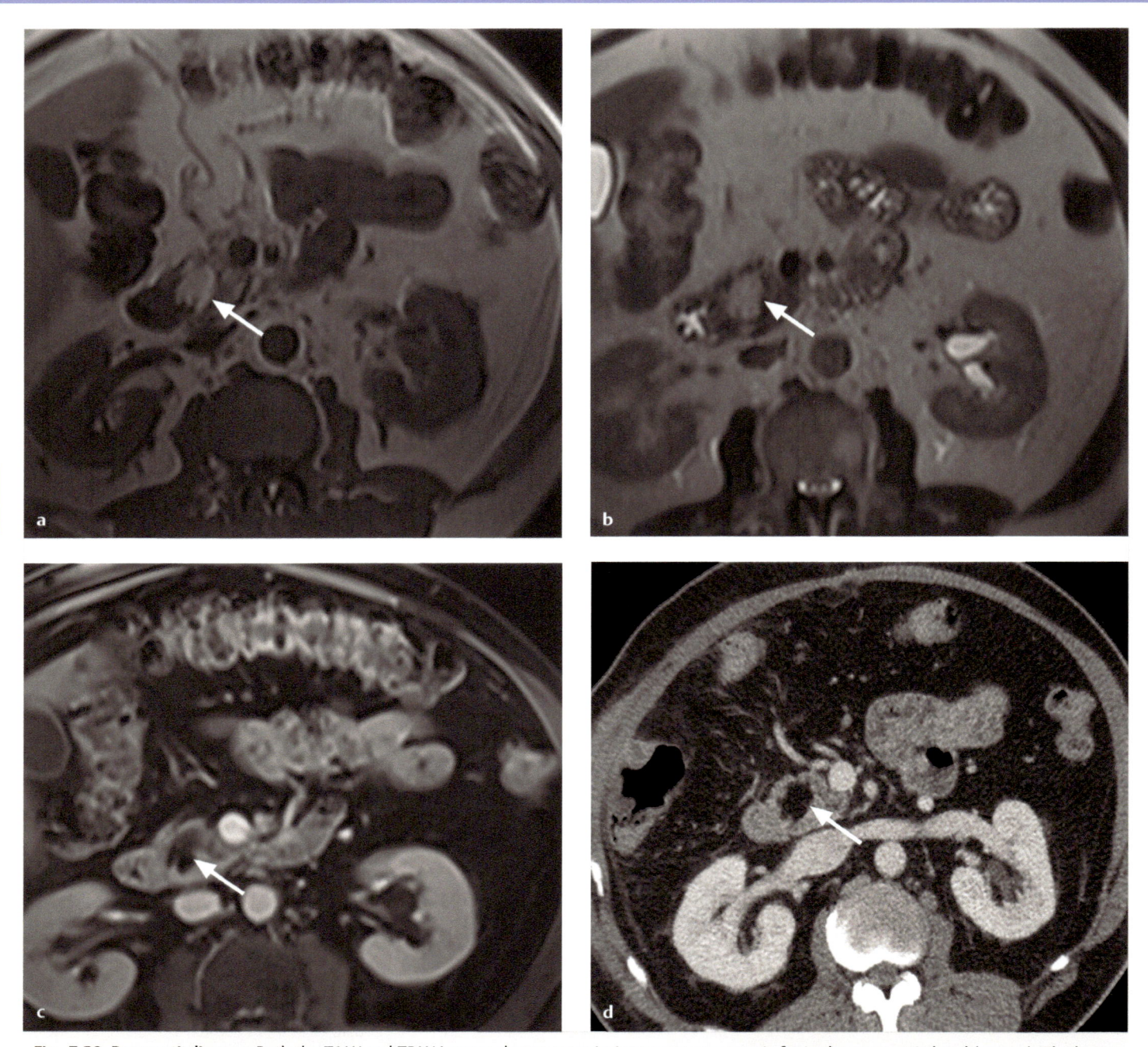

Fig. 7.29 Pancreatic lipoma. Both the T1W and T2W images show a mass isointense to mesenteric fat in the pancreatic head (arrows). The lesion does not enhance ([c], arrow) and fat suppression nulls its signal, similar to the mesenteric fat. The lesion shows typical negative attenuation values on CT ([d], arrow), proving that it contains fat. (a) Unenhanced T1W image. (b) T2W image. (c) T1W image after administration of contrast medium. (d) CT.

▶ **Imaging signs.** At ultrasound, fatty replacement of the parenchyma leads to increased echogenicity of the pancreas (▶ Fig. 7.30). CT may show negative attenuation values throughout the pancreas, indicating complete fatty replacement (▶ Fig. 7.31). Pancreatic lipomatosis in many patients is associated with enlargement of the organ, known as lipomatous pseudohypertrophy (▶ Fig. 7.32). The pancreas appears hyperintense in all MR sequences in which fat shows high signal intensity (e.g., T2W TSE images and T1W sequences without fat suppression). The high signal intensity in the pancreas can be reduced by fat suppression (▶ Fig. 7.33). Pancreatic cysts in cystic fibrosis are usually small.

▶ **Clinical features.** Pulmonary symptoms chiefly determine the patient's general health status and prognosis. Endocrine pancreatic insufficiency leads to diabetes mellitus, while exocrine insufficiency leads to recurrent diarrhea with maldigestion and weight loss.

▶ **Differential diagnosis.** Atrophy of the pancreas may develop in a setting of chronic pancreatitis. In this case, however, CT will usually show small calcifications within the parenchyma. The pancreas may also become atrophic with ageing. This condition is also associated with diffuse fatty infiltration (lipomatosis) of the pancreas, but this change is much less pronounced than in cystic fibrosis and affects older individuals, unlike the pediatric age group

7.4 Generalized Pancreatic Changes

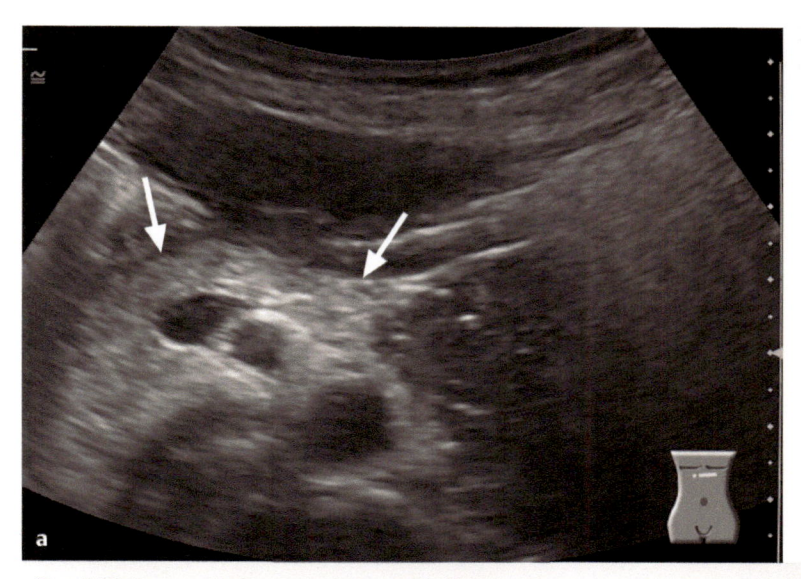

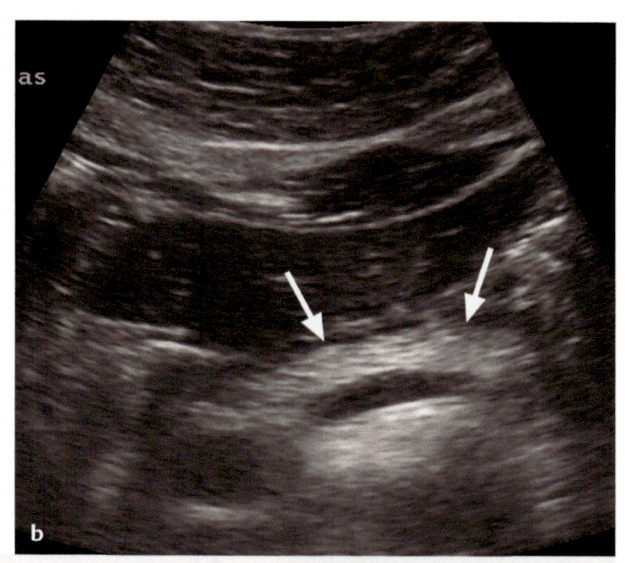

Fig. 7.30 Pancreatic lipomatosis in cystic fibrosis. The pancreas shows markedly increased echogenicity (arrows). **(a)** Patient 1. **(b)** Patient 2.

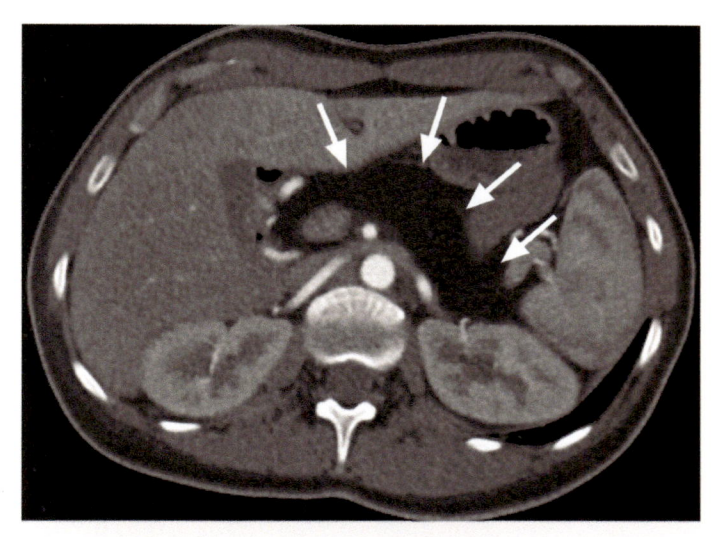

Fig. 7.31 Cystic fibrosis with pancreatic lipomatosis. Axial CT scan in a 34-year-old woman shows diffuse fatty replacement of the pancreas (arrows).

affected by cystic fibrosis. Primary hemochromatosis may lead to pancreatic atrophy but is accompanied by increased density of the liver parenchyma on unenhanced CT and decreased signal intensity in almost all MRI sequences. Pseudohypertrophy of the pancreas, on the other hand, is pathognomonic for cystic fibrosis.

7.4.3 Primary Hemochromatosis

▶ **Brief definition.** Primary hemochromatosis follows an autosomal recessive inheritance and is characterized by deficiency of "hemochromatosis protein," which is necessary in the synthesis of hepcidin. This hormone inhibits excessive iron absorption in the small intestine. The absence of hepcidin permits unrestrained iron absorption from food, leading to an iron overload in the body. This iron is stored intracellularly in the liver, heart, skin, and synovium and in endocrine glands including the pancreas.

▶ **Imaging signs.** Accumulation of iron in the liver and pancreas leads to increased echogenicity of these organs on ultrasonography. Attenuation values on CT are significantly increased (▶ Fig. 7.34). MRI shows decreased signal intensity in the organs that accumulate iron. The spleen, meanwhile, remains unchanged in all modalities.

▶ **Clinical features.** Patients with primary hemochromatosis develop hepatic cirrhosis and diabetes mellitus and experience skin discoloration ("bronze diabetes"). Iron deposits in the joints incite an inflammatory reaction with associated arthralgia, which is frequently the earliest complaint.

▶ **Differential diagnosis.** In secondary hemochromatosis (also called hemosiderosis), an iron overload caused by chronic hemolysis and blood transfusions, extracellular iron accumulation occurs mainly in the reticuloendothelial system; thus the liver and spleen are affected while the pancreas is spared for some time (▶ Fig. 7.35). Pancreatic iron deposition occurs only in the late stage of the disease (▶ Fig. 7.36).

> **Note**
>
> Primary hemochromatosis is characterized by intracellular iron storage; the pancreas and liver are affected, while the spleen is spared. Hemosiderosis (secondary hemochromatosis), on the other hand, is associated with iron storage in the reticuloendothelial system, and therefore the liver and spleen are affected. Iron deposition in the pancreas does not occur during the early years of the disease.

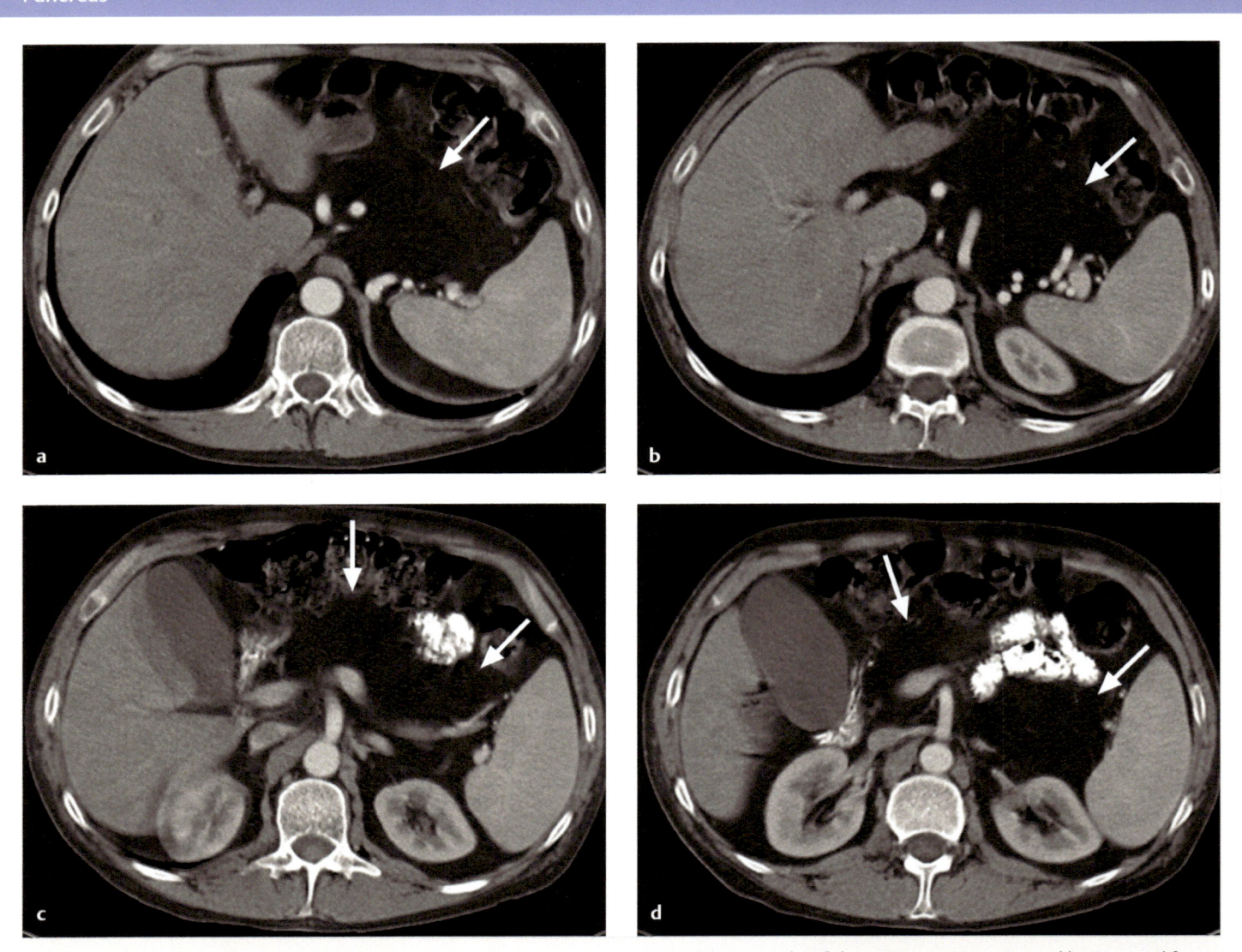

Fig. 7.32 **Pseudohypertrophy of the pancreas in cystic fibrosis.** Lipomatous pseudohypertrophy of the pancreas is accompanied by increased fatty tissue in the pancreatic bed (arrows). Contrast-enhanced multidetector CT of the pancreas in contiguous 5-mm slices from cranial (**a**) to caudal (**d**). At all levels the pancreas is diffusely enlarged and shows fat attenuation, appearing almost "black" in the images (arrows). Attenuation measurements indicate negative (fat-equivalent) HU values. (**a**) Cranial scan. (**b**) Scan at a lower level, contiguous to (**a**). (**c**) Scan at a lower level, contiguous to (**b**). (**d**) Caudal scan.

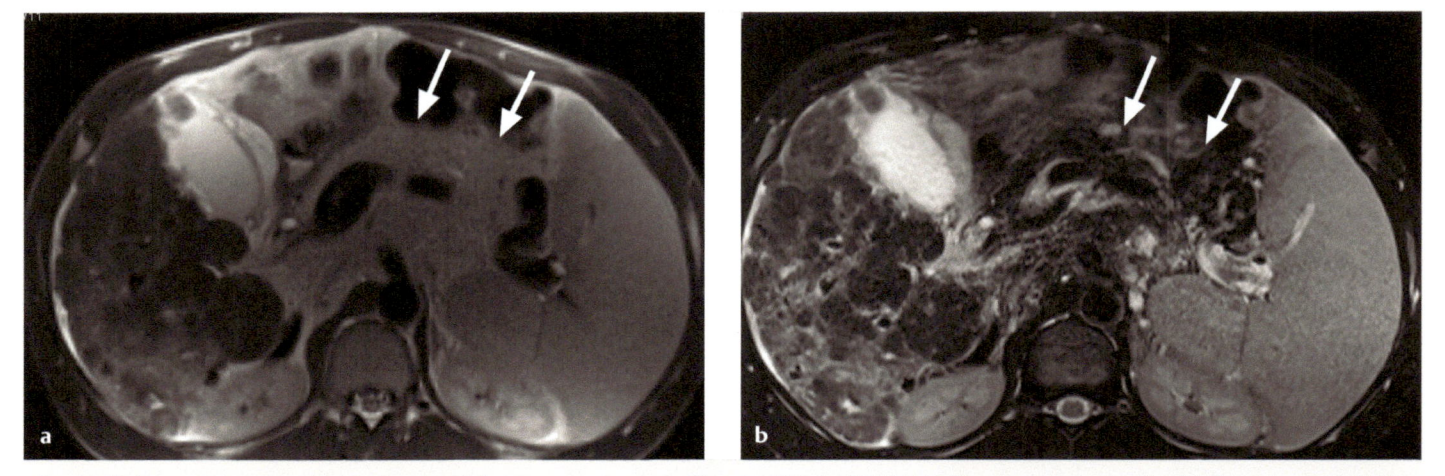

Fig. 7.33 **Lipomatous pseudohypertrophy of the pancreas in cystic fibrosis.** MRI. (**a**) T2W HASTE sequence shows a bright signal (arrows). (**b**) In the fat-suppressed sequence, the signal intensity of the pseudohypertrophy (arrows) is almost completely suppressed.

7.4 Generalized Pancreatic Changes

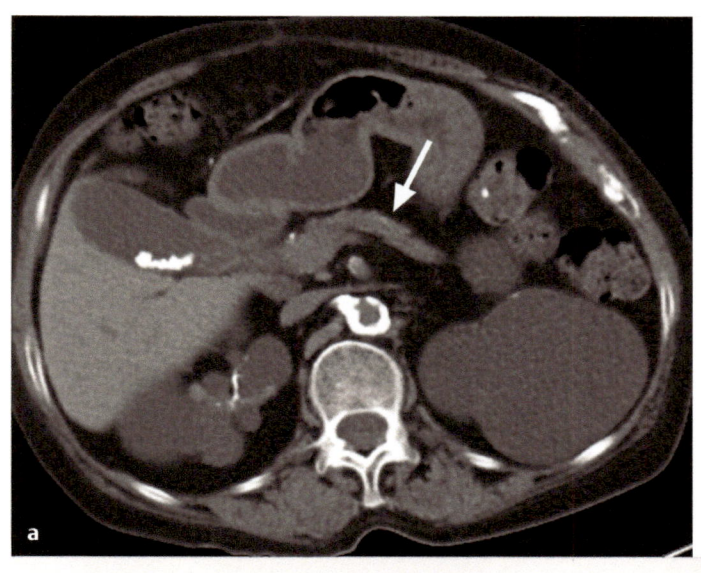

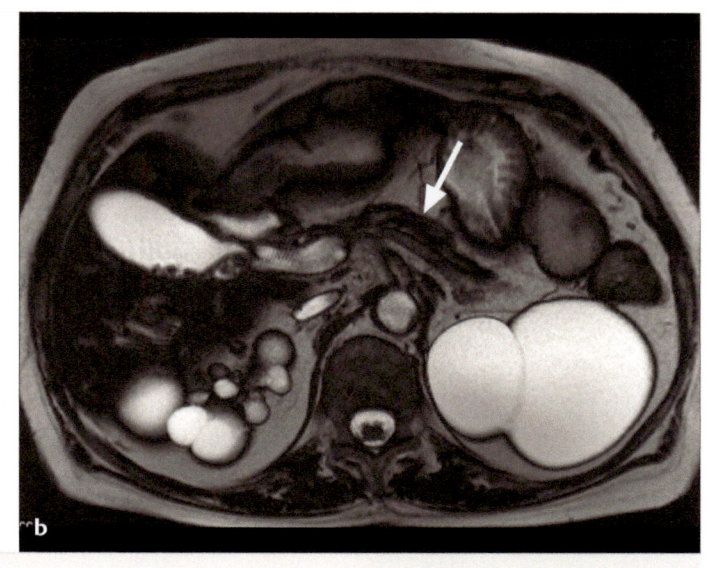

Fig. 7.34 Primary hemochromatosis. (a) Unenhanced CT shows increased density of the atrophic pancreas (arrow) and the liver. **(b)** T2W MR image shows decreased signal intensity of the atrophic pancreas.

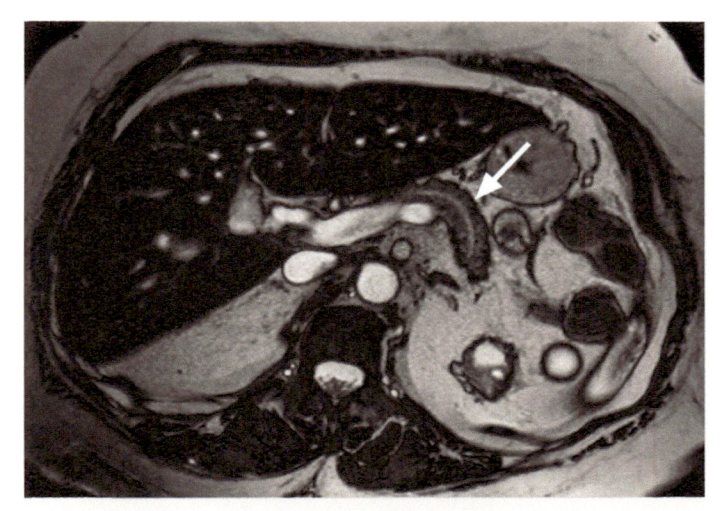

Fig. 7.35 Hemosiderosis (secondary hemochromatosis) caused by blood transfusions. In this T2W sequence, the liver shows markedly decreased signal intensity, while the pancreas shows normal signal intensity (arrow).

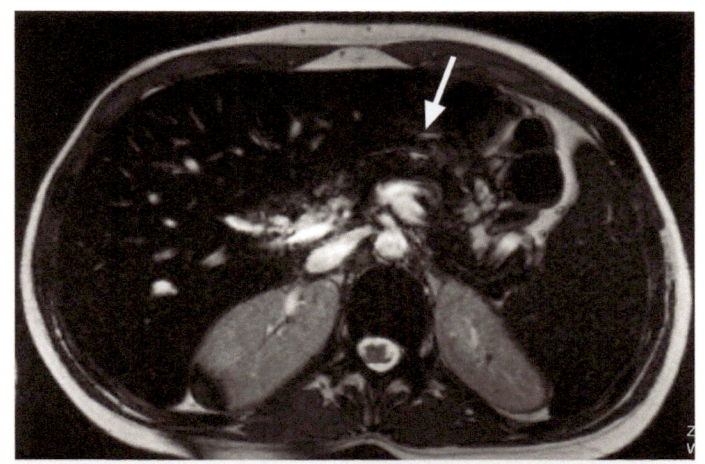

Fig. 7.36 Hemosiderosis in β-thalassemia. In the late stage of the disease, the pancreas also shows decreased signal intensity (arrow) like the liver and spleen. The kidneys exhibit normal signal intensity.

Bibliography

[1] Schünke M, Schulte E, Schumacher U, eds. Prometheus, Lernatlas der Anatomie: Hals und innere Organe. Stuttgart: Thieme; 2005:214–217. Illustrated by M. Voll/K. Wesker

[2] Grenacher L, Klauss M. Computed tomography of pancreatic tumors [in German]. Radiologe. 2009; 49(2):107–123

[3] Richter GM, Wunsch C, Schneider B, et al. [Hydro-CT in detection and staging of pancreatic carcinoma]. Radiologe. 1998; 38(4):279–286

[4] Vitale GC, Vitale M, Vitale DS, Binford JC, Hill B. Long-term follow-up of endoscopic stenting in patients with chronic pancreatitis secondary to pancreas divisum. Surg Endosc. 2007; 21(12):2199–2202

[5] Brambs H-J. Erkrankungen des Pankreas. In: Freyschmidt J, Feuerbach S, eds. Handbuch diagnostische Radiologie: Gastrointestinales System. Berlin: Springer; 2007:627–631

[6] Lehman GA, Sherman S. Diagnosis and therapy of pancreas divisum. Gastrointest Endosc Clin N Am. 1998; 8(1):55–77

[7] Floemer F, Buitrago C, Steinbrich W. [Pancreas anulare as an incidental finding in multidetector computer tomography for symptomatic abdominal aortic aneurysm]. RoFo Fortschr Geb Rontgenstr Nuklearmed. 2006; 178(4):448–450

[8] Frossard JL, Steer ML, Pastor CM. Acute pancreatitis. Lancet. 2008; 371 (9607):143–152

[9] van Santvoort HC, Bollen TL, Besselink MG, et al. Describing peripancreatic collections in severe acute pancreatitis using morphologic terms: an international interobserver agreement study. Pancreatology. 2008; 8(6):593–599

[10] Alsfasser G, Rau BM, Klar E. Scoring of human acute pancreatitis: state of the art. Langenbecks Arch Surg. 2013; 398(6):789–797

[11] Knaus WA, Draper EA, Wagner DP, Zimmerman JE. APACHE II: a severity of disease classification system. Crit Care Med. 1985; 13(10):818–829

[12] Ranson JH, Rifkind KM, Roses DF, Fink SD, Eng K, Spencer FC. Prognostic signs and the role of operative management in acute pancreatitis. Surg Gynecol Obstet. 1974; 139(1):69–81

[13] Vincent JL, Moreno R, Takala J, et al. The SOFA (Sepsis-related Organ Failure Assessment) score to describe organ dysfunction/failure. On behalf of the Working Group on Sepsis-Related Problems of the European Society of Intensive Care Medicine. Intensive Care Med. 1996; 22(7):707–710

[14] Banks PA, Bollen TL, Dervenis C, et al. Acute Pancreatitis Classification Working Group. Classification of acute pancreatitis–2012: revision of the Atlanta classification and definitions by international consensus. Gut. 2013; 62(1):102–111

[15] Bradley EL, III. A clinically based classification system for acute pancreatitis. Summary of the International Symposium on Acute Pancreatitis, Atlanta, GA, September 11 through 13, 1992. Arch Surg. 1993; 128(5):586–590

[16] Thoeni RF. The revised Atlanta classification of acute pancreatitis: its importance for the radiologist and its effect on treatment. Radiology. 2012; 262(3):751–764

[17] Hoffmeister A, Mayerle J, Beglinger C, et al. Chronic Pancreatitis German Society of Digestive and Metabolic Diseases (DGVS). [S3-Consensus guidelines on definition, etiology, diagnosis and medical, endoscopic and surgical management of chronic pancreatitis German Society of Digestive and Metabolic Diseases (DGVS)]. Z Gastroenterol. 2012; 50(11):1176–1224

[18] Dufour MC, Adamson MD. The epidemiology of alcohol-induced pancreatitis. Pancreas. 2003; 27(4):286–290

[19] Braganza JM, Lee SH, McCloy RF, McMahon MJ. Chronic pancreatitis. Lancet. 2011; 377(9772):1184–1197

[20] Lévy P, Mathurin P, Roqueplo A, Rueff B, Bernades P. A multidimensional case-control study of dietary, alcohol, and tobacco habits in alcoholic men with chronic pancreatitis. Pancreas. 1995; 10(3):231–238

[21] Whitcomb DC, Gorry MC, Preston RA, et al. Hereditary pancreatitis is caused by a mutation in the cationic trypsinogen gene. Nat Genet. 1996; 14(2):141–145

[22] Lowenfels AB, Maisonneuve P, Cavallini G, et al. International Pancreatitis Study Group. Pancreatitis and the risk of pancreatic cancer. N Engl J Med. 1993; 328(20):1433–1437

[23] Yoshida K, Toki F, Takeuchi T, Watanabe S, Shiratori K, Hayashi N. Chronic pancreatitis caused by an autoimmune abnormality. Proposal of the concept of autoimmune pancreatitis. Dig Dis Sci. 1995; 40(7):1561–1568

[24] Rehnitz C, Klauss M, Singer R, et al. Morphologic patterns of autoimmune pancreatitis in CT and MRI. Pancreatology. 2011; 11(2):240–251

[25] American Cancer Society. Key statistics for pancreatic cancer. Available at: http://www.cancer.org/cancer/pancreaticcancer/detailedguide/pancreatic-cancer-key-statistics. Accessed June 7, 2016

[26] Robert Koch Institut. Gesellschaft der epidemiologischen Krebsregister in Deutschland e.V., eds. Krebs in Deutschland 2005/2006. Häufigkeiten und Trends. 7th ed. Berlin: Robert Koch Institut; 2010:40–43

[27] Genkinger JM, Spiegelman D, Anderson KE, et al. A pooled analysis of 14 cohort studies of anthropometric factors and pancreatic cancer risk. Int J Cancer. 2011; 129(7):1708–1717

[28] Zheng W, McLaughlin JK, Gridley G, et al. A cohort study of smoking, alcohol consumption, and dietary factors for pancreatic cancer (United States). Cancer Causes Control. 1993; 4(5):477–482

[29] Neoptolemos JP, Stocken DD, Friess H, et al. European Study Group for Pancreatic Cancer. A randomized trial of chemoradiotherapy and chemotherapy after resection of pancreatic cancer. N Engl J Med. 2004; 350(12):1200–1210

[30] Schünke M, Schulte E, Schumacher U., eds. Prometheus. LernAtlas der Anatomie: Innere Organe. 2nd ed. Stuttgart: Thieme; 2009. Illustrated by M. Voll/K. Wesker

[31] Wagner M, Redaelli C, Lietz M, Seiler CA, Friess H, Büchler MW. Curative resection is the single most important factor determining outcome in patients with pancreatic adenocarcinoma. Br J Surg. 2004; 91(5):586–594

[32] Wittekind C, Meyer HJ. TNM-Klassifikation maligner Tumoren – Pankreas. 7th ed. Weinheim: Wiley-Blackwell; 2010:122–125

[33] Bipat S, Phoa SS, van Delden OM, et al. Ultrasonography, computed tomography and magnetic resonance imaging for diagnosis and determining resectability of pancreatic adenocarcinoma: a meta-analysis. J Comput Assist Tomogr. 2005; 29(4):438–445

[34] Furukawa H, Kosuge T, Mukai K, et al. Helical computed tomography in the diagnosis of portal vein invasion by pancreatic head carcinoma: usefulness for selecting surgical procedures and predicting the outcome. Arch Surg. 1998; 133(1):61–65

[35] Lehmann KJ, Diehl SJ, Lachmann R, Georgi M. Value of dual-phase-helical CT in the preoperative diagnosis of pancreatic cancer–a prospective study [in German]. RoFo Fortschr Geb Rontgenstr Nuklearmed. 1998; 168(3):211–216

[36] Zeman RK, Cooper C, Zeiberg AS, et al. TNM staging of pancreatic carcinoma using helical CT. AJR Am J Roentgenol. 1997; 169(2):459–464

[37] Klauss M, Mohr A, von Tengg-Kobligk H, et al. A new invasion score for determining the resectability of pancreatic carcinomas with contrast-enhanced multidetector computed tomography. Pancreatology. 2008; 8(2):204–210

[38] Li H, Zeng MS, Zhou KR, Jin DY, Lou WH. Pancreatic adenocarcinoma: the different CT criteria for peripancreatic major arterial and venous invasion. J Comput Assist Tomogr. 2005; 29(2):170–175

[39] Li H, Zeng MS, Zhou KR, Jin DY, Lou WH. Pancreatic adenocarcinoma: signs of vascular invasion determined by multi-detector row CT. Br J Radiol. 2006; 79(947):880–887

[40] D'Onofrio M, Barbi E, Dietrich CF, et al. Pancreatic multicenter ultrasound study (PAMUS). Eur J Radiol. 2012; 81(4):630–638

[41] Ariyama J, Suyama M, Satoh K, Wakabayashi K. Endoscopic ultrasound and intraductal ultrasound in the diagnosis of small pancreatic tumors. Abdom Imaging. 1998; 23(4):380–386

[42] Helmstaedter L, Riemann JF. Pancreatic cancer—EUS and early diagnosis. Langenbecks Arch Surg. 2008; 393(6):923–927

[43] Spier BJ, Johnson EA, Gopal DV, et al. Predictors of malignancy and recommended follow-up in patients with negative endoscopic ultrasound-guided fine-needle aspiration of suspected pancreatic lesions. Can J Gastroenterol. 2009; 23(4):279–286

[44] Prokesch RW, Chow LC, Beaulieu CF, Bammer R, Jeffrey RB, Jr. Isoattenuating pancreatic adenocarcinoma at multi-detector row CT: secondary signs. Radiology. 2002; 224(3):764–768

[45] Adler G, Seufferlein T, Bischoff SC, et al. S3-Guidelines "Exocrine pancreatic cancer" 2007 [in German]. Z Gastroenterol. 2007; 45(6):487–523

[46] Grenacher L, Klauss M, Dukic L, et al. Diagnosis and staging of pancreatic carcinoma: MRI versus multislice-CT—a prospective study [in German]. RoFo Fortschr Geb Rontgenstr Nuklearmed. 2004; 176(11):1624–1633

[47] Vincent A, Herman J, Schulick R, Hruban RH, Goggins M. Pancreatic cancer. Lancet. 2011; 378(9791):607–620

[48] Kessler CM. The link between cancer and venous thromboembolism: a review. Am J Clin Oncol. 2009; 32(4) Suppl:S3–S7

[49] Bubendorf L, Feichter GE, Obermann EC, et al. Pathologie: Zytopathologie. Berlin: Springer; 2011:397–410

[50] Nöldge G, Weber MA, Ritzel RA, Werner MJ, Kauczor HU, Grenacher L. Invasive diagnostic procedures for insulinomas of the pancreas [in German]. Radiologe. 2009; 49(3):224–232

[51] Vick C, Zech CJ, Höpfner S, Waggershauser T, Reiser M. Imaging of neuroendocrine tumors of the pancreas [in German]. Radiologe. 2003; 43(4):293–300

[52] Okabayashi T, Shima Y, Sumiyoshi T, et al. Diagnosis and management of insulinoma. World J Gastroenterol. 2013; 19(6):829–837

[53] Herold G, ed. Innere Medizin: eine vorlesungsorientierte Darstellung, unter Berücksichtigung des Gegenstandskataloges für die Ärztliche Prüfung. Köln: Herold; 2009:469–483

[54] Kim SH, Lee JM, Han JK, et al. Intrapancreatic accessory spleen: findings on MR Imaging, CT, US and scintigraphy, and the pathologic analysis. Korean J Radiol. 2008; 9(2):162–174

[55] Wang YX. Superparamagnetic iron oxide based MRI contrast agents: Current status of clinical application. Quant Imaging Med Surg. 2011; 1(1):35–40

[56] Fernández-del Castillo C, Warshaw AL. Cystic tumors of the pancreas. Surg Clin North Am. 1995; 75(5):1001–1016

[57] Berland LL, Silverman SG, Gore RM, et al. Managing incidental findings on abdominal CT: white paper of the ACR incidental findings committee. J Am Coll Radiol. 2010; 7(10):754–773

[58] Sahani DV, Kadavigere R, Saokar A, Fernandez-del Castillo C, Brugge WR, Hahn PF. Cystic pancreatic lesions: a simple imaging-based classification system for guiding management. Radiographics. 2005; 25(6):1471–1484

[59] Buerke B, Heindel W, Wessling J. [Differential diagnosis and radiological management of cystic pancreatic lesions]. RoFo Fortschr Geb Rontgenstr Nuklearmed. 2010; 182(10):852–860

[60] Capella C, Solda E, Klöppel G, et al. Serous cystic neoplasms of the pancreas. In: Hamilton S, Lauri A, Kleihues P, Sobin LH, eds. Pathology and genetics of tumours of the digestive system—World Health Organization Classification of tumours. Lyon: IARC Press; 2000:231–232

[61] Brugge WR, Lauwers GY, Sahani D, Fernandez-del Castillo C, Warshaw AL. Cystic neoplasms of the pancreas. N Engl J Med. 2004; 351(12):1218–1226

[62] Strobel O, Z'graggen K, Schmitz-Winnenthal FH, et al. Risk of malignancy in serous cystic neoplasms of the pancreas. Digestion. 2003; 68(1):24–33
[63] D'Angelica M, Brennan MF, Suriawinata AA, Klimstra D, Conlon KC. Intraductal papillary mucinous neoplasms of the pancreas: an analysis of clinicopathologic features and outcome. Ann Surg. 2004; 239(3):400–408
[64] Salvia R, Fernández-del Castillo C, Bassi C, et al. Main-duct intraductal papillary mucinous neoplasms of the pancreas: clinical predictors of malignancy and long-term survival following resection. Ann Surg. 2004; 239(5):678–685, discussion 685–687
[65] Sohn TA, Yeo CJ, Cameron JL, et al. Intraductal papillary mucinous neoplasms of the pancreas: an updated experience. Ann Surg. 2004; 239(6):788–797, discussion 797–799
[66] Gourgiotis S, Ridolfini MP, Germanos S. Intraductal papillary mucinous neoplasms of the pancreas. Eur J Surg Oncol. 2007; 33(6):678–684
[67] Murakami Y, Uemura K, Hayashidani Y, Sudo T, Sueda T. Predictive factors of malignant or invasive intraductal papillary-mucinous neoplasms of the pancreas. J Gastrointest Surg. 2007; 11(3):338–344
[68] Campbell F, Azadeh B. Cystic neoplasms of the exocrine pancreas. Histopathology. 2008; 52(5):539–551
[69] Goh BK, Tan YM, Yap WM, et al. Pancreatic serous oligocystic adenomas: clinicopathologic features and a comparison with serous microcystic adenomas and mucinous cystic neoplasms. World J Surg. 2006; 30(8):1553–1559
[70] Tanaka M, Fernández-del Castillo C, Adsay V, et al. International Association of Pancreatology. International consensus guidelines 2012 for the management of IPMN and MCN of the pancreas. Pancreatology. 2012; 12(3):183–197
[71] Tipton SG, Smyrk TC, Sarr MG, Thompson GB. Malignant potential of solid pseudopapillary neoplasm of the pancreas. Br J Surg. 2006; 93(6):733–737
[72] Lee SY, Thng CH, Chow PKh. Lipoma of the pancreas, a case report and a review of the literature. World J Radiol. 2011; 3(10):246–248
[73] Sener SF, Fremgen A, Menck HR, et al. Pancreatic cancer: a report of treatment and survival trends for 100 313 patients diagnosed from 1985–1995, using the National Cancer Database. J Am Coll Surg. 1999; 189:1–7
[74] Zhang HM, Yao F, Liu GF, et al. The differences in imaging features of malignant and benign branch duct type of Intraductal Papillary Mucinous Tumor. Eur J Radiol. 2011; 80:744–748

8 Gastrointestinal Tract

Thomas C. Lauenstein and Lale Umutlu

8.1 Anatomy

8.1.1 Position and Divisions

All portions of the gastrointestinal tract—the esophagus, stomach, duodenum, jejunum, ileum, colon, and rectum—have the same general wall structure, which is adapted somewhat for specific regions. The wall layers that occur in all parts of the gastrointestinal tract are reviewed in ▶ Table 8.1.

The esophagus is a hollow muscular tube, approximately 25 cm long, located in the mediastinum between the pharynx and stomach. It consists of three parts:
- The cervical part.
- The thoracic part.
- The abdominal part.

The esophagus has three physiologic constrictions (▶ Fig. 8.1):
- *The upper esophageal constriction* includes the upper esophageal sphincter behind the cricoid cartilage.
- *The middle esophageal constriction* occurs where the esophagus is compressed by the aortic arch and tracheal bifurcation.
- *The lower esophageal constriction* is located at the level of the diaphragm.

The mucosal lining of the esophagus (squamous epithelium) is marked by a pattern of longitudinal folds.

The stomach occupies an asymmetrical position in the left upper quadrant of the abdomen (▶ Fig. 8.2). It curves from the gastroesophageal junction (cardia) to the gastric outlet (pylorus). The upper part of the stomach is formed by the fundus, which is continuous with the main part, or body, of the stomach. The portion of the stomach proximal to the pylorus is called the antrum. The stomach has characteristic longitudinal rugal folds that start in the proximal fundus and run distally to the antrum. The rugal folds are prominent in the empty stomach and are effaced as the stomach becomes distended.

The small intestine can be divided into three parts: the duodenum, jejunum, and ileum (▶ Fig. 8.3):

Table 8.1 Wall layers of the gastrointestinal tract, listed from inside to outside

Layers	Functions
Mucosa	
• Epithelium	Superficial protection, hormone production, glandular cells (except for the esophagus)
• Lamina propria	Mobility, lymphatic tissue
• Muscularis mucosae	Fine control of mucosal folds
Submucosa	Mobility, lymphatic tissue, Meissner plexus
Muscularis propria	Mixing and transport actions: myenteric plexus (Auerbach's plexus) between circular and longitudinal muscle layers
• Circular layer	
• Longitudinal layer	
Adventitia	Connective tissue, incorporates the gastrointestinal tract into surrounding tissues
Subserosa	Present only in intraperitoneal portions of the gastrointestinal tract
Serosa	Present only in intraperitoneal portions of the gastrointestinal tract
• Lamina propria of serosa	
• Mesothelium	

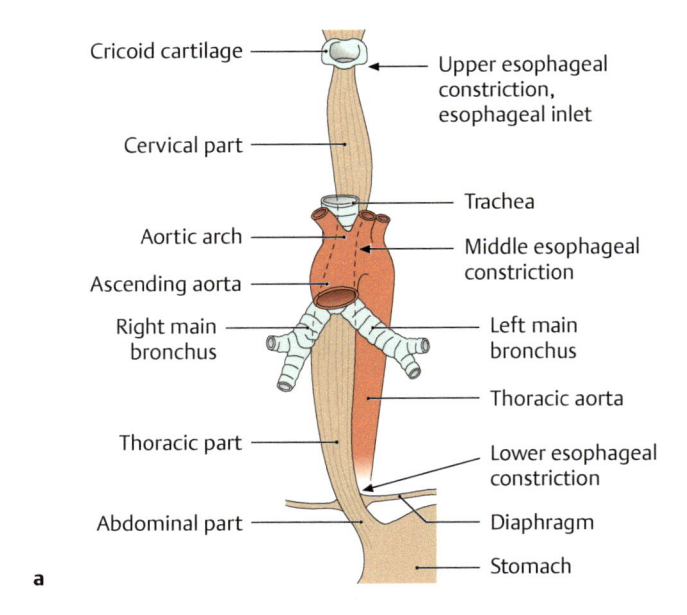

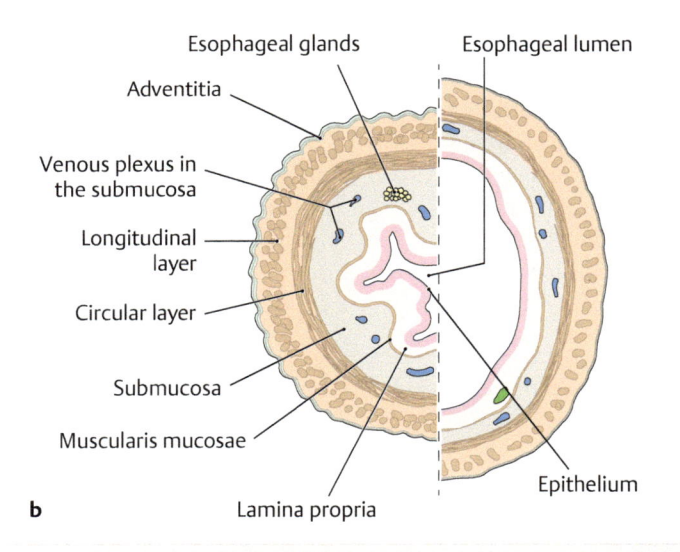

Fig. 8.1 Anatomy of the esophagus. (a) The trachea is anterior to the esophagus. The three physiologic constrictions are shown. (b) Structure of the esophageal wall in the contracted state (left) and relaxed state (right). (Reproduced from Schünke M, Schulte E, Schumacher U. Prometheus. LernAtlas der Anatomie: Innere Organe. Illustrated by M. Voll/K. Wesker. 2nd ed. Stuttgart: Thieme; 2009.)

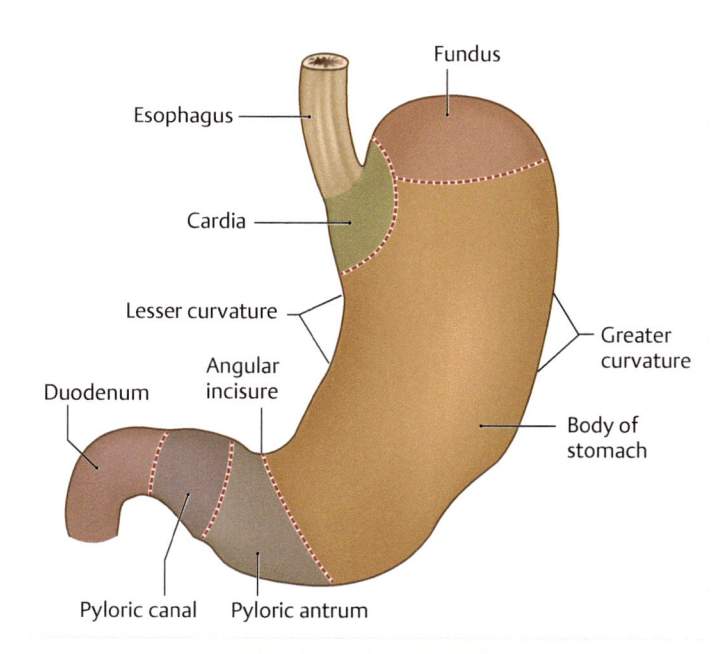

Fig. 8.2 Anatomy of the stomach. Schematic diagram.

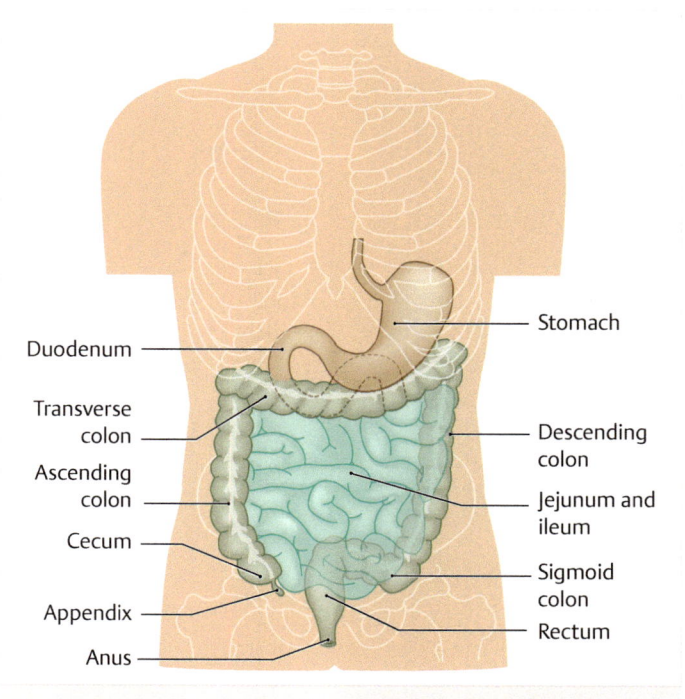

Fig. 8.3 Anatomy of the small and large intestine. Schematic diagram.

- *Duodenum*: The duodenum is approximately 25 cm long, receives the common bile duct and pancreatic duct at the papilla of Vater, and merges with the jejunum at the ligament of Treitz. The C-shaped duodenum consists (from oral to aboral) of a superior part, a descending part, a horizontal part, and an ascending part. The inner surface of the duodenum is almost completely devoid of folds. The descending part has a short longitudinal fold, or plica, on which the pancreatic duct and common bile duct open at the papilla of Vater.
- *Jejunum*: The jejunum is in the left upper quadrant of the abdomen and is approximately 2.0 to 2.5 meters long. Together with the ileum, its function is to absorb nutrients from ingested food. The mucosal lining of the jejunum is marked by transverse, crescent-shaped folds (Kerckring's folds, valvulae conniventes).
- *Ileum*: The ileum is located in the mid- and lower abdomen and is approximately 3 m long. Small mucosal folds are present only in its proximal portion. Instead, the ileum has nodular areas of lymphatic tissue (Peyer's patches) on the side opposite the mesentery, which are grossly visible from the outside through the bowel wall. The ileum joins with the large intestine at the ileocecal valve.

The large intestine can be divided into three parts:
- Cecum.
- Colon.
- Rectum (see ▶ Fig. 8.3).

The colon, in turn, consists of several segments:
- Ascending colon.
- Transverse colon.
- Descending colon.
- Sigmoid colon.

Note

The gastrointestinal tract has both intraperitoneal and retroperitoneal portions. The following portions are retroperitoneal:
- Duodenum (except for the ascending part.)
- Ascending colon.
- Descending colon.
- Rectum.

The total length of the colon ranges from 100 to 170 cm. The wall structure of the colon is markedly different from that of the small intestine and rectum. It is characterized by three separate, longitudinal bands of smooth muscle fibers in the colon wall (teniae coli). Another feature is an alternation between sacculations of the colon wall (haustra) and crescent-shaped constrictions (semilunar folds). The rectum is characterized by several transverse mucosal folds. The middle and most prominent transverse fold, called Kohlrausch's fold, is situated approximately 5 to 8 cm proximal to the anus and marks the start of the retroperitoneal part of the rectum. Viewed in longitudinal section, the muscular layer of the rectum is not bundled into teniae as in the colon but forms a uniform longitudinal coat. Viewed in cross section, the muscular layer of the rectum is thickened above the anus to form a constricting ring, the internal anal sphincter.

8.1.2 Imaging Landmarks

▶ **Radiographic landmarks.** ▶ Fig. 8.4 shows the radiographic landmarks for the esophagus, and ▶ Fig. 8.5 shows the landmarks

Gastrointestinal Tract

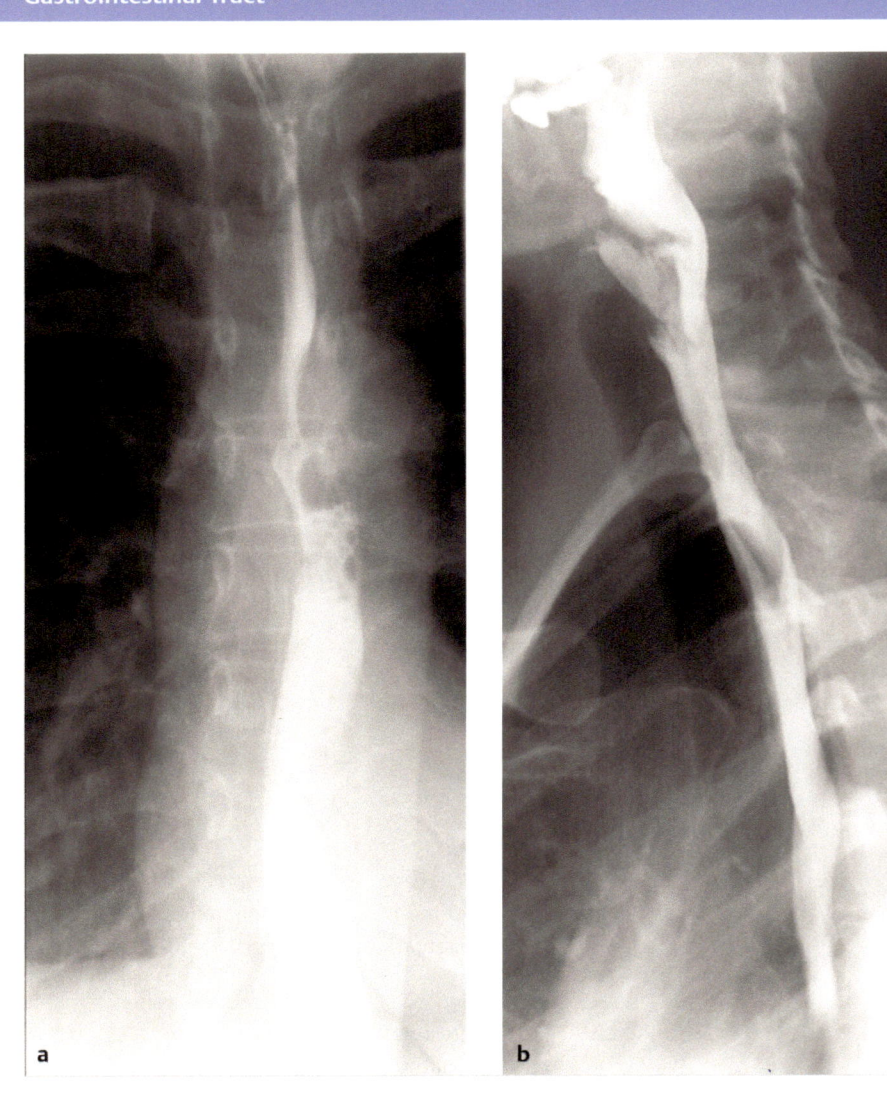

Fig. 8.4 Anatomy of the esophagus. Oral contrast examination. **(a)** AP projection. **(b)** Lateral projection.

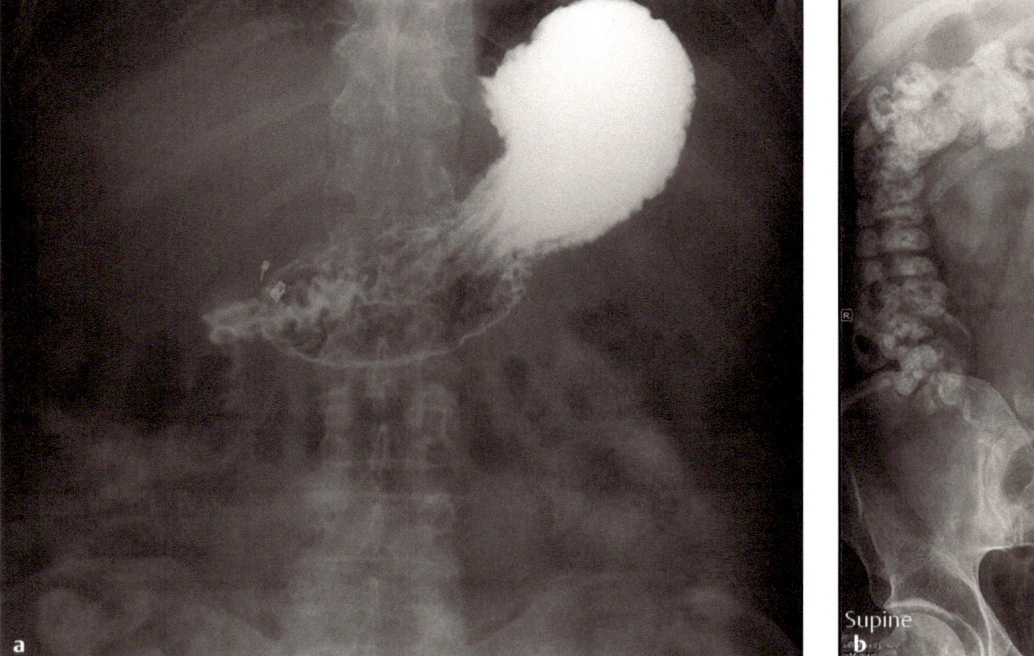

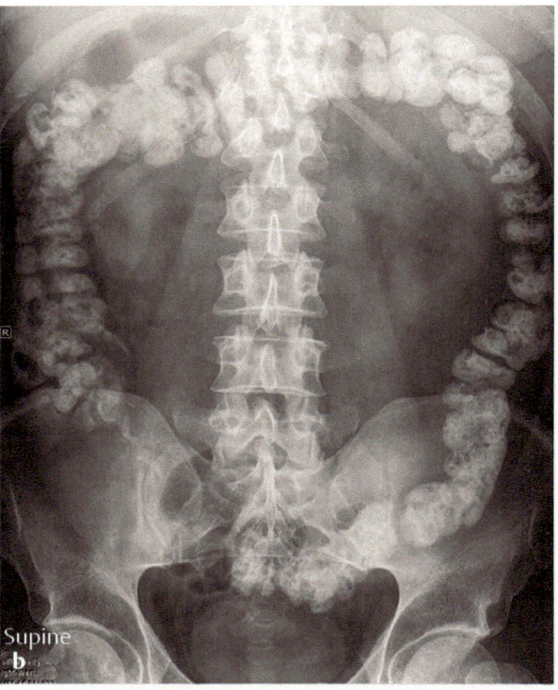

Fig. 8.5 Anatomy of the stomach and large intestine. (a) Anatomy of the stomach in the left upper abdomen after oral administration of contrast medium. **(b)** Anatomy of the ascending, transverse and descending colon after rectal administration of contrast medium.

for the gastrointestinal tract. In most cases, delineation of the gastrointestinal tract requires the administration of contrast material such as certain barium compounds or iodinated contrast media.

▶ **Sonographic landmarks.** Ultrasound displays the typical stratified wall structure of the gastrointestinal tract, consisting of the hypoechoic mucosa, hyperechoic submucosa, and hypoechoic muscularis propria (▶ Fig. 8.6).

▶ **Landmarks in CT and MRI.** As in conventional radiography, gastrointestinal structures are demonstrated more clearly by CT and MRI when orally and/or rectally administered contrast media are used. Without contrast medium, portions of the stomach and bowel are often in a collapsed state and are poorly delineated from neighboring structures. Moreover, diagnostic evaluation of the gastrointestinal wall is significantly more difficult without contrast material. The esophagus descends between the trachea and the aorta in the posterior superior mediastinum. Its distal portion borders on the left atrium. The anterior stomach wall is in contact with the liver on the left side and the spleen on the right side. The stomach relates posteriorly to the pancreas and inferiorly to the transverse colon (▶ Fig. 8.7). Imaging landmarks for the small and large intestine are illustrated in ▶ Fig. 8.8 and ▶ Fig. 8.9.

8.2 Imaging

8.2.1 Radiography

Fluoroscopic examination with oral contrast medium still has a major role in imaging studies of the esophagus.

> **Caution**
>
> The use of barium contrast medium is contraindicated in patients with a suspected esophageal perforation. Also, a water-soluble iodinated iso-osmotic contrast medium should be used if there is a risk of aspiration (test with a sip of water).

Disease of the gastrointestinal tract have a diverse etiology that mainly includes inflammations, infections, and tumors. The indications for a plain abdominal radiograph, which should be taken in the supine or left lateral decubitus (LLD) position, are limited to a few conditions such as bowel obstruction (▶ Fig. 8.10) or suspected free air originating from a perforation or dehiscent suture line (▶ Fig. 8.11). Abdominal radiographs may also be obtained to evaluate the transit of oral contrast medium and check for lesions that could delay gastrointestinal transit, such as tumors or bowel adhesions.

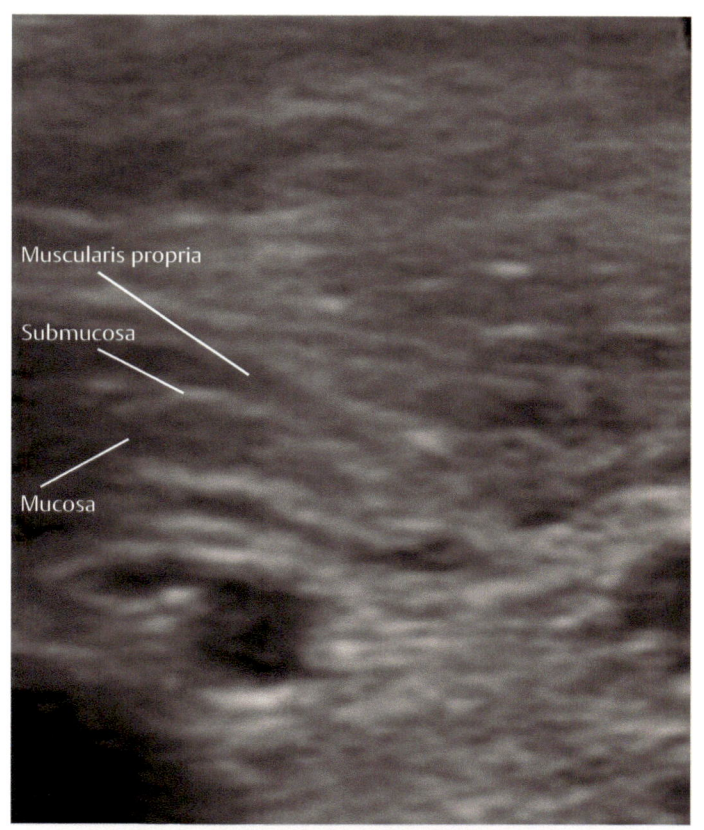

Fig. 8.6 Gastrointestinal wall. Ultrasound appearance. The mucosa is hypoechoic, the submucosa is hyperechoic, and the muscularis propria is hypoechoic.

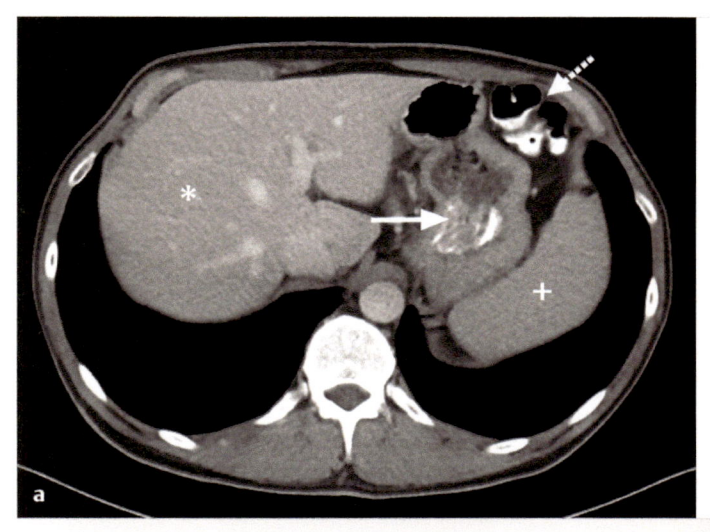

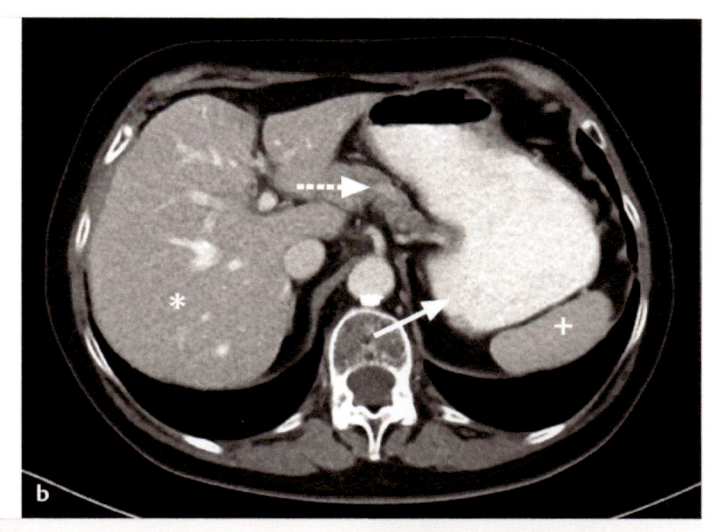

Fig. 8.7 Stomach and adjacent organs. Axial CT scans. **(a)** Solid arrow, stomach; dashed arrow, colon; cross, spleen; asterisk, liver. **(b)** Solid arrow, stomach; dashed arrow, pancreas: cross, spleen; asterisk, liver.

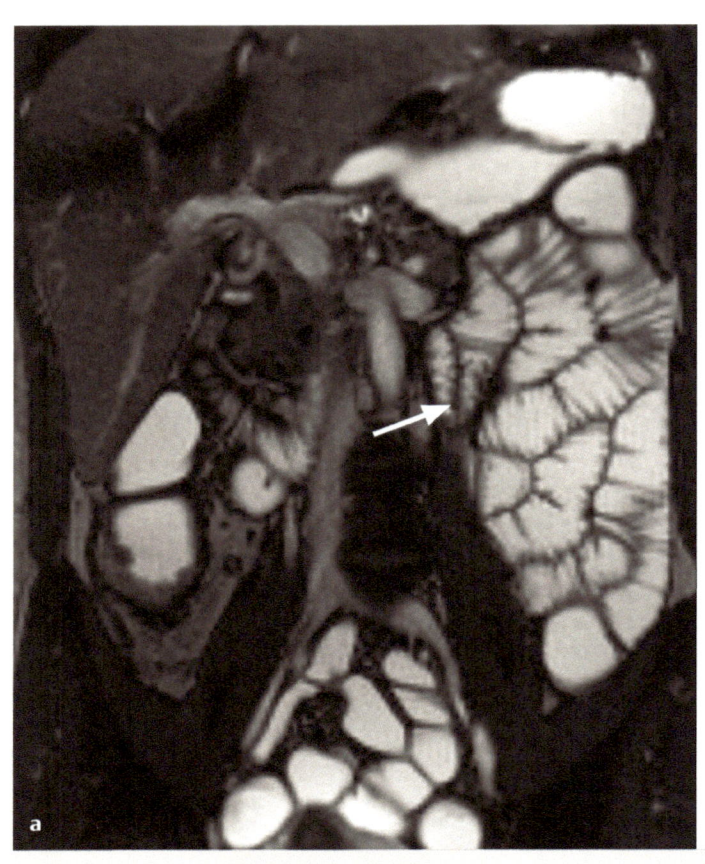

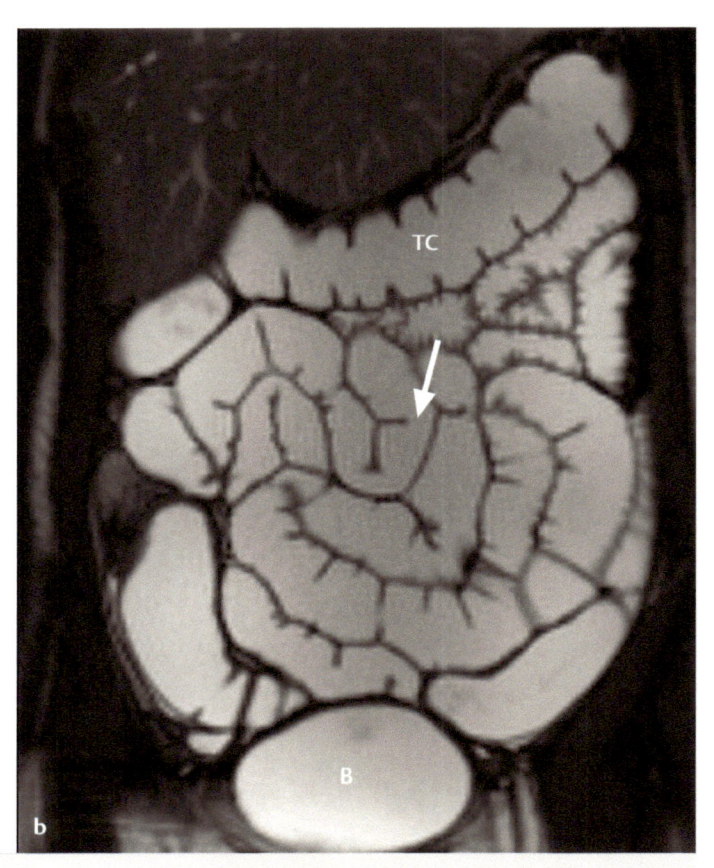

Fig. 8.8 Sectional imaging landmarks for the small intestine. Coronal MR images. **(a)** The jejunum (arrow). **(b)** The ileum (arrow). The transverse colon (TC) and urinary bladder (B) are also shown.

8.2.2 Computed Tomography and Magnetic Resonance Imaging

Computed tomography (CT) is the imaging modality of choice for acute clinical diagnosis and for staging. Magnetic resonance imaging (MRI) is preferred for nonacute indications (e.g., follow-ups).

Note

With few exceptions, sectional imaging modalities like CT and MRI have replaced conventional radiographs in the evaluation of gastrointestinal diseases.

8.2.3 Contrast Media

The use of oral or rectal contrast media often provides great diagnostic benefit:
- They help define the wall of the gastrointestinal tract and delineate it from the lumen.
- They help in distinguishing bowel from mesenteric or retroperitoneal structures.

Conventional imaging studies employ barium-containing or iodinated media as positive contrast agents. Barium-based media should not be used in patients with a suspected perforation of the gastrointestinal tract, as they could incite a severe peritonitis. Recent studies have shown that negative contrast media such as mannitol or mineral water (1 liter ingested over a 30-minute period) are better than positive media for evaluating the intestinal wall on CT. Gastrografin, a water-soluble radiopaque contrast medium, should be used in patients with a suspected perforation because contrast extravasation into the free abdominal cavity would be indistinguishable from ascites if a negative medium was used. Water-based contrast media (e.g., mannitol solutions) can also be used in MRI.

8.3 Diseases of the Esophagus

8.3.1 Achalasia

▶ **Brief definition.** Achalasia is a functional disorder of the smooth muscle of the lower esophageal sphincter secondary to degenerative changes in the myenteric plexus. It results in a failure of lower esophageal sphincter relaxation during swallowing. The prevalence of achalasia is approximately 10:100,000 population per year, with a peak age of incidence in the third and fourth decades.

Note

Achalasia progresses in three stages:
- Hypermotile stage.
- Hypomotile stage.
- Amotile stage.

During the first stage, the proximal part of the esophagus increases its motility in an effort to surmount the increased distal resistance. Further progression is marked by increasing damage to the esophageal muscles and diminished contractions.

8.3 Diseases of the Esophagus

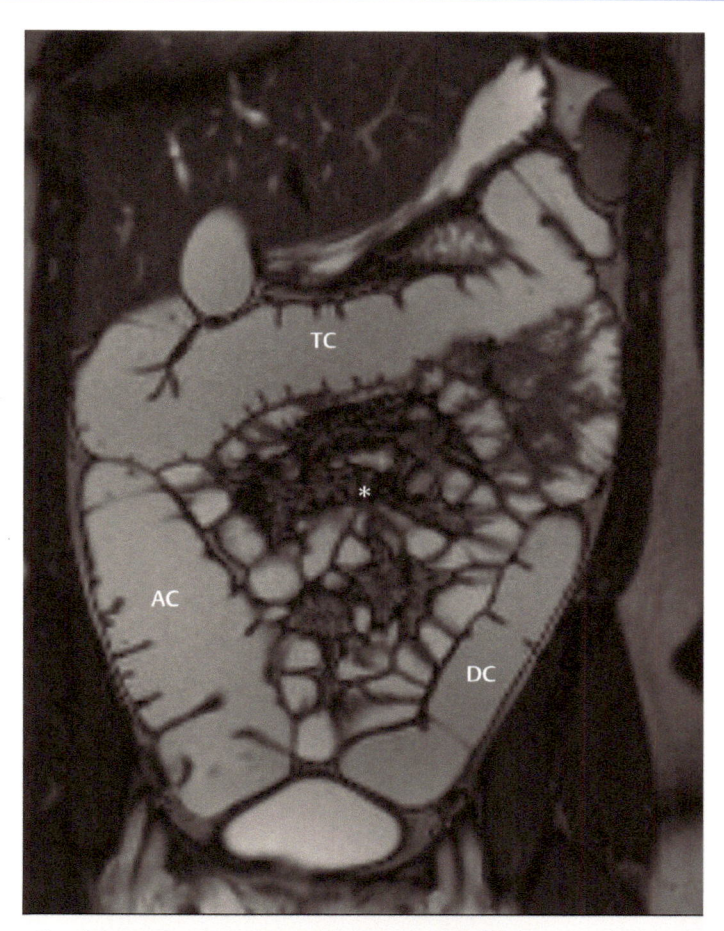

Fig. 8.9 Sectional imaging of the colon. Limbs of the colon displayed by T2 W MRI. The asterisk indicates small bowel loops and mesenteric structures enclosed by the colon. AC, ascending colon; DC, descending colon; TC, transverse colon.

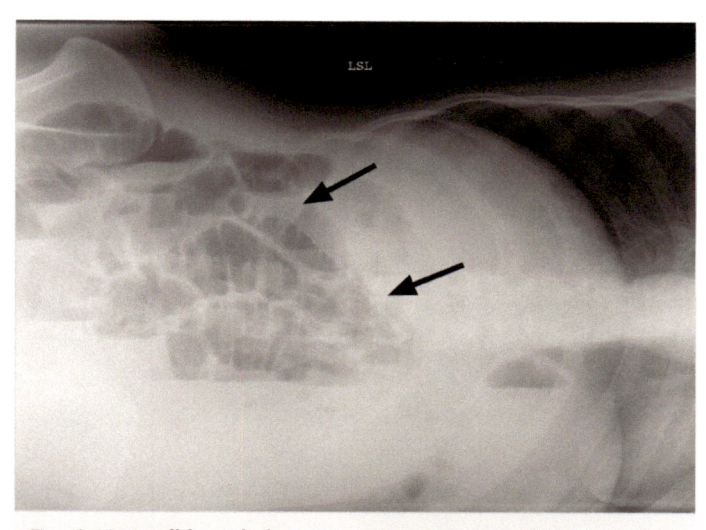

Fig. 8.10 Small-bowel obstruction. Conventional radiograph in left lateral decubitus shows moderately distended small-bowel loops with multiple air–fluid levels (arrows) consistent with a small-bowel obstruction.

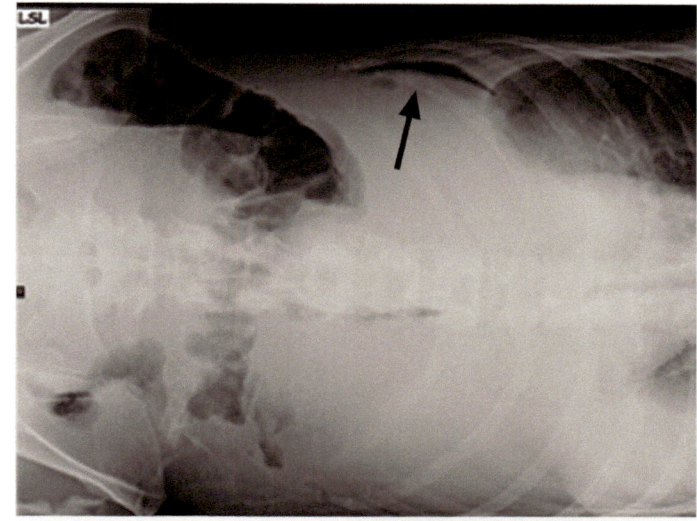

Fig. 8.11 Free air. Free air is visible along the dome of the liver (arrow) in a patient with a perforated bowel.

▶ Imaging signs. Fluoroscopic imaging (▶ Fig. 8.12) shows dilatation of the thoracic esophagus with funnel-shaped or "bird-beak" narrowing of the distal esophagus. The passage of contrast medium through the gastroesophageal junction is greatly delayed.

▶ Clinical features. Patients typically present with dysphagia, which is usually associated with regurgitation (and possible aspiration) and retrosternal pain. Initial treatment consists of pharmacologic agents such as calcium-channel blockers to reduce the muscle tone of the lower esophageal sphincter. Other treatment options are balloon dilation (which may be repeated as required), endoscopic botulinum injection, and surgery.

▶ Differential diagnosis. It is important to exclude a secondary cause of lower esophageal narrowing, such as a malignant tumor. In this case, however, a mass lesion would be found at imaging, whereas primary achalasia would not be associated with a detectable mass. The differential diagnosis also includes scleroderma, which is distinguished by generalized dilatation and dysmotility of the esophagus.

▶ Key points. Before achalasia is diagnosed, it is important to exclude a different cause of esophageal obstruction, particularly a malignant tumor.

8.3.2 Esophageal Diverticula

▶ Brief definition. Esophageal diverticula are outpouchings that involve one or more layers of the esophageal wall. Two main types are distinguished:
- *Pulsion diverticula*: These are pseudodiverticula that result from increased intraluminal pressure and involve the herniation of mucosa and submucosa through the muscularis propria.
- *Traction diverticula*: These are true diverticula that involve the herniation of all wall layers. They usually result from pulling forces on the outer aspect of the esophagus.

Pulsion diverticula are far more common than traction diverticula. Esophageal diverticula are classified by their location (▶ Fig. 8.13):
- *Zenker's diverticulum*: a pulsion diverticulum caused by weakness of the cervical esophagus just above the cricopharyngeus muscle.

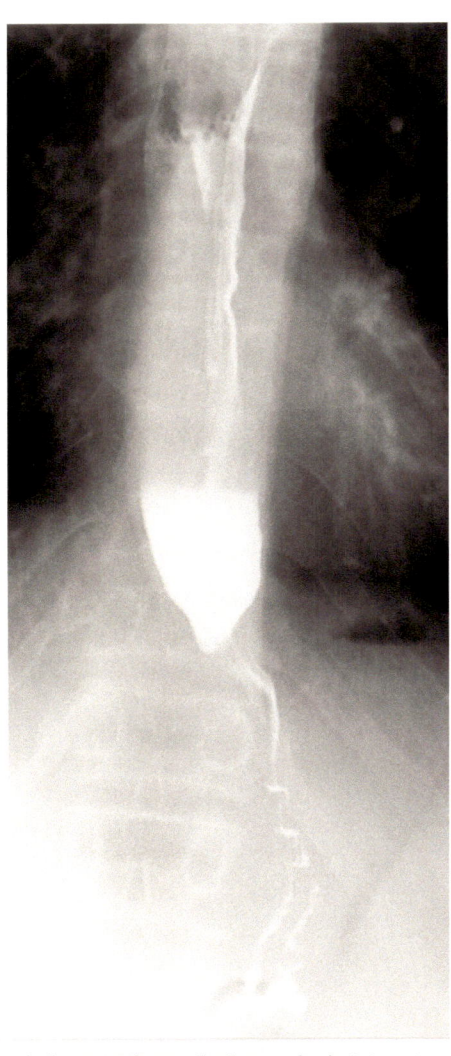

Fig. 8.12 Achalasia. Radiograph after oral administration of contrast medium. The distal esophagus is tapered with a "champagne glass" appearance.

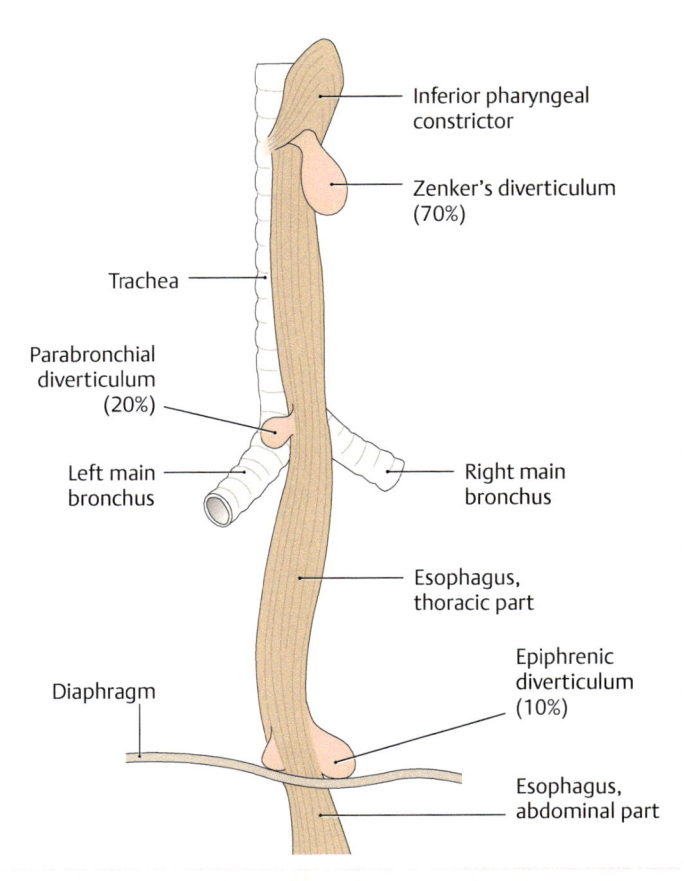

Fig. 8.13 Location and frequency distribution of esophageal diverticula. Schematic diagram. (Reproduced from Schünke M, Schulte E, Schumacher U. Prometheus. LernAtlas der Anatomie: Innere Organe. Illustrated by M. Voll/K. Wesker. 2nd ed. Stuttgart: Thieme; 2009.)

- *Parabronchial diverticulum*: a traction diverticulum usually caused by inflammation of lymph nodes with subsequent scarring and adhesion of matted nodes to the esophagus.
- *Epiphrenic diverticulum*: a pulsion diverticulum of the distal esophagus that results from a swallowing disorder in which the intraluminal pressure is raised before the food bolus enters the stomach.

▶ **Imaging signs.** Most esophageal diverticula are clearly detectable as outpouchings in the oral contrast study. The examination should always be performed in two stages. After the contrast medium bolus has been swallowed and has passed through the esophagus, contrast medium will tend to pool in the diverticulum, and the retained contrast medium will remain visible for some time (▶ Fig. 8.14).

▶ **Clinical features.** Esophageal diverticula are usually asymptomatic, but some patients complain of dysphagia and a foreign-body sensation. Foul breath odor may result from retained food residues in the diverticulum. Complications such as fistulation or rupture are rare. Very large, symptomatic diverticula should be surgically removed.

▶ **Differential diagnosis.** Diverticula have very typical imaging features, so generally there is no need to consider other possible entities. Hiatal hernias can sometimes mimic diverticula on sectional images, but differentiation is easily accomplished by oral contrast examination.

▶ **Key points.** Esophageal diverticula are usually asymptomatic. Oral contrast examination is diagnostic.

8.3.3 Esophageal Varices

▶ **Brief definition.** Esophageal varices are enlarged submucosal vessels in the esophageal wall that develop in response to portal hypertension. The portal hypertension, usually secondary to hepatic cirrhosis, stimulates the development of collateral blood flow (through the short gastric veins to the esophageal veins), causing enlargement of the esophageal vessels and the development of a portocaval shunt.

▶ **Imaging signs.** Contrast-enhanced CT or MRI can clearly demonstrate the convoluted varices in or on the esophageal wall (▶ Fig. 8.15). On fluoroscopic examination with oral contrast medium, esophageal varices appear as tortuous, longitudinal filling defects in the esophageal lumen (▶ Fig. 8.16).

▶ **Clinical features.** Esophageal varices may be clinically silent initially. Very large varices may lead to narrowing or obstruction

8.3 Diseases of the Esophagus

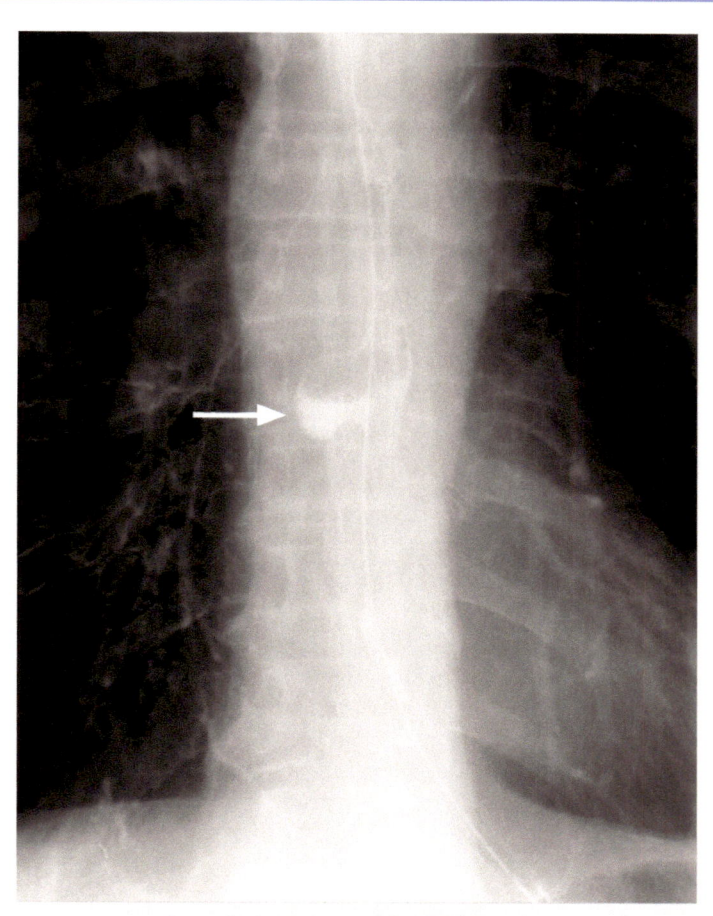

Fig. 8.14 Parabronchial esophageal diverticulum. Contrast medium has been retained in a diverticulum (arrow) following oral contrast examination.

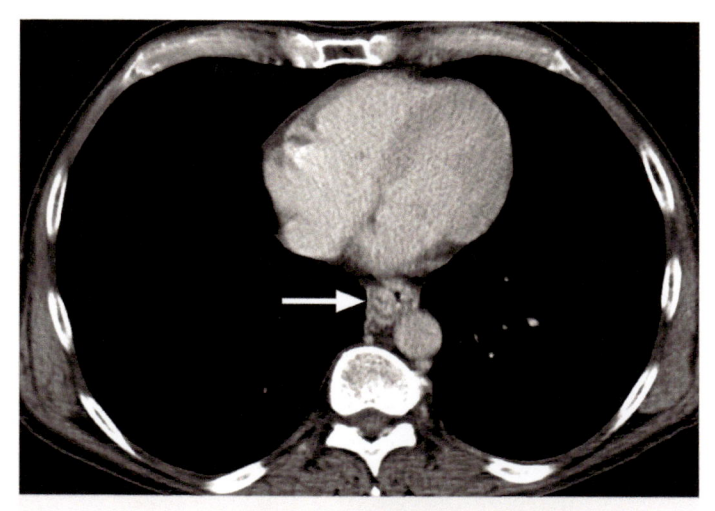

Fig. 8.15 Varices in and on the esophageal wall. Axial CT scan shows marked enhancement and tortuosity of the varices (arrow).

of the esophageal lumen. It is common to find associated signs of portal hypertension such as splenomegaly or ascites.

Note
Rupture and bleeding of the thin-walled esophageal varices is a life-threatening complication that requires prompt endoscopic sclerotherapy.

If sclerotherapy cannot be undertaken right away, a Sengstaken–Blakemore tube with an inflatable balloon can be passed down the esophagus as a temporizing measure. The mortality rate of acute variceal hemorrhage is 30%. In patients with recurrent bleeding, a transjugular intrahepatic portosystemic shunt can be placed to lower the portal venous pressure and reduce the bleeding risk.

▶ **Differential diagnosis.** Only a few entities need to be considered in the differential diagnosis. Hiatal hernias may resemble esophageal varices on sectional images but will generally contain air–fluid levels. Other masses such as esophageal carcinoma or mediastinal lymph nodes do not display the typical longitudinal orientation or tortuosity of esophageal varices. Another helpful differentiating criterion is given by the fact that esophageal varices almost always occur in a setting of hepatic cirrhosis.

▶ **Key points.** Esophageal varices have a characteristic imaging appearance with a very limited differential diagnosis.

8.3.4 Esophageal Atresia and Tracheoesophageal Fistula

▶ **Brief definition.** Esophageal atresia is a congenital interruption of the esophagus, usually with an associated tracheoesophageal fistula. Esophageal atresia has a reported prevalence of 1 in 3,000 to 4,000 neonates. The most common form, accounting for 90% of cases, is Vogt type IIIb (▶ Table 8.2, ▶ Fig. 8.17). Esophageal atresia is usually combined with other anomalies in the VACTERL association:
- V: vertebral anomalies.
- A: anal atresia.
- C: cardiac anomalies.
- TE: tracheoesophageal fistula.
- R: renal anomalies.
- L: limb deformities.

▶ **Imaging signs.** Findings on plain chest and abdominal radiographs are variable, depending on the type of atresia. Types I, II, and IIIa are associated with an air-free abdomen, while types IIIb and IIIc are characterized by air in the upper abdomen. It is common to find pulmonary changes due to aspiration. Oral administration of contrast medium demonstrates pooling of contrast medium within a blind pouch.

▶ **Clinical features.** Clinical manifestations include coughing and drooling in neonates, with a deterioration of clinical status. Suspicion of esophageal atresia can be confirmed by introducing a gastric tube. If atresia is present, the tube cannot be passed into the stomach, and gastric juices cannot be aspirated (▶ Fig. 8.18). Treatment is surgical and consists of an end-to-end anastomosis of the esophagus or reconstruction by an esophagoplasty. Surgery includes the repair of tracheoesophageal fistulas.

▶ **Differential diagnosis.** The differential diagnosis includes high-grade esophageal strictures or stenoses, but these lesions are rare in neonates.

▶ **Key points.** Radiological findings depend on the type of atresia. It is also important to look for possible associated anomalies.

Gastrointestinal Tract

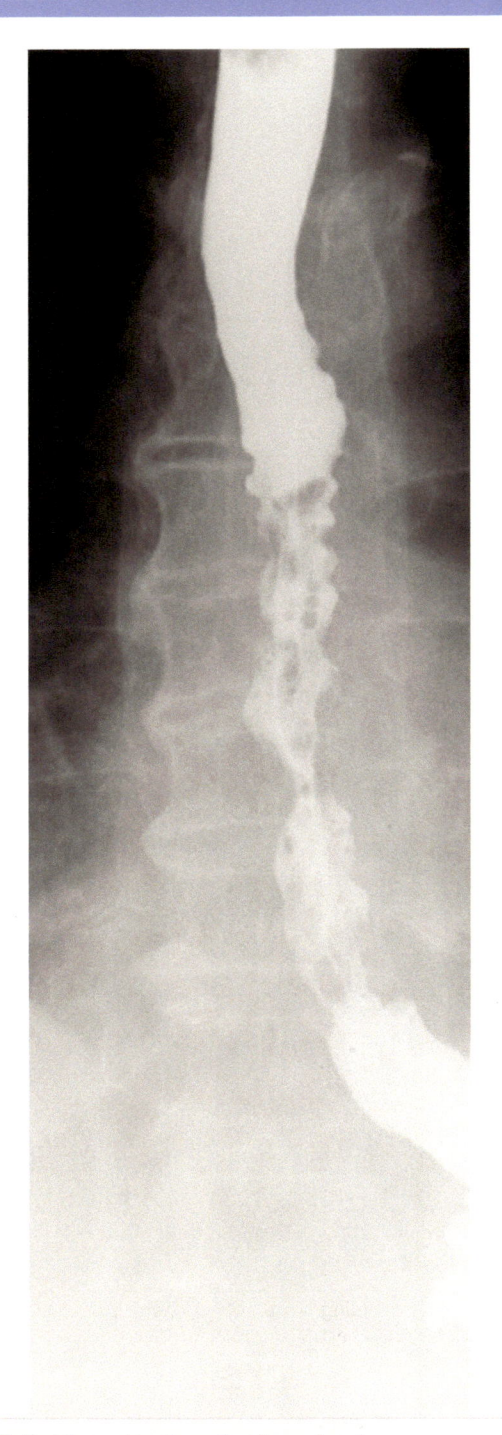

Fig. 8.16 Esophageal varices. Esophageal varices appear as longitudinal filling defects on oral contrast examination.

Table 8.2 Vogt classification of esophageal atresia

Type	Description
I	Aplasia
II	Atresia without a fistula
IIIa	Atresia with a proximal fistula
IIIb	Atresia with a distal fistula
IIIc	Combination of types IIIa and IIIb
IV	Tracheoesophageal fistula without atresia (H-type fistula)

▶ **Imaging signs.** Plain radiography and sectional imaging demonstrate an intrathoracic or retrocardiac mass that is partially air-filled and is closely related to the diaphragm (▶ Fig. 8.21).

▶ **Clinical features.** Hiatal hernia is usually asymptomatic, but loss of the functional esophageal sphincter may lead to increased gastroesophageal reflux. This can produce symptoms of reflux disease such as heartburn, regurgitation, and pain. Barrett's esophagus will develop in approximately 10% of patients with reflux disease. This condition results from chronic inflammation of the esophagus due to acid reflux and is characterized by a metaplasia that transforms the nonkeratinized stratified squamous epithelium of the esophagus into a single layer of columnar epithelium. Barrett's esophagus is considered a precancerous condition with a 40-fold increase in cancer risk relative to the normal population. In addition, large hernias may compromise pulmonary ventilation. Axial sliding hernia with concomitant reflux disease can be treated by fundoplication. Paraesophageal hernias should be surgically repaired because of the risk of incarceration or volvulus.

▶ **Differential diagnosis.** The differential diagnosis includes other masses of the posterior mediastinum such as neurogenic tumors or pericardial cysts, but these lesions do not contain air. Bronchogenic cysts may be difficult to distinguish from hiatal hernia because they may also contain air if they communicate with the bronchial tree or esophagus. Oral contrast examination can reliably differentiate these conditions, however.

▶ **Key points.** Hiatal hernias are a common finding in older patients and are usually asymptomatic.

8.3.5 Hiatal Hernia

▶ **Brief definition.** A hiatal hernia occurs when portions of the stomach herniate into the chest through the esophageal hiatus of the diaphragm. Two main types are distinguished:
- *Axial sliding hernia*: In this type the gastric cardia slides through the esophageal hiatus into the mediastinum (▶ Fig. 8.19). The gastroesophageal junction is intrathoracic.
- *Paraesophageal hernia*: Portions of the stomach herniate through the esophageal hiatus alongside the esophagus. The gastroesophageal junction is intra-abdominal. The extreme form is an "upside-down stomach" (▶ Fig. 8.20).

8.3.6 Esophageal Carcinoma

▶ **Brief definition.** Esophageal carcinoma is a malignant tumor of the esophagus. The two main types are squamous cell carcinoma (70–80% of cases) and adenocarcinoma (20–30%). The risk of developing squamous cell carcinoma is increased in smokers, heavy drinkers, and patients with achalasia. Adenocarcinoma often develops in patients with a Barrett's esophagus. The peak age of incidence is in the sixth and seventh decades.

▶ **Imaging signs.** The contrast swallow study shows irregular narrowing of the esophageal lumen, sometimes with associated ulceration of the esophageal mucosa (▶ Fig. 8.22). Sectional imaging can define the depth of mediastinal invasion and provide

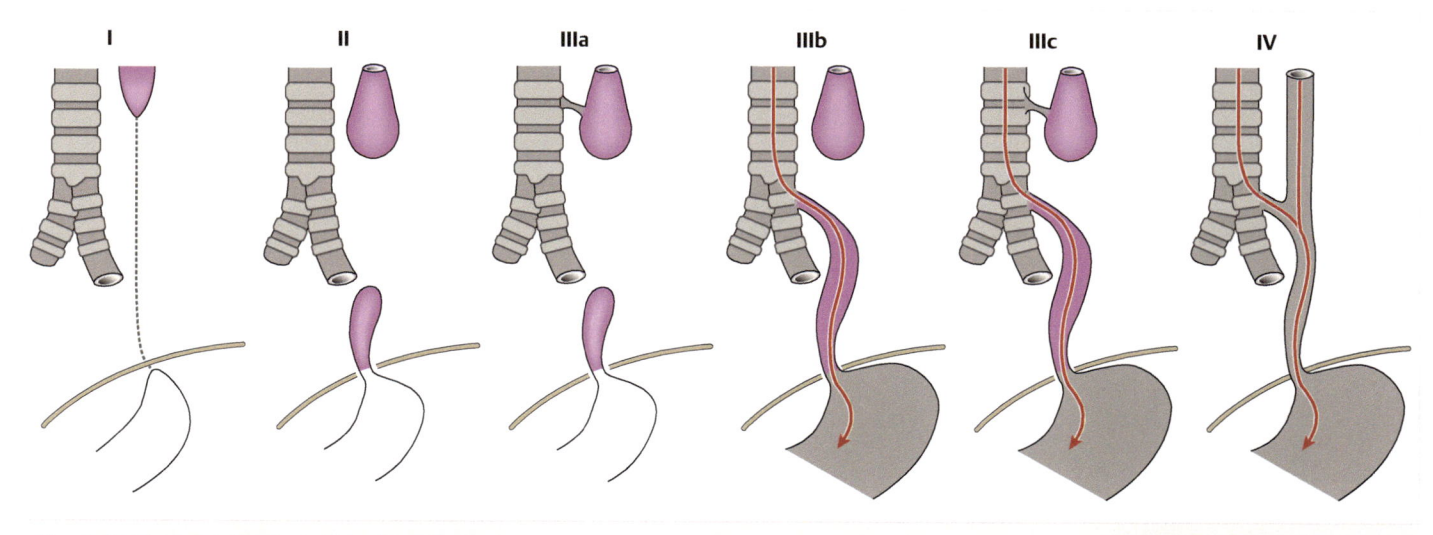

Fig. 8.17 Vogt classification of esophageal atresia.

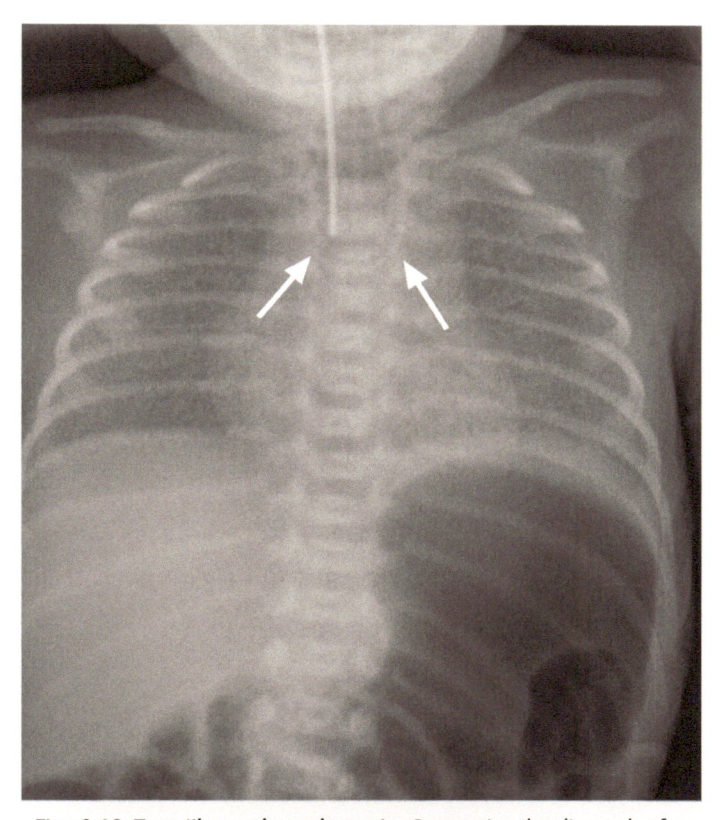

Fig. 8.18 Type IIb esophageal atresia. Conventional radiograph of a newborn shows a stomach tube doubled back in an esophageal blind pouch (arrows). The air-filled stomach suggests the presence of a tracheoesophageal fistula.

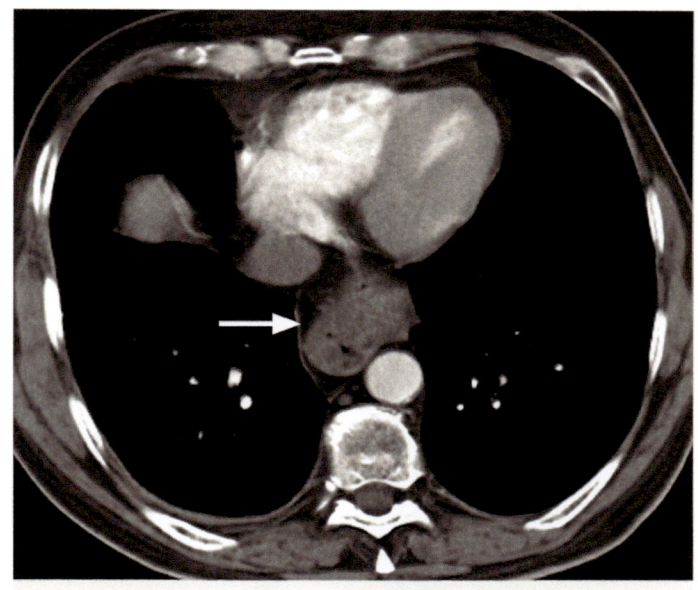

Fig. 8.19 Para-axial sliding hernia. CT shows displacement of the gastric cardia into the chest (arrow).

▶ **Differential diagnosis.** The differential diagnosis includes esophageal strictures due to other causes (e.g., peptic strictures) and achalasia, which is distinguished by a smooth, less irregular mucosal lining. Other tumors of the esophagus, such as leiomyomas, are rare.

▶ **Key points.** The primary tumor can be clearly visualized in a contrast swallow study. CT is used mainly for the staging of disease.

information on lymph node status and possible distant metastasis (▶ Fig. 8.23).

▶ **Clinical features.** Esophageal carcinoma is associated with dysphagia and weight loss. The TNM classification of esophageal carcinoma is shown in ▶ Table 8.3. Treatment options (surgery, chemoradiotherapy) are determined by the UICC (Union for International Cancer Control) stage of the disease (▶ Table 8.4).

8.4 Diseases of the Gastroduodenum

Because many pathologic changes in the stomach and duodenum occur at the mucosal level, imaging studies are often less rewarding than endoscopy. Nevertheless, imaging plays a crucial role in

Gastrointestinal Tract

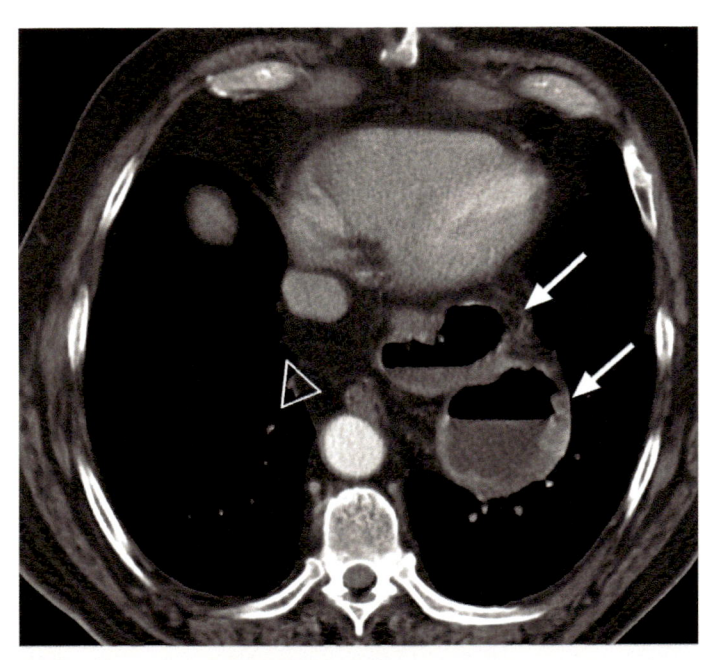

Fig. 8.20 Paraesophageal hernia with an "upside-down stomach." The esophagus (open arrowhead) is visible in the same section as intrathoracic portions of the herniated stomach (arrows).

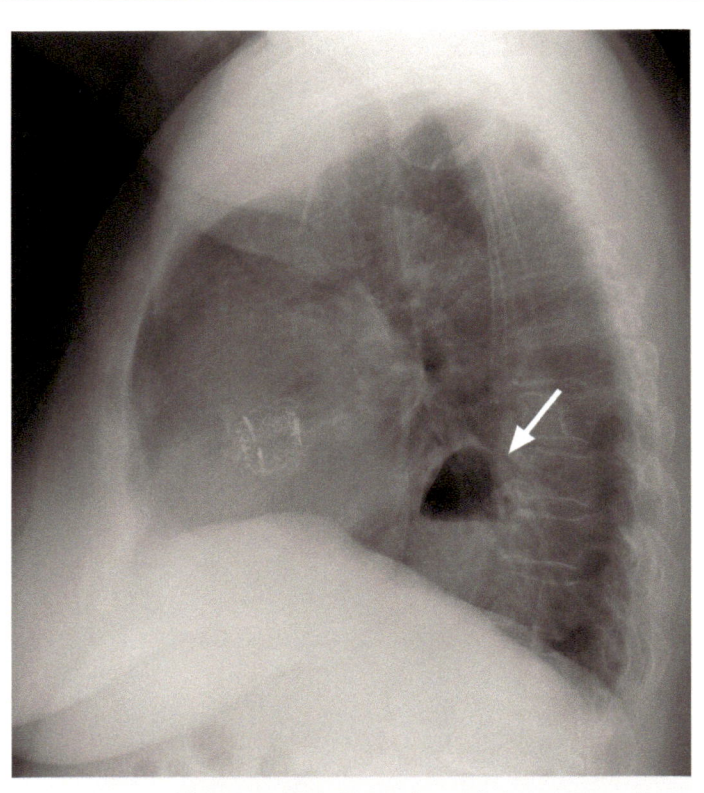

Fig. 8.21 Hiatal hernia. Lateral chest radiograph demonstrates the hiatal hernia as a partially air-filled retrocardiac mass (arrow). Previous aortic valve replacement is noted as an incidental finding.

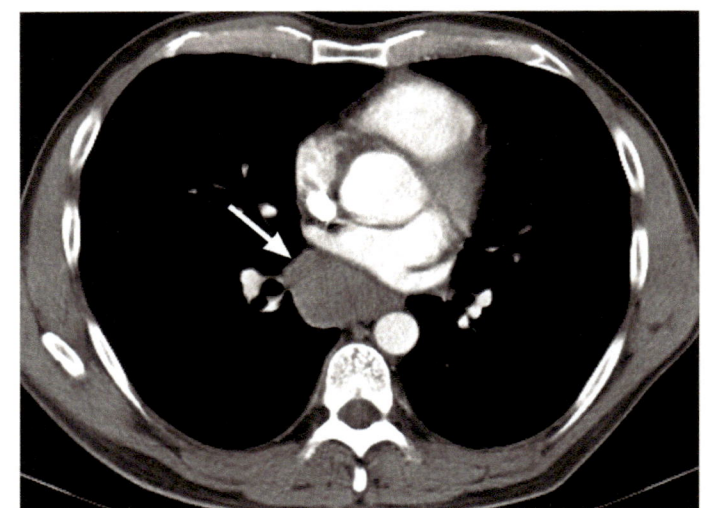

Fig. 8.23 Large esophageal carcinoma. CT can accurately define the extent of tumor involvement (arrow).

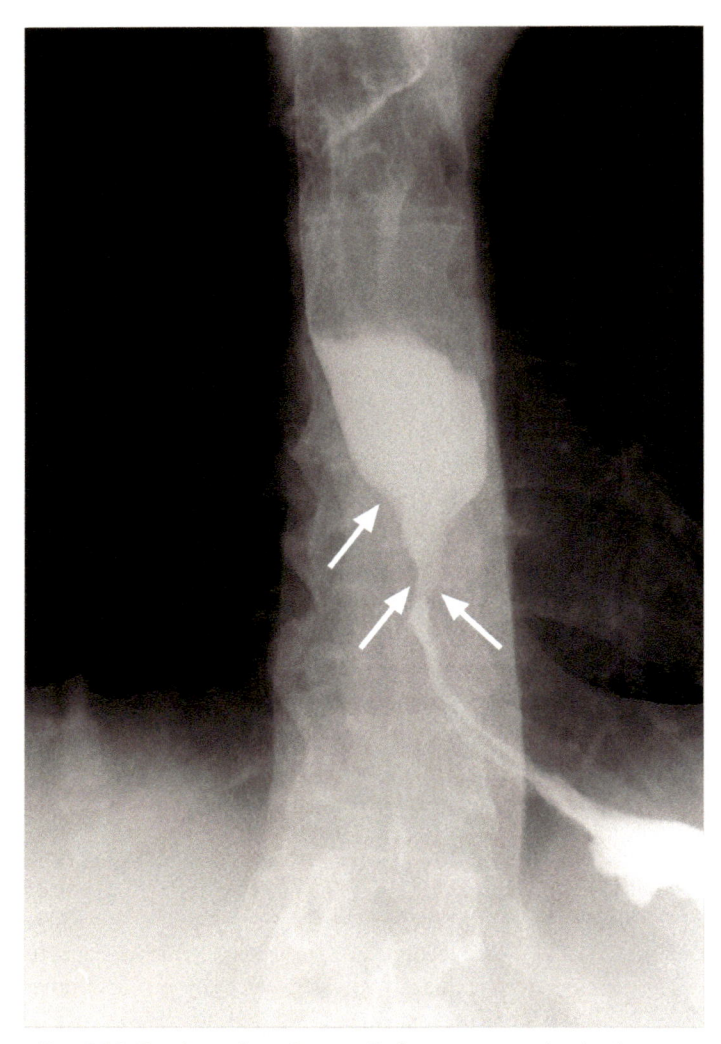

Fig. 8.22 Esophageal carcinoma. Oral contrast examination in a patient with esophageal carcinoma shows dilatation of the proximal esophagus and irregular narrowing of the distal esophagus caused by the tumor (arrows).

emergency situations (acute abdomen, suspected perforation) and the staging of malignant disease.

8.4.1 Hypertrophic Pyloric Stenosis

▶ **Brief definition.** This condition is a narrowing of the gastric outlet due to thickening of the circular muscle layer and swelling of the mucosa. The disorder occurs predominantly in male infants 3 to 7 weeks old. Its prevalence in the western population is estimated at 1 in 800 infants. Pyloric stenosis is virtually unknown in the Asian and African populations. The etiology of hypertrophic pyloric stenosis is not yet fully understood.

Table 8.3 TNM classification of esophageal carcinoma

Designation	Description
Primary tumor	
Tis	Carcinoma in situ (high-grade dysplasia)
T1	Tumor invades the lamina propria or submucosa
T2	Tumor invades the muscularis propria
T3	Tumor invades the adventitia
T4	Tumor invades adjacent structures
Lymph nodes	
N0	No regional lymph node metastasis
N1	Regional lymph node metastasis
Distant metastasis	
M0	No distant metastasis
M1	Distant metastasis

Table 8.4 UICC staging system for esophageal carcinoma

Stage	Groupings
I	T1 N0 M0
IIa	T2–3 N0 M0
IIb	T1–2 N1 M0
III	T3 N1 M0 or T4 N0–1 M0
IV	T1–4 N0–1 M1

▶ **Imaging signs.** Ultrasound demonstrates hyperperistalsis of the strongly fluid-distended stomach. The pyloric canal is elongated (>16 mm) with thickened musculature (>4 mm) and a small lumen (▶ Fig. 8.24). Thoracic and abdominal radiographs show a large stomach and an under-aerated small intestine. Pulmonary changes due to aspiration are a common finding.

▶ **Clinical features.** Pyloric stenosis impairs the passage of gastric contents, and infants typically present with projectile vomiting after feeding. The loss of gastric acid leads to metabolic hyperchloremic alkalosis. Physical examination may reveal a palpable pyloric mass ("palpable olive").

▶ **Differential diagnosis.** Narrowing of the gastric outlet may also result from a tumor or from scarring due to ulcerative disease. However, these conditions would affect a different age group than hypertrophic pyloric stenosis, and an underlying disease (tumor, inflammation) would also be present.

▶ **Key points.** Hypertrophic pyloric stenosis presents typical ultrasound imaging features that are usually diagnostic when correlated with clinical findings.

8.4.2 Diverticula

▶ **Brief definition.** A gastric or duodenal diverticulum is an outpouching of the wall layers in the upper gastrointestinal tract. Diverticula of the stomach are most commonly located in the gastric cardia (▶ Fig. 8.25). Duodenal diverticula are often located in the descending part of the duodenum (▶ Fig. 8.26).

▶ **Imaging signs.** Air–fluid levels are commonly found in diverticula. When barium or another oral contrast medium is administered, fluoroscopy or conventional radiography will often show contrast medium pooling in the diverticulum. On sectional imaging by CT or MRI, a diverticulum will show only peripheral enhancement after IV injection of contrast medium, while the central (air- or fluid-filled) areas do not enhance. This effect is more clearly appreciated with a negative contrast medium such as mannitol solution than with a positive contrast medium like barium or an iodinated medium.

▶ **Clinical features.** Most diverticula are asymptomatic and do not require treatment. However, the infection of a diverticulum (diverticulitis) may cause significant symptoms such as pain. Treatment options range from antibiotic therapy to surgery, depending on the severity of symptoms.

▶ **Differential diagnosis.** Diverticula at certain sites can mimic masses of the stomach, duodenum, or other organs. These include tumors of the adrenal gland, spleen, or pancreas. Abscesses may also resemble diverticula. The two imaging hallmarks—the pooling of swallowed contrast medium in the diverticular lumen and peripheral enhancement after IV injection of contrast medium—are important imaging clues that distinguish diverticula from other lesions of the gastric or duodenal wall.

▶ **Key points.** Diverticula are rare, benign lesions of the upper gastrointestinal tract. The use of oral or IV contrast media is helpful in differentiating diverticula from tumors and abscesses.

8.4.3 Peptic Ulcer Disease

▶ **Brief definition of peptic ulcer disease (PUD).** A peptic ulcer is a defect in the gastric or duodenal wall that penetrates past the level of the mucosa and submucosa to involve deeper wall layers. The pathogenesis of ulcer disease involves an imbalance between protective and aggressive factors (e.g., gastritis, *Helicobacter pylori* infection, use of NSAIDs, stressful situations such as intensive care). Peptic ulcers are most commonly located in the lesser curvature of the stomach or the duodenal bulb.

▶ **Imaging signs.** Fluoroscopy with contrast medium usually shows a well-circumscribed area of contrast medium pooling in the ulcer niche. With a perforated ulcer, free air can be detected by a plain abdominal radiograph in LLD or by CT (▶ Fig. 8.27).

▶ **Clinical features.** While a gastric ulcer typically causes epigastric pain during a meal, the symptoms of a duodenal ulcer usually occur on an empty stomach and are relieved by a meal. Possible complications include bleeding and perforation. The latter constitutes an emergency with an acute abdomen that requires immediate surgical treatment.

▶ **Differential diagnosis.** Differentiation is required mainly from malignant diseases of the gastrointestinal tract: carcinoma, gastrointestinal stromal tumor (GIST), and lymphoma. Often this

Gastrointestinal Tract

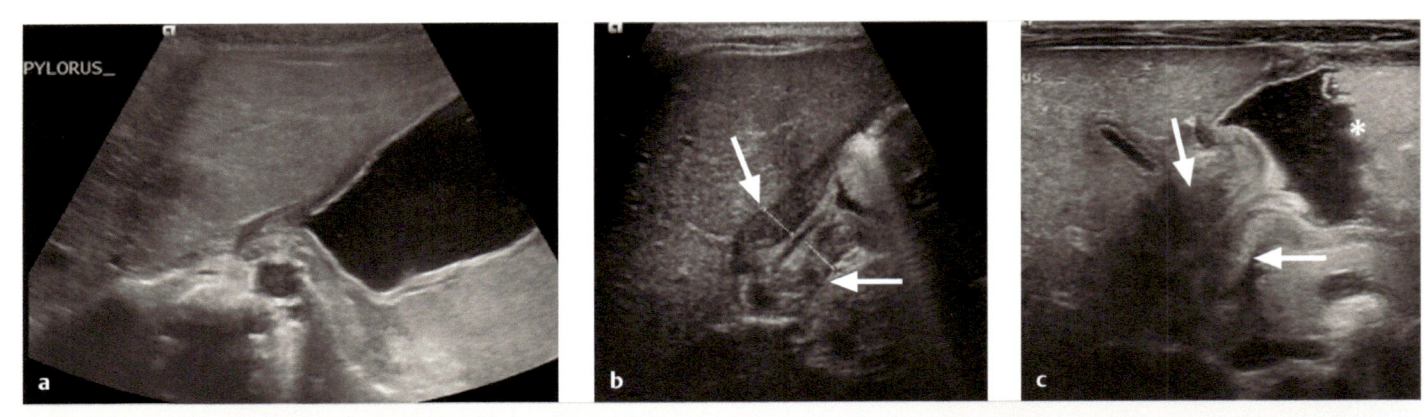

Fig. 8.24 **Pyloric stenosis.** Ultrasound appearance. (a) Infant with a normal pylorus. (b) Infant with pyloric stenosis. The scan shows marked thickening of the muscular layer at the gastric outlet (arrows). (c) Same infant as in [b]. This scan also shows a thickened muscular layer at the gastric outlet (arrows) and a distended, fluid-filled gastric bubble (asterisk).

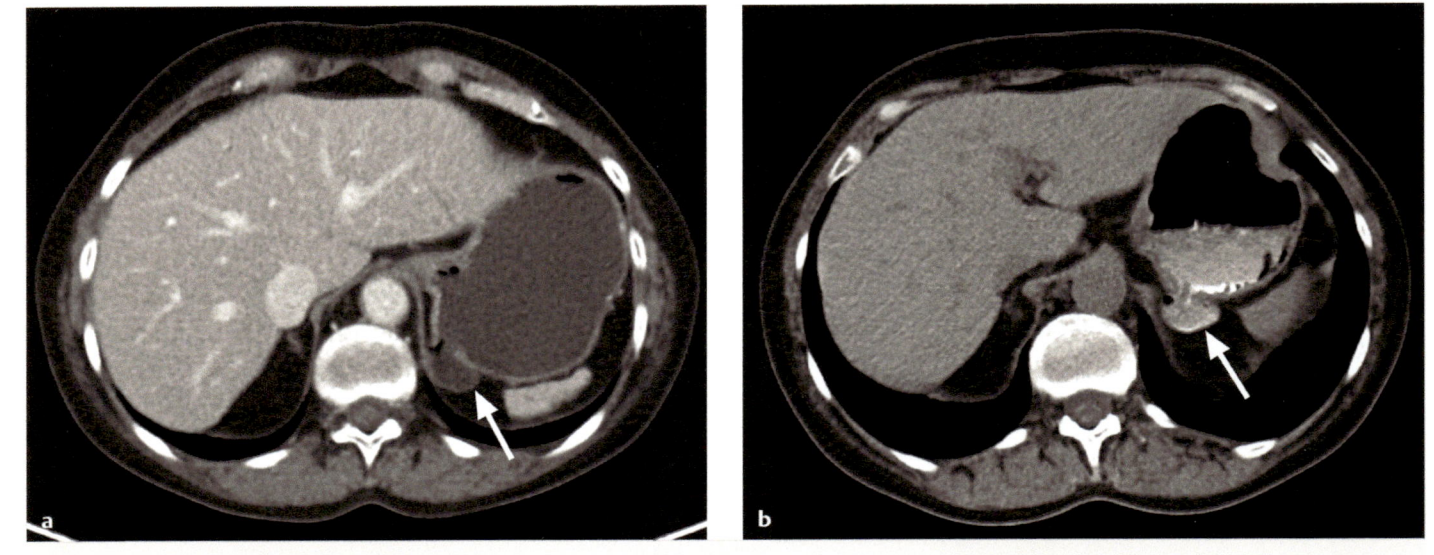

Fig. 8.25 **Diverticulum of the gastric cardia.** CT appearance. (a) Water-filled diverticulum (arrow). (b) Diverticulum filled with oral contrast medium (arrow).

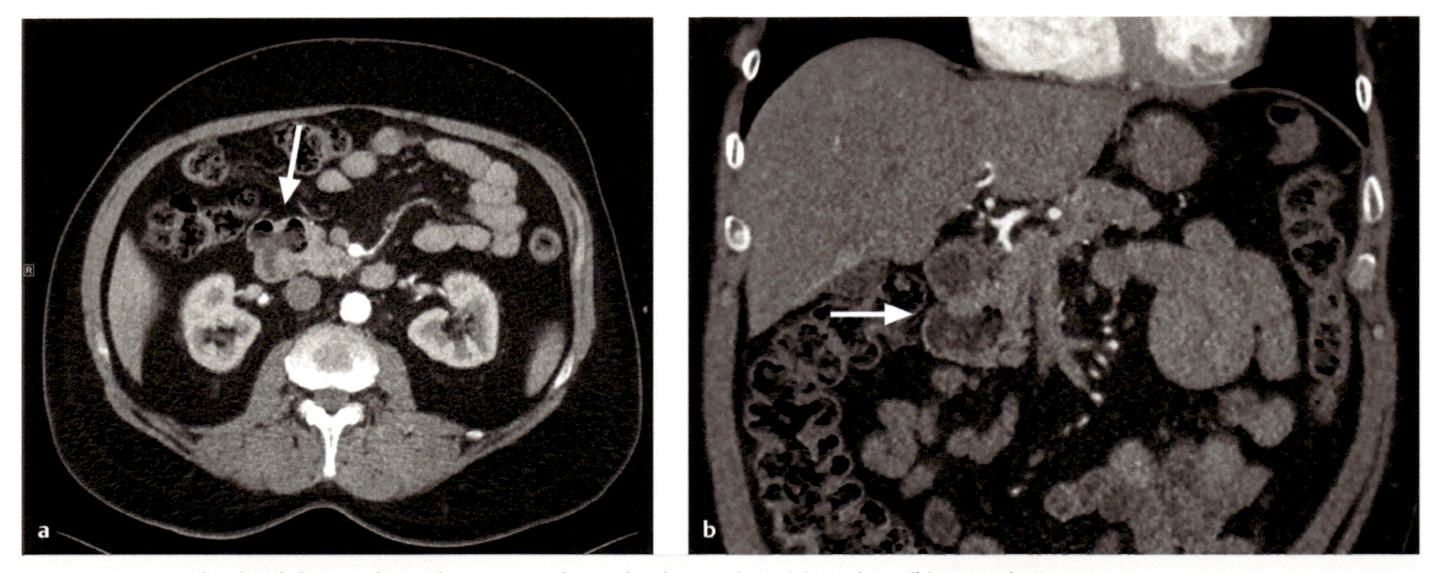

Fig. 8.26 **Large duodenal diverticulum.** The arrows indicate the diverticulum. (a) Axial CT. (b) Coronal CT.

8.4 Diseases of the Gastroduodenum

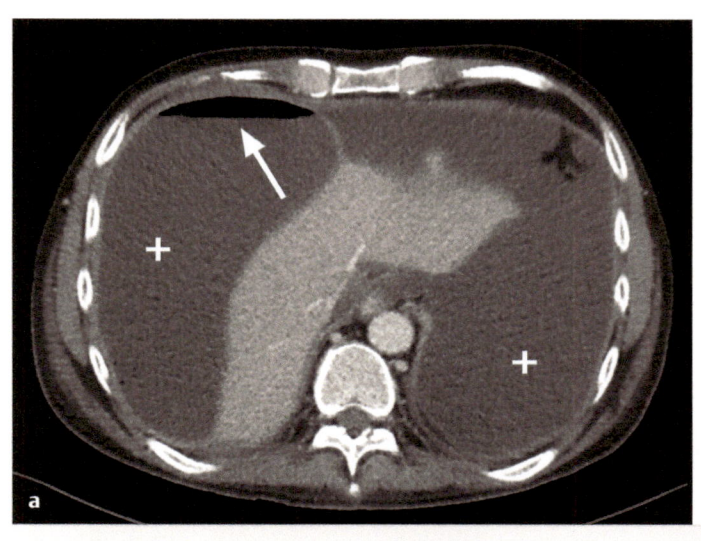

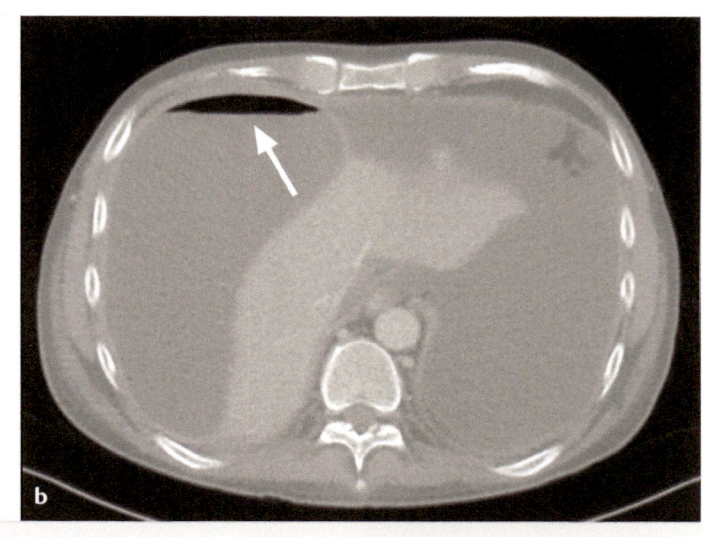

Fig. 8.27 **Perforated ulcer.** Free intra-abdominal air ([a], [b], arrows) is detected on axial CT in a patient with a perforated ulcer. A significant volume of ascites ([a], crosses) is also present. (a) Soft tissue window. (b) Lung window.

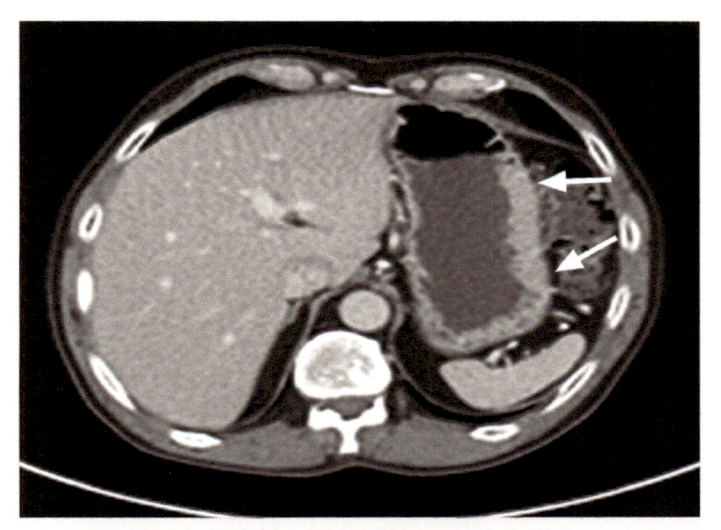

Fig. 8.28 **Zollinger–Ellison syndrome.** CT reveals marked hypertrophy of the gastric rugal folds (arrows).

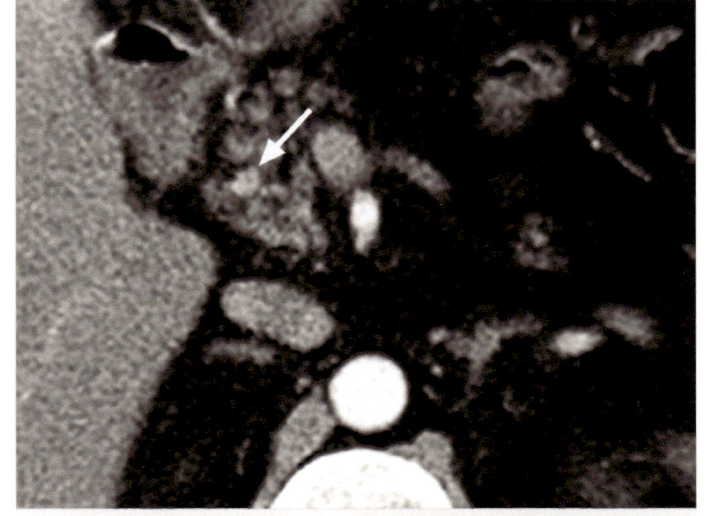

Fig. 8.29 **Zollinger–Ellison syndrome.** Contrast-enhanced CT in the arterial phase shows a hypervascular gastrinoma in the head of the pancreas (arrow).

cannot be accomplished with imaging alone and requires further investigation, usually by endoscopy.

▶ **Key points.** Imaging is of limited value in the diagnosis of ulcer disease and is inferior to endoscopy. Imaging is of greater value in advanced stages of ulcer disease and in patients with a perforated gastrointestinal ulcer.

> **Caution**
> If a perforated ulcer is suspected, the use of barium contrast medium is contraindicated due to the risk of peritonitis.

8.4.4 Zollinger–Ellison Syndrome

▶ **Brief definition.** Zollinger–Ellison syndrome is the clinical presentation that results from an overproduction of gastrin. It is characterized by a triad of gastroduodenal ulcers, hypergastrinemia, and the presence of a gastrinoma in the pancreas or duodenum.

▶ **Imaging signs.** Excessive gastrin secretion stimulates increased acid production, leading to hyperplasia of the gastric parietal cells. Thus, ulcerations are accompanied by diffuse thickening of the mucosal folds in the stomach and duodenum (▶ Fig. 8.28). The gastric-secreting primary tumor can be identified by sectional imaging and usually shows increased arterial enhancement (▶ Fig. 8.29).

▶ **Clinical features.** The clinical manifestations of Zollinger–Ellison syndrome are closely related to the symptoms of ulcer disease described above and often include diarrhea in addition to pain.

▶ **Differential diagnosis.** The differential diagnosis includes gastritis from other causes and tumors of the stomach and duodenum.

Gastrointestinal Tract

The detection of a gastrinoma in the duodenum or pancreas often leads to the diagnosis of Zollinger–Ellison syndrome.

▶ **Key points.** Zollinger–Ellison syndrome presents mixed features of ulceration and mucosal hyperplasia.

8.4.5 Gastrointestinal Stromal Tumors

▶ **Brief definition.** A gastrointestinal stromal tumor (GIST) is a tumor that originates from smooth muscle cells and is located in the submucosa. Although GISTs can occur anywhere in the digestive tract, they have a predilection for the stomach (60%) and small intestine (30%). Peak occurrence is in the sixth and seventh decades.

▶ **Imaging signs.** A characteristic feature of GISTs is a submucosal location that spares the overlying mucosa. This provides a useful criterion of differentiation from gastric carcinoma (▶ Fig. 8.30). Because the tumor is very vascular, it often shows increased enhancement during the arterial phase of contrast-enhanced CT or MRI. The tumor may grow exophytically, and necrotic areas may develop, especially in larger tumors. On MRI, GISTs are isointense in T1 W images and hypo- to isointense in T2 W images.

▶ **Clinical features.** Some GISTs are asymptomatic. Others become symptomatic through a mass effect or as a result of ulceration and bleeding. The tumor can metastasize to the liver, lung, and peritoneal cavity. Besides surgical resection, chemotherapy with imatinib mesylate, a tyrosine kinase inhibitor, has become an established treatment in cases where metastasis has occurred. The TNM classification of GISTs is shown in ▶ Table 8.5.

Note
Frequently, GISTs do not show an initial size reduction in response to imatinib mesylate therapy. A more common response is increasing tumor necrosis with an associated fall of attenuation values on CT. The tumor may even respond with initial enlargement due to necrosis, intralesional hemorrhage, or mucoid degeneration. For this reason, traditional RECIST or WHO criteria should not be used in evaluating treatment response. The Choi criteria should be applied (▶ Table 8.6).

▶ **Differential diagnosis.** Differentiation is required mainly from gastric carcinoma, which invariably affects the mucosa and generally is less vascular than GIST. Differentiation from lymphoma may be difficult. Intramural lipoma can also mimic a GIST, but the determination of the lesion's fat content by CT or MRI should suggest the correct diagnosis.

▶ **Key points.** GISTs are distinguished by their primary involvement of the submucosa.

8.4.6 Lymphoma

▶ **Brief definition.** Lymphomas of the gastrointestinal tract are predominantly non-Hodgkin's lymphomas of the B cell line. Mucosa-associated lymphoid tissue (MALT) lymphomas are a subtype that most commonly occurs in the stomach of patients with chronic *Helicobacter pylori* infection. Additionally there may be secondary involvement of the gastrointestinal tract by primary nodal (extraintestinal) non-Hodgkin's lymphoma.

▶ **Imaging signs.** Gastrointestinal lymphomas are characterized by diffuse thickening of the gastric or intestinal wall with loss of

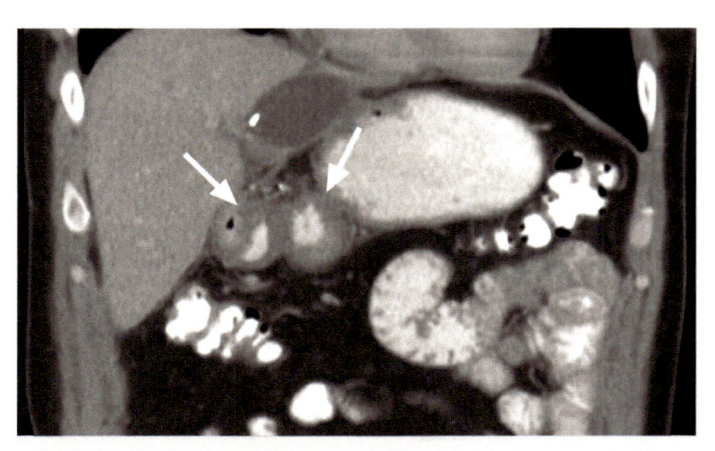

Fig. 8.30 GIST. Coronal reformatted CT image shows tumor involvement of the gastric wall in the antral and pyloric region (arrows), sparing the mucosa (hypervascular zone bordering the lumen).

Table 8.5 TNM classification of gastrointestinal stromal tumors

Designation	Description
Primary tumor	
T1	Tumor ≤ 2 cm
T2	Tumor > 2 cm but ≤ 5 cm
T3	Tumor > 5 cm but ≤ 10 cm
T4	Tumor > 10 cm in greatest dimension
Lymph nodes	
N0	No regional lymph node metastasis
N1	Regional lymph node metastasis
Distant metastasis	
M0	No distant metastasis
M1	Distant metastasis

Table 8.6 Choi response criteria for gastrointestinal stromal tumor (GIST)

Level of response	Criteria
Complete response	Disappearance of all target lesions
Partial response	≥ 10% decrease in tumor size or ≥ 15% decrease in tumor attenuation on CT; no new lesions
Stable disease	Neither partial response, complete response, nor progressive disease
Progressive disease	≥ 10% increase in tumor size; does not meet the criteria for partial response based on tumor attenuation

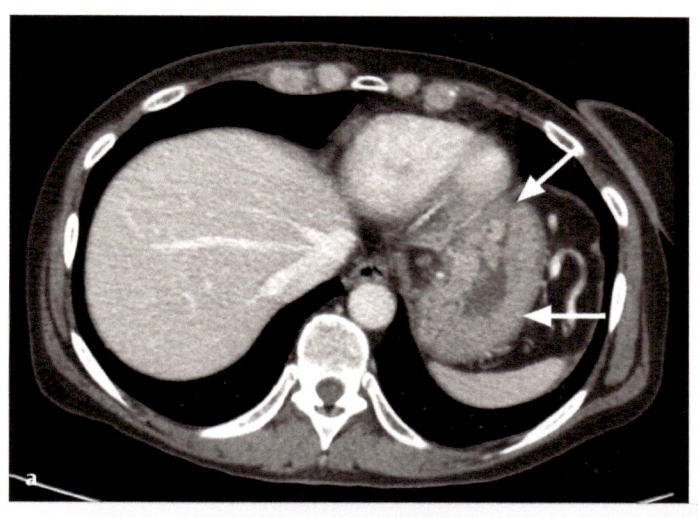

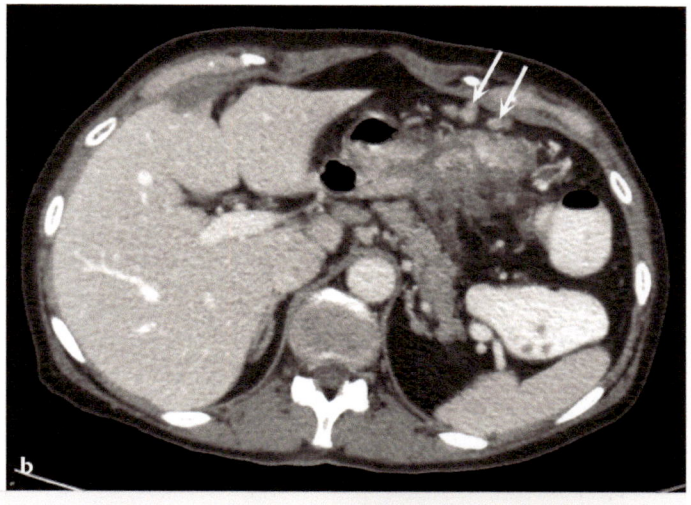

Fig. 8.31 **Gastric lymphoma.** CT appearance. (a) Marked thickening of the gastric wall (arrows). (b) Locoregional lymphadenopathy (arrows).

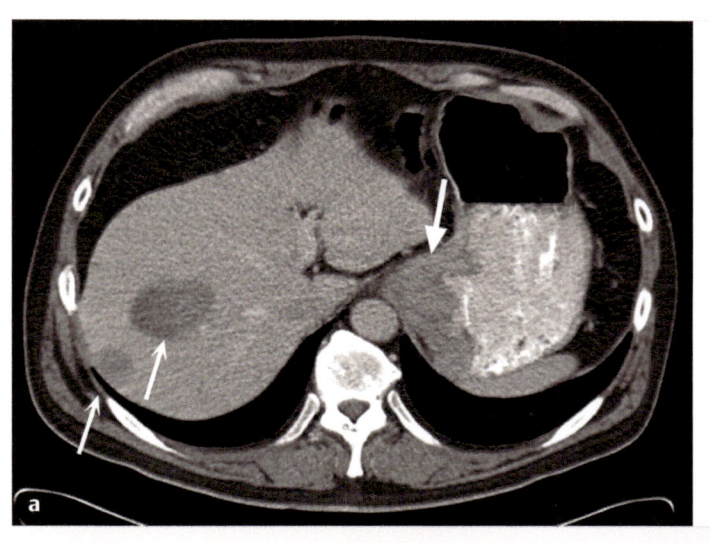

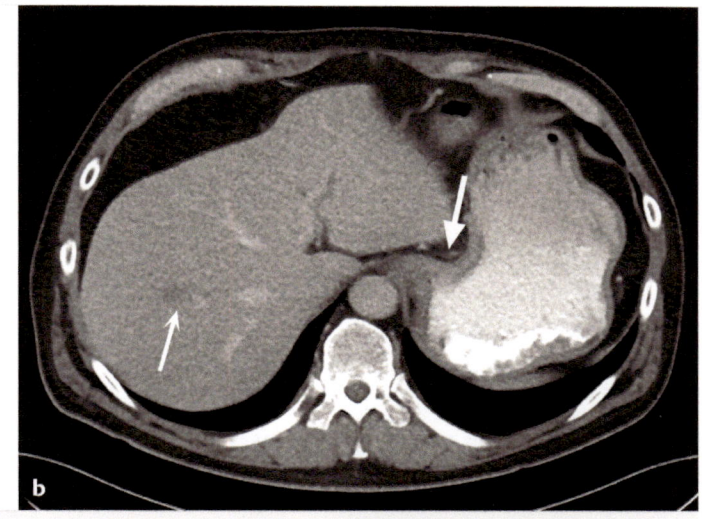

Fig. 8.32 **Gastric carcinoma.** (a) Axial CT shows pronounced thickening of the cardial wall due to carcinoma involvement (heavy arrow). Metastases are noted in the right lobe of the liver (light arrow). (b) The wall thickening shows significant response to neoadjuvant chemotherapy (heavy arrow). There is significant correlative regression of the metastases in the hepatic right lobe (light arrow).

normal fold patterns (▶ Fig. 8.31). Sectional imaging studies are superior to conventional radiographs in their ability to detect the transmural and peri-intestinal component of the disease. Thus, regional lymph node involvement is detectable by CT and MRI.

▶ **Clinical features.** The clinical presentation is usually nonspecific and may include pain, nausea, and weight loss. Obstruction may occur with larger tumors. Treatment options include medical therapy as well as the (partial) resection of tumors that have caused mechanical obstruction.

▶ **Differential diagnosis.** Diffuse involvement of the gastric and intestinal wall is a hallmark of lymphomas and an important differentiating criterion from focal neoplasms (carcinoma, GIST). The involvement of other lymphatic organs such as the spleen is also suggestive of lymphoma.

▶ **Key points.** Lymphomas of the stomach and bowel tend to cause diffuse involvement rather than a focal tumor mass.

8.4.7 Gastric Carcinoma

▶ **Brief definition.** Gastric carcinoma is a malignant neoplasm of the stomach wall. It is the third most common gastrointestinal malignancy after colorectal carcinoma and pancreatic adenocarcinoma. Besides genetic factors, the etiology of gastric carcinoma involves environmental factors such as nutritional habits. Histologically, more than 90% of gastric cancers are adenocarcinomas. The peak age of incidence is in the sixth and seventh decades.

▶ **Imaging signs.** CT imaging should employ negative oral contrast media such as water to provide good delineation between the gastric wall and lumen, which barium-containing or iodinated contrast media do not provide. CT can demonstrate a combination of polypoid masses and ulcerations (▶ Fig. 8.32). It is also common to find wall thickening and, with transmural tumors, the invasion of perigastric soft tissues. The staging of gastric carcinoma is of major importance in routine practice and should include the evaluation of perigastric lymph node status by contrast-enhanced CT or MRI. These studies can also supply information on possible hepatic and distant metastases.

▶ **Clinical features.** The symptoms of gastric carcinoma may be absent or nonspecific in early stages. Later symptoms may include weight loss, pain, and anemia. The final diagnosis is established by endoscopic biopsy. Gastric carcinoma can metastasize by direct spread, by the lymphogenous route (left supraclavicular lymph nodes, also called sentinel nodes), or by the hematogenous route (liver). Ovarian metastasis, also called a Krukenberg's tumor, is a very common occurrence with gastric carcinoma. Its route of metastasis is still uncertain. Transperitoneal spread was once the favored hypothesis, but this mechanism is inconsistent with the fact that ovarian metastases are located in the stroma and skip the greater omentum. Today it is believed that Krukenberg's tumors arise by hematogenous spread. Treatment options are partial or total gastrectomy, depending on tumor stage, and may include adjuvant chemotherapy or radiation.

▶ **Differential diagnosis.** Besides other gastric tumors (GIST, lymphoma), ulcerations can also mimic gastric carcinoma. Differentiation is difficult by imaging alone and usually requires endoscopy with biopsy and subsequent histology.

▶ **Key points.** Radiological techniques are used mainly for staging gastric carcinoma in routine situations and are less useful for primary diagnosis.

8.5 Diseases of the Jejunum and Ileum

8.5.1 Meckel's Diverticulum

▶ **Brief definition.** A Meckel's diverticulum is a remnant of the omphalomesenteric duct (vitelline duct) and is present in approximately 2% of the population. A Meckel's diverticulum in children is located in the ileum about 50 cm proximal to the ileocecal valve, while the average distance in adults is 1 meter. This discrepancy is explained by the growth of mesenteric structures during the first and second decades of life.

▶ **Imaging signs.** A Meckel's diverticulum is most commonly found in the right lower quadrant of the abdomen. It appears on fluoroscopy or CT as an approximately 5-cm pouch in contact with the ileum (▶ Fig. 8.33). Inflammation may cause thickening of the diverticular wall, increased wall enhancement after IV injection of contrast medium (e.g., on CT or MRI), and edema of the diverticular wall and adjacent organs.

▶ **Clinical features.** Meckel's diverticula are usually asymptomatic. The acute inflammation of a Meckel's diverticulum may produce symptoms that mimic appendicitis. Symptoms of small-bowel obstruction may also occur. Ectopic pancreatic tissue or gastric mucosa within the diverticulum may cause complications due to ulceration and bleeding.

▶ **Differential diagnosis.** Meckel's diverticulitis requires differentiation from other inflammatory processes in the right lower quadrant such as appendicitis, Crohn's disease, and infectious enteritis. Differentiation from appendicitis may be very difficult with imaging alone. In clinical practice, a definitive diagnosis of Meckel's diverticulum is often delayed until surgery. Crohn's disease is ultimately a histological diagnosis.

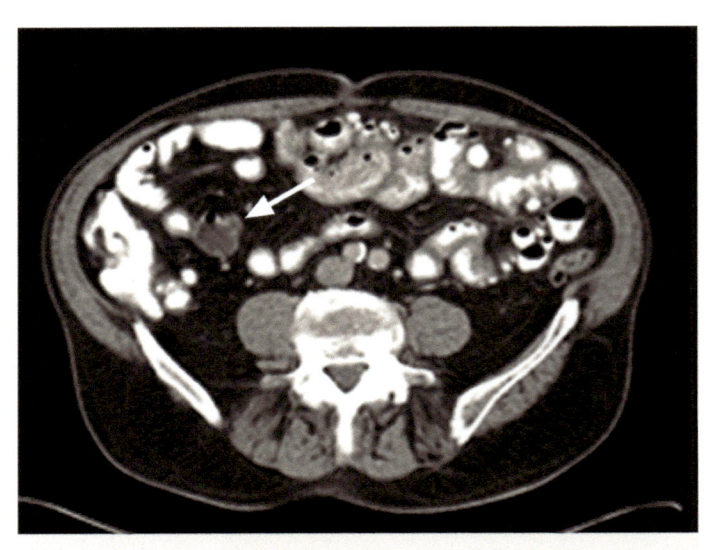

Fig. 8.33 Meckel's diverticulum. CT reveals a fluid-filled mass several centimeters in diameter (arrow) on the small intestine in the right mid- to lower abdomen.

▶ **Key points.** Meckel's diverticulum is often an incidental finding. Clinical symptoms are usually the result of inflammation.

Note
"Meckel's diverticulum is frequently suspected, often looked for, and seldom found." (Charles W. Mayo)

8.5.2 Intestinal Obstruction

▶ **Brief definition.** Intestinal obstruction (bowel obstruction) refers to an absence or delay of intestinal transit. The cause may be mechanical or paralytic:
- *Mechanical bowel obstruction*: Intestinal transit is blocked due to narrowing or occlusion of the bowel lumen. The most frequent causes are adhesions (▶ Fig. 8.34), hernias, and tumors.
- *Paralytic (adynamic) ileus*: This is a failure of enteric transit in the absence of a mechanical obstruction. The ileus can be classified etiologically as postoperative, posttraumatic, or inflammatory.

▶ **Imaging signs.** The LLD abdominal radiograph in a patient with intestinal obstruction shows dilated bowel loops with air–fluid levels. The position of the air–fluid levels on the abdominal radiograph is helpful for distinguishing a mechanical obstruction from paralytic ileus: With a mechanical obstruction, the air–fluid levels are at different heights in the same loop of bowel because of peristaltic motion. This sign is absent in ileus, where the air–fluid levels in the same loop are at the same height. CT, which often must be performed without oral contrast medium due to clinical requirements, reveals a similar pattern. With a mechanical bowel obstruction, a transition point is found at the site of the obstruction. The bowel proximal to that point shows typical

8.5 Diseases of the Jejunum and Ileum

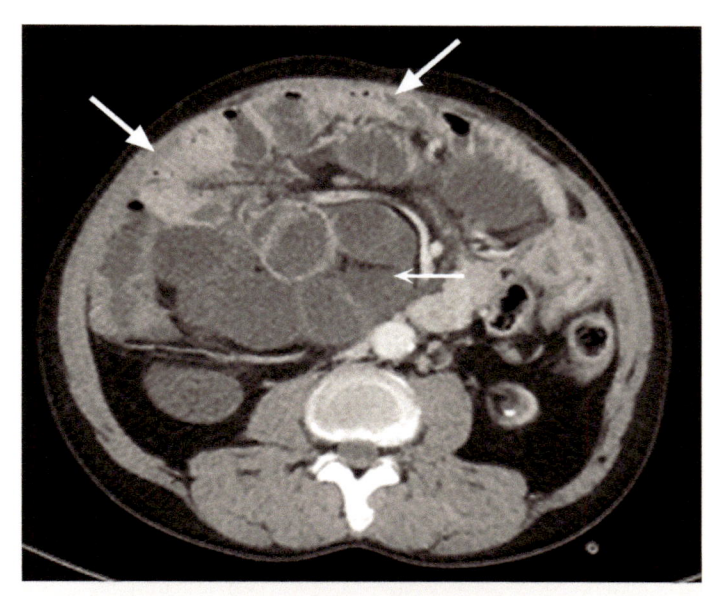

Fig. 8.34 Small-bowel obstruction. CT shows distended and separated small-bowel loops (light arrow) caused by the postoperative adhesion of small-bowel loops to the abdominal wall (heavy arrows).

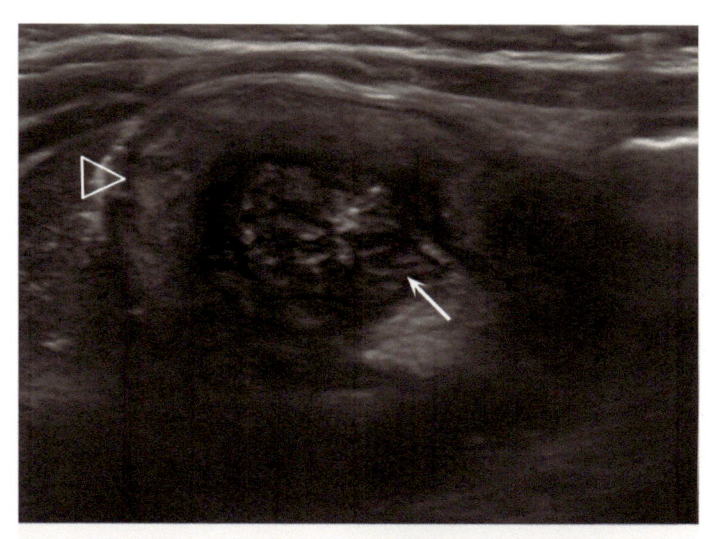

Fig. 8.35 Intussusception. Ultrasound appearance. Arrow, small intestine; open arrowhead, large intestine.

dilatation with fluid levels, while the distal bowel loops tend to be empty and collapsed. Ileus presents a different pattern: there is no transition point, and the bowel dilatation and fluid levels are ubiquitous.

▶ **Clinical features.** Symptoms vary considerably with the degree of severity. Abdominal pain, vomiting, and nausea are frequently experienced. The fully developed presentation of intestinal obstruction is an acute abdomen; intestinal ischemia is a potential complication. Treatment also varies with the form and severity of the condition, ranging from gastric intubation and parenteral nutrition to emergency surgery for a complete obstruction.

▶ **Differential diagnosis.** The imaging features of intestinal obstruction are characteristic and strongly constrain the differential diagnosis. Etiology is a more important consideration within the clinical context, i.e., referring the obstruction to a mechanical or paralytic cause.

▶ **Key points.** Intestinal obstruction can often be diagnosed on a conventional LLD radiograph, but CT is more precise in detecting and identifying the cause of the obstruction.

8.5.3 Intussusception

▶ **Brief definition.** Intussusception is the invagination ("telescoping") of one part of the intestinal tract into a more distal part. The intussusception of small intestine into the large intestine requires treatment. Infants and small children are most commonly affected (ca. 95% of cases). Most cases of intussusception are directly preceded by gastroenteritis with reactive lymphadenopathy. The enlarged lymph nodes act as a fulcrum over which the intussusception occurs and creates a barrier to normal peristalsis. Intussusception is the second leading cause (after appendicitis) of an acute abdomen in the pediatric age group. The most common type is an ileocolic intussusception. By contrast, an intussusception between portions of the small intestine (enteroenteric) has little if any pathologic significance. Enteroenteric intussusceptions and their spontaneous reduction are frequently observed in abdominal ultrasound examinations. Intussusception in adults is considerably rarer. Many cases in this age group have an underlying mechanical cause such as a neoplasm.

▶ **Imaging signs.** Ultrasound is the imaging modality of first choice for suspected intussusception in children (▶ Fig. 8.35). The target pattern characteristic of intussusception is usually found in the right mid- or upper abdomen. The target pattern may also be found in the mid-upper abdomen (transverse colon), depending on the level of the intussusception. The target pattern is usually greater than 4 cm in diameter. By contrast, enteroenteric intussusceptions usually produce very small target patterns less than 2 cm in diameter. On conventional barium contrast examination, intussusceptions have a coiled-spring appearance caused by trapping of the contrast medium between the invaginated bowel loops. Various stages can be distinguished on sectional imaging:
- The bowel loops initially form a target pattern in the early stage (▶ Fig. 8.36).
- Later the bowel wall assumes a masslike appearance due to edema.
- Imaging in the late stage shows features of intestinal obstruction.

▶ **Clinical features.** The intussusception initially causes compression of entrapped venous and then arterial mesenteric vessels. This leads to ischemia, which may progress to necrosis and perforation. The clinical picture is marked by acute onset of pain with accompanying nausea and vomiting. The patient exhibits peritonism with muscular guarding and rigidity. Often an elongated, tubular mass is palpable through the abdominal wall. If adequate treatment is not provided at this stage, a "silent interval" follows in which nausea, vomiting, and pain are diminished. Children appear tired and apathetic. This stage may be misinterpreted as

Gastrointestinal Tract

improvement. The late stage is often characterized by the passage of bloody, mucoid stools due to incipient necrosis of the bowel wall, and untreated cases will progress to perforation. Treatment within 24 hours of symptom onset consists of hydrostatic reduction by water enemas or air insufflation under sonographic control or by contrast enema or air insufflation under fluoroscopic control (▶ Fig. 8.37). If the attempt at reduction is initially unsuccessful, sedating the child will increase the chance of success by decreasing muscular rigidity.

Note
Reduction of the intussusception under sedation should be discontinued after three failed attempts as it is highly unlikely that the procedure will subsequently be successful.

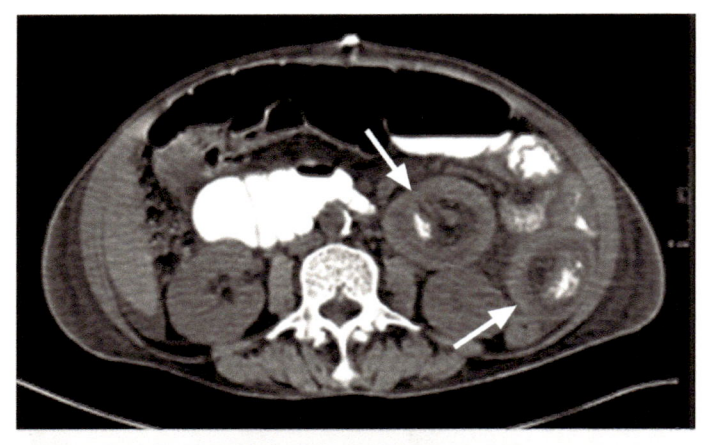

Fig. 8.36 Intussusception of the small intestine. Target patterns (arrows) on axial CT.

The success rate depends in part on how long the intussusception has been present. If conservative therapy is unsuccessful, rapid surgical intervention is needed and may include resection of necrotic bowel wall.

▶ **Differential diagnosis.** Intussusception must be differentiated from tumor-related thickening of the bowel wall, but the clinical presentation and acute symptom onset of intussusception should suggest the correct diagnosis.

▶ **Key points.** Intussusception is a condition of acute onset that occurs predominantly in infants and small children as a sequel to gastroenteritis.

8.5.4 Mesenteric Ischemia

▶ **Brief definition.** Narrowing or occlusion of the mesenteric arteries or veins decreases the flow of oxygen-rich blood to the intestine. With a venous occlusion, this results from impaired drainage and damming back of blood into the arteries, with a consequent reduced inflow of fresh blood. Vascular occlusion may be caused by a thrombus or embolus (acute) or may be secondary to severe atherosclerosis (chronic). Vessels may also be narrowed by a mechanical process such as tumor encasement.

▶ **Imaging signs.** A major goal of imaging is to diagnose the changes in the vascular bed (e.g., the vascular occlusion) using (CT) angiographic methods (▶ Fig. 8.38). Additionally, sectional imaging in particular can detect changes in the bowel wall itself. These may include edematous thickening of the bowel wall and signs of intestinal obstruction (see ▶ Fig. 8.38). Later stages are characterized by pneumatosis intestinalis, a collection of gas in the bowel wall (▶ Fig. 8.39), which may allow small gas bubbles to pass into the portal venous system.

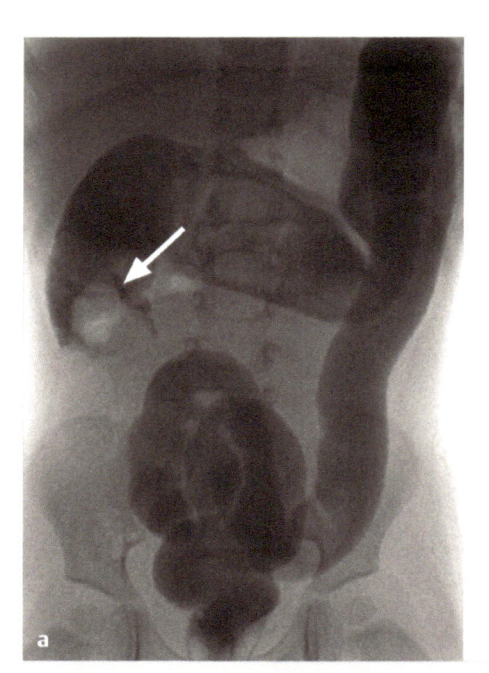

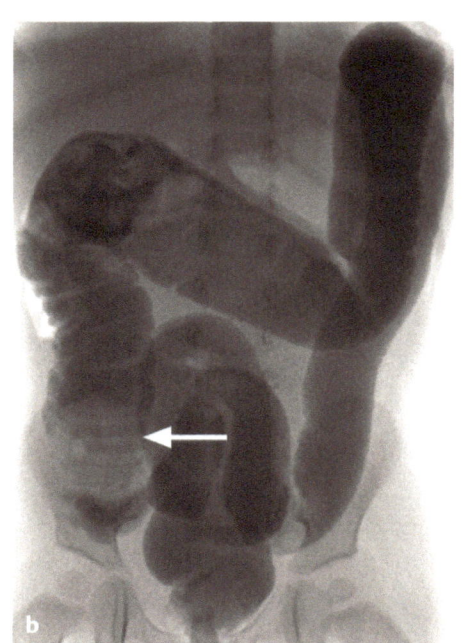

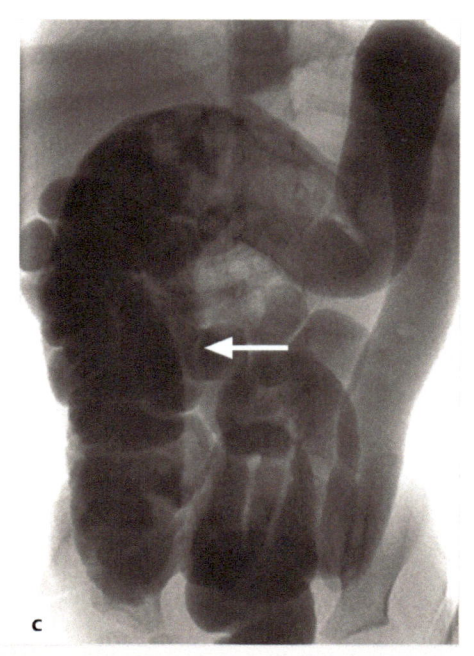

Fig. 8.37 Reduction of an ileocolic intussusception in a small child. (a) Contrast medium has reached the intussusceptum (arrow). (b) The contrast medium is pushing the intussusceptum (arrow) out of the colon. (c) Subsequent passage of contrast medium into the terminal ileum (arrow) confirms a successful reduction.

8.5 Diseases of the Jejunum and Ileum

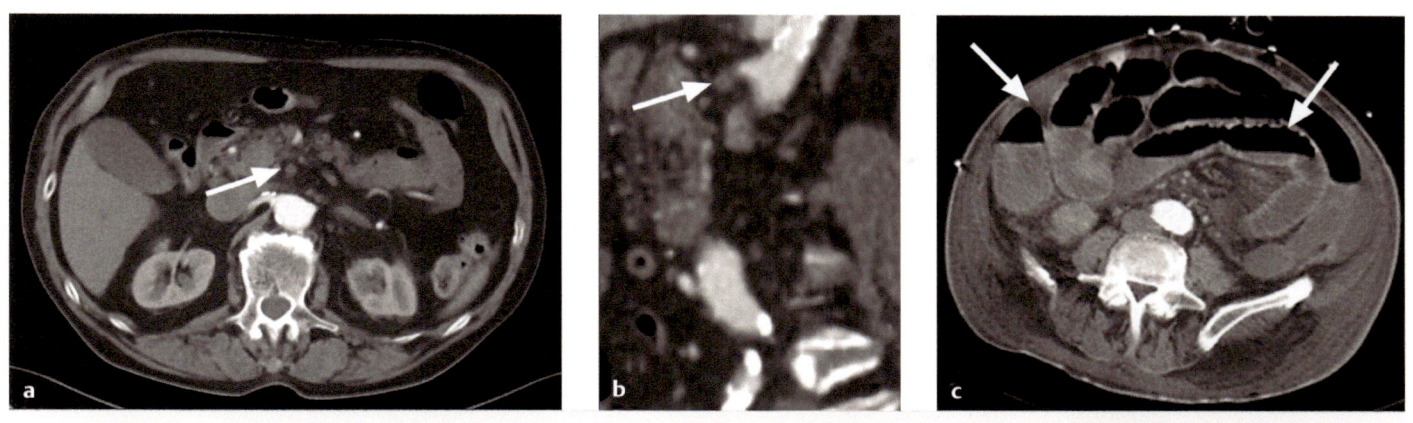

Fig. 8.38 Acute occlusion of the superior mesenteric artery. (a) Axial CT. The arrow indicates the site of arterial occlusion. (b) Sagittal CT. The arterial occlusion (arrow) is also visible in this plane of section. (c) Axial CT. The arrows indicate distended, wall-thickened small-bowel loops with multiple air–fluid levels, consistent with an ischemic small-bowel obstruction.

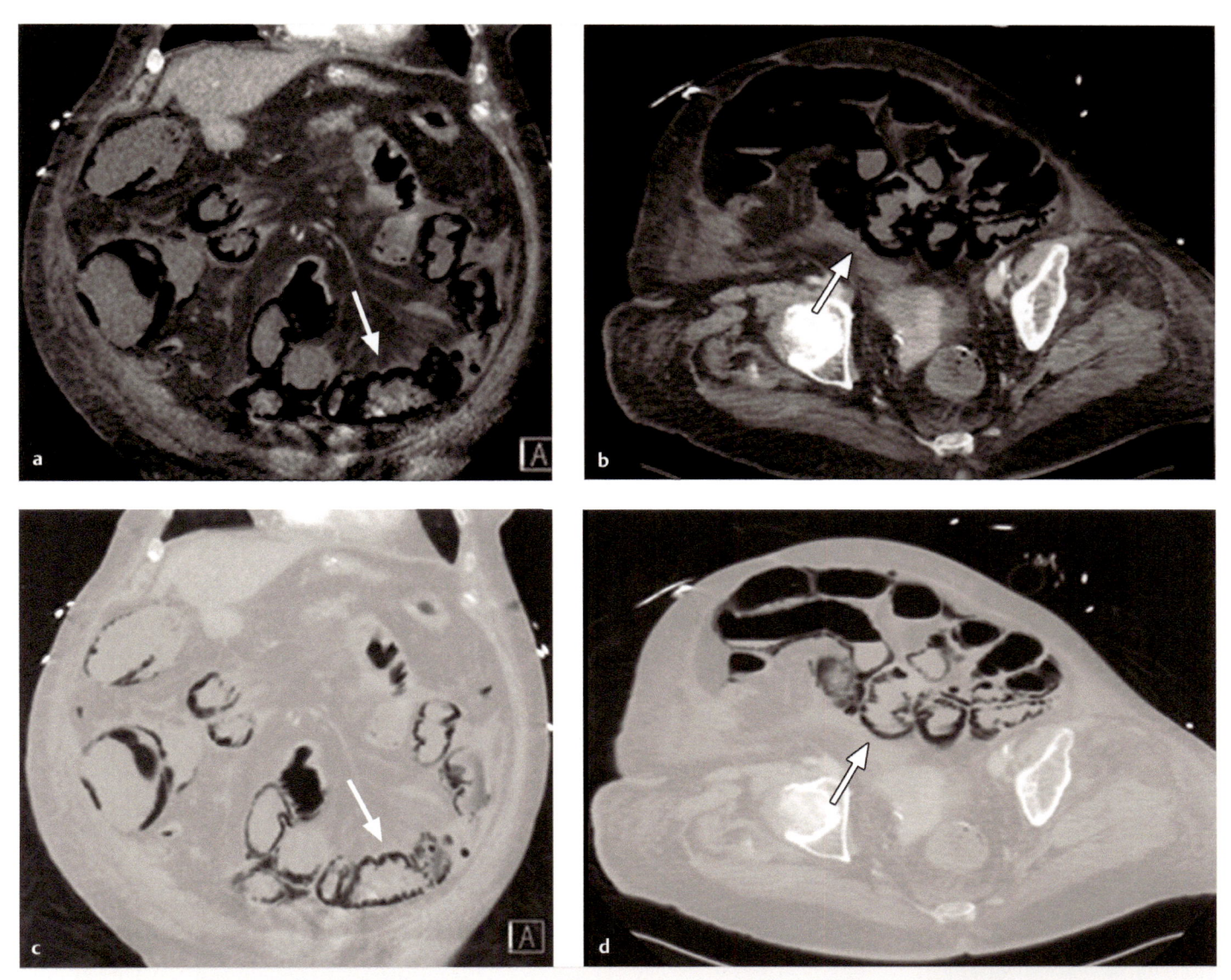

Fig. 8.39 Pronounced pneumatosis intestinalis throughout the gastrointestinal tract. The arrows indicate the pneumatosis. (a) CT with a soft tissue window (section 1). (b) CT with a soft tissue window (section 2). (c) CT with a lung window (section 1). (d) CT with a lung window (section 2).

> **Caution**
>
> Some pathologic changes in small mesenteric vessels are not detectable by imaging. This applies to nonocclusive mesenteric ischemia—narrowing at the arteriolar and capillary level that often occurs as a result of cardiovascular surgery, sepsis, or catecholamine therapy.

▶ **Clinical features.** Chronic mesenteric ischemia is characterized by abdominal pain after meals. The clinical manifestations of acute mesenteric ischemia often progress in three phases:
- *Initial phase*: abdominal pain and guarding.
- *Latent phase*: diminution of clinical symptoms and intestinal peristalsis.
- *Late phase*: intestinal necrosis, obstruction, and peritonitis, with a high mortality rate.

Anticoagulation is usually unsuccessful in the treatment of acute mesenteric ischemia. A more effective strategy is exploratory laparotomy with resection of the necrotic bowel.

▶ **Differential diagnosis.** Bowel wall thickening may also occur in the setting of chronic inflammatory bowel disease, allergies, and malignancies. The sudden onset of symptoms is more typical of acute mesenteric ischemia, however.

▶ **Key points.** Whenever mesenteric ischemia is suspected, it is important to evaluate both vascular and parenchymal changes. This is best accomplished with CT scans in the arterial and portal venous phases of enhancement.

> **Note**
>
> Acute mesenteric ischemia is an emergency situation that requires immediate diagnosis and treatment. The mortality rate is high when diagnosis is delayed.

8.5.5 Hemorrhage

▶ **Brief definition.** Intestinal hemorrhage is acute or chronic bleeding into the intestinal lumen originating from mesenteric vessels. Besides ulcerations and varices in the upper gastrointestinal tract, inflammatory or neoplastic changes and angiodysplasia have major causal significance in bleeding distal to the ligament of Treitz.

▶ **Imaging signs.** Catheter-based angiography is of great value in the investigation of gastrointestinal hemorrhage, as it can also be used therapeutically. Thus, digital subtraction angiography (DSA) can locate the bleeding site and, in the same sitting, provide transcatheter access for endovascular occlusion by coil embolization (▶ Fig. 8.40). This technique allows for superselective embolization as close to the bleeding site as possible. Embolization should not be done with particles or a liquid agent, as these materials could cause small vessel occlusion leading to necrosis of the bowel wall. Coil embolization greatly reduces this risk. DSA may be of limited diagnostic value, however, as intestinal peristalsis and low contrast resolution may cause a hemorrhage to be missed if the bleeding rate is less than 1 mL/min. On the other hand, noninvasive CT can provide acceptable diagnostic accuracy even at low bleeding rates, but it cannot be used therapeutically. When CT scanning is done prior to the surgical treatment of intestinal bleeding, for example, the protocol should always include imaging in a (portal) venous enhancement phase in addition to the arterial phase (▶ Fig. 8.41).

▶ **Clinical features.** Patients may present with hematemesis (vomiting of blood) or melena (tarry stool) due to upper gastrointestinal hemorrhage, or with hematochezia (fresh blood in the stool) due to lower gastrointestinal hemorrhage. Severe acute bleeding may lead to hypovolemic shock. With a chronic (slow) hemorrhage, the dominant clinical features are those of anemia.

▶ **Differential diagnosis.** Extravasation of contrast medium into the bowel lumen is diagnostic of gastrointestinal hemorrhage. However, it can be difficult to determine etiology (inflammatory, neoplastic, or varicose) from imaging findings alone.

▶ **Key points.** In patients with gastrointestinal hemorrhage, initial localization of the bleeding site is usually done endoscopically (gastroscopy or colonoscopy). A small-bowel hemorrhage often cannot be verified endoscopically, however, and imaging procedures assume a major role.

8.5.6 Crohn's Disease

▶ **Brief definition.** Crohn's disease is a chronic inflammatory bowel disease that commonly often involves the distal ileum and ascending colon but may occur anywhere in the digestive tract. It is characterized by a transmural, segmental, and discontinuous ("skip lesions") inflammatory process in the bowel wall. The etiology and pathogenesis of Crohn's disease are not fully understood but may relate to a combination of immunologic, infectious, and genetic factors. The incidence is 2 or 3 per 100,000 population per year, with a prevalence of 300 to 500:100,000 population per year. Initial manifestations of Crohn's disease typically appear in the second or third decade but also have a second age peak in the sixth decade.

▶ **Imaging signs.** Similarly to the entities described above, there has been a change in diagnostic imaging strategies for Crohn's disease. The double-contrast examination of the small intestine using the Sellink technique has been replaced by CT in acute clinical settings and by MRI for more elective indications. The bowel wall is markedly thickened in affected areas and shows increased enhancement on CT or MRI after IV injection of contrast medium (▶ Fig. 8.42). The transmural inflammatory process often leads to abscess formation as well as formation of fistulas between the bowel and adjacent structures (e.g., enteroenteric, enterovesical, enterocutaneous; ▶ Fig. 8.43). Other typical findings on contrast-enhanced images are prominent peri-intestinal lymph nodes and accentuated mesenteric vessels, which form parallel lines that create the "comb sign" (see ▶ Fig. 8.43).

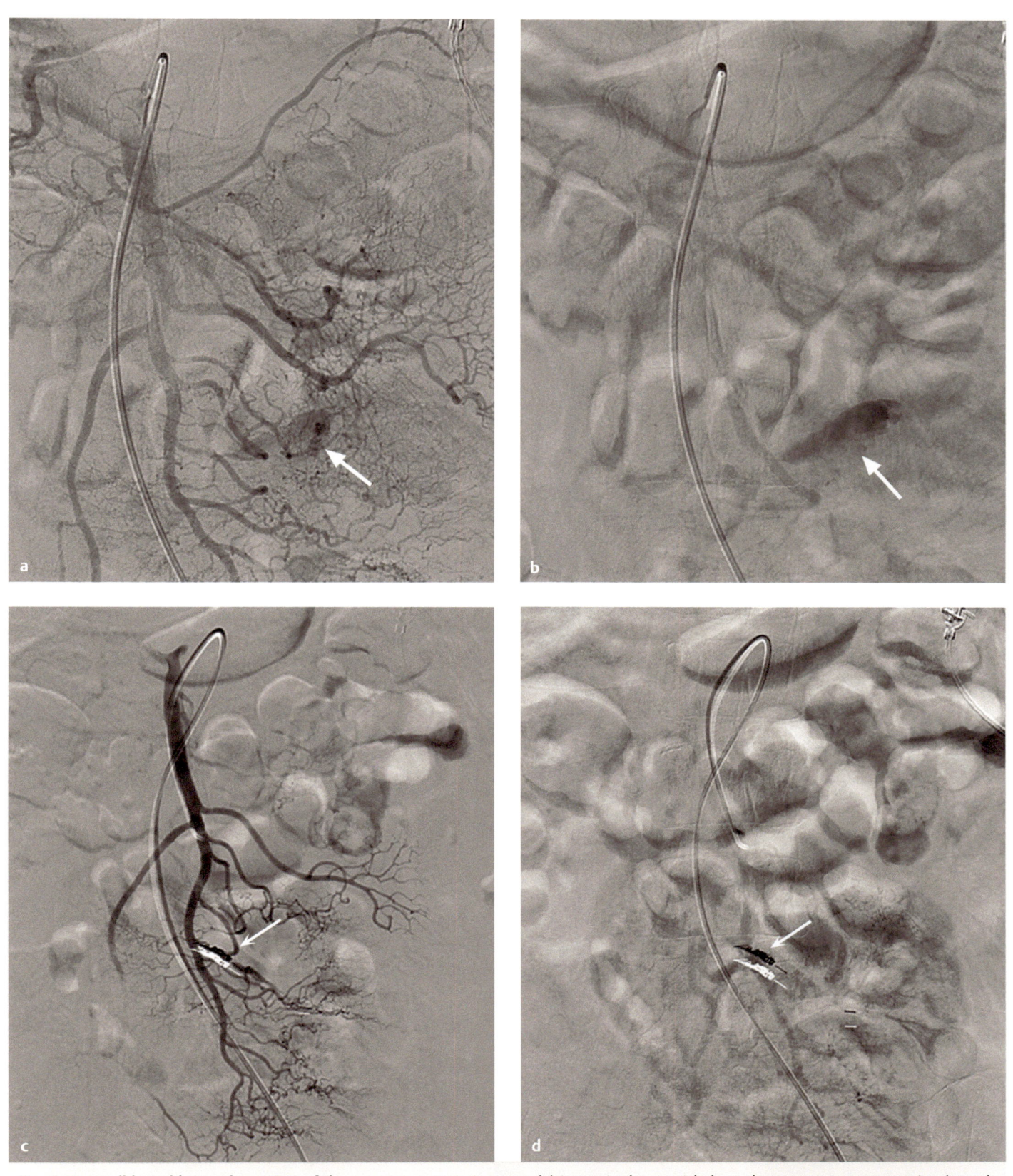

Fig. 8.40 Small-bowel hemorrhage. DSA of the superior mesenteric artery. **(a)** Image in the arterial phase shows contrast extravasation (arrow). **(b)** Contrast extravasation (arrow) is still visible in the late phase. **(c)** Arterial phase image after vascular branch embolization with coils (arrow) shows absence of contrast extravasation. **(d)** Image in the late phase after embolization (arrow) confirms that the bleeding site has been occluded.

Gastrointestinal Tract

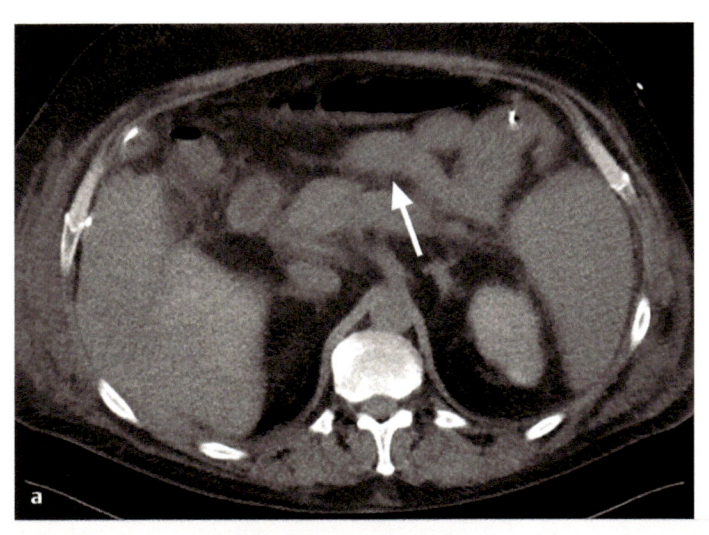

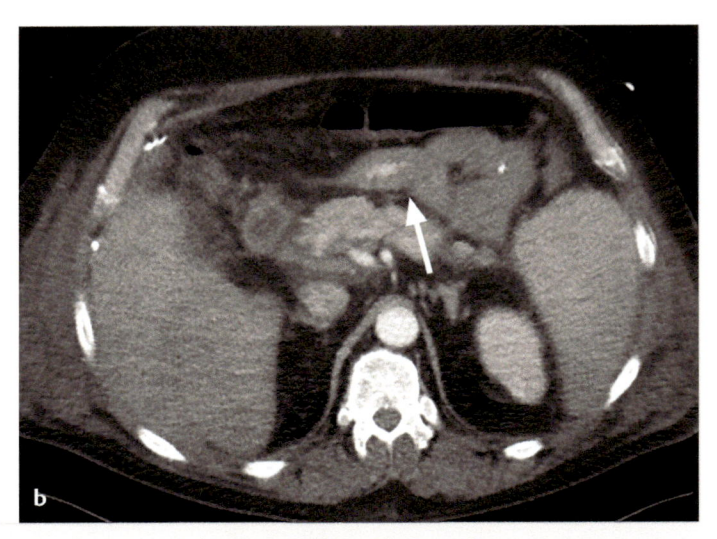

Fig. 8.41 Small-bowel hemorrhage. CT appearance. **(a)** Precontrast phase. For comparison, the arrow indicates the site of contrast extravasation shown in panel [b]. **(b)** Image in the portal venous phase after IV injection of contrast medium displays contrast extravasation into the bowel lumen (arrow).

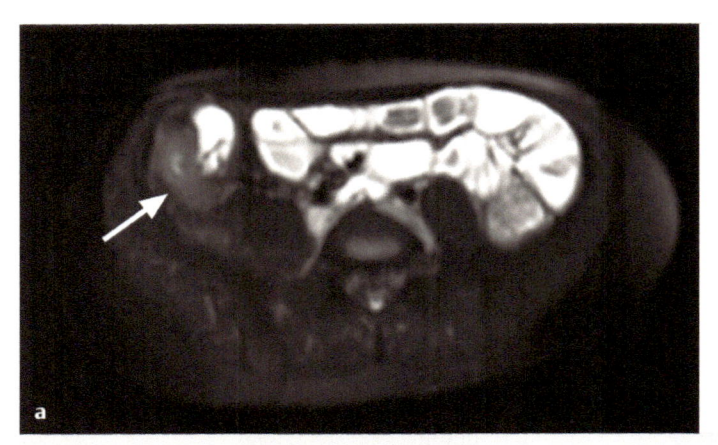

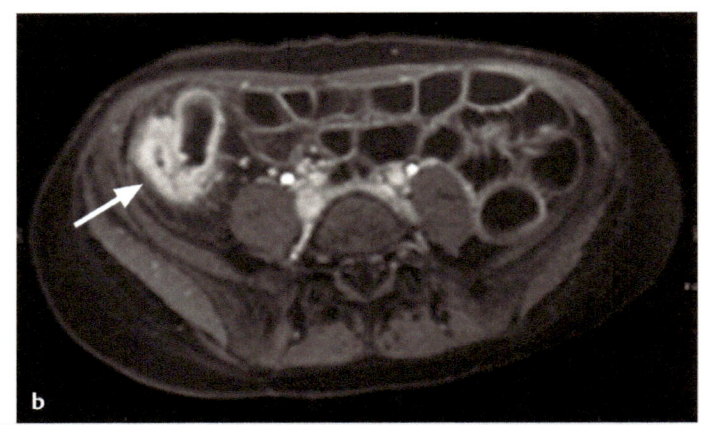

Fig. 8.42 Acute exacerbation of Crohn's disease. MRI. **(a)** Fat-saturated T2W image shows edematous wall thickening in the terminal ileum (arrow). **(b)** T1W image after administration of contrast medium shows marked enhancement at the corresponding site (arrow).

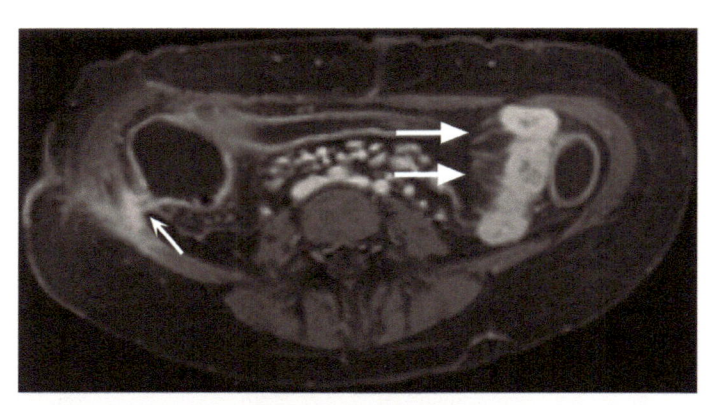

Fig. 8.43 Crohn's disease. Contrast-enhanced MRI shows markedly wall-thickened bowel loops in the left midabdomen accompanied by a typical comb sign (heavy arrows). An enterocutaneous fistula is also visible in the right midabdomen (light arrow).

Caution

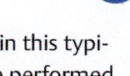

On account of concerns about radiation exposure in this typically young age group, CT examinations should be performed only in the acute stage of the disease (e.g., to exclude abscess formation).

MRI has become the diagnostic modality of choice at many centers. Ultrasound is also commonly used, especially in pediatric patients (▶ Fig. 8.44). Edema formation signifying an acute inflammatory process can be clearly identified in fat-saturated T2W MR images (see ▶ Fig. 8.42).

▶ **Clinical features.** Crohn's disease usually presents with nonspecific symptoms such as fatigue, diarrhea, and weight loss. The

8.5 Diseases of the Jejunum and Ileum

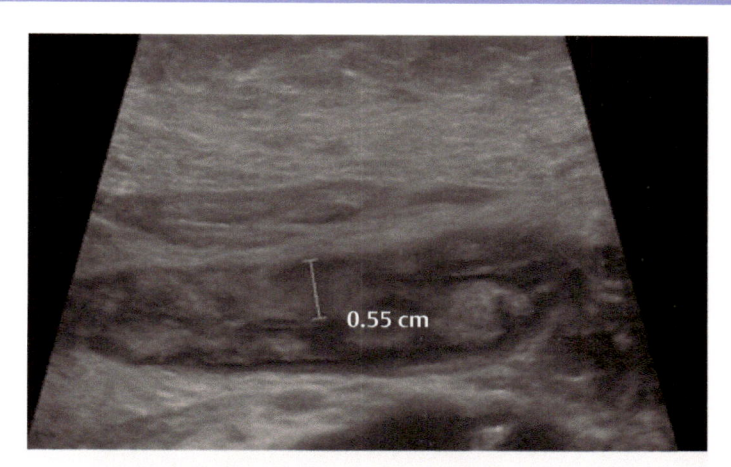

Fig. 8.44 **Crohn's disease.** Ultrasound scan shows definite thickening of the ileal wall (marker).

Table 8.7 Differences between Crohn's disease and ulcerative colitis

Criteria	Crohn's disease	Ulcerative colitis
Location	Any part of the gastrointestinal tract	Rectum and colon
Level of inflammation	All wall layers	Mucosa
Spread	Discontinuous (skip lesions)	Continuous, retrograde
Ileal involvement	Common	Rare (backwash ileitis)
Rectal involvement	Rare	Always
Extraintestinal changes	Common	Rare
Complications	Abscess and fistula	Toxic megacolon

acute stage is marked by abdominal pain and fever. This may be followed by symptoms of bowel obstruction due to a stenosing inflammatory process. Treatment of an acute exacerbation is based on pharmacologic immune suppression. Abscesses should be treated surgically or by interventional drain placement. Non-acute or fibrotic changes in the intestinal wall are managed by resection of the affected bowel.

▶ **Differential diagnosis.** The differential diagnosis includes ulcerative colitis, which presents as a non-transmural, continuous inflammatory process that starts from the rectum and spreads proximally to the rest of the large intestine. Differentiation of Crohn's disease from ulcerative colitis can be particularly difficult if the colitis spreads to the terminal ileum ("backwash ileitis"). The features of Crohn's disease and ulcerative colitis are contrasted in ▶ Table 8.7. Infectious forms of enteritis (e.g., due to *Yersinia* infection or tuberculosis) may have imaging features that are indistinguishable from those of Crohn's disease. Differentiation is aided by clinical correlation and disease progression (e.g., favorable response to antibiotics).

▶ **Key points.** Crohn's disease is a histological diagnosis. Imaging findings may be suggestive but cannot establish an initial diagnosis. Imaging does play a key role in follow-up, however. The modalities of choice for elective examinations are ultrasound and MRI. CT is preferred in patients with a suspected loop abscess as it can provide guidance for percutaneous drain insertion.

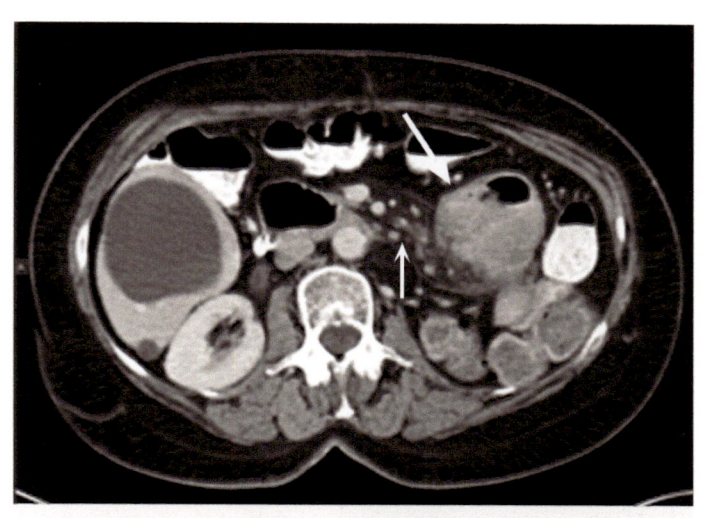

Fig. 8.45 **Large carcinoma of the small intestine.** Axial CT. The heavy arrow indicates the small bowel carcinoma. There is associated imbibition of adjacent fat and mesenteric lymphadenopathy (light arrow).

8.5.7 Adenocarcinoma

▶ **Brief definition.** Adenocarcinoma is a malignant tumor of the small bowel that usually arises from benign adenomatous precursors (polyps). The incidence of small-bowel carcinoma has been rising significantly and now averages 1.5:100,000 population per year. The peak age of incidence is 60 years.

▶ **Imaging signs.** Sectional imaging shows a mass that encircles and constricts the bowel lumen (▶ Fig. 8.45). On reaching a certain size, the tumor develops necrotic areas that create a heterogeneous appearance on CT and MRI. After IV administration of contrast medium, adenocarcinoma shows delayed enhancement relative to unaffected bowel wall.

▶ **Clinical features.** The clinical signs of adenocarcinoma are nonspecific and include abdominal pain and weight loss. Erosive changes may lead to bleeding with subsequent anemia. If the tumor obstructs the intestinal lumen, symptoms of bowel obstruction will develop. The tumor metastasizes by the lymphogenous route (adjacent lymph node stations) and the hematogenous route, with a predilection for the liver. The TNM classification is shown in ▶ Table 8.8.

▶ **Differential diagnosis.** The differential diagnosis should include other tumors of the small intestine:
- *Lymphoma*: Lymphoma usually shows diffuse, long-segment involvement of small-bowel loops; bowel obstruction tends to be a late complication.
- *Carcinoid tumors*: Carcinoid tumors are hypervascular and show greater arterial-phase enhancement than adenocarcinoma.
- *GIST*: This tumor does not involve the gastrointestinal mucosa but arises from the submucosa, resulting in a smooth margin on the luminal side. By contrast, adenocarcinoma arises in the

Gastrointestinal Tract

mucosal cells, and the tumor surface facing the bowel lumen often has a fissured appearance.

▶ **Key points.** On the whole, malignant tumors of the small intestine are less common than malignancies of the large intestine. Nevertheless, they are important in the differential diagnosis of tumors and inflammatory processes. The principal characteristics of small bowel tumors are reviewed in ▶ Table 8.9.

8.5.8 Carcinoid Tumors

▶ **Brief definition.** Carcinoid, or carcinoid tumor, is a collective term for various tumors that arise from the neuroendocrine system. The principal sites of occurrence are in the gastrointestinal tract and pancreas. The term "carcinoid" has been replaced with "neuroendocrine tumor" in the WHO classification (▶ Table 8.10), although the traditional term is often still used for tumors at gastrointestinal sites. Carcinoid tumors arise from enterochromaffin Kulchitsky's cells in the crypts of Lieberkuhn. While malignant forms most commonly involve the ileum, benign carcinoid tumors occur mainly in the vermiform appendix. Patients over 50 years of age are predominantly affected.

▶ **Imaging signs.** Sectional imaging shows a well-defined tumor of the small intestine that often displays fingerlike extensions into the mesentery (▶ Fig. 8.46). Tumor calcifications are a common finding on CT scans. Increasingly, carcinoid tumors are diagnosed by PET-CT using the carcinoid-specific tracers DOTATOC, DOTANOC, or DOTATATE (▶ Fig. 8.47).

Note
Because of the hypervascularity of the tumor and possible metastases, the sectional imaging protocol should always include an arterial enhancement phase whenever a carcinoid tumor is suspected.

▶ **Clinical features.** Frequently the tumor runs a protracted, indolent clinical course. Over time, especially if hepatic metastasis has occurred, the patient may develop "carcinoid syndrome" caused by the formation of serotonin. This syndrome is characterized by diarrhea, bronchial constriction or asthma, and flushing with a reddish-blue discoloration of the face and upper body. Treatment includes surgical resection of the tumor. Gastrointestinal carcinoid tumors have an excellent prognosis in the absence of metastasis. Even if hepatic metastases develop and a palliative situation arises, patients may survive for several years.

▶ **Differential diagnosis.** Differentiation from other small-bowel tumors, especially lymphoma and adenocarcinoma, may be difficult. Lymphomas, however, usually show diffuse involvement of the bowel. Adenocarcinomas are usually hypovascular; thus, the detection of hypervascular hepatic metastases may suggest the correct diagnosis of a carcinoid tumor.

▶ **Key points.** Carcinoid is a rare tumor of the distal ileum and appendix but should still be considered in the differential diagnosis of intestinal masses along with other tumors and inflammatory processes.

Table 8.8 TNM classification of small bowel adenocarcinoma

Designation	Description
Primary tumor	
T1a	Tumor invades the lamina propria
T1b	Tumor invades the submucosa
T2	Tumor invades the muscularis propria
T3	Tumor invades through the muscularis propria into the subserosa
T4	Tumor invades the mesentery or other organs
Lymph nodes	
N0	No regional lymph node metastasis
N1	Metastasis in 1–3 regional lymph nodes
N2	Metastases in 4 or more regional lymph nodes
Distant metastasis	
M0	No distant metastasis
M1	Distant metastasis

Table 8.9 Distinguishing features of small bowel tumors.

Tumor	Distinguishing features
Lymphoma	Diffuse or long segmental wall thickening, prominent adenopathy
GIST	Located in the submucosa
Adenocarcinoma	Arises from the mucosa, grows by infiltration, hypovascular
Carcinoid	Hypervascular tumor + hepatic metastases

Abbreviation: GIST, gastrointestinal stromal tumor.

Table 8.10 WHO classification of neuroendocrine tumors[1]

WHO 1980	WHO 2000	WHO 2010
Carcinoid	Well differentiated neuroendocrine tumor	G1 neuroendocrine tumor (carcinoid tumor)
	Well differentiated neuroendocrine carcinoma	G2 neuroendocrine tumor
	Poorly differentiated (small-cell) neuroendocrine carcinoma	G3 (small- or large-cell) neuroendocrine carcinoma
Mucocarcinoid	Mixed endocrine–exocrine carcinoma	Mixed adenoneuroendocrine carcinoma
Mixed carcinoid-adenocarcinoma		
Pseudotumoral lesion	Tumorlike lesion	Hyperplastic and preneoplastic lesion

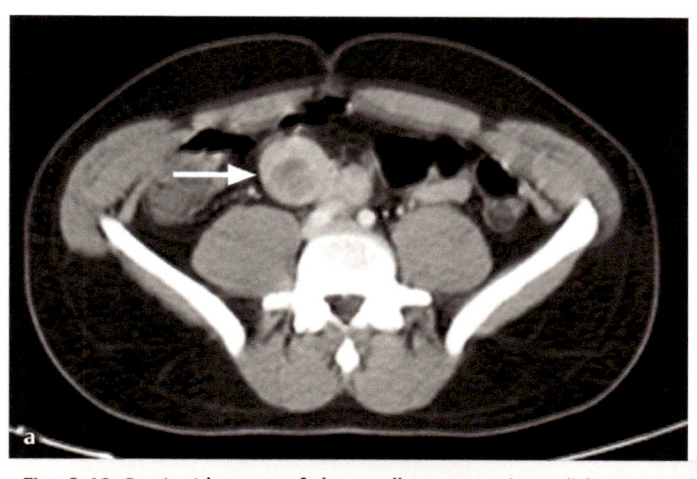

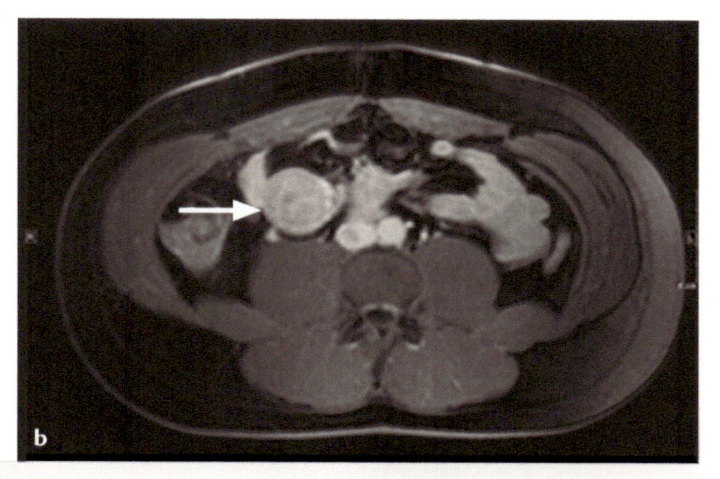

Fig. 8.46 **Carcinoid tumor of the small intestine.** (Partial) hypervascularization of the tumor (arrows). **(a)** Contrast-enhanced CT. **(b)** Contrast-enhanced MRI.

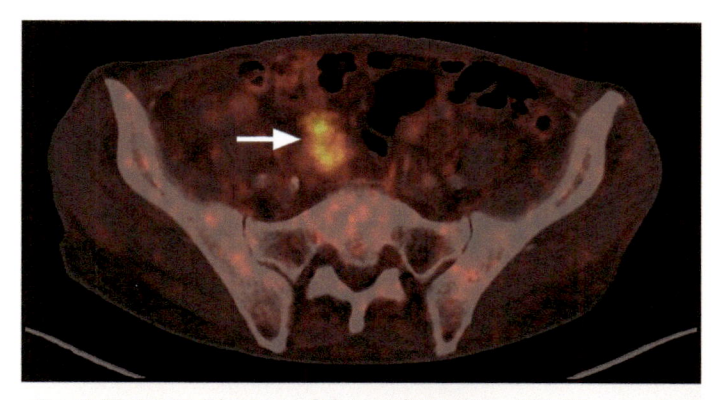

Fig. 8.47 **Carcinoid tumor of the small intestine.** PET-CT scan using the tracer gallium Ga 68 DOTATOC. Strong tracer uptake provides accurate localization of the tumor (arrow).

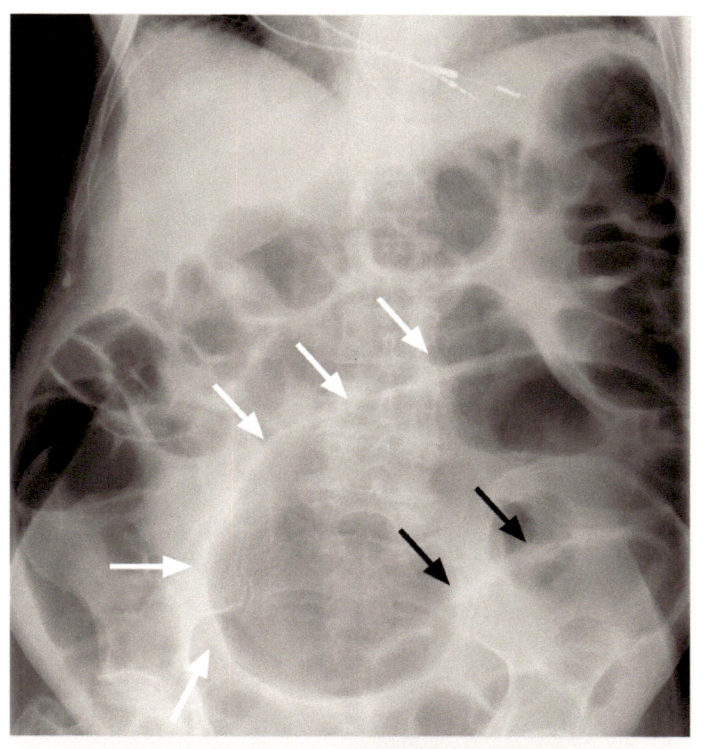

Fig. 8.48 **Sigmoid volvulus.** Conventional abdominal radiograph shows a markedly dilated small bowel loop (white arrows) and a typical coffee bean sign caused by an apposed bowel loop (black arrows).

8.6 Diseases of the Colon and Rectum

8.6.1 Volvulus

▶ **Brief definition.** Volvulus refers to the twisting or torsion of an organ, especially the twisting of a bowel segment on its mesenteric root. Accordingly, volvulus can occur only in a bowel segment that has a mesenteric pedicle. The sigmoid colon is most frequently affected, followed by the cecum. Sigmoid volvulus is particularly common among older patients in the seventh decade of life. After colon cancer, volvulus is the second leading cause of large bowel obstruction.

▶ **Imaging signs.** A plain abdominal radiograph can show dilated colon loops forming an "inverted U" shape in the sigmoid colon. This feature is called the "coffee bean sign" for its resemblance to an oversized coffee bean (▶ Fig. 8.48). The twisting of mesenteric structures can produce the "whirlpool sign" on CT scans (▶ Fig. 8.49).

▶ **Clinical features.** Volvulus may have an acute onset or may occur as a protracted event. The main clinical findings are pain, bloating, and vomiting due to the obstructive effect of the volvulus. If the torsion compresses and obstructs intestinal vessels, it may lead to ischemia with subsequent bowel necrosis and perforation. An early stage of sigmoid volvulus may be treatable by placement of a rectal tube and barium enema. Otherwise volvulus is an indication for surgical detorsion.

▶ **Differential diagnosis.** The differential diagnosis starts with paralytic ileus, which is distinguished by the generalized dilatation of bowel loops with absence of a focal colonic obstruction. Colon carcinoma is another possibility, but the tumor causes narrowing of the colon lumen, appearing on images as the "apple core sign." Strictures in a setting of chronic diverticulitis may also cause large-bowel obstruction. In this case the clinical course suggests the correct diagnosis (prior history of diverticulitis).

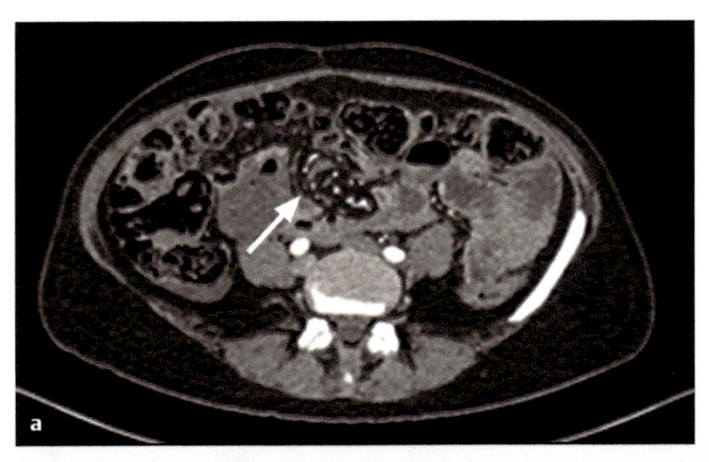

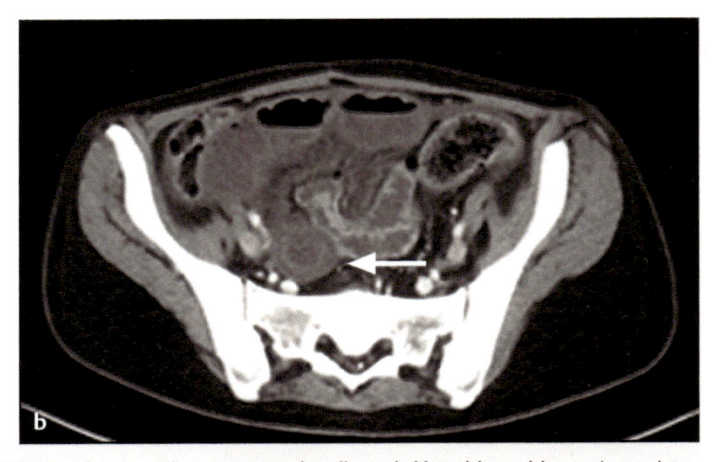

Fig. 8.49 Volvulus. CT. (a) Twisting of the mesenteric root (arrow). (b) Whirlpool sign with accentuated walls and dilated bowel loops (arrow).

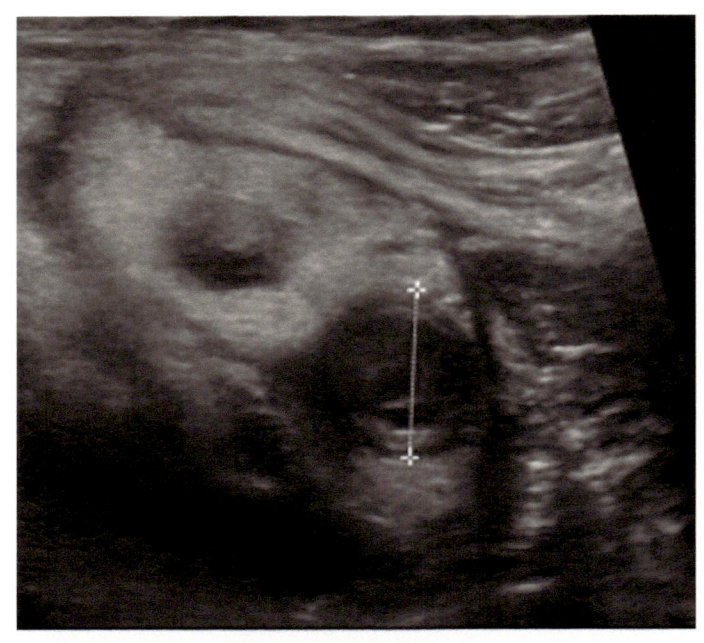

Fig. 8.50 Acute appendicitis. Ultrasound scan shows marked wall thickening and edema of the appendix (marker).

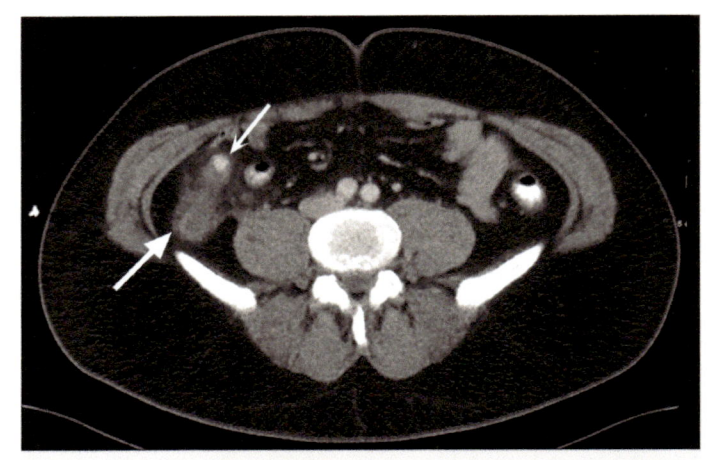

Fig. 8.51 Acute appendicitis. CT shows marked enlargement of the appendix (heavy arrow) and imbibition of locoregional fat. The light arrow points to an appendicolith, which is frequently present.

▶ **Key points.** Besides colon carcinoma, volvulus should be considered as a potential cause of large-bowel obstruction, especially in elderly patients.

8.6.2 Appendicitis

▶ **Brief definition.** Appendicitis is an inflammation of the vermiform appendix caused by intestinal flora (e.g., secondary to luminal bowel obstruction by adhesions or fecoliths) or by the hematogenous spread of infection. Appendicitis is most common in the pediatric age group.

▶ **Imaging signs.** Both ultrasound and CT are suitable modalities for diagnosing appendicitis. There is no general consensus on the diagnostic algorithm (CT versus ultrasound), and different CT protocols are followed at different institutions (with or without IV or oral contrast medium). Ultrasound shows edematous swelling of the appendix with a thickened, spongy wall (▶ Fig. 8.50). CT shows focal thickening of the appendix with an associated inflammatory reaction in adjacent fat (▶ Fig. 8.51). Fluid collections can often be found in the right lower quadrant and cul-de-sac. A radiopaque appendicolith is detectable in up to 40% of patients (see ▶ Fig. 8.51). The CT protocol should include a lung window setting to detect possible extraintestinal air that would signify a perforation.

▶ **Clinical features.** The classic presentation consists of periumbilical pain that later localizes to the McBurney point in the right lower quadrant. Associated features are nausea, vomiting, diarrhea, and fever, but patients may also present with nonspecific signs and symptoms.

▶ **Differential diagnosis.** Clinical and radiological differentiation from other inflammatory processes such as Crohn's disease or infectious enteritis can be difficult, but generally these processes are not confined to the appendix. The differential diagnosis in females should include gynecological disorders such as hemorrhagic ovarian cyst and ovarian torsion. These conditions are distinguished by corresponding radiological changes in the adnexa. Additionally, tumors of the appendix (e.g., carcinoma, carcinoid, or lymphoma) can mimic the imaging features of an inflammatory process. Nevertheless, the clinical picture should be sufficient to differentiate these conditions from appendicitis.

8.6 Diseases of the Colon and Rectum

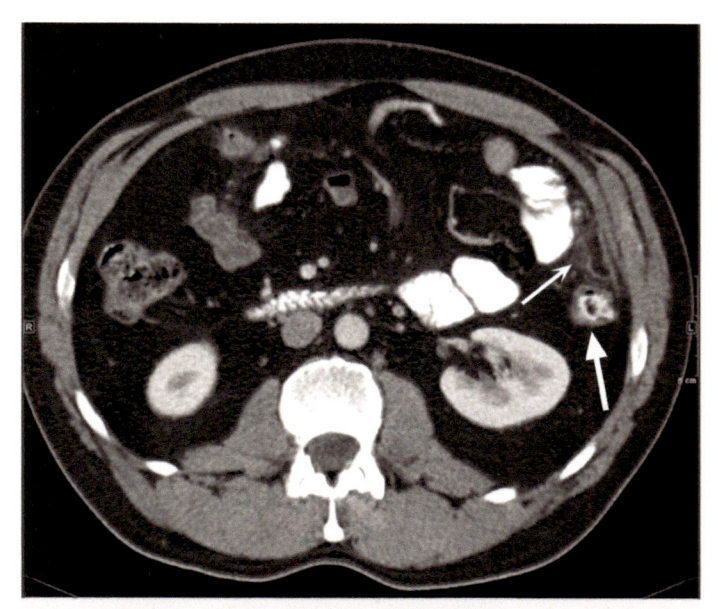

Fig. 8.52 **Epiploic appendagitis.** CT demonstrates an oval-shaped mass of fat attenuation with surrounding edema (light arrow) and reactive wall thickening of the sigmoid colon (heavy arrow).

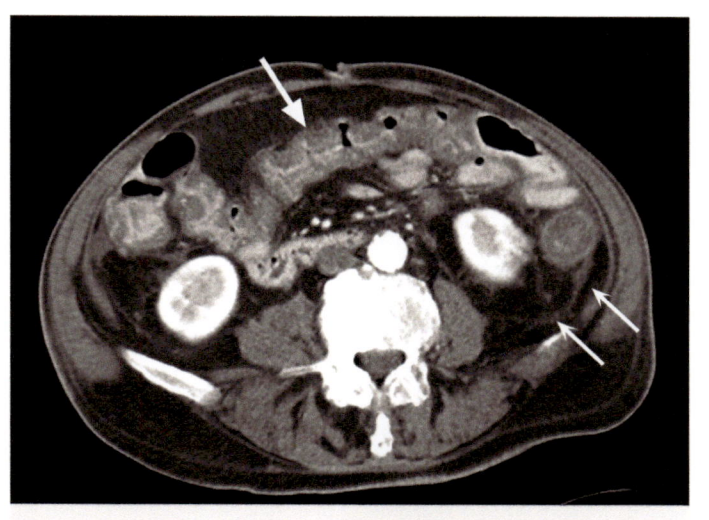

Fig. 8.53 **Pseudomembranous colitis.** CT shows a typical accordion sign (heavy arrow) with accompanying edema of adjacent fat (light arrows).

▶ **Key points.** Appendicitis is an illustrative model for the imaging characteristics of gastrointestinal inflammations. It exhibits wall thickening associated with edema of adjacent fat and fluid collections.

8.6.3 Epiploic Appendagitis

▶ **Brief definition.** The epiploic appendages (appendices) are fatty protrusions several centimeters large arising from the taeniae of the colon. Torsion or infarction of these appendages leads to focal peritoneal irritation. Epiploic appendagitis most commonly affects young, obese patients in the second to fourth decades.

▶ **Imaging signs.** CT reveals an ovoid mass of fat density adjacent to the colon with surrounding edema. The mass shows marked peripheral enhancement after IV injection of contrast medium (▶ Fig. 8.52).

▶ **Clinical features.** Patients typically present with an acute abdomen of sudden onset. The symptoms will usually regress spontaneously within a few days, so treatment consists of conservative analgesic therapy.

▶ **Differential diagnosis.** Clinical differentiation is required from appendicitis and diverticulitis. The presence of an ovoid, fatty pericolic mass is sufficient to distinguish epiploic appendagitis from other conditions.

▶ **Key points.** Epiploic appendagitis is a rare disorder. With a correct diagnosis, patients can be spared unnecessary invasive treatment.

8.6.4 Pseudomembranous Colitis

▶ **Brief definition.** Use of antibiotics or chemotherapy may disrupt the normal intestinal flora, allowing colonization by resistant bacteria such as *Clostridium difficile*. Clostridia produce toxins that can incite an inflammatory reaction in the colon. Several days usually pass before patients on antibiotics exhibit symptoms of pseudomembranous colitis.

Note
The disease is called "pseudomembranous colitis" because fibrin deposits form a characteristic pseudomembrane on the colonic mucosa that is visible at endoscopy.

▶ **Imaging signs.** CT is the imaging modality of choice as it has a positive predictive value of 90%. The inflammatory changes in pseudomembranous colitis may occur anywhere in the colon, although the right hemicolon is most commonly affected. Imaging reveals nodular thickening of the colon wall. Sectional imaging after oral administration of contrast medium shows a typical accordion sign (▶ Fig. 8.53) produced by contrast medium trapped between the thickened haustral folds.

▶ **Clinical features.** Pseudomembranous colitis presents clinically with diarrhea and systemic inflammatory signs. Besides imaging, the diagnosis is established by laboratory detection of *Clostridium difficile* toxins. Metronidazole is the therapeutic agent of choice after discontinuation of the initial antibiotics. With prompt diagnosis and proper therapy, the prognosis is very good.

▶ **Differential diagnosis.** The differential diagnosis includes other forms of colitis (e.g., with an ischemic or inflammatory cause), but those are excluded by noting a prior history of antibiotic use. Crohn's disease is distinguished from pseudomembranous colitis by its skip lesions and frequent involvement of the terminal ileum.

▶ **Key points.** The radiological accordion sign is pathognomonic for pseudomembranous colitis when interpreted in the clinical context of antibiotic use.

8.6.5 Ulcerative Colitis

▶ **Brief definition.** Ulcerative colitis and Crohn's disease are among the most common representatives of chronic inflammatory bowel disease. The period prevalence of ulcerative colitis is approximately 50:100,000 population per year, with an incidence of

Gastrointestinal Tract

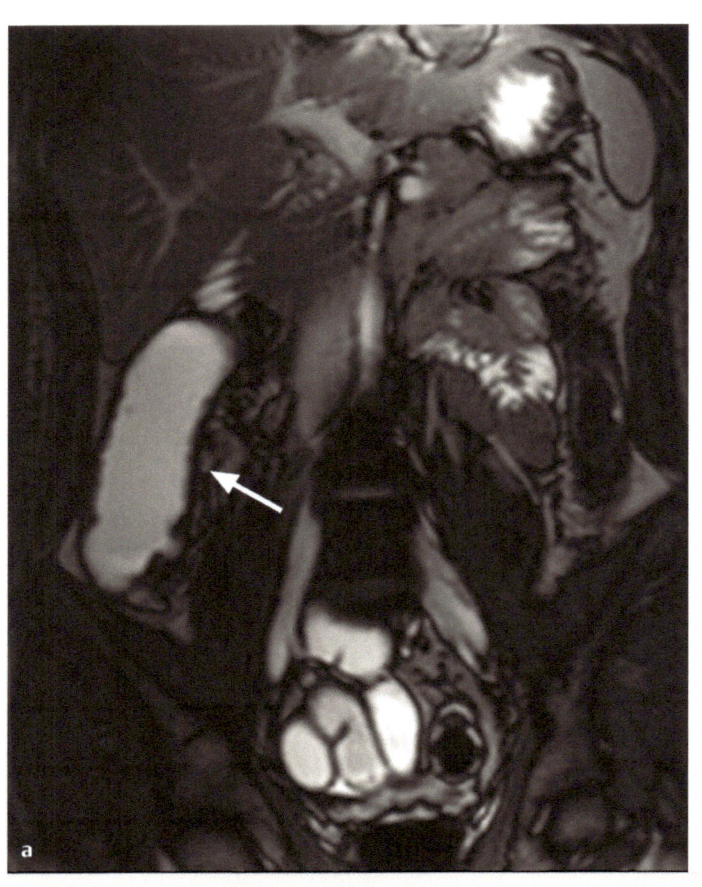

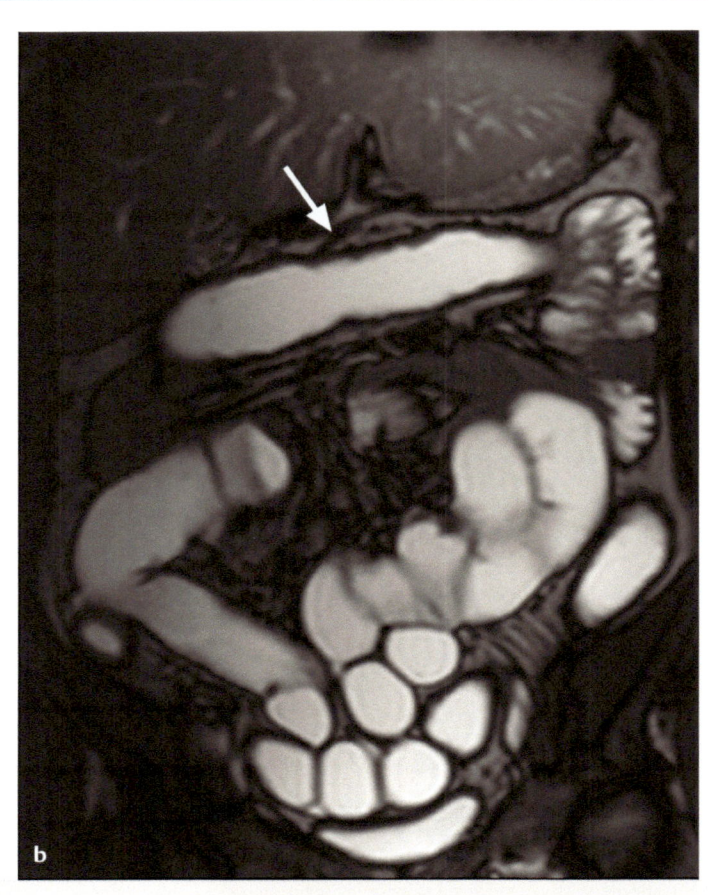

Fig. 8.54 Advanced ulcerative colitis. T2 W MRI. **(a)** Typical loss of haustral markings in the ascending colon (arrow). **(b)** Typical loss of haustral markings in the transverse colon (arrow). Islands of mucosa appear as small pseudopolyps.

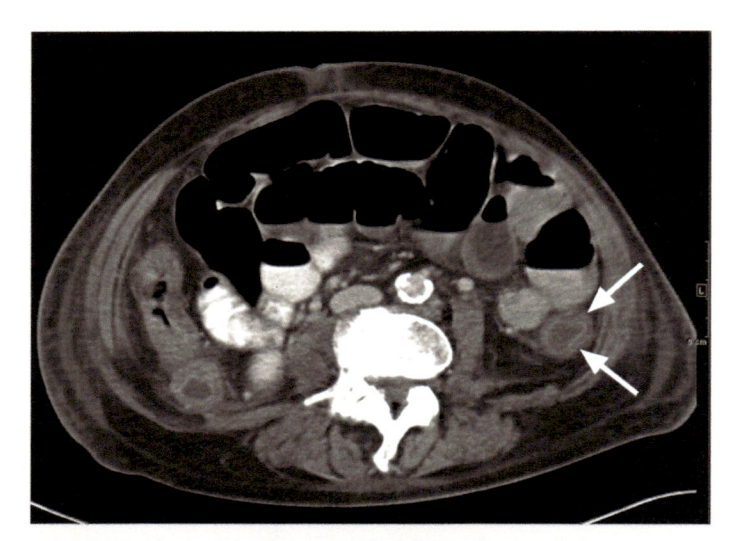

Fig. 8.55 Ulcerative colitis. Typical wall stratification (halo sign, arrows): The mucosa and the muscularis propria both show marked enhancement while the intermediate layer, the submucosa, is hypodense (due to edema, fatty degeneration).

4 to 10:100,000 population per year. There are many parallels with Crohn's disease. The etiology and pathogenesis of both diseases are not fully understood and probably involve a multifactorial process (genetics, environmental influences, psychosocial factors). The peak age of incidence of ulcerative colitis is between the second and fourth decades, similar to that of Crohn's disease. Ulcerative colitis spreads in retrograde fashion from the rectum to the colon and causes ulcerations in the mucosa. Involvement of the terminal ileum (backwash ileitis) may also be present.

8.6.6 Imaging Signs

Because ulcerative colitis is an inflammation of the mucosa, sectional imaging has limited sensitivity in early stages of the disease. Consequently, the disease is usually diagnosed by colonoscopy with biopsies taken at multiple sites. Later stages show a loss of normal haustral markings ("lead pipe" or "garden hose" colon) demonstrable by CT or MRI (▶ Fig. 8.54). On sectional imaging after IV injection of contrast medium, the bowel wall shows a halo sign (▶ Fig. 8.55) with increased enhancement of the mucosa (due to inflammation), decreased enhancement of the middle layer (due to edema or fatty infiltration), and increased enhancement of the outer bowel wall (muscularis propria). Mucosal islands, appearing as pseudopolyps, may also be found. As in Crohn's disease, fat-saturated T2 W MRI has major importance along with contrast-enhanced images. This protocol can clearly detect (peri)intestinal edema (signifying an active inflammatory process) as an area of high signal intensity.

8.6.7 Clinical Features

The major symptom is bloody diarrhea with mucus, in severe cases accompanied by inflammatory manifestations with fever, abdominal pain, and weight loss. There may also be intestinal complications such as megacolon (> 10 cm in diameter) and an increased risk of perforation. Patients with ulcerative colitis have

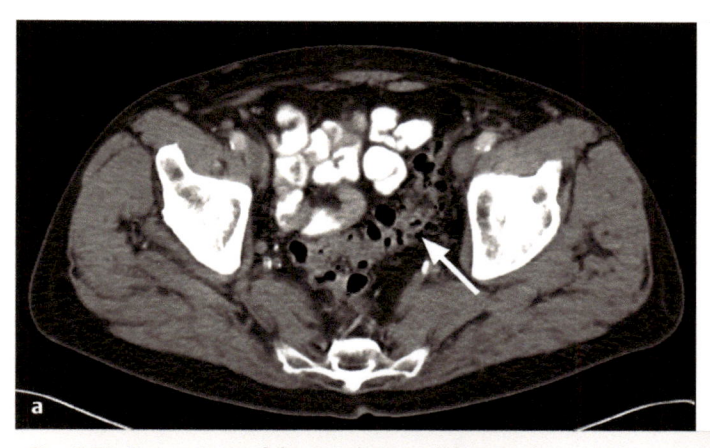

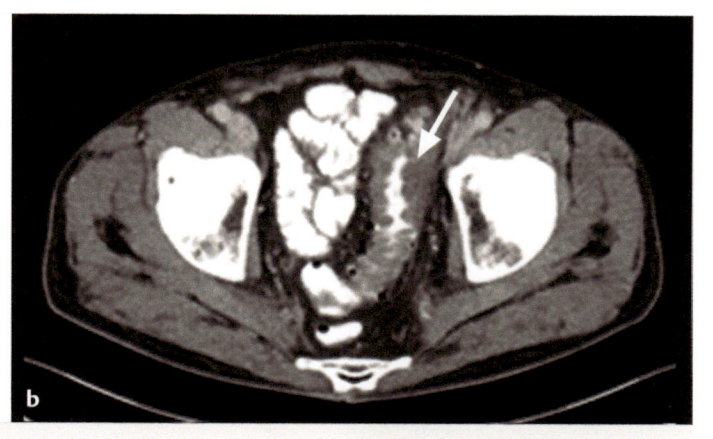

Fig. 8.56 Comparison of diverticulosis and diverticulitis. CT appearance. While diverticulosis consists of small, air-filled outpouchings in the colon wall, diverticulitis is associated with marked thickening of the bowel wall. **(a)** Patient with diverticulosis of the sigmoid colon (arrow). **(b)** Patient with sigmoid diverticulitis (arrow).

a markedly increased risk of developing colorectal cancer. There may also be extraintestinal complications such as primary sclerosing cholangitis. Ulcerative colitis patients are also susceptible to HLA-B27-associated diseases from the rheumatoid group.

Note
Approximately two-thirds of patients with primary sclerosing cholangitis also have ulcerative colitis. However, only about 5% of patients with ulcerative colitis have primary sclerosing cholangitis.

As well as medical treatment with immunosuppressive agents, surgical colectomy is an option in severe cases with epithelial dysplasia or when drug therapy is contraindicated.

▶ **Differential diagnosis.** Ulcerative colitis is not always distinguishable from Crohn's disease by imaging. Even differentiation by histopathology may be challenging. Typical distinguishing features from Crohn's disease are listed in ▶ Table 8.7. The differential diagnosis also includes other forms of colitis (with an inflammatory or ischemic cause) and diverticulitis, but these diseases spare the rectum and the inflammatory process is focal or segmental in its extent.

▶ **Key points.** Because ulcerative colitis is an inflammation of the mucosa, sectional imaging has only limited sensitivity, especially in early stages of the disease.

8.6.8 Diverticulosis and Diverticulitis

▶ **Brief definition.** Colonic diverticula are small acquired herniations through the muscular layers of the large intestine. The sigmoid colon is a site of predilection, but diverticula may occur in any part of the large bowel. The incidence of colonic diverticulosis increases with age and is associated with a lifelong preference for low-fiber foods and chronic constipation. The inflammation of one or more diverticula is usually secondary to impaction of stool in the diverticulum and related bacterial infection.

▶ **Imaging signs.** CT is the imaging modality of choice and should employ rectal administration of a positive contrast agent (not barium-containing) to differentiate perforation from ascites. *Diverticulosis* appears as multiple stool- or contrast medium–filled outpouchings of the bowel wall (▶ Fig. 8.56). *Diverticulitis* is characterized by a thickened colon wall with edematous stranding of adjacent fat (see ▶ Fig. 8.56). Intramural or pericolic abscesses appear as fluid collections with gas inclusions and increased peripheral enhancement after IV injection of contrast medium.

Note
The rectal administration of a positive contrast agent permits an accurate diagnosis of bowel perforation based on extraintestinal contrast pooling. CT performed for suspected diverticulitis should include lung window settings to facilitate the detection of free air from a perforation.

▶ **Clinical features.** Most patients with diverticulosis are asymptomatic. When clinical symptoms arise, they usually result from diverticulitis with a classic triad of abdominal pain (left lower quadrant pain with sigmoid diverticulitis), fever, and leukocytosis. The early stage is managed conservatively with antibiotics. An abscess is treated by CT- or ultrasound-guided drainage. Perforated diverticulitis is an acute indication for surgery.

▶ **Differential diagnosis.** The differential diagnosis of diverticulitis includes other inflammatory processes of the colon such as Crohn's disease and infectious or ischemic colitis. The latter diseases are distinguished by an absence of visible diverticula and, while diverticulitis is a focal inflammatory process, the other diseases tend to involve a greater length of bowel.

▶ **Key points.** Diverticulitis is a common cause of acute abdomen in older patients. CT is a fast and accurate method for establishing the diagnosis.

8.6.9 Colorectal Carcinoma

▶ **Brief definition.** Colorectal carcinoma is one of the most common malignancies in the western world, with a peak age of incidence in the seventh decade. Approximately 95% of these tumors are adenocarcinomas, which develop from benign polypoid

Gastrointestinal Tract

Table 8.11 TNM classification of colorectal carcinoma

Designation	Description
Primary tumor	
Tis	Carcinoma in situ, intraepithelial or invasion of the lamina propria
T1	Tumor invades the submucosa
T2	Tumor invades the muscularis propria
T3	Tumor invades the subserosa or perirectal fat
T4	Tumor invades the peritoneum (4a) or adjacent organs (4b)
Lymph nodes	
N0	No regional lymph node metastasis
N1	Metastasis in 1–3 pericolic or perirectal lymph nodes
N2	Metastases in 4 or more pericolic or perirectal lymph nodes
Distant metastasis	
M0	No distant metastasis
M1	Distant metastasis

Table 8.12 Dukes staging system for colorectal carcinoma

Stage	Groupings
I	T1–2 N0 M0
IIa	T3 N0 M0
IIb	T4a N0 M0
IIc	T4b N0 M0
IIIa	T1–2 N1 M0
IIIb	T3–4 N1 M0
IIIc	T3–4 N2 M0
IV	T1–4 N0–2 M1

- *Colon carcinoma*: The colon is both intra- and extraperitoneal. It is drained by tributaries of the portal vein, so the liver is a frequent site of initial metastasis.
- *Rectal carcinoma*: The rectum is partially extraperitoneal and lacks a serosa, so it is common for rectal cancers to invade adjacent tissues. The rectum is drained by tributaries of the internal iliac vein. Consequently, the lung is a common initial site of hematogenous metastasis from rectal carcinoma.

The TNM classification of colorectal carcinoma is shown in ▶ Table 8.11. The Dukes staging system (▶ Table 8.12) is used to determine prognosis and direct treatment.

▶ **Imaging signs**
- *Colon carcinoma*: On classic fluoroscopic imaging with rectal administration of contrast medium, colon carcinoma typically appears as an annular filling defect that resembles an apple core or napkin ring (▶ Fig. 8.57). Abrupt luminal narrowing with a "shoulder" at the junction with normal adjacent bowel is responsible for the apple core appearance. (PET-)CT or MRI shows marked focal thickening of the colon wall, which may cause luminal obstruction (▶ Fig. 8.58). Peri-intestinal lymph node metastasis and hepatic metastases are also common findings at the time of initial diagnosis. If colon carcinoma is suspected, bowel preparation is recommended before imaging to ensure that stool particles will not obscure the tumor.
- *Rectal carcinoma*: This tumor has a similar imaging appearance to colon carcinoma, except that it is more locally invasive. MRI can precisely define the tumor margins and invasion depth, which is of major importance for staging and therapeutic decision making (▶ Fig. 8.59). This is why pretherapeutic high-resolution MRI of the rectum is prescribed in current guidelines. Imaging is performed with a surface coil (wrap-around body coil). T2-weighted sequences without fat suppression are essential.

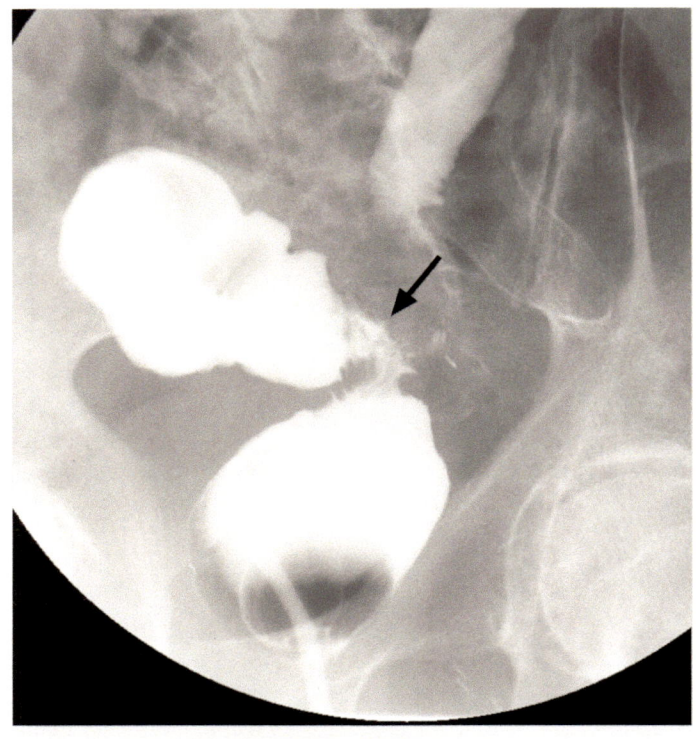

Fig. 8.57 Carcinoma of the sigmoid colon. Conventional radiograph with rectal contrast shows circumferential narrowing of the colon lumen ("apple core" or "napkin ring" sign).

Note

At many centers, virtual colonography using sectional imaging (CT or MRI) and image postprocessing software provides an alternative to endoscopy in the early detection and evaluation of colorectal cancer. This can be combined with simultaneous abdominal staging (e.g., to exclude hepatic metastases). Current guidelines for rectal carcinoma recommend the use of high-resolution MRI to differentiate between T2 and T3 tumors.

adenomas. The transformation of adenoma to carcinoma (the "adenoma–carcinoma sequence") takes an average of 3 to 5 years. Patients with familial polyposis and chronic inflammatory bowel disease are at increased risk for developing colorectal carcinoma. Clinically and anatomically, it is important to distinguish between colon carcinoma and rectal carcinoma:

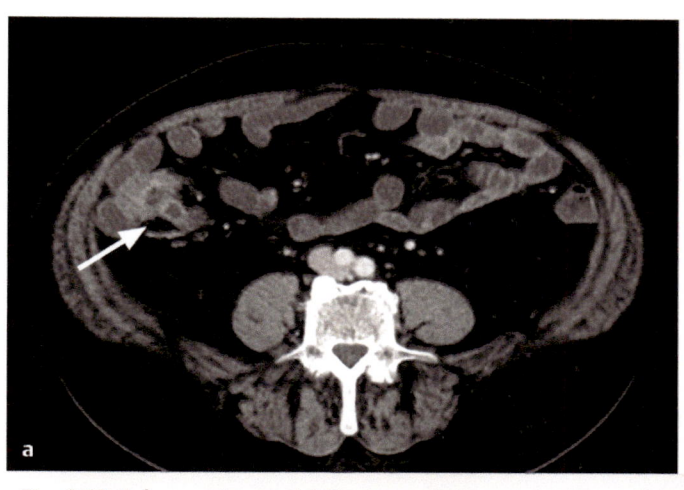

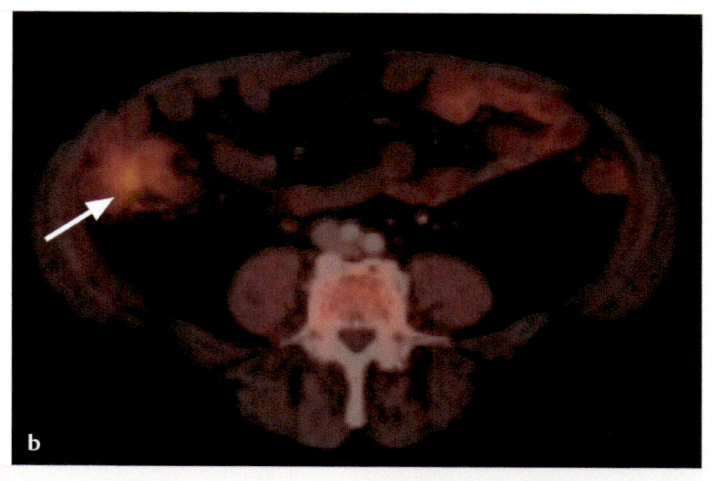

Fig. 8.58 Colon carcinoma. (a) Carcinoma in the proximal ascending colon (arrow). (b) Abnormal tracer uptake or glucose utilization in a PET-CT fusion image (arrow).

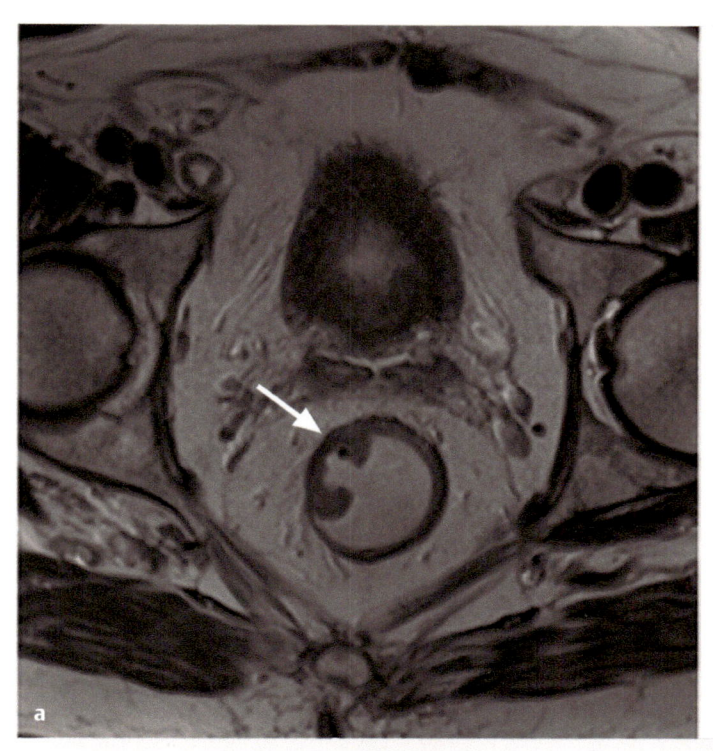

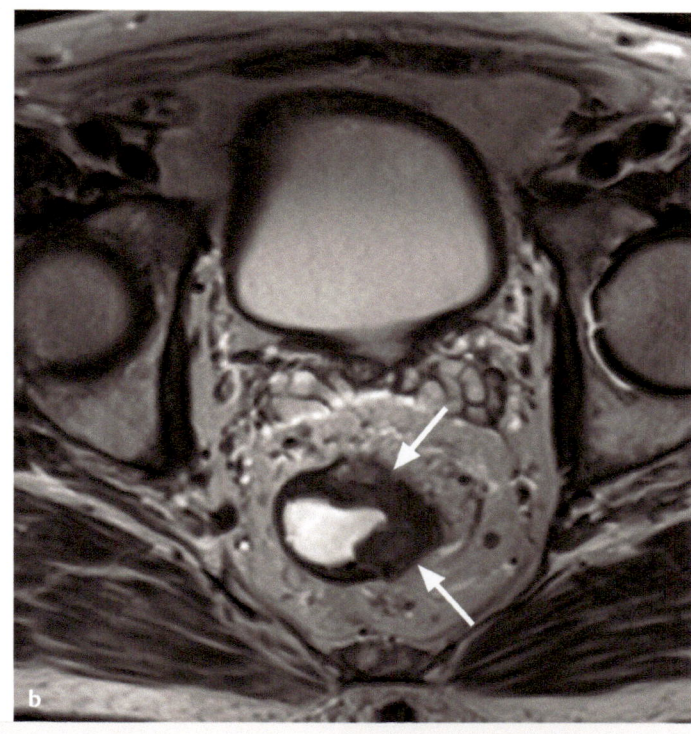

Fig. 8.59 Rectal carcinomas at different stages. Axial T2 W MR images. (a) Patient with stage T2 rectal carcinoma: invasion depth extends to the muscularis propria (arrow). (b) Patient with stage T3 rectal carcinoma: tumor has invaded the perirectal fat (arrows).

▶ **Clinical features.** B symptoms (weight loss, night sweats) may be combined with intestinal symptoms such as paradoxical diarrhea, constipation, and bowel obstruction by stenosing lesions. Many patients also have hematochezia or melena. The treatment of colorectal carcinoma includes surgical resection combined with pre- and/or postoperative radiation or chemotherapy.

▶ **Differential diagnosis.** Differentiation is mainly required from focal infectious or ischemic forms of colitis and diverticulitis. Besides bowel wall thickening, however, these disorders also cause signs of inflammation with pericolic edema, abscess formation, or perforation.

▶ **Key points.** The sectional imaging of colorectal carcinoma should always include the evaluation of common sites for hematogenous and lymphogenous metastasis.

8.6.10 Ogilvie's Syndrome

Ogilvie's syndrome is a colonic pseudo-obstruction caused by loss of autonomic innervation to the bowel due to functional compromise of the ganglia. It is named for Sir William Ogilvie, who first described the syndrome.

▶ **Imaging signs.** Abdominal radiography or sectional imaging shows an atonic, markedly dilated colon with no signs of a mechanical obstruction (▶ Fig. 8.60).

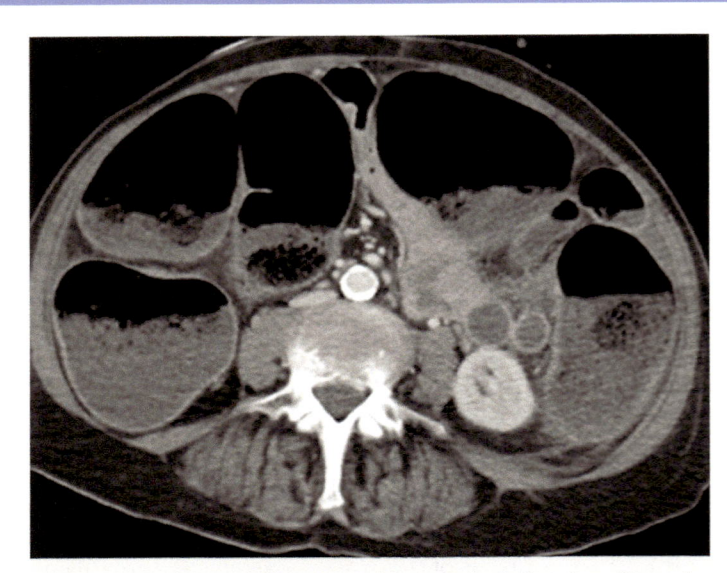

Fig. 8.60 Ogilvie's syndrome. CT shows marked dilatation of bowel loops in the absence of a mechanical obstruction.

▶ **Clinical features.** Ogilvie's syndrome is a rare disorder that occurs predominantly in older patients. It may develop after a surgical procedure or in the setting of another serious illness. Colic, bloating, and constipation are the clinical triad of Ogilvie's syndrome. Conservative treatment should be tried first (nasogastric decompression, correction of electrolyte imbalance, parasympathomimetic drugs). If these measures are unsuccessful, surgical treatment (cecostomy) is indicated.

▶ **Differential diagnosis.** Colonic pseudo-obstruction requires differentiation mainly from mechanical bowel obstruction, which is also associated with markedly dilated bowel loops. The latter condition is distinguished by the presence of a mechanical obstruction and requires a prompt decision for surgical intervention.

▶ **Key points.** Ogilvie's syndrome is characterized by an acute onset of symptoms and the absence of a mechanical bowel obstruction.

Bibliography

[1] Schott M, Klöppel G, Raffel A, Saleh A, Knoefel WT, Scherbaum WA. Neuroendocrine neoplasms of the gastrointestinal tract. Dtsch Arztebl Int. 2011; 108 (18):305–312
[2] Adamek HE, Lauenstein TC, eds. MRT in der Gastroenterologie. Stuttgart: Thieme; 2010
[3] Anzidei M, Napoli A, Zini C, Kirchin MA, Catalano C, Passariello R. Malignant tumours of the small intestine: a review of histopathology, multidetector CT and MRI aspects. Br J Radiol. 2011; 84(1004):677–690
[4] Byrne AT, Geoghegan T, Govender P, Lyburn ID, Colhoun E, Torreggiani WC. The imaging of intussusception. Clin Radiol. 2005; 60(1):39–46
[5] Dave-Verma H, Moore S, Singh A, Martins N, Zawacki J. Computed tomographic enterography and enteroclysis: pearls and pitfalls. Curr Probl Diagn Radiol. 2008; 37(6):279–287
[6] Erturk SM, Mortelé KJ, Oliva MR, Barish MA. State-of-the-art computed tomographic and magnetic resonance imaging of the gastrointestinal system. Gastrointest Endosc Clin N Am. 2005; 15(3):581–614, x
[7] Fidler J. MR imaging of the small bowel. Radiol Clin North Am. 2007; 45 (2):317–331
[8] Gourtsoyanni S, Gourtsoyannis NC, Papanikolaou N. Small bowel. In: Gourtsoyiannis NC, eds. Clinical MRI of the Abdomen. Heidelberg: Springer; 2011
[9] Grenacher L, Hansmann J. [Radiological imaging of the upper gastrointestinal tract. Part II. The stomach]. Radiologe. 2007; 47(1):71–88
[10] Kim KW, Ha HK. MRI for small bowel diseases. Semin Ultrasound CT MR. 2003; 24(5):387–402
[11] Lauenstein TC. MR colonography In: Gourtsoyiannis NC, eds. Clinical MRI of the Abdomen. Heidelberg: Springer; 2011
[12] Lauenstein TC, Goyen M, Eds. Gastrointestinale MRT: Theorie und Praxis. Berlin: ABW Verlag; 2009
[13] Long BW. Colorectal cancer imaging. Radiol Technol. 2004; 75(3):215–229, quiz 230–232
[14] McSweeney SE, O'Donoghue PM, Jhaveri K. Current and emerging techniques in gastrointestinal imaging. J Postgrad Med. 2010; 56(2):109–116
[15] Maglinte DD. Small bowel imaging—a rapidly changing field and a challenge to radiology. Eur Radiol. 2006; 16(5):967–971
[16] Masselli G, Gualdi G. CT and MR enterography in evaluating small bowel diseases: when to use which modality? Abdom Imaging. 2013; 38 (2):249–259
[17] Nicolaou S, Kai B, Ho S, Su J, Ahamed K. Imaging of acute small-bowel obstruction. AJR Am J Roentgenol. 2005; 185(4):1036–1044
[18] Reimer P, Schima W, Lauenstein TC, et al. Abdomen: liver, spleen, biliary system, pancreas and GI tract. In: Reimer P, Parizel PM, Meaney JFM, Stichnoth FA, eds. Clinical MR Imaging. Heidelberg: Springer; 2010
[19] Rockey DC. Computed tomographic and magnetic resonance colonography: challenge for colonoscopy. Dig Dis. 2012; 30 Suppl 2:60–67
[20] Sailer J, Zacherl J, Schima W. MDCT of small bowel tumours. Cancer Imaging. 2007; 7:224–233
[21] Sandrasegaran K, Maglinte DD, Howard TJ, Kelvin FM, Lappas JC. The multifaceted role of radiology in small bowel obstruction. Semin Ultrasound CT MR. 2003; 24(5):319–335
[22] Sarma D, Longo WE, NDSG. Diagnostic imaging for diverticulitis. J Clin Gastroenterol. 2008; 42(10):1139–1141
[23] Schaefer O, Baumann T, Treier M, Langer M. Diagnostic imaging of inflammatory and tumorous diseases of the colon [in German]. Radiologe. 2006; 46 (8):703–719, quiz 720
[24] Schünke M, Schulte E, Schumacher U., eds. Prometheus. LernAtlas der Anatomie: Innere Organe. 2nd ed. Stuttgart: Thieme; 2009. Illustrated by M. Voll/K. Wesker
[25] Schreyer AG. New imaging methods for bowel imaging [in German]. Praxis (Bern 1994). 2006; 95(50):1975–1978
[26] Schreyer AG, Seitz J, Feuerbach S, Rogler G, Herfarth H. Modern imaging using computer tomography and magnetic resonance imaging for inflammatory bowel disease (IBD) AU1. Inflamm Bowel Dis. 2004; 10(1):45–54
[27] Sinha R, Murphy P, Hawker P, Sanders S, Rajesh A, Verma R. Role of MRI in Crohn's disease. Clin Radiol. 2009; 64(4):341–352
[28] Tennyson CA, Semrad CE. Advances in small bowel imaging. Curr Gastroenterol Rep. 2011; 13(5):408–417
[29] Virmani V, Khandelwal A, Sethi V, Fraser-Hill M, Fasih N, Kielar A. Neoplastic stomach lesions and their mimickers: spectrum of imaging manifestations. Cancer Imaging. 2012; 12:269–278

9 Spleen and Lymphatic System

Christoph Thomas

9.1 Introduction

The organs of the lymphatic system are the spleen, lymph nodes, thymus, and tonsils. Except where they are concentrated in these organs, the cells of the immune system are diffusely distributed throughout the body and are interconnected by blood vessels and lymphatic pathways.

9.2 Spleen

9.2.1 Anatomy

The spleen is an intraperitoneal organ located just below the diaphragm in the left upper quadrant of the abdomen. It is protected laterally by the ribs and it borders on the stomach, the left kidney, the left lobe of the liver, and the left colic flexure. The pancreatic tail often extends into the splenic hilum. The normal spleen measures 4 cm × 7 cm × 11 cm and weighs an average of 150 g (range of ca. 100–250 g). The spleen is held in place by two fibrous peritoneal attachments, the gastrosplenic ligament and splenorenal ligament. Because of these attachments, mechanical manipulations can lead to injury of the splenic capsule.[1]

The spleen derives its blood supply from the splenic artery, which arises from the celiac trunk and often runs a very tortuous course along the superior border of the pancreas to the splenic hilum. Before entering the spleen, the splenic artery usually divides into several branches that pierce the splenic capsule separately, accompanied by veins.[1]

Trabeculae emerge from the fibrous capsule and extend into the spleen, subdividing the splenic parenchyma and forming a framework that contains the red and white pulp. Arterial blood from the trabecular arteries, located within the trabeculae, flows through the white pulp, which contains lymphoid follicles, and is channeled from there to the red pulp, which is permeated by sinusoidal veins.[1] This unique architecture imparts a heterogeneous "tiger stripe" appearance to the splenic parenchyma on CT and MR images acquired in the arterial phase, when enhancement occurs predominantly in the white pulp (see ▶ Fig. 9.1, ▶ Fig. 9.2).[2] This pattern should not be mistaken for pathology. With images acquired in the venous phase, on the other hand, enhancement occurs predominantly in the red pulp, creating a homogeneous appearance on sectional images.

Consistent with its role in the immune system, some hematopoiesis (lymphocytes and plasma cells) takes place within the spleen. Another function of the spleen is the removal of old, damaged erythrocytes from the circulation.[1] It also functions as a reservoir for blood storage.

Note
The normal dimensions of the spleen are 4 cm × 7 cm × 11 cm.

Caution
Inhomogeneous enhancement of the spleen on arterial-phase images is normal.

9.2.2 Imaging
Radiography

Because of the lack of soft tissue contrast, conventional radiographs are not useful for evaluating the spleen.

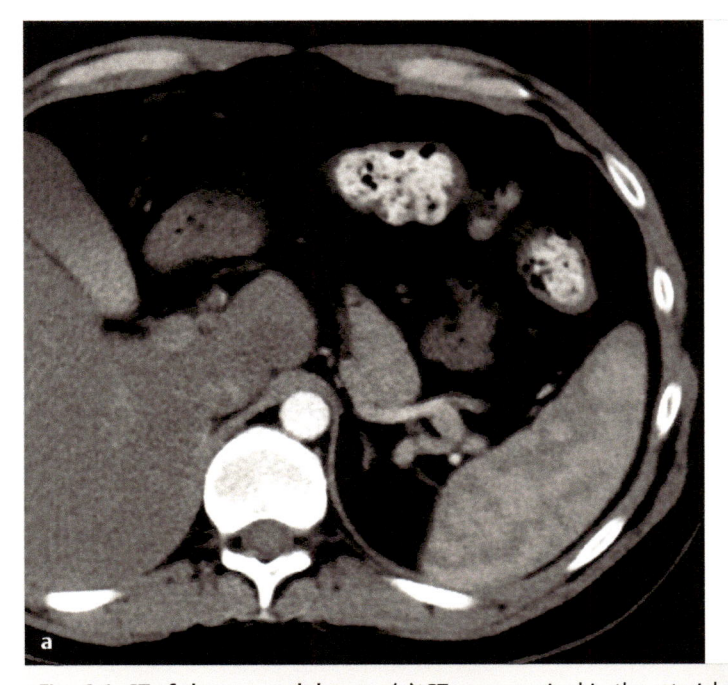

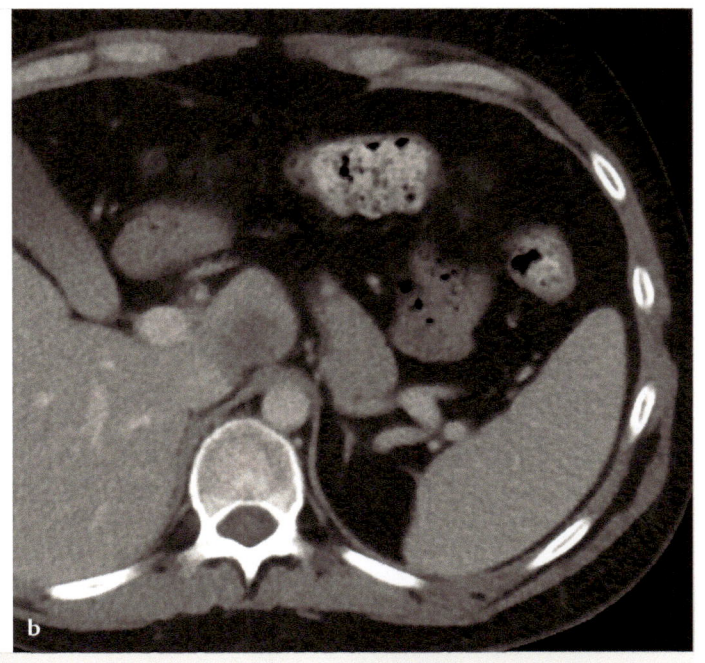

Fig. 9.1 CT of the upper abdomen. (a) CT scan acquired in the arterial phase of enhancement. The spleen has a typical inhomogeneous "tiger stripe" appearance. **(b)** CT scan in the venous phase of enhancement. The spleen has a homogeneous appearance.

Spleen and Lymphatic System

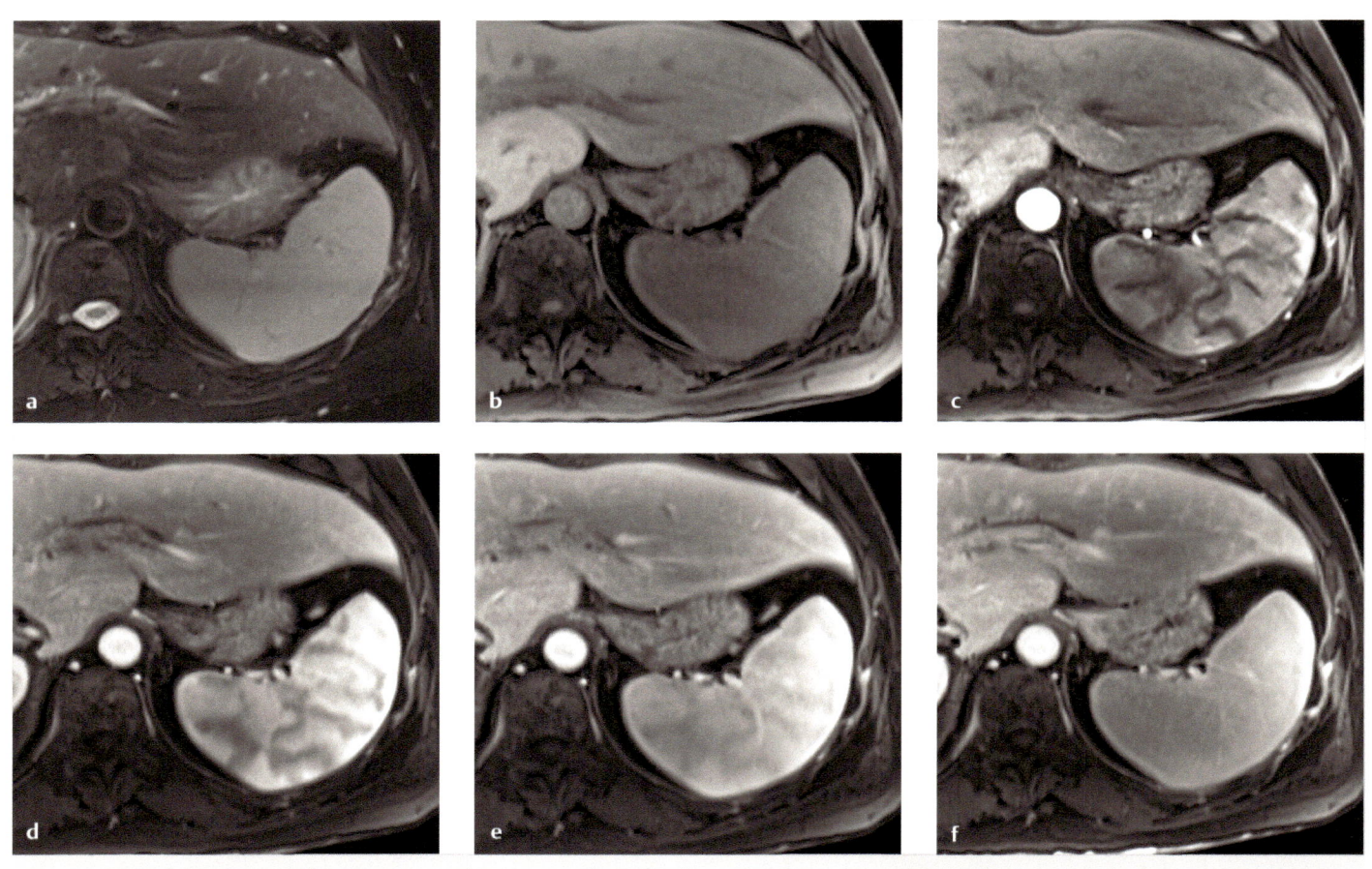

Fig. 9.2 MRI of the upper abdomen at 3.0 T. This patient is known to have partial portal vein thrombosis (not shown). This condition slows the blood flow through the spleen, delaying the enhancement dynamics of the splenic parenchyma. Standard T1 W and T2 W sequences are shown along with enhancement dynamics. Images in the dynamic series (**b–f**) were acquired at approximately 30-second intervals. (**a**) Fat-saturated T2 W TSE sequence. (**b**) Unenhanced T1 W 3D GRE sequence. (**c**) Early arterial T1 W 3D GRE sequence. (**d**) Late arterial T1 W 3D GRE sequence. (**e**) Early venous T1 W 3D GRE sequence. (**f**) Late venous T1 W 3D GRE sequence.

Ultrasound

Ultrasound is considered the standard modality for initial imaging evaluation of the spleen (▶ Fig. 9.3). It can be used to determine the size and shape of the spleen, evaluate parenchymal lesions, and exclude injuries.[3]

The spleen should be scanned with a low-frequency probe (e.g., 3.5 MHz) with the patient in the supine position. Because splenic ultrasound requires an intercostal approach, it may be helpful to have the patient elevate the arm to spread the ribs apart. Due to the subphrenic location of the spleen and the presence of air in the costodiaphragmatic recess, it is often difficult to define all portions of the spleen with ultrasound. The acoustic window can be optimized by scanning at end expiration or during slow expiration.[3]

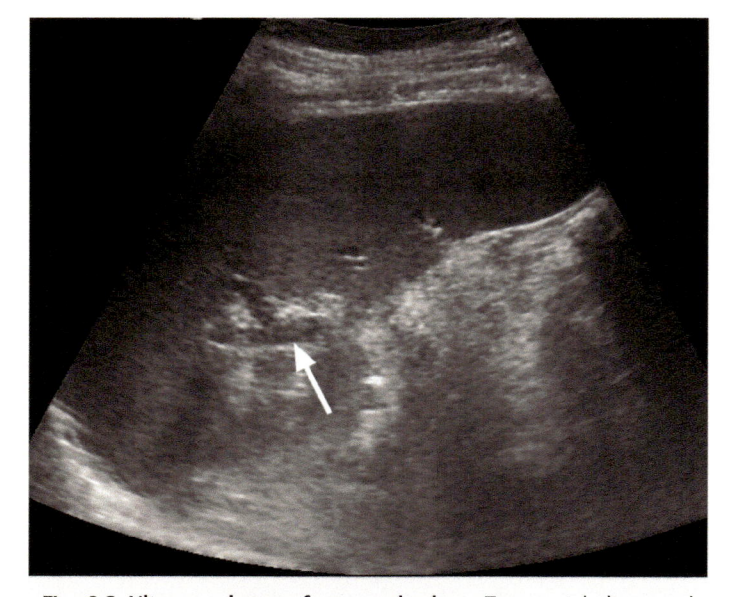

Fig. 9.3 Ultrasound scan of a normal spleen. Transcostal ultrasound scan in a 39-year-old man displays the spleen in its greatest longitudinal dimension. The scan also depicts the splenic vein in the splenic hilum (arrow). The spleen in this patient measures approximately 13 cm, but this is not considered abnormal given the otherwise normal configuration of the organ (homogeneous parenchyma, tapered borders).

Computed Tomography

CT usually permits a more precise evaluation of the spleen than ultrasound owing to its high spatial resolution and because it is independent of acoustic windows and the experience of the examiner.

Because of its vascular architecture, the spleen shows a very inhomogeneous enhancement pattern (▶ Fig. 9.1) when imaged in the arterial phase approximately 30 seconds after IV bolus injection. A normal spleen will then show homogeneous enhancement

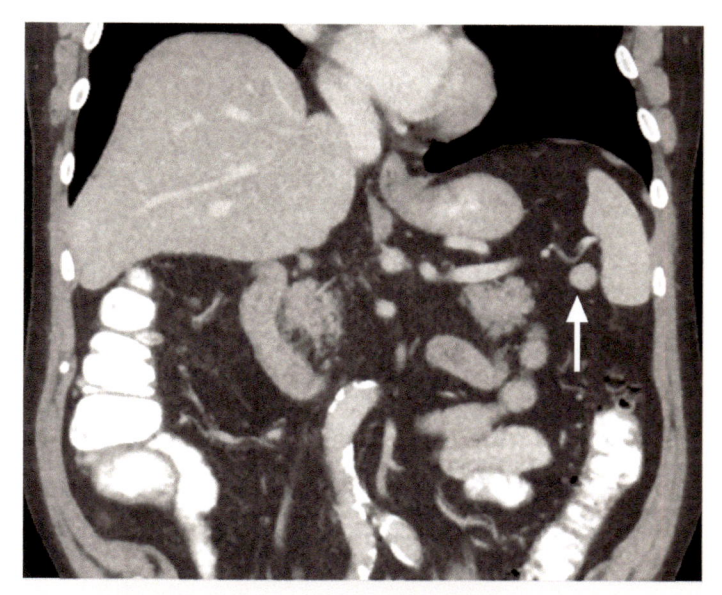

Fig. 9.4 Accessory spleen. Contrast-enhanced CT of the abdomen in a 68-year-old man (coronal reformatted image). An accessory spleen (arrow) is noted in the splenic hilum as an incidental finding.

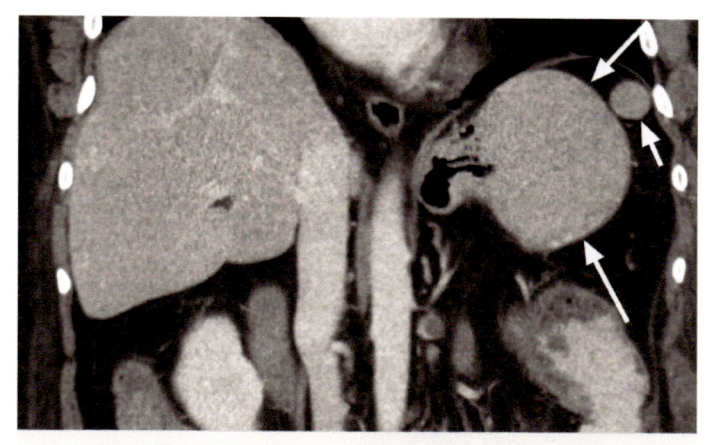

Fig. 9.5 Splenosis in a 53-year-old man who had a splenectomy in his youth because of abdominal trauma. The current CT examination was for staging of rectal carcinoma. Besides the opacified stomach (long arrows), the image shows a rounded mass in the left upper quadrant (short arrow) consistent with a focus of splenosis.

when imaged in the portal venous phase approximately 60 to 90 seconds after bolus injection.

Magnetic Resonance Imaging

MRI is useful for the further characterization of focal lesions detected in the spleen, for example by differentiating metastases and hemangiomas. The iron content of the spleen can also be evaluated with MRI, which is useful in the quantification of hemochromatosis.

The full range of sequences ordinarily used for upper abdominal imaging can also be used for the spleen:
- T1 W and fat-saturated T2 W sequences to bring out anatomical details.
- Diffusion-weighted imaging (DWI) sequences and enhancement dynamics for identification and characterization of lesions (▶ Fig. 9.2), e.g., for differentiating metastases, hemangiomas, and cysts.
- T2*W GRE sequences and double-echo sequences to evaluate splenic iron content.
- Magnetic resonance angiography (MRA) techniques to evaluate the vessels supplying and draining the spleen.

9.2.3 Anomalies and Normal Variants

Accessory Spleen

▶ **Brief definition.** Approximately 30% of individuals have one or more small accessory spleens (up to approximately 4 cm in diameter) in addition to the main spleen. Accessory spleens are usually located close to the spleen, e.g., in the gastrosplenic ligament, splenic hilum, or greater omentum (▶ Fig. 9.4).[4] An accessory spleen consists of ectopic splenic tissue that has developed apart from the main spleen.

▶ **Imaging signs.** Accessory spleens have the same density or intensity as the main spleen in sectional imaging studies.

▶ **Clinical features.** Accessory spleens are not pathologic in the true sense. The majority are asymptomatic, although a few may become symptomatic due to torsion and rupture.

▶ **Differential diagnosis**
- Splenosis (implantation of ectopic splenic tissue in the peritoneal cavity after abdominal trauma or surgery; ▶ Fig. 9.5).[5]
- Tumors (e.g., pancreatic, adrenal, renal, or gastric).
- Metastases (especially peritoneal deposits).
- Polysplenia.

▶ **Pitfalls.** An accessory spleen may be misinterpreted as a malignant mass.

Note

An accessory spleen should be considered whenever an intraparietal mass is discovered close to the spleen.

Asplenia and Polysplenia

▶ **Brief definition.** Very rarely, and usually in association with other congenital anomalies (fetal heterotaxy syndrome), the spleen may be congenitally absent (asplenia in right isomerism) or may consist of multiple unfused spleens (polysplenia in left isomerism).[6,7] Some authors also define splenectomy as a form of asplenia.

▶ **Imaging signs**
- *Asplenia syndrome (right isomerism)*: bilateral right-sidedness. Asplenia may be accompanied by a number of other anomalies such as severe, usually cyanotic cardiac anomalies, bilateral trilobed lungs, esophageal varices, gastric hypoplasia or duplication, annular pancreas, Hirschsprung's disease, anal atresia, ectopic liver and gallbladder, and urogenital tract anomalies. Approximately 80% of affected children die before 1 year of age.
- *Polysplenia syndrome (left isomerism)*: Besides multiple small spleens, patients often have severe cardiac anomalies, bilateral bilobed lungs, esophageal or duodenal atresia,

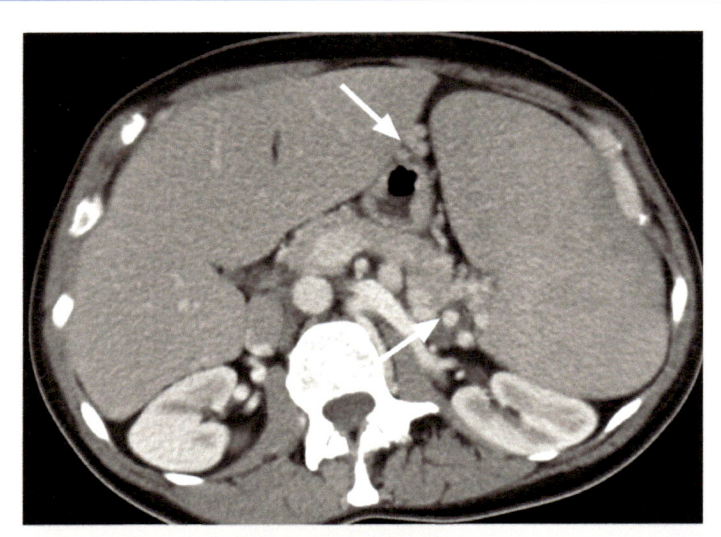

Fig. 9.6 Splenomegaly. CT of the upper abdomen in a 54-year-old man with hepatosplenomegaly in a setting of osteomyelofibrosis. The spleen has a slightly inhomogeneous, nodular appearance with rounded surface contours. Collaterals have developed in the splenic hilum and perigastric region (arrows) in response to portal hypertension. The displacement and deformation of the left kidney underscores the chronic nature of the disease.

tracheoesophageal fistulas, pancreatic anomalies, duplicated stomach, and short bowel syndrome or malrotation. There is frequent intrahepatic interruption of the inferior vena cava with azygos continuation. With an approximately 50% mortality rate before age 1 year, polysplenia syndrome has a somewhat better prognosis than asplenia syndrome, but only 10% of affected children survive to adolescence.

▶ **Clinical features.** Polysplenia and asplenia in the setting of heterotaxy syndromes are associated with cardiopulmonary, gastrointestinal, and hepatic anomalies.

▶ **Differential diagnosis.** If there are no additional anomalies, a diagnosis of polysplenia or asplenia is unlikely. Polysplenia requires differentiation from splenosis and multiple accessory spleens. Prior splenectomy should be included in the differential diagnosis of asplenia.

▶ **Pitfalls.** There is a risk of confusing splenosis or accessory spleens with polysplenia.

9.2.4 Diseases

Differential Diagnosis of Splenomegaly

▶ **Brief definition.** Splenomegaly refers to abnormal enlargement of the spleen.

▶ **Imaging signs.** As noted earlier, the normal dimensions of the spleen are 4 cm × 7 cm × 11 cm. Nevertheless, significant variations of physiologic splenic size may be encountered in practice. Even spleens with a greatest dimension of 12 or 13 cm may still be considered normal, depending on the patient's constitution. Splenomegaly is diagnosed when the volume of the spleen is 500 cm³ or more.[5] As well as sheer size, it is also important to evaluate the morphology of the spleen. The poles of a normal

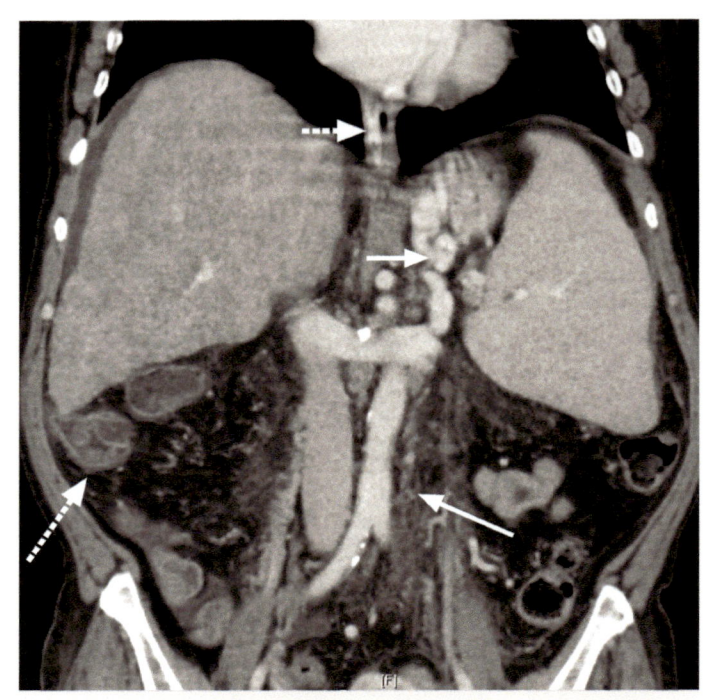

Fig. 9.7 Alcoholic cirrhosis of the liver. Abdominal CT in a 53-year-old man. Coronal reformatted image with venous contrast enhancement shows numerous signs of portal hypertension: splenomegaly, varicose anastomoses about the splenic hilum (short arrow), esophageal varices (short dashed arrow), thickening of the cecal wall due to congestive enteropathy (long dashed arrow), increased density of the mesenteric root due to fluid permeation (long arrow), and some perihepatic ascites.

spleen are sharply tapered, whereas they are rounded and blunted in splenomegaly (▶ Fig. 9.6).

▶ **Clinical features.** Splenomegaly in itself is usually asymptomatic. Very large spleens may exert a mass effect on adjacent structures. Otherwise the clinical findings depend on the cause of the splenomegaly.

▶ **Differential diagnosis.** Splenomegaly may have a variety of causes. It is helpful to divide the potential causes into five etiologic categories[5,8]:
- *Congestion*: congestion may be due, for example, to portal vein or splenic vein thrombosis, hepatic cirrhosis, diffuse high-grade tumor invasion of the liver, hepatic vein thrombosis (Budd–Chiari syndrome), or right heart failure. Imaging in these cases shows portocaval anastomoses as evidence of portal hypertension (dilatation of the splenic and portal veins, esophageal and fundic varices, recanalized umbilical vein with a caput medusae, splenorenal shunts, shunting via the hepatic and splenic capsule, and so on; ▶ Fig. 9.7, ▶ Fig. 9.8).
- *Hematologic*: possible causes of splenomegaly in this category are leukemias, hemoglobinopathies, polycythemia vera, and osteomyelofibrosis. The underlying cause is a redistribution of hematopoietic bone marrow from the medullary cavities to the spleen.
- *Inflammatory or infectious*: viral infections such as mononucleosis, HIV, and tuberculosis as well as granulomatous diseases such as sarcoidosis and rheumatoid disorders may be associated with splenomegaly. Viral infections may incite a general immune

9.2 Spleen

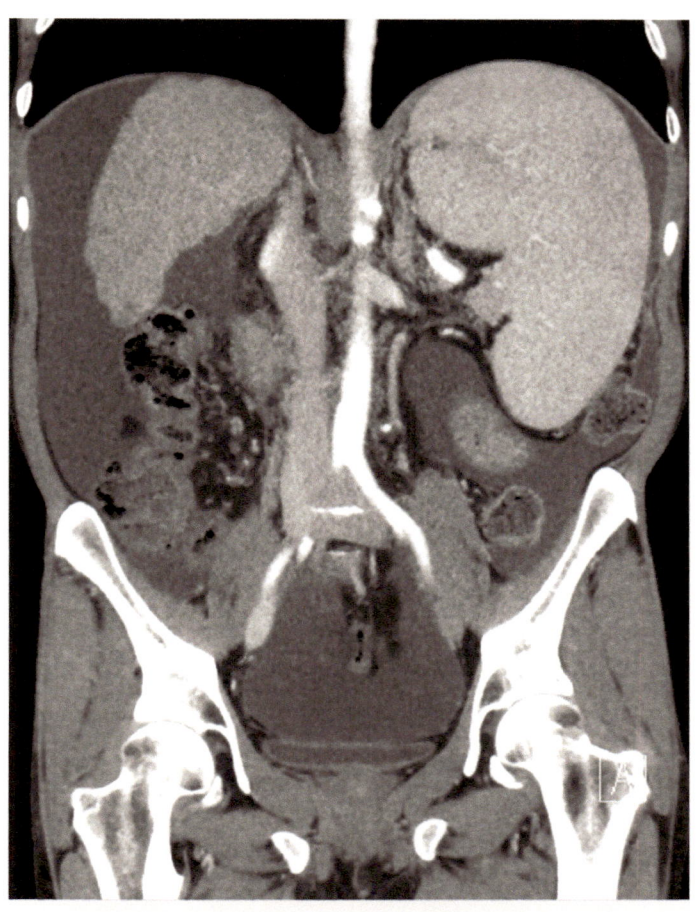

Fig. 9.8 Alcoholic cirrhosis of the liver. Abdominal CT in a 43-year-old man. Coronal reformatted image with venous contrast enhancement shows a nodular liver surface, splenomegaly, and ascites.

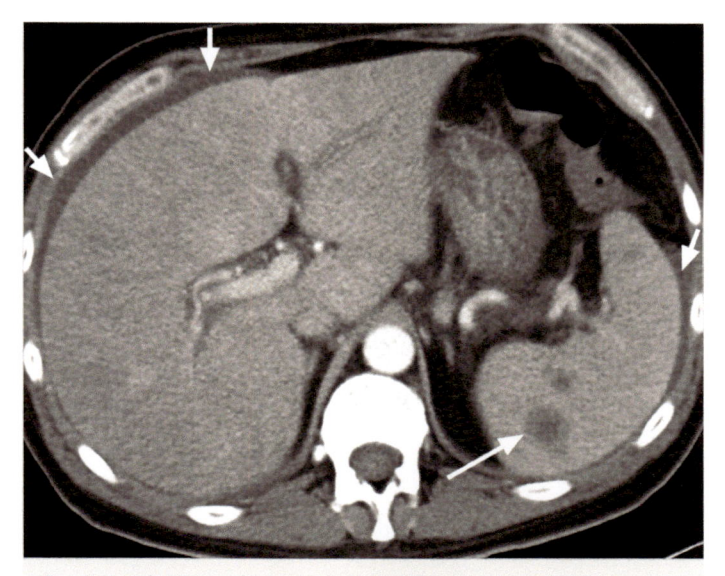

Fig. 9.9 Splenic involvement by lymphoma in a 41-year-old man who underwent allogeneic bone marrow transplantation for acute myeloid leukemia and Epstein–Barr virus–associated lymphoproliferative disease. Abdominal CT in the venous phase shows hypodense splenic lesions with faint margins (long arrow) and heterogeneous enhancement of the liver with periportal edema, consistent with lymphomatous involvement. There is also ascites (short arrows).

- *Masses*: splenomegaly due to lymphoma, metastases, or cysts. Malignant infiltration of the spleen may be a unifocal, multifocal, or diffuse process (see ▶ Fig. 9.9, ▶ Fig. 9.10, ▶ Fig. 9.11). Cysts are a rare cause of splenomegaly.
- *Deposition disorders*: hemochromatosis, amyloidosis, and other storage diseases can lead to splenomegaly.

▶ **Pitfalls.** A slightly enlarged spleen with a normal shape may be mistaken for splenomegaly.

▶ **Key points.** Splenomegaly may have hemodynamic, hematologic, infectious/immunologic, oncologic, or deposition-related causes.

Note

Look for signs of portal hypertension when splenomegaly is present.

Splenic Infarction

▶ **Brief definition.** Splenic infarction results from the segmental (frequent) or global (rare) infarction of arterial vessels in the splenic parenchyma. Possible causes are emboli (atrial fibrillation, atherosclerosis, foreign bodies, septic embolism), hematologic disorders with increased cellularity or coagulability, and specific changes that can cause splenomegaly.[9]

▶ **Imaging signs.** Splenic infarcts usually appear as peripheral wedge-shaped areas on sectional images (▶ Fig. 9.12). They are hypodense on contrast-enhanced CT and are frequently isoechoic on ultrasound. Acute infarcts on MRI are hyperintense in T2W sequences due to the presence of hemorrhage and edema. Chronic infarcts are usually hypointense. Over time there may be

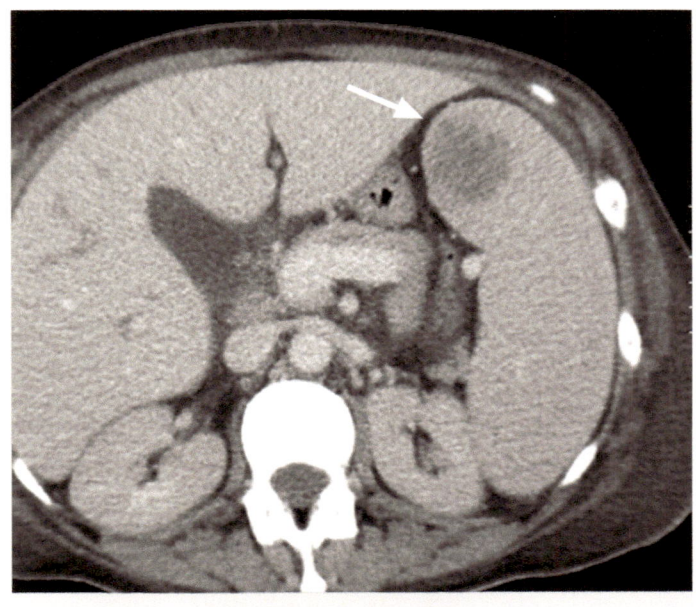

Fig. 9.10 Splenic involvement by lymphoma in a 67-year-old woman with non-Hodgkin's lymphoma. Axial CT of the upper abdomen demonstrates focal splenic involvement (arrow).

activation, causing a relatively homogeneous splenomegaly, whereas granulomatous diseases often cause a nodular infiltration of the spleen with possible associated calcifications. Splenomegaly may be a permanent condition after certain viral diseases (typically Epstein–Barr virus).

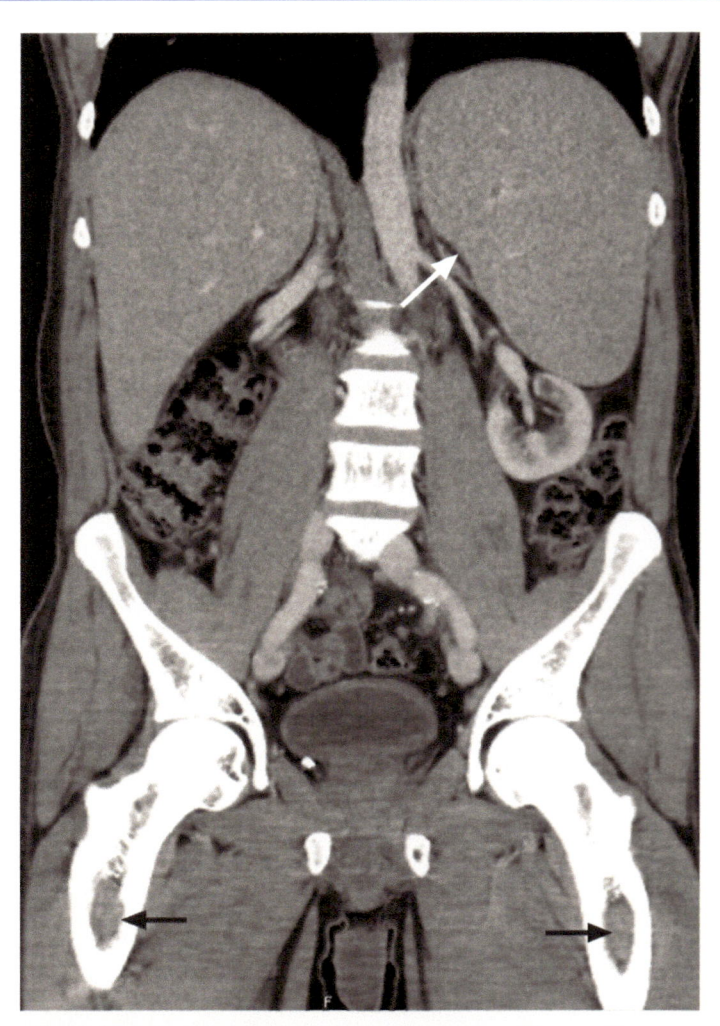

Fig. 9.11 Splenic involvement by lymphoma in a 57-year-old man with marginal zone lymphoma. Coronal reformatted abdominal CT image with venous contrast enhancement shows diffuse infiltration of the spleen with splenomegaly (white arrow) accompanied by homogeneous bone marrow infiltration in both femurs (black arrows).

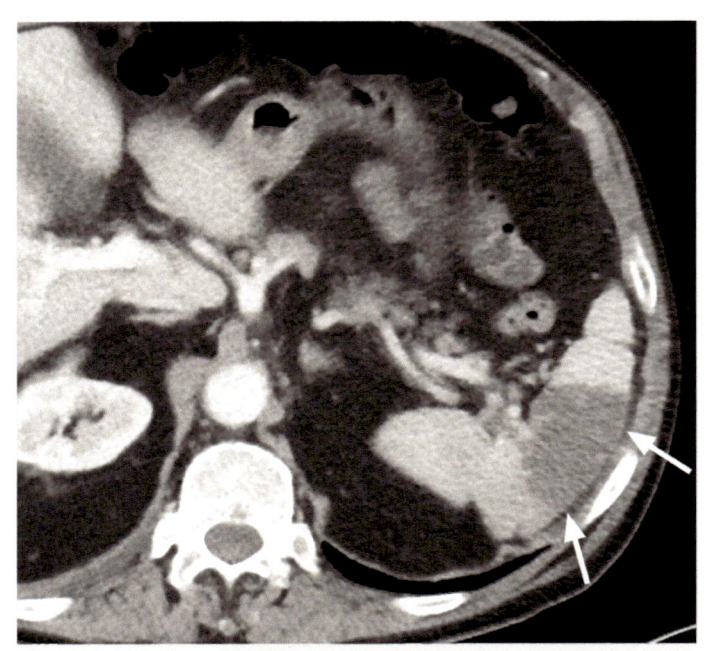

Fig. 9.12 Splenic infarction in a 63-year-old man with left upper quadrant pain. Abdominal CT with venous contrast enhancement shows a hypodense, wedge-shaped perfusion defect in the spleen (arrows) with no parenchymal scarring or constriction. This finding is most consistent with an acute splenic infarction.

a regression of affected regions with capsular constriction, and cysts may also form (see ► Fig. 9.13).

▶ **Clinical features.** Acute splenic infarction may be manifested by upper abdominal pain. There may also be periembolic symptoms such as fever and chills.[10] These symptoms are self-limiting and should last no longer than one week. As a rule, there is no need for treatment. Splenectomy may be considered if symptoms are severe.

▶ **Differential diagnosis.** The differential diagnosis of splenic infarction should include abscesses, masses, cysts, and splenic injury.

▶ **Pitfalls.** A splenic infarct may be mistaken for a laceration of the spleen.

▶ **Key points.** Splenic infarcts typically appear as peripheral, wedge-shaped parenchymal lesions.

> **Note**
>
> A possible embolic source should be investigated in all cases of suspected splenic infarction.

Splenic Cysts

▶ **Brief definition.** An etiologic distinction is made between (true) dysontogenetic cysts and secondary (acquired) cysts. Dysontogenetic cysts result from an error of mesothelial migration and have an endothelial cyst wall.[5] They comprise approximately 10 to 25% of all splenic cysts.[11] Acquired cysts, on the other hand, usually develop from infarcts or colliquative hematomas and have a fibrous wall. Dysontogenetic and acquired cysts are not distinguishable by imaging, and such a distinction would have no clinical implications in most patients.

▶ **Imaging signs.** Cysts typically have a thin wall and smooth margins. Ultrasound shows an echo-free mass with posterior acoustic enhancement. CT shows well-circumscribed hypodense lesions that do not enhance after IV injection of contrast medium (► Fig. 9.14). Hemorrhagic cysts may show uniform high attenuation on CT (► Fig. 9.15). Mural calcification is occasionally noted in splenic cysts (► Fig. 9.13).

▶ **Clinical features.** Splenic cysts are usually asymptomatic. Large cysts may exert capsular tension that causes upper abdominal pain. Over time, splenic cysts may undergo intracystic hemorrhage, rupture, or infection. Symptomatic cysts are treated surgically.

▶ **Differential diagnosis**
- Abscesses and echinococcal cysts (usually thick-walled).
- Metastases (usually show enhancement).
- Infiltration by lymphoma (usually shows enhancement, indistinct margins).
- Intrasplenic pseudocysts (arising from the pancreatic tail; associated signs of pancreatitis).

▶ **Key points.** Splenic lesions with smooth margins and fluid attenuation are usually cysts.

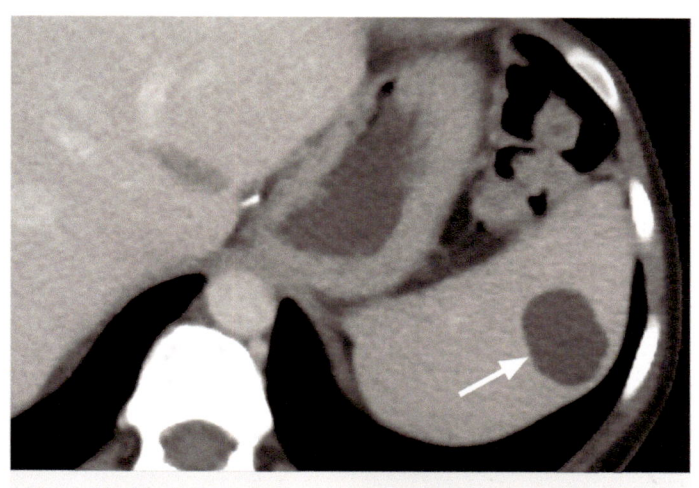

Fig. 9.14 **Splenic cyst** discovered during melanoma staging in a 35-year-old woman. Abdominal CT with venous contrast enhancement shows a well-circumscribed, homogeneous lesion of the spleen (arrow) with no peripheral rim enhancement and fluid-equivalent attenuation values (comparable to gastric contents), most consistent with a dysontogenetic cyst.

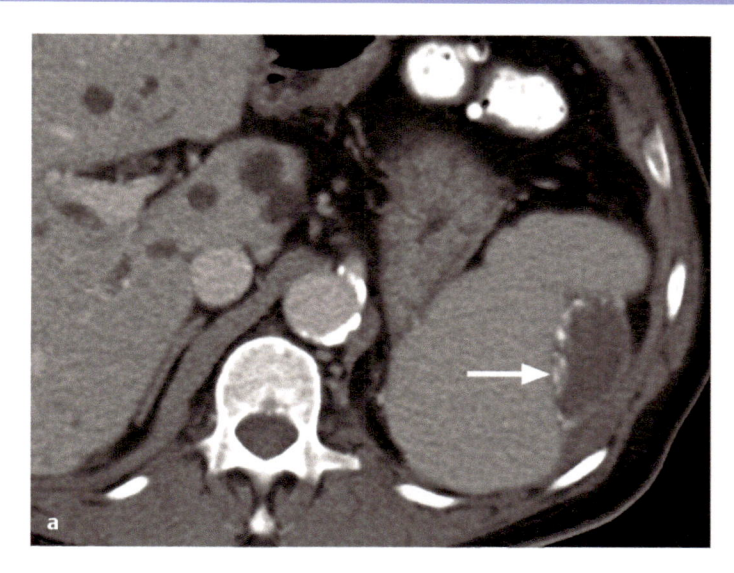

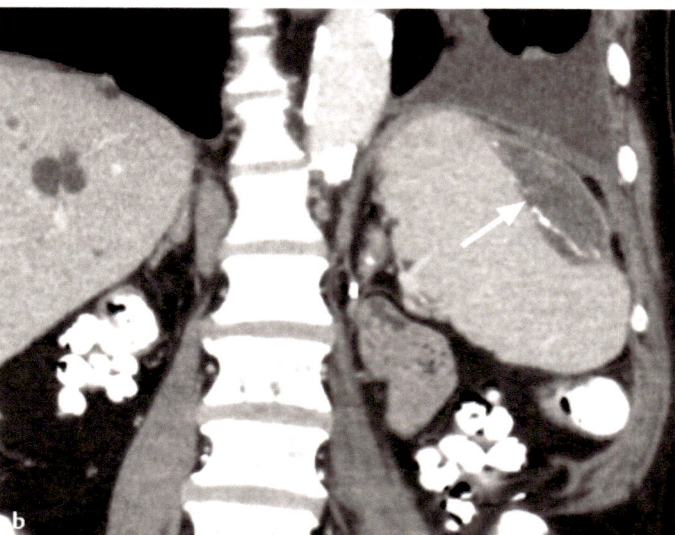

Fig. 9.13 **Calcified splenic cyst** in a 67-year-old man. Abdominal CT incidentally detects a splenic defect with a rim-calcified cystic lesion (arrows), most likely secondary to a partial infarction of the spleen that occurred years earlier. The differential diagnosis would also include previous splenic trauma. Multiple hepatic lesions and a left pleural effusion are also noted as incidental findings. (a) Axial CT scan. (b) Coronal reformatted image with venous contrast.

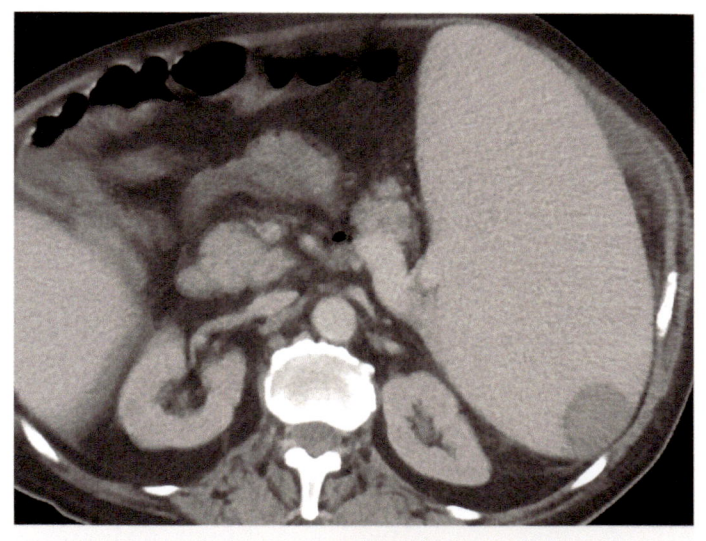

Fig. 9.15 **Hemorrhagic splenic cyst** in a 66-year-old woman with chronic myeloid leukemia and acute thrombocytopenia resulting in poor coagulation status. The patient suffered a cerebral hemorrhage several days before the examination. Whole-body CT shows splenomegaly and a hyperattenuating splenic cyst with intracystic hemorrhage, most likely due to the patient's hemorrhagic diathesis.

Splenic Abscess

▶ **Brief definition.** A splenic abscess is a localized collection of pus within the splenic capsule. Formation of abscesses in the spleen is most commonly due to hematogenous spread from a primary focus such as infectious endocarditis. Another potential cause is superinfection of cysts, infarcts, or hematomas. The main causative organisms are bacteria, fungi, and parasites (echinococci).

▶ **Imaging signs.** Splenic abscesses appear as rounded lesions with indistinct margins and peripheral enhancement. Abscesses are hypoechoic on ultrasound with ill-defined margins and internal echoes. The lesions are hypodense on CT with non-water-equivalent attenuation values. Often they have an intensely enhancing rim that has undergone inflammatory changes (▶ Fig. 9.16, ▶ Fig. 9.17). Echinococcal cysts in particular, as well as bacterial abscesses, appear as loculated lesions with internal septa and possible fine mural calcifications. The septa are usually well defined by ultrasound but often are not visualized on CT. Gas inclusions (from anaerobes) are occasionally detectable within abscesses.

▶ **Clinical features.** The dominant clinical findings are those of the underlying infectious disease. Patients are often septic and seriously ill.

▶ **Differential diagnosis**
- Splenic infarction.
- Tumor, metastasis, or lymphoma.
- Splenic injury.

Spleen and Lymphatic System

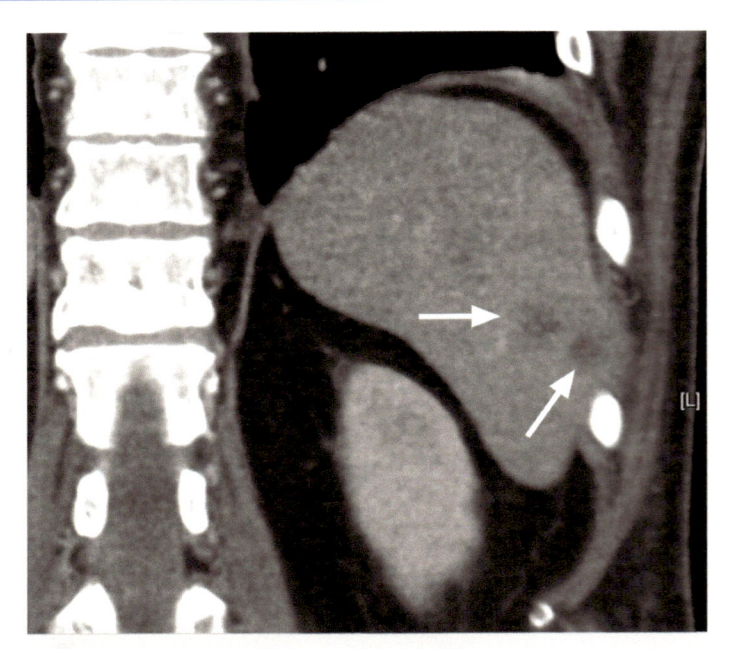

Fig. 9.16 Splenic abscesses in an immunosuppressed 61-year-old man (status post bone marrow transplantation for acute myeloid leukemia). Coronal reformatted image from abdominal CT with venous contrast, performed for localization of an infectious focus, shows multiple faint hypodensities in the spleen surrounded by areas of slightly increased enhancement (arrows), consistent with abscesses.

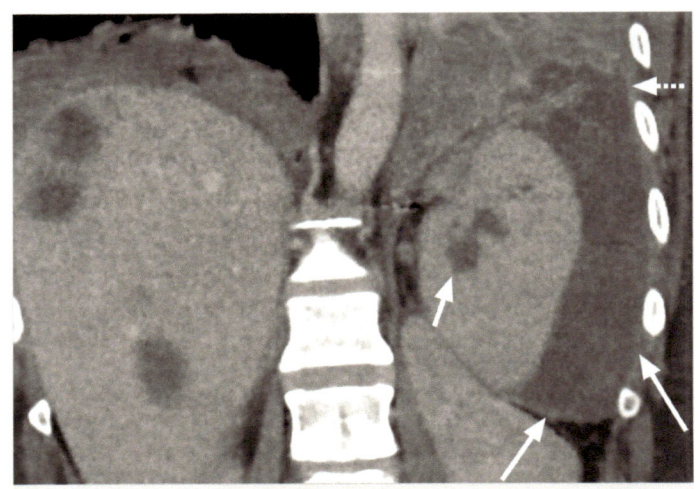

Fig. 9.17 Splenic abscess in a seriously ill, immunosuppressed 52-year-old woman. Coronal reformatted image from abdominal CT with venous contrast enhancement shows hypodense lesions with indistinct margins in the liver and spleen, consistent with multiple abscesses (short arrow). The abscess has broken through the splenic capsule, resulting in an extensive purulent collection around the spleen (long arrows). Pus has penetrated the diaphragm (dashed arrow) with associated pleural empyema.

An abscess is often indistinguishable from a malignant process on the basis of morphological imaging features alone. The differential diagnosis should be considered within the clinical context, and serial examination may be necessary to rule out alternative diagnoses.

▶ **Pitfalls.** There is potential for confusion with infarction, lymphoma, or metastasis.

▶ **Key points.** Splenic abscesses produce heterogeneous findings. Clinical findings should always be included in the evaluation.

> **Note**
>
> Abscesses are difficult to distinguish from lymphomas, infarcts, and metastases on the basis of imaging findings alone.

Neoplastic Diseases

Primary Splenic Tumors and Lymphoma

▶ **Brief definition.** Benign neoplasms are to be distinguished from malignancies. The most common benign splenic tumor is hemangioma, followed by lymphangioma and hamartoma. The most common malignant tumor of the spleen is lymphoma. Other possible tumor entities are angiosarcoma, leiomyosarcoma, fibrosarcoma, and epithelioid tumors.

▶ **Imaging signs.** Imaging alone cannot provide a specific diagnosis in most cases. Nevertheless, different entities do exhibit characteristic patterns on imaging:
- *Hemangioma*: Hemangiomas are well-circumscribed lesions that typically show uniform high echogenicity at ultrasound. CT often shows an "iris diaphragm" sign marked by intense, inhomogeneous enhancement in the arterial phase and a gradual progression to isointensity with surrounding tissue in later phases, typically proceeding in a centripetal pattern (▶ Fig. 9.18).
- *Lymphangioma*: Lymphangiomas have a cystic appearance and are often multiple.
- *Hamartoma*: Splenic hamartomas show nonspecific features and often appear as large, inhomogeneously enhancing lesions. Calcifications and fat may be present within the lesion.
- *Lymphoma*: Splenic lymphoma is a very heterogeneous lesion that shows diffuse and focal patterns of infiltration (▶ Fig. 9.9, ▶ Fig. 9.10, ▶ Fig. 9.11).
- *Angiosarcoma*: Angiosarcomas have irregular margins and are frequently nodular. There may be intralesional hemorrhage and calcifications.

▶ **Clinical features.** Neoplasms of the spleen do not have a typical clinical presentation.

▶ **Differential diagnosis.** Differentiation is required from metastases, hematomas, abscesses, infarcts, cysts, and granulomatous diseases (e.g., sarcoidosis, tuberculosis).

▶ **Pitfalls.** Making a premature diagnosis of a particular entity is a common error. The range of differential diagnoses should be known and carefully considered.

▶ **Key points.** Primary splenic tumors and lymphomas comprise a very heterogeneous group of diseases. In the majority of cases, imaging alone cannot differentiate them from one another with an acceptable degree of confidence.

Splenic Metastases

▶ **Brief definition.** Metastasis to the spleen is relatively rare compared with other sites and is most common with melanoma

9.2 Spleen

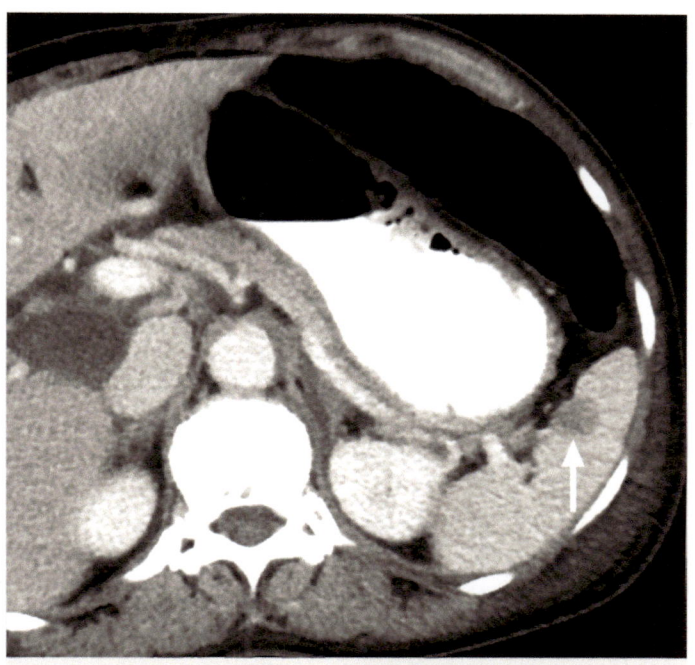

Fig. 9.19 Splenic metastasis in a 67-year-old woman with metastatic ovarian carcinoma. Staging CT of the abdomen in the venous phase shows a relatively sharply circumscribed, enhancing mass in the spleen (arrow) that is most likely a metastasis. Since the lesion is based on the capsule, peritoneal implantation would also be a possibility.

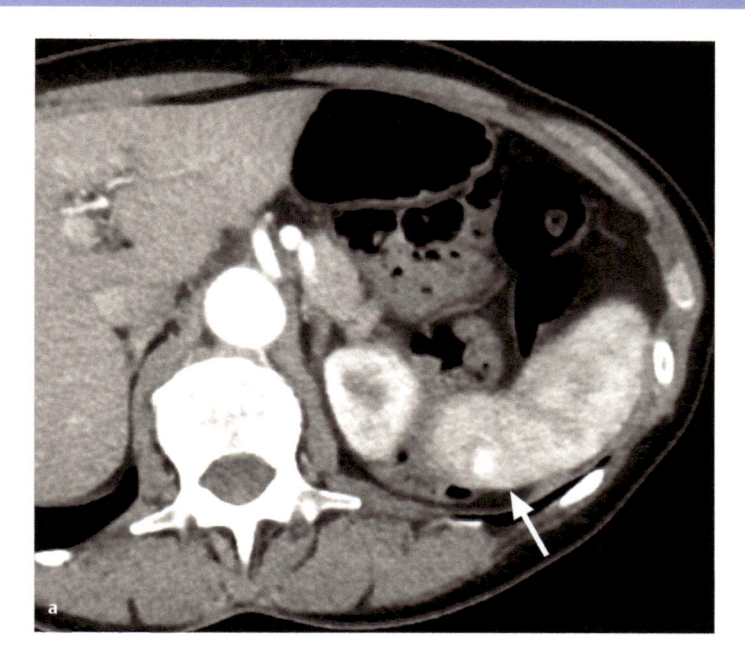

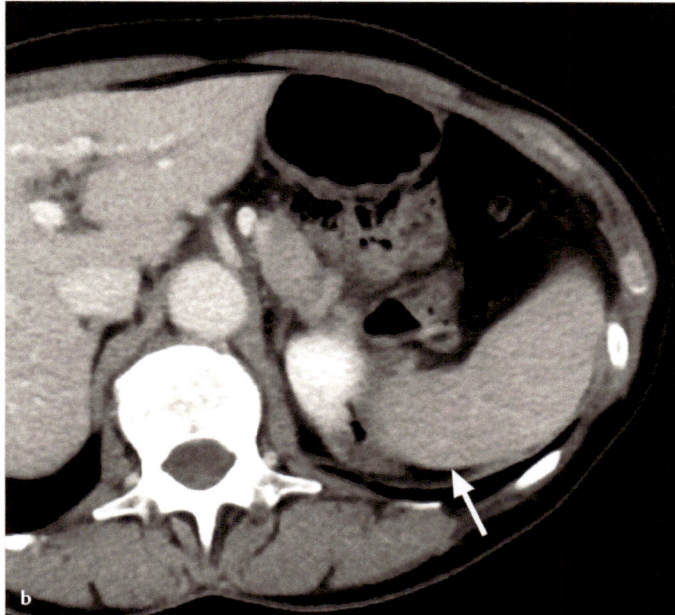

Fig. 9.18 Splenic hemangioma. Staging CT in a 71-year-old woman with breast cancer. **(a)** CT scan of the upper abdomen with arterial contrast enhancement shows a hyperdense splenic mass (arrow). **(b)** Scan with venous contrast enhancement. The splenic mass was no longer visualized and showed no further changes over time. These findings are most consistent with hemangioma. The differential diagnosis would include an arteriovenous shunt.

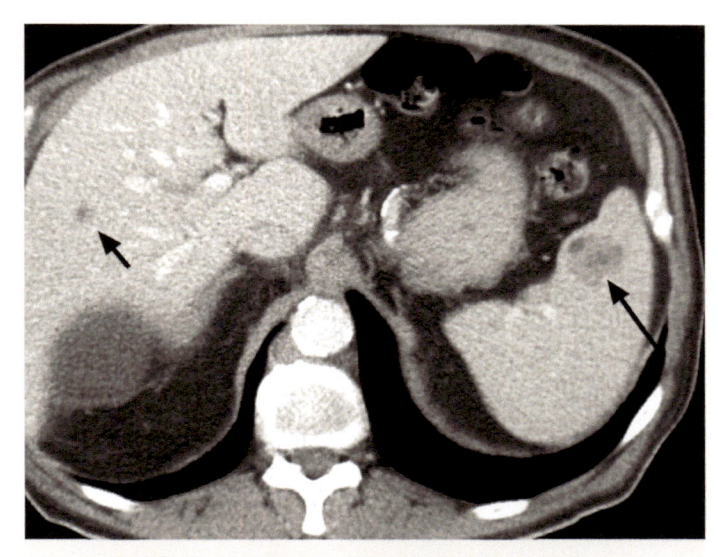

Fig. 9.20 Splenic metastasis in a 65-year-old man with known malignant melanoma. Axial CT of the abdomen with venous contrast (for tumor staging) shows an inhomogeneously enhancing splenic mass (long arrow) that is most likely a metastasis. Additional lesions are noted in the liver (short arrow).

and lung cancer. Generally the route of metastasis is hematogenous; peritoneal seeding may also occur.

▶ **Imaging signs.** Metastases do not display uniform imaging features. They may be solitary or multiple, typically showing indistinct margins and low echogenicity on ultrasound scans. On CT the lesions usually have a hypodense center with indistinct margins and enhance after IV injection of contrast medium (▶ Fig. 9.19, ▶ Fig. 9.20).

▶ **Clinical features.** Most patients are clinically asymptomatic. Infarction or capsular invasion may be associated with upper abdominal pain.

▶ **Differential diagnosis.** The differential diagnosis includes all benign and malignant splenic tumors, involvement by lymphoma, abscesses, and granulomatous diseases.

▶ **Pitfalls.** The "tiger stripe" appearance of the spleen in the arterial phase can mimic pathology.

▶ **Key points.** Splenic metastases are rare. Clinical correlation and differential diagnoses should be considered in their evaluation.

Splenic Rupture

▶ **Brief definition.** Splenic rupture (synonyms: splenic laceration or fracture, subcapsular splenic hematoma) denotes a parenchymal injury to the spleen that may or may not be associated with capsular injury.

▶ **Imaging signs.** CT is the most sensitive modality for evaluating splenic injury and is routinely indicated in patients with blunt abdominal trauma.[12] It is definitely superior to ultrasound in this regard, especially in emergency settings where examination conditions are often unfavorable. Both CT and ultrasound can detect hypodense hematomas in the splenic parenchyma. Capsular injury appears as a discontinuity in the splenic capsule. Active extrasplenic or intrasplenic hemorrhage appears on CT as hypodense contrast extravasation ("contrast plume") or pseudoaneurysms within the parenchyma. Additionally, CT will usually show hematomas of variable size around the spleen in the form of hemoperitoneum or even copious free intra-abdominal fluid (▶ Fig. 9.21). Increased CT attenuation values in the fluid (> 30 HU) indicate the presence of blood constituents, analogous to the increased echogenicity of the fluid that is seen at ultrasound. Contrast-enhanced ultrasound has also been used increasingly in recent years for the detection of splenic injuries.[13] Various classification schemes have been devised for splenic injuries. Ultimately, however, these classifications are of limited value as they do not have therapeutic implications.

▶ **Clinical features.** The spleen is the most frequently injured abdominal organ that requires surgery. Splenic injuries typically result from blunt abdominal and thoracic trauma. The main clinical findings are upper abdominal pain and possible hypotension. Delayed splenic rupture is a feared condition in which an initial splenic hematoma is followed within days by rupture of the splenic capsule. Nevertheless, given the problems associated with postsplenectomy syndrome, conservative therapy is preferred over splenectomy whenever possible, especially in children.[7]

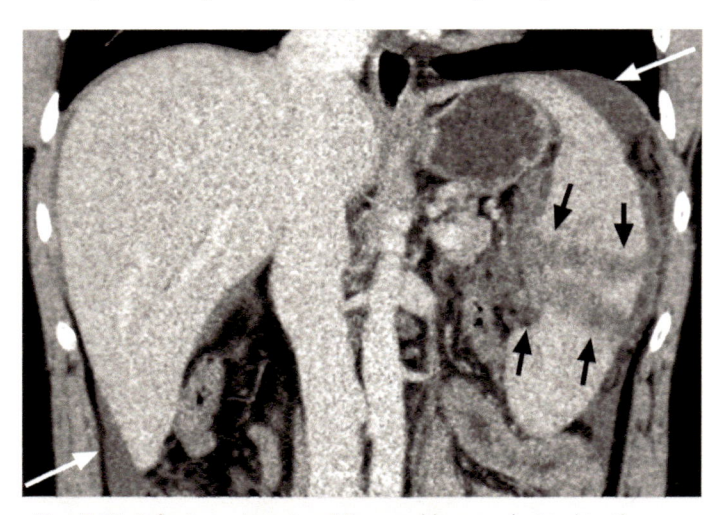

Fig. 9.21 Splenic rupture in a 28-year-old man admitted to the emergency room with blunt abdominal trauma (from motor vehicle accident). Coronal reformatted CT image in the venous phase of enhancement shows extensive parenchymal lesions of the spleen extending into the hilar region (short arrows). The image also shows hyperdense free fluid around the liver and spleen, consistent with hemoperitoneum (long arrows).

Active bleeding sites can be embolized using interventional endovascular technique.[14,15]

▶ **Differential diagnosis**
- Splenic abscess.
- Splenic infarction (wedge-shaped hypodensity).
- Lymphoma and other tumors.
- Physiologic notching of the splenic capsule by the diaphragm crus.

▶ **Pitfalls.** There is a risk of underestimating subtle signs of splenic injury in patients with a trauma history. Given the risk of delayed rupture, these signs should prompt a recommendation for appropriate patient surveillance.

▶ **Key points.** Splenic rupture is a life-threatening injury. At present, patient surveillance is increasingly favored as an alternative to splenectomy.

Splenic Artery Aneurysm

▶ **Brief definition.** Splenic artery aneurysm is a visceral artery aneurysm in the course of the splenic artery.

▶ **Imaging signs.** CT and MRI show a mass with the same enhancement and signal characteristics as the splenic artery. Duplex ultrasound may detect a flow signal but is often limited by overlying air in the stomach. Invasive angiography (digital subtraction angiography; DSA) can also demonstrate a splenic artery aneurysm and can define its feeding and draining vessels. CT angiography (CTA) or MR angiography (MRA) is indicated for precise size determination and treatment planning; CT is usually preferred owing to its higher spatial resolution (▶ Fig. 9.22).

▶ **Clinical features.** Most splenic artery aneurysms are asymptomatic. Symptomatic aneurysms cause upper abdominal pain, indicating a need for treatment. Rupture of a splenic artery aneurysm may cause life-threatening hemorrhage into the omental bursa and free abdominal cavity. Based on the guidelines of the German Society for Vascular Surgery, splenic artery aneurysms larger than 2 cm are considered an absolute indication for treatment, as are symptomatic, progressively enlarging, and ruptured aneurysms.[16] Due to the significant perioperative trauma of median laparotomy and a perioperative mortality rate of up to 3%, endovascular occlusion has become the current treatment of choice.[16] Endovascular treatment may employ a covered endoluminal stent, coils, or ethylene vinyl alcohol copolymer embolization, depending on the morphology of the aneurysm.[17] Endovascular treatment may be challenging or infeasible in some cases due to a distal aneurysmal site or tortuosity of vessels. Open surgical treatment options include resection of the aneurysm with end-to-end anastomosis of the proximal and distal segments or the use of vascular or prosthetic interposition grafts.

▶ **Pitfalls.** Partially thrombosed splenic artery aneurysms may be mistaken for pancreatic tumors.[18]

Note

Splenic artery aneurysms larger than 2 cm are considered at high risk for rupture and therefore require treatment.

9.3 Lymph Nodes
9.3.1 Anatomy

Lymph nodes function as immunologic filtering stations along the lymphatic pathways. There are many hundreds of lymph nodes in the human body—their exact number is unknown. Normal lymph nodes can range from a few millimeters to more than 1 cm in size.

Lymph nodes are invested by a fibrous capsule. Trabeculae extend from the capsule into the interior of the lymph node, dividing it into several segments. Afferent lymphatic vessels pierce the capsule at multiple sites and convey the lymph to the marginal sinuses. From there the lymph flows past the central lymph follicles, where it interacts with the lymphocytes. Lymph nodes have a central hilum with an artery, vein, and efferent lymphatic vessel.

9.3.2 Imaging

Ultrasound, MRI, and CT can all provide a purely morphological evaluation of lymph nodes. All three modalities can determine the dimensions of a lymph node along multiple axes and can differentiate between cortex and hilum. The principal morphological criteria for identifying lymph node pathology are:
- Round or globular shape (instead of oval).
- Enlarged short-axis diameter (>1 cm).
- Absence of the hilum due to tumor invasion.
- Central necrosis.
- Increased enhancement (▶ Fig. 9.23) or an abnormal flow pattern on duplex ultrasound.

While these criteria are often used successfully to identify gross malignant lymphadenopathy, to date there has been little success in detecting micrometastases within lymph nodes using imaging techniques. Thus, limitations of sensitivity and specificity tend to restrict the efficacy of ultrasound, CT, and MRI in the detection of early lymphadenopathy.

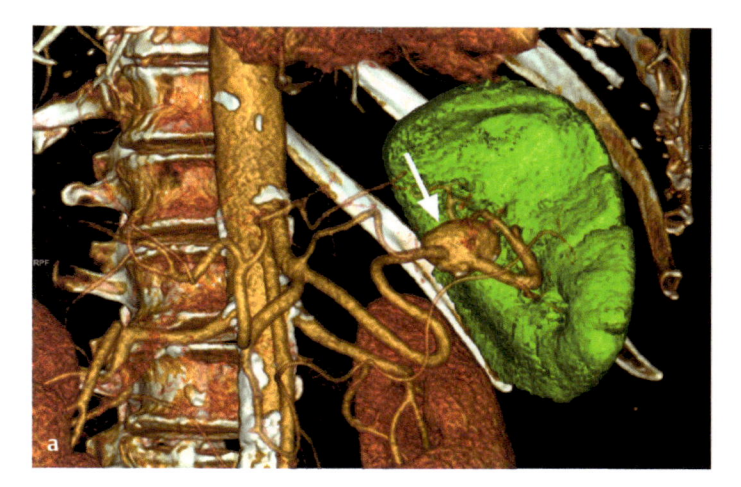

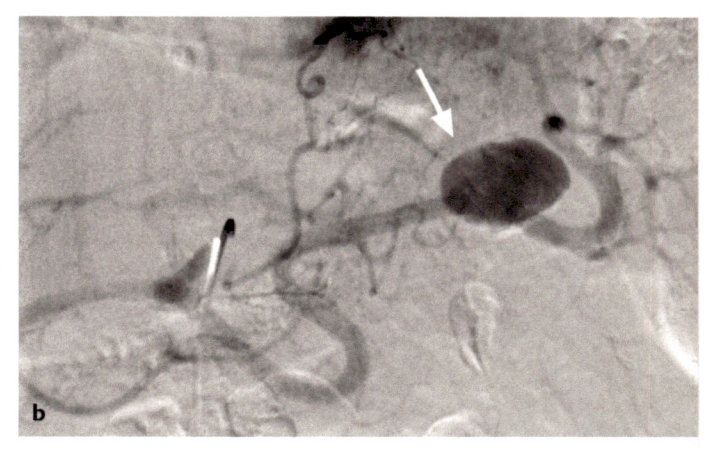

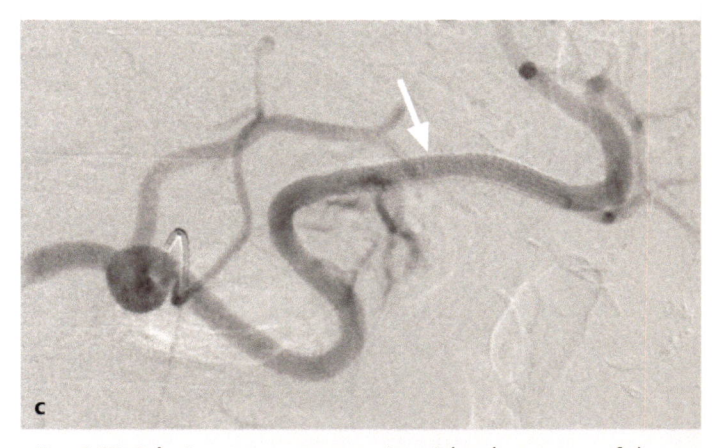

Fig. 9.22 **Splenic artery aneurysm.** A peripheral aneurysm of the splenic artery (arrow) was detected incidentally in a 62-year-old man. The aneurysm is definitely larger than 2 cm, indicating a need for treatment. **(a)** Volume-rendered CTA. **(b)** DSA with an angiographic catheter in the celiac trunk. **(c)** The aneurysm was selectively catheterized and excluded from the circulation by the interventional placement of an intravascular stent.

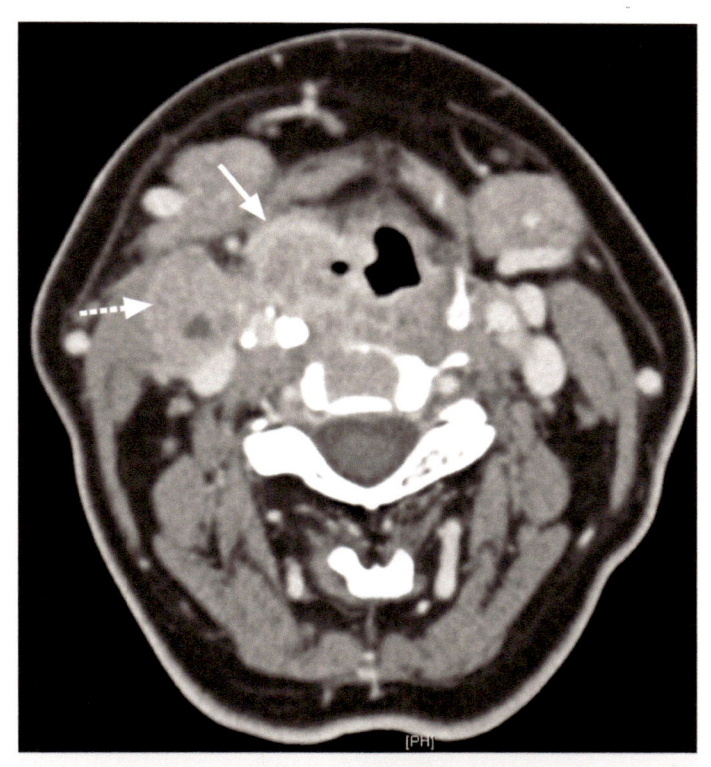

Fig. 9.23 **Lymph node metastasis** in a 50-year-old woman with a mass in the right hypopharynx. Contrast-enhanced CT of the neck shows a large mass with central liquefaction and an enhancing rim in the region of the right hypopharynx (arrow), and a markedly enlarged lymph node with central liquefaction (dashed arrow), consistent with a nodal metastasis.

Spleen and Lymphatic System

> **Note**
> All imaging modalities have low sensitivity and specificity for detecting micrometastases in lymph nodes.

Ultrasound

Ultrasound is well suited for the evaluation of superficial lymph nodes owing to its high spatial resolution (▶ Fig. 9.24). As well as displaying morphological features, color duplex ultrasound can also evaluate lymph node perfusion.

Chest Radiography

Despite their low sensitivity, PA and lateral chest radiographs (p. 2) are often the initial imaging study performed for the exclusion of mediastinal or hilar lymphadenopathy. Lymph node calcifications are also detectable on radiographs.

Computed Tomography

CT is the standard modality used to evaluate for lymph node enlargement. Its strength lies in its ability to define even deeply seated lymph nodes without artifacts. It is often possible to differentiate the cortex and hilum. CT can also enable evaluation of blood flow based on assessment of enhancement characteristics. Nevertheless, CT has limited sensitivity and specificity for detecting malignant lymphadenopathy, especially in the absence of nodal enlargement.

Magnetic Resonance Imaging

MRI, like CT, can provide a whole-body screening examination for lymph node enlargement. While MRI is often inferior to CT in its spatial resolution, the variations in tissue contrast with MRI allow for a detailed evaluation. In addition to gadolinium-based contrast media, superparamagnetic iron oxide (SPIO) particles were used in the past as investigational contrast agents for evaluating lymph node infiltration. At the time of publication (2018), however, these agents are no longer available on the market. Like CT, MRI has limited sensitivity and specificity in the detection of malignant lymphadenopathy.

Positron Emission Tomography–Computed Tomography

^{18}F-FDG PET-CT is the only imaging technique that can detect a focal increase of metabolic activity in lymph nodes. It is thus considered the most sensitive technique for the diagnosis of malignant lymphadenopathy (▶ Fig. 9.25).

9.3.3 Diseases

Differential Diagnosis of Lymph Node Enlargement

Enlarged lymph nodes are found in the following diseases:
- *Reactive lymphadenopathy*: Localized or generalized inflammatory diseases are often associated with the reactive enlargement and hyperperfusion of lymph nodes. Affected nodes have a demonstrable hilum. A well-known clinical example is cervical lymphadenopathy in infectious diseases.
- *Granulomatous lymphadenopathy*.
- *Lymph node abscess*: Bacterial infections may lead to abscess formation in lymph nodes with typical associated imaging signs (indistinct margins, faint hypodense or non-echo-free liquefaction with a hyperperfused wall and perifocal reaction). A special case is tuberculous lymphadenitis (▶ Fig. 9.26).
- Castleman's disease (p. 370).

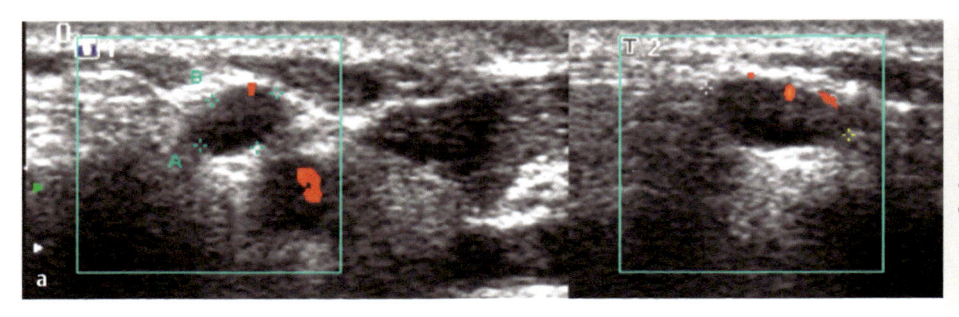

Fig. 9.24 Sonography of the cervical lymph nodes in a melanoma patient. (a) Normal morphological findings (oval shape, not enlarged, homogeneous echogenicity). (b) Lymph nodes suspicious for metastasis (rounded shape, abnormal enlargement, inhomogeneous echogenicity, increased perfusion).

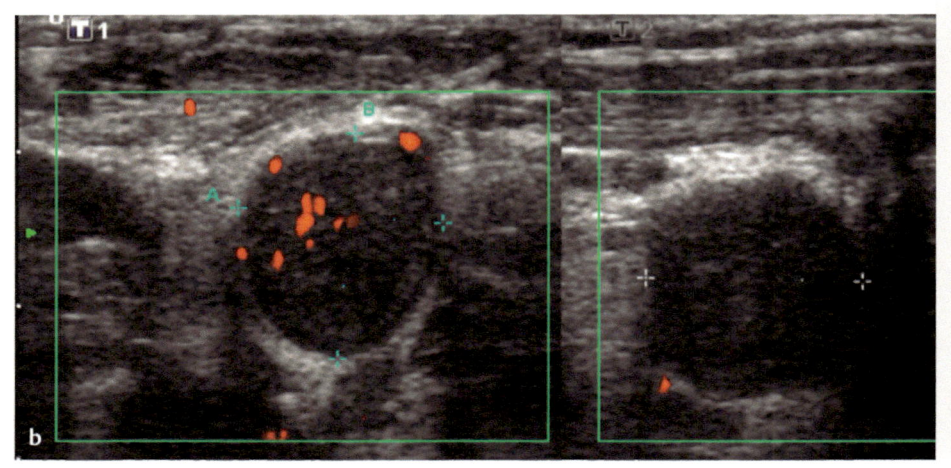

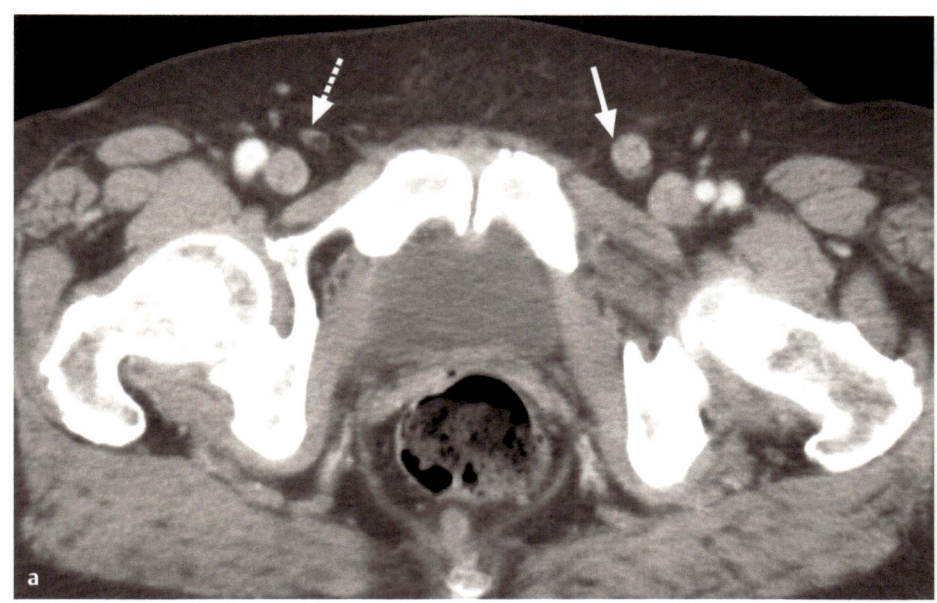

Fig. 9.25 CT and PET-CT of the lymph nodes in a melanoma patient. **(a)** CT shows abnormal enlargement of an inguinal lymph node on the left side (arrow). A normal lymph node with a fatty hilum (dashed arrow) is visible on the opposite side. **(b)** ^{18}F-FDG PET-CT. The color-coded PET image superimposed over the CT scan shows focal hypermetabolism in the lymph node (arrow).

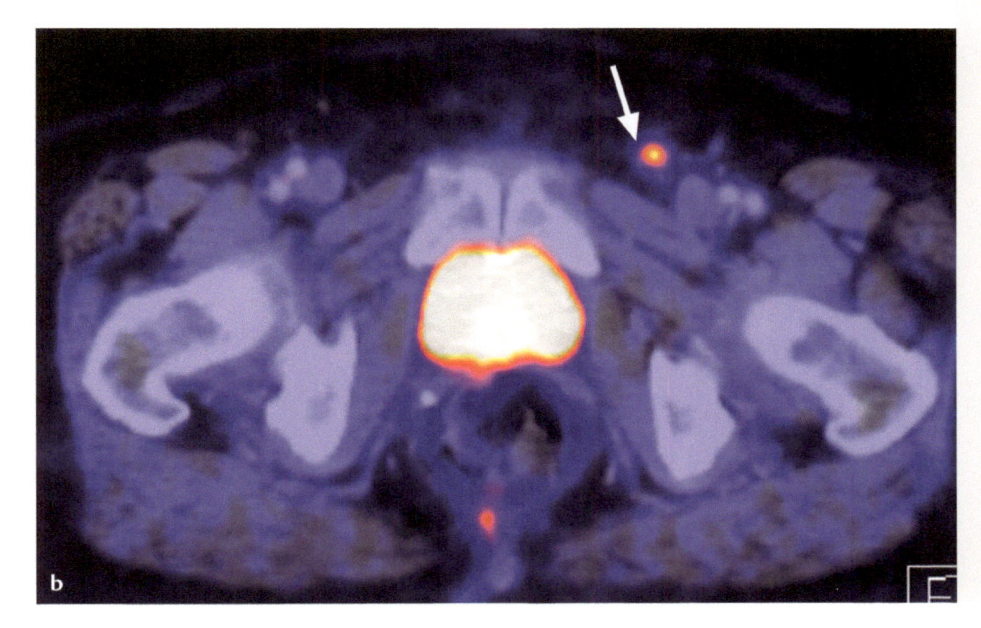

- *Metastases*: Almost all malignancies may give rise to lymphogenous metastasis involving locoregional lymph nodes (▶ Fig. 9.27).
- *Malignant lymphoma*: See below (p. 367).

Malignant Lymphoma

▶ **Brief definition.** Malignant lymphomas are defined as neoplasms arising in the cells of the lymphatic system. The two main histological categories are Hodgkin's and non-Hodgkin's lymphoma. Most lymphomas in their early stages involve lymph nodes and other organs of the lymphatic system and then spread in their later stages to involve extralymphatic organs as well (e.g., bone marrow and liver). There are forms that show primary end-organ involvement on initial diagnosis (multiple myeloma with primary involvement of bone marrow, primary lymphoma of the CNS, MALT lymphoma, cutaneous B-cell lymphoma).
- *Hodgkin's lymphoma*: Hodgkin's lymphomas are monoclonal B-cell lymphomas that contain multinucleated Sternberg giant cells and mononuclear Hodgkin's cells. They have a bimodal age peak around 30 and 60 years of age. The Ann Arbor system is used for the staging of Hodgkin's lymphoma (▶ Table 9.1).
- *Non-Hodgkin's lymphoma*: Non-Hodgkin's lymphomas are malignant lymphomas of the B cell and T cell lines. Approximately 30% of non-Hodgkin's lymphomas have a leukemic presentation. They are staged according to the Ann Arbor system for non-Hodgkin's lymphoma (▶ Table 9.2).

The following are some of the principal forms of non-Hodgkin's lymphoma:
- *Chronic lymphocytic leukemia*: This disease occurs mainly in elderly patients (with a rising incidence up to age 80 years). It has an indolent onset and is one of the most common non-Hodgkin's lymphomas. It is a B-cell lymphoma that takes a leukemic course. Imaging shows lymphadenopathy and hepatosplenomegaly.
- *Hairy cell leukemia*: This is a low-grade B-cell non-Hodgkin's lymphoma that infiltrates the medullary cavity, leading to

Spleen and Lymphatic System

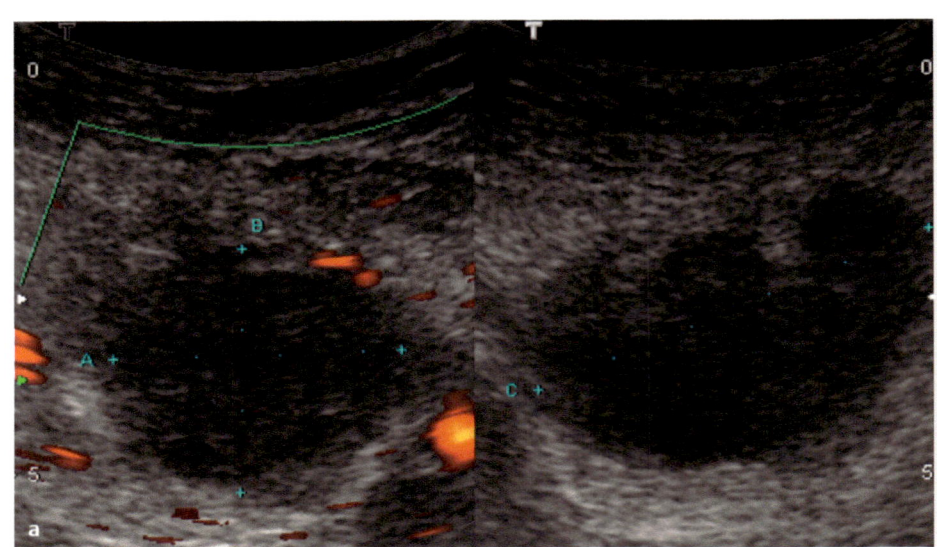

Fig. 9.26 Tuberculous lymphadenitis in a 23-year-old woman with a right axillary mass. **(a)** Initial color Doppler scan shows a slightly enlarged lymph node with partial central liquefaction and indistinct margins. **(b)** Further investigation by CT reveals multiple enlarged lymph nodes with intense rim enhancement in the right axillary and subclavicular regions, consistent with tuberculous lymphadenitis. Histology and microbiology (not shown) showed a granulomatous inflammation with caseating necrosis and isolated acid-fast rods. The polymerase chain reaction (PCR) was positive for *Mycobacterium tuberculosis*. **(c)** Ultrasound scans after 2 months' tuberculostatic therapy continue to show markedly enlarged subclavicular lymph nodes with increased liquefaction.

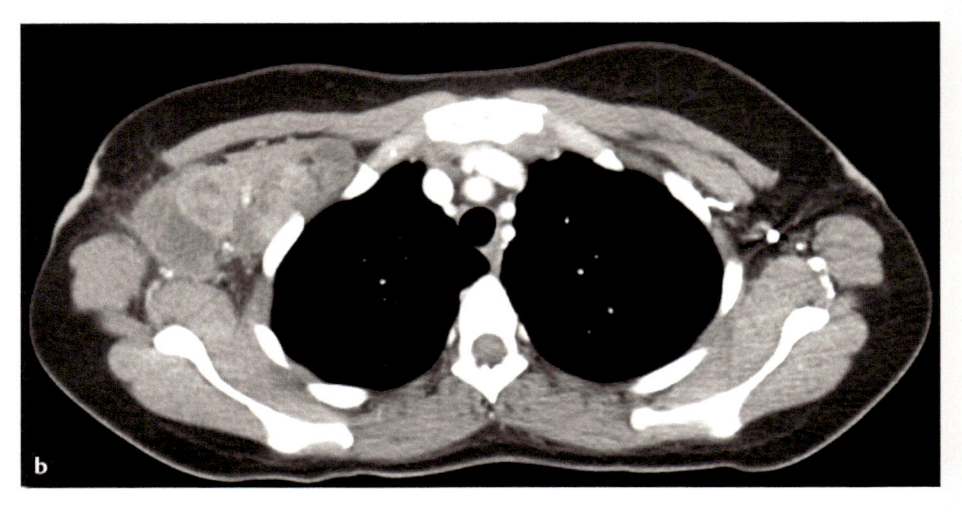

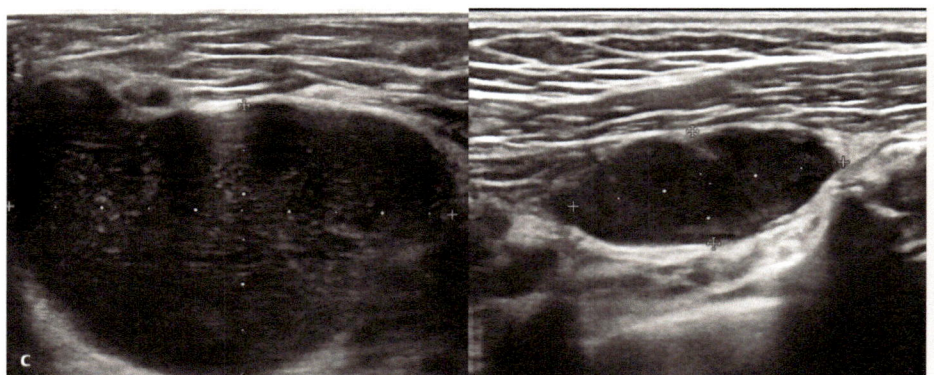

pancytopenia and splenomegaly in the form of hypersplenia syndrome. Hairy cell leukemia is rare with a peak incidence around 60 years of age.

- *Cutaneous T-cell lymphoma*: Known representatives of cutaneous T-cell lymphomas are mycosis fungoides and Sezary's syndrome. As well as pure cutaneous and lymph node involvement, advanced stages of mycosis fungoides also undergo systemic spread to various organs. Cutaneous lymphomas are most common in elderly patients.
- *Marginal zone lymphoma and MALT lymphoma*: Marginal zone lymphomas are indolent B-cell lymphomas that arise from the marginal zone of B-cell follicles and are capable of proliferating in nonlymphatic tissues. Marginal zone lymphomas may be of nodal, extranodal, or splenic origin. Extranodal marginal zone lymphomas may be mucosa-associated (MALT lymphoma), bronchus-associated (BALT lymphoma), or skin-associated (SALT lymphoma; ▶ Fig. 9.28, ▶ Fig. 9.29). A special subtype is *Helicobacter pylori*–associated MALT lymphoma of the stomach, but MALT lymphomas may develop anywhere in the body (see ▶ Fig. 9.28). MALT lymphomas are the most common lymphomas of the gastrointestinal tract. Imaging in patients with gastric or intestinal involvement may show thickening of the stomach or bowel wall (if visible signs are present). MALT lymphomas generally have a good prognosis.

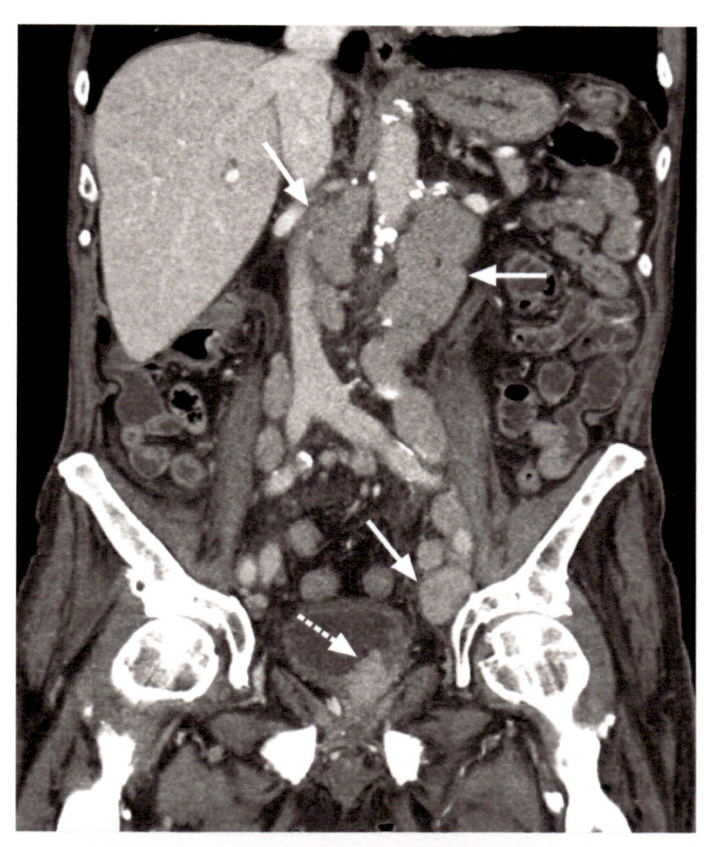

Fig. 9.27 Lymph node metastases from prostatic carcinoma.
A 73-year-old man with known prostate cancer underwent contrast-enhanced abdominal CT for tumor staging. Coronal reformatted image reveals bladder invasion (dashed arrow) by the primary tumor and multiple enlarged retroperitoneal lymph nodes (para-aortic, iliac; solid arrows). As well as lymph node metastases, the differential diagnosis of this case should include lymphoma.

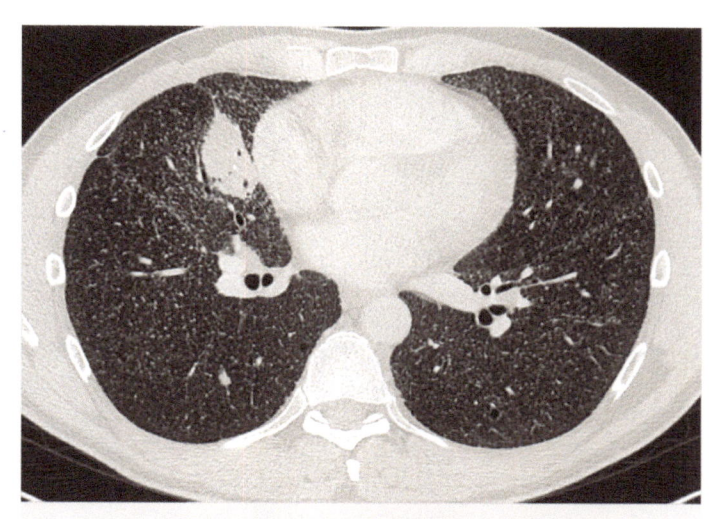

Fig. 9.28 Pulmonary MALT lymphoma. Primary pulmonary MALT lymphoma in a 48-year-old man in treatment. Thoracic axial CT with a lung window setting displays the lymphoma as a solid mass in the middle lobe of the right lung. Disseminated micronodular lesions are also noted throughout the lung parenchyma.

Table 9.1 Ann Arbor staging system for Hodgkin's lymphoma

Stage	Description
I	Involvement of one lymph node region (stage I N) or one extranodal site (stage I E)
II	Involvement of two or more lymph node regions on the same side of the diaphragm (stage II N) or localized extranodal sites with stage II criteria on the same side of the diaphragm (stage II E)
III	Involvement of lymph node regions or extranodal sites on both sides of the diaphragm
IV	Disseminated involvement of one or more extralymphatic organs

Table 9.2 Ann Arbor staging system for non-Hodgkin's lymphoma

Stage	Description
I	Involvement of one lymph node region (stage I N) or one extranodal site (stage I E)
II	Involvement of two or more lymph node regions on the same side of the diaphragm (stage II N) or localized extranodal sites with stage II criteria on the same side of the diaphragm (stage II E)
III	Involvement of lymph node regions or extranodal sites on both sides of the diaphragm
III1	Subphrenic involvement limited to splenic, celiac and portal lymph nodes
III2	Subphrenic involvement with para-aortic, mesenteric, iliac and/or inguinal lymph node involvement
IV	Disseminated involvement of one or more extralymphatic organs

- *Burkitt's lymphoma*: Burkitt's lymphoma is an aggressive, B-lymphoblastic lymphoma. Three variants are distinguished:
  - *Endemic* variant occurs in tropical Africa, where 95% of cases are Epstein–Barr virus–associated. Children are predominantly affected. Typical sites of occurrence are the mandible and maxilla.
  - *Sporadic* type is rarely Epstein–Barr virus–associated. Children are frequently affected as in the endemic type, but internal organs are more commonly involved than facial bones.
  - *Immunodeficiency-associated* variant typically affects HIV patients but may also occur in immunosuppressed patients.
- *Diffuse large B-cell lymphoma*: This is the most common type of non-Hodgkin's lymphoma and is considered a high-grade malignancy. It occurs mainly in elderly patients (median age approximately 70 years). Extranodal involvement is common.
- *Mantle cell lymphoma*: Mantle cell lymphoma is considered the most aggressive non-Hodgkin's lymphoma and has a very poor prognosis. Imaging shows multiple sites of lymphadenopathy, often accompanied by splenomegaly. Median patient age is 65 years.
- *Multiple myeloma*: See below (p. 370).
- *Immunocytoma (Waldenström disease)*: Immunocytoma, like plasmacytoma, is characterized by the formation of monoclonal antibodies, but osteolytic lesions are not observed. Immunocytoma is rarer than plasmacytoma and occurs predominantly in older patients.

Spleen and Lymphatic System

▶ **Imaging signs.** Ultrasound, CT, and MRI show the following signs (▶ Fig. 9.30, ▶ Fig. 9.31):
- Lymphadenopathy (CT, ultrasound, radiographs).
- Splenomegaly (inhomogeneous, nodular infiltration is also possible).
- Hepatomegaly.
- Extranodal involvement.

18F-FDG PET-CT can supply additional information on the metabolic activity of an affected lymph node and is therefore increasingly used for initial staging and for monitoring treatment response in lymphoma patients.

▶ **Clinical features.** The typical clinical features of lymphomas consist of classic B symptoms (fever, night sweats, weight loss, reduced exercise tolerance, possible itching). Palpable lymph node swelling, usually in the neck, often directs attention to the disease. Mediastinal lymphadenopathy may lead to a persistent cough. Later stages of the disease may be marked by hepatomegaly, splenomegaly, and a variety of symptoms due to organ involvement. Impaired hematopoiesis may also give rise to associated symptoms.

▶ **Differential diagnosis.** Lymph node enlargement may occur in any of the following conditions:
- Infection, especially viral infection.
- Metastasis.
- Tuberculosis.
- Castleman's disease.
- Sarcoidosis.

Note

Imaging studies in lymphoma patients are used mainly for staging the extent of disease.

Castleman's Disease

▶ **Brief definition.** Castleman's disease is a rare lymphoproliferative disorder of unknown cause characterized by multiple enlarged lymph nodes (▶ Fig. 9.32). Involvement of human herpesvirus 8 has been suggested. The disease may occur in a unicentric or a multicentric form.

▶ **Clinical features.** Patients may exhibit lymphoma-like B symptoms due to the production of cytokines.

Sarcoidosis

Sarcoidosis (p. 20) is discussed in Chapter 1, Mediastinum.

Multiple Myeloma

▶ **Brief definition.** Multiple myeloma, also called plasmacytoma, is a B-cell non-Hodgkin's lymphoma resulting from the monoclonal proliferation of malignant plasma cells.[19] It initially involves the bone marrow, and various patterns of involvement are distinguished. Infiltration of the bone marrow often leads to the development of potentially painful osteolytic lesions, which may compromise the stability of the skeleton. Extraosseous manifestations may also occur. The median patient age is 65 years.

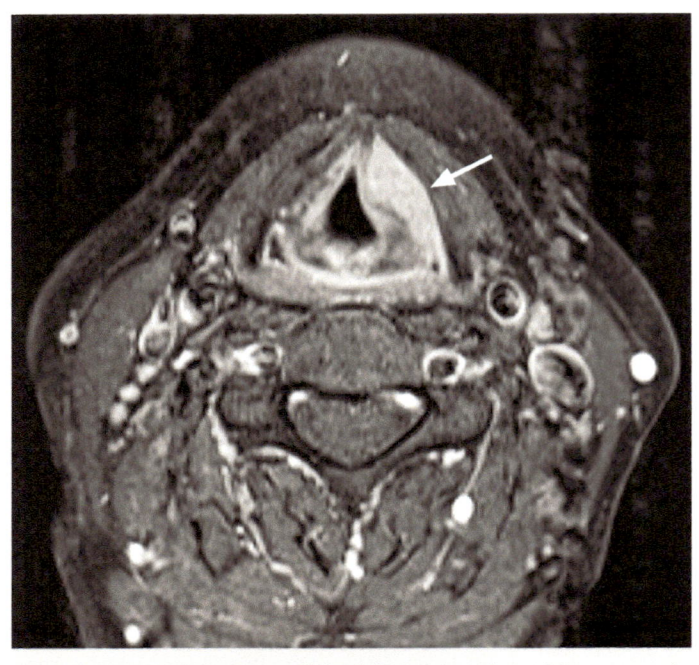

Fig. 9.29 **MALT lymphoma of the left vocal cord.** Axial fat-saturated T1W MRI sequence after IV injection of contrast medium shows a homogeneously enhancing mass in the left vocal cord (arrow).

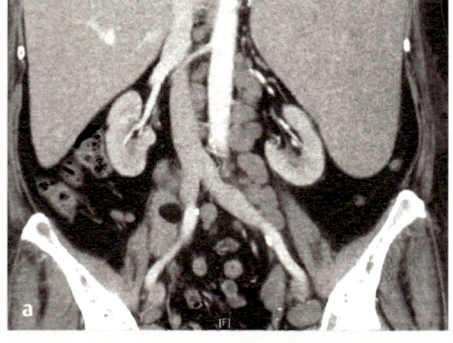

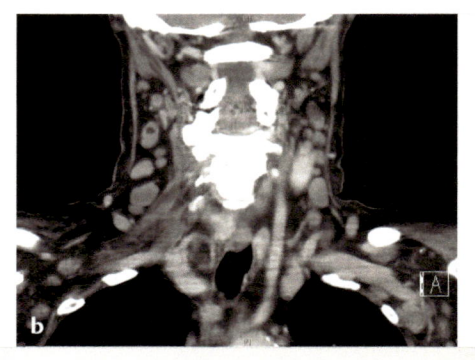

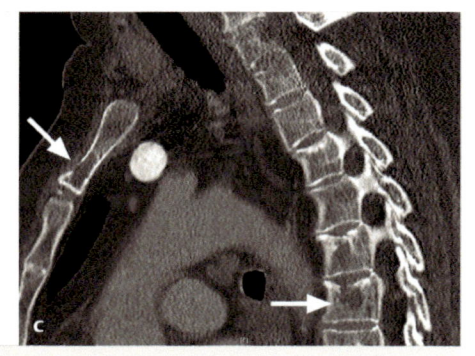

Fig. 9.30 **B-cell non-Hodgkin's lymphoma.** Whole-body CT in a 64-year-old woman with diffuse large-B-cell non-Hodgkin's lymphoma shows ubiquitous lymphadenopathy (illustrated here for retroperitoneal and cervical nodes) and diffuse splenic involvement. Bone marrow infiltration with osteolytic areas (arrows) is also found. (a) Coronal pelvis. (b) Coronal neck and shoulder girdle. (c) Sagittal neck and shoulder girdle with a bone window.

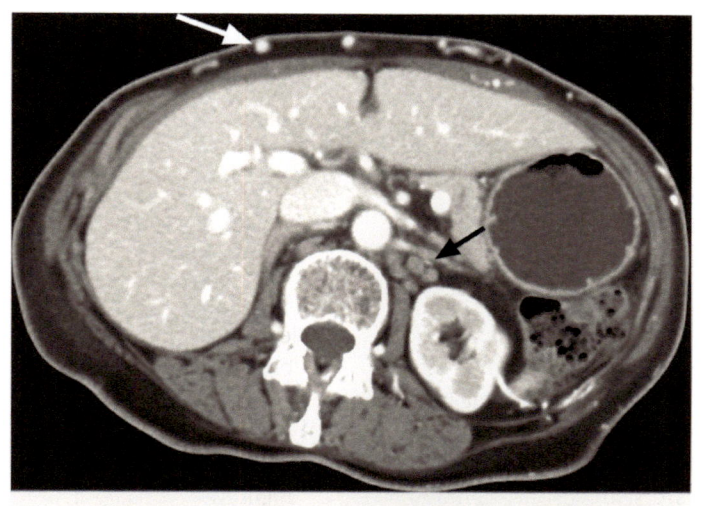

Fig. 9.32 Castleman's disease. CT in a 53-year-old woman shows an increase in the number of retroperitoneal lymph nodes (black arrow) and venous collaterals in the abdominal wall (white arrow) due to obstruction of the superior vena cava by a large mediastinal mass (not shown).

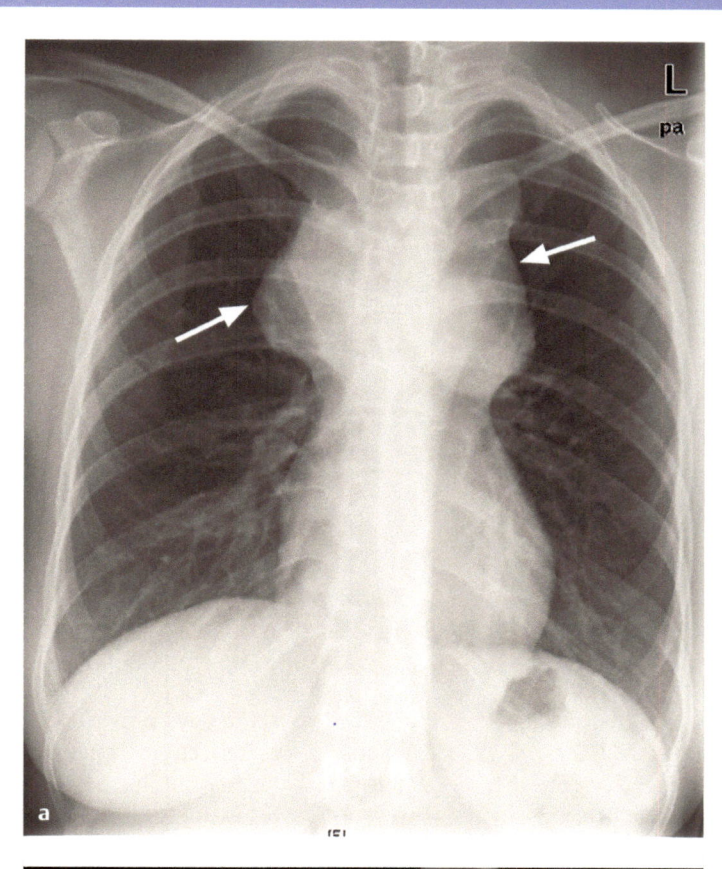

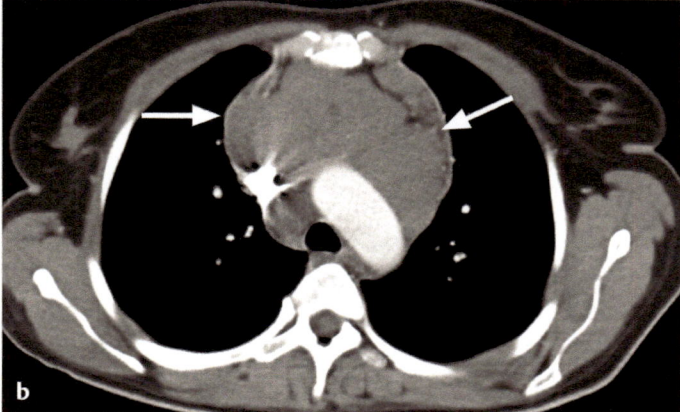

Fig. 9.31 Hodgkin's disease in a 38-year-old woman with B symptoms. (a) Conventional radiograph shows massive widening of the upper mediastinum (arrows). (b) Correlative CT shows pronounced mediastinal and cervical lymphadenopathy (arrows). Histology indicated Hodgkin's disease (not shown). No lymphomas were found below the diaphragm (not shown), indicating stage II disease.

▶ **Imaging signs.** A standard radiographic skeletal survey (frontal and lateral skull and cervico-thoraco-lumbar spine, and AP views of the chest, pelvis, and proximal limb bones) is still recommended in guidelines worldwide, due to its excellent availability and low cost. Conventional radiographs show osteolytic lesions in cases where only 35 % of the bone is left. Thus they have a far lower sensitivity compared to CT or MRI. Osteolytic lesions, especially in the skull and pelvis, typically appear as punched-out lucencies without sclerotic margins ("buckshot skull"). Focal lytic lesions in the long bones may be accompanied by other findings such as endosteal thinning of the cortex (endosteal scalloping) or moth-eaten destructive changes that indicate osteolytic activity. Conventional radiography has limited sensitivity and specificity compared with modern sectional imaging techniques, and CT has replaced the standard skeletal survey at many centers.[20] Multidetector-row spiral CT scanners have become widely available and can cover the entire axial skeleton, skull, and proximal limbs in a single acquisition while the patient lies supine with the arms resting above the head. In patients who are in pain, this can be a major advantage over time-consuming radiographs that require multiple position changes.[21] Because of its high intrinsic bone contrast, CT scans can be acquired with low-dose technique and without IV administration of contrast medium. Multiplanar reconstructions in coronal and sagittal projections can provide nonsuperimposed views of the entire skeleton with high sensitivity for osteolytic lesions (▶ Fig. 9.33, ▶ Fig. 9.34). The stability of specific skeletal regions can also be evaluated more accurately than on conventional radiographs. Additionally, the medullary cavities of the long bones can be evaluated and plasma cell nests that have not yet caused osteolysis can be identified. CT is also a valuable tool for therapeutic monitoring. Within in limitations (difficulty in evaluating parenchymal abdominal organs), CT can also be used to evaluate extramedullary sites of disease. Although MRI cannot directly visualize bone structures as can CT, its intrinsically high soft-tissue contrast allows for sensitive detection of plasma cell nests in bone marrow, before osteolytic changes have occurred. ^{18}F-FDG PET-CT can highlight sites of increased glucose metabolism that would indicate focal infiltration of the medullary cavity.

> **Note**
>
> MRI and ^{18}F-FDG PET-CT are considered the most sensitive techniques for the detection of bone marrow infiltration by multiple myeloma.

Several patterns of involvement can be distinguished with MRI:
- Multifocal involvement.
- Diffuse homogeneous involvement.
- Salt-and-pepper pattern (micronodular involvement with remaining islets of fatty bone marrow).

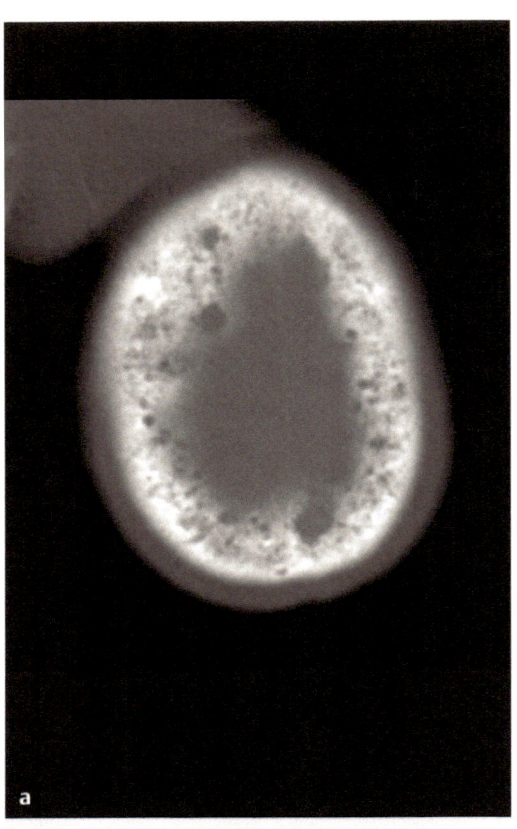

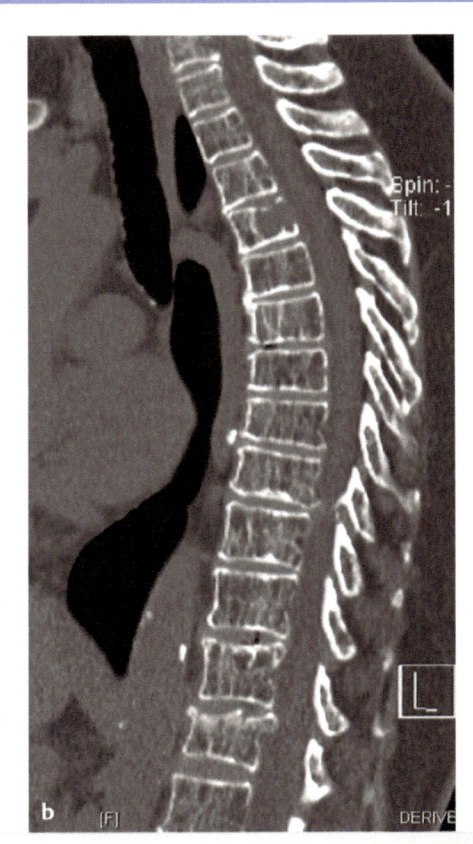

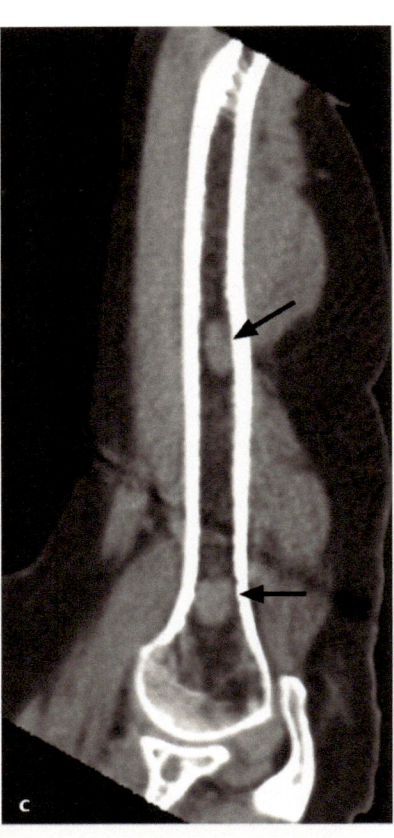

Fig. 9.33 Multiple myeloma. Typical CT findings: multiple osteolytic lesions in the calvaria and axial skeleton and nodular infiltration of the medullary cavities in the humeri (arrows in [c]). **(a)** Skull. **(b)** Axial skeleton. **(c)** Humerus.

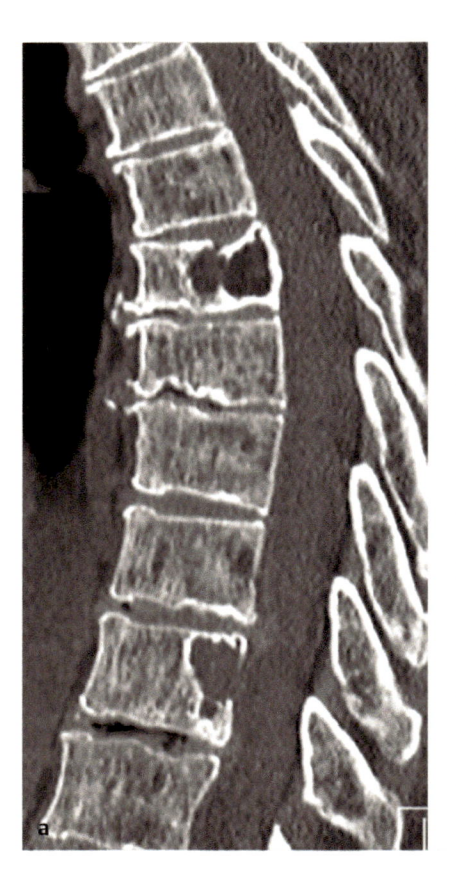

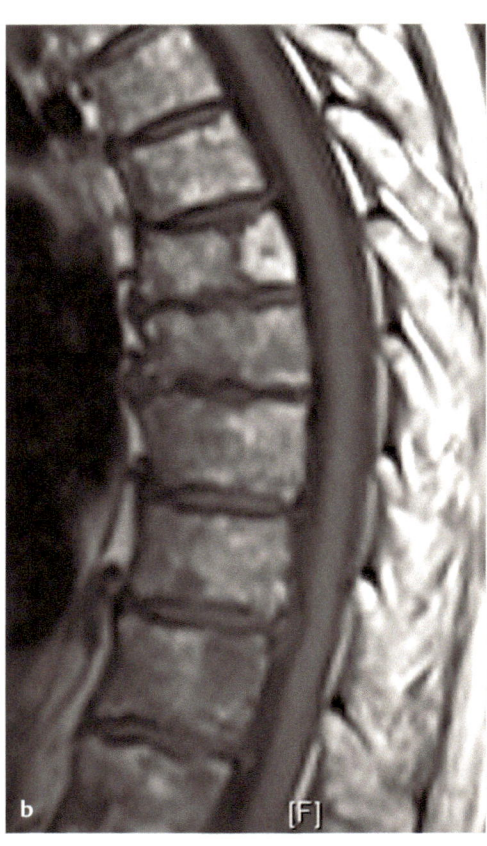

Fig. 9.34 Multiple myeloma. Spinal images in a woman with multiple myeloma. The upper osteolytic lesion appears hypodense on CT and hyperintense on MRI, indicating fatty degeneration in an older lesion with no acute infiltration. The lower lesion is hyperdense on CT and hypointense on MRI. This finding is consistent with cellular infiltration and suggests active disease.

Because radionuclide uptake does not occur in multiple myelomas, bone scintigraphy is not useful for their diagnosis.

▶ **Clinical features.** The degenerated plasma cells produce monoclonal immunoglobulins or only light chains that may lead to renal failure, polyneuropathy, and hyperviscosity syndromes as a result of protein overload in the blood. The plasma cells nests in the bone marrow crowd out the physiologic bone marrow, leading to anemia, thrombocytopenia, and leukopenia. Lytic bone lesions lead to bone pain, pathologic fractures, and hypercalcemia.

▶ **Differential diagnosis.** Skeletal metastasis is far more common than multiple myeloma and should be considered first in the differential diagnosis of multiple osteolytic lesions.

Bibliography

[1] Drenckhahn D, ed. Benninghoff, Drenckhahn: Anatomie. München: Urban & Fischer; 2008
[2] Reiser M, Kuhn F. Debus J. Radiologie. Stuttgart: Thieme; 2006
[3] Hofer M. Sono Grundkurs. Stuttgart: Thieme; 2005
[4] Mortelé KJ, Mortelé B, Silverman SG. CT features of the accessory spleen. AJR Am J Roentgenol. 2004; 183(6):1653–1657
[5] Federle MP, Brooke JR, Woodward PJ, et al. Diagnostic Imaging Abdomen. Salt Lake City (UT): Amirsys; 2010
[6] Elsayes KM, Narra VR, Mukundan G, Lewis JS, Jr, Menias CO, Heiken JP. MR maging of the spleen: spectrum of abnormalities. Radiographics. 2005; 25(4): 967–982
[7] Olthof DC, van der Vlies CH, Joosse P, van Delden OM, Jurkovich GJ, Goslings JC, PYTHIA Collaboration Group. Consensus strategies for the nonoperative management of patients with blunt splenic injury: a Delphi study. J Trauma Acute Care Surg. 2013; 74(6):1567–1574
[8] Bowdler AJ. Splenomegaly and hypersplenism. Clin Haematol. 1983; 12(2): 467–488
[9] Argiris A. Splenic and renal infarctions complicating atrial fibrillation. Mt Sinai J Med. 1997; 64(4–5):342–349
[10] Hatipoglu AR, Karakaya K, Karagülle E, Turgut B. A rare cause of acute abdomen: splenic infarction. Hepatogastroenterology. 2001; 48(41):1333–1336
[11] Urrutia M, Mergo PJ, Ros LH, Torres GM, Ros PR. Cystic masses of the spleen: radiologic-pathologic correlation. Radiographics. 1996; 16(1):107–129
[12] Becker CD, Poletti PA. The trauma concept: the role of MDCT in the diagnosis and management of visceral injuries. Eur Radiol. 2005; 15 Suppl 4:D105–D109
[13] Tang J, Li W, Lv F, et al. Comparison of gray-scale contrast-enhanced ultrasonography with contrast-enhanced computed tomography in different grading of blunt hepatic and splenic trauma: an animal experiment. Ultrasound Med Biol. 2009; 35(4):566–575
[14] Haan JM, Biffl W, Knudson MM, et al. Western Trauma Association Multi-Institutional Trials Committee. Splenic embolization revisited: a multicenter review. J Trauma. 2004; 56(3):542–547
[15] Haan JM, Bochicchio GV, Kramer N, Scalea TM. Nonoperative management of blunt splenic injury: a 5-year experience. J Trauma. 2005; 58(3):492–498
[16] Vorstand der Deutschen Gesellschaft für Gefäßchirurgie (DGG). Leitlinie "Diagnostik und Therapie der Aneurysmen des Truncus coeliacus, der A. lienalis, hepatica und mesenterica"; 2011
[17] Belli AM, Markose G, Morgan R. The role of interventional radiology in the management of abdominal visceral artery aneurysms. Cardiovasc Intervent Radiol. 2012; 35(2):234–243
[18] Nagamatsu H, Takahashi K, Ueo T, et al. A case of splenic artery aneurysm simulating a pancreas tumor. Nihon Shokakibyo Gakkai zasshi. 2011; 108(8):1420–1427
[19] Herold G. Innere Medizin. Köln: Herold; 2012
[20] Horger M, Claussen CD, Bross-Bach U, et al. Whole-body low-dose multidetector row-CT in the diagnosis of multiple myeloma: an alternative to conventional radiography. Eur J Radiol. 2005; 54(2):289–297
[21] Horger M, Kanz L, Denecke B, et al. The benefit of using whole-body, low-dose, nonenhanced, multidetector computed tomography for follow-up and therapy response monitoring in patients with multiple myeloma. Cancer. 2007; 109(8):1617–1626

10 Adrenal Glands

Andreas Saleh

10.1 Anatomy

The left adrenal gland is located anteromedial to the upper pole of the left kidney. The right adrenal gland is located at a slightly higher level (see ▶ Fig. 10.1, ▶ Fig. 10.2, ▶ Fig. 10.3).

10.2 Imaging

10.2.1 Ultrasound

Adults

The right adrenal gland is consistently definable with transabdominal ultrasound in adults, whereas the left adrenal gland is not. The region of the left adrenal gland can be visualized but the gland itself cannot be positively identified in most cases. As a result, masses of the adrenal gland cannot be confidently excluded with ultrasound.

Note

If an adrenal mass is detected with ultrasound, there are no sonographic criteria that can narrow the differential diagnosis. Given these limitations, targeted ultrasound scanning of the adrenal glands is almost never indicated in adults.

Nevertheless, the adrenal region should still be located and identified during a complete abdominal ultrasound examination. If the adrenal glands are not specifically examined, masses up to 3 cm in size could be overlooked, especially on the left side. On the right side, the inferior vena cava provides a landmark for orientation. The gland is surveyed from above downward in transverse scans, which can be acquired through an intercostal window. The right adrenal gland is located to the right of and behind the vena cava. The left adrenal gland can be imaged with a flank scan that displays the aorta, spleen, and kidney in one image. The left adrenal region is identified in the triangle between these landmarks and is scanned using the same technique as on the right side.

Note

Ultrasound is the imaging modality of first choice for evaluating the adrenal glands in children.

Children

In children the adrenal glands can be clearly visualized on both sides, especially in newborns. The limbs of the neonatal adrenal glands are on average 1.6 cm long and 3 mm wide. The hypoechoic

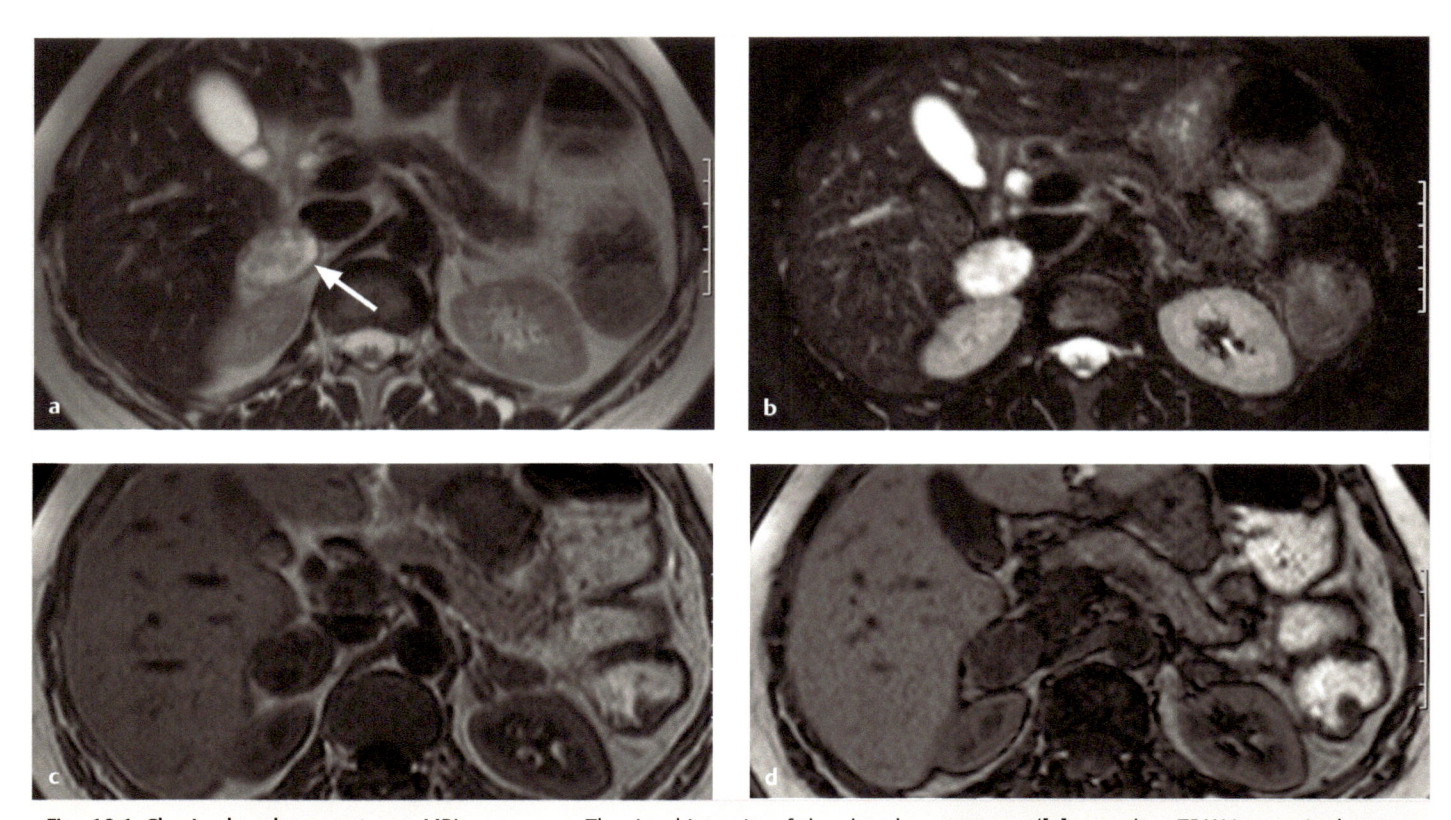

Fig. 10.1 **Classic pheochromocytoma.** MRI appearance. The signal intensity of the pheochromocytoma ([a], arrow) on T2W images is almost as high as that of bile and CSF. This is particularly evident in the fat-suppressed images (b). The opposed-phase image (d) does not show loss of signal intensity. Note also the relatively central location of the adrenal mass in the body. (a) T2W image. (b) Fat-saturated T2W image. (c) In-phase image. (d) Opposed-phase image.

10.2 Imaging

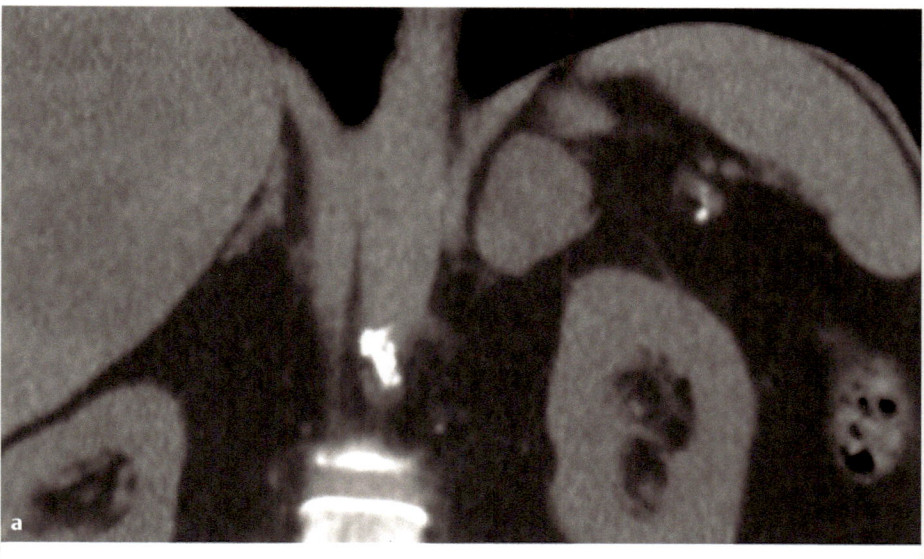

Fig. 10.2 Nonfunctioning incidentaloma of the left adrenal gland. The mass is 3.6 cm in its longest dimension. Note in **(a)** the different relationships of the right and left adrenal glands to the corresponding kidney.
(a) Unenhanced CT. The mass has an attenuation value of 23 HU, which is not diagnostic of adrenal adenoma. **(b)** In-phase image. The lesion is isointense to spleen.
(c) Opposed-phase image. The lesion is hypointense to spleen. This identifies the mass as a (lipid-poor) adenoma. Adrenalectomy was still performed, however, and confirmed the diagnosis.

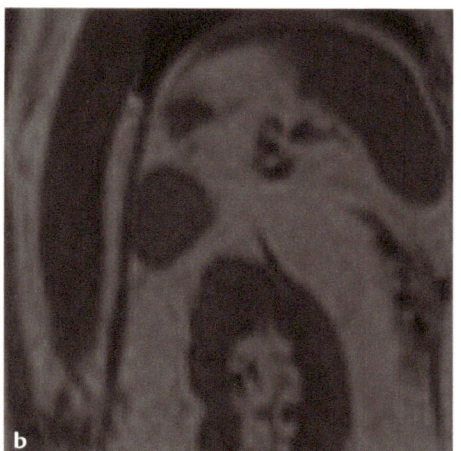

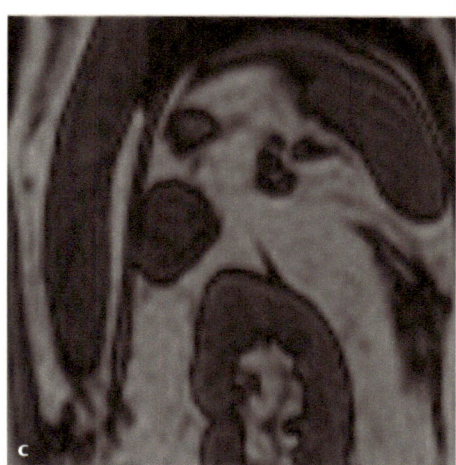

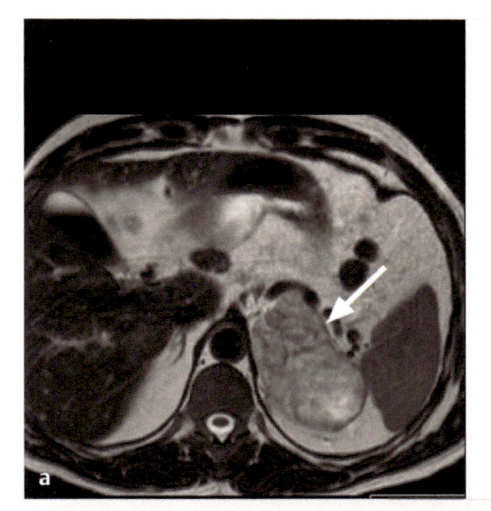

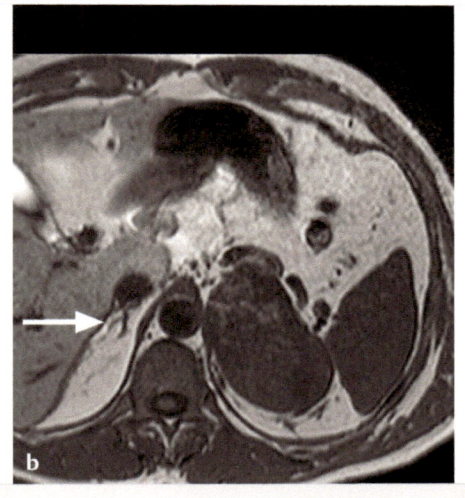

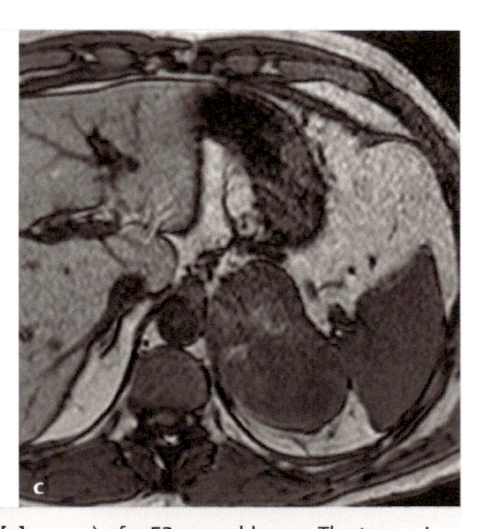

Fig. 10.3 Adrenocortical carcinoma. A mass was detected incidentally in the left adrenal gland ([a], arrow) of a 52-year-old man. The tumor is inhomogeneous and does not show loss of signal intensity in opposed-phase images **(c)**. Its margins are not infiltrative and there is no evidence of metastasis. Because the mass was large (7.4 cm) and its features were not typical of adenoma, adrenalectomy was performed. Histology indicated adrenocortical carcinoma T2 N0 M0. Note the position of the adrenal glands, especially on the (unaffected) right side ([b], arrow). The affected adrenal gland is located almost in the midline. **(a)** T2W image. **(b)** In-phase image. **(c)** Opposed-phase image.

adrenal cortex and the echogenic medulla are clearly distinct from each other at this time (see ▶ Fig. 10.4). The volume of the adrenal glands decreases by 50% during the first 6 weeks after birth. If the limbs of the adrenal glands in a 6-week-old child are more than 2 cm long and more than 5 mm wide, resembling the large adrenal glands of a newborn, it is very likely than an adrenogenital syndrome is present. The decline in adrenal gland volume is paralleled by an increasing loss of corticomedullary differentiation. By

Adrenal Glands

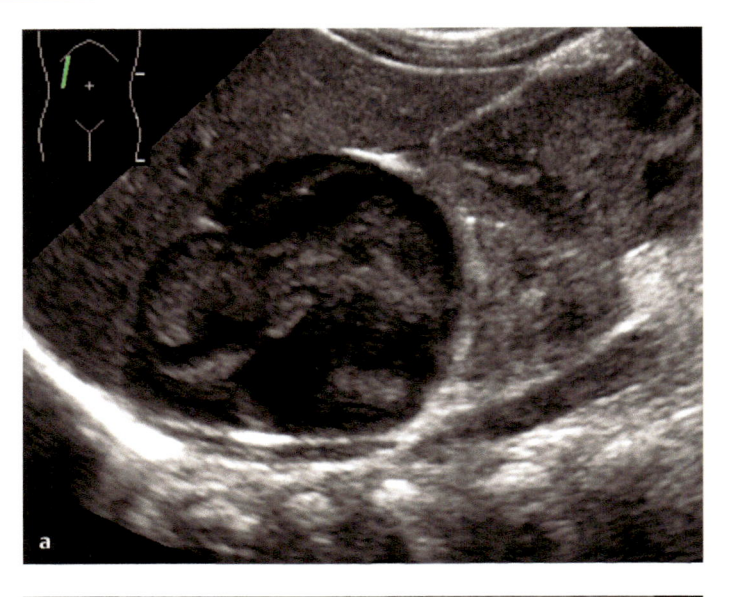

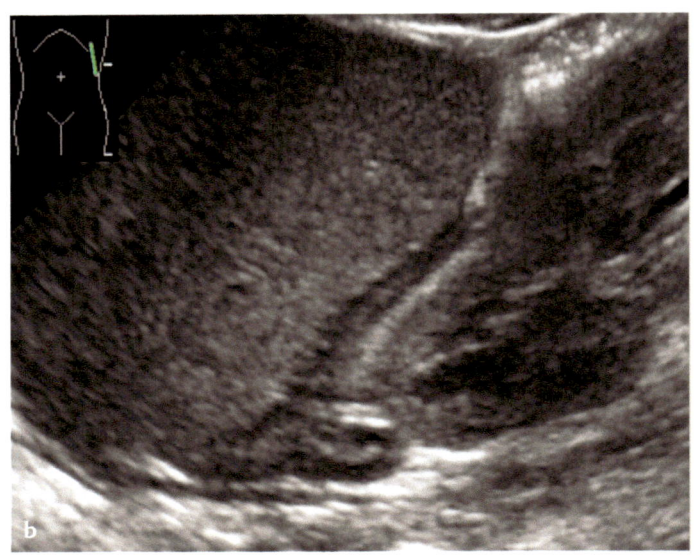

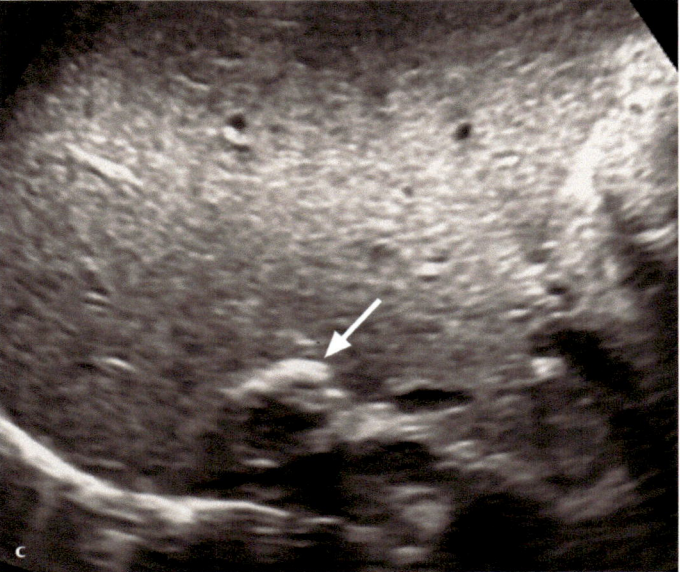

Fig. 10.4 **Adrenal hematoma** in a preterm infant (36 weeks' gestation). The newborn was macrosomic with a birth weight of 4,110 g. (**a**) Routine ultrasound scan reveals a mass in the right adrenal gland, presumed to be a hematoma due to absence of vascularity on color duplex (not shown). (**b**) The left adrenal gland appears normal for age, with very good corticomedullary differentiation. (**c**) Follow-up at 6 weeks shows a calcified residual mass (arrow) on the right side.

12 months of age, the sonographic morphology of the adrenal glands is practically the same as in adults. The limbs of the adrenal glands appear hypoechoic with no corticomedullary differentiation.

10.2.2 Computed Tomography

Three CT techniques are available for evaluating the adrenal glands:
- Measurement of mean attenuation.
- Percentage of pixels with negative attenuation values (histogram analysis).
- Measurement of contrast medium washout.

Attenuation measurement of an adrenal mass and histogram analysis exploit the high fat content of most adenomas. An adrenal mass with a CT attenuation of 10 HU or less is definitely an adenoma. This technique has 100% specificity, i.e., there are no false-positives for adenoma and there is no chance of mistaking an adenoma for a metastasis. However, only about 70% of adenomas have a sufficiently high lipid content to produce a CT attenuation of 10 HU or less. Histogram analysis, determination of contrast medium washout, and chemical shift imaging are methods that are designed to diagnose these lipid-poor adenomas despite their low fat content.

A histogram analysis does not involve computing the arithmetic mean of attenuation values in the region of interest as in ordinary densitometry. Instead, the frequencies of the attenuation values are plotted and the percentage of pixels with negative attenuation values within the adrenal mass or region of interest is determined. Most picture archiving and communication system (PACS) software does not have this capability, but histogram analysis can be performed at the diagnostic console of the CT system. If more than 10% of the pixels in the adrenal mass have negative attenuation values, the mass is definitely an adenoma.

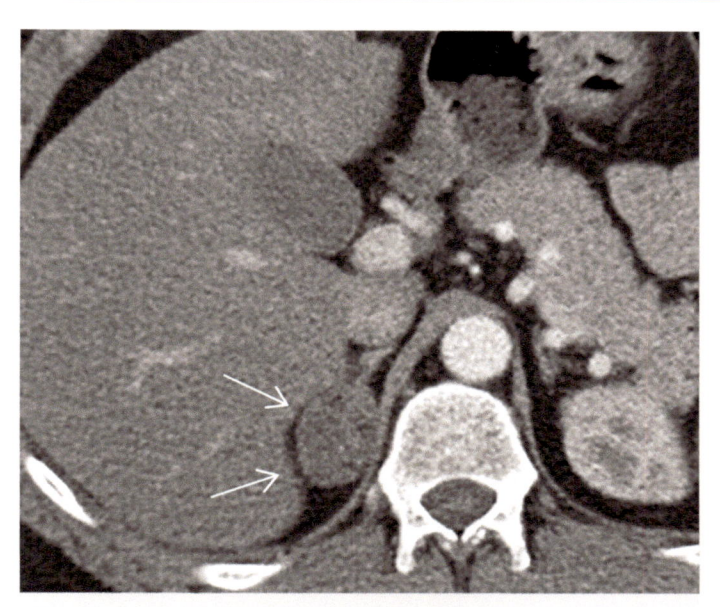

Fig. 10.5 CT in suspected hepatocellular carcinoma. An indeterminate hepatic lesion (not shown) was found in a patient with alcoholic cirrhosis of the liver. CT demonstrates a 3.5-cm mass in the right adrenal gland (arrows). Unenhanced CT is not available. The adrenal mass has an attenuation of 28 HU in the arterial phase of enhancement. Histogram analysis shows 15% negative pixels, positively identifying the mass as adenoma.

Histogram analysis increases the sensitivity of unenhanced CT for the diagnosis of adenomas from 70% to 85%.[1]

Frequently, only contrast-enhanced images are initially available. If these images show the necessary attenuation threshold (less than 10 HU, at least 10% negative pixels), then this is sufficient for a diagnosis of adenoma (▶ Fig. 10.5). Use of contrast does not alter the 100% specificity; it changes only the sensitivity, due to so-called pseudoenhancement, which is naturally lower than in unenhanced CT. Nevertheless, even the analysis of contrast-enhanced scans can often eliminate the need to proceed with unenhanced CT or MRI.

If an adenoma is very lipid-poor, all techniques based on the detection of a high fat content (CT attenuation, histogram analysis, chemical shift imaging) will fail. One way to diagnose lipid-poor adenomas is with dynamic CT.[2] This technique exploits the fact that adenomas and nonadenomas differ in their enhancement whereas lipid-rich and lipid-poor adenomas have the same washout characteristics. Adenomas enhance more rapidly and intensely than nonadenomas and show faster washout. Contrast washout is determined with a 10-minute delayed scan. If unenhanced CT is available, the absolute washout can be calculated as follows:

$$\text{Absolute washout} = \frac{\text{portal venous CT(HU)} - \text{10min CT (HU)}}{\text{portal venous CT(HU)} - \text{unenhanced CT(HU)}}$$

If only contrast-enhanced series are available, the relative washout can be determined using the formula:

$$\text{Relative washout} = \frac{\text{portal venous CT(HU)} - \text{10min CT (HU)}}{\text{portal venous CT(HU)}}$$

An absolute washout greater than 60% or a relative washout greater than 40% indicates adenoma.

> **Caution**
>
> Even nonadenomas may show very high washout of enhancement. The specificity of dynamic CT in differentiating adenomas and nonadenomas is only about 90%.[3]

This means that a degree of relative uncertainty exists when an adenoma is diagnosed.

10.2.3 Positron Emission Tomography–Computed Tomography

Targeted PET imaging of the adrenal glands is rarely done but may be appropriate in selected investigations such as the detection or exclusion of pheochromocytoma (p. 382). More commonly, the adrenal glands are evaluated as part of a FDG PET staging examination in tumor patients. In this case the FDG uptake of the adrenal glands is compared with that of the liver. An analysis of standardized uptake values does not add significant information.

> **Caution**
>
> False-positive and false-negative PET findings are not uncommon in the adrenal glands.

False-negative findings may have various causes. If the primary tumor does not have increased glucose metabolism, its metastases will not show increased FDG uptake. Tumors smaller than 1 cm often escape PET detection, as do tumors with intralesional hemorrhage or necrosis. False-positive findings are most common with adenomas that have increased glucose metabolism. The reasons for this metabolic increase are unclear. Hormonally active adenomas and hormonally inactive adenomas do not differ in their FDG uptake. If the FDG uptake of adrenal lesions is slightly higher than that of the liver, evaluation of the CT component with densitometry and possible histogram analysis may be helpful.[4] In some cases this can establish adenoma and avoid a false-positive PET diagnosis (▶ Fig. 10.6). Occasionally a false-negative PET diagnosis can also be avoided if an adrenal metastasis is so small that it does not present as a mass and is detectable only by its greatly increased metabolism (▶ Fig. 10.7).

10.2.4 Magnetic Resonance Imaging

MRI techniques also exploit the high lipid content of adenomas. The lipid component is detected not by fat-suppression methods but by chemical shift imaging. Due to the different precession frequencies of water and lipid protons, there is a point in time at which the signal intensities from lipid and water protons add together (in phase) and another at which the signals from lipid and water protons are subtracted (opposed phase). A T1 W double-echo sequence is used to generate both in-phase and opposed-phase images by suitable selection of the echo times for sampling (at 1.5 T, in-phase at 1.5, 4.6, 9.2 and 13.8 ms; opposed-phase at 2.3, 6.9 and 11.5 ms; the values will vary at different field

Adrenal Glands

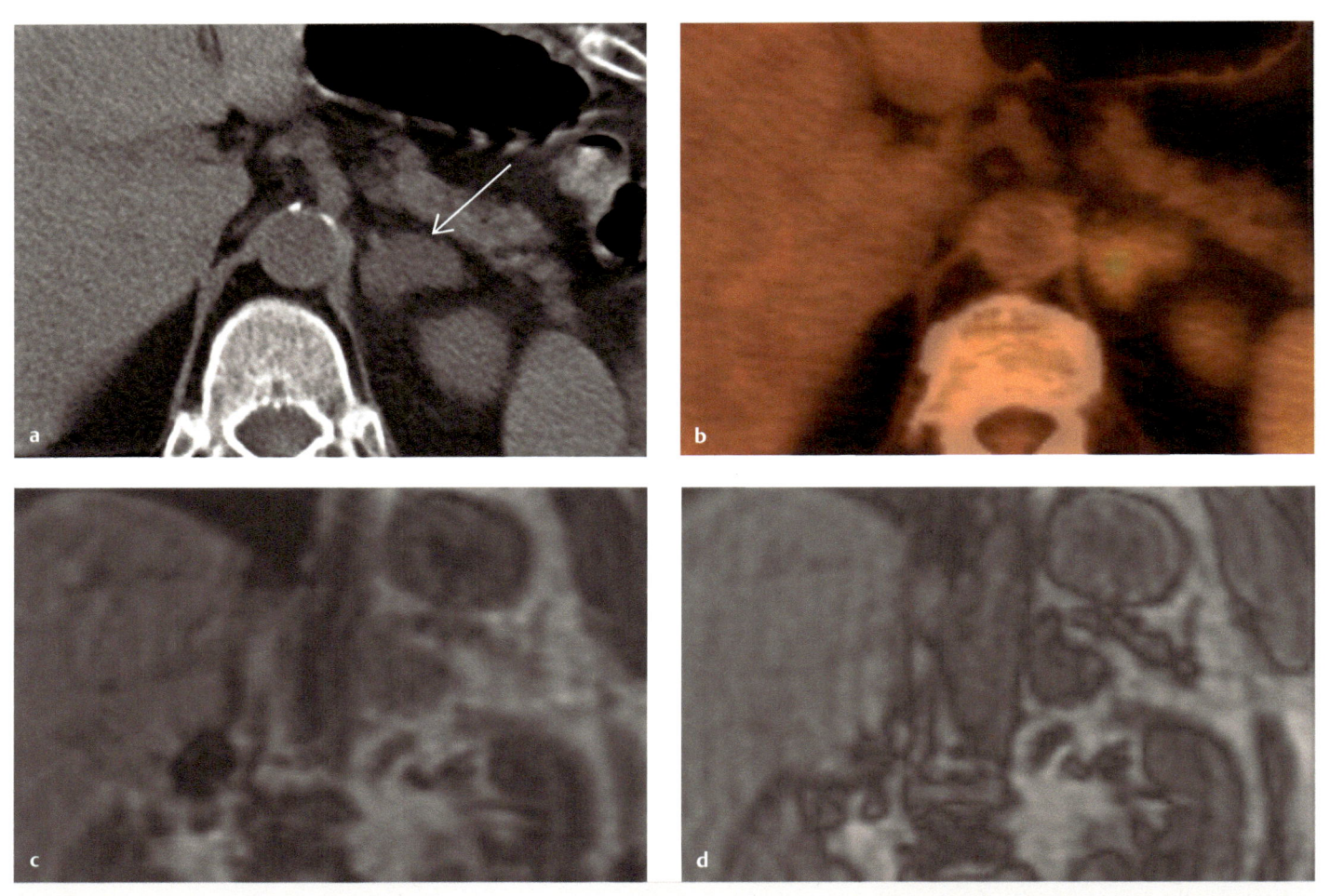

Fig. 10.6 PET-CT in a patient with lung cancer (cT3 cN1 Mx). (a) Staging CT demonstrates a mass in the left adrenal gland (arrow). **(b)** Glucose metabolism of the left adrenal mass on FDG PET-CT is suspicious for malignancy, with a maximum standardized uptake value of 4.1. The unenhanced CT attenuation of the mass is 6 HU, however. **(c)** In-phase image. **(d)** Opposed-phase image shows marked loss of signal intensity, indicating a false-positive PET scan.

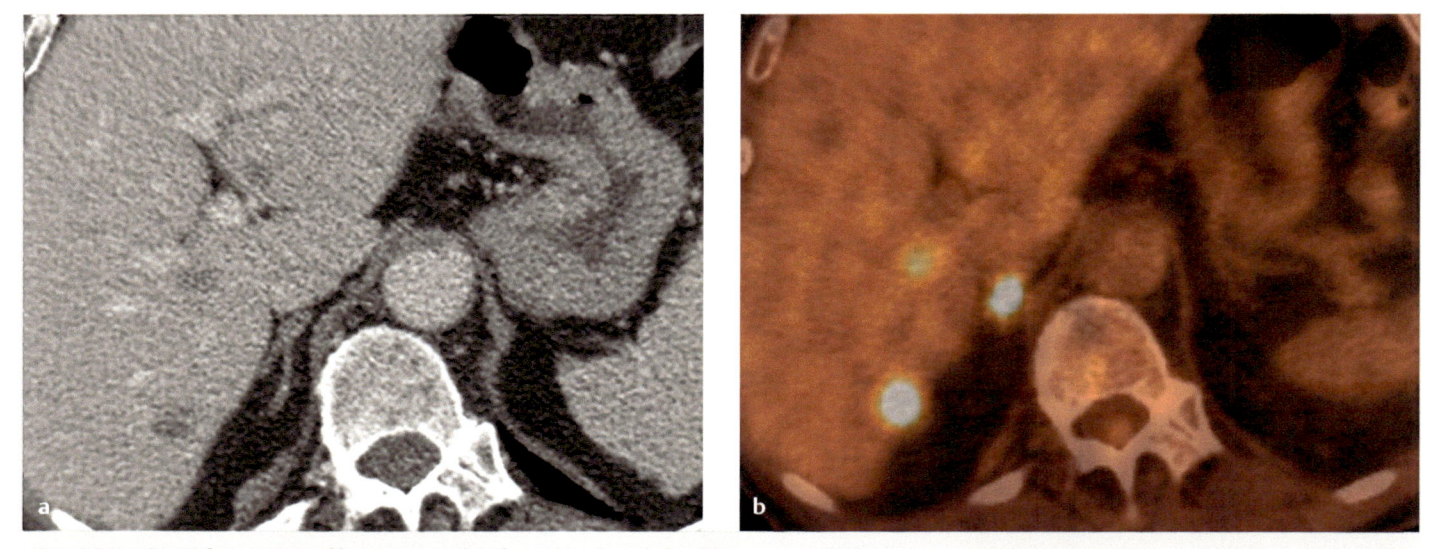

Fig. 10.7 PET-CT for staging of lung cancer. (a) The right adrenal gland has a normal CT appearance. **(b)** Increased glucose metabolism of the right adrenal gland is suspicious for malignancy, however. Two metabolically active hepatic metastases are noted as incidental findings.

strengths). The signal intensities of the adrenal mass in the in-phase image are compared with a reference tissue (e.g., liver or spleen). If a definite loss of signal intensity is seen in the opposed-phase image, this indicates a significant lipid component and confirms a diagnosis of adenoma (▶ Fig. 10.8). In routine clinical settings, this technique can yield acceptable results without taking ROI measurements or calculating ratios; the subjective impression of the radiologist is entirely satisfactory.

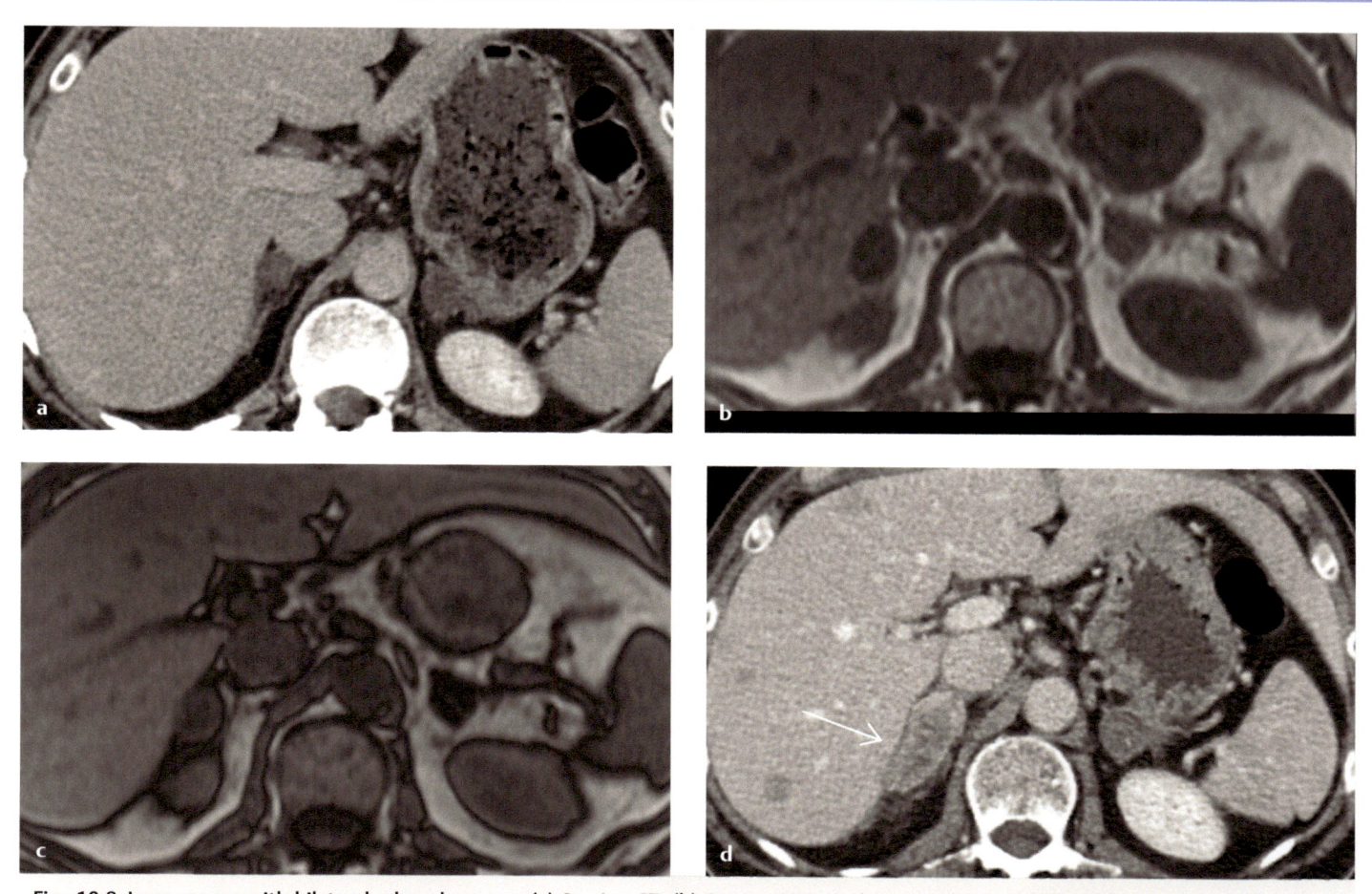

Fig. 10.8 Lung cancer with bilateral adrenal masses. (a) Staging CT. (b) Staging MRI, in-phase image. The left adrenal gland is hyperintense to spleen, while the right adrenal gland is isointense to spleen. (c) Staging MRI, opposed-phase image. The left adrenal gland is hypointense to spleen, while the right adrenal gland is still isointense. This confirms the adenoma in the left adrenal gland. An adenoma was not confirmed on the right side. (d) CT 2 months later shows enlargement of the right (metastatic) adrenal gland (arrow), but not of the left. New hepatic metastases are noted as incidental findings.

Note

In the case of lipid-poor adenomas with a CT attenuation greater than 10 HU, chemical shift MRI can diagnose the adenomas with a sensitivity of 67% and specificity of 100%.[5] Thus, chemical shift imaging is superior to the measurement of CT attenuation on unenhanced CT.

It should be noted, however, that adrenal metastases from clear-cell renal cell carcinoma may contain so much fat that they show loss of signal intensity in opposed-phase images. This limitation has become clinically important now that the ipsilateral adrenal gland is no longer routinely removed as part of a tumor nephrectomy. Very rarely, metastases from hepatocellular carcinoma or liposarcoma may also show decreased signal intensity in the opposed-phase image.

Other MR techniques have no practical significance, so the imaging protocol for adenoma detection is generally quite short, consisting of a T2W sequence plus T1W in-phase and opposed-phase sequences. Administration of contrast medium is unnecessary, as different adrenal pathologies do not show consistent, significant differences in their enhancement characteristics. Diffusion-weighted (DW) images do not aid in differential diagnosis. More detailed MRI protocols are necessary only for malignant lesions associated with local organ invasion and metastasis.

10.2.5 Adrenal Vein Sampling

Adrenal vein blood sampling is done almost exclusively in patients with primary hyperaldosteronism to determine whether autonomous overproduction of aldosterone is unilateral or bilateral. The adrenal veins are catheterized through a transvenous, inguinal approach under imaging guidance. Aldosterone and cortisol in the adrenal venous blood are compared with levels in peripheral blood drawn from the inguinal sheath, for example. The left adrenal vein opens into the left renal vein. The right adrenal vein opens directly into the inferior vena cava and is therefore more difficult to catheterize (see ▶ Fig. 10.9b, c). Technical details can be found in the relevant literature.[6]

10.3 Diseases

10.3.1 Incidentalomas

▶ **Brief definition.** An incidentaloma of the adrenal gland is a clinically silent adrenal mass more than 1 cm in diameter that is detected incidentally in an imaging examination.[7] The incidence of these lesions is approximately 1% in abdominal CT examinations.

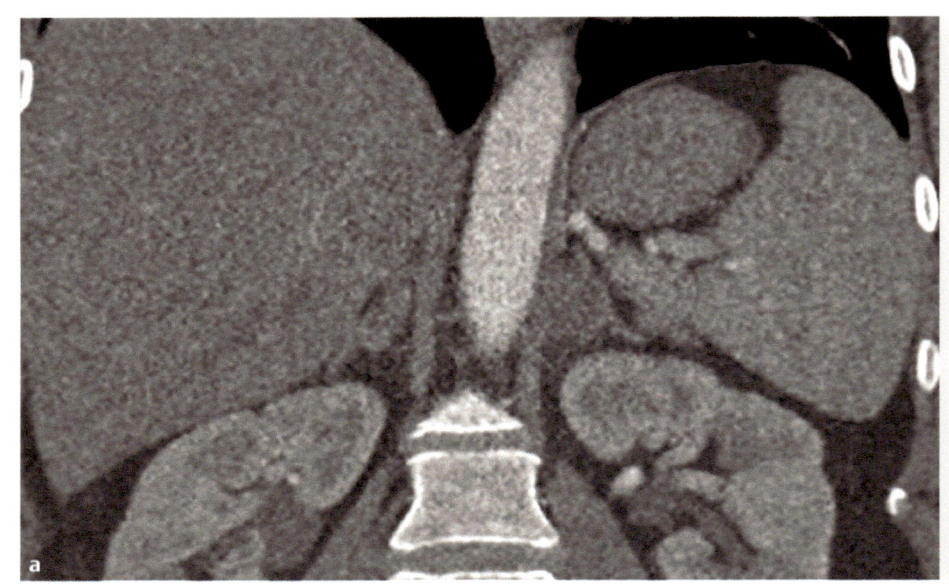

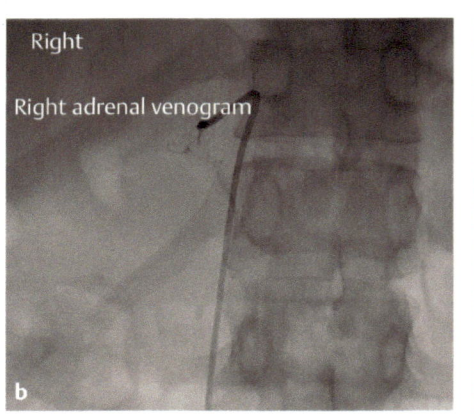

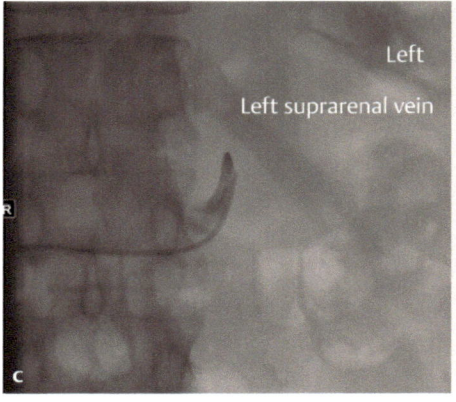

Fig. 10.9 Arterial hypertension in primary hyperaldosteronism. CT findings (a) do not permit a definite management decision, so selective adrenal vein sampling is performed (b, c). The ratio of aldosterone to cortisol is 22 for the right adrenal gland, 393 for the left adrenal gland, and 27 for peripheral blood. The test shows a massive increase on the left side and suppression on the right side with a selectivity index greater than 6 for the right adrenal vein. This means that left adrenalectomy is indicated for an aldosterone-producing adenoma on the left side. Left adrenalectomy was subsequently performed and was followed by clinical recovery with a normalization of laboratory values. (a) CT demonstrates a right adrenal adenoma measuring 24 mm × 11 mm and a left adrenal adenoma measuring 28 mm × 21 mm. (b) Venous blood sampling from the right adrenal vein. (c) Venous blood sampling from the left adrenal vein.

▶ **Imaging signs.** The term "incidentaloma" is a tentative working diagnosis that is replaced by a definitive diagnosis once a suitable work-up has been completed. Laboratory tests are done first to exclude subclinical hypercortisolism, pheochromocytoma, and primary hyperaldosteronism. Once subclinical hormonal dysfunction has been excluded, an oncologic work-up should begin. This includes measuring the size of the incidentaloma and determining whether its imaging features are consistent with adenoma. Both criteria are used to estimate the likelihood that the incidentaloma is an adrenocortical carcinoma.[8] Adrenocortical carcinomas smaller than 4 cm are extremely rare. If a lesion of this size has imaging features typical of adenoma, the finding is sufficient to exclude adrenocortical carcinoma. Most adrenocortical carcinomas are larger than 6 cm. Approximately 25% of adrenal masses of this size are adrenocortical carcinomas. Consequently, incidentalomas of this size are always surgically removed, regardless of their imaging features. Even with incidentalomas in the 4 to 6 cm size range that have adenoma-type imaging features, there is still a significant risk of adrenocortical carcinoma, and adrenalectomy is indicated. It is more difficult to find evidence-based criteria for managing incidentalomas smaller than 4 cm with adenoma-type imaging features, and for incidentalomas in the 4 to 6 cm range with adenoma-type features. In both cases the lesions are most likely adenomas, but there is a small degree of residual uncertainty. Because there are no current study data on the most effective way to resolve this uncertainty, management decisions should be made case by case. Yearly biochemical follow-ups for a 5-years are recommended for unresected tumors (▶ Fig. 10.10).

▶ **Pitfalls**
- Occasionally the term "incidentaloma" is used synonymously with "benign adrenal mass." This is inaccurate. *Incidentaloma* refers only to an adrenal mass that has been detected incidentally: by definition, it is uncertain whether the lesion is benign or malignant. Algorithms have been developed specifically for making this determination.
- The most common radiological error is to describe the incidentaloma without investigating it further. The necessary endocrine work-up is very often omitted, and it is equally common to omit differentiating studies such as histogram analysis and chemical shift imaging. Thus the lesion remains unidentified, even though its identity could often be established with a proper work-up.
- The differential diagnosis of incidentaloma is usually limited to a possible metastasis. The question of greatest interest, however, is whether the incidentaloma could be adrenocortical carcinoma, since patients could benefit from the resection of that lesion but not from the resection of a metastasis.
- Incidentalomas smaller than 4 cm that have adenoma-type imaging features are commonly resected. This is a mistake, because nonfunctioning adenomas have no pathologic significance.

10.3 Diseases

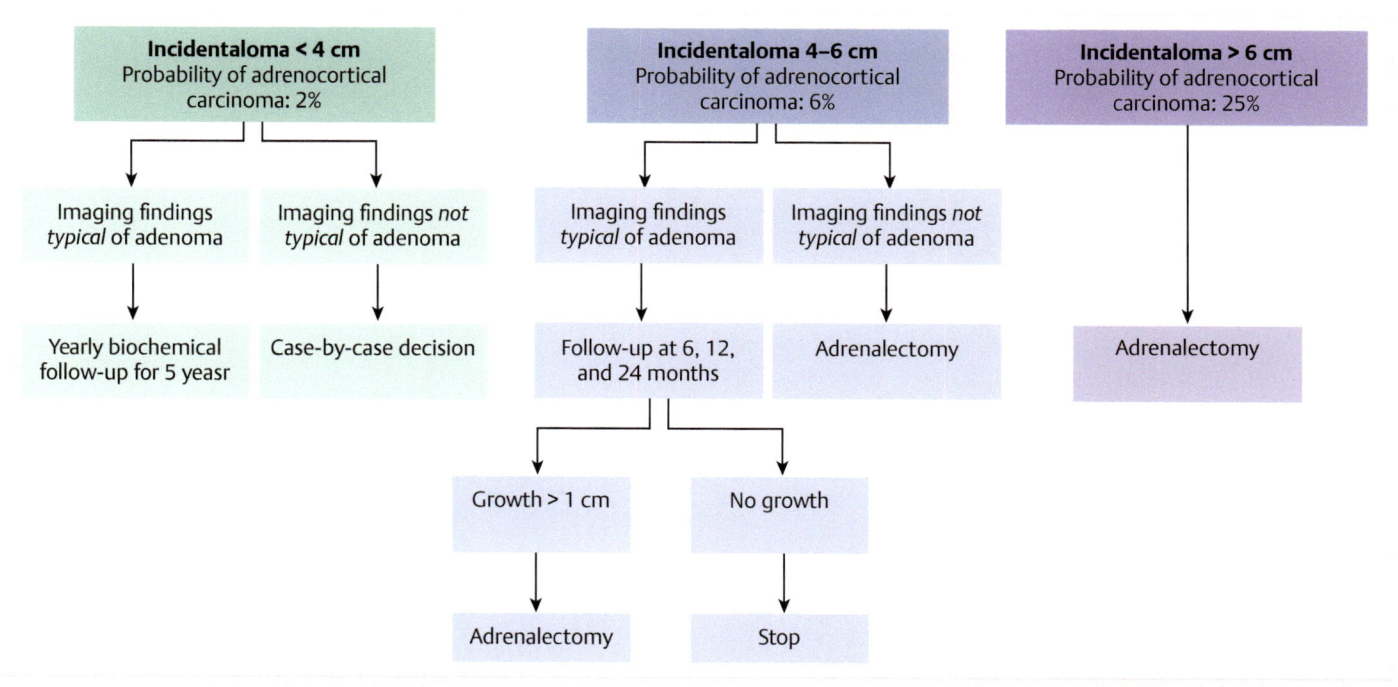

Fig. 10.10 Algorithm for the management of incidentalomas.

- ▶ **Key points.** Incidentalomas are incidentally detected adrenal masses. Algorithms are available for their endocrinologic and oncologic investigation. "Incidentaloma" is unacceptable as a definitive diagnosis.

10.3.2 Functional Disorders

Hypercortisolism

- ▶ **Brief definition.** Endogenous hypercortisolism is caused in 20% of cases by the overproduction of cortisol (ACTH-independent Cushing's syndrome) and in 80% of cases by the overproduction of adrenocorticotropic hormone (ACTH-dependent Cushing's syndrome). ACTH-independent Cushing's syndrome is caused by a cortisol-producing adrenal adenoma in two-thirds of cases and by an adrenocortical carcinoma in one-third of cases. Besides these unilateral forms of ACTH-independent Cushing's syndrome, there are very rare bilateral forms: micronodular ACTH-independent adrenal hyperplasia and macronodular ACTH-independent adrenal hyperplasia.

- ▶ **Selection of modalities.** Because many adrenocortical carcinomas have already metastasized at the time of diagnosis, CT has significant advantages over MRI as a staging examination. At the same time, a cortisol-producing adenoma can be elegantly demonstrated by MRI. In the very rare cases of bilateral hypersecretion, both CT and MRI should be employed.

- ▶ **Imaging signs.** Cortisol-producing adenomas average 3.5 cm in diameter (2.0–7.0 cm) and are lipid-rich with an unenhanced CT attenuation less than 10 HU.[9] Cortisol-producing carcinomas, in contrast, average 14.5 cm in size (7.5–21.0 cm) and are lipid-poor; their solid portions have an unenhanced CT attenuation greater than 10 HU. Approximately 90% of carcinomas contain necrotic areas. With micronodular hyperplasia, the adrenal glands are not generally enlarged but exhibit nodules no larger than 4 mm that are well defined because the adrenal gland between the nodules is thin due to the down-regulation of ACTH. The nodules are hypointense on T1W and T2W images because of their pigment content. With macronodular hyperplasia, the nodules are larger than 5 mm and the adrenal glands have the same appearance as in bilateral hyperplasia. The bilateral forms show loss of signal intensity in opposed-phase images; this is a strong diagnostic indicator in patients with ACTH-independent hypercortisolism.

- ▶ **Clinical features.** The clinical symptoms of hypercortisolism are caused by the metabolic effects of the increased cortisol. Typical manifestations are obesity, moon facies, glucose intolerance, muscle weakness, hypertension, altered mental status, hirsutism, impotence, and fractures.

Hyperaldosteronism

- ▶ **Brief definition.** This condition results from excessive aldosterone secretion due to an aldosterone-producing adrenal adenoma or bilateral hyperplasia of the adrenal glands. Although it was once thought that 80% of cases were due to adenoma and 20% to bilateral hyperplasia, today it is believed that these percentages are reversed.

> **Note**
>
> The role of radiology in hyperaldosteronism is to determine whether its cause is unilateral overproduction (adenoma) or bilateral overproduction (hyperplasia). This cannot be determined from morphological findings alone (i.e., sectional imaging).

- ▶ **Selection of modalities.** Conn adenomas are small lesions with an average diameter of 1.5 cm (0.5–3.5 cm). The principal nodule in bilateral hyperplasia may be mistaken for an adenoma. Even if an adenoma is diagnosed, it is uncertain whether it is actually producing aldosterone. The prevalence of adrenal adenomas is very high. It is quite possible for a nonfunctioning adenoma

Adrenal Glands

to be present in bilateral hyperplasia. Morphological lesion detection requires the highest possible spatial resolution. This is accomplished best and most easily with CT, and accordingly this modality should always be used in primary hyperaldosteronism. Selective bilateral adrenal vein sampling is also indicated (▶ Fig. 10.9). The ratio of aldosterone to cortisol is determined for diagnosis of the laterality of aldosterone secretion. With an aldosterone-producing adenoma, the aldosterone:cortisol ratio should be elevated relative to that in the peripheral blood; the ratio in the contralateral (suppressed) adrenal gland should be lower than in the peripheral blood.[10] Venous blood sampling from the right adrenal vein is technically challenging, even for experienced examiners, and selective bilateral sampling is successful in only 70 to 90% of cases. CT is therefore an essential study.

▶ **Clinical features.** Primary hyperaldosteronism is the most common form of secondary hypertension and is present in 5 to 10% of hypertensive patients.

▶ **Pitfalls.** A common error is to refer patients with arterial hypertension for adrenal CT scans without a preliminary diagnosis of primary hyperaldosteronism.

> **Caution**
>
> The most common radiological error is overlooking Conn adenomas. Because they are often quite small, they may elude the untrained eye in images reconstructed with a 5-mm slice thickness, for example. This error can be avoided by evaluating thin slices (≤ 2 mm) and coronal and sagittal images reconstructed from isotropic voxels.

Another common mistake is to omit selective adrenal venous blood sampling. It has been shown that the results of adrenal vein sampling disagree with CT results in 38% of cases.[11] If only CT results were used to determine laterality, adrenalectomy would be performed in 15% of cases based on the incorrect assumption of an aldosterone-producing adenoma when bilateral hyperplasia is actually present. Relying on CT alone in these cases would result in unnecessary surgery. In 19% of cases, patients would be inappropriately excluded from adrenalectomy based on an erroneous diagnosis of bilateral hyperplasia when they actually have a surgically curable aldosterone-producing adenoma. In 4% of cases adrenalectomy would be performed on the wrong side; i.e., an adrenal gland with a nonfunctioning adenoma would be removed while leaving intact the contralateral adrenal gland with a (very small) aldosterone-producing adenoma.

▶ **Key points.** Primary hyperaldosteronism is diagnosed by laboratory tests, not by imaging. CT examination of the adrenal glands is combined with selective adrenal vein sampling to differentiate an aldosterone-producing adenoma (an indication for adrenalectomy) from bilateral adrenal hyperplasia (not an indication for adrenalectomy).

Pheochromocytoma

▶ **Brief definition.** Pheochromocytomas are catecholamine-producing neuroendocrine tumors that arise from the chromaffin cells of the adrenal medulla or extra-adrenal paraganglia.

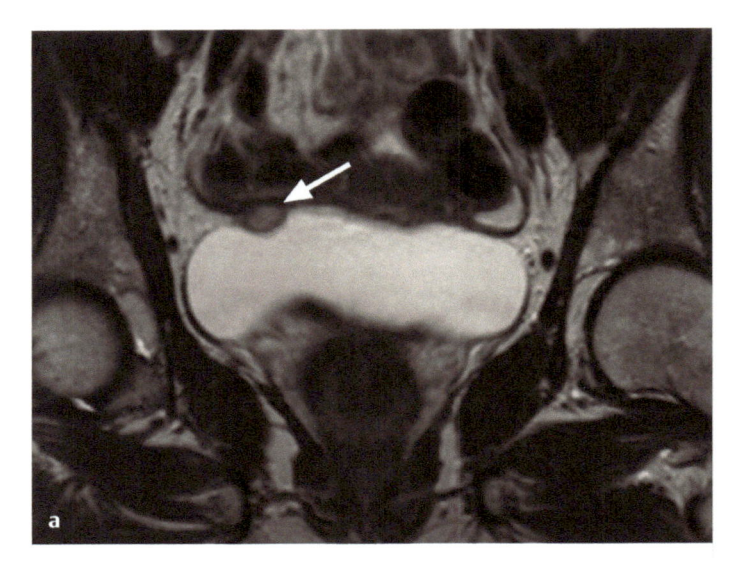

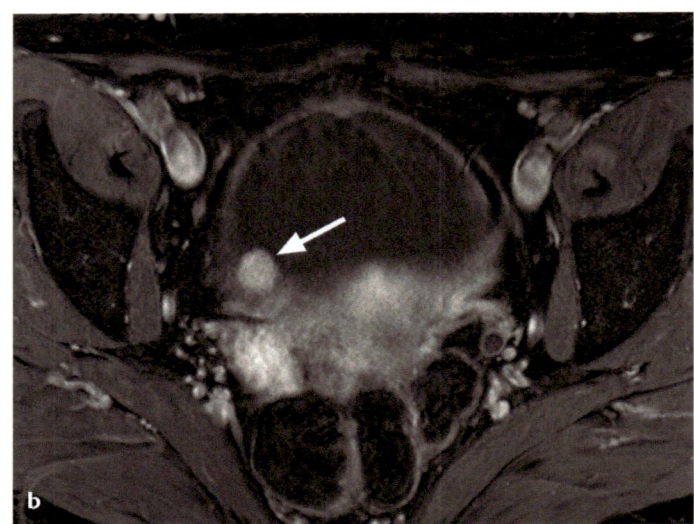

Fig. 10.11 Pheochromocytoma in the bladder wall. The lesion was detected incidentally at ultrasound. Definitive diagnosis was established by histology. (a) Coronal T2W image shows a moderately hyperintense mass in the roof of the bladder (arrow). (b) Axial T1W after IV injection of contrast medium shows intense, homogeneous enhancement (arrow).

Extra-adrenal pheochromocytomas are also called paragangliomas. Glomus tumors of the head and neck region (carotid body, glomus vagale, glomus jugulare) also are referred to as paragangliomas but almost never produce catecholamines. Catecholamine-producing pheochromocytomas are almost invariably located in the abdomen (▶ Fig. 10.11). Pheochromocytomas may be sporadic or hereditary in their occurrence, a distinction that is very important clinically. Sporadic cases are most commonly diagnosed between 40 and 50 years of age and tend to be solitary. Hereditary cases (multiple endocrine neoplasia, von Hippel–Lindau syndrome, neurofibromatosis type 1, familial paragangliomas) are also diagnosed in children and are often multifocal.[12]

▶ **Selection of modalities.** Once a pheochromocytoma has been diagnosed from laboratory tests, it is localized by imaging studies that supply functional information (MIBG [metaiodobenzylguanidine] scintigraphy) and anatomical details. Anatomical visualization can be accomplished with MRI and CT. Preparation for administration of contrast medium by alpha and beta blockade is no longer

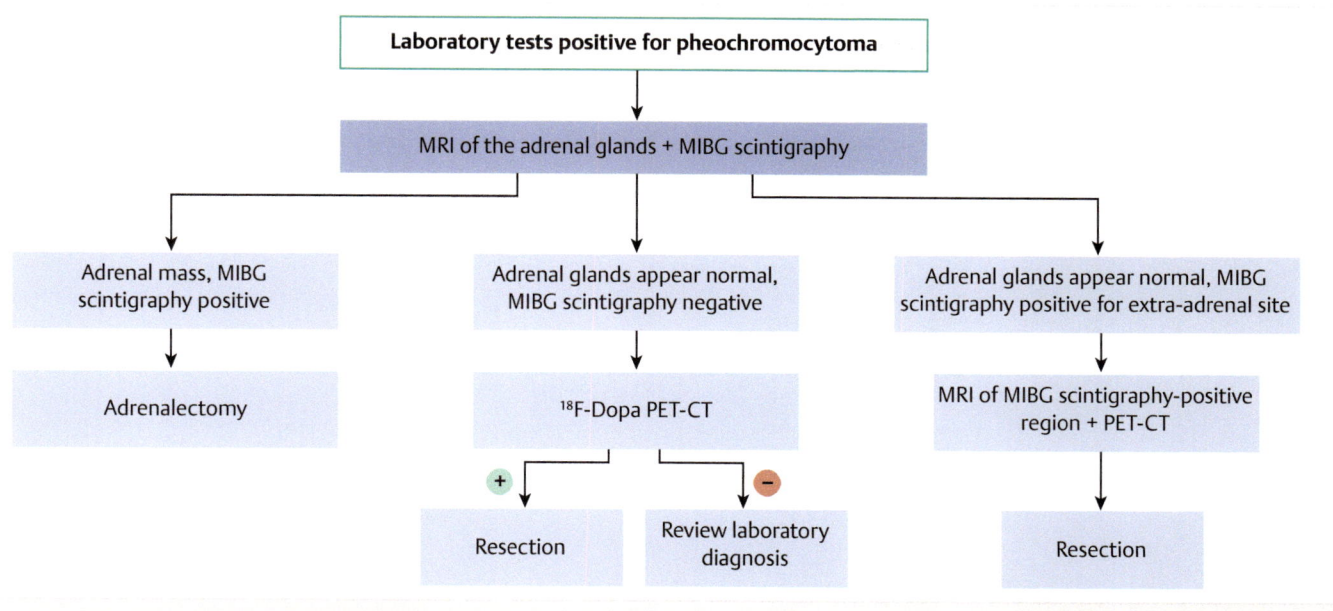

Fig. 10.12 Simplified diagnostic algorithm for pheochromocytoma.

necessary owing to the use of nonionic contrast media. PET has advantages over other diagnostic techniques in the investigation of malignant, extra-adrenal, and hereditary pheochromocytomas. The preferred tracer may be FDG, ^{18}F-DOPA, or perhaps both, depending on the situation.[13] A simplified flowchart for the diagnostic investigation of pheochromocytoma is shown in ▶ Fig. 10.12.

▶ **Imaging signs.** Sporadic pheochromocytomas are always large, with an average diameter of 5.5 cm. Hereditary pheochromocytomas may be very small. Pheochromocytomas present as nonadenomas on CT, i.e., their attenuation on unenhanced CT is greater than 10 HU and they do not show rapid washout of enhancement. Pheochromocytomas may contain large necrotic areas and may even have a cystic appearance, or they may be solid. From 10 to 20% of pheochromocytomas contain calcifications. Pheochromocytomas may contain areas of pure fat, causing them to be mistaken for adenomas or myelolipomas—an error that is preventable by adding laboratory tests and nuclear medicine scans. Pheochromocytomas also have the MRI characteristics of nonadenomas, showing no loss of signal intensity in the opposed-phase image relative to the in-phase image. They typically show high signal intensity on T2W images. Approximately 10% of lesions are isointense to CSF and 33% are hyperintense to liver and spleen (▶ Fig. 10.1). At least half of all pheochromocytomas have complex signal characteristics with T2-hyperintense components but an inhomogeneous pattern that is not

▶ **Clinical features.** Owing to frequent use of imaging studies and the screening of patients with a familial or genetic risk, asymptomatic pheochromocytomas are being diagnosed with greater frequency. Approximately 5% of all incidentalomas are pheochromocytomas, and approximately 25% of all pheochromocytomas are found in screenings for a different disease. It is difficult to diagnose pheochromocytoma from clinical signs and symptoms. No more than 0.5% of all patients with arterial hypertension have a pheochromocytoma. The hypertension in these cases may be persistent or may occur as intermittent hypertensive crises. Other possible symptoms are tachycardia, pallor, headache, anxiety, nausea, hyperglycemia, and weight loss.

▶ **Differential diagnosis.** If the basic rule of combining functional and anatomical imaging is followed, it is usually unnecessary to consider other possible diagnoses. There have been only anecdotal reports of false-positive MIBG findings due to adrenocortical carcinoma or infection. False-negative MIBG findings are also very rare.

Note

As a general rule, a negative MIBG scan excludes pheochromocytoma, while a positive MIBG scan confirms it.

Benign and malignant pheochromocytoma can be differentiated only by the detection of metastases (▶ Fig. 10.13). Not even a pathologist can make this differentiation. After the removal of a benign-appearing pheochromocytoma, therefore, patients with sporadic pheochromocytoma should remain in follow-up for at least 10 years, while patients with possible hereditary pheochromocytoma should be followed for life. Regular imaging is unnecessary for follow-up; clinical and laboratory follow-ups are satisfactory.

Note

A pheochromocytoma is diagnosed not by imaging but by laboratory tests. The role of imaging is not to establish the diagnosis but to localize a pheochromocytoma already diagnosed from laboratory tests.

▶ **Pitfalls.** Another common error is to omit functional imaging, generally in the form of MIBG scintigraphy. An adrenal mass is found, and the patient is referred for surgery. It is not unusual in such cases for patients with a classic diagnosis of "pheochromocytoma" to undergo surgery only to find that

Adrenal Glands

findings, the region of interest is imaged by MRI. If MIBG scintigraphy is negative, PET-CT should be performed. Barring significant comorbidity, pheochromocytoma is treated by surgical resection.

Virilization

▶ **Brief definition.** Virilization refers to the excessive and premature development of male secondary sex characteristics. The clinical presentation depends on patient gender and the onset of androgen overproduction. Boys and girls may be affected. Possible causes are:
- Adrenogenital syndrome.
- Androgen-producing adrenal adenoma.
- Androgen-producing adrenocortical carcinoma.
- Extra-adrenal pathology (e.g., polycystic ovaries or androgen-producing gonadal tumors).

Note

The role of imaging in virilization is to exclude or detect surgically treatable sources of androgen overproduction. The adrenal glands and gonads are examined.

▶ **Selection of modalities.** Newborns are examined with ultrasound. MRI of the adrenal glands is recommended in children and young adults due to radiation safety concerns; CT is also suitable in older adults. The ovaries are examined by transvaginal ultrasound. Ultrasound is also used for testicular imaging.

▶ **Imaging signs.** Adrenogenital syndrome is based on an autosomal recessive enzyme defect that affects steroid synthesis. The secretion of ACTH is up-regulated due to a deficiency of cortisol and possibly aldosterone. The ACTH excess greatly increases the production of androgens and stimulates growth of the adrenal glands. When children are diagnosed at birth, their adrenal glands appear normal but enlarged. A finding that one limb of an adrenal gland is more than 20 mm long and more than 4 mm wide is considered strong evidence of congenital adrenal hyperplasia. If an adrenogenital syndrome goes untreated (by steroid replacement) for a long period, the adrenal glands may lose their normal configuration and resemble tumors, although these changes will generally regress with steroid replacement. Some 80% of children with adrenocortical carcinoma present with virilization symptoms, compared with only 20 to 30% of adults.

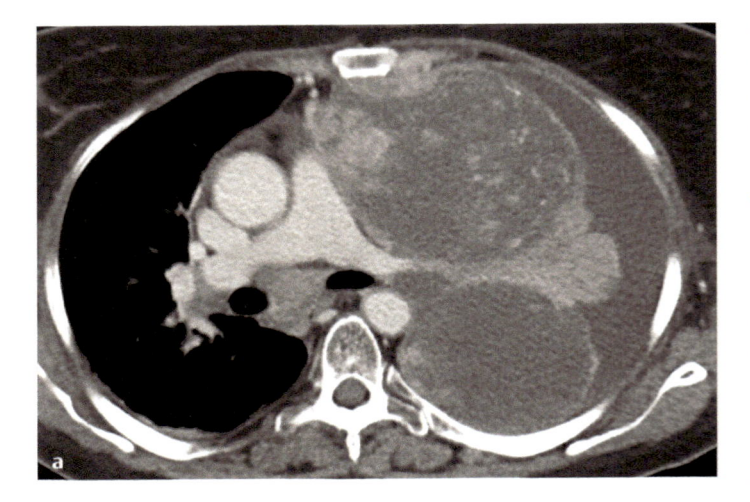

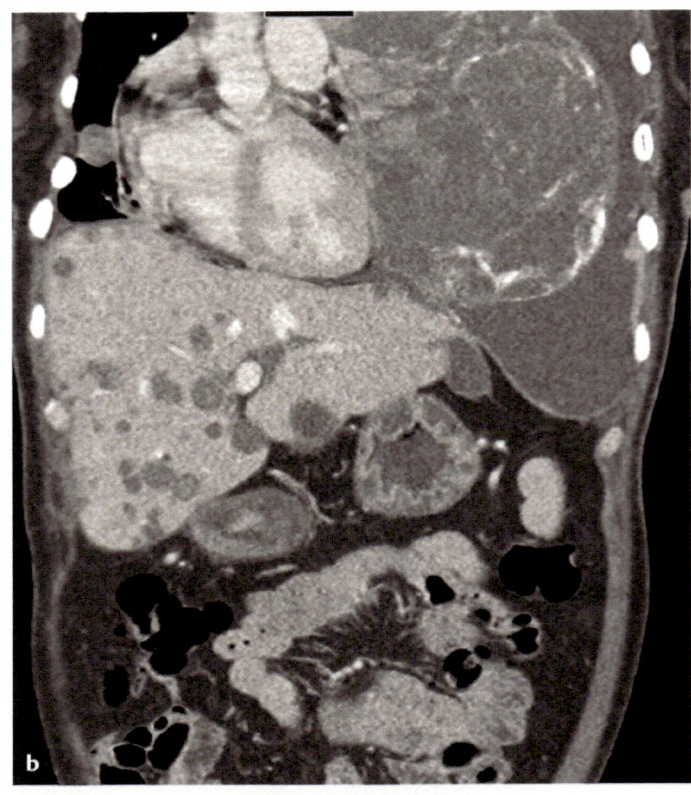

Fig. 10.13 **Metastatic pheochromocytoma.** Almost the entire left hemithorax is occupied by tumor and malignant effusion. CT shows bilateral hilar lymph node metastasis, multiple pulmonary metastases in the right lung, and multiple hepatic metastases. Skeletal metastases are not shown. (a) Axial image. (b) Coronal image.

histology refutes the diagnosis. Another risk of this practice is that it may fail to detect multifocality or metastasis. MIBG scintigraphy is definitely indicated if the likelihood of malignancy is relatively high, as in the case of large tumors (> 5 cm) and extra-adrenal occurrence. MIBG scintigraphy is also essential if the tumor is relatively small (< 3 cm), as the small size makes the presence of a sporadic pheochromocytoma unlikely. A third error, not uncommon, is the biopsy of a pheochromocytoma, provoking a hypertensive crisis.[14]

▶ **Key points.** Pheochromocytoma is diagnosed by laboratory testing. The next step is a localizing study by MIBG scintigraphy and MRI of the adrenal glands. With positive extra-adrenal MIBG

▶ **Clinical features.** An androgen excess that is already present at birth leads to female pseudohermaphroditism in girls, characterized by virilization of the external genitalia. The clitoris is hypertrophic but the uterus, ovaries, fallopian tubes, and vagina are present. Boys with a congenital androgen excess appear normal at birth but within 6 months manifest signs of premature development (precocious pseudopuberty) with penile hypertrophy. Girls and boys experience excessive growth of facial and body hair (hirsutism), deepening of the voice, acne, adult body odor, and accelerated skeletal maturation.

▶ **Pitfalls.** The common practice of referring children with virilization symptoms for ultrasound scans of the adrenal glands and gonads has seldom led to catastrophic results, but only because androgen-producing tumors are extremely rare. Ultrasound is the imaging modality of choice for evaluating the adrenal glands in newborns but it is inadequate in all other patients.

▶ **Key points.** Congenital adrenal hyperplasia can be diagnosed sonographically, and the underlying hormonal disorders are detected in laboratory tests. If it is necessary to exclude an androgen-producing adrenal tumor in an older child or adult, sectional imaging (MRI or CT) is required.

Adrenocortical Insufficiency

▶ **Brief definition.** The loss of adrenal function is a rare disorder manifested by a loss of adrenocortical hormones, whereas loss of the adrenal medulla (which secretes catecholamines) can be compensated by other sympathetic nervous centers. Destruction of the adrenal glands themselves is known as primary adrenocortical insufficiency; it leads to a failure of cortisol and aldosterone secretion and to the hypersecretion of ACTH. The absence of adrenal stimulation due to a failure of ACTH secretion is termed secondary adrenocortical insufficiency. Adrenocortical insufficiency in the western world is caused by autoimmune adrenalitis in approximately 80% of cases. Worldwide, the most frequent cause of adrenal gland destruction is infection, usually tuberculosis.

▶ **Selection of modalities.** Imaging studies are of secondary importance in the work-up of adrenocortical insufficiency, which is diagnosed by the determination of cortisol and ACTH levels. Autoimmune adrenalitis can be diagnosed by the detection of corresponding antibodies. The adrenal glands are examined sonographically in small children; otherwise, CT is the imaging modality of choice.

▶ **Imaging signs.** In patients with chronic adrenocortical insufficiency due to autoimmune adrenalitis or infection, the adrenal glands are atrophic and often contain calcifications. In acute adrenocortical insufficiency, both adrenal glands are enlarged or expanded by a tumor or hematoma.

▶ **Clinical features.** In the acute form of adrenocortical insufficiency (addisonian crisis), the lack of mineralocorticoids leads to dehydration, hypotension, oliguria, and shock. Gastrointestinal complaints with abdominal pain, nausea, and stool changes are often misdiagnosed as gastroenteritis. The chronic form of adrenocortical insufficiency (Addison's disease) also causes gastrointestinal symptoms and hypotension along with fatigue syndrome and characteristic hyperpigmentation of the skin and mucous membranes.

▶ **Pitfalls.** Adrenal function cannot be assessed by imaging. Physicians often fall into mechanistic thinking and assume (or fear) that a bilateral adrenal process must signify adrenal insufficiency. In reality this almost never happens, despite the relatively high frequency of bilateral adrenal hematomas and bilateral adrenal metastases, since more than 90% of the adrenocortical tissue would have to be destroyed before clinical symptoms appeared. An exception is Waterhouse–Friderichsen syndrome, when bleeding into the adrenal glands due to meningococcal sepsis, for example, leads to acute adrenocortical insufficiency.

▶ **Key points.** Adrenocortical insufficiency is diagnosed from clinical signs and laboratory test results. In some cases imaging can help determine the etiology of primary adrenal insufficiency.

10.3.3 Tumors

Adrenal Cysts

▶ **Brief definition.** Adrenal cysts are very rare. Their pathogenic classification as endothelial, epithelial, parasitic, or pseudocystic is of no clinical importance.

> **Note**
>
> An adrenal cyst may be a cystic neoplasm even in the absence of detectable solid components.[15]

Cystic neuroblastomas, adenomas, pheochromocytomas, and adrenocortical carcinomas may be encountered. Possible calcification of the cyst wall is not a useful criterion for differentiating cystic neoplasms from nonneoplastic cysts. Adrenal cysts may be detected incidentally (cystic incidentaloma) or may be symptomatic.

▶ **Clinical features.** The most common symptom is pain. As with solid incidentalomas, diagnosis begins with endocrine tests, chiefly to exclude a pheochromocytoma (▶ Fig. 10.14). Symptomatic or hormonally active cysts are surgically removed. Cysts larger than 6 cm should also be removed. Cysts in the range of 4 to 6 cm should at least be followed. Asymptomatic cysts smaller than 4 cm with nonsuspicious imaging features do not require further action. Needle aspiration of an adrenal cyst is never indicated.

Adrenal Myelolipoma

▶ **Brief definition.** Myelolipomas are benign tumorlike lesions composed of pure fatty tissue with embedded hematopoietic cells heaving the features of bone marrow or extramedullary hematopoiesis. Approximately 85% of myelolipomas originate in the adrenal gland, and most are unilateral. It is less common to find bilateral adrenal myelolipomas or extra-adrenal myolipomas, which may occur at a variety of sites.

▶ **Selection of modalities.** If its fatty component is dominant, myelolipoma has a pathognomonic ultrasound appearance characterized by smooth outer margins and a uniformly echogenic tumor matrix. Otherwise both CT and MRI are excellent for identifying the typical fatty component of myelolipoma (▶ Fig. 10.15). Diagnostic accuracy depends greatly on the proportion of the myeloid component. In many cases myelolipomas have a lipoma-like appearance with only a subtle myeloid component.[16] Strictly speaking, the differentiation between lipoma and myelolipoma is not possible, but neither is it necessary. If there are no clinical symptoms, neither entity has significant implications. Because adrenal myelolipoma is far more common than lipoma, it is always reasonable to assume a myelolipoma. If this is a confident diagnosis in an asymptomatic patient, no surgery or follow-up is needed. The remote possibility of intralesional hemorrhage does not justify adrenalectomy. The more dominant the myeloid component and the less conspicuous the fatty component, the less certain is the "dogma" that the detection of mature fat proves

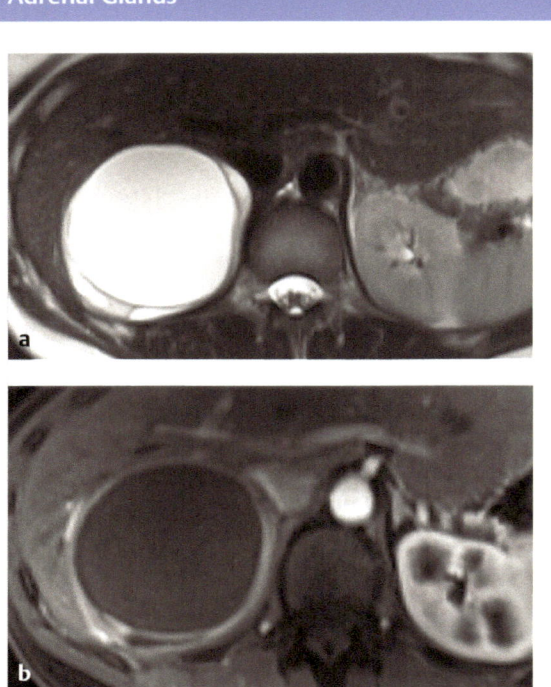

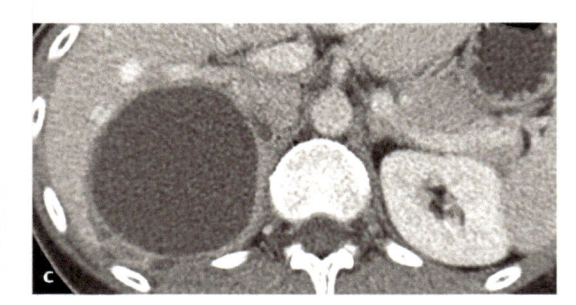

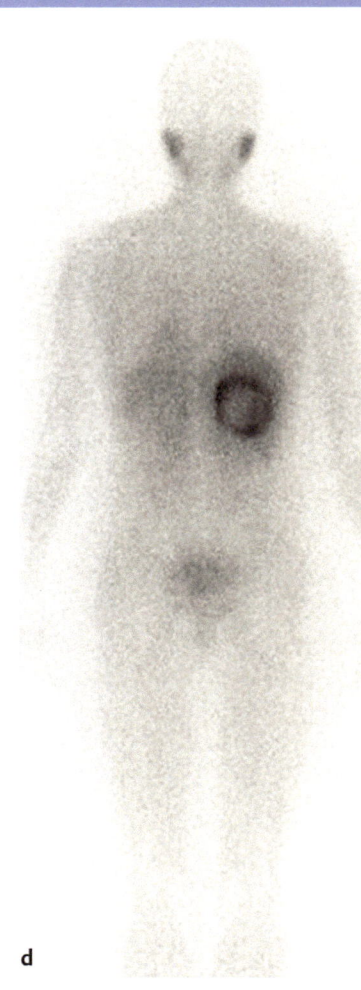

Fig. 10.14 **Cystic pheochromocytoma** in a patient with a 4-year history of paroxysmal complaints lasting 15 to 30 minutes: tachycardia, blood pressure elevation, pallor, nausea, vomiting, and headache. Plasma and urinary metanephrine and normetanephrine levels were markedly elevated. MIBG scintigraphy (**d**) shows a ring pattern of tracer uptake in the right upper quadrant. CT (**c**) and MRI (**a, b**) show a 9-cm cystic mass with an enhancing, solid-appearing rim. (**a**) T2W image. (**b**) T1W image after injection of contrast medium. (**c**) CT after injection of contrast medium. (**d**) MIBG (metaiodobenzylguanidine) scintigraphy.

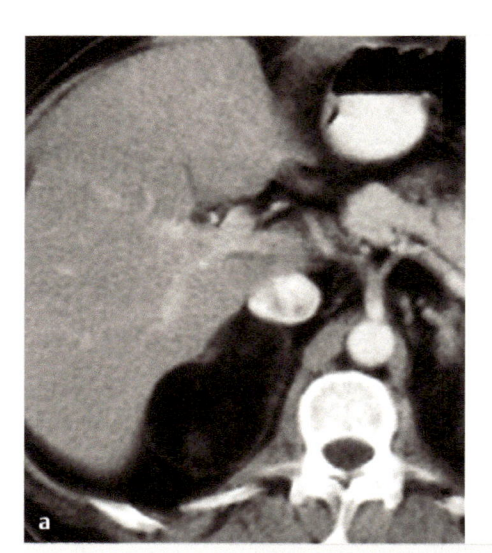

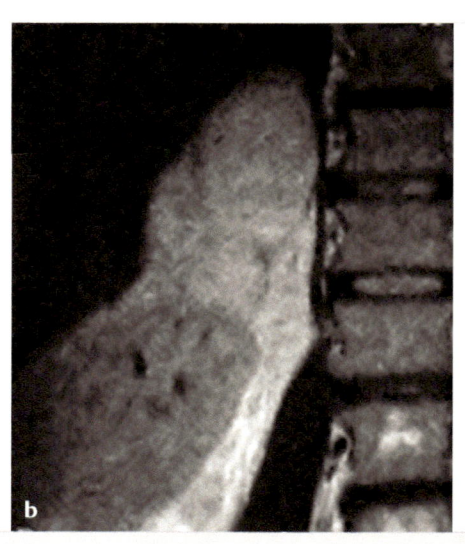

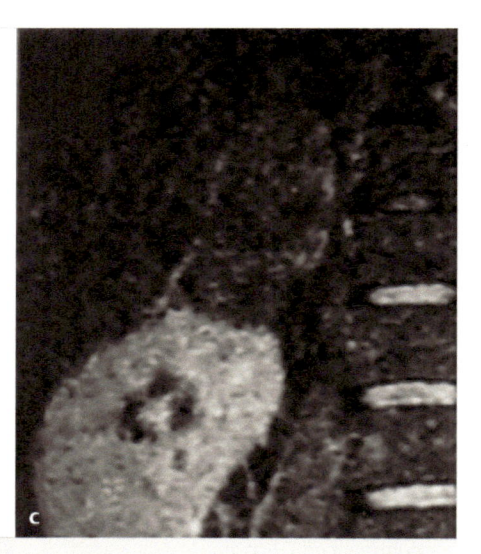

Fig. 10.15 **Myelolipoma of the right adrenal gland consisting mostly of fat.** (**a**) CT shows fat-equivalent attenuation values. (**b**) On T2W MRI the myelolipoma has approximately the same signal intensity as retroperitoneal fat. (**c**) Frequency-selective fat saturation causes equal suppression of the myelolipoma and of retroperitoneal fat.

that the adrenal lesion is benign. There are case reports of fat occurring in adenomas, pheochromocytoma, and adrenocortical carcinoma. For lesions larger than 6 cm, therefore, there is a valid rationale for adrenalectomy. Percutaneous biopsy could be considered for smaller lesions, although this procedure is very rarely indicated for adrenal lesions. In the case of myelolipoma, however, it may be considered under the circumstances stated above, since the detection of hematopoietic cells is pathognomonic and serves to distinguish the tumor from adrenocortical carcinoma or liposarcoma.

▶ **Imaging signs.** Myelolipomas generally range in size from 2 to 10 cm but may be considerably larger. On ultrasound, myelolipoma shows relatively homogeneous echogenicity with marked posterior acoustic shadowing. On CT, the detection of pure fatty tissue with attenuation values of −50 to −90 HU is diagnostic of myelolipoma. The fat is detectable on MRI by its high signal intensity on T1W and T2W images combined with fat-saturated sequences.

▶ **Clinical features.** Adrenal myelolipoma is diagnosed at approximately 50 years of age on average, and most patients are asymptomatic. Myelolipomas themselves do not cause endocrine dysfunction, but there are case reports of "collision tumors," meaning two different entities occurring in the same adrenal gland. Intralesional hemorrhage in an adrenal myelolipoma is a very rare complication.

▶ **Pitfalls.** Adrenal myelolipoma is unrelated to renal angiomyolipoma. The "myelo" in myelolipoma refers to bone marrow, while the "myo" in angiomyolipoma refers to muscle tissue.

Adrenal Adenomas

▶ **Brief definition.** Adrenal adenomas are benign neoplasms of the adrenal cortex; they may develop in any of the layers comprising the adrenal cortex. Adrenocortical adenomas are very common and have a prevalence of approximately 25% in autopsy series. They may be hormonally active (functioning) or inactive (nonfunctioning).

▶ **Selection of modalities.** The main role of adrenal imaging is to confirm that an adrenal lesion is an adenoma. Almost all methods are based on detecting the high lipid content of adenomas, as described earlier in Chapter 10.3.1 (p. 379) (▶ Fig. 10.2). Recommendations on the use of cutoff values claim a 100% diagnostic specificity, indicating a 0% rate of false-positive diagnoses. In other words, if the radiologist says a lesion is adenoma, it is adenoma. Conversely, the sensitivity of adenoma detection is less than 100%, so there is a potential for false-negative diagnosis. This means that some adenomas (lipid-poor!) are diagnosed as nonadenomas on CT or MRI.

A second basic rule in adrenal imaging is not to try to differentiate between benign and malignant adrenal lesions but rather between adenoma (benign) and nonadenoma (benign or malignant). Pheochromocytomas, for example, are predominantly benign, but histologically and radiologically they are nonadenomas and cannot be positively distinguished from, say, adrenocortical carcinoma or metastasis by CT or MRI.

> **Note**
>
> Findings that prove adenoma:
> - Unenhanced CT attenuation less than 10 HU.
> - More than 10% negative pixels in the region of interest based on histogram analysis.
> - Significant loss of signal intensity in opposed-phase images relative to in-phase images.

▶ **Imaging signs.** Studies indicate that adenomas show greater contrast enhancement than nonadenomas and that the washout of enhancement is more rapid in adenomas than in nonadenomas. No imaging or nuclear medicine technique can discriminate between functionally active and inactive adenomas. This can be done only by adrenal vein sampling with the determination of hormone titers.

▶ **Pitfalls.** Adrenal adenoma and myelolipoma both have a typically high fat content, but their patterns of fat distribution are different: The fat in adenomas is located within the cytoplasm and is detectable by in-phase and opposed-phase MRI. In the case of myelolipoma, portions of the lesion consist of pure fat and are detectable by frequency-selective fat saturation, for example. The application of frequency-selective fat saturation to adrenal adenoma will not cause signal suppression like that in the fatty components of myelolipoma. A loss of signal intensity on opposed-phase images can occur only if lipid and water protons make similar contributions to signal intensity. Frequency-selective fat saturation can suppress MR signal intensity only if lipid protons contribute most of the signal.

Adrenal Metastases

▶ **Brief definition.** The adrenal glands are a common site of metastasis, most notably from primary tumors of the lung, breast, skin (melanoma), kidney, liver, thyroid gland, and colon. If staging examination reveals an adrenal mass that may be a metastatic deposit, it is essential to establish a definitive diagnosis, generally by histological examination. This is because curative therapy is no longer an option in patients with metastatic stage IV disease, and resection of the primary tumor is usually withheld. Since benign adrenal adenomas are common, an adrenal mass coexisting with a primary tumor does not necessarily indicate a metastatic stage of disease. In patients with non–small cell lung cancer, for example, only about one-third of adrenal masses found at staging examination are actually metastatic. In patients with renal cell carcinoma, fewer than half of ipsilateral adrenal masses are metastatic. Thus, a final diagnosis must be established to ensure that the potentially curative resection of a primary tumor is not mistakenly withheld. If an adenoma is not proven by imaging, this can generally be accomplished by CT-guided biopsy.

▶ **Selection of modalities.** CT is the most commonly used staging modality. Unenhanced CT is not available in most cases, making it more difficult to evaluate the fat content of an indeterminate adrenal lesion. If the lesion is an extremely lipid-rich adenoma, a CT attenuation value less than 10 HU may be found in the hepatic arterial phase, for example. But in most cases even lipid-rich adenomas will have an attenuation greater than 10 HU due to IV administration of contrast medium. Doubts can often be resolved by a histogram analysis showing more than 10% negative pixels, which positively identifies the lesion as adenoma. If this is unsuccessful, the work-up should be supplemented by either unenhanced CT or chemical shift MRI.

▶ **Imaging signs.** In contrast to adrenocortical carcinoma, there is no relationship between the size of an adrenal lesion and the likelihood that it is metastatic. Moreover, homogeneity or nonhomogeneity cannot differentiate adenoma from metastasis. Both entities are generally homogeneous until they have grown large enough to develop regressive changes. As noted earlier in connection with adrenal adenomas (p. 387), adenomas and nonadenomas of the adrenal gland have approximately the same attenuation values on routine contrast-enhanced CT. This is because adenomas have a lower primary density but show greater enhancement than nonadenomas.

▶ **Key points.** Adrenal masses detected during tumor staging are very often benign. Before curative treatment is withheld, a potential metastasis should be histologically confirmed unless there is other convincing evidence of metastatic disease. All noninvasive options for confirming adenoma should be exhausted before proceeding with an invasive diagnostic procedure.

Neuroblastoma

▶ **Brief definition.** Neuroblastoma, ganglioneuroblastoma, and ganglioneuroma are tumors of the sympathetic nervous system that develop from cells of the primitive neural crest. As long as these precursor cells are undifferentiated, they are called neuroblasts. Cells that have differentiated are called ganglion cells. An undifferentiated malignant tumor composed of neuroblasts is called a neuroblastoma. A differentiated benign tumor composed of mature ganglion cells is called a ganglioneuroma. A tumor that contains mature and immature cells is called a ganglioneuroblastoma. This group of neuroectodermal tumors is also referred to as neuroblastic tumors or ganglioglioma-ganglioneuroblastoma-neuroblastoma complex; these terms refer to the cellular origin of the different tumors. Some of these tumors show many similarities on diagnostic imaging, but clinically they are very diverse. Given their common origin, the tumors have identical potential sites of occurrence anywhere within the distribution of the sympathetic ganglia. Approximately 35% of neuroblastomas occur in the adrenal gland; the rest may occur anywhere along the sympathetic trunk from the neck to the pelvis.

▶ **Selection of modalities.** The standard practice is to examine the affected region with ultrasound and MRI. Approximately 75% of neuroblastomas are located in the abdomen. In these cases the MRI protocol should include at least coronal and axial T2W sequences, an axial T1W sequence, and an axial fat-suppressed T1W sequence after administration of contrast medium. This is considered the minimal protocol. The author recommends a more detailed protocol that also includes fat-suppressed T2W and DWI sequences, with the same sequences acquired before and after injection of contrast medium. A complete staging work-up will also include chest radiographs, ultrasound scans of the neck, abdomen, and brain (if the fontanelle is still open), and MIBG scintigraphy (▶ Fig. 10.16). Additional studies (cranial MRI, bone scintigraphy, skeletal radiography) are performed only in selected cases. CT is expressly not recommended.

▶ **Imaging signs.** Neuroblastoma has an average size of 8 cm at the time of diagnosis. In newborns, the tumor tends to undergo hemorrhagic necrosis and may have a purely cystic appearance. In older children the tumor is more frequently solid and somewhat inhomogeneous due to calcifications, small hemorrhages, and necrosis. It shows moderate contrast enhancement. Abdominal vessels are displaced and stretched by the tumor. The staging of neuroblastoma is based on the International Neuroblastoma Staging System (▶ Table 10.1),[17] which takes into account clinical, radiological, and surgical findings.

▶ **Clinical features.** Most children are 1 to 5 years of age (average 22 months) when diagnosed. They present with a painless abdominal mass or signs suggestive of metastasis such as periorbital ecchymosis or bone pain. Approximately 70% of children have metastatic disease at the time of diagnosis.

▶ **Differential diagnosis.** Ganglioneuroblastoma and ganglioneuroma have the same imaging appearance as neuroblastoma and require histological differentiation. A prevertebral abscess can mimic a neuroblastic tumor arising from the sympathetic trunk (▶ Fig. 10.17). Hematoma in newborns requires differentiation from neuroblastoma (▶ Fig. 10.4). This is aided by epidemiology: nontraumatic adrenal hematomas occur almost exclusively in the neonatal period. They may be unilateral or bilateral. At ultrasound they are initially echogenic and appear solid, resembling neuroblastoma. Over time they may liquefy and mimic a cystic neuroblastoma. Definitive resolution of the hematoma takes weeks or months and calcifications often form, just as in neuroblastoma. Thus, the differentiation of hematoma from neuroblastoma is difficult on the basis of a snapshot view of the process at any given time. If the lesion more closely resembles a hematoma, ultrasound follow-up is indicated. Otherwise the investigation of a neonatal adrenal mass that is not definitely a hematoma should follow this protocol:
- Children under 3 months of age:
  - Inspection of the skin.
  - Laboratory tests.
  - Ultrasound imaging of the brain, neck, and abdomen.
- Children over 3 months of age:
  - MRI of the affected region.
  - MIBG scintigraphy.
  - Bone marrow aspiration.
  - Tumor biopsy.

Wilms's tumor is an important differential diagnosis in older children. In many cases multiplanar reconstructions will help localize the tumor origin to the kidney; this differs from neuroblastoma, which displaces the kidney. Often enough, however, it is difficult to attribute the tumor to a specific organ. Differentiation may be aided by noting that Wilms's tumor is rarely calcified and metastasizes to the lung in approximately 20% of cases, whereas neuroblastoma rarely shows pulmonary metastasis. Wilms's tumor often shows direct extension into the renal vein and inferior vena cava; this does not occur with neuroblastoma. Wilms's tumor displaces blood vessels, while neuroblastoma tends to encase them.

Adrenal Hematoma

▶ **Brief definition.** Spontaneous adrenal hematomas occur almost exclusively in the neonatal period. babies that are large for gestational age are most commonly affected. The hematomas may be unilateral or bilateral. Posttraumatic adrenal hematomas usually result from blunt abdominal trauma but may also occur as a complication of ACTH therapy, anticoagulant drugs, or sepsis.

▶ **Selection of modalities.** Ultrasound is the imaging modality of choice in neonates and children. Color duplex ultrasound is used initially to differentiate adrenal hematoma from neoplastic changes such as neuroblastoma (p. 388). Remaining doubts are resolved by MRI and, if necessary, MIBG scintigraphy. CT is

10.3 Diseases

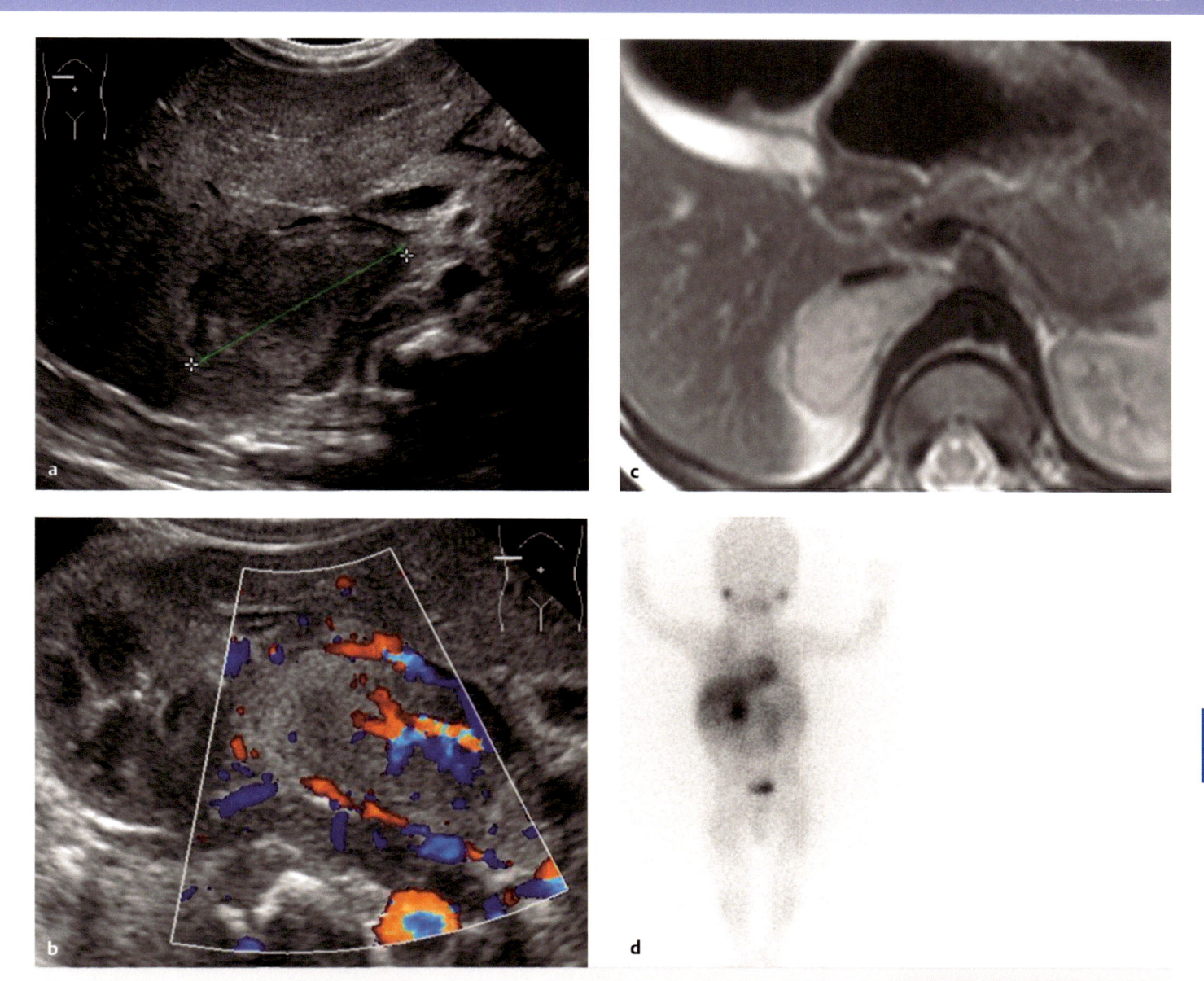

Fig. 10.16 Neuroblastoma in a full term newborn. (a) Routine ultrasound scan demonstrates a 2.6-cm mass in the right adrenal gland. (b) Color duplex scan shows vascularity that is suspicious for neonatal neuroblastoma. (c) MRI was performed in accordance with the staging protocol. (d) Staging MIBG scintigraphy was also performed, showing uptake in the adrenal neuroblastoma. There is no evidence of metastasis.

Table 10.1 International neuroblastoma staging system

Stage	Description
1	Localized tumor confined to the area of origin. Complete gross excision, with or without microscopic residual disease. Identifiable ipsilateral and contralateral lymph nodes negative microscopically
2A	Unilateral tumor with incomplete gross excision. Identifiable ipsilateral and contralateral lymph nodes negative microscopically
2B	Unilateral tumor with incomplete gross excision. Positive ipsilateral lymph nodes. Identifiable contralateral lymph nodes negative microscopically
3	Tumor infiltrating across the midline with or without regional lymph node involvement. Unilateral tumor with contralateral regional lymph node involvement. Midline tumor with bilateral regional lymph node involvement
4	Dissemination of tumor to distant lymph nodes, bone, bone marrow, liver, and/or other organs (except as defined in stage 4S)
4S	Localized primary tumor as defined for Stage 1 or 2. Dissemination limited to liver, skin and/or bone marrow. By definition, only children < 1 year old are affected. Fewer than 10% tumor cells in bone marrow, and MIBG scintigraphy negative for bone marrow

Abbreviation: MIBG, metaiodobenzylguanidine.

HU. It does not enhance after IV administration of contrast medium. Adrenal hematomas are usually confined to the adrenal gland, although adjacent stranding may be seen. Retroperitoneal or even intraperitoneal fluid collections are a less common finding.

Note
The main clinical significance of adrenal hematomas is that they require differentiation from neoplasms.

▶ **Clinical features.** Adrenal hematoma itself is generally asymptomatic. Even bilateral hematomas do not cause adrenal insufficiency (p. 385) as a rule.

▶ **Differential diagnosis.** Neuroblastoma is an important differential diagnosis in newborns. In adults with no definite trauma history, the differential diagnosis should include bilateral adenomas, metastases, lymphomas, or even hyperplasia if findings are less pronounced. A simple but very effective rule for differentiating hematoma from neoplasm is that hematomas become smaller over time. Thus, ultrasound follow-ups should employ standard scan planes to allow for reproducible size measurements.

Adrenocortical Carcinoma

▶ **Brief definition.** Adrenocortical carcinoma is a rare aggressive malignancy arising from cells of the adrenal cortex.

▶ **Imaging signs.** The work-up of an incidentally detected adrenal mass that may be adrenocortical carcinoma is covered in Chapter 10.3.1 (p. 379). CT is the preferred staging modality for more advanced adrenocortical carcinoma that has invaded adjacent structures (T3) or organs (T4) or has metastasized. Bone scintigraphy is also performed, and conventional radiographs should be obtained if uptake is noted outside the CT scan volume. On average, adrenocortical carcinomas are larger than 11 cm at the time of diagnosis.[18] They are inhomogeneous due to hemorrhage and necrosis, and 30% of the tumors contain calcifications. Even smaller adrenocortical carcinomas always have imaging features that are not typical of adenoma (▶ Fig. 10.3). There have been no reports of adrenocortical carcinoma with a CT attenuation less than 13 HU. The T stage in the TNM system reflects the growth characteristics of the tumor (▶ Table 10.2). As the tumor enlarges, its margins become infiltrative with respect to surrounding fat. Later the tumor invades adjacent organs and structures including the renal vein and inferior vena cava (▶ Fig. 10.18). In 30% of cases the carcinoma has already metastasized to lung, liver, and bone at the time of initial diagnosis.

▶ **Clinical features.** Adrenocortical carcinoma has a bimodal age distribution with peaks in childhood and in the fourth to fifth decades. Detailed biochemical testing will show that virtually all adrenocortical carcinomas are hormonally active, but only some patients develop signs or symptoms of a hormonal excess. Approximately 60% of patients present with a rapidly progressive Cushing's syndrome or virilization. Adrenocortical carcinoma is the most frequent cause of Cushing's syndrome in children. Patients with a nonfunctioning adrenocortical carcinoma may present with abdominal fullness, nausea, and vomiting.

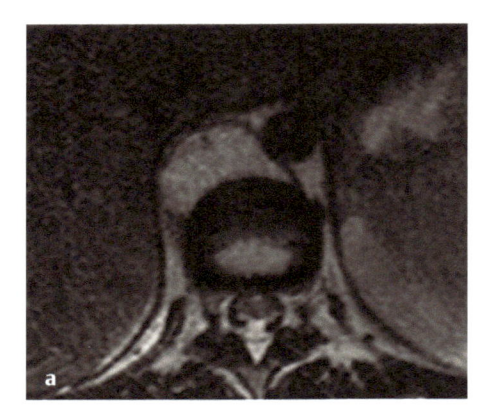

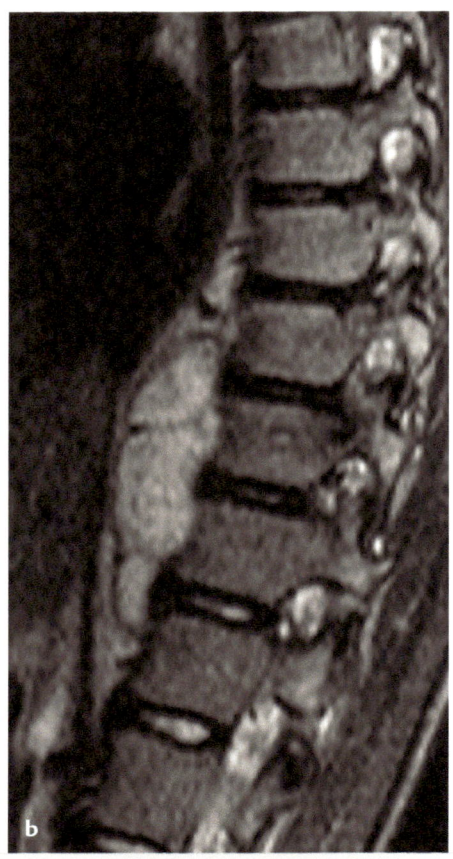

Fig. 10.17 Prevertebral abscess in a 13-year-old girl with inflammatory signs, recurrent febrile episodes, and back pain. MRI demonstrates a prevertebral mass that resembles a neuroblastic tumor. However, detailed image analysis shows that the mass is posterior to the anterior longitudinal ligament, while the sympathetic trunk and the tumors arising from it are anterior to the anterior longitudinal ligament. Tumor markers were negative. Blood culture was positive for brucellosis. The lesion resolved completely in response to antibiotic therapy. **(a)** T2 W MRI. **(b)** STIR (short tau inversion recovery) image.

generally used in adults and in patients who have sustained high-impact trauma.

▶ **Imaging signs.** Spontaneous adrenal hematoma in newborns and traumatic adrenal hematoma have the same appearance on ultrasound. An acute hemorrhage is isoechoic or hyperechoic. The hematoma becomes hypoechoic with passage of time. A pseudocyst and/or calcifications may eventually develop. Color duplex ultrasound shows absence of vascularity. On CT, the hematoma is hyperdense in the acute phase with attenuation values of 50 to 90

10.3 Diseases

Table 10.2 TNM classification of adrenocortical carcinoma

Designation	Description
Primary tumor	
T1	Tumor 5 cm or less in greatest dimension, no extra-adrenal invasion
T2	Tumor more than 5 cm in greatest dimension, no extra-adrenal invasion
T3	Tumor of any size with local invasion, but not invading adjacent organs
T4	Tumor of any size with invasion of adjacent organs or extension into the renal vein (inferior vena cava)
Lymph nodes	
N0	No regional lymph node metastasis
N1	Regional lymph node metastasis
Distant metastasis	
M0	No distant metastasis
M1	Distant metastasis

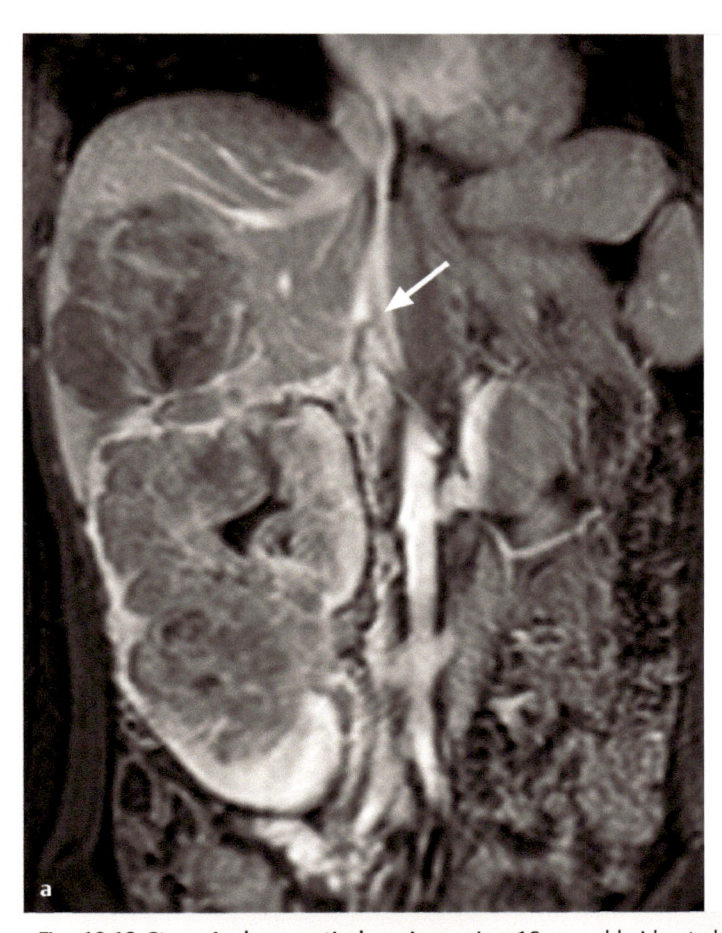

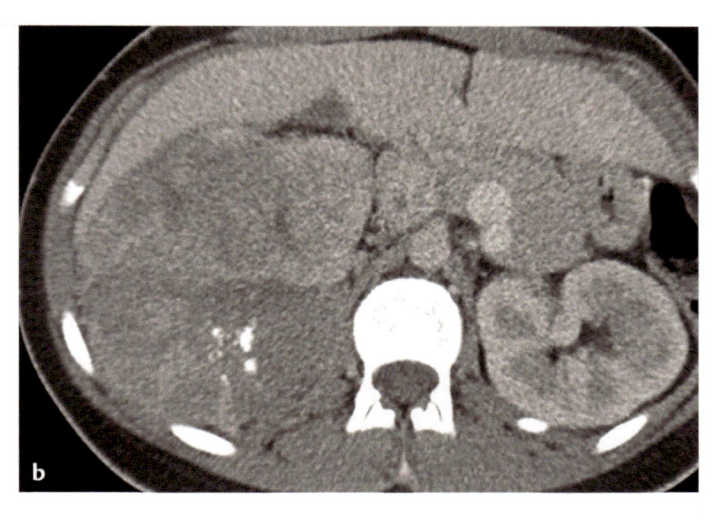

Fig. 10.18 **Stage 4 adrenocortical carcinoma** in a 16-year-old girl noted to have a palpable abdominal mass during investigation of Crohn disease. (a) T1 W MRI after injection of contrast medium shows a 24-cm tumor that has invaded the liver and kidney, with extension into the inferior vena cava (arrow). (b) CT reveals intratumoral necrotic areas and calcifications.

Bibliography

[1] Ho LM, Paulson EK, Brady MJ, Wong TZ, Schindera ST. Lipid-poor adenomas on unenhanced CT: does histogram analysis increase sensitivity compared with a mean attenuation threshold? AJR Am J Roentgenol. 2008; 191(1):234–238

[2] Blake MA, Kalra MK, Sweeney AT, et al. Distinguishing benign from malignant adrenal masses: multi-detector row CT protocol with 10-minute delay. Radiology. 2006; 238(2):578–585

[3] Caoili EM, Korobkin M, Francis IR, et al. Adrenal masses: characterization with combined unenhanced and delayed enhanced CT. Radiology. 2002; 222(3):629–633

[4] Perri M, Erba P, Volterrani D, et al. Adrenal masses in patients with cancer: PET/CT characterization with combined CT histogram and standardized uptake value PET analysis. AJR Am J Roentgenol. 2011; 197(1):209–216

[5] Haider MA, Ghai S, Jhaveri K, Lockwood G. Chemical shift MR imaging of hyperattenuating (> 10 HU) adrenal masses: does it still have a role? Radiology. 2004; 231(3):711–716

[6] Daunt N. Adrenal vein sampling: how to make it quick, easy, and successful. Radiographics. 2005; 25 Suppl 1:S143–S158

[7] Fischer E, Beuschlein F. Inzidentalom und subklinische Funktionsstörungen der Nebenniere. Dtsch Med Wochenschr. 2013; 138(8):375–380

[8] Grumbach MM, Biller BMK, Braunstein GD, et al. Management of the clinically inapparent adrenal mass ("incidentaloma"). Ann Intern Med. 2003; 138(5):424–429

[9] Rockall AG, Babar SA, Sohaib SA, et al. CT and MR imaging of the adrenal glands in ACTH-independent Cushing syndrome. Radiographics. 2004; 24(2):435–452

[10] Mulatero P, Bertello C, Sukor N, et al. Impact of different diagnostic criteria during adrenal vein sampling on reproducibility of subtype diagnosis in patients with primary aldosteronism. Hypertension. 2010; 55(3):667–673

[11] Kempers MJE, Lenders JWM, van Outheusden L, et al. Systematic review: diagnostic procedures to differentiate unilateral from bilateral adrenal abnormality in primary aldosteronism. Ann Intern Med. 2009; 151(5):329–337

[12] Lenders JWM, Eisenhofer G, Mannelli M, Pacak K. Phaeochromocytoma. Lancet. 2005; 366(9486):665–675

[13] Taïeb D, Timmers HJ, Hindié E, et al. European Association of Nuclear Medicine. EANM 2012 guidelines for radionuclide imaging of phaeochromocytoma and paraganglioma. Eur J Nucl Med Mol Imaging. 2012; 39(12):1977–1995

[14] Vanderveen KA, Thompson SM, Callstrom MR, et al. Biopsy of pheochromocytomas and paragangliomas: potential for disaster. Surgery. 2009; 146(6):1158–1166

[15] Erickson LA, Lloyd RV, Hartman R, Thompson G. Cystic adrenal neoplasms. Cancer. 2004; 101(7):1537–1544

[16] Rao P, Kenney PJ, Wagner BJ, Davidson AJ. Imaging and pathologic features of myelolipoma. Radiographics. 1997; 17(6):1373–1385

[17] Brodeur GM, Pritchard J, Berthold F, et al. Revisions of the international criteria for neuroblastoma diagnosis, staging, and response to treatment. J Clin Oncol. 1993; 11(8):1466–1477

[18] Fassnacht M, Kroiss M, Allolio B. Update in adrenocortical carcinoma. J Clin Endocrinol Metab. 2013; 98(12):4551–4564

11 Kidney and Urinary Tract

Ulrike I. Attenberger, Johanna Nissen, and Metin Sertdemir

11.1 Kidney

11.1.1 Imaging

Ultrasound

Ultrasound imaging is widely used for examining the kidneys and urinary tract, especially in the emergency work-up of hydronephrosis (▶ Fig. 11.1) and its prevention. The advent of contrast-enhanced ultrasound imaging has significantly increased the sensitivity of this modality in the evaluation of renal masses.[1]

Radiography

The sectional imaging modalities, CT and MRI, have increasingly replaced conventional radiography in recent years because they can provide detailed views that are not obscured by superimposed structures. Today the use of conventional radiography and fluoroscopy is limited to selected applications such as evaluation of the urethra, especially in male patients.

Voiding Cystourethrography

Voiding cystourethrography is an excellent study for investigating reflux in the pediatric age group.

Computed Tomography

Computed tomography (CT) is the modality of choice for imaging the kidneys, investigating masses, and numerous other applications. The imaging protocol varies considerably depending on the indication.

Following the publication by Smith et al. in 1996, the excretory urogram, which had been the mainstay for the diagnostic investigation of urolithiasis up to that time, was increasingly replaced by modern low-dose CT. When used in a low-dose protocol, CT provides a sensitivity of 96%, specificity of 99%, and diagnostic accuracy of 98% in the detection of urinary stones.[2,3] A modern low-dose CT protocol employs a tube voltage in the range of 100 to 140 kV. Because the CT imaging of urinary stones involves the detection of high-contrast structures, radiation dose reduction is achieved principally by reducing the tube current, time product which ranges from approximately 20 to 40 mAs.

The size, shape, location, and even the composition of urinary stones can be evaluated with CT.[2] In patients with known radiopaque stones, follow-up examinations based on a combination of plain radiographs and ultrasound scans can provide sensitivity of 58 to 100% and specificity of 37 to 100%.[4,5,6,7]

The introduction of dual-energy technology has taken us beyond simple stone detection to characterization of stones in terms of chemical composition. This is particularly important with regard to further management, in as much as uric acid stones (15% of all stones) are treated medically whereas magnesium ammonium phosphate stones (struvite stones, infection stones; 11% of total) are often treatable by extracorporeal shockwave lithotripsy. On the other hand, calcium phosphate stones (9% of total) and cysteine stones (1% of total) are relatively resistant to treatment by shockwave lithotripsy. Dual-energy CT technology can differentiate uric acid stones from non-uric acid stones with high accuracy on the basis of differences in their X-ray attenuation at different tube voltages.[10,11] Several studies have also shown that dual-energy CT can differentiate cysteine stones from magnesium ammonium phosphate stones.[12,13,14] Dual-energy CT acquires two data sets from the same anatomical region at different X-ray energies (80 and 140 kV or 100 and 150 kV). Stone discrimination is based on the principle that the attenuation properties of different tissue components of high atomic number [and hence high nuclear charge] differ from each other as a function of the applied tube voltage. In multiphase examinations of the kidneys with contrast medium, the voltage-dependent differentiation of calcium and iodine also enables us to omit the acquisition of an unenhanced phase because a "virtual unenhanced series" can be generated from the dual-energy CT data sets.

Another advantage of CT over excretory urography is the ability to image the renal parenchyma and ureters in a single examination. In patients with abdominal trauma, CT permits a rapid diagnostic evaluation for hemorrhage and ureteral injury. The main disadvantages of CT relate to cumulative radiation exposure from multiphase protocols and the use of iodinated contrast medium in patients with impaired renal function. However, further technical advances in CT with regard to detector technology and iterative reconstruction techniques that provide diagnostic images despite lower doses of contrast medium and lower radiation dose will eliminate most of these limitations in the years ahead.

A multiphase protocol should be used in the investigation of renal masses. An unenhanced spiral acquisition permits accurate evaluation of enhancement in postcontrast acquisitions, since renal masses may already be hyperdense on precontrast scans. The same tube voltage and current should be used in all phases

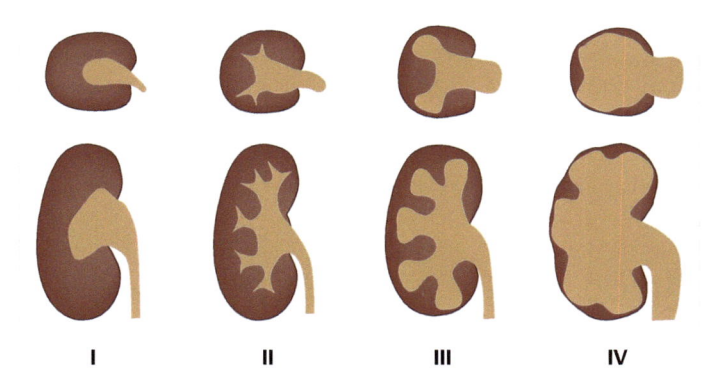

Fig. 11.1 Radiological grades of hydronephrosis. Grade I: dilatation of the renal pelvis without dilatation of the calyces; no parenchymal atrophy. Grade II: dilatation of the renal pelvis and calyces; papillary tips are preserved, no blunting of the fornices, no parenchymal atrophy. Grade III: marked dilatation of the renal pelvis and calyces; signs of parenchymal atrophy (flattening of papillae and blunting of fornices). Grade IV: gross dilatation of the pelvicalyceal system with loss of borders between the renal pelvis and calyces; almost complete atrophy of the renal parenchyma ("hydronephrotic sac").

to ensure that later measurements of attenuation values will not be distorted and unevaluable due to a different signal-to-noise ratios. Assuming that constant scan parameters are maintained, an attenuation increase of 10 HU is considered the threshold value for contrast enhancement.

In contrast-enhanced imaging of the kidneys, various phases are distinguished in both CT and MRI:
- *Corticomedullary (arterial) phase*: This phase begins approximately 20 to 30 seconds after injection of contrast medium, depending on the cardiac stroke volume. The arteries are clearly depicted in this phase, and veins are also defined owing to the high volume of renal blood flow. Malignant tumors such as renal cell carcinoma are hyperperfused, and most are clearly visualized in the arterial phase.
- *Venous phase*: This phase begins approximately 50 seconds after injection of contrast medium. The late venous phase begins at approximately 90 seconds.
- *Parenchymal (nephrographic) phase*: This phase is reached approximately 100 seconds after injection of contrast medium. The parenchymal phase is best for detecting malignant tumors, as hypervascular tumors appear hypodense at this time. Consequently, this is the only mandatory phase that is stipulated in current recommendations.
- *Urographic phase*: This delayed phase, characterized by the renal excretion of contrast medium, begins approximately 5 minutes after injection of contrast medium. Contrast medium fills the renal pelvis at this time, allowing urographic phase imaging.

Note
In CT the urographic phase can be combined with the nephrographic phase to reduce radiation exposure. This is done by injecting an initial contrast bolus of approximately 40 mL immediately after the unenhanced series. A second bolus with the rest of the contrast dose is injected 5 minutes later. Spiral acquisition is started after a delay of 100 seconds and displays the nephrographic phase for the renal parenchyma, while the renal pelvis and ureter are already opacified from the first bolus.

Magnetic Resonance Imaging

A standard magnetic resonance imaging (MRI) protocol for the kidney and urinary tract should consist of the following sequences:
- *T2W sequences*: Coronal T2W sequences can detect inflammatory changes such as a psoas abscess in the retroperitoneum. Axial T2W sequences, with their black-blood information, are particularly useful for excluding a possible tumor thrombus in the renal vein secondary to advanced renal cell carcinoma. Additionally, T2W sequences can supply key diagnostic information on pheochromocytoma and renal cysts owing to their specific signal characteristics. They are also excellent for the visualization of lymph nodes.
- *T1W sequences*: In-phase and opposed-phase GRE sequences are useful for the detection of cytoplasmic lipid (not always grossly visible) and thus for the evaluation of lesions such as adrenal adenoma (p. 387). In these sequences, images are acquired at two different points in time—once when the lipid and water protons are in phase (in-phase image) and once when they are out of phase (opposed-phase image). Newer 3D GRE techniques such as VIBE (volume-interpolated breath-hold examination) or LAVA (liver acquisition with volume acceleration) make it possible to cover a large imaging volume, such as the entire kidneys in the arterial or nephrographic/urographic phase during one acquisition of less than 30 seconds' duration. These techniques also permit the sequential acquisition of a complete dynamic series (unenhanced, arterial phase, nephrographic phase, late venous phase, and urographic phase). Three-dimensional volumes can be acquired for multiplanar reconstructions, which are very helpful for identifying normal variants. A 3-T scanner can achieve slice thicknesses of 2 mm owing to the higher intrinsic signal intensities in the higher field. A 1.5-T scanner can achieve a slice thickness of 3 mm with a good signal-to-noise ratio.
- *Diffusion-weighted imaging (DWI)*: DWI employs two additional diffusion gradients for the measurement of brownian molecular motion. This supplies information on tissue cellularity, i.e., the density of cells in a particular tissue entity or mass. Various authors have shown that determination of the apparent diffusion coefficient (ADC) in DWI can discriminate among different tissue entities based on differences in their cellularity.[15,16] The ADC has become a useful indicator in oncologic and other routine settings, especially in the diagnosis of pyelonephritis and the exclusion of renal abscess.[15,17]

11.1.2 Anatomy and Congenital Variants

Anatomy

The kidneys are retroperitoneal organs located adjacent to the spinal column in the lumbar recess. They are encapsulated by Gerota's fascia. This renal fascia is open medially and encloses the perirenal space, which is occupied by perirenal fat. The space outside Gerota's fascia is called the pararenal space. Gerota's fascia acts as a barrier to the spread of pathologic processes such as collections of extrapancreatic fluid due to pancreatitis or the spread of hematoma due to renal hemorrhage (▶ Fig. 11.2). The renal hilum is normally rotated slightly forward. The ureters descend on the psoas muscle (a useful imaging landmark) into the pelvis, cross over the common iliac artery and vein, and open at the trigone in the bladder fundus. The bladder trigone is a triangular region in the bladder wall located between the ureteral orifices and the origin of the urethra. The wall structure prevents any creasing of the bladder wall in this region, which keeps the orifices patent even in an empty bladder and maintain urinary drainage.

Caution
Note that the twelfth rib crosses the kidneys at a 45° angle, and that the left kidney is usually 1 to 2 cm higher than the right kidney and is 1 cm longer. Because of this, close attention should be paid to the posterior costodiaphragmatic recess during percutaneous renal biopsy so as to avoid accidental puncture of the pleura.

Generally the renal parenchyma is approximately 1.5 cm thick. The cortex and medulla are clearly differentiated from each other

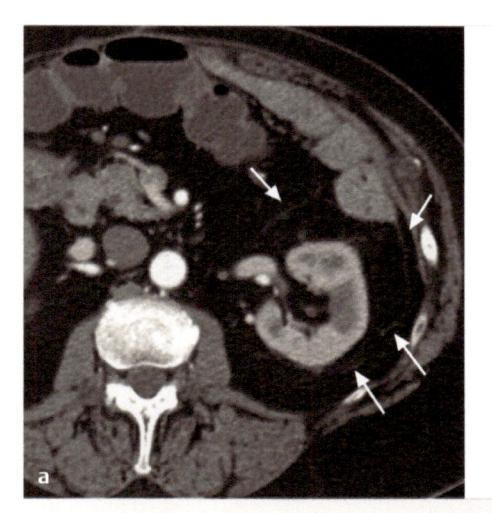

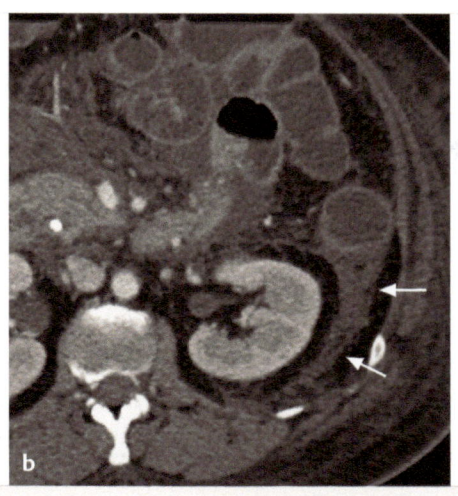

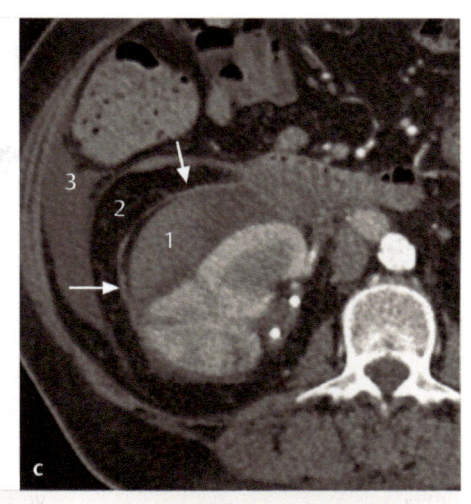

Fig. 11.2 Gerota's fascia. (a) Normal anatomy of the kidney. The renal axis is rotated slightly posteriorly, with the hilum facing somewhat medially. The Gerota's fascia is visible as an extremely fine line (arrows). The fascia almost completely envelopes the kidney and is open on the medial side. The Gerota's fascia encloses the perirenal space, which is occupied by perirenal fat. Outside the fascia is the pararenal space, which is occupied by pararenal fat. **(b)** Acute necrotizing pancreatitis. Extrapancreatic fluid collections surround the Gerota's fascia (arrows) without penetrating it. **(c)** Renal hemorrhage. The hematoma fills the perirenal space within the Gerota's fascia. Some blood has spilled from the medial fascial opening, through which the renal hilum also emerges. The hematoma does not fill the pararenal space (arrows). 1, perirenal space within the Gerota's fascia; 2, retroperitoneal pararenal space outside the Gerota's fascia; 3, peritoneal cavity.

after IV administration of contrast medium (see ▶ Fig. 11.2). The renal cortex contains the glomeruli, tubules, and vessels, while the medulla (pyramids) contains the collecting ducts and is less vascular. Cortical extensions, called the renal columns, pass between the pyramids to the renal pelvis. Prominent renal columns may be mistaken for masses, especially on ultrasound scans. They can be identified by tracing them back to their origin and noting their continuity with the renal cortex.[18]

Congenital Variants

We can better understand possible variants in the anatomy and position of the kidneys by considering their development during the embryonic period.[18] An important factor in renal development is the nephrogenic cord, which arises from the intermediate mesoderm and subdivides into cervical, thoracic, lumbar, and sacral segments. The nephrogenic cord undergoes three developmental phases, which proceed successively in a craniocaudal direction:
- *Pronephros*: The cervical segment of the nephrogenic cord develops into the pronephros, which is nonfunctioning and normally regresses with further development.
- *Mesonephros*: The pronephros is succeeded by the mesonephros, which forms in the thoracic and upper lumbar region. The mesonephros fuses with the pronephros to form the wolffian (mesonephric) duct. The wolffian duct develops an outpouching, the ureteral bud, from which the ureter, pyelocalyceal system, and collecting ducts are formed. The stalk of the ureteral bud later becomes the ureter.
- *Metanephros*: The actual kidney is formed by the fusion of the metanephrogenic blastema (which is the lower lumbar and sacral portion of the nephrogenic cord) with the ureteral bud. The ureteral bud divides and stimulates the proliferation and differentiation of the metanephrogenic blastema.

Renal Agenesis

Renal agenesis, or congenital absence of the kidney, occurs when the ureteral bud fails to interact with the metanephrogenic blastema, eliminating the normal inductive effect of the ureteral bud. Renal agenesis is commonly associated with other genital anomalies.

Bifid Ureter and Duplex Ureter

Premature branching or division of the ureteral bud—before the ureteral bud reaches the metanephrogenic blastema—may lead to duplication of the ureter. In the case of a bifid ureter, the two ureters unite before draining into the bladder through a common orifice. The formation of two ureteral buds from the wolffian duct leads to a duplex ureter. In this case the duplicated ureters drain into the bladder through separate orifices. The upper (extra) ureteral bud induces formation of the upper renal pole while the lower (normal) ureteral bud induces formation of the lower pole. If the wolffian duct is incorporated into the bladder floor as far as the origin of the lower ureteral bud, the upper bud will continue to migrate caudally with the rest of the wolffian duct. This leads to a crossing of the ureters, and the extra upper ureter may terminate at an abnormally low level, inserting, for example, into the urethra, vagina, or vas deferens. In the great majority of cases, however, both ureters open into the bladder.

Note

The crossed position of duplicated ureters is known as the Weigert–Meyer law: the upper-pole ureter always inserts into the bladder below the lower-pole ureter.

Positional Variants

The metanephros ascends from the pelvic region to the lumbar region during embryonic development. The metanephros also rotates during its ascent. The renal pelvis moves from an anterior to a medial orientation. Failure of the metanephros to ascend normally may lead to alterations of renal position ranging from

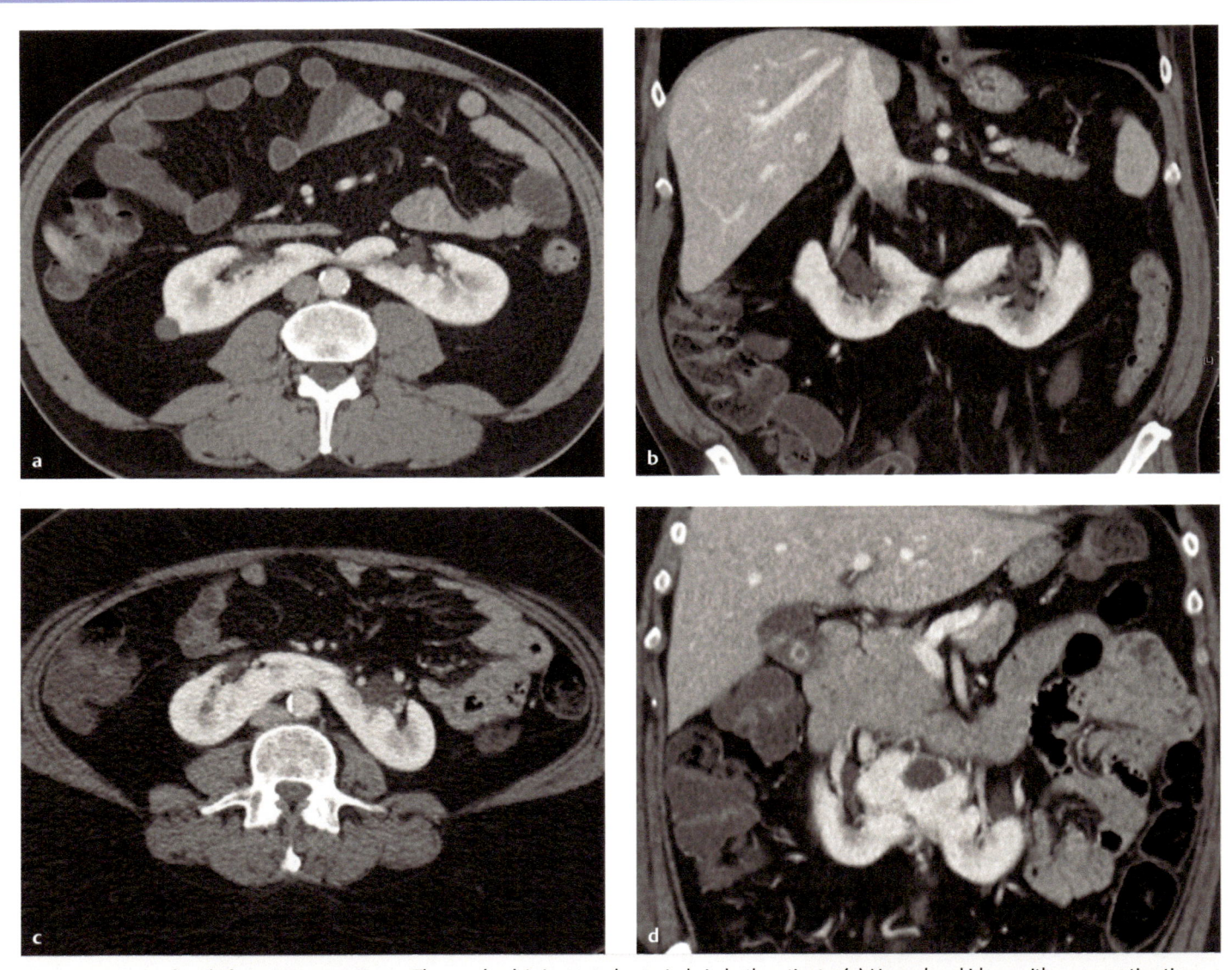

Fig. 11.3 Horseshoe kidneys in two patients. The renal pelvis is rotated anteriorly in both patients. (a) Horseshoe kidney with a connective tissue isthmus (axial CT). (b) Horseshoe kidney with a connective tissue isthmus (coronal reformatted image). (c) Horseshoe kidney with a parenchymal isthmus (axial CT). (d) Horseshoe kidney with a parenchymal isthmus (coronal reformatted image).

pelvic kidneys to malrotated kidneys with the renal hilum directed anteriorly.

Horseshoe Kidney

Horseshoe kidney results from the fusion of the two kidneys at their lower poles (▶ Fig. 11.3, ▶ Fig. 11.4). The fused area may consist purely of connective tissue or of functional renal parenchyma.

Accessory Renal Arteries

As the kidney ascends to the lumbar level, its vascular supply also changes. It is supplied initially by branches of the iliac artery, then by segmental branches of the lower aorta, and it finally receives its definitive supply from segmental branches at the level of the second lumbar segment. The persistence of one or more precursor vessels leads to the presence of accessory renal arteries (e.g., an accessory lower-pole artery, ▶ Fig. 11.5). The renal artery divides at the hilum into segmental arteries. As a rule, four segmental arteries run anterior to the renal pelvis and one posterior (▶ Fig. 11.6). The interlobar arteries that arise from the segmental arteries enter the kidney through the renal columns, run lateral to the pyramids, and branch first into arcuate arteries and then into interlobular arteries. A knowledge of this branching pattern is helpful in performing a percutaneous nephrostomy or renal biopsy. The safest route for placing a nephrostomy tube is to pass the catheter through the papillary tips into the renal pelvis.

11.1.3 Diseases

Masses

Cystic Renal Masses

▶ **Brief definition.** Cysts are the most common renal changes detectable by imaging. Simple renal cysts are fluid-filled spaces with a fibrous wall. They may be solitary, multiple, unilateral, or bilateral and may be symptomatic or have no pathologic significance. At least one renal cyst can be found in approximately 50% of the population over 50 years of age.[19] Renal cysts may also show intralesional hemorrhage or internal septa, in which case they are classified as complex cysts. A crucial differentiation is between renal cysts and renal cell carcinoma, which often has a

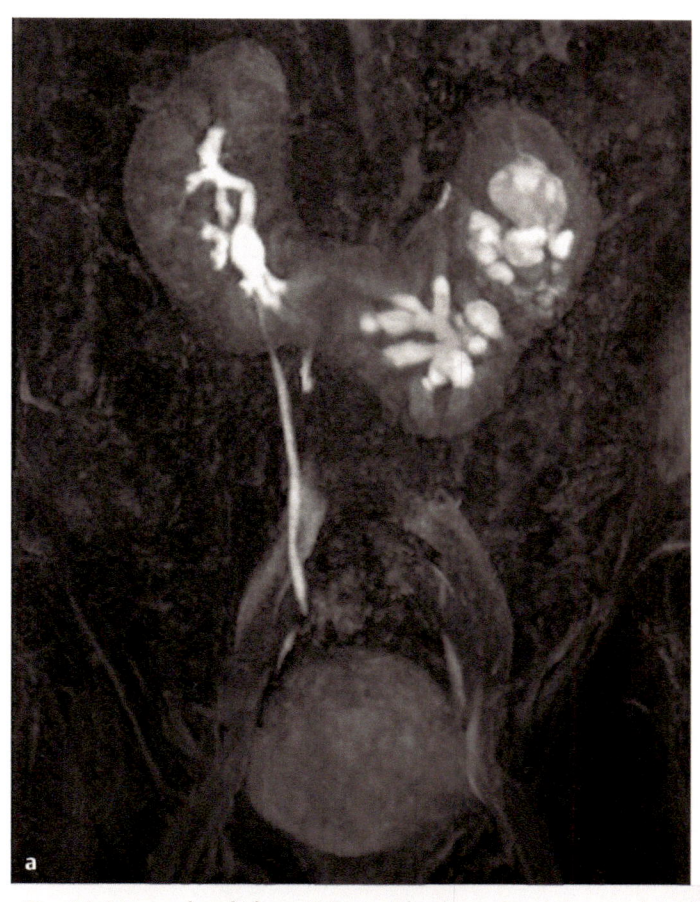

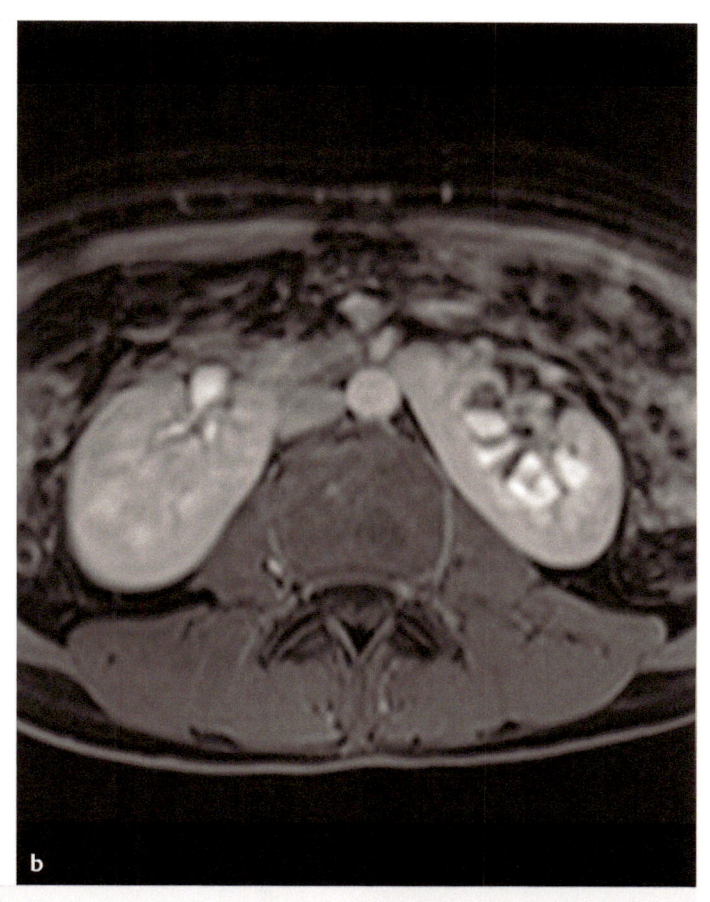

Fig. 11.4 Horseshoe kidney. Patient with a horseshoe kidney and duplicated left pelvicalyceal system. **(a)** Coronal maximum intensity projection. **(b)** Axial T1 W sequence after IV administration of contrast medium displays the inferior mesenteric artery, which has obstructed the ascent of the embryonic kidneys.

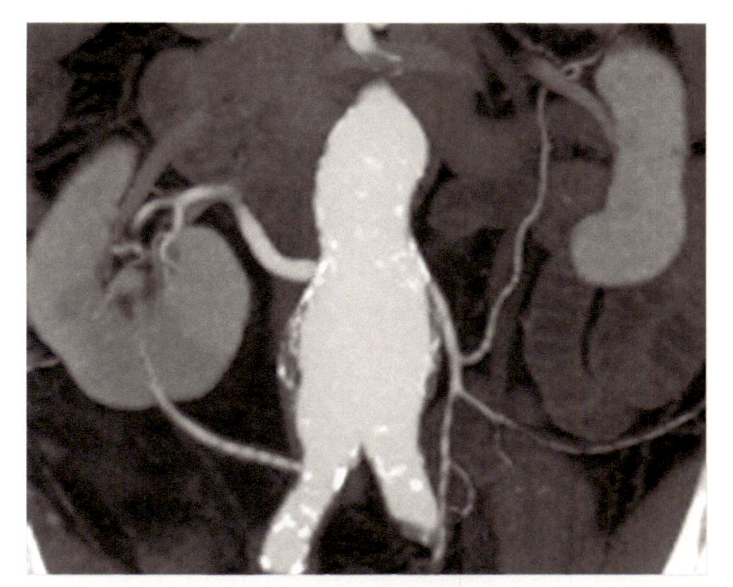

Fig. 11.5 Accessory lower pole artery in a 60-year-old man with an infrarenal aortic aneurysm. An accessory lower-pole artery arises from the right common iliac artery due to abnormal renal ascent.

> **Caution**
>
> The original Bosniak classification is based on morphological imaging criteria visible on CT scans. It has been shown that the original classification is applicable to MRI,[21] with the caveat that the greater soft tissue contrast on MRI may lead to overestimation of cyst category.[22]

cystic appearance. The Bosniak classification,[20] introduced in 1986, is helpful for characterizing renal cysts in terms of their malignancy risk, or the possible presence of renal cell carcinoma, and thus for standardizing their clinical management.

The use of high-resolution MRI sequences in a 3-T field, such as a 3D GRE sequence with fat suppression after IV administration of contrast medium, may improve the detection of hypervascular septa at a maximum resolution of 2 mm. This makes MRI particularly useful for monitoring lesions with a potential for malignant change.

▶ **Imaging signs.** Simple renal cysts appear sonographically as well-circumscribed, echo-free lesions with posterior acoustic enhancement. Inspissated proteinaceous or hemorrhagic contents can produce internal echoes of variable amplitude. Ultrasound may also show variable internal septa or polypoid masses. The different Bosniak categories are associated with the following imaging findings:

- *Bosniak type 1 cysts*: Type 1 cysts are isodense to water on CT, with attenuation values in the range 0 to 20 HU. They have a thin (< 1 mm), nonenhancing capsule (▶ Fig. 11.7). On MRI they are hypointense in T1 W sequences and homogeneously

Kidney and Urinary Tract

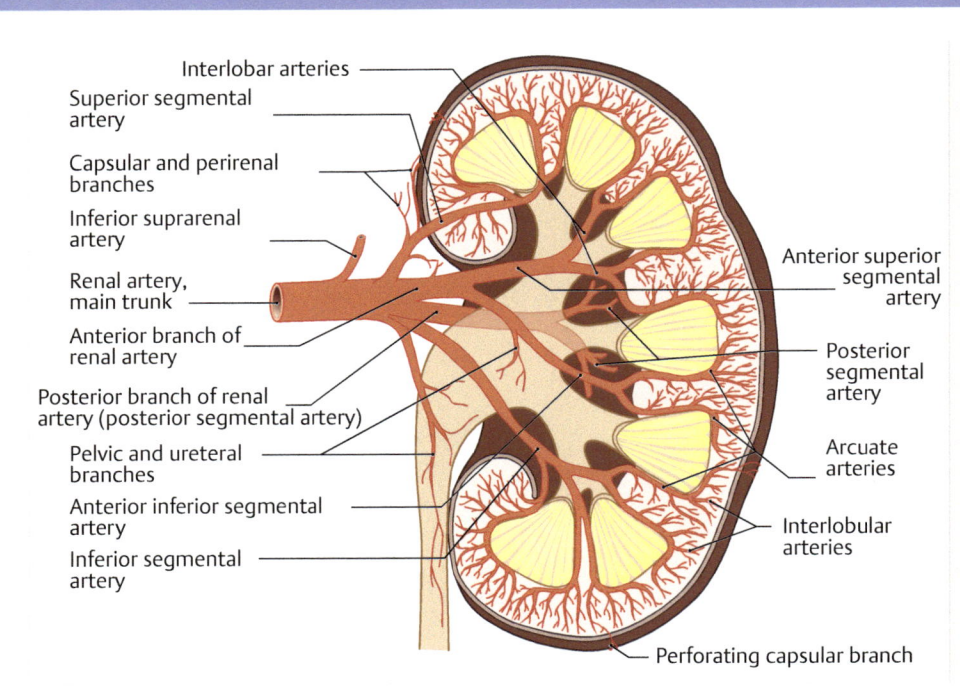

Fig. 11.6 Arterial anatomy of the kidney. In most cases there are four segmental arteries anterior to the renal pelvis and one posterior. The papillary apices are avascular and provide good access sites for the introduction of a nephrostomy catheter.

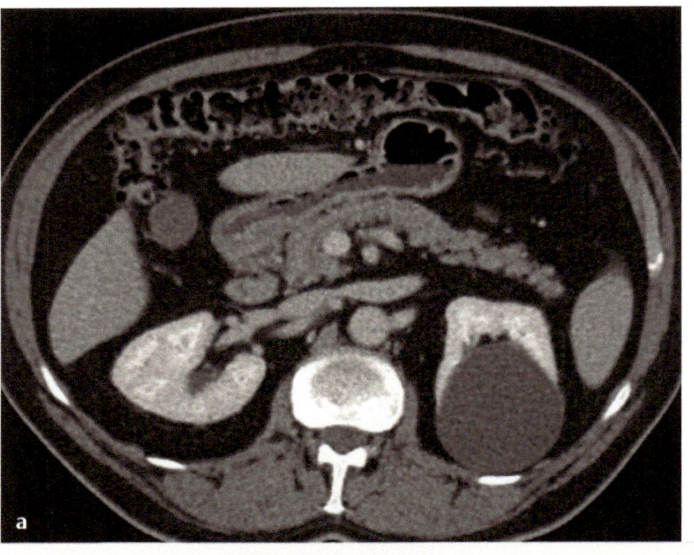

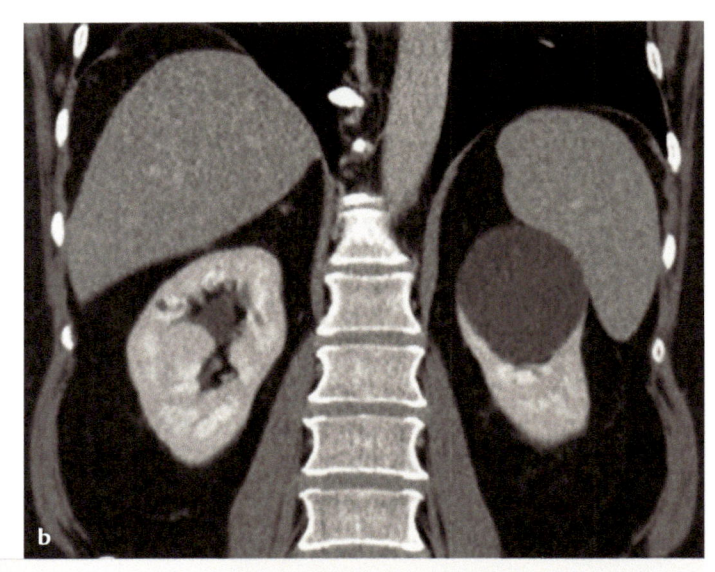

Fig. 11.7 Simple renal cyst without calcifications or septa (Bosniak type 1). CT, nephrographic phase. (a) Axial image. (b) Coronal image.

hyperintense in T2W sequences (▶ Fig. 11.8). As on CT, contrast enhancement is not observed. Bosniak type 1 cysts have no malignant potential and therefore do not require follow-up or surgical removal.
- *Bosniak type 2 cysts*: These cysts have relatively high CT attenuation (> 20 HU) compared with type 1 cysts. They contain thin septa (< 1 mm). They may exhibit fine mural or septal calcifications but are minimally complex and nonenhancing. They may be hypointense or hyperintense in T1W MRI sequences, depending on the presence of intracystic hemorrhage (cyst diameter < 3 cm). Their T2W signal intensity is also variable, depending on the same factors. Type 2 cysts do not enhance (▶ Fig. 11.9) and have no risk of malignant transformation.
- *Bosniak type 2F cysts*: These are cystic lesions with a thickened, irregular cyst wall and septa. Nodular calcifications may be present but have no soft-tissue elements and do not enhance (▶ Fig. 11.10, ▶ Fig. 11.11). Cysts with hemorrhagic contents larger than 3 cm in diameter are also classified as Bosniak type 2F. The malignancy risk is 0 to 10%. Patients with a type 2F cyst should be followed (the "F" stands for "follow up"). Currently there are no uniform standards for setting follow-up intervals. O'Malley et al. recommend an initial follow-up at 6 months and, if there has been no change, two subsequent 1-year follow-ups and a final follow-up at 2 years.[22]
- *Bosniak type 3 cysts*: Both imaging modalities show a thickened, irregular wall with septa (▶ Fig. 11.12) Irregular mural calcifications may also be present. There is contrast enhancement that exceeds 15 HU on CT relative to unenhanced images. The malignancy risk is approximately 50%, and therefore surgical removal is advised.
- *Bosniak type 4 cysts*: Cysts in this category are clearly malignant cystic lesions with solid components and contrast enhancement (▶ Fig. 11.13, ▶ Fig. 11.14). The risk of malignancy is 100% and surgical removal is indicated.

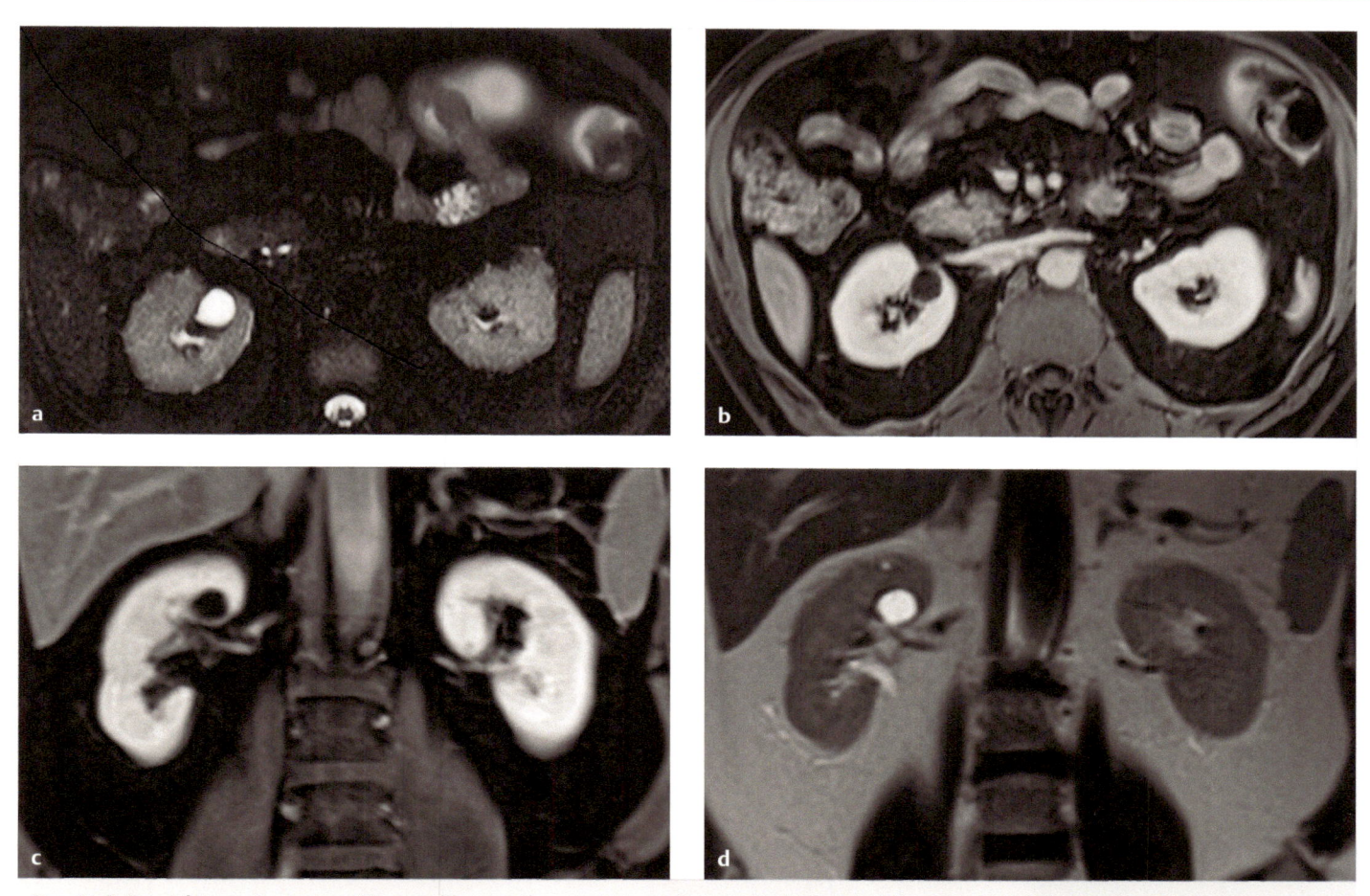

Fig. 11.8 Bosniak type 1 cyst in a 57-year-old man. Characteristic cystic mass in the upper pole of the right kidney is hyperintense in the T2 W sequence and hypointense in the T1 W sequence. The absence of septa and enhancement positively identifies the cyst as Bosniak type 1. **(a)** Axial T2 W image. **(b)** Axial T1 W image, venous phase. **(c)** Coronal T1 W image, venous phase. **(d)** Coronal T2 W image.

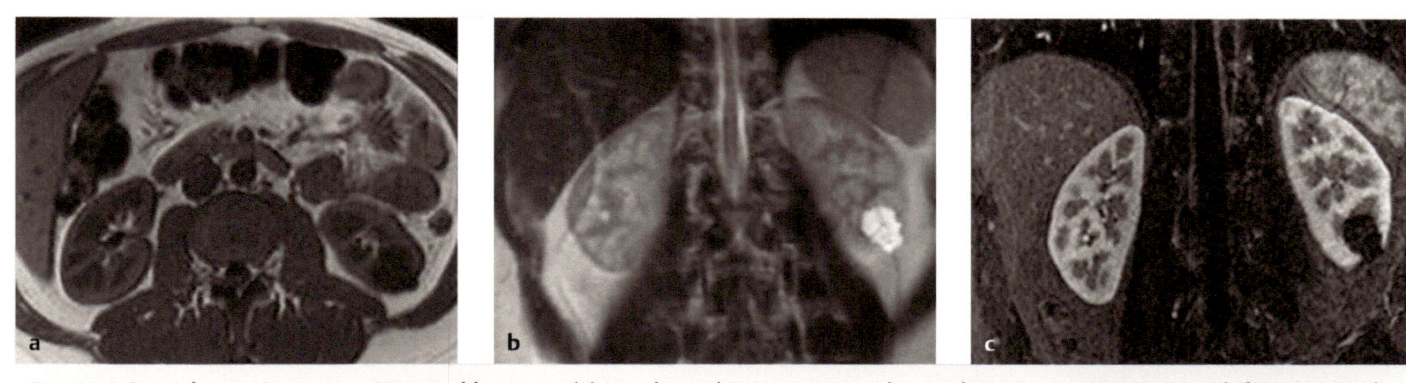

Fig. 11.9 Bosniak type 2 cyst in a 46-year-old woman. **(a)** Unenhanced T1 W sequence shows a hypointense cystic mass with fine septa in the lower pole of the left kidney. **(b)** The mass appears hyperintense in the T2 W sequence. **(c)** T1 W sequence after administration of contrast medium. The septa do not enhance.

▶ **Clinical features.** Uncomplicated renal cysts are usually asymptomatic and are detected incidentally during a routine ultrasound examination, for example. Large renal cysts may cause flank pain due to renal displacement.

▶ **Differential diagnosis.** Congenital renal cysts, which are classified as Potter type I to IV, require differentiation from the renal cysts described above.

Cystic Renal Diseases

Cystic renal diseases include a number of genetically mediated diseases that have different manifestations:
- Autosomal recessive polycystic kidney disease (ARPKD).
- Autosomal dominant polycystic kidney disease (ADPKD).
- Medullary cystic disease or juvenile nephronophthisis.
- Medullary sponge kidney.
- Congenital nephrotic syndrome.
- Familial hypoplastic glomerulocystic disease.

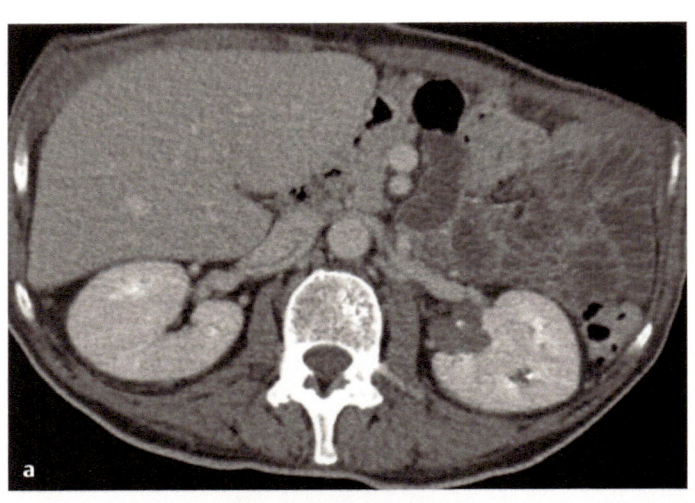

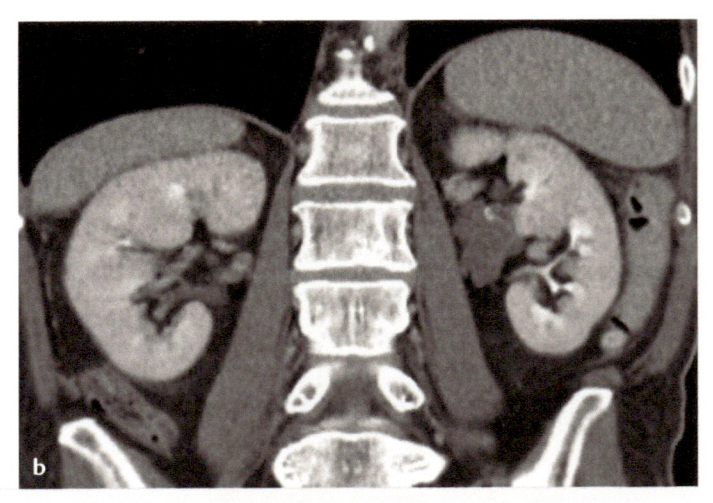

Fig. 11.10 **Septated renal cyst with calcifications (Bosniak type 2F).** CT, urographic phase. Left renal cyst shows absence of enhancement. (a) Axial image. (b) Coronal image.

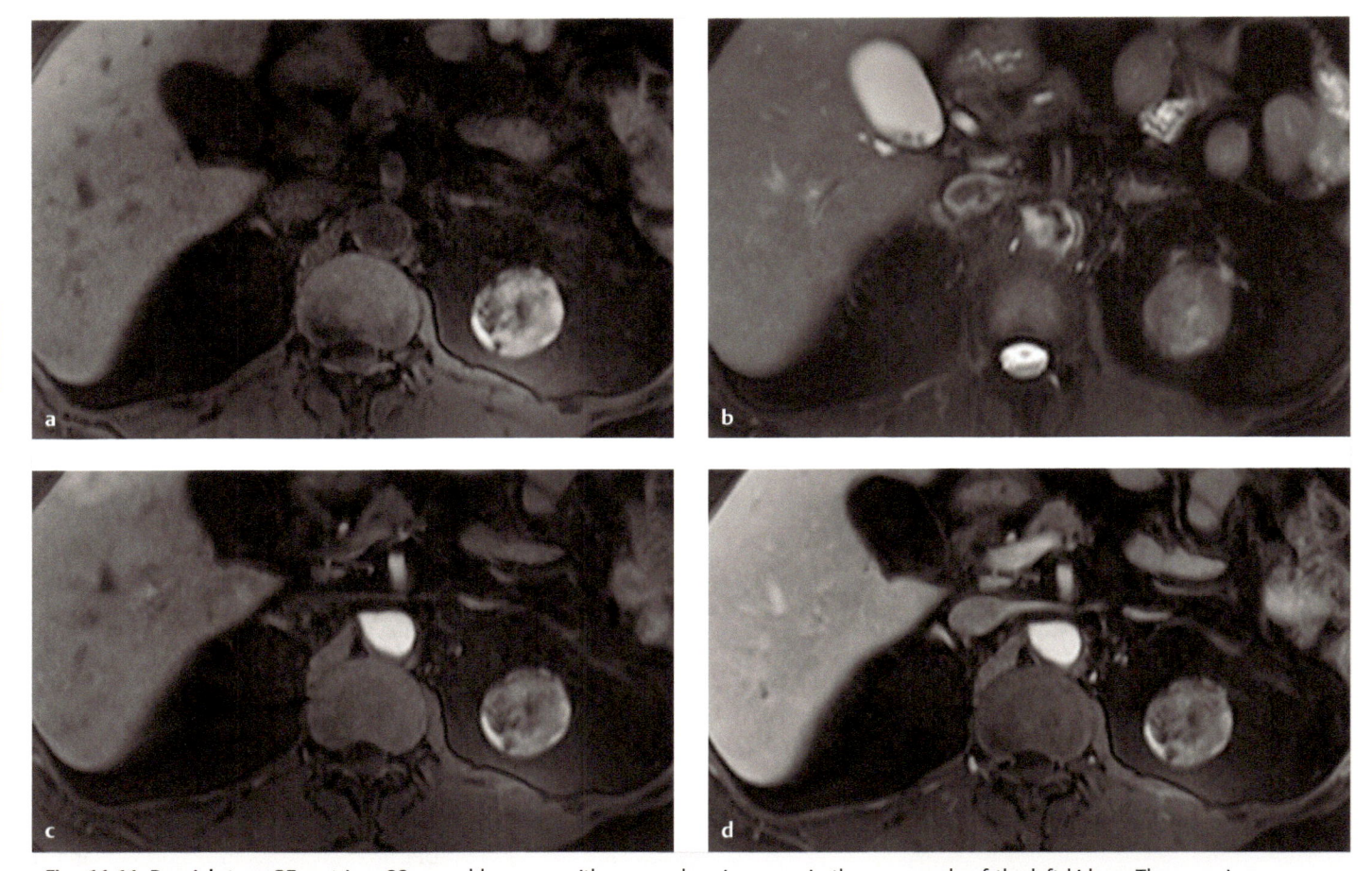

Fig. 11.11 **Bosniak type 2F cyst** in a 66-year-old woman with a nonenhancing mass in the upper pole of the left kidney. The mass is heterogeneously hyperintense in the unenhanced T1W sequence and heterogeneously hypointense in the T2W sequence. (a) Unenhanced T1W image. (b) T2W image. (c) T1W image after administration of contrast medium, early arterial phase. (d) T1W image after administration of contrast medium, venous phase.

- Malformation syndromes such as von Hippel–Lindau syndrome or tuberous sclerosis.
- Multicystic renal dysplasia.
- Sporadic glomerulocystic renal disease.

The Potter classification is based on histological examination of the site of cyst origin.

Polycystic Kidney Disease (Infantile Form)

ARPKD is further differentiated by the affected gene locus, each of which loci is associated with a different clinical presentation:

- *Neonatal form*: Even prenatally, both kidneys are greatly enlarged and echogenic due to myriad tiny cysts that are too small to be resolved with ultrasound. There is oligohydramnios

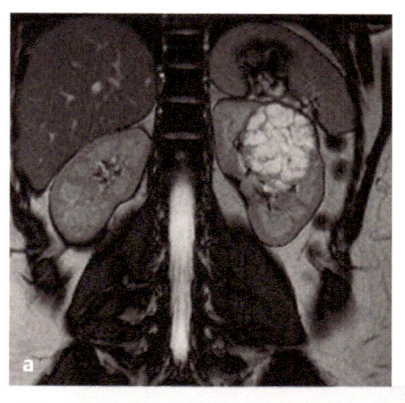

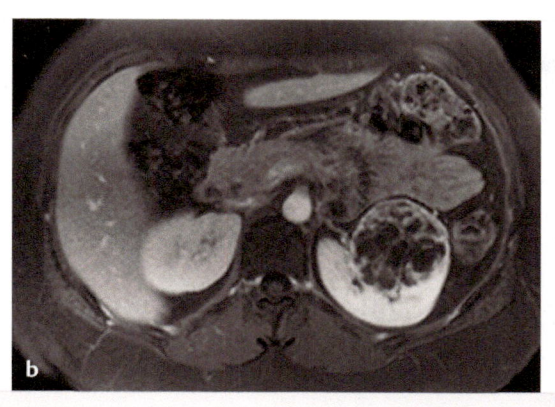

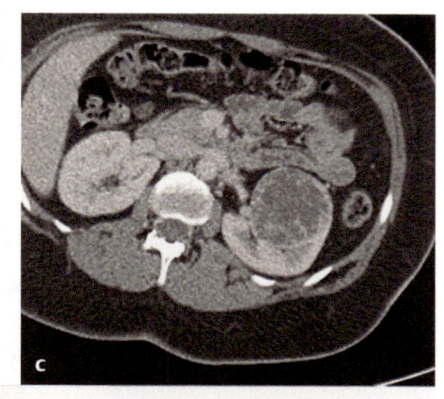

Fig. 11.12 Bosniak type 3 cyst. A cystic mass with multiple internal septa and irregular septal thickening is detected in the left kidney of a 68-year-old man. The mass has high T2W signal intensity and enhances after IV administration of contrast medium. **(a)** T2W sequence. **(b)** T1W sequence after administration of contrast medium. **(c)** Axial CT (portal venous phase).

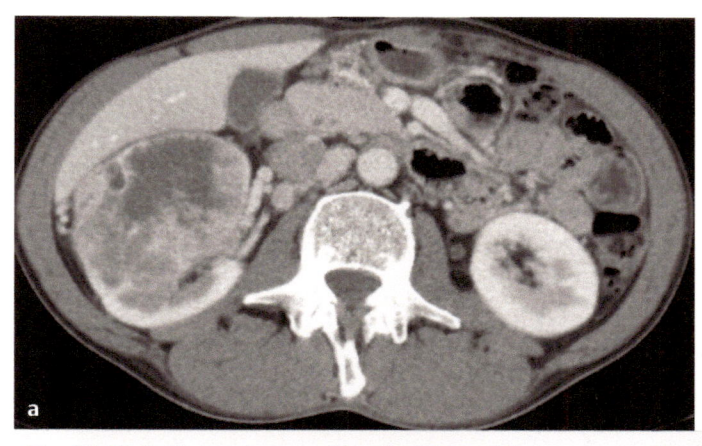

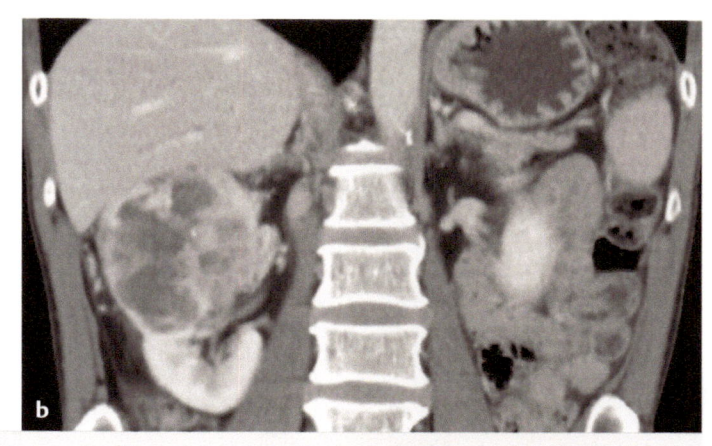

Fig. 11.13 Cystic renal mass with enhancing solid components (Bosniak type 4). CT, nephrographic phase. **(a)** Axial image. **(b)** Coronal image.

due to intrauterine renal failure, and the decreased amniotic fluid volume leads to pulmonary hypoplasia. Oligohydramnios may also lead to clubbing of the feet and cranial deformities.
- *Intermediate form*: Renal failure and renal hypertension develop during the first year of life.
- *Juvenile form*: The dominant clinical finding is hepatic fibrosis leading to portal hypertension with esophageal varices. The kidneys are echogenic and slightly enlarged due to the presence of multiple small cysts.

Polycystic Kidney Disease (Adult Form, Potter Type III)

▶ **Brief definition.** Autosomal dominant polycystic kidney disease (ADPKD; Potter type III) is an autosomal dominant disease characterized by prominent cysts in one or both kidneys. Cysts are also present in the pancreas, spleen, or liver. An association with cerebral berry aneurysms is also found in ADPKD patients. The cystic renal degeneration is often marked by a combination of simple and complex cysts. In contrast to acquired polycystic kidney disease (e.g., in dialysis patients), the risk of malignant transformation is not significantly increased.

▶ **Imaging signs.** The kidneys are permeated by multiple cysts (▶ Fig. 11.15), making it difficult or impossible to detect residual, original renal parenchyma. The kidneys are markedly enlarged due to the presence of numerous cysts. It is common to find simple cysts coexisting with partially complex cysts with hemorrhagic changes (▶ Fig. 11.16). The cysts themselves are radiologically indistinguishable from acquired simple cysts and benign cysts. Bilateral multicystic permeation of the kidneys is characteristic. Because ADPKD is a systemic disease, other organs are also affected. In addition to renal cysts, multiple cysts are most commonly found in the liver but may also occur in the pancreas and spleen.

▶ **Clinical features.** ADPKD usually becomes symptomatic in adulthood. Complaints include hematuria (usually due to self-limiting intracystic hemorrhage), recurrent urinary tract infections, microalbuminuria, hypertension, progressive impairment of renal function, nonspecific abdominal complaints or back pain, and a possible increase in abdominal circumference. Progressive renal failure and uremia usually develop after 40 years of age. Some patients with cystic kidneys remain asymptomatic until renal failure supervenes, leading to delays in diagnosis and genetic counseling.

Kidney and Urinary Tract

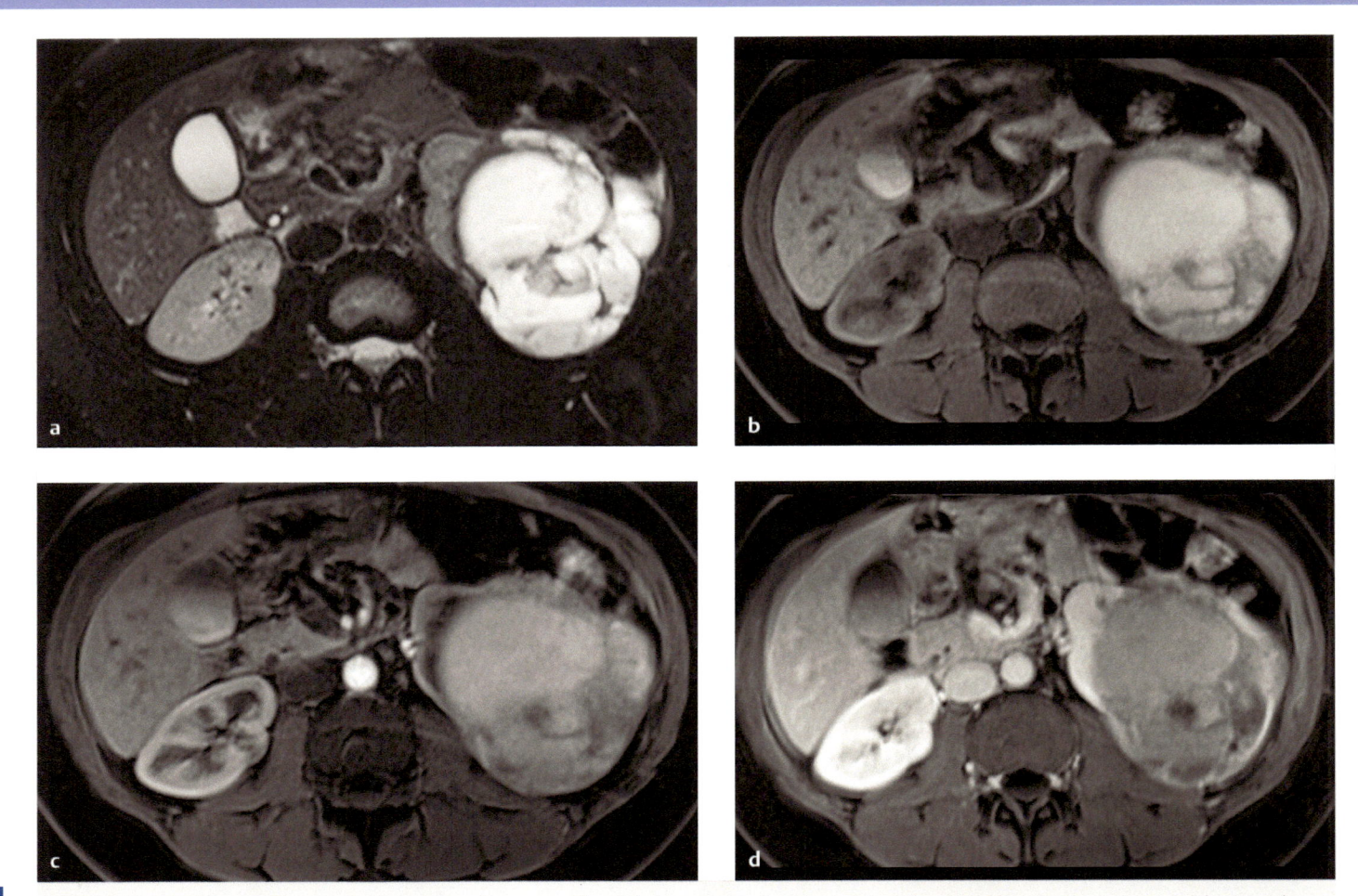

Fig. 11.14 Bosniak type 4 cyst. An irregular cystic mass with solid components is detected in a 74-year-old man. The mass is predominantly hyperintense in the T2 W and T1 W sequences, consistent with intracystic hemorrhage. The T1 W sequence after administration of contrast medium shows heterogeneous enhancement. **(a)** Axial T2 W sequence. **(b)** Axial unenhanced T1 W sequence. **(c)** Axial T1 W sequence, early arterial phase. **(d)** Axial T1 W sequence, venous phase.

▶ **Differential diagnosis**
- Acquired renal cysts.
- Complex renal cysts.

Medullary Sponge Kidney

Medullary sponge kidney is caused by cystic dilatation of the collecting ducts in the medullary pyramids; the cortex is unaffected. The findings may be confined to one pyramid or one segment. Initial manifestations of the disease appear in adolescence and consist of recurrent pyelonephritis, hematuria, or flank pain due to urolithiasis.

Medullary Cystic Kidney Disease

This disease is divided into a juvenile form (also called juvenile nephronophthisis, autosomal recessive) and an adult form (autosomal dominant). The medullary cysts are accompanied by renal atrophy culminating in renal failure.

Solid Renal Masses

Solid renal masses can be divided into two groups according to their origin:
- *Epithelial tumors*: adenoma, oncocytoma, renal cell carcinoma.
- *Mesenchymal tumors*: angiomyolipoma, medullary fibroma, liposarcoma, leiomyosarcoma, hemangiopericytoma.

Oncocytoma

▶ **Brief definition.** Oncocytoma is a benign, very slow-growing solid renal tumor[24,25] that arises from the epithelium of the renal collecting ducts and contains eosinophilic cells. The peak incidence is in the fifth through seventh decades, with a 2:1 ratio of males to females. Average tumor size at the time of diagnosis is approximately 6 cm. From 3 to 7% of all renal tumors are oncocytomas.

▶ **Imaging signs.** Oncocytoma appears on CT as a homogeneously enhancing mass. Often it contains a central stellate or spoked-wheel nonenhancing scar that suggests a diagnosis of oncocytoma (▶ Fig. 11.17). A corresponding pattern can be seen on MRI (▶ Fig. 11.18).

▶ **Clinical features.** Oncocytomas are usually asymptomatic, and most are detected incidentally by imaging during a work-up for other conditions. Large oncocytomas may become symptomatic due to organ displacement, presenting with nonspecific abdominal or flank pain. The clinical presentation is indistinguishable from that of renal cell carcinoma.

▶ **Differential diagnosis.** Oncocytoma closely resembles renal cell carcinoma in its imaging features. Even biopsy cannot always differentiate these entities.

11.1 Kidney

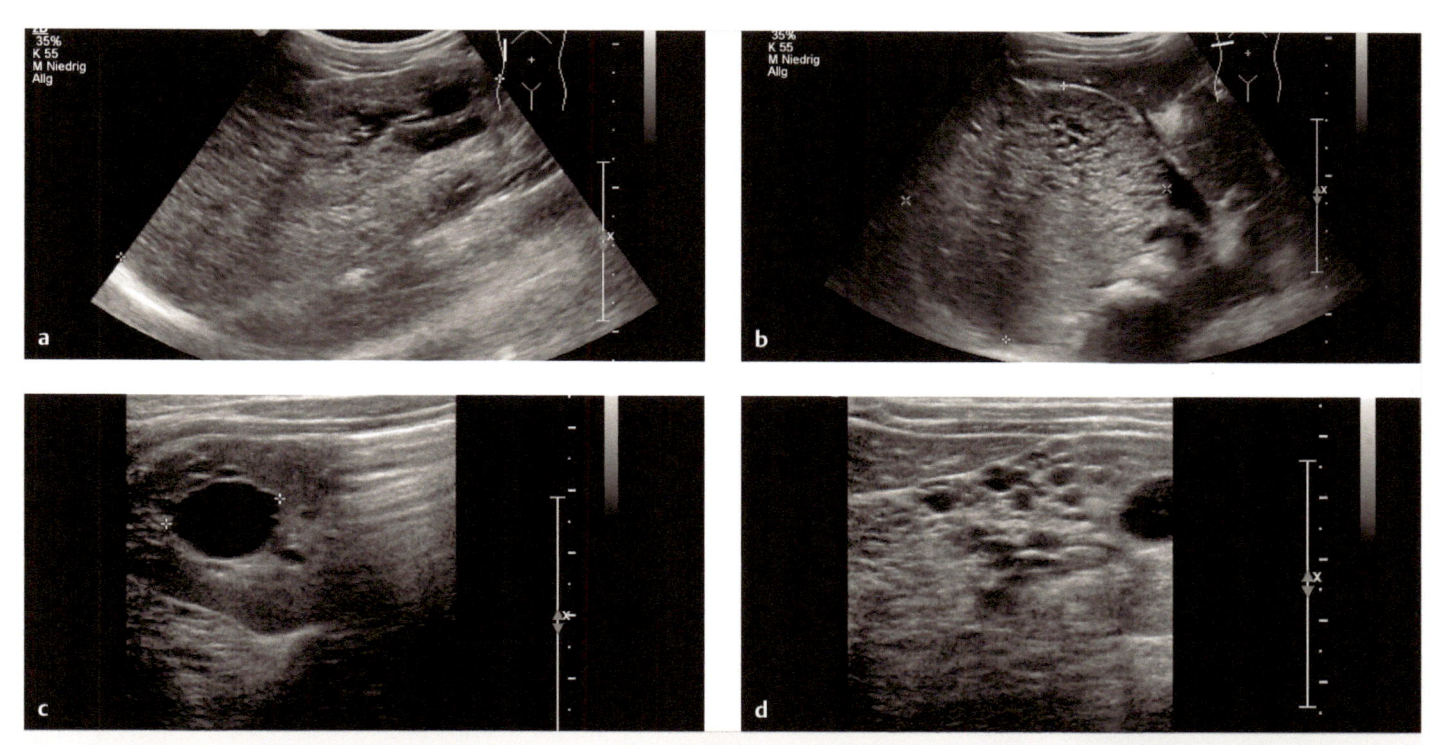

Fig. 11.15 **Cystic renal degeneration** in a 4-year-old girl with histologically confirmed cystic kidney disease. Ultrasound shows an inhomogeneous region in the upper pole of the right kidney (a) with multiple small, echo-free cysts (c, d) coexisting with larger cysts (b). (a) Longitudinal scan from the posterior side (curved array transducer). (b) Transverse scan from the posterior side (curved array transducer). (c) Transverse scan from the posterior side (linear transducer). (d) Longitudinal scan from the posterior side (linear transducer).

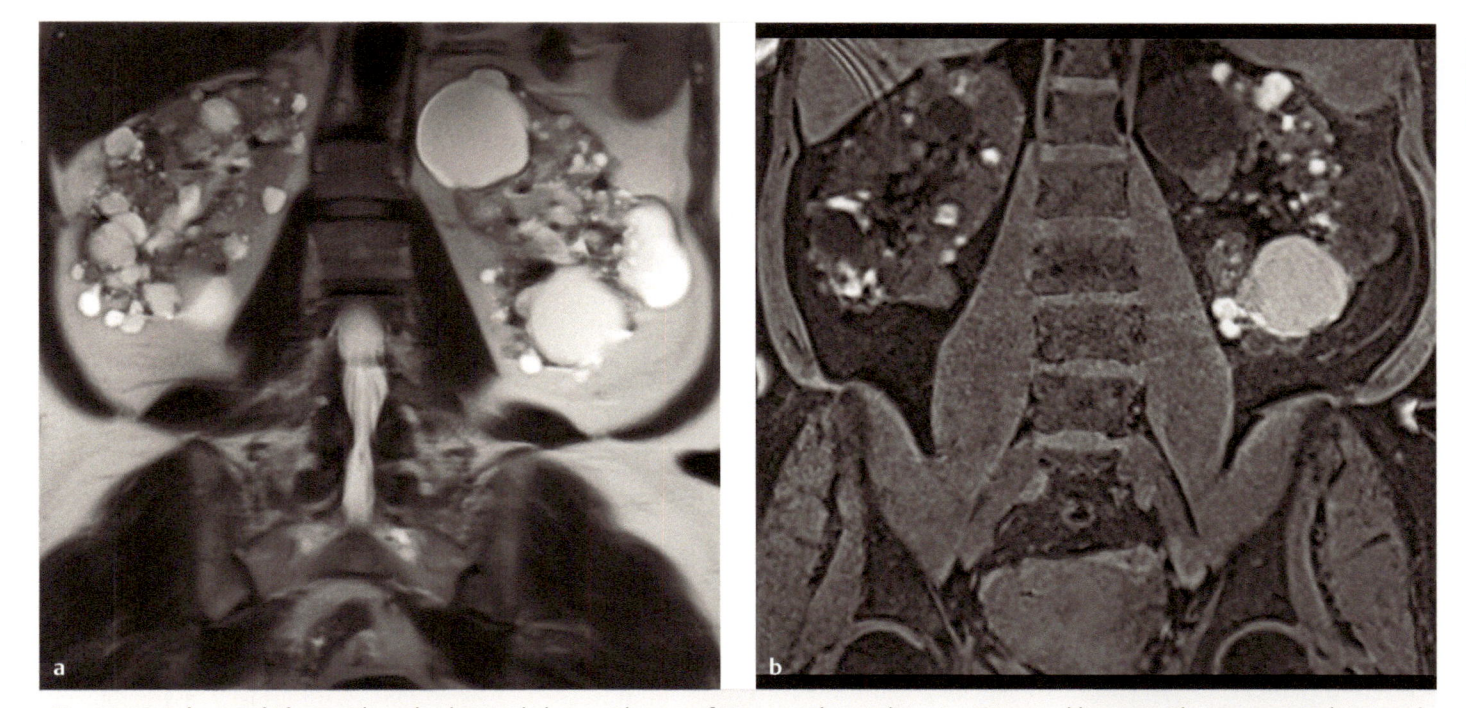

Fig. 11.16 **Polycystic kidneys.** Bilateral polycystic kidneys with areas of intracystic hemorrhage in a 74-year-old woman. The cysts appear hypo- and isointense in the T2W sequence (a) and hyperintense in the T1W sequence (b).

Note

A solitary, homogeneous mass with a central spoked-wheel structure is an indication for partial (or complete) nephrectomy due to the problem of differentiating oncocytoma from renal cell carcinoma.

Angiomyolipoma

▶ **Brief definition.** Angiomyolipomas are benign hamartomas composed of mature fat, smooth muscle, and thick-walled vessels. They originate from perivascular cells. The peak age of incidence is in the fifth and sixth decades. Females predominate over males by approximately 4:1. Patients with tuberous

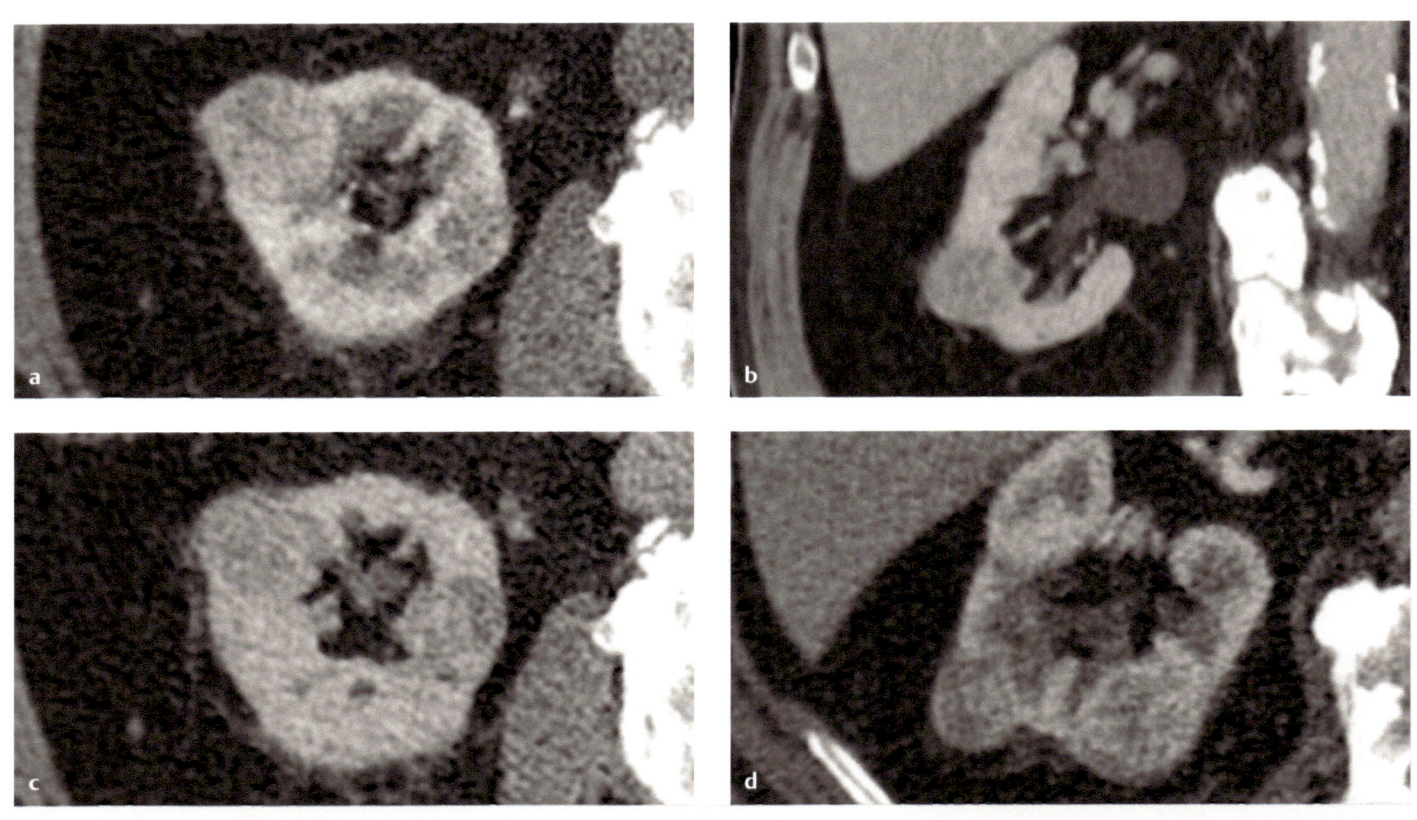

Fig. 11.17 **Multiple oncocytomas in an 87-year-old man.** The largest of the lesions shows a classic, nonenhancing central scar that contrasts with the surrounding enhancing portion of the mass. **(a)** CT, arterial phase. **(b)** CT, coronal reformatted image. **(c)** CT, nephrographic phase. **(d)** CT, excretory phase.

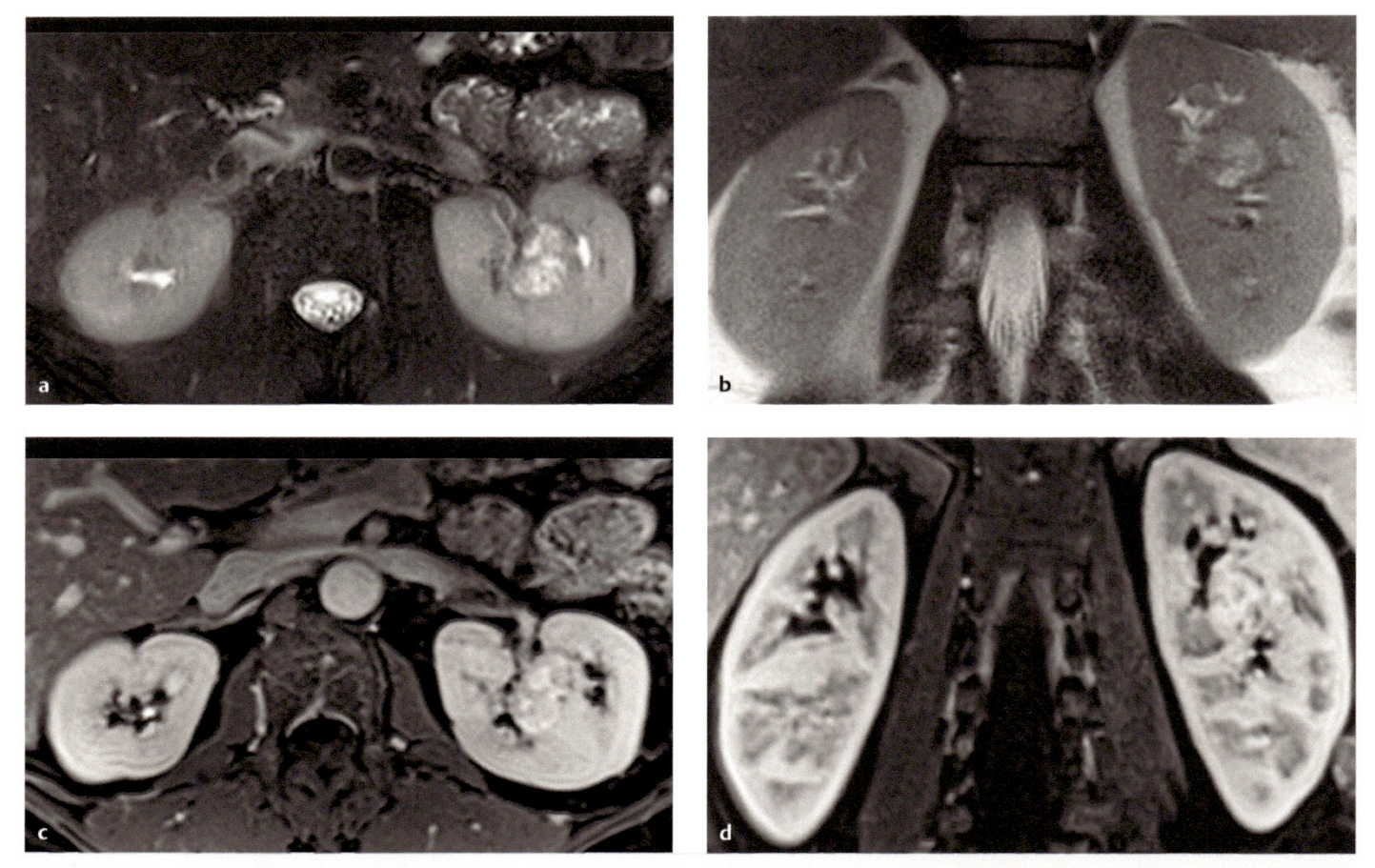

Fig. 11.18 **Renal oncocytoma** in a 42-year-old man with a T2-hyperintense mass in the midportion of the left kidney. The mass enhances in the T1 W sequence and has a central nonenhancing scar. **(a)** Axial T2 W sequence. **(b)** Coronal T2 W sequence. **(c)** Axial fat-suppressed T1 W sequence, venous phase. **(d)** Coronal fat-suppressed T1 W sequence, venous phase.

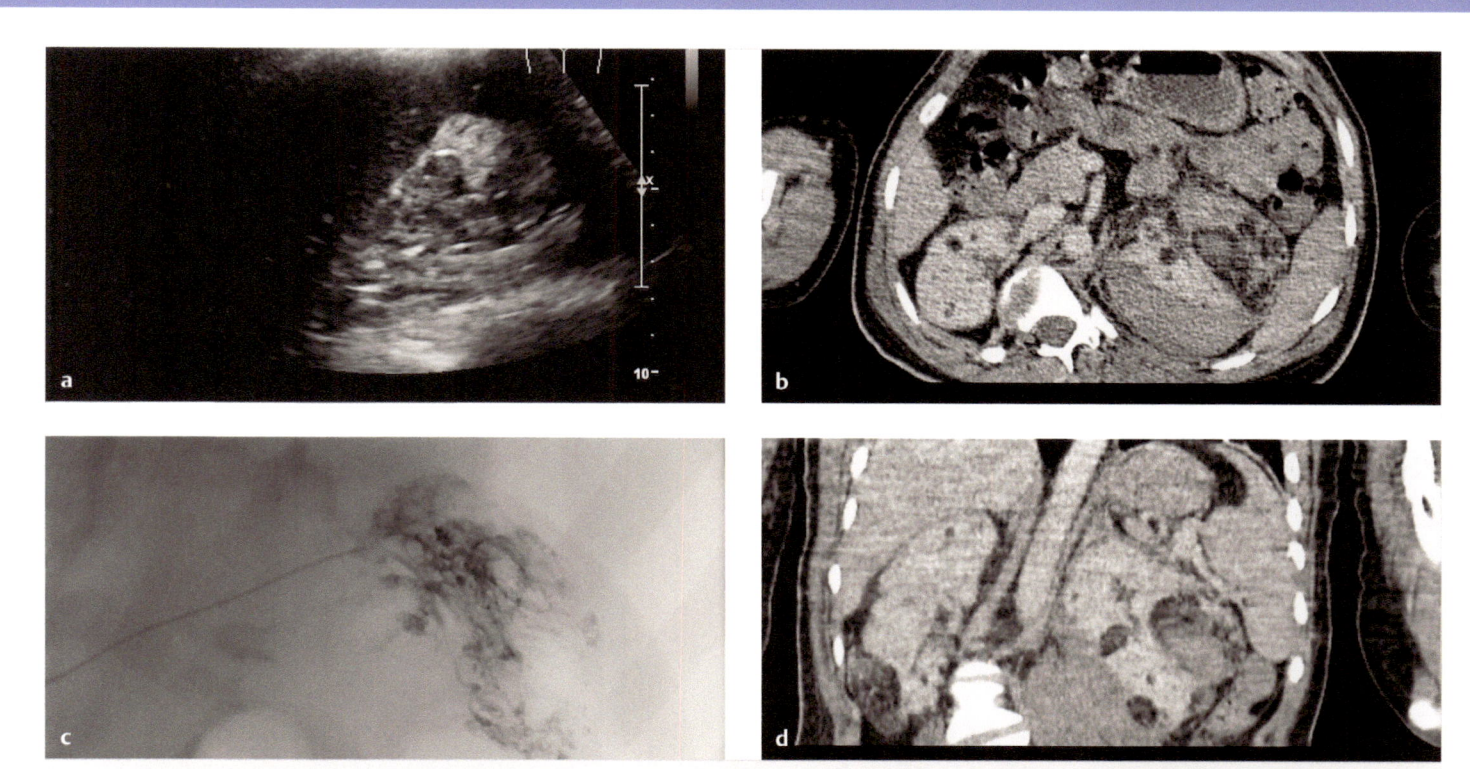

Fig. 11.19 Renal angiomyolipoma and Wunderlich's syndrome in a 21-year-old man with known tuberous sclerosis. His hemoglobin level fell from 14 to 7 mg/dL. **(a)** Ultrasound scan shows an inhomogeneous kidney with loss of corticomedullary differentiation and an echogenic hemorrhage with some degree of perirenal spread. **(b)** Axial CT shows bilateral renal masses, some with fat attenuation, with a left perirenal hematoma. **(c)** Left renal angiogram demonstrates multiple corkscrewlike feeder vessels to the angiomyolipoma with active bleeding from one feeder. **(d)** Coronal CT.

sclerosis are at increased risk for angiomyolipoma (present in 80% of cases), and frequently both kidneys are affected. Both sexes are represented equally in this group, and the peak age of incidence is 30 years. Approximately 80% of angiomyolipomas occur sporadically, however. The risk of intratumoral hemorrhage increases with tumor size (past 4 cm). Spontaneous retroperitoneal hemorrhage occurring in association with angiomyolipoma is known as Wunderlich's syndrome (▶ Fig. 11.19, ▶ Fig. 11.20). The growth of angiomyolipomas is presumed to be hormone-dependent, and the risk of rupture is increased in pregnancy. Prophylactic excision, ablation, or embolization is generally recommended for tumors 4 cm or more in diameter. Tumors smaller than 4 cm can be managed by yearly imaging follow-up. The growth rate of sporadic angiomyolipomas is 5% per year. Tumors in patients with tuberous sclerosis have a 20% annual growth rate.

▶ **Imaging signs.** Angiomyolipomas appear sonographically as hyperechoic masses with a posterior acoustic shadow, resulting in a large overlap of findings with renal cell carcinoma (▶ Fig. 11.21). The appearance of angiomyolipoma on CT and MRI depends on the proportion of intratumoral fat. Grossly detectable fat with CT attenuation less than −20 HU is diagnostic. On MRI, angiomyolipomas are hyperintense in T2 W and T1 W sequences. There is loss of signal intensity in fat-suppressed sequences (▶ Fig. 11.22). Linear hypointensities are consistent with flow voids caused by blood flow in larger vessels within the mass. If CT and MRI show areas of definite fat attenuation or signal intensity within the tumor, angiomyolipoma is the most likely diagnosis because it is extremely rare for there to be fat in renal cell carcinoma.

▶ **Clinical features.** Smaller angiomyolipomas are asymptomatic and are usually detected incidentally during a routine ultrasound examination. Angiomyolipomas may present with flank pain due to lesion growth or (intratumoral) hemorrhage (see also Wunderlich's syndrome).

▶ **Differential diagnosis**
- Renal cell carcinoma (especially the clear cell and papillary types).
- Liposarcoma.
- Lipoma.

▶ **Pitfalls.** Approximately 5% of all angiomyolipomas do not contain fat detectable by CT or MRI. These lipid-poor angiomyolipomas are indistinguishable from renal cell carcinoma and require treatment by enucleation. Small angiomyolipomas may also be very difficult to distinguish from renal cell carcinoma.[26]

Lymphoma

▶ **Brief definition.** Like other organs, the kidneys are subject to involvement by lymphoma (more common with non-Hodgkin's lymphoma than Hodgkin's lymphoma). Primary renal lymphoma is very rare.

▶ **Imaging signs.** Renal involvement by lymphoma may present as a solitary focus or multiple foci. Diffuse lymphomatous infiltration of the kidney may also occur, resulting in renal enlargement. There may also be invasion from contiguous retroperitoneal lymphoma. Renal lymphoma has a homogeneous imaging appearance and shows less contrast enhancement than healthy renal tissue (▶ Fig. 11.23, ▶ Fig. 11.24).

Kidney and Urinary Tract

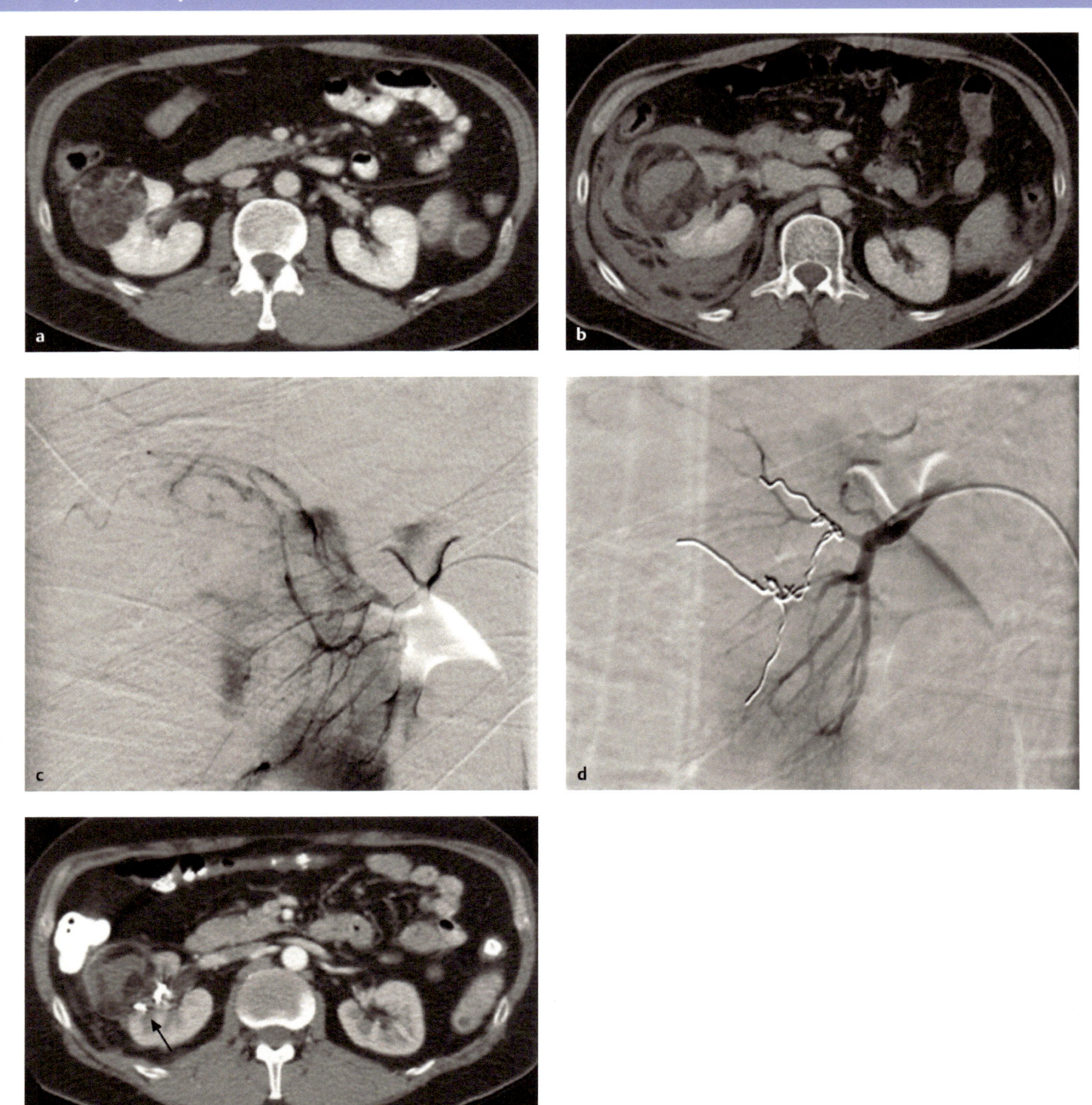

Fig. 11.20 Angiomyolipoma in a 45-year-old man. (a) CT shows characteristic density in the nephrographic phase. (b) Wunderlich's syndrome: acute retroperitoneal hemorrhage. (c) Angiography before coil embolization. (d) Angiography after coil embolization of the tumor-feeding vessels. (e) CT in the nephrographic phase 3 months after embolization. The hematoma has been reabsorbed. The coils can be identified (arrow).

▶ **Clinical features.** As well as flank pain and hematuria, primary renal lymphoma presents with the same B symptoms as systemic lymphoma, including unexplained fever, night sweats, unexplained weight loss, and reduced exercise tolerance. Other features are hypercalcemia and hyperuricemia culminating in renal failure.

▶ **Differential diagnosis**
- Renal infarction.
- Nephritis.

▶ **Pitfalls.** The presence of a cortical rim sign (i.e., a subcapsular enhancing rim with little or no enhancement elsewhere in the kidney) favors a differential diagnosis of renal infarction. Capsular vessels in this case are sufficient to maintain blood flow to the subcapsular renal parenchyma despite an infarction caused by renal artery occlusion or embolism.

Renal Cell Carcinoma

▶ **Brief definition.** The following main types of renal cell carcinoma are distinguished:
- *Clear cell carcinoma* (approximately 70–80% of all renal cell carcinomas).
- *Papillary renal cell carcinoma* (approximately 10–15% of all renal cell carcinomas).
- *Chromophobe renal cell carcinoma* (approximately 4–11% of all renal cell carcinomas).
- *Bellini duct carcinoma* (very rare, less than 1% of all renal cell carcinomas).
- *Unclassifiable renal cell carcinoma* (approximately 10% of all renal cell carcinomas).

Renal cell carcinomas constitute 85% of all malignant renal tumors. Approximately 10% are urothelial carcinomas of the pelvicalyceal system, and approximately 2% are renal sarcomas. Consistent with its epithelial cell origin, renal cell carcinoma arises from the renal tubules or collecting ducts. Risk factors are nicotine abuse, obesity, hypertension, diabetes mellitus, cystic renal degeneration, renal failure, and von Hippel–Lindau syndrome. On the risk factor profile, males currently predominate over females by a 2:1 ratio. The peak age of incidence of renal cell carcinoma is in the fifth to seventh decades. There are an estimated 64,000 new cases of renal cell carcinoma per year in the United States alone.

▶ **Imaging signs.** The sonographic features of renal cell carcinoma are highly variable. The tumor may be hypoechoic, isoechoic, or hyperechoic to healthy renal parenchyma. Some lesions have cystic components or cysts with solid central components. The different types present the following imaging signs:
- *Clear cell carcinoma*: This type appears as an enhancing heterogeneous mass on both CT and MRI (▶ Fig. 11.25). MRI findings depend on the presence and degree of intralesional hemorrhage or necrosis: the lesion may be isointense, hypointense, or hyperintense in T1 W sequences and heterogeneously hyperintense in T2 W sequences with a hypointense pseudocapsule. There may be disruption of the pseudocapsule, indicating fat infiltration. Cystic degeneration is found in 4 to 15% of cases.
- *Papillary renal cell carcinoma*: This lesion appears homogeneously hypointense in T2 W sequences (▶ Fig. 11.26). It shows relatively little enhancement and is also subject to necrotic and hemorrhagic changes.
- *Chromophobe renal cell carcinoma, Bellini duct carcinoma, and unclassifiable renal cell carcinoma*: These types are similar to clear cell carcinoma in their imaging characteristics.

The TNM classification of renal cell carcinoma is shown in ▶ Table 11.1.

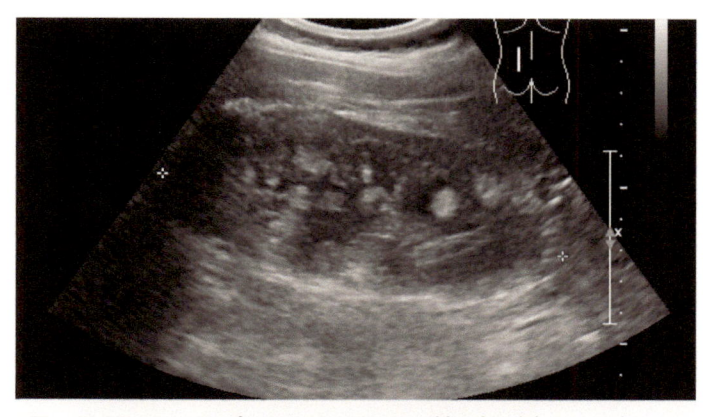

Fig. 11.21 Angiomyolipoma in a 13-year-old girl with known tuberous sclerosis. The left kidney is permeated by multiple echogenic masses.

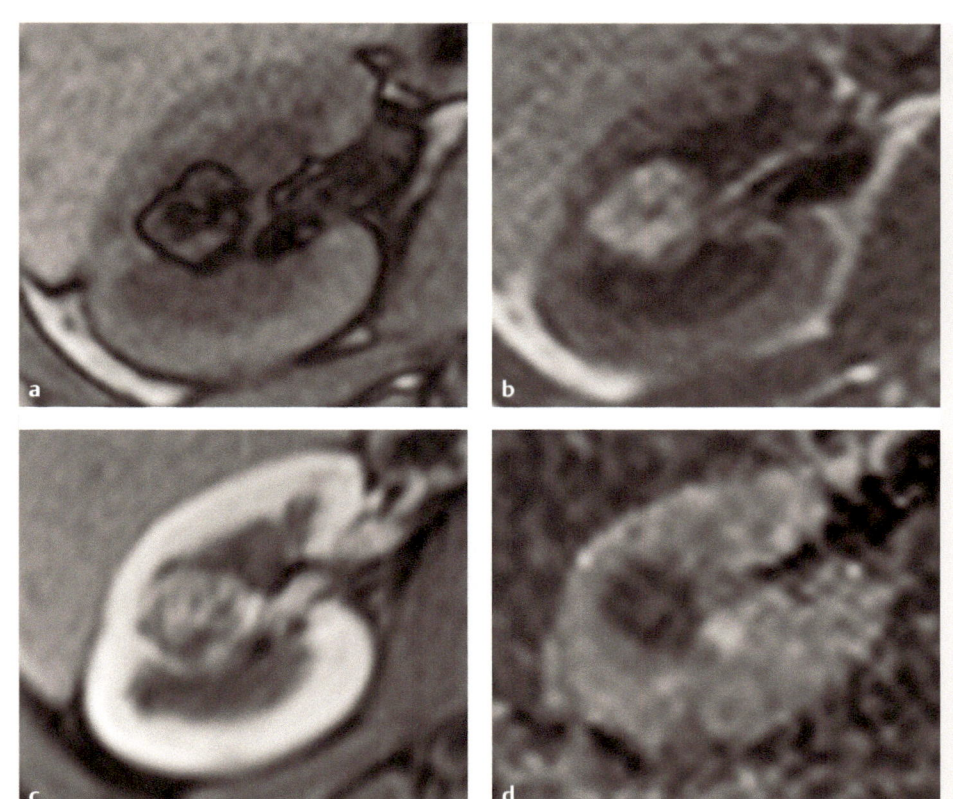

Fig. 11.22 Angiomyolipoma in a 66-year-old man with a heterogeneously enhancing mass on T1 W MRI (c) in the midportion of the right kidney with restricted diffusion (d). The mass is markedly hyperintense in the in-phase image (b) and shows significant loss of signal intensity (> 50%) in the opposed-phase image (a). This establishes the presence of cytoplasmic fat.
(a) Opposed-phase image. (b) In-phase image.
(c) T1 W image after administration of contrast medium. (d) ADC map.

Kidney and Urinary Tract

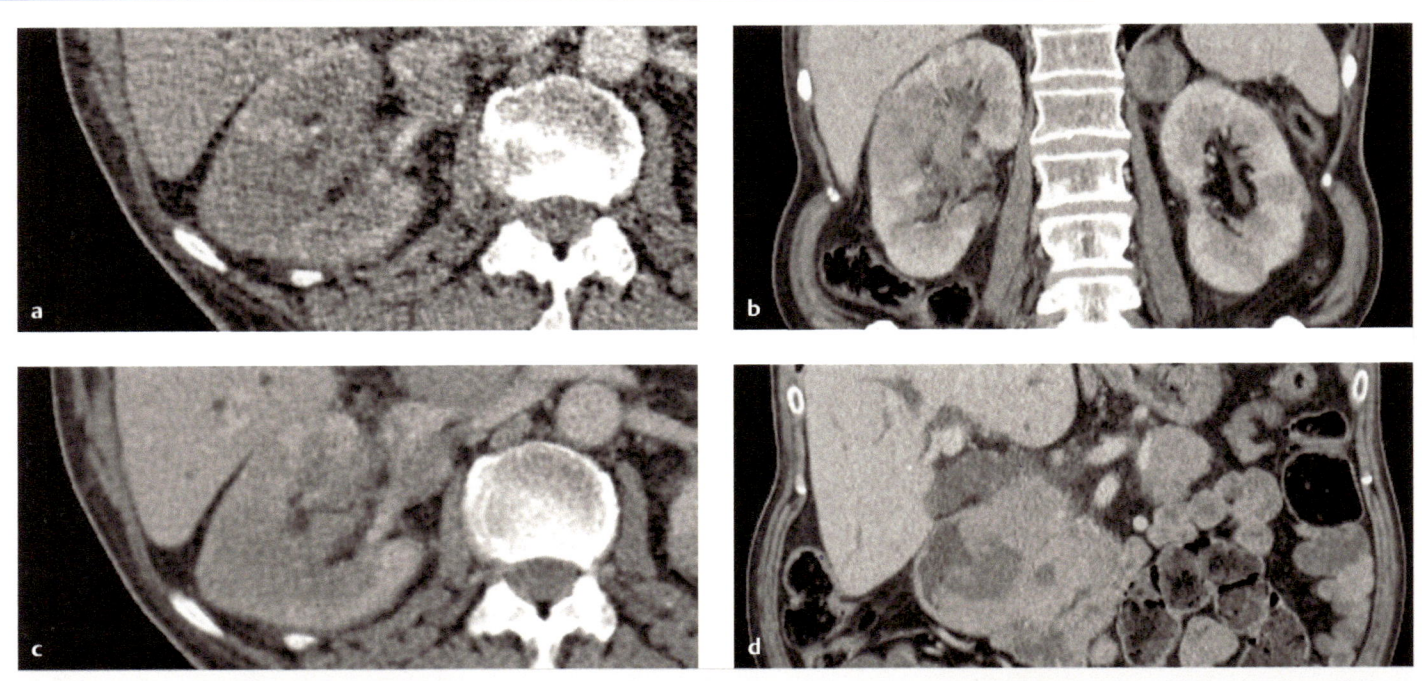

Fig. 11.23 Renal involvement by lymphoma in a 71-year-old man with known B-cell lymphoma. Laboratory tests showed elevated cholestase parameters and lipase activity. CT shows hypodense renal lesions that are not hypervascular in the early arterial phase (**a**) and show only faint, homogeneous enhancement in the portal venous phase (**b, c**). Lymphomatous involvement of the pancreas and duodenum is also present, causing obstructed biliary drainage and cholestasis. (**a**) Axial CT, early arterial phase. (**b**) Coronal CT, venous phase. (**c**) Axial CT, venous phase. (**d**) Coronal reformatted CT, venous phase.

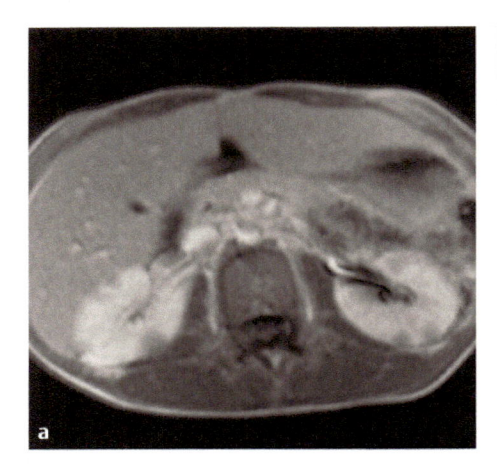

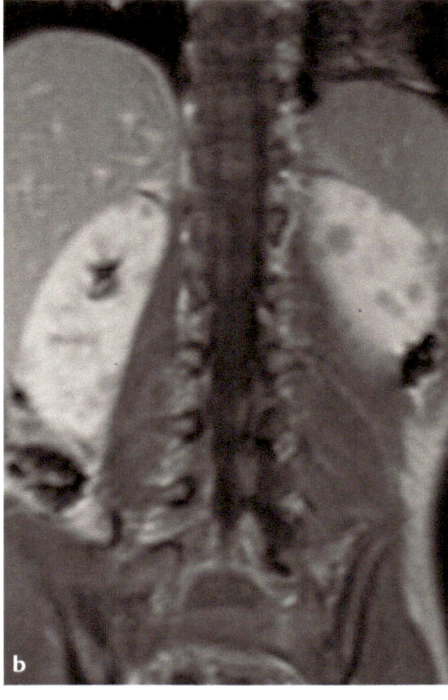

Fig. 11.24 Renal involvement by lymphoma in a 24-year-old woman with histologically confirmed non-Hodgkin's lymphoma. MRI shows multiple bilateral renal masses that are hypointense to normal renal parenchyma in the contrast-enhanced T1W sequence. (**a**) Axial image. (**b**) Coronal image.

▶ **Clinical features.** Because renal cell carcinomas are usually asymptomatic in their initial stage, they are detected incidentally during routine sonography or other imaging studies. Tumors at an advanced stage present with nonspecific symptoms such as weight loss, unexplained fever, fatigue, and anemia. Abdominal pain and gross hematuria may also be present, depending on tumor size.

Note

When findings are reported, it is important for surgical planning to describe the relationship of the renal cell carcinoma to the renal pelvis and vessels.

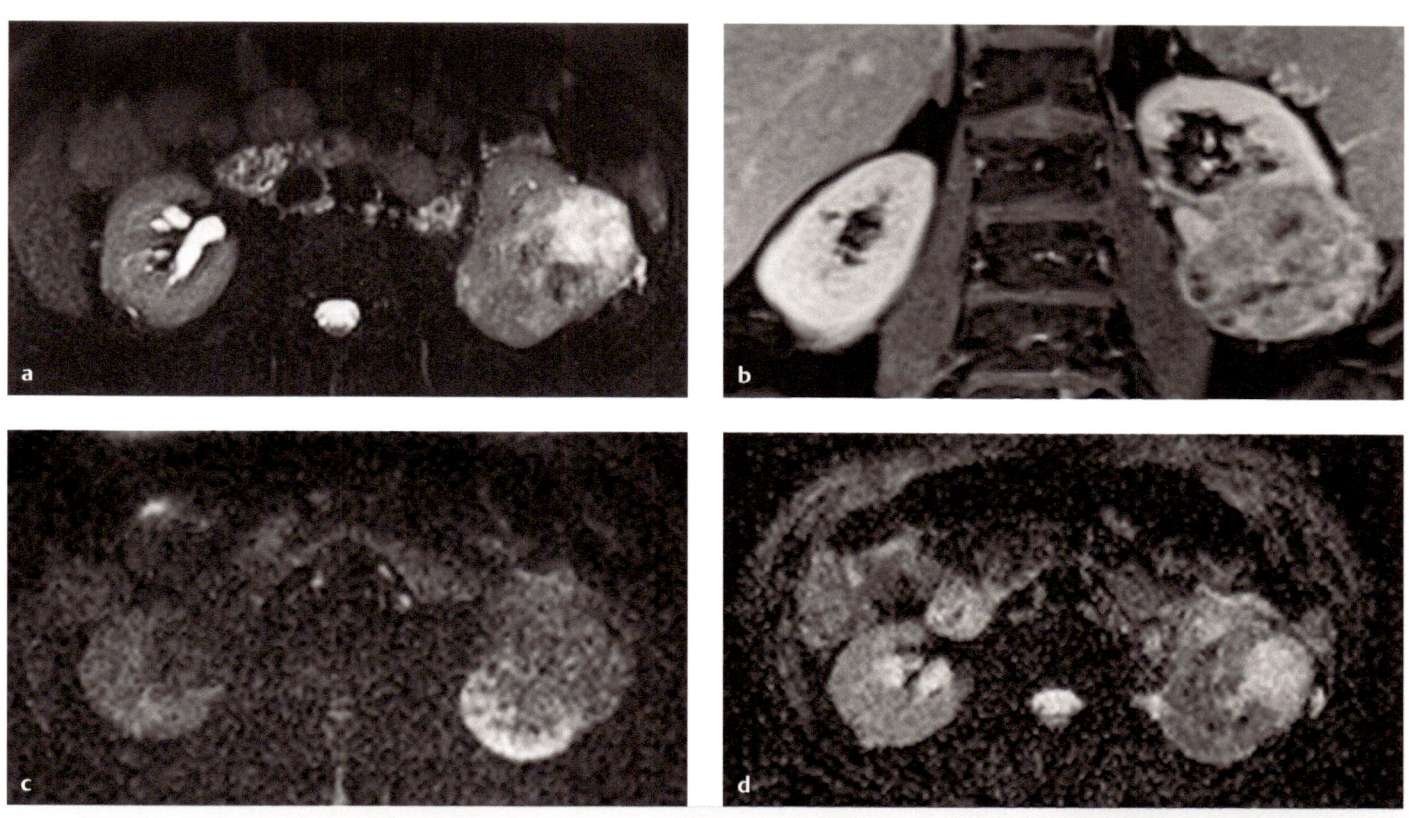

Fig. 11.25 Renal cell carcinoma (clear cell type) in a 42-year-old man with a mass in the lower pole of the left kidney. The mass is heterogeneously hyperintense in the T2W sequence (a) and shows marked heterogeneous enhancement in the postcontrast T1W sequence (b). The solid components (posteromedial) show significant restricted diffusion (c, d). (a) T2W image. (b) T1W after administration of contrast medium. (c) Diffusion-weighted image. (d) ADC map.

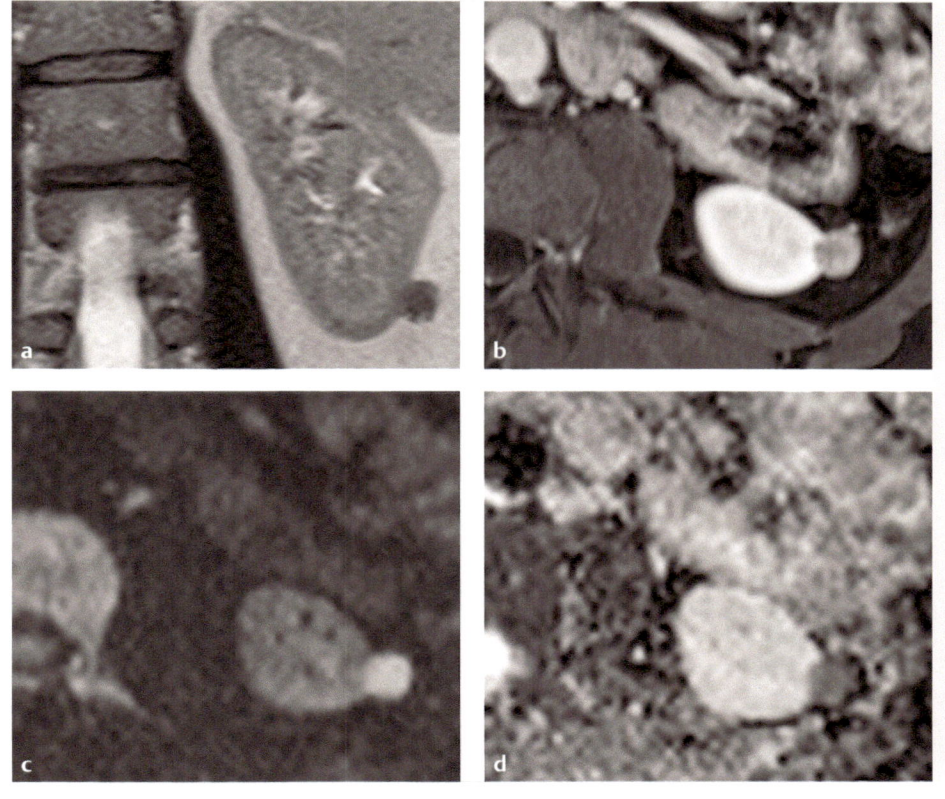

Fig. 11.26 Renal cell carcinoma (papillary type). Exophytic mass in the lower pole of the left kidney is hypointense in the T2W sequence (a) and shows moderate enhancement in the postcontrast T1W sequence (b) and restricted diffusion (c, d). (a) T2W image. (b) T1W image after administration of contrast medium. (c) Diffusion-weighted image. (d) ADC map.

Table 11.1 TNM classification of renal cell carcinoma[27]

Designation	Description
Primary tumor	
TX	Primary tumor cannot be assessed
T0	No evidence of primary tumor
T1	Tumor ≤ 7 cm in greatest dimension, limited to the kidney
• T1a	Tumor ≤ 4 cm in greatest dimension, limited to the kidney
• T1b	Tumor > 4 cm but ≤ 7 cm in greatest dimension, limited to the kidney
T2	Tumor > 7 cm in greatest dimension, limited to the kidney
• T2a	Tumor > 7 cm but ≤ 10 cm in greatest dimension, limited to the kidney
• T2b	Tumor > 10 cm in greatest dimension, limited to the kidney
T3	Tumor extends into major veins or perinephric tissues but not into the ipsilateral adrenal gland and not beyond the Gerota's fascia
• T3a	Tumor grossly extends into the renal vein or its segmental (muscle-containing) branches, or tumor invades perirenal and/or renal sinus fat but not beyond the Gerota's fascia
• T3b	Tumor grossly extends into the vena cava below the diaphragm
• T3c	Tumor grossly extends into the vena cava above the diaphragm or invades the wall of the vena cava
T4	Tumor invades beyond the Gerota's fascia (including contiguous extension into the ipsilateral adrenal gland)
Regional lymph nodes	
NX	Regional lymph nodes cannot be assessed
N0	No regional lymph node metastasis
N1	Metastasis in a single regional lymph node
N2	Metastasis in more than one regional lymph node
Distant metastasis	
MX	Distant metastasis cannot be assessed
M0	No distant metastasis
M1	Distant metastasis

Pediatric Tumors

Nephroblastoma

▶ **Brief definition.** Nephroblastoma, also known as Wilms's tumor, is a malignant dysontogenetic tumor composed of primitive nephroblastic tissue. It arises from persistent embryonic cells of the metanephrogenic blastema. Nephroblastoma is the most common renal tumor in children and adolescents, with a prevalence of 1:100,000. Most nephroblastomas occur before 4 years of age. An associated anomaly is Beckwith–Wiedemann syndrome (also known as omphalocele-macroglossia-gigantism syndrome).

▶ **Imaging signs.** Nephroblastoma may reach an enormous size by the time of diagnosis, causing displacement of surrounding structures. Generally the initial imaging study is ultrasonography, which shows an echogenic mass with a pseudocapsule (compressed renal parenchyma) arising from the kidney (▶ Fig. 11.27). The guidelines of the German Association of Scientific Medical Societies (AWMF) and also most other national and international societies recommend MRI as the second imaging study after ultrasound. Nephroblastoma has an inhomogeneous MRI appearance in both T1W and T2W sequences. Small areas of intratumoral hemorrhage (hyperintense in unenhanced T1W images) may be detected in some cases. Nephroblastoma shows heterogeneous enhancement after IV administration of contrast medium (▶ Fig. 11.28). Most guidelines recommend plain chest radiographs in two planes to exclude pulmonary metastases. Suspicious findings should be investigated further by spiral CT. International Society of Pediatric Oncology (SIOP) criteria are used for the staging of nephroblastoma (▶ Table 11.2).

▶ **Clinical features.** Children typically present with a painless abdominal mass. There is rarely hematuria or hypertension. If the tumor is relatively small, it may sometimes be detected incidentally during an ultrasound examination for a different indication.

11.1 Kidney

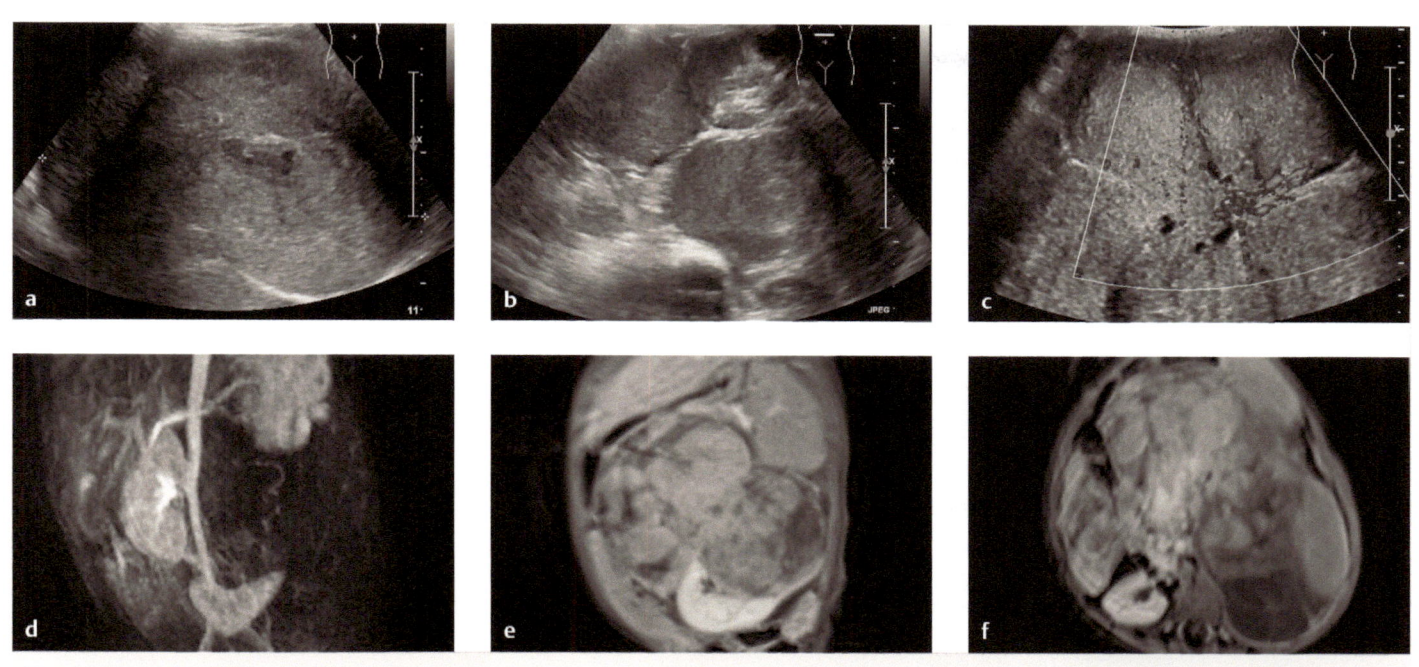

Fig. 11.27 Nephroblastoma. (a) Ultrasound shows a large, well-circumscribed mass of heterogeneous echogenicity in the left upper quadrant. (b) The mass crosses the midline. (c) Color Doppler scan shows predominantly peripheral vascularity. (d) Time-resolved MR angiography with interleaved stochastic trajectories (TWIST) shows slight aortic displacement to the right and perfused normal renal parenchyma, which is displaced inferiorly. (e) Contrast-enhanced T1W image shows a lobulated mass arising from the left kidney. (f) The mass crosses the midline.

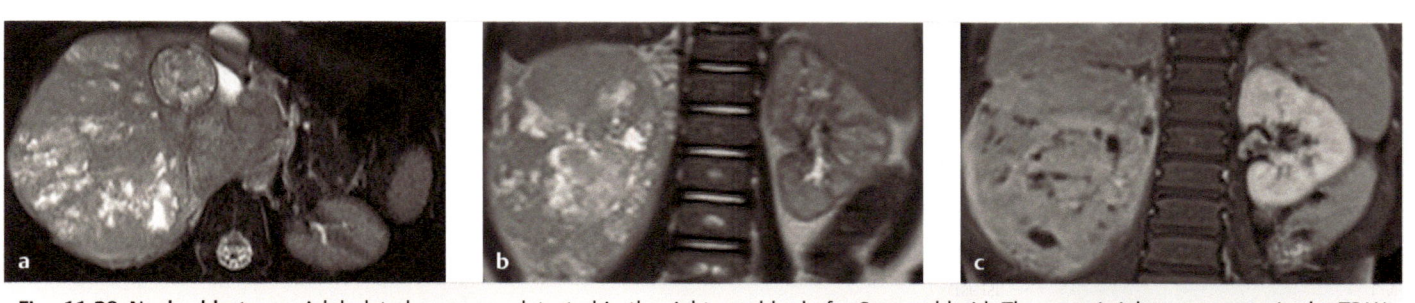

Fig. 11.28 Nephroblastoma. A lobulated mass was detected in the right renal bed of a 6-year-old girl. The mass is inhomogeneous in the T2W sequences (a, b) and enhances intensely in the T1W sequence (c). (a) Axial T2W sequence. (b) Coronal T2W sequence. (c) T1W sequence after administration of contrast medium.

Table 11.2 SIOP staging system for nephroblastoma

Stage	Description
I	Tumor is limited to the kidney; the renal capsule may be infiltrated with the tumor, but it does not reach the outer surface; the tumor is completely resectable
II	Tumor extends beyond the kidney or penetrates through the renal capsule but is completely resectable; abdominal lymph nodes are not involved
III	Incomplete excision of the tumor, which extends beyond resection margins; no hematogenous metastasis; tumor rupture before surgery or intraoperatively; any abdominal lymph nodes are involved
IV	Hematogenous metastases or lymph node metastases outside the abdominopelvic region
V	Bilateral renal involvement at diagnosis

Abbreviation: SIOP, International Society of Pediatric Oncology.

Note

Nephroblastoma detected by imaging in children from 6 months to 16 years of age but not confirmed histologically should be treated with cytostatic therapy to reduce tumor size. Percutaneous or open tumor biopsy would carry a risk of inoculation metastasis and peritoneal seeding. Histological confirmation and determination of histological subtype (low-grade, standard risk, high-grade) are then done within the framework of tumor nephrectomy following chemotherapy.

Untreated cases have a grave prognosis. Standard treatment modalities are chemotherapy, surgery, and radiotherapy. Preoperative chemotherapy increases the number of patients who come to surgery with stage 1 disease. Postoperative therapy is then geared toward the stage achieved by chemotherapy and the histological subtype.

▶ **Differential diagnosis**
- Mesoblastic nephroma.
- Neuroblastoma (displaces the kidney inferiorly).
- Renal lymphoma.

▶ **Pitfalls.** If the origin of the mass is uncertain, especially in the case of large masses, it may be helpful to evaluate the surrounding healthy renal parenchyma. If compressed renal tissue is found on or around the tumor, this confirms that the mass has a renal origin. This is also evidenced by destruction of the renal pelvis.

Neuroblastoma

▶ **Brief definition.** Neuroblastoma is a malignant embryonic tumor of the sympathetic nervous system. Accordingly, neuroblastomas occur not only in the adrenal gland (adrenal medulla, 48% of neuroblastomas) but also at sites along the cervical, thoracic, and abdominal sympathetic trunk and in the paraganglia. The second most common site of occurrence after the adrenal bed is the extra-adrenal retroperitoneum (25% of neuroblastomas). Neuroblastoma is the most common extracranial solid tumor in children. Based on data from the SEER database, the incidence of neuroblastoma in children under 14 years of age in the United States is about 10.5/100,000 (population at risk). Because neuroblastomas are embryonic tumors, most are diagnosed during the first years of life: approximately 40% in the first 12 months, and 90% of patients are younger than age 6 at the time of diagnosis. The incidence declines with increasing age.

▶ **Imaging signs.** As with almost all pediatric tumors, ultrasound is the initial imaging study used to define the primary tumor and evaluate locoregional lymph nodes. This is followed by detailed imaging with MRI, which is superior to other modalities for detecting intraspinal extension of neuroblastoma through the neural foramina. MIBG (metaiodobenzylguanidine) scintigraphy is used to screen for metastases. Neuroblastoma appears sonographically as an echogenic mass with inhomogeneities due to necrosis, cystic changes, intratumoral hemorrhage, and calcifications (▶ Fig. 11.29). In some cases, the intraspinal extension of tumor through the neural foramina is already detectable on initial ultrasound. On MRI, neuroblastomas are heterogeneous even on unenhanced images. They are hyperintense in T2 W sequences and hypointense in T1 W sequences. Extensions into adjacent neural foramina may be apparent. Calcifications are a more common finding in neuroblastoma than in nephroblastoma. Unlike nephroblastomas, neuroblastomas are characterized by invasive growth and vascular encasement (▶ Fig. 11.30). Neuroblastoma is classified into four stages in the International Neuroblastoma Staging System (INSS, ▶ Table 11.3).

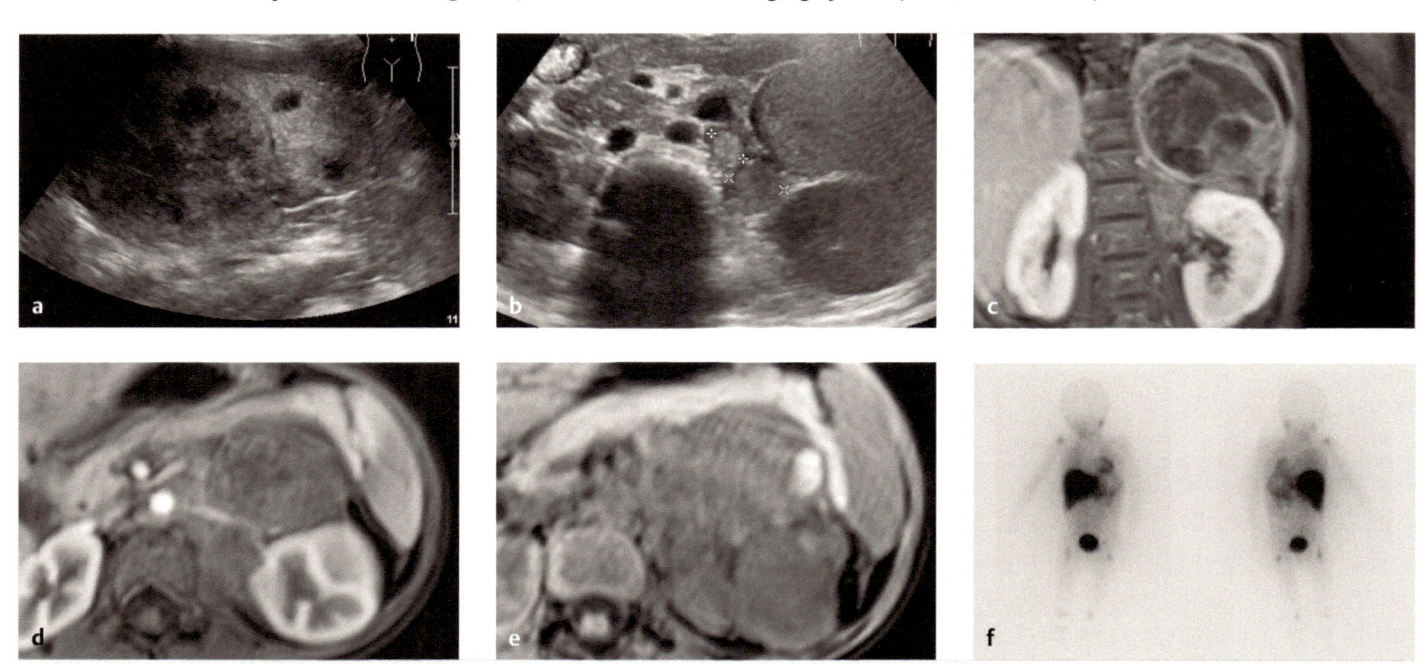

Fig. 11.29 Neuroblastoma. (a) Ultrasound shows a left-upper-quadrant mass of heterogeneous echogenicity that includes echo-free and necrotic components. (b) Sonographic view of para-aortic lymph node metastases. (c) Coronal T1 W sequence after administration of contrast medium. The mass is delineated from the kidney, which is displaced inferiorly, and shows heterogeneous enhancement. (d) Axial T1 W sequence after administration of contrast medium. The mass encases the renal vessels. (e) Axial T1 W sequence before administration of contrast medium. Hyperintense components in the unenhanced image represent intratumoral hemorrhage. (f) MIBG scan depicts the primary tumor in the left upper quadrant along with sites of skeletal metastasis, including the right humerus.

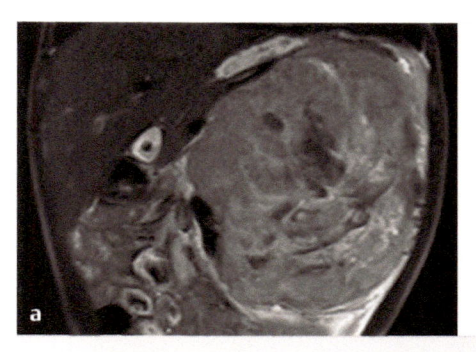

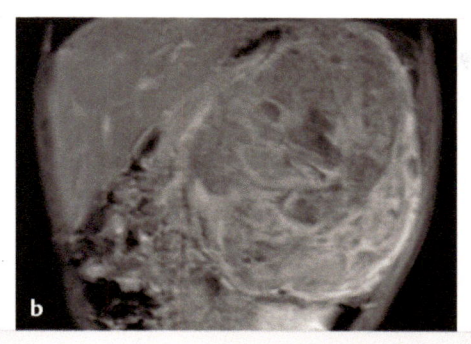

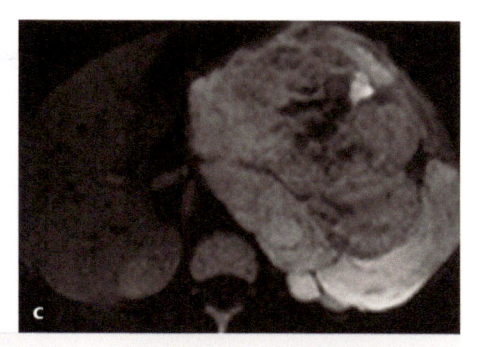

Fig. 11.30 Neuroblastoma. (a) T2W image shows a heterogeneous mass with areas of intralesional hemorrhage and necrosis in the left upper and midabdomen. (b) T1W image after administration of contrast medium shows inhomogeneous enhancement. Branches of the celiac trunk can be seen passing through the mass. This finding is characteristic of neuroblastoma. (c) DWI shows restricted diffusion.

Table 11.3 International Neuroblastoma Staging System (INSS) for neuroblastoma

Stage	Description
I	Completely resectable tumor confined to the area of origin
II	Incompletely resectable tumor that does not cross the midline
III	Tumor infiltrating across the midline or contralateral lymph node involvement
IV	Distant metastasis

▶ **Clinical features.** There may be urinary tract obstruction, depending on tumor size. Intraspinal tumor extension through the neural foramina leads to corresponding neurologic symptoms. Patients with an advanced tumor stage present with (nonspecific) B symptoms such as lethargy and fever.

▶ **Differential diagnosis**
- Wilms's tumor.
- Adrenal hemorrhage.
- Ganglioneuroblastoma.
- Ganglioneuroma.

▶ **Pitfalls.** Vessels may be encased by tumor. This imaging finding in children under 6 years old is strongly suggestive of neuroblastoma. The second most important differential diagnosis in this age group, nephroblastoma, tends to displace rather than encase vessels. Similarly, benign masses such as ganglioneuromas do not encase vessels.

Inflammatory Changes
Acute and Chronic Pyelonephritis

▶ **Brief definition.** Pyelonephritis is the most common bacterial infection of the kidney. The most frequent causes is ascending cystitis. The main causative organism is *Escherichia coli*, which suppresses ureteral peristalsis and creates a route for retrograde infection of the kidney. A special form is emphysematous pyelonephritis, a rare necrotizing infection of the renal parenchyma with gas production. Diabetes mellitus is the principal risk factor (90% of patients) for the development of emphysematous pyelonephritis. The main causative organism of emphysematous pyelonephritis is again *Escherichia coli*. The disease has a high mortality rate and requires immediate intervention.

▶ **Imaging signs.** According to the S3 guidelines of the AWMF and the ACR appropriateness criteria, imaging is unnecessary in the diagnostic work-up of uncomplicated pyelonephritis in adults. Ultrasound is the modality of choice for the investigation of complicating factors. Other imaging modalities are necessary only to address specific questions that may be raised by sonographic findings, and the preferred modality will depend on the nature of the questions raised. Vesicoureteral reflux is the most frequent cause of pyelonephritis in small children. Patients with repeated episodes of pyelonephritis should be evaluated for reflux by sonography or voiding cystourethrography in an infection-free interval (▶ Fig. 11.31, ▶ Table 11.4). Voiding cystourethrography should be performed by doctors experienced in the use of fluoroscopic equipment, as the gonadal dose from this examination may be relatively high. The fluoroscopic equipment should allow for pulsed exposure and the storage of fluoroscopic images (last-image-hold in the fluoroscopic sequence, to reduce the number of frames needed for documentation).

> **Note**
>
> Children with suspected pyelonephritis should undergo ultrasound examination to exclude possible anomalies associated with urinary tract obstruction.

The kidney may be swollen to twice its normal size in the acute stage of pyelonephritis. A hallmark of pyelonephritis is the spreading of inflammation past the papillary tips and tubules into the renal cortex. The interstitial edema associated with pyelonephritis raises the tissue pressure, leading to vascular constriction followed by wedge-shaped defects (▶ Fig. 11.32). In contrast, a hematogenous infection leads to peripheral lesions distributed in the cortex. Thus, the sectional imaging of pyelonephritis displays a spoked-wheel pattern of wedge-shaped parenchymal changes that show less enhancement than the surrounding parenchyma (▶ Fig. 11.33). The infected kidney is enlarged relative to the opposite side. Areas that have undergone inflammatory changes appear hypointense in the ADC map. This results from restricted diffusion due to the inflammatory reaction (▶ Fig. 11.34). Delayed excretion is also noted in the inflammatory areas. This may be associated with inflammatory perirenal

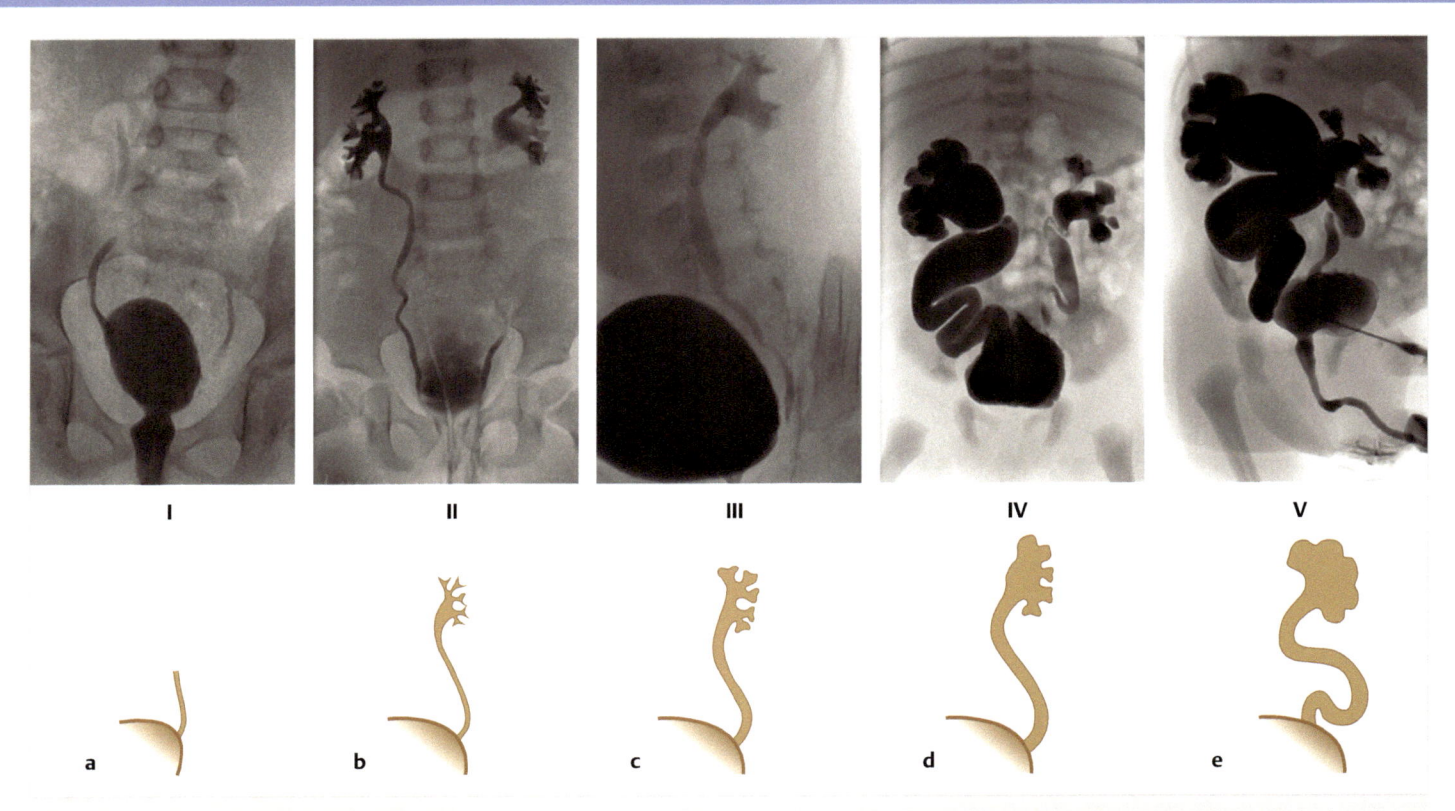

Fig. 11.31 Grades of vesicoureteral reflux in the International Reflux Study Group classification. Diagrammatic representation (below) and sample images (above). In addition to the AP view, the ureters are each displayed in a rotated view (c). The urethra is completely visualized (e) and should be evaluated for the presence of a urethral valve. (If a transurethral catheter was used for intravesical contrast instillation, it should be removed for this purpose.) (a) Grade I. (b) Grade II. (c) Grade III. (d) Grade IV (right side). (e) Grade IV (left side).

Table 11.4 International Reflux Study Group grading system for vesicoureteral reflux. Reflux is also classified as low-pressure or high-pressure reflux based on its occurrence at rest or only during micturition

Grade	Description
I	Reflux into the ureter only
II	Reflux into the collecting system, without dilatation
III	Reflux into the collecting system with mild dilatation, slight ureteral tortuosity, and little or no blunting of the fornices
IV	Moderate dilatation and/or tortuosity of the ureter and moderate dilatation of the renal pelvis and calyces, with complete obliteration of the sharp angle of the fornices but maintenance of the papillary impressions
V	Gross dilatation and tortuosity of the ureter, with gross dilatation of the renal pelvis and calyces and absence of papillary impressions

changes such as imbibition of perirenal fat and a thin perirenal fluid film. Progression of inflammation may even lead to abscess formation, characterized by round to oval-shaped honeycomb areas with peripheral rim enhancement and restricted diffusion (▶ Fig. 11.35). Emphysematous pyelonephritis is distinguished from other diseases by the presence of gas collections.

▶ Clinical features. The initiating event is often an acute upper urinary tract infection that is clinically silent. Progression of the untreated infection leads to pyelonephritis, which presents with flank pain and systemic signs such as fever, chills, lethargy, and dysuria. There are also acute forms of pyelonephritis that cause nonspecific gastrointestinal complaints. Chronic pyelonephritis—apart from acute flares with symptoms like those of acute pyelonephritis—is usually manifested by nonspecific symptoms such as weight loss and fatigue. The advanced stage is marked by organ damage leading to renal failure.

▶ Differential diagnosis. The differential diagnosis of pyelonephritis includes trauma, infarction, and malacoplakia. Malacoplakia (▶ Fig. 11.36) is a rare inflammatory disorder characterized by nodular plaque formation. It occurs predominantly in immunosuppressed patients and those with diabetes mellitus and lymphoma. MRI demonstrates renal enlargement and heterogeneous enhancement. The renal parenchyma shows inhomogeneous signal characteristics in T2W sequences. Malacoplakia is treatable with antibiotics.

▶ Pitfalls. Pyelonephritis may be misinterpreted as renal infarction. In contrast to pyelonephritis, the renal infarct appears as a wedge-shaped area that does not show contrast enhancement except for the subcapsular cortex.

Xanthogranulomatous Pyelonephritis

▶ Brief definition. Xanthogranulomatous pyelonephritis is a chronic granulomatous bacterial infection of the kidney resulting from chronic obstruction of the pelvicalyceal system. The chronic

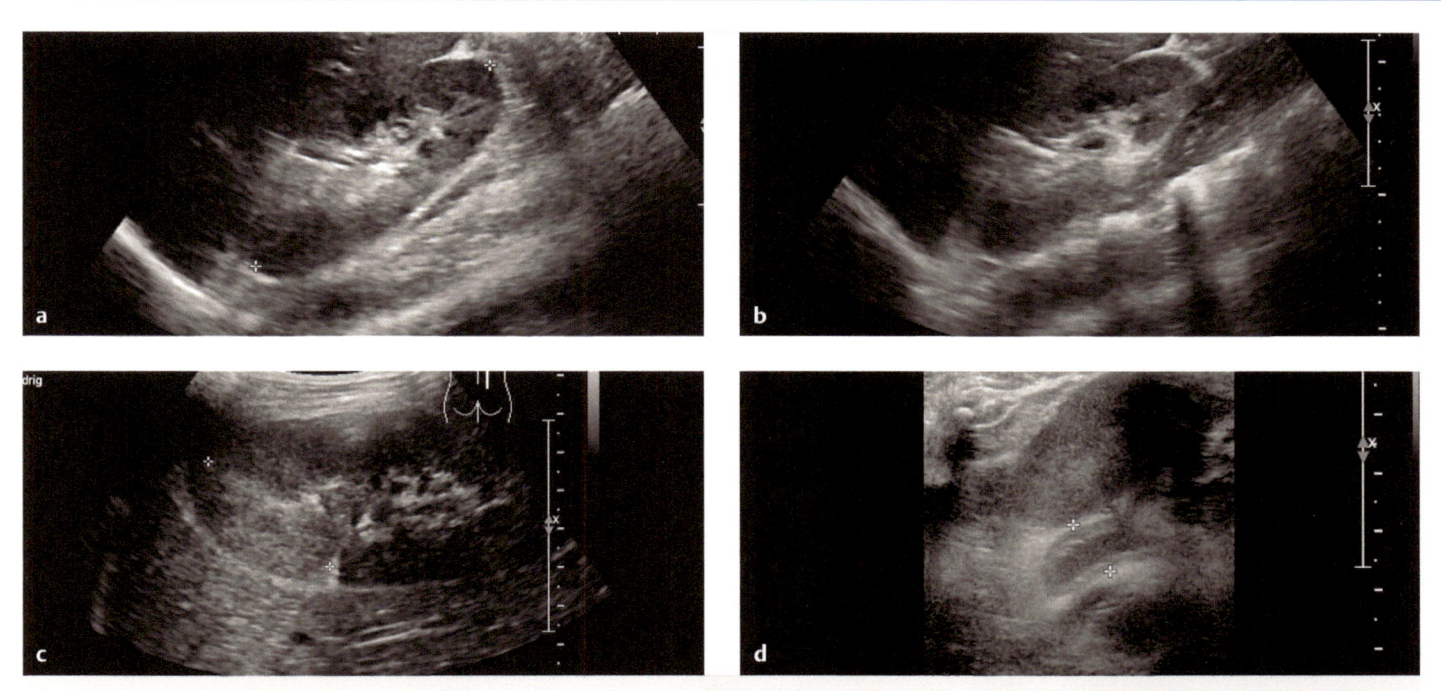

Fig. 11.32 Pyelonephritis. Ultrasound scans show an echogenic, wedge-shaped area in the upper portion of the right kidney (**a, c**) and marked thickening of the renal pelvic wall (positive urothelial sign [**b, d**]). (**a**) Transhepatic scan from the anterior side (curved array transducer). (**b**) Transhepatic scan from the anterior side (curved array transducer). (**c**) Scan from the posterior side (curved array transducer). (**d**) Scan from the posterior side (linear transducer).

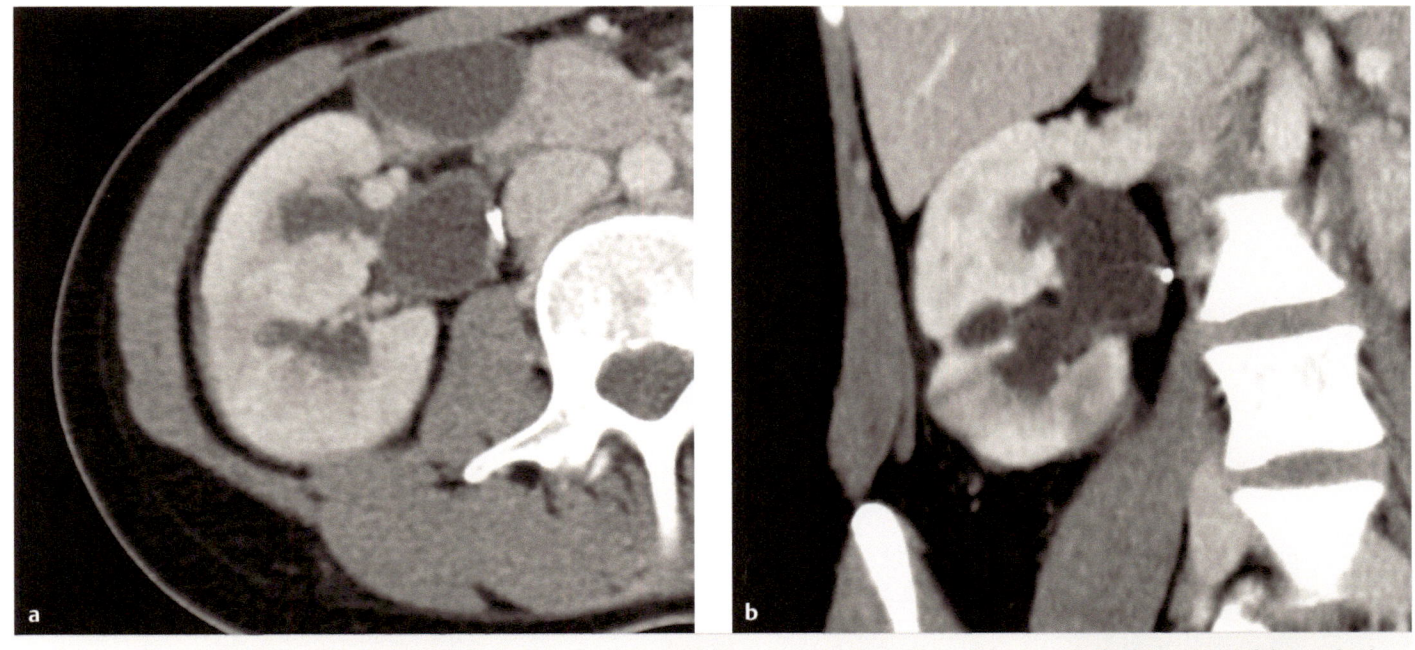

Fig. 11.33 Pyelonephritis in a patient with dilatation of the right pelvicalyceal system. (**a**) Axial CT shows thickening and enhancement of the renal pelvic wall. (**b**) Coronal reformatted image shows faint, wedge-shaped hypoenhancing areas in the renal lower pole with loss of corticomedullary differentiation.

obstruction leads to dilatation of the calyces, which are filled with cellular debris and pus, and to parenchymal atrophy.

▶ **Imaging signs.** Imaging typically demonstrates a large calculus in the renal pelvis with associated calyceal dilatation and possible hilar lymphadenopathy. The renal outline is enlarged. These findings are well depicted by ultrasound. MRI or CT shows relative hypoperfusion of the renal parenchyma (▶ Fig. 11.37). Xanthogranulomatous pyelonephritis is hyperintense in T2 W sequences and iso- to hypointense in T1 W sequences (▶ Fig. 11.38).

▶ **Clinical features.** The clinical presentation of xanthogranulomatous pyelonephritis is nonspecific. Typical symptoms are flank pain and nonspecific signs such as fever, weight loss, and chills. Other findings are positive urine cultures and a possible flank mass. The treatment of choice is surgical resection.

Kidney and Urinary Tract

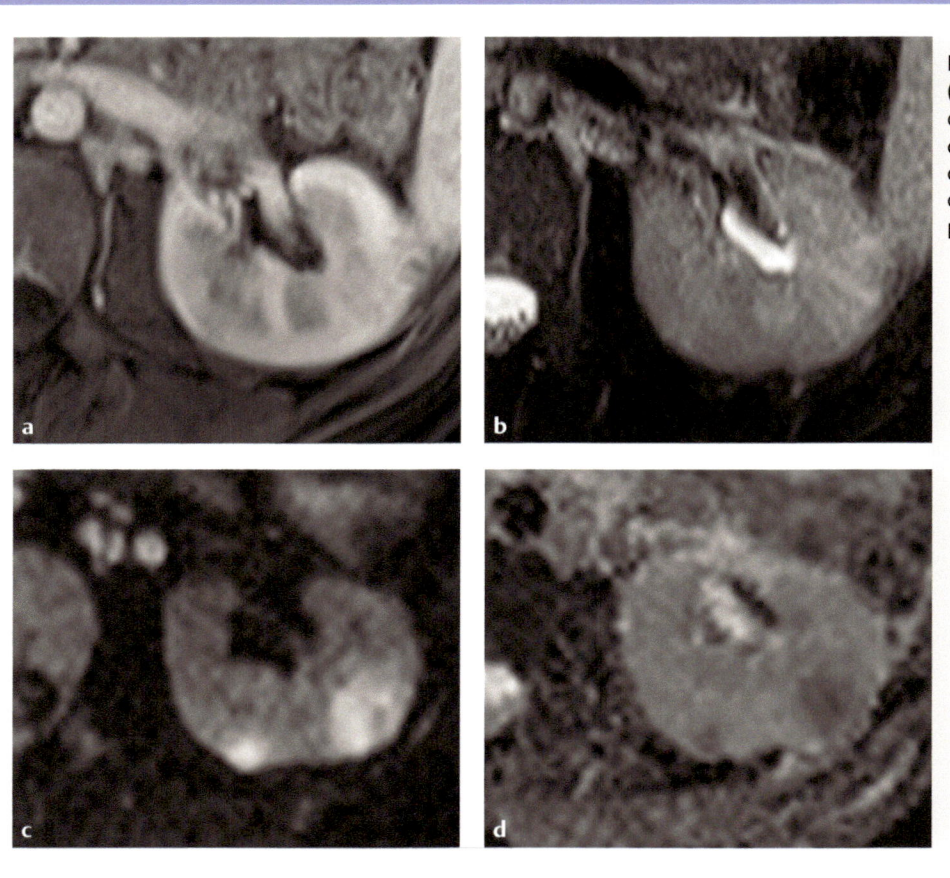

Fig. 11.34 **Pyelonephritis** in a 21-year-old man. (a) T1W sequence after administration of contrast medium shows wedge-shaped areas of decreased perfusion. (b) T2W sequence shows corresponding hyperintensity. (c) DWI shows corresponding restricted diffusion in the mid-portion of the left kidney. (d) ADC map.

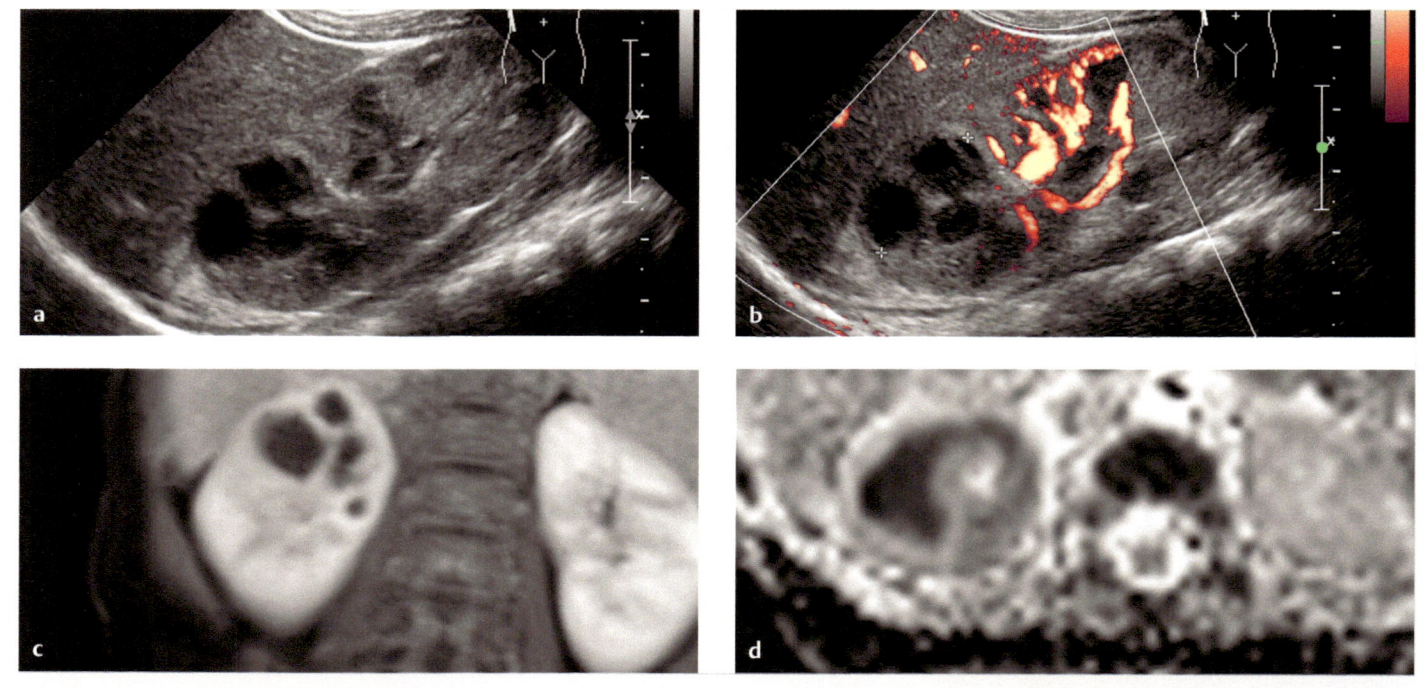

Fig. 11.35 **Renal abscess** in a 4-month-old child with elevated temperature (38.5 °C). (a) Ultrasound demonstrates a hypoechoic loculated mass with central echo-free areas in the upper pole of the right kidney. (b) Color and power Doppler imaging shows absence of vascularity. (c) Coronal T1W sequence shows central hypointense components. (d) ADC map shows a mass with low ADC values.

▶ **Differential diagnosis**
- Urothelial carcinoma.
- Lymphoma.

▶ **Pitfalls.** A common error is to misinterpret the mass effect of xanthogranulomatous pyelonephritis as urothelial carcinoma (▶ Fig. 11.39). The presence of a calculus occluding the proximal ureter suggests the correct diagnosis.

Vascular Changes

Atherosclerotic Renal Artery Stenosis

▶ **Brief definition.** In 90% of cases, renal artery stenosis is caused by focal acquired atherosclerotic changes in the vessel wall, which typically involve the ostial portion of the artery. The stenosis occurs within a setting of generalized atherosclerosis.

11.1 Kidney

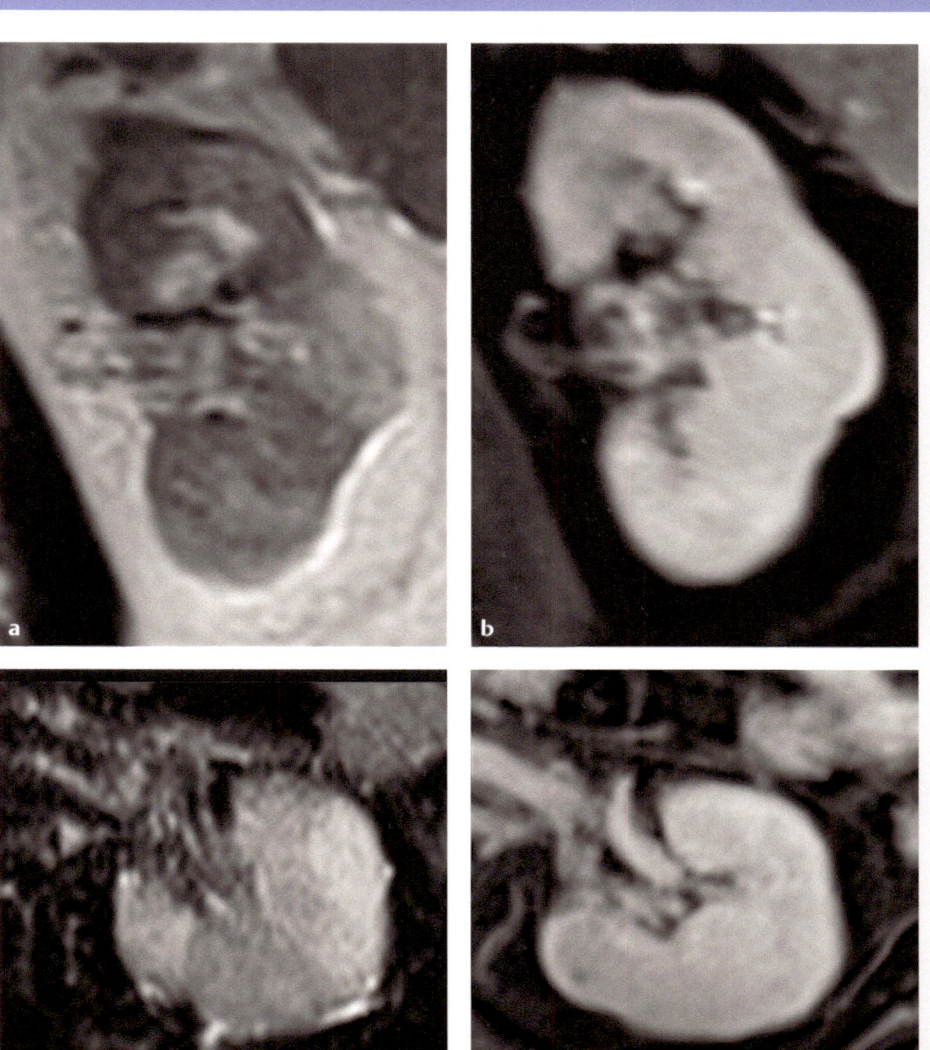

Fig. 11.36 Malacoplakia in a 73-year-old man. **(a)** T2W sequence demonstrates lobular, hyperintense parenchymal changes in the left kidney. **(b)** Coronal T1W sequence after administration of contrast medium shows absence of definite enhancement. **(c)** diffusion-weighted imaging (ADC map) shows mild restricted diffusion. **(d)** Corresponding axial T1W sequence after administration of contrast medium.

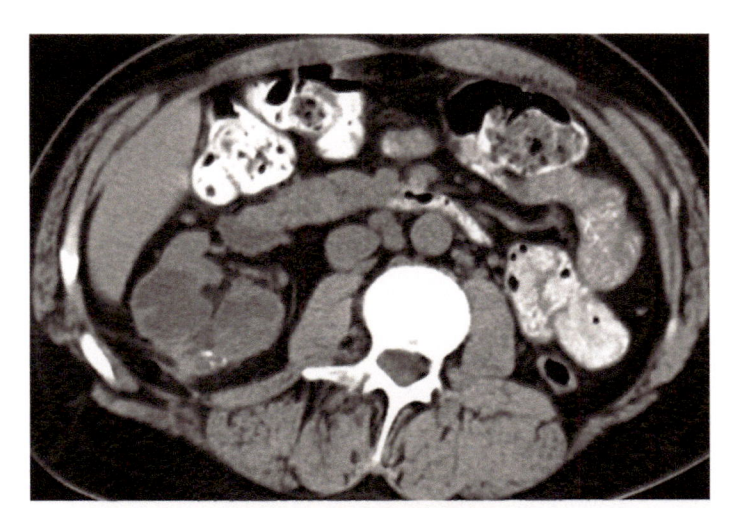

Fig. 11.37 Xanthogranulomatous pyelonephritis. Unenhanced CT shows typical expansion and decreased density.

For example, 45% of patients with peripheral arterial occlusive disease are also found to have renal artery stenosis. The prevalence of atherosclerotic renal artery stenosis in autopsy studies is 4.3%.[28,29] Renal artery stenosis is the leading cause of secondary hypertension, which is provoked by the renin–angiotensin system in response to decreased renal blood flow. Hemodynamically significant renal artery stenosis additionally leads to deterioration of renal function.

▶ **Imaging signs.** Conventional angiography has been replaced almost completely as a diagnostic modality by Doppler ultrasound and MRA; today it is used only during the interventional therapy of renal artery stenosis. The imaging hallmark is focal luminal narrowing that predominantly involves the proximal third of the renal artery. Renal artery stenosis is graded according to the percentage of vessel narrowing. Based on current guidelines, renal artery stenosis is diagnosed when luminal narrowing exceeds 50%. The stenosis is classified as hemodynamically significant when luminal narrowing exceeds 70%. Narrowing greater than 95 to 99% is defined as preocclusive renal artery stenosis (▶ Fig. 11.40).

▶ **Clinical features.** Hemodynamically significant narrowing of the renal artery is usually manifested by arterial hypertension. It may also lead to impaired renal function, otherwise unexplained pulmonary edema, and heart failure.

▶ **Differential diagnosis.** Differentiation is required from fibromuscular dysplasia.

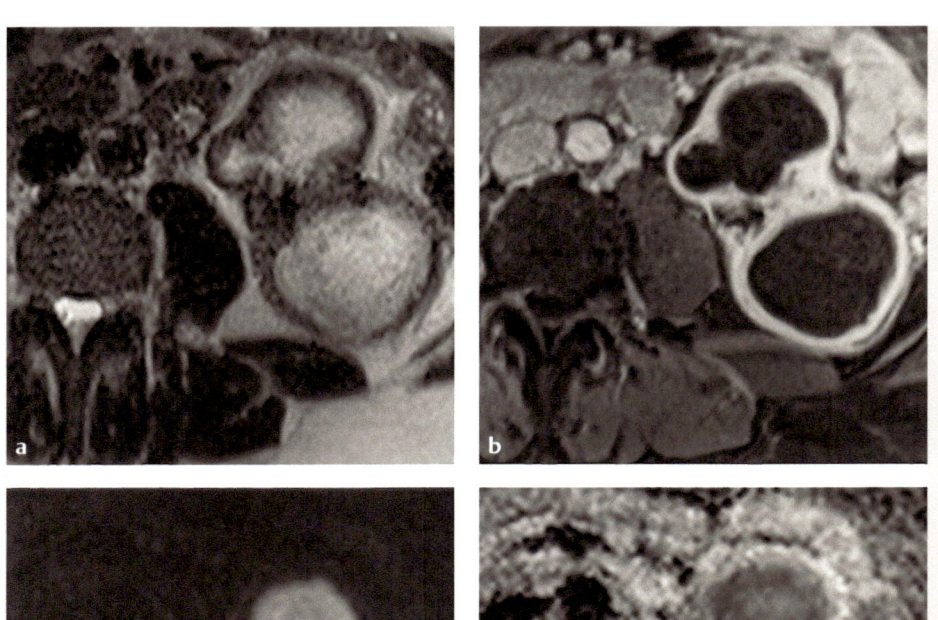

Fig. 11.38 Xanthogranulomatous pyelonephritis in a 77-year-old woman. **(a)** Axial T2 W image. The left kidney is enlarged and hyperintense. **(b)** Axial T1 W image after administration of contrast medium shows hydronephrosis with enhancement. **(c)** Significant diffusion restriction on diffusion-weighted imaging. **(d)** ADC map.

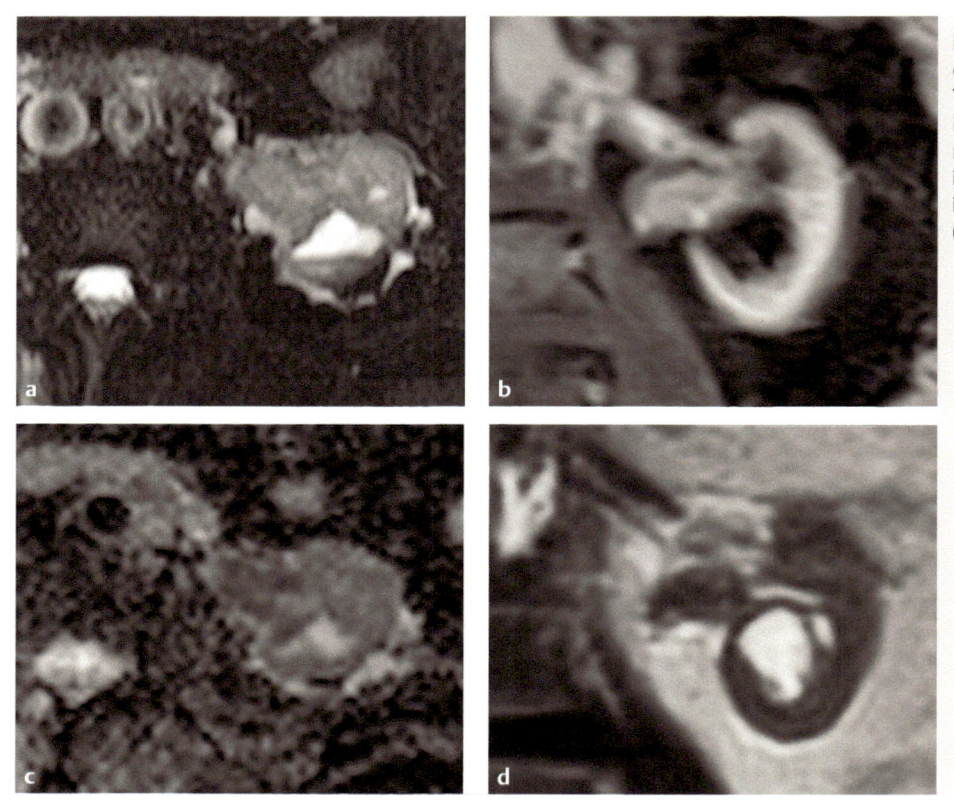

Fig. 11.39 Urothelial carcinoma in a 63-year-old woman with a hypointense filling defect in T2 W sequences **(a, d)** and slight enhancement in T1 W sequences **(b)**. Restricted diffusion is noted in the left renal pelvis **(c)**. **(a)** Axial T2 W image. **(b)** Coronal T1 W image after administration of contrast medium. **(c)** ADC map. **(d)** Coronal T2 W image.

Fibromuscular Dysplasia

▶ **Brief definition.** Fibromuscular dysplasia is the second leading cause of renal artery stenosis after atherosclerosis. Unlike atherosclerotic renal artery stenosis, fibromuscular dysplasia is a congenital rather than an acquired vessel wall disease that most commonly affects the media. Fibromuscular dysplasia is characterized by the proliferation of connective tissue and smooth muscle cells due to a still-unknown cause, leading to areas of circumscribed wall thickening that narrow the vessel lumen and alternate with sites of wall thinning. The intimal form of the disease, predominantly affecting the intimal layer of the vessel wall, is less common. Fibromuscular dysplasia is most prevalent in young women.

▶ **Imaging signs.** The classic imaging sign is an alternation of vascular stenoses and dilatations. This creates a "string of beads" appearance that is pathognomonic for fibromuscular dysplasia. In contrast to atherosclerotic renal artery stenosis, the vascular changes in fibromuscular dysplasia involve the distal two-thirds of the renal artery. MRA has a sensitivity of 93 to 97% in the diagnosis of fibromuscular dysplasia (▶ Fig. 11.41).

▶ **Clinical features.** Renal artery stenosis due to fibromuscular dysplasia has the same clinical presentation as atherosclerotic renal artery stenosis.

▶ **Differential diagnosis**
- Renal artery aneurysm.
- Atherosclerotic renal artery stenosis.

▶ **Pitfalls.** Acquisitions with a spatial resolution that is too low (> 1 mm³ voxel size) and/or an acquisition time that is too long (> 25–30 seconds, depending on the patient's breath-holding ability) limit diagnostic accuracy due to insufficient spatial resolution and the increased risk of respiratory motion artifacts during a long acquisition.

11.1.4 Renal Transplantation

Preoperative Evaluation

Live kidney donation has become a subject of major interest. The role of sectional imaging in the preoperative evaluation of a potential renal donor lies in the exclusion of tumors and the assessment of vascular changes, especially the detection of accessory or aberrant renal arteries and veins. These findings can improve surgical planning and minimize the risk of intraoperative complications. Delayed imaging of the ureters in the urographic phase is useful for detecting congenital ureteral variants or an aberrant course.

Postoperative Period

The indications for imaging in the postoperative period include the detection of vascular complications such as renal artery stenosis, renal vein thrombosis, or ureteral stenosis. Ultrasound and MRI are the most frequently used modalities. MRI is also useful for detecting renal transplantation complications such as

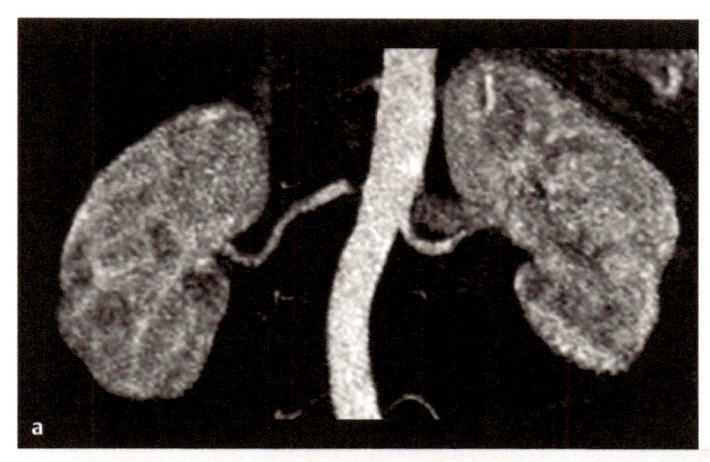

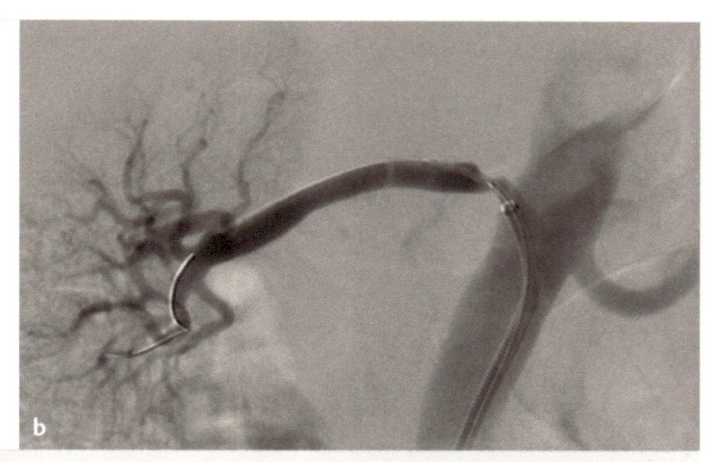

Fig. 11.40 **Renal artery stenosis.** High-grade, proximal atherosclerotic stenosis of the right renal artery in a 74-year-old man. (a) CT angiography. (b) Digital subtraction angiography.

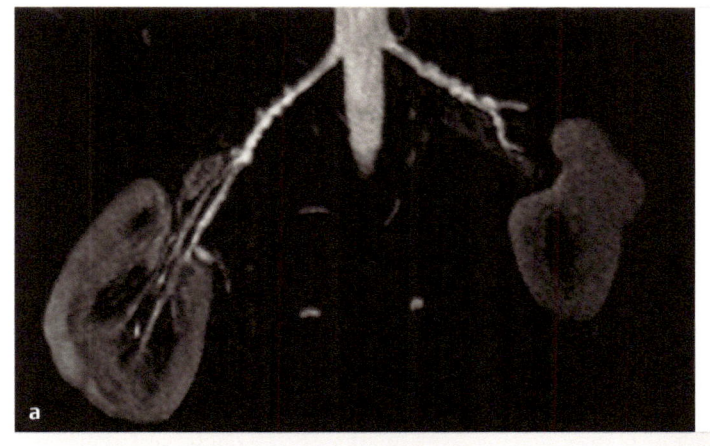

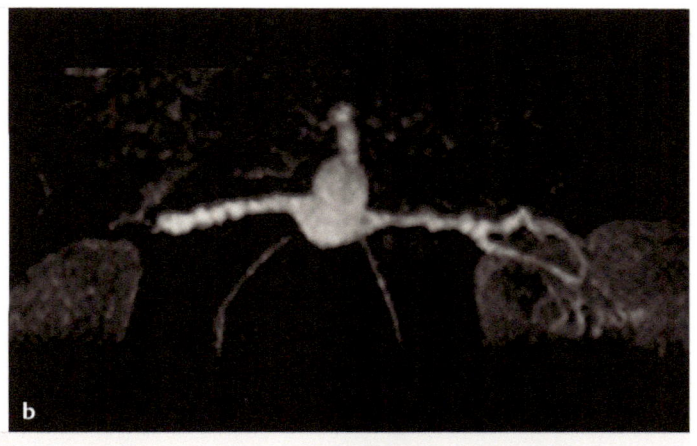

Fig. 11.41 **Fibromuscular dysplasia.** Classic string-of-beads sign in both renal arteries caused by alternating dilatations and stenoses in a 22-year-old woman. (a) Coronal MRA, maximum intensity projection. (b) Axial MRA, maximum intensity projection.

Kidney and Urinary Tract

lymphoceles, lymphoproliferative disorder, and granulomatous diseases owing to its excellent soft tissue contrast. Fluid collections such as urinomas, hematomas, lymphoceles, and abscesses show intermediate hyperintensity in T2 W sequences. While lymphoceles do not enhance, abscesses tend to show rim enhancement. Hematomas do not enhance but are hyperintense in the fat-saturated T1 W sequence before administration of contrast medium.

Acute allograft rejection does not have a morphological correlate on MR images. Contrast pooling in the medulla will be found in patients with acute tubular necrosis.

11.2 Urinary Tract

11.2.1 Retroperitoneal Masses

▶ **Brief definition.** As well as the entities described above, the differential diagnosis of retroperitoneal masses includes perirenal lymphoma, retroperitoneal fibrosis (Ormond's disease), lymph node metastasis (e.g., from renal cell carcinoma or from cancers of the bladder, uterus, or prostate), xanthogranulomatous pyelonephritis, and sarcoma. Other possibilities are neuroectodermal tumors such as paragangliomas, extra-adrenal pheochromocytoma, and germ cell tumors (teratoma). The most common tumor entity is liposarcoma. Retroperitoneal fibrosis (Ormond's disease) is a rare disease with a male predilection. It is idiopathic in 70% of cases and drug-related in 10% of cases (e.g., β-blockers). The rest have an association with lymphomas, aneurysms, and retroperitoneal hematomas. Ormond's disease is bilateral in more than 50% of cases.

▶ **Imaging signs**
- *Retroperitoneal fibrosis*: Benign retroperitoneal fibrosis (Ormond's disease) is characterized sonographically by hyperechoic para-aortic and interaortocaval tissue. CT shows tissue proliferation at these sites (▶ Fig. 11.42). The ureters are displaced medially (medialized) by fibrosis. On MRI, the fibrotic tissue has a signal intensity that is intermediate between that of fat and muscle. Postcontrast images show moderate enhancement (▶ Fig. 11.43). This contrasts with malignant retroperitoneal fibrosis, which is hyperintense in fat-suppressed T2 W sequences and shows only slight gadolinium enhancement. The great vessels (abdominal aorta and inferior vena cava) are often ensheathed by retroperitoneal fibrosis but are not occluded. Unlike lymphomas, retroperitoneal fibrosis does not have a lobular outline. While benign retroperitoneal fibrosis shows bilateral encasement and medialization of the ureters, malignant retroperitoneal fibrosis often affects the ureter on one side only. Morphological imaging criteria are insufficient for positive differentiation between malignant and benign retroperitoneal fibrosis.
- *Lymph node metastases*: Metastatic lymph nodes do not show specific echogenicity (ultrasound), density (CT), or signal characteristics (MRI) in any of the sectional modalities. They are characterized mainly by their enlargement (para-aortic and paracaval nodes > 15 mm, retrocrural nodes > 6 mm). Enlarged lymph nodes generally show homogeneous enhancement on CT scans. On MRI they have homogeneous, intermediate signal intensity in T1 W sequences and are hyperintense in T2 W sequences.
- *Liposarcoma and lipoma*: The signal characteristics of liposarcomas depend mainly on the proportion of fatty tissue and on tumor grade. Lipomas, on the other hand, are homogeneously hyperintense in T1 W sequences without fat saturation and show variable hyperintensity in T2 W sequences. A key differentiating criterion at imaging is the nodular enhancement that occurs in dedifferentiated liposarcoma.

Caution
Note that well-differentiated liposarcomas are very similar to lipomas in their signal characteristics.

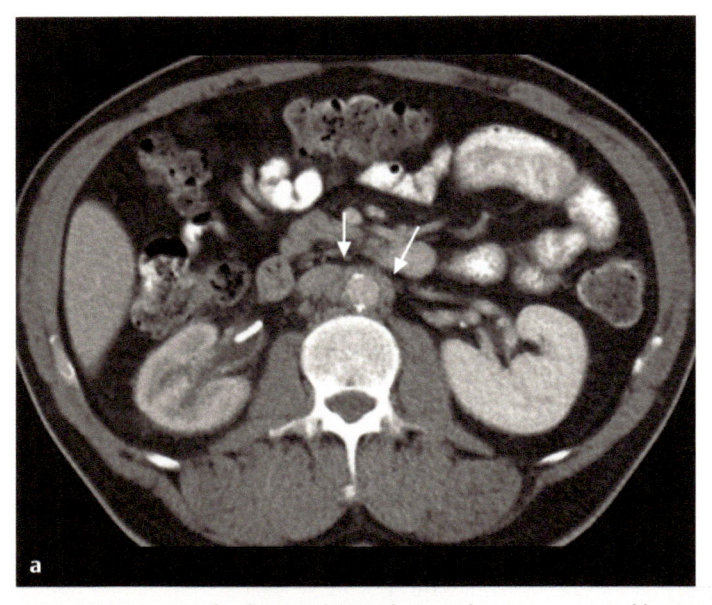

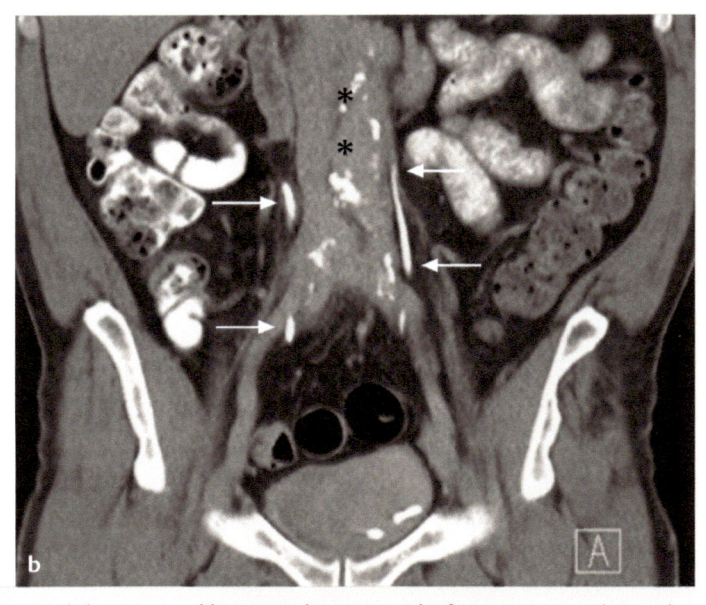

Fig. 11.42 Ormond's disease. (a) CT shows a density at a typical location around the aorta and between the aorta and inferior vena cava (arrows). (b) Coronal maximum intensity projection in the urographic phase shows medialization of both ureters (arrows). The asterisks mark a density between the aorta and inferior vena cava. The right ureter has been stented with a double-J catheter to relieve hydronephrosis.

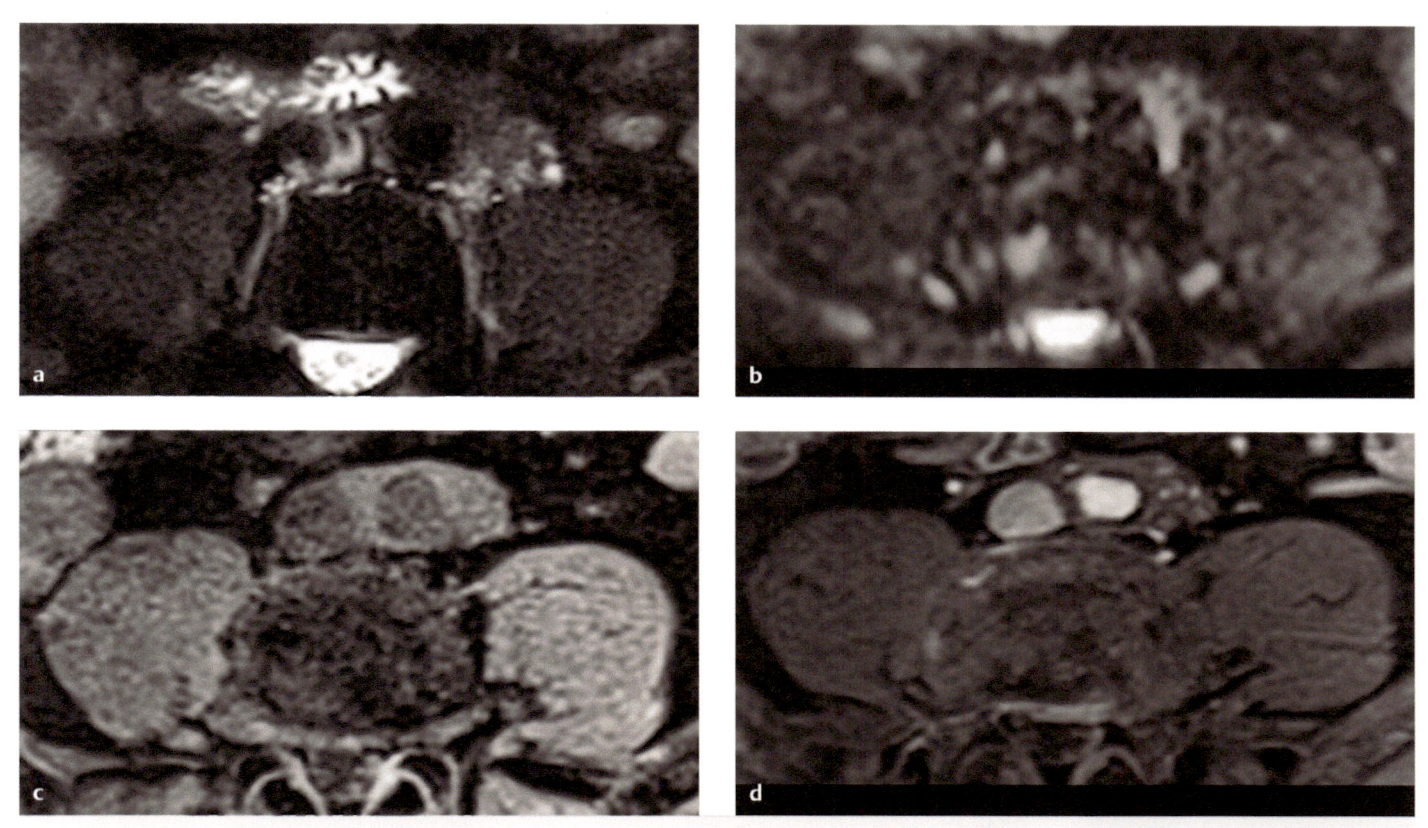

Fig. 11.43 Ormond's disease in a 66-year-old woman. (a) T2W sequence demonstrates a hypointense para-aortic soft tissue mass. (b) Diffusion-weighted imaging does not show restricted diffusion. (c) Unenhanced T1W sequence. The soft tissue mass appears isointense. (d) T1W sequence after administration of contrast medium shows no enhancement.

▶ **Clinical features**
- *Retroperitoneal fibrosis*: Ormond's disease often presents with nonspecific back or flank pain that does not vary with changes of position. Urinary tract obstruction and uremia may occur in the advanced stage. Lower extremity edema and/or gross hematuria may also be encountered in Ormond's disease.
- *Liposarcoma*: This tumor does not become symptomatic until an advanced stage, when symptoms result mainly from the displacement of adjacent organs. Besides nonspecific abdominal complaints, which may consist of pain and digestive disorders, paresthesias may also occur depending on the tumor location.

▶ **Differential diagnosis**
- Benign retroperitoneal fibrosis.
- Malignant retroperitoneal fibrosis.
- Lymphoma.
- Lipoma.
- Differentiated liposarcoma.

11.2.2 Congenital Variants

▶ **Brief definition.** As described under the anatomy and congenital variants of the kidney (p. 394), a range of possible anatomical variants may be encountered. Examples are complete or incomplete duplication of the ureters, duplex ureter, and bifid ureter, with an associated duplex kidney on the affected side.

▶ **Imaging signs.** A duplex kidney has parenchymal bands that define two separate renal pelvises drained by two ureters (▶ Fig. 11.44). The renal pelvises may be of different sizes, and there may be variable dilatation of the renal pelvis and ureter depending on the drainage configuration and possible combined anomalies (▶ Fig. 11.45). The upper-pole ureter is more likely to have a ureterocele (▶ Fig. 11.46) or ectopic insertion. Vesicoureteral reflux is more commonly found in the lower moiety. With a bifid ureter, on the other hand, the Y-shaped pathway may permit the recirculation of urine from the upper to the lower moiety, leading to different calibers of the ureteral segments (▶ Fig. 11.47).

▶ **Differential diagnosis**
- Bifid ureter (▶ Fig. 11.48).
- Duplex ureter (▶ Fig. 11.49).

▶ **Pitfalls.** A common error is to start the last sequence of the excretory phase or urodynamic study too soon, at a time when the excretory portion of the urinary tract is not yet fully opacified. Differentiation of a bifid ureter from a duplex ureter may be difficult if the bifid ureters unite at a low level. The physiologic constriction of the ureter at the level where it crosses over the iliac vessels is often misinterpreted as abnormal narrowing.

11.2.3 Bladder Masses

▶ **Brief definition.** In the classification of bladder masses, primary masses arising from the bladder itself must be differentiated from secondary processes that infiltrate the bladder from adjacent organs or metastasize to the bladder from more distant sites. Lung cancer, breast cancer, and melanoma are the tumors that most commonly metastasize to the bladder. The most common primary bladder tumor is urothelial carcinoma, which arises from the

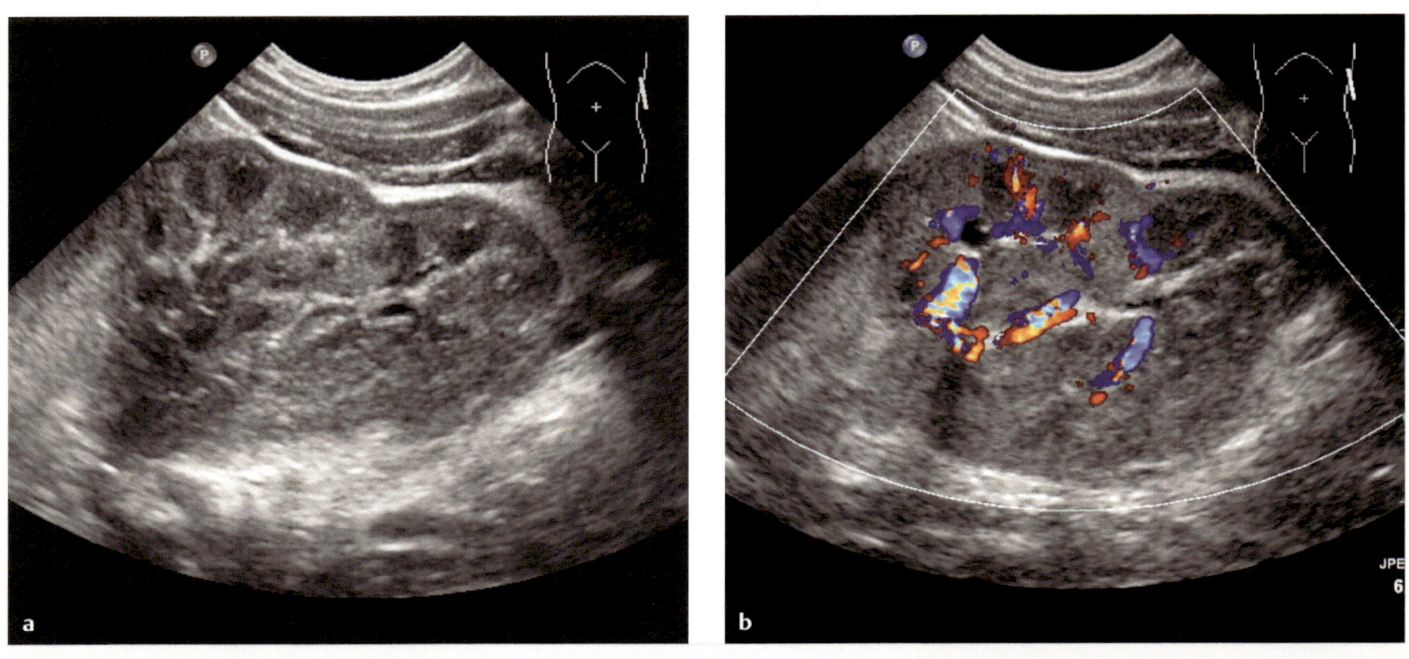

Fig. 11.44 **Duplex kidney.** (a) Ultrasound scan shows the bulging outlines of the left kidney with a central parenchymal band. (b) Color Doppler scan shows a duplicated vascular supply.

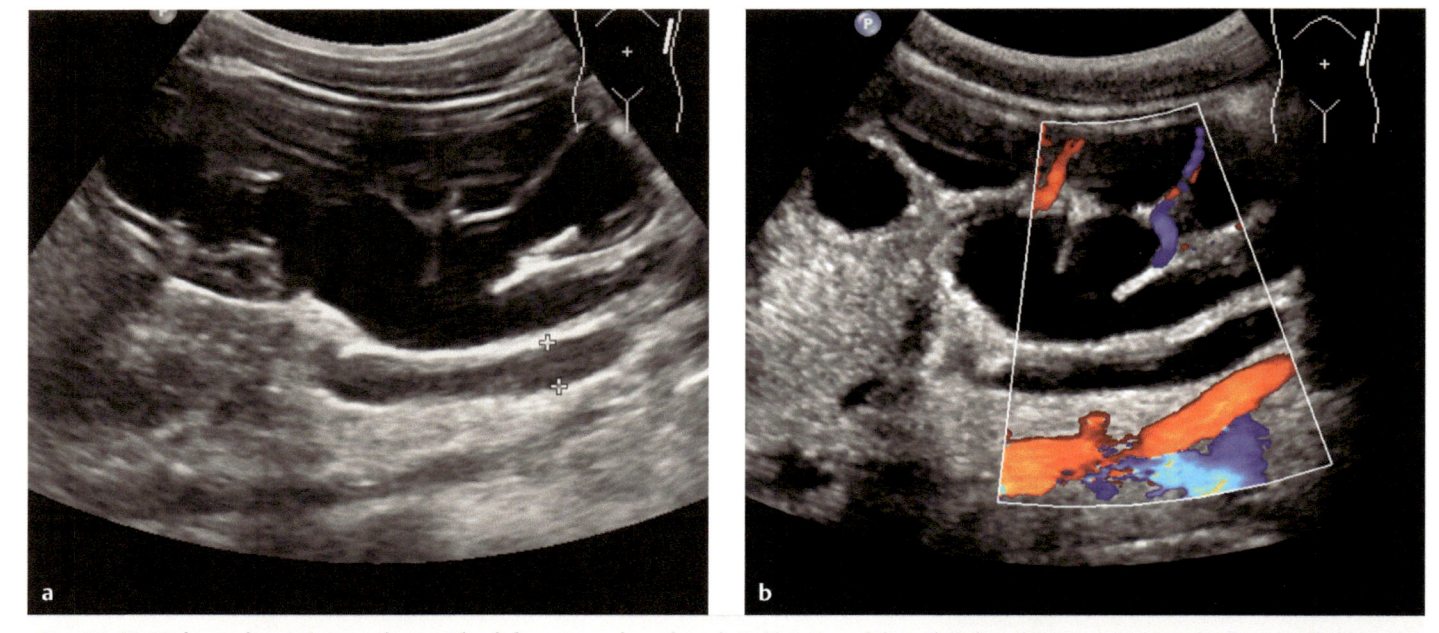

Fig. 11.45 **Hydronephrosis** in a newborn with a left ureterocele and grade 3 dilatation of the pelvicalyceal system. (a) B-mode ultrasound. (b) Color Doppler scan.

bladder epithelium. Adenocarcinoma and squamous cell carcinoma are much less common. Squamous cell cancers are often triggered by infection with schistosomes (*Schistosoma haematobium*). Rarely, non-Hodgkin's lymphoma may present as primary extranodal disease involving the bladder. These lesions are indistinguishable from primary urothelial carcinoma by imaging alone.[30] Other possible entities are mesenchymal tumors such as leiomyoma, neurofibroma, rhabdomyosarcoma, and fibrosarcoma.

▶ **Imaging signs.** The bladder should be well distended for sonographic examination. Thickening of the bladder wall to more than 2.5 mm in children or more than 7 mm in adults is considered pathologic in a well-distended bladder. Tumors of the bladder may appear as areas of (irregular) wall thickening (e.g., sessile bladder carcinoma) or as a polypous mass. Bladder carcinomas are isoechoic to the bladder wall and usually present an undulating surface. Rhabdomyosarcomas of the bladder tend to show homogeneous high echogenicity. Both tumors are commonly located in the trigone region. If gross hematuria is present, the vascularity of the lesion can be assessed with color Doppler ultrasound to differentiate between a tumor and possible blood clot. Additionally, movement of the mass in response to the patient's

11.2 Urinary Tract

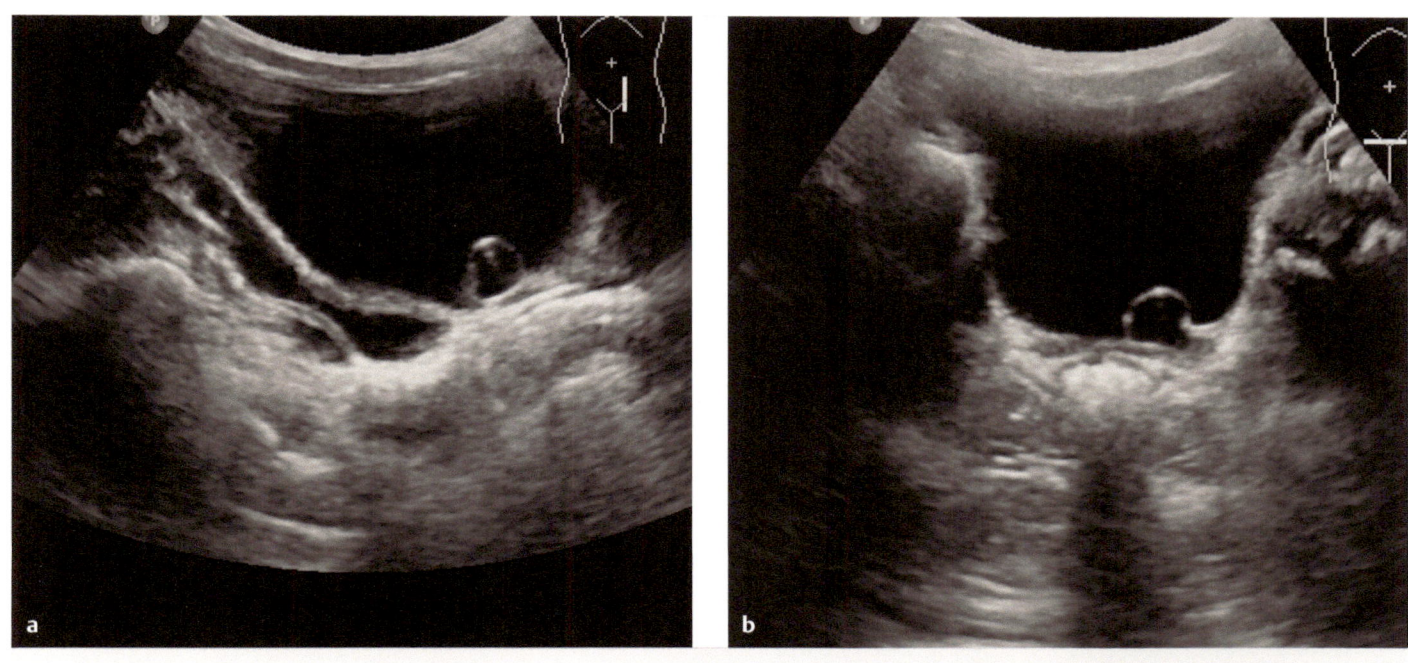

Fig. 11.46 **Orthotopic ureterocele.** Ultrasound findings. (a) Dilatation of the left ureter. (b) Orthotopic ureterocele on the left side.

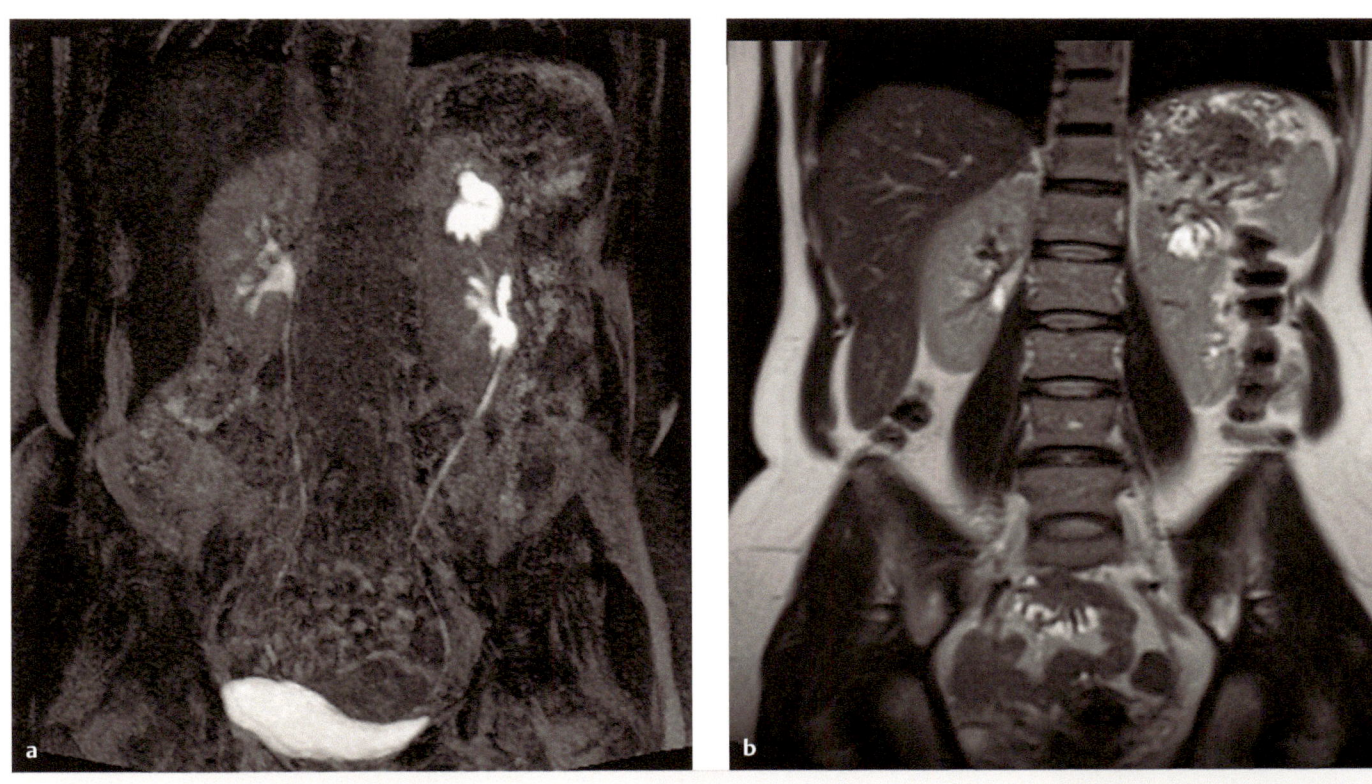

Fig. 11.47 **Duplex kidney.** MRI demonstrates two separate renal pelvises at the upper and lower poles of the left kidney. (a) T1W image, delayed phase (urographic or excretory phase). (b) T2W image, delayed phase.

changes of position is a helpful criterion for identifying a nonneoplastic foreign body or blood clot. The bladder wall shows only slight enhancement on postcontrast CT. A bladder carcinoma will generally show greater enhancement than unaffected wall areas and may protrude exophytically into the bladder lumen (▶ Fig. 11.50). The healthy bladder wall has intermediate signal intensity in T1W sequences and low signal intensity in T2W sequences. The different layers that make up the bladder wall cannot be differentiated from one another. Bladder carcinomas are demarcated in T2W sequences as iso- or hypointense lesions (▶ Fig. 11.51). If the outer layer of the bladder wall is delineated as an uninterrupted T2-hypointense line, this indicates a stage T1 or T2 tumor that does not extend beyond the bladder wall. The complete interruption of this

Kidney and Urinary Tract

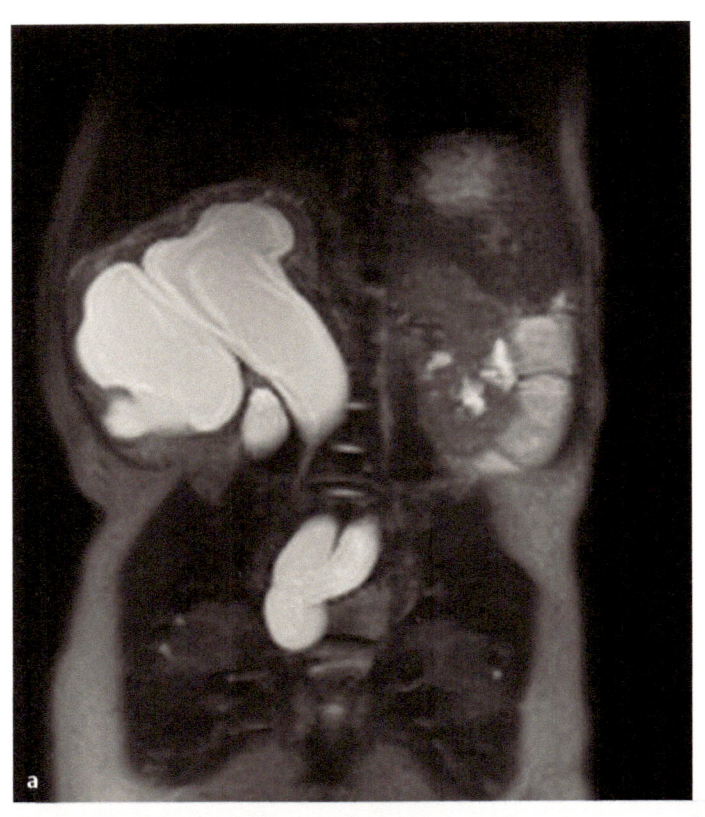

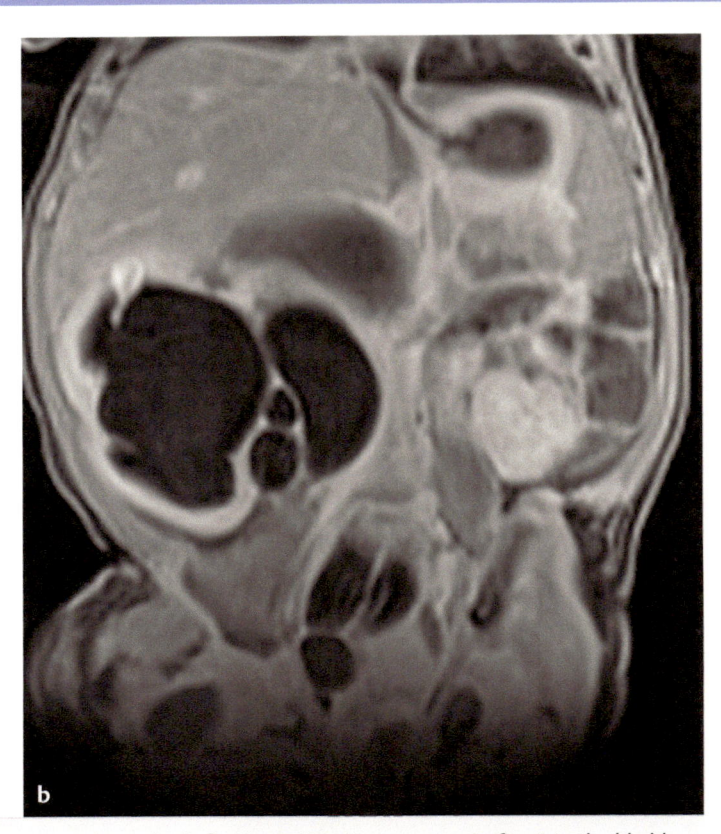

Fig. 11.48 Bifid ureter. Coronal HASTE sequences demonstrate two right ureters that unite before inserting via a common orifice into the bladder. **(a)** Coronal T2 W sequence. **(b)** Coronal T1 W sequence, venous phase.

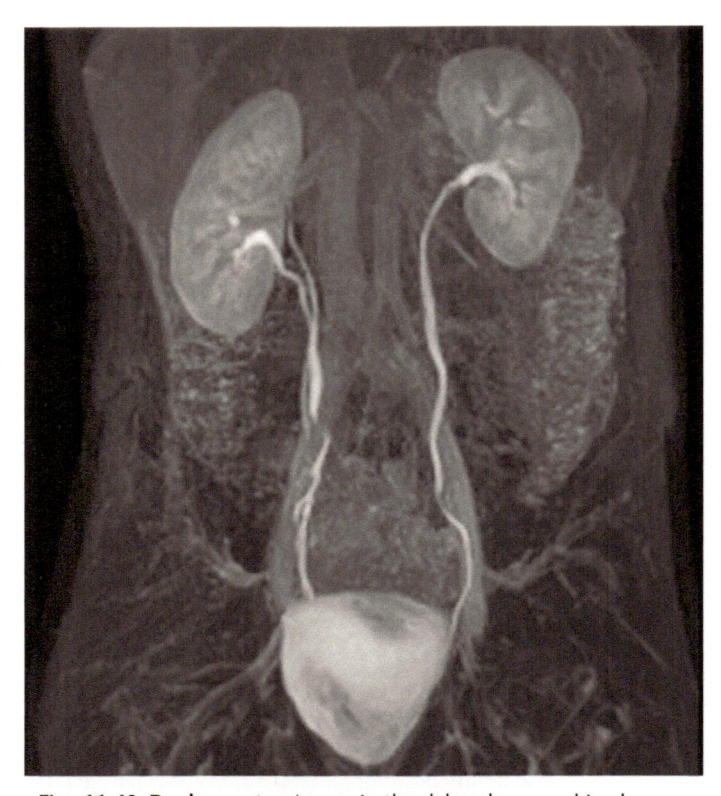

Fig. 11.49 Duplex ureter. Image in the delayed urographic phase reveals two ureters on the right side. Unlike a bifid ureter, the duplex ureters insert separately into the bladder.

hypointense line indicates a stage T3b lesion. Tumors confined to the bladder wall cannot be distinguished from perifocal edema or adjacent inflammatory changes in unenhanced sequences.[31] Administration of contrast medium permits a more accurate differential diagnosis.[32]

▶ **Clinical features**
- *Bladder carcinoma*: Painless hematuria, which may be intermittent, is accompanied by signs such as pollakiuria and dysuria. More advanced stages of bladder carcinoma present with non-specific B symptoms (night sweats and weight loss), hydronephrosis, flank and bone pain, and in some cases a palpable lower abdominal mass.
- *Rhabdomyosarcoma*: This tumor presents similar symptoms that may include dysuria and pollakiuria, lower abdominal pain, hematuria, and possible urinary retention, depending on tumor size.

▶ **Differential diagnosis**
- Inflammatory pseudotumor.
- Metastasis.
- Bladder infiltration from surrounding structures.
- Mesenchymal tumors.

▶ **Pitfalls.** A potential mass may not be definable unless the bladder lumen is adequately distended.

11.2.4 Urothelial Carcinoma of the Upper Urinary Tract

▶ **Brief definition.** Urothelial carcinoma most commonly occurs in the bladder, but 5% of these tumors arise in the ureter or pelvicalyceal system. Hematuria is a typical clinical sign. Upper-tract urothelial carcinomas are bilateral in 2 to 4% of cases.

11.2 Urinary Tract

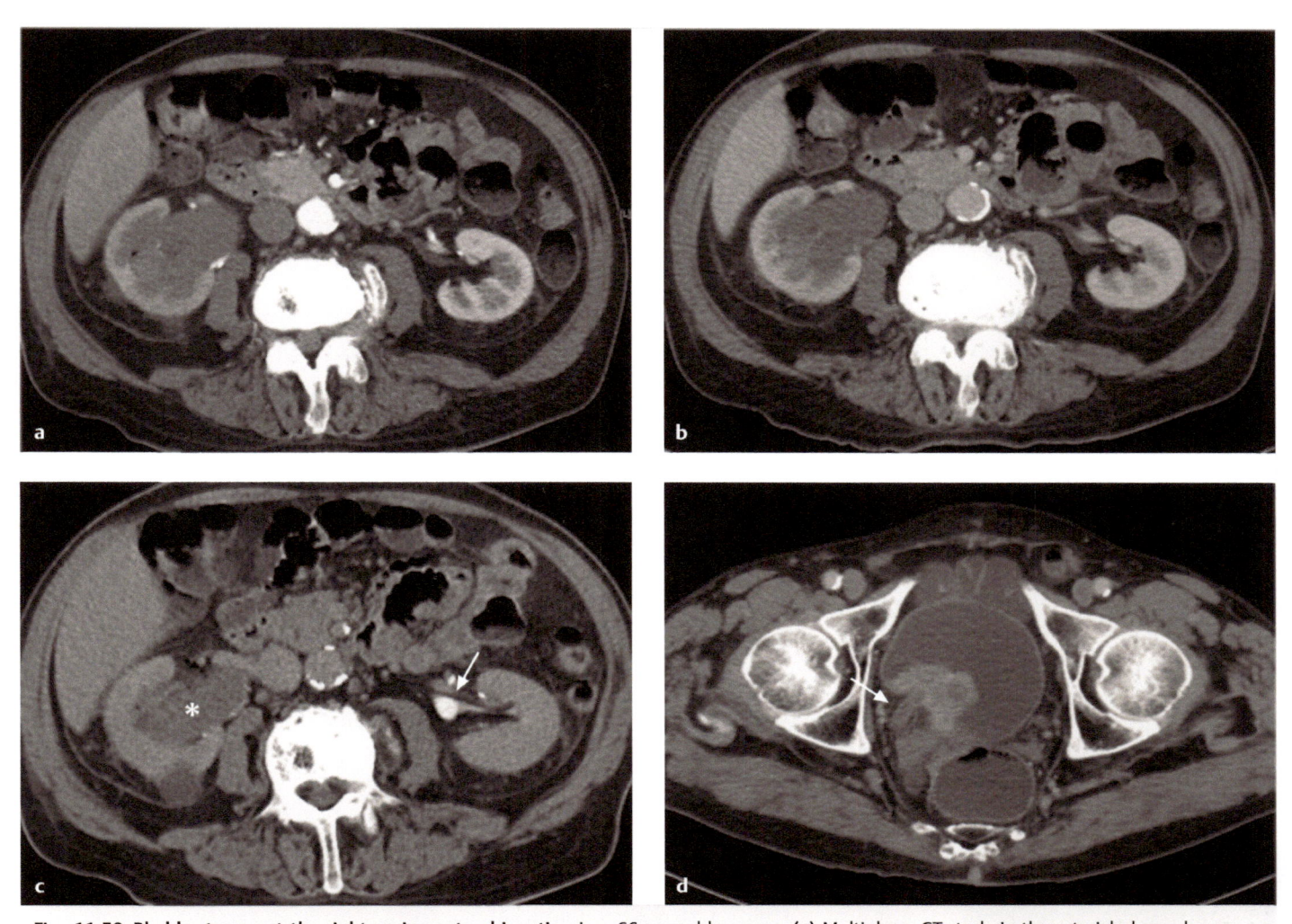

Fig. 11.50 Bladder tumor at the right vesicoureteral junction in a 66-year-old woman. **(a)** Multiphase CT study in the arterial phase shows significant hydronephrosis on the right side. Parenchymal enhancement of the right kidney is decreased relative to the left kidney. **(b)** CT, venous phase. The discrepancy is less pronounced in this phase. **(c)** CT, urographic phase. Renal contrast excretion is absent on the right side. The enlarged renal pelvis (asterisk) shows no increase in density, while contrast medium fills the left renal pelvis (arrow). **(d)** The exophytic tumor protrudes into the bladder lumen and encases the orifice of the right ureter, which is dilated due to obstructed outflow (arrow).

▶ **Imaging signs.** A urothelial carcinoma of the renal pelvis appears sonographically as a hypoechoic, polypous intraluminal mass that fills the renal pelvis and basically forms a pelvic "cast." Most of these tumors have a homogeneous echo pattern. Necrosis or calcifications appear as hypoechoic or hyperechoic areas, respectively, giving the mass a heterogeneous appearance. Unlike pseudotumors such as blood clots, the tumor has a vascular supply that is detectable with color Doppler ultrasound. Urothelial carcinoma shows intermediate, heterogeneous enhancement on postcontrast CT. The mass may be located in the region of the ureteropelvic junction. With a mass located directly in the renal pelvis, axial CT may show loss of the typical C-shaped configuration of the hilum (▶ Fig. 11.52). The tumor shows intermediate signal intensity in T2W sequences and enhances in postcontrast sequences. Associated periureteral edema is often present.

▶ **Clinical features.** The clinical manifestations of upper urinary tract tumors may include flank pain, renal or ureteral colic, and hematuria. Advanced tumors present with B symptoms (e.g., fever, weight loss, lethargy) and hydronephrosis.

▶ **Differential diagnosis**
- Squamous cell carcinoma.
- Adenocarcinoma.
- Papilloma.
- Tuberculosis.
- Malacoplakia.
- Leukoplakia.
- Ureteritis cystica.

▶ **Pitfalls.** Because lesions are multifocal in 25 to 30% of cases, all portions of the urinary tract should be evaluated.

11.2.5 Ureteral Stones

▶ **Brief definition.** Urinary stones (calculi) are formed in the renal collecting system and may then move from the kidney into the ureter.

▶ **Imaging signs.** CT shows a structure of calcific density in the pelvicalyceal system or ureter (▶ Fig. 11.53). CT and MR images in the delayed urographic phase show a rounded or oval filling defect. Stones appear sonographically as an echogenic structure with an associated acoustic shadow (▶ Fig. 11.54).

Kidney and Urinary Tract

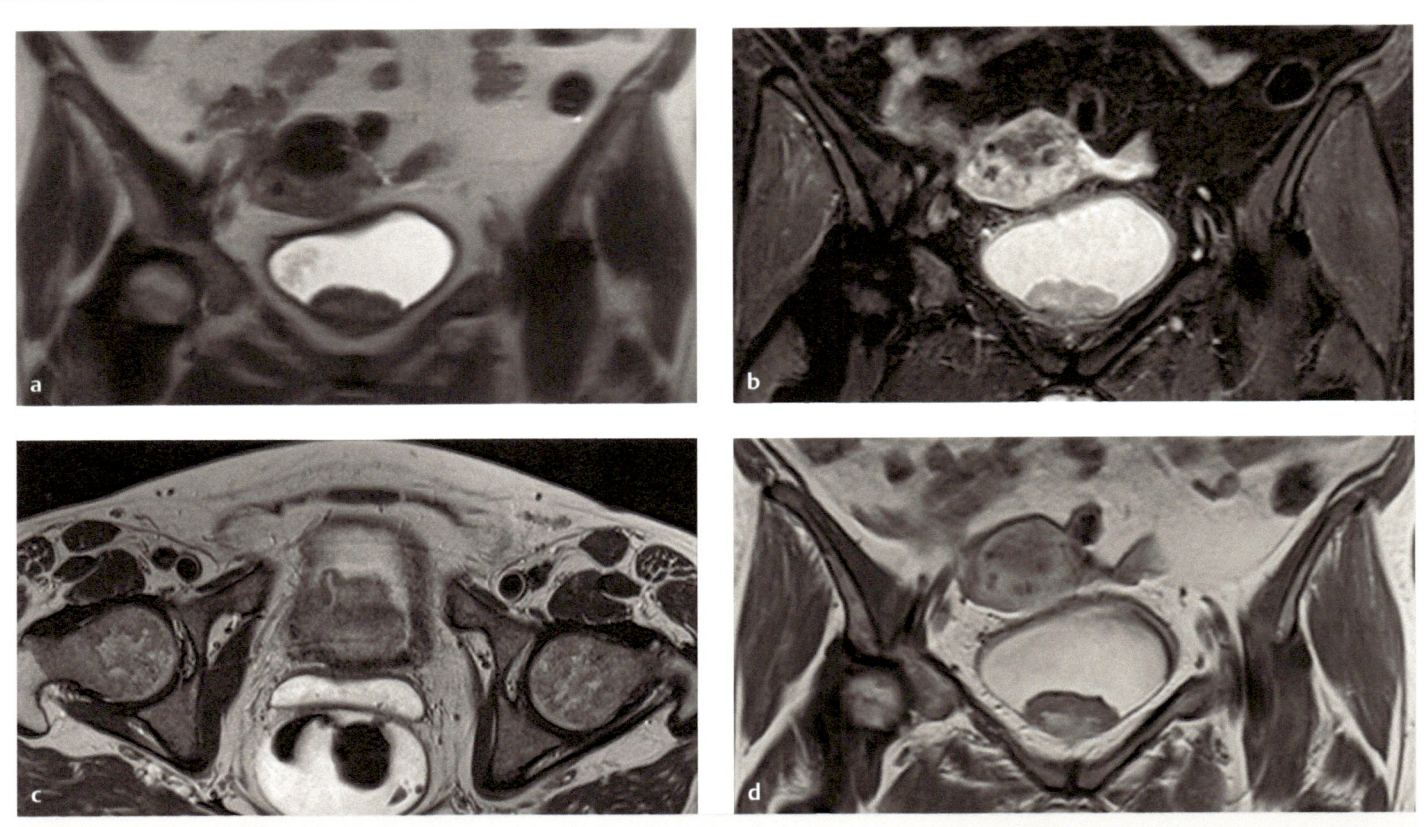

Fig. 11.51 **Bladder carcinoma.** Lobulated mass in the bladder is iso-to hypointense in the T2 W sequences and hyperintense in the STIR sequence (a–c) and heterogeneously hypointense with enhancement in the postcontrast T1 W sequence (d). (a) Coronal T2 W sequence. (b) Coronal STIR sequence. (c) Axial T2 W sequence. (d) Coronal T1 W sequence after administration of contrast medium.

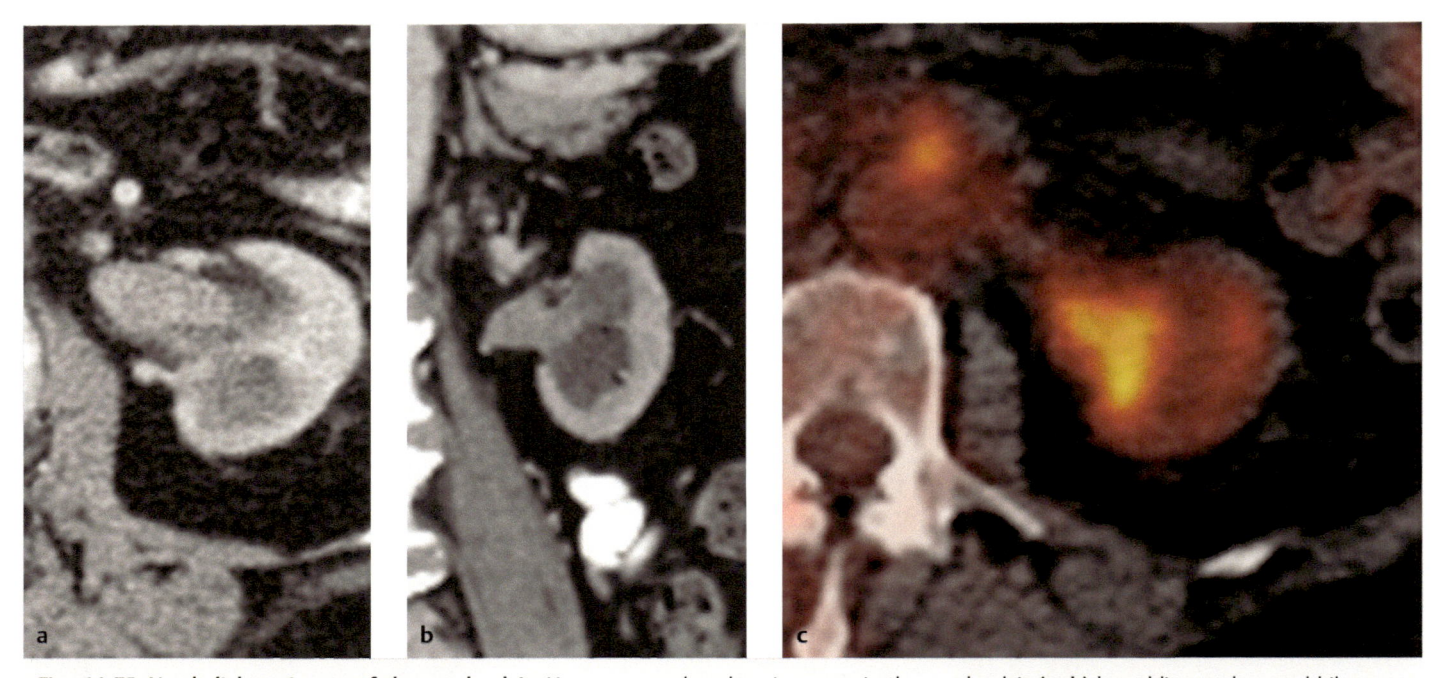

Fig. 11.52 **Urothelial carcinoma of the renal pelvis.** Homogeneously enhancing mass in the renal pelvis (a, b) has obliterated normal hilar structures (a). FDG PET-CT image shows increased uptake in the mass (c). (a) Axial CT, venous phase. (b) Coronal reformatted image, venous phase. (c) FDG PET-CT.

▶ **Clinical features.** The clinical presentation of ureteral stones depends on their location. Stones in the middle third of the ureter or at the junction of the middle and lower thirds are associated with colicky pain in the back and lateral lower abdomen. With stones at a lower level, the pain radiates to the inguinal and genital regions. The colicky pain is sometimes associated with nausea, vomiting, and constipation.

11.2 Urinary Tract

▶ **Differential diagnosis**
- Xanthogranulomatous nephritis.
- Vessel wall calcification.

▶ **Pitfalls.** Vessel wall–associated calcifications or phleboliths in the lesser pelvis or calcified pelvic lymph nodes may be misinterpreted as ureteral stones.

11.2.6 Urachal Cysts

▶ **Brief definition.** Persistence of the urachus postnatally results in a patent channel between the bladder and umbilicus, which presents clinically with umbilical drainage. If the urachus is partially obliterated, the residual portion may remain patent, forming a urachal cyst. If the persistent portion is located just past the origin of the urachus from the bladder, a bladder diverticulum is formed, which may lead to lithiasis or recurrent episodes of cystitis. Very rarely, a urachal cyst may become superinfected. The treatment of choice is drain insertion or surgical excision.

▶ **Imaging signs.** All modalities display a cordlike connection between the bladder and umbilicus. If superinfection occurs, the wall is thickened and shows contrast enhancement on CT and MRI (▶ Fig. 11.55).

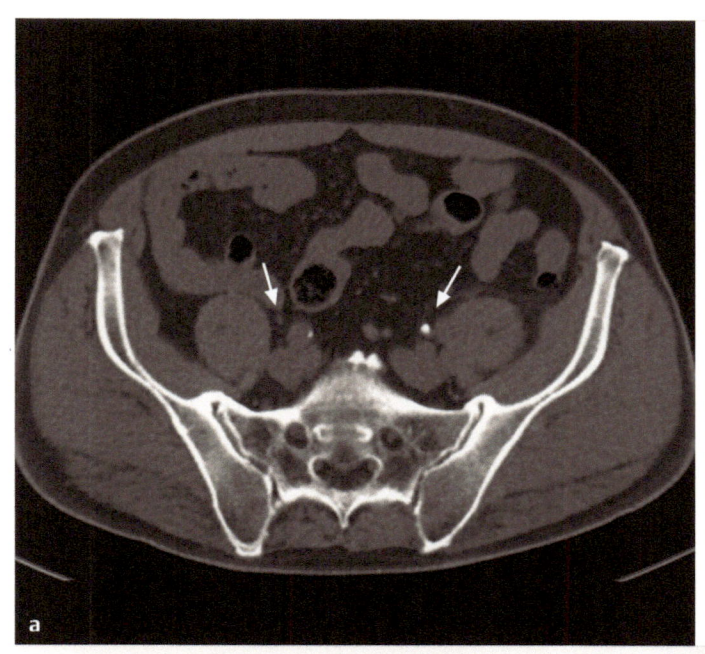

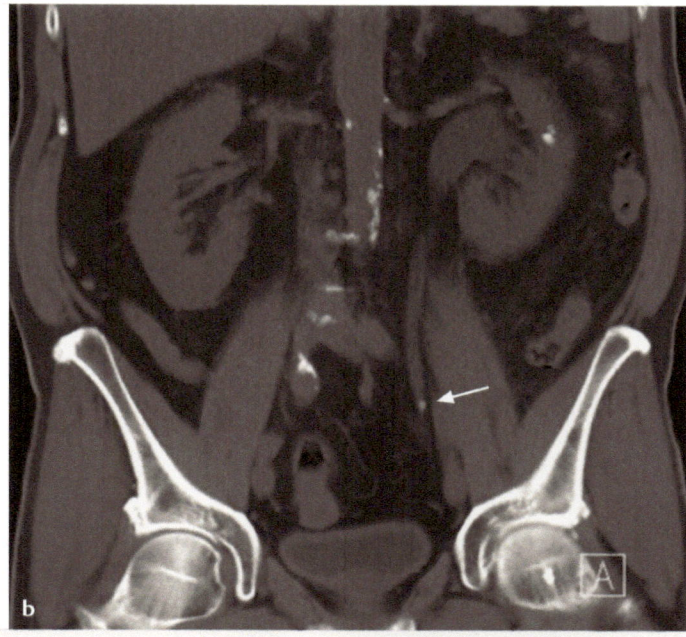

Fig. 11.53 Urolithiasis. Patient with a calculus in the proximal left ureter ([a, b]; arrows). Unenhanced CT shows a round, circumscribed mass of calcific density at the center of the ureter with associated grade 2 hydronephrosis. (a) Axial image. (b) Coronal image.

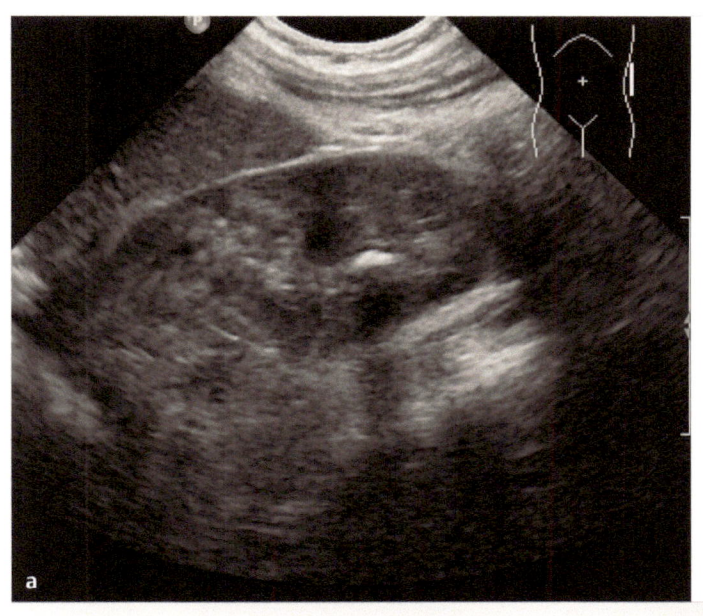

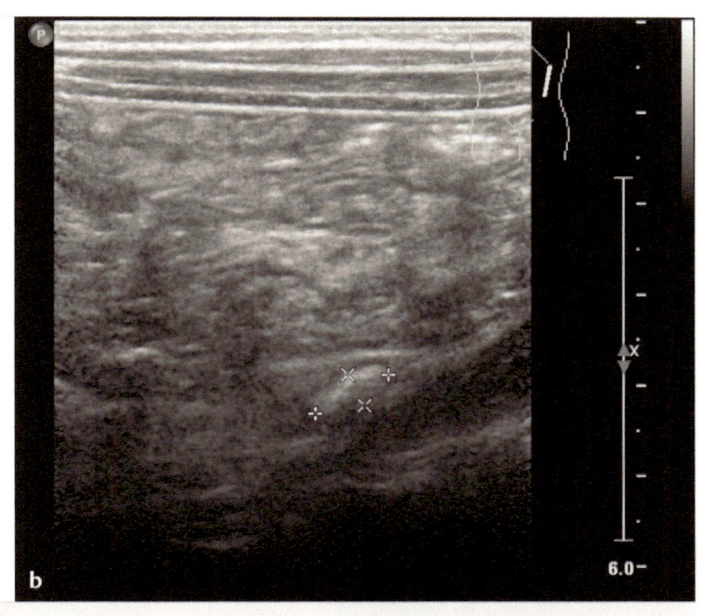

Fig. 11.54 Urolithiasis. (a) Ultrasound scan of a kidney stone that was initially in the left renal pelvis. The stone is hyperechoic and casts an acoustic shadow. (b) The patient later became symptomatic, presenting with colicky left flank pains. Ultrasound now shows that the stone is in the left ureter.

Kidney and Urinary Tract

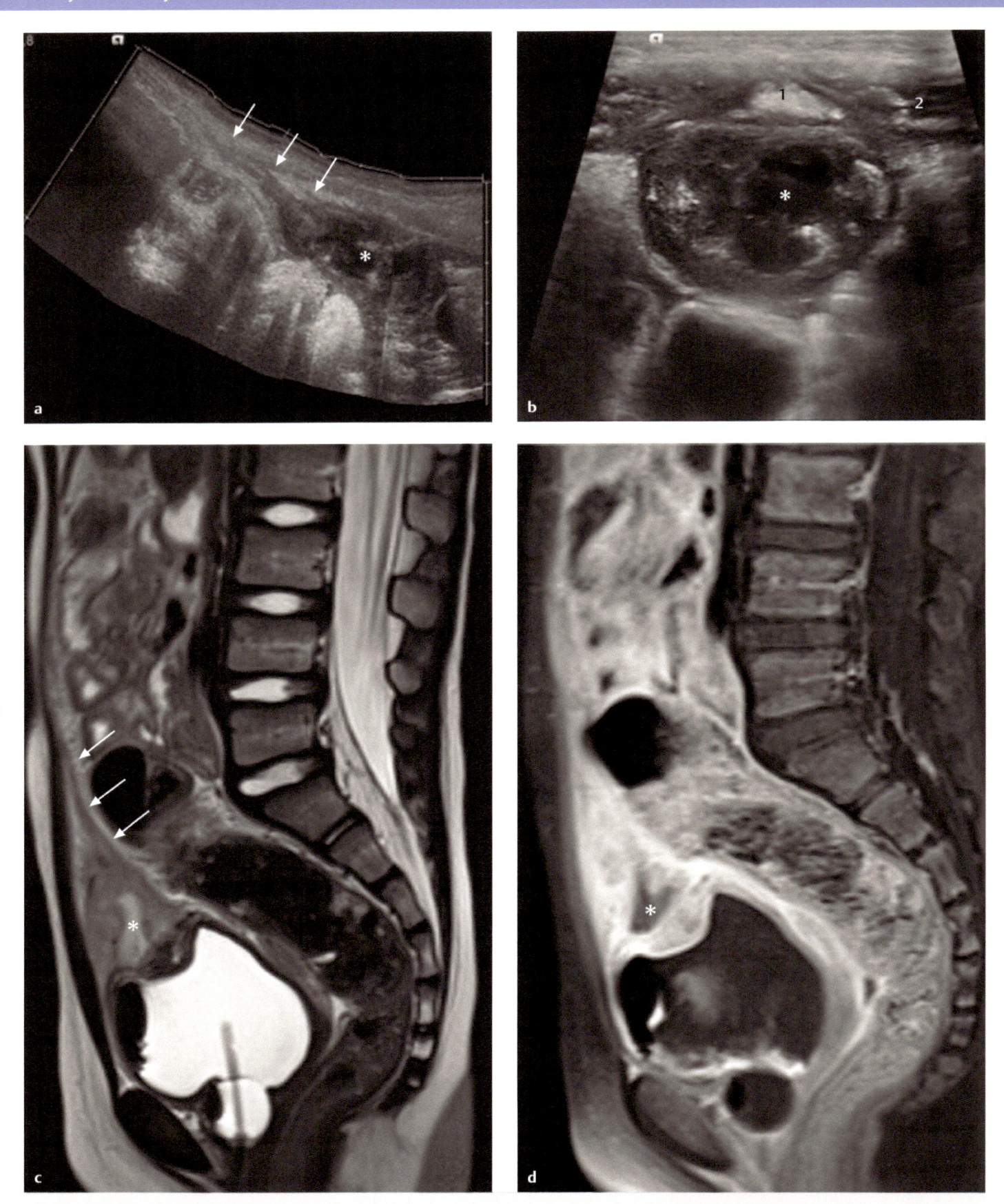

Fig. 11.55 **Infected urachal cyst** in a 5-year-old girl. (a) Panoramic ultrasound scan shows the infected cyst (asterisk) with a thickened wall. The cyst communicates with the umbilicus (arrows). (b) Axial ultrasound scan displays the relationship of the cyst (asterisk) to the linea alba (1) and rectus muscle (2). (c) Preoperative T2 W MRI. The sequence demonstrates the urachus (arrows) and the cyst (asterisk). (d) Preoperative fat-suppressed T1 W image after IV administration of contrast medium shows enhancement in the cyst wall (asterisk).

Bibliography

[1] Fan L, Lianfang D, Jinfang X, Yijin S, Ying W. Diagnostic efficacy of contrast-enhanced ultrasonography in solid renal parenchymal lesions with maximum diameters of 5 cm. J Ultrasound Med. 2008; 27(6):875–885

[2] Motley G, Dalrymple N, Keesling C, Fischer J, Harmon W. Hounsfield unit density in the determination of urinary stone composition. Urology. 2001; 58(2):170–173

[3] Smith RC, Verga M, McCarthy S, Rosenfield AT. Diagnosis of acute flank pain: value of unenhanced helical CT. AJR Am J Roentgenol. 1996; 166(1):97–101

[4] Boulay I, Holtz P, Foley WD, White B, Begun FP. Ureteral calculi: diagnostic efficacy of helical CT and implications for treatment of patients. AJR Am J Roentgenol. 1999; 172(6):1485–1490

[5] Chowdhury FU, Kotwal S, Raghunathan G, Wah TM, Joyce A, Irving HC. Unenhanced multidetector CT (CT KUB) in the initial imaging of suspected acute renal colic: evaluating a new service. Clin Radiol. 2007; 62(10):970–977

[6] Ege G, Akman H, Kuzucu K, Yildiz S. Acute ureterolithiasis: incidence of secondary signs on unenhanced helical CT and influence on patient management. Clin Radiol. 2003; 58(12):990–994

[7] El-Nahas AR, El-Assmy AM, Mansour O, Sheir KZ. A prospective multivariate analysis of factors predicting stone disintegration by extracorporeal shock wave lithotripsy: the value of high-resolution noncontrast computed tomography. Eur Urol. 2007; 51(6):1688–1693, discussion 1693–1694

[8] Parekattil SJ, White MD, Moran ME, Kogan BA. A computer model to predict the outcome and duration of ureteral or renal calculous passage. J Urol. 2004; 171(4):1436–1439

[9] Takahashi N, Kawashima A, Ernst RD, et al. Ureterolithiasis: can clinical outcome be predicted with unenhanced helical CT? Radiology. 1998; 208(1):97–102

[10] Deveci S, Coşkun M, Tekin MI, Peşkircioglu L, Tarhan NC, Ozkardeş H. Spiral computed tomography: role in determination of chemical compositions of pure and mixed urinary stones—an in vitro study. Urology. 2004; 64(2):237–240

[11] Dretler SP, Spencer BA. CT and stone fragility. J Endourol. 2001; 15(1):31–36

[12] Hillman BJ, Drach GW, Tracey P, Gaines JA. Computed tomographic analysis of renal calculi. AJR Am J Roentgenol. 1984; 142(3):549–552

[13] Lell MM, Panknin C, Saleh R, et al. Evaluation of coronary stents and stenoses at different heart rates with dual source spiral CT (DSCT). Invest Radiol. 2007; 42(7):536–541

[14] Scheffel H, Stolzmann P, Frauenfelder T, et al. Dual-energy contrast-enhanced computed tomography for the detection of urinary stone disease. Invest Radiol. 2007; 42(12):823–829

[15] Manenti G, Di Roma M, Mancino S, et al. Malignant renal neoplasms: correlation between ADC values and cellularity in diffusion weighted magnetic resonance imaging at 3 T. Radiol Med (Torino). 2008; 113(2):199–213

[16] Paudyal B, Paudyal P, Tsushima Y, et al. The role of the ADC value in the characterisation of renal carcinoma by diffusion-weighted MRI. Br J Radiol. 2010; 83(988):336–343

[17] Vivier PH, Sallem A, Beurdeley M, et al. MRI and suspected acute pyelonephritis in children: comparison of diffusion-weighted imaging with gadolinium-enhanced T1-weighted imaging. Eur Radiol. 2014; 24(1):19–25

[18] Sadler WT. Medizinische Embryologie: Die normale menschliche Entwicklung und ihre Fehlbildungen. Stuttgart: Thieme; 2008

[19] Terada N, Arai Y, Kinukawa N, Yoshimura K, Terai A. Risk factors for renal cysts. BJU Int. 2004; 93(9):1300–1302

[20] Bosniak MA. The current radiological approach to renal cysts. Radiology. 1986; 158(1):1–10

[21] Israel GM, Bosniak MA. Renal imaging for diagnosis and staging of renal cell carcinoma. Urol Clin North Am. 2003; 30(3):499–514

[22] O'Malley RL, Godoy G, Hecht EM, Stifelman MD, Taneja SS. Bosniak category IIF designation and surgery for complex renal cysts. J Urol. 2009; 182(3):1091–1095

[23] Smith AD, Remer EM, Cox KL, et al. Bosniak category IIF and III cystic renal lesions: outcomes and associations. Radiology. 2012; 262(1):152–160

[24] Alamara C, Karapanagiotou EM, Tourkantonis I, et al. Renal oncocytoma: a case report and short review of the literature. Eur J Intern Med. 2008; 19(7):e67–e69

[25] Zippel L. Zur Kenntnis der Onkozyten. Virchows Arch Path Anat. 1942; 308:360

[26] Kim JK, Kim SH, Jang YJ, et al. Renal angiomyolipoma with minimal fat: differentiation from other neoplasms at double-echo chemical shift FLASH MR imaging. Radiology. 2006; 239(1):174–180

[27] Sobin LH, Compton CC. TNM seventh edition: what's new, what's changed: communication from the International Union Against Cancer and the American Joint Committee on Cancer. Cancer. 2010; 116(22):5336–5339

[28] Missouris CG, Buckenham T, Cappuccio FP, MacGregor GA. Renal artery stenosis: a common and important problem in patients with peripheral vascular disease. Am J Med. 1994; 96(1):10–14

[29] Reiser M. Magnetic Resonance Tomography. Berlin: Springer; 2008

[30] Yeoman LJ, Mason MD, Olliff JF. Non-Hodgkin's lymphoma of the bladder—CT and MRI appearances. Clin Radiol. 1991; 44(6):389–392

[31] Hricak H, White S, Vigneron D, et al. Carcinoma of the prostate gland: MR imaging with pelvic phased-array coils versus integrated endorectal–pelvic phased-array coils. Radiology. 1994; 193(3):703–709

[32] Jager GJ, Barentsz JO, Ruijter ET, de la Rosette JJ, Oosterhof GO. Primary staging of prostate cancer. Eur Radiol. 1996; 6(2):134–139

[33] Benz-Bohm G, ed. RRR Kinderradiologie. 2nd ed. Stuttgart: Thieme; 2005

[34] Günther RW, Thelen M. Interventionelle Radiologie. Stuttgart: Thieme; 1996

[35] Kawashima A, Vrtiska TJ, LeRoy AJ, Hartman RP, McCollough CH, King BF, Jr. CT urography. Radiographics. 2004; 24 Suppl 1:S35–S54, discussion S55–S58

12 Female Pelvis

Céline D. Alt

12.1 Anatomy

12.1.1 External and Internal Genitalia

The female external genitalia (vulva) extend from the mons pubis across the introitus (opening of the urethra and vagina) to the perineum. The internal genitalia consist of the uterine corpus, cervix, vagina, fallopian tubes, and ovaries. The pelvic organs are invested by peritoneum. Anterior to the uterus, the peritoneal cavity extends between the uterine isthmus and posterior bladder wall to form the vesicouterine pouch. The rectouterine pouch, called also the cul-de-sac or pouch of Douglas, is the extension of the peritoneal cavity between the rectum and the cervix and posterior uterine wall (▶ Fig. 12.1).

Because the female internal genitalia are stabilized within the pelvis by suspensory ligaments, the uterus is subject to a number of positional variants that are influenced by the degree of bladder and rectal distention. In approximately 90% of cases the uterus occupies an anteflexed and anteverted position. The size of the uterus is also variable and depends upon age, hormonal status, pregnancy, and any prior radiation exposure.

The main parts of the uterus are the corpus (body), fundus, isthmus, and cervix (▶ Fig. 12.2). The uterine corpus is composed of three layers:
- *Endometrium*: the inner mucosal layer, whose thickness depends on age and hormonal status.
- *Myometrium*: the middle muscular layer, separated from the endometrium by a very thin junctional zone (the inner myometrium).
- *Perimetrium*: a thin peritoneal layer.

The vagina is located between the urethra, the bladder, and the rectum. Its superior portions are the anterior and posterior fornices. It terminates distally at the vaginal orifice. The approximately

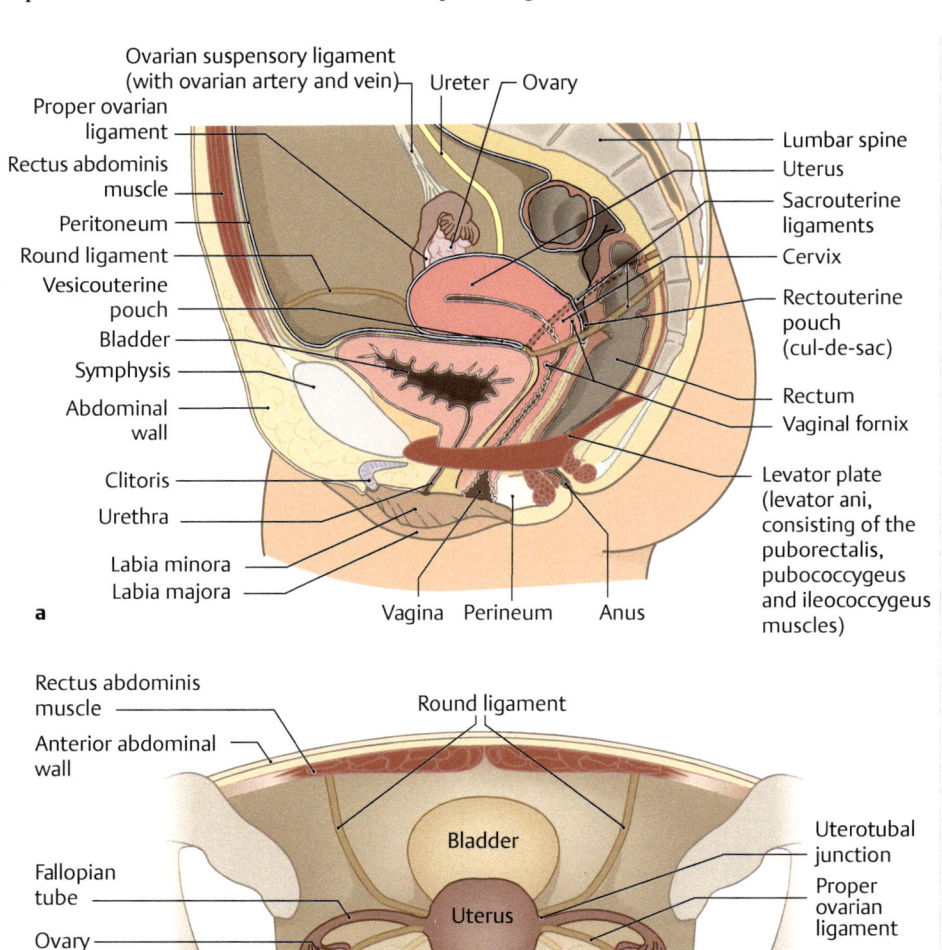

Fig. 12.1 Lateral and axial views of the female pelvis. (a) Diagram illustrating the position of the pelvic organs, the peritoneal pouches, the major suspensory ligaments, and the pelvic floor muscles for orientation and reporting. (b) Cross section through the female pelvis to display the relationships of the organs and suspensory ligaments.

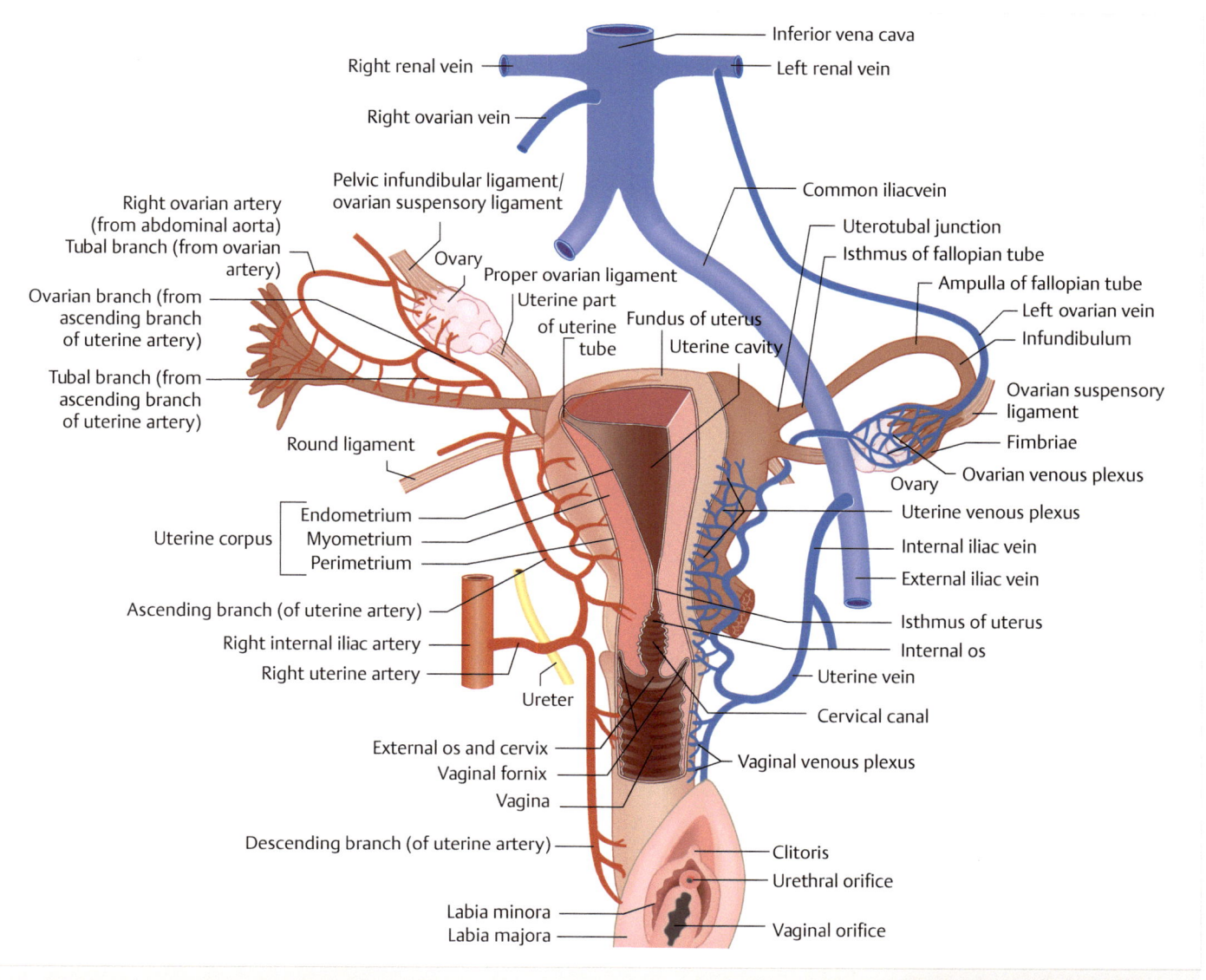

Fig. 12.2 Anterior view of the female pelvic organs. Diagrammatic representation of the arterial blood supply and venous drainage of the pelvic organs.

10-cm-long muscular tube of the vagina is surrounded by connective tissue—the paracolpium.

The fallopian tubes (uterine tube, salpinx) are each approximately 10 to 14 cm long and 1 to 4 mm in diameter. Each of the paired fallopian tubes arises from a superiorly tapered extension of the uterine cavity called the intramural or interstitial part of the tube. The narrow proximal tubal segment, called the isthmus, widens laterally to form the ampulla before terminating at the fimbriated end close to the ovary. An open communication exists between the fallopian tube and the abdominal cavity. The tube runs at almost a 90° angle at its junction with the uterine corpus; this area is called the uterotubal junction or uterine horn. Each of the fallopian tubes lies lateral to the uterus and is attached to the uterine broad ligament via the mesosalpinx (see ▶ Fig. 12.2).[1,2]

The ovaries are paired gonads located within the ovarian fossa on the lateral wall of the lesser pelvis (within the bifurcation of the common iliac artery). Structures in close relation to the ovary are the obturator nerve, ureter, external iliac vein, internal iliac artery and vein, umbilical artery, and obturator artery. Each ovary measures approximately 4 cm × 2 cm × 1 cm, has an ovoid shape, and is attached to the back of the uterine broad ligament by the mesovarium. The ovary is attached to the uterus at the level of the uterine horns by the proper ovarian ligament, and it is bound to the pelvic sidewall by the ovarian suspensory ligament (infundibulopelvic ligament; see ▶ Fig. 12.2).[1,2,3]

The ovarian stroma consists of two zones:[1]
- *Cortex*: The ovarian cortex contains follicles at various stages of maturity and also the corpora lutea.
- *Medulla*: The ovarian medulla is composed of connective tissue, smooth muscle cells, and elastic fibers and is traversed by blood vessels, lymphatics, and nerves.

The zonal anatomy of the ovary is less clearly defined in postmenopausal women than in women of reproductive age. The postmenopausal ovaries are frequently atrophic, and the stroma undergoes increasing fibrous transformation.

The fallopian tube and ovary are often referred to collectively as the adnexa.

12.1.2 Suspensory Apparatus

The pelvic organs are held in place by a suspensory apparatus consisting of various ligaments, connective tissue, and smooth muscle cells (see ▶ Fig. 12.1).
- *Broad ligament*: The broad ligament is a transverse reflection of peritoneum that attaches the uterus to the pelvic sidewall and envelops the fallopian tubes and ovaries.
- *Round ligament*: This superiorly placed ligament originates at the uterine horns, curves along the pelvic sidewall, then passes through the inguinal canal and inserts into the labia majora.
- *Cardinal ligament (transverse cervical ligament)*: The cardinal ligament is located at the base of the broad ligament. It is considered part of the parametria and is traversed by the ureter and blood vessels on each side.
- *Parametria*: The parametria are suspensory structures that include the pubocervical fascia (pubocervical ligament, pubovesical ligament), which runs anteriorly along the bladder to the pubis, and the sacrouterine (rectouterine) ligament, which runs posteriorly along the rectum to the sacrum.

12.1.3 Pelvic Floor

The lesser pelvis is bounded inferiorly by the pelvic floor, which stretches between the symphysis, the pubic rami, and the ischial tuberosities. It consists of a total of three layers, which are formed by several muscles that blend together and function chiefly to suspend the pelvic organs and prevent descent of the pelvic floor[2]:
- *Superior layer (posterior portion of the pelvic floor)*: This layer forms the pelvic diaphragm and contains the coccygeus muscle and the levator ani comprising portions of the ileococcygeus, pubococcygeus, and puborectalis muscles.
- *Urogenital diaphragm (anterior portion of the pelvic floor)*: This is a fibrous layer composed of tough connective tissue stretching between the pubic rami and the ischia and containing the deep transverse perineal muscle (m. transversus perinei profundus) and, at its inferior border, the superficial transverse perineal muscle (m. transversus perinei superficialis).
- *Inferior layer (sphincter plane)*: This layer consists of the external pelvic floor muscles and perineal muscles and contains the external anal sphincter, bulbospongiosus, and ischiocavernosus muscles (see ▶ Fig. 12.1).

12.1.4 Blood Supply

The female pelvic organs receive most of their arterial blood supply from the paired ovarian arteries, each of which arises directly from the infrarenal abdominal aorta and runs retroperitoneally down the psoas muscle and along the ovarian suspensory ligament to the ovary (supplying the ovary and fallopian tube). The ovarian artery runs over the uterine artery, which arises from the internal iliac artery on the corresponding side, and passes distally into the uterine broad ligament, crossing anterior to the ureter. At the cervical level it divides into two tortuous branches, an ascending branch (supplying the ovary, fallopian tube, and uterus) and a descending branch (supplying the vagina and cervical ring).

Blood is collected by venous plexuses on the cervix, vagina, uterus, and ovary, from which it drains chiefly through the internal iliac veins. The ovarian vein opens directly into the inferior vena cava on the right side; on the left side it opens into the left renal vein (see ▶ Fig. 12.2).[2]

12.1.5 Lymphatic Drainage

Because the lymphatic vessels in the pelvis form an arborizing system composed of multiple trunks, vessels, and anastomoses, the lymphatic return from the female pelvic organs drains to various groups of lymph nodes, some of which are not directly adjacent to the organ[3]:
- Lymph from the *ovary* and *distal fallopian tube* drains primarily to upper para-aortic lymph nodes and to pelvic or inguinal lymph nodes.[4]
- Lymph from the *uterine corpus* and *proximal fallopian tube* can drain primarily to locoregional parametrial lymph nodes, iliac and sacral lymph node groups, directly to para-aortic lymph nodes at the level of the renal vein, or to inguinal lymph nodes.
- Lymph from the *cervix* drains primarily to parametrial, sacral, and iliac nodal groups.
- Lymph from the *upper two-thirds of the vagina* drains primarily to iliac lymph nodes above the inguinal ligament, while the lower one-third of the vagina and the vulva are drained primarily by inguinal and femoral lymph nodes.[3,5]

Caution

An understanding of the various lymph node groups is relevant in patients with pelvic malignancies to avoid missing lymph node metastases that could potentially alter the treatment strategy.

12.2 Imaging

If the pelvic examination and ultrasound scans yield equivocal findings, more detailed imaging studies should be performed for the exclusion of malignancy or the staging of confirmed disease.

The sectional imaging modality of choice is MRI because of its excellent soft-tissue contrast, high level of detail, and variable sequence options, which can supply a diagnosis even without IV administration of contrast medium (▶ Fig. 12.3).

CT is definitely inferior to MRI for imaging the pelvic organs because of its relatively poor soft tissue contrast. Its main role is in planning radiotherapy, the detection of distant metastases, or the acute investigation of unexplained pelvic pain. If abdominal images are available from a CT examination for a nongynecologic indication, venous-phase images of the pelvic organs may provide useful information (▶ Fig. 12.4).

PET is most rewarding in the detection of recurrence or occult metastasis.[6,7]

Note

Image interpretation and reporting should always follow a structured routine to ensure that all questions of gynecologic interest are addressed. Especially in the evaluation of a primary tumor, all criteria that may influence tumor staging should be taken into account and noted in the report.

12.2 Imaging

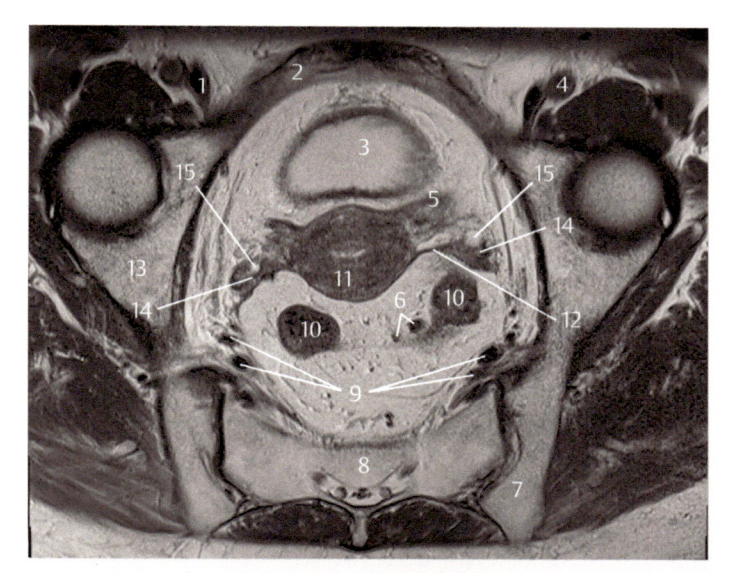

Fig. 12.3 Axial MR image of the female pelvis. Unenhanced T2 W sequence to display anatomical relationships. 1, femoral vein; 2, symphysis; 3, bladder; 4, femoral artery; 5, round ligament; 6, diverticulum; 7, ilium; 8, sacrum; 9, iliac vessels; 10, sigmoid colon; 11, uterine corpus; 12, proper ovarian ligament; 13, acetabulum; 14, ovary; 15, follicle.

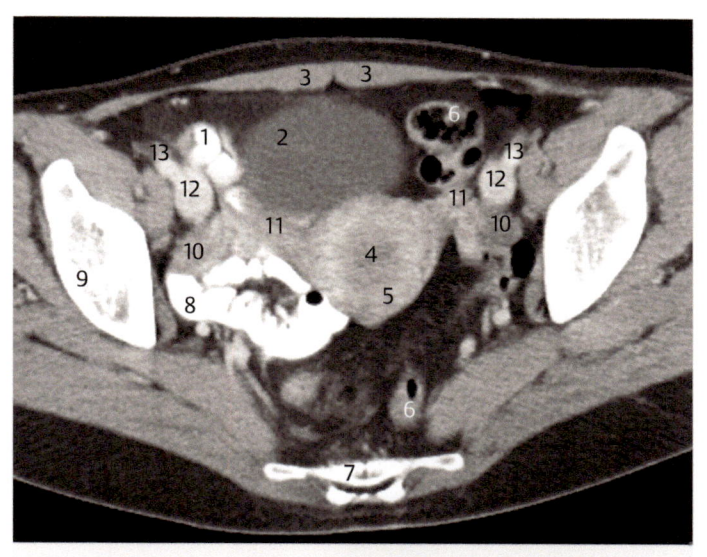

Fig. 12.4 Axial CT scan of the female pelvis. Venous-phase scan to display anatomical relationships. 1, small-bowel loops; 2, bladder; 3, rectus abdominis; 4, uterine cavity; 5 uterine corpus; 6, bowel; 7, sacrum; 8, small bowel; 9, roof of acetabulum; 10, ovary; 11, fallopian tube; 12, femoral vein; 13, femoral artery.

12.2.1 Transabdominal Ultrasound

Transabdominal ultrasound scanning provides an overview of the internal genitalia using the distended bladder as an acoustic window. Bladder distention also displaces loops of small bowel out of the lesser pelvis, which is essential for evaluating the ovaries.

An abdominal transducer is acceptable in most patients. In girls, young women, or very thin patients, a linear-array transducer with a tissue harmonic imaging option can provide better spatial resolution of the pelvic organs, with some reduction in scanning depth.

12.2.2 Magnetic Resonance Imaging

Patients are imaged in the supine position with a high-resolution surface coil. Patient preparations should include the following:
- *Moderate bladder distention*: A moderately distended bladder permits a more accurate evaluation of the bladder wall and posterior fat plane. The distended bladder also moves to a more upright position in the lesser pelvis, which simplifies anatomical orientation for angled sequences.
- *Administration of butylscopolamine to immobilize the bowel*: An antiperistaltic agent is given to minimize motion artifacts. Contraindications are raised intraocular pressure and cardiac arrhythmias, in which case glucagon is an acceptable substitute (*contraindicated in patients with diabetes mellitus*).
- *Vaginal distention*: When in a physiologically collapsed state, the vagina is distended with 20 to 40 mL of (sterile) ultrasound gel to improve the visualization of vaginal structures and the cervix. Intravaginal gel is also helpful in hysterectomized patients, as it can improve the detection of vaginal stump recurrence.

Unenhanced high-resolution T2 W TSE sequences are essential for morphological evaluation of the female pelvic organs. The pelvic protocol should always include a contrast-enhanced fat-saturated T1 W sequence, which will add significant information in almost any investigation.[8,9,10,11] Where available, the use of a DWI sequence with *b* values of 800 to 1000 is also recommended for staging the primary tumor and lymph nodes.[12,13,14] A fat-saturated T2 W sequence is helpful for evaluating inflammatory changes or fistulas, especially in cases where IV contrast medium cannot be used. An axial unenhanced T1 W sequence or proton-density sequence is used for lymph node detection. An unenhanced fat-saturated T1 W sequence is recommended for the differentiation of fatty or hemorrhagic components (particularly relevant for an ovarian mass).[15]

Note

Evaluation of the female pelvic organs requires organ-specific angulation of the MRI sequences. The image orientation may have to be adjusted during the examination (as bladder distention increases).

Sagittal sequences should be prescribed in axial paramedian slices to obtain longitudinal sections of the uterine corpus and cervix in one plane. The axial oblique slices should always be individually adjusted for organ position and indication and may not correspond to the axial or coronal planes of the body axis.[8]

The longitudinal axis through the lumen of interest serves as the reference standard for organ-specific angulation of the MRI sequences. The prescribed images are angled perpendicular to the reference organ (for axial, short-axis views) or parallel to it (for coronal views). In this way the reference organ should present a ring or "doughnut" appearance in the axial sections (▶ Table 12.1, ▶ Fig. 12.5). For anatomical orientation, the angled oblique scans can be preceded by a fast T2 W sequence in axial and coronal planes relative to the cardinal body axis.

Female Pelvis

12.2.3 Computed Tomography

Multidetector CT can quickly scan the body region of interest in axial sections with submillimeter resolution, and the acquired data can be processed into multiplanar reformatted images with essentially the same resolution.[16] The examination should be performed with IV administration of contrast medium. Nevertheless, even in the recommended venous phase of enhancement, soft-tissue contrast is still inferior to that of unenhanced MRI.

12.2.4 Differential Diagnosis

A knowledge of differential diagnoses is helpful in selecting the proper imaging modality, allowing for protocol modifications and thereby simplifying the diagnostic procedure. Good history taking is essential. In women who present with lower abdominal pain, it is important to describe the pain characteristics, the onset and duration of the pain, its location, and any previous operations or diseases. Some important considerations in the differential diagnosis of acute or chronic lower abdominal pain are listed below:

- Acute lower abdominal pain:[17,18]
  - Ruptured ovarian cyst.
  - Hemorrhagic ovarian cyst.
  - Pelvic inflammatory disease.
  - Tubo-ovarian abscess.
  - Adnexal torsion.
  - Acute necrosis of a pedunculated leiomyoma due to torsion.
  - Ectopic pregnancy.
  - Appendicitis.
  - Diverticulitis.
  - Urinary tract infection.
  - Ureteral colic.
- Chronic lower abdominal pain:[19]
  - Endometriosis.
  - Uterine adenomyosis.
  - Leiomyomas.
  - Polyps.
  - Chronic inflammation.
  - Adhesions.
  - Pelvic varicosity.
  - Retroverted uterus.
  - Anomalies.
  - Adnexal mass.
  - Neoplasm.
  - Ascites due to malignancy.

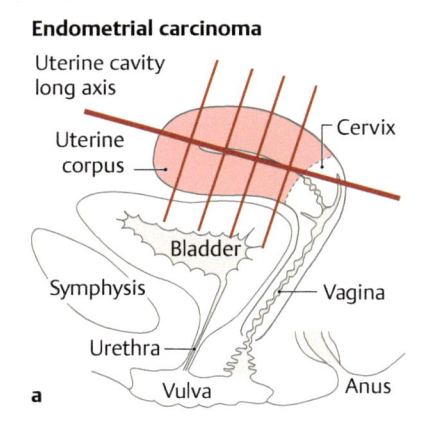

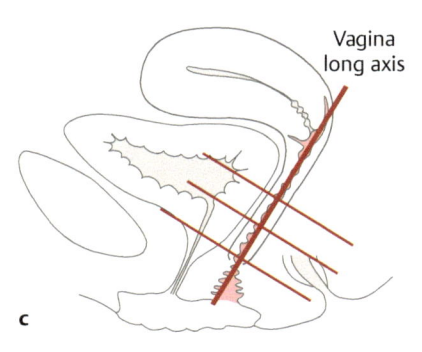

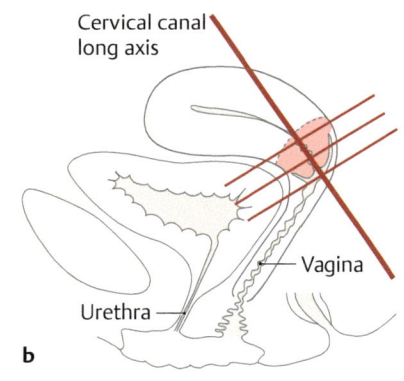

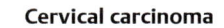

Table 12.1 Reference axes for organ-specific image orientation in axial and coronal MRI

Organ, indication	Structures that define the longitudinal reference axis for image orientation
Endometrium, uterine corpus	Corpus lumen
Cervix	Cervical canal
Vagina, tumor recurrence after hysterectomy	Vaginal canal, vaginal stump
Vulva	Distal urethra at the level of the introitus
Ovary	Parallel to the corpus lumen, especially for localizing masses to the ovary or uterus

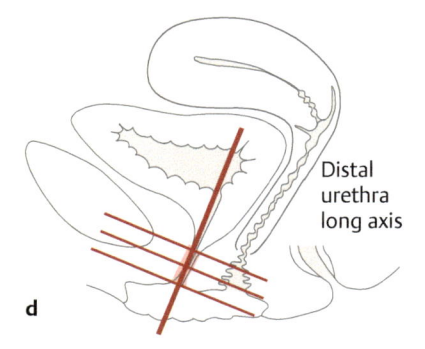

Fig. 12.5 MRI planes angled relative to specific pelvic organs. Thick lines denote the longitudinal axis for prescribing perpendicular axial slices (thin lines) and parallel coronal slices.

12.3 Congenital Anomalies

Congenital anomalies of the female genitalia may be caused by genetic defects or exposure to exogenous agents. They result from a failure or deficiency of formation such as deficient growth, failure of canalization, or incomplete fusion of the müllerian ducts.[20] The anomalies are often detected in routine pediatric examinations, whereupon the diagnosis is usually confirmed by transabdominal ultrasound or fluoroscopic examination after retrograde administration of contrast medium. If necessary, MRI may be helpful for the more detailed characterization of complex anomalies.

> **Note**
>
> Given the close proximity of the internal genitalia and urinary tract, genital malformations are commonly associated with urinary tract anomalies, which should also be investigated.[20]

12.3.1 Bicornuate Uterus, Uterus Didelphys, and (Sub)Septate Uterus

▶ **Brief definition.** Abnormalities of differentiation that occur between weeks 9 and 12 of gestation lead to various duplication anomalies of the uterus and vagina. The following disorders are distinguished:[20]
- Anomalies that involve absent or incomplete fusion of the müllerian ducts—especially a bicornuate unicollis or bicollis uterus (uterus bicornis unicollis or bicollis) and uterus didelphys.
- Anomalies that involve absent or incomplete reabsorption of the septum after normal fusion of the müllerian ducts—especially a (sub)septate uterus and arcuate uterus

▶ **Imaging signs** (▶ Fig. 12.6)
- Failure of fusion:
  - A bicornuate unicollis uterus has two uterine cavities that open into one cervix. The central myometrium extends to the internal os.
  - A bicornuate bicollis uterus has two uterine cavities and two cervices (▶ Fig. 12.7). The central myometrium extends to the external os.
  - Uterus didelphys involves a complete duplication of the uterus with one horn each, two separate cervices, and a possible double vagina (double uterus with a double vagina or vaginal septum).
- Absent or incomplete septal reabsorption:
  - In a septate uterus, the septum extends to the cervix.
  - In a subseptate uterus, the septum is present only within the uterine cavity.
  - In an arcuate uterus, the fundus bulges into the uterine cavity.

▶ **Clinical features.** Most women are asymptomatic, but the anomalies are frequently associated with reproductive failure and pregnancy loss.

12.3.2 Hymenal Atresia

▶ **Brief definition.** If perforation of the hymen—which separates the vagina from the urogenital sinus during development—fails to occur, the hymenal epithelium is transformed into fibrous connective tissue that obstructs outflow from the uterus. Hymenal atresia is the most common congenital anomaly with otherwise normal formation of the internal genitalia. The reported incidence ranges from 1:1,000 to 1:16,000.[5,21,22]

▶ **Imaging signs.** The vagina is distended by mucus, blood, and blood breakdown products. The diagnosis of hymenal atresia can

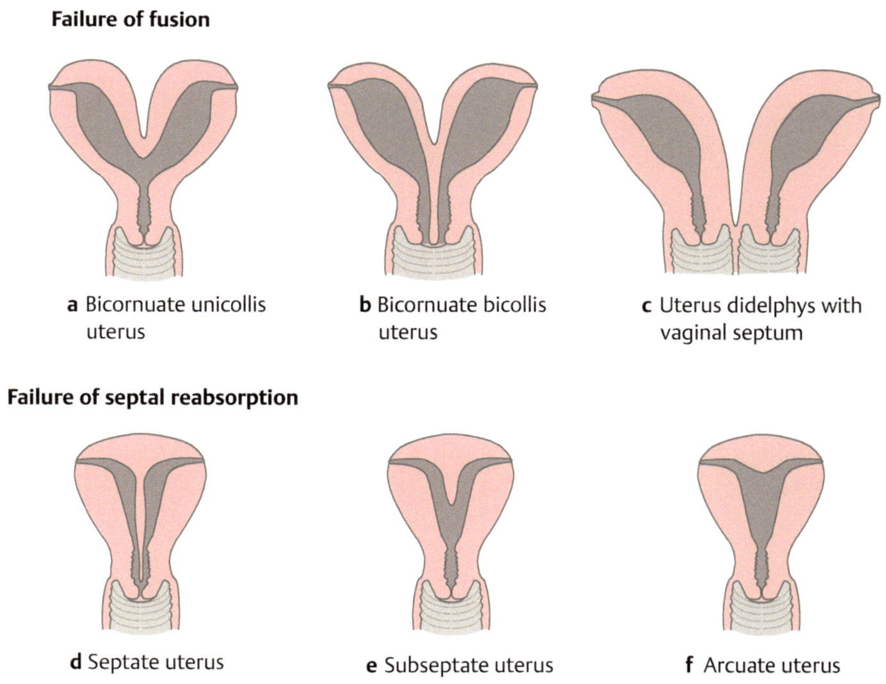

Failure of fusion

a Bicornuate unicollis uterus
b Bicornuate bicollis uterus
c Uterus didelphys with vaginal septum

Failure of septal reabsorption

d Septate uterus
e Subseptate uterus
f Arcuate uterus

Fig. 12.6 Uterine anomalies. (a–c) Anomalies due to incomplete fusion of the müllerian ducts. (d–f) Anomalies due to absent or incomplete septal reabsorption.

Female Pelvis

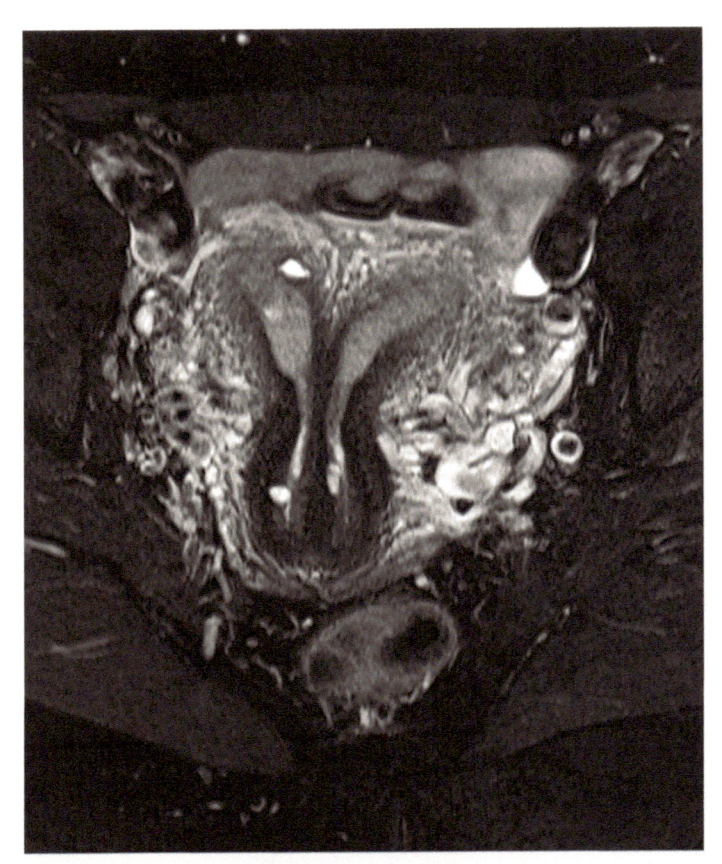

Fig. 12.7 Bicornuate bicollis uterus. Fat-saturated axial T2W image reveals two uterine horns and two cervices. The central myometrium extends to the external os, creating the characteristic pattern of a bicornuate bicollis uterus. A small corpus cyst and two small cervical cysts (nabothian follicles) are incidental findings without pathologic significance.

be confirmed by transabdominal ultrasound (limited penetration depth) or high-resolution MRI without contrast medium (for surveying the whole lesser pelvis).

▶ **Clinical features.** Young girls may complain of monthly colicky pains or may present with an acute abdomen. Complaints first appear after menarche and result from the accumulation of blood first in the vagina (hematocolpos), then in the uterus (hematometra), and finally in the fallopian tube (hematosalpinx) due to the obstructive effect of the imperforate hymen. There may be associated dysuria, urinary retention, and constipation. Girls are asymptomatic as infants, as only mucus is retained in the vagina (mucocolpos).[20]

12.3.3 Uterovaginal Agenesis

▶ **Brief definition.** The incidence of this autosomal disorder, also known as Mayer–Rokitansky–Küster–Hauser syndrome, is approximately 1:5,000 female births. The syndrome is characterized by a rudimentary uterus and fallopian tubes with vaginal aplasia. But because the ovaries develop normally and have normal function, the external genitalia are female. This condition is often associated with renal anomalies, usually in the form of a horseshoe kidney, as well as skeletal malformations (e.g., fused cervical vertebrae or rudimentary vertebral bodies).[20]

▶ **Clinical features.** Girls with uterovaginal agenesis become symptomatic at puberty, presenting with primary amenorrhea.

▶ **Imaging signs.** The rudimentary development of the uterus and vagina is detectable with transabdominal ultrasound. If necessary, unenhanced high-resolution MRI of the pelvis is helpful in confirming the diagnosis, as it provides a survey view of the lesser pelvis and demonstrates normal development of both ovaries.

12.4 Diseases

12.4.1 Inflammatory Changes

▶ **Brief definition.** Pelvic inflammatory disease in women may be caused by a primary infection of the uterus, fallopian tube, or ovaries with microorganisms (especially chlamydia, mycobacteria, gram-negative bacteria, or gonococci) leading to salpingitis, endometritis, pyosalpinx, or even a tubo-ovarian abscess. Bacterial colonization during or after menstruation, in the postpartum period, or after gynecologic or other surgical procedures may provoke an acute inflammatory process; or inflammation may spread from an adjacent organ to the internal genitalia, usually secondary to appendicitis or diverticulitis. Infection may spread from the fallopian tubes to the peritoneal cavity or may disseminate by the lymphogenous or hematogenous route, as in tuberculosis (p. 437), for example. If an inflammation becomes chronic (due to a silent course or recurrent inflammations), it may lead to tubal or other adhesions with secondary complications such as infertility or ectopic pregnancy.[11]

▶ **Imaging signs.** The initial imaging study of choice is ultrasound.

> **Caution**
>
> Abdominal CT is often used as a survey study in the acute setting. But since most patients are young women, MRI should generally be favored over CT.[11,23]

Imaging signs on CT and MRI:
- *Endometritis*: The endometrium is thickened and the uterine cavity is filled with fluid. Concomitant myometritis is often present and is manifested by edematous thickening of the myometrium.
- *Hydrosalpinx, hematosalpinx, and pyosalpinx*: Hydrosalpinx, caused by tubal obstruction due to postinflammatory adhesions, endometriosis, or even a malignant process, is characterized by fluid retention with dilatation of the tubal lumen, which may be several centimeters in diameter or may assume a C- or S-shaped configuration (▶ Fig. 12.8). With *hematosalpinx*, the dilated tubal lumen is hyperechoic on ultrasound and shows increased attenuation on CT and increased T1W signal intensity on unenhanced MRI. Superinfection leads to *pyosalpinx*, appearing as a distended tube with hypervascular wall thickening. The intraluminal fluid may be heterogeneous, depending on its protein content. An air–fluid level is pathognomonic but not always detectable.[23]
- *Salpingitis and oophoritis*: In salpingitis, the fallopian tube is edematous and the wall shows intense enhancement. Frequently the lumen is not dilated. The surrounding tissue shows inflammatory imbibition. In oophoritis the ovary is enlarged and shows loss of corticomedullary differentiation. There is usually surrounding free fluid.[11,23]

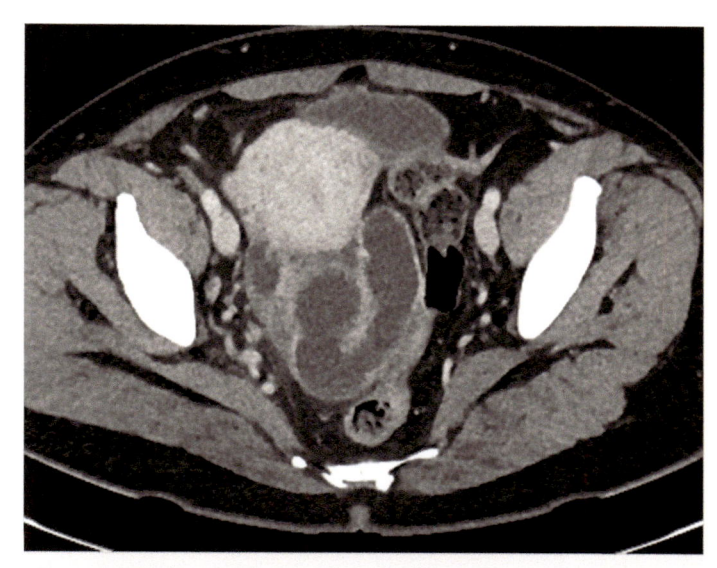

Fig. 12.8 Hydrosalpinx. Venous CT reveals a C-shaped, fluid-filled structure with prominent walls and contrast enhancement posterior to the homogeneously enhancing uterus, consistent with a distended fallopian tube (hydrosalpinx).

- *Tubo-ovarian complex (adnexitis) and tubo-ovarian abscess*:
  ○ Tubo-ovarian complex typically presents as a fluid-filled multicystic mass. The fallopian tube and ovary can still be differentiated.
  ○ A tubo-ovarian abscess, on the other hand, appears as a thick-walled mass that is poorly delineated from the uterus and small-bowel loops and may include both cystic and solid components, internal septa, and possible gas collections. It enhances intensely due to the inflammatory component.[24,25] Imbibition is often seen in the fatty tissue around the primary inflammatory process. Possible associated findings are adhesions, thickening of the uterosacral ligaments, reactive lymphadenopathy, and free fluid in the lesser pelvis.[11,26,27]

Note

Tubo-ovarian abscess may closely resemble ovarian carcinoma in its imaging appearance. However, primary ovarian carcinoma is not associated with a dilated fallopian tube and usually lacks a perifocal inflammatory reaction. Differentiation is aided by imaging an additional plane that shows continuity of the abscess with a dilated fallopian tube.[25,28]

▶ **Clinical features.** Women with acute pelvic inflammatory disease often present with lower abdominal pain, fever, and positive serum markers for infection. In approximately 20% of cases, however, the patient may be afebrile with a white blood count that is within normal limits.[11] The rupture of a tubo-ovarian abscess may incite a life-threatening peritonitis.[25] The secondary involvement of surrounding structures may cause bowel obstruction or an intraperitoneal abscess. Chronic inflammation often leads to nonspecific lower abdominal complaints and may cause back pain due to adhesions.

▶ **Differential diagnosis**[29]
- Appendicitis.
- Diverticulitis.
- Urinary tract infection.
- Ectopic pregnancy.
- Endometriosis.
- Hemorrhagic corpus luteum cyst.
- Uterine leiomyomas.
- Ovarian cancer.
- Fallopian tube cancer.

Hydrosalpinx in particular requires differentiation from the following:
- Cystic ovarian tumor.
- Ileus (but ultrasound shows peristalsis).
- Pelvic varicosities (ultrasound shows intraluminal echoes and Doppler blood flow; the veins enhance on postcontrast CT and MRI).
- Epithelial stromal tumor of the ovary.

▶ **Key points.** The MRI protocol for female pelvic inflammatory disease should include the following sequences:
- High-resolution, thin-slice (3–4 mm) T2 W TSE sequence in at least two planes.
- Unenhanced axial T1 W sequence.
- Fat-saturated axial T2 W sequence.
- Contrast-enhanced and fat-saturated T1 W sequence in two planes.

Tuberculosis of the Genital Tract

The fallopian tubes are the most common primary site of involvement by tuberculosis in the female pelvis, and the involvement is usually bilateral. Spread to adjacent genital organs may occur by the hematogenous or the lymphogenous route. On the whole, only 1.3% of women with tuberculosis develop genital tract involvement.[23,27]

▶ **Imaging signs**
- *Tubercular salpingitis*: The fallopian tubes are dilated, with no evidence of obstruction, and their walls are thickened. The tubes may show an S-shaped or string-of-beads configuration and enhance intensely after IV administration of contrast medium.
- *Tubercular tubo-ovarian abscess*: This lesion appears as a solid or mixed cystic–solid ovarian mass, possibly with small nodules and septa within the cystic portion. Calcifications are sometimes seen. Other findings are free fluid, thickening of the peritoneum with peritoneal nodules, and areas of mesenteric and omental soft-tissue infiltration.[27] On MRI the abscess has heterogeneous signal intensity in T2 W sequences (hypointense solid component, hyperintense cystic component, hypointense nodules). The abscess is hypointense to moderately hyperintense in T1 W sequences, depending on its protein content. The solid components, septa, and peritoneum show intense enhancement. Ascites, which shows very high T2 W signal intensity, is permeated by thin septa of low T2 W signal intensity.[27]

▶ **Clinical features.** Patients complain of acute or chronic lower abdominal pain or vaginal bleeding. Peritonism is detected in approximately one-half of patients. Infertility or an elevated CA 125 level may also be found. In most cases, however, genital

Female Pelvis

tuberculosis is detected incidentally in curettage material or during laparoscopic biopsy.[30]

▶ **Differential diagnosis**
- Ovarian carcinoma.
- Peritoneal metastases.

Vaginal Fistulas

▶ **Brief definition.** Vaginal fistulas may occur as a result of surgery (especially hysterectomy), inflammatory bowel disease, malignancy, or radiotherapy, or in the setting of a congenital anomaly.

▶ **Imaging signs.** Because fistulas may be quite extensive and may even form a complex, branched network of burrowing tracts, MRI is the modality of choice for obtaining an overall view. The rectal or vaginal introduction of fluid or ultrasound gel facilitates detection, especially of small-caliber tracts. The fistulous tract is very hyperintense in the fat-saturated T2 W sequence. The surrounding tissue may show an inflammatory reaction, depending on activity, and will then show increased signal intensity. Fluid collections or abscesses may also be found (▶ Fig. 12.9).

▶ **Clinical features.** The clinical presentation depends on inflammatory activity, location, and the structures that communicate with the vagina through the fistulous tract. Vesicovaginal, rectovaginal, enterovaginal, and colovaginal fistulas are commonly found.

▶ **Key points.** A thin-slice (fat-saturated) T1 W sequence in two planes is recommended for the detection of vaginal fistulas. The axial plane is angled relative to the vagina, and a sagittal or coronal sequence may have to be added for complete visualization. Fistula imaging is also aided by a thin-slice, contrast-enhanced T1 W sequence with fat saturation.

12.4.2 Benign Lesions and Pseudotumors

Cysts of the Uterus, Vulva, and Vagina

▶ **Brief definition.** Cysts may arise in the endometrium or cervix (nabothian follicles) and from the Bartholin's glands (Bartholin's cysts) or vaginal Gartner's ducts (Gartner's duct cysts). They are incidental imaging findings.

▶ **Imaging signs.** When imaged sonographically, simple cysts have smooth margins and are devoid of internal echoes. On MRI they are hypointense in unenhanced T1 W sequences and very hyperintense in T2 W sequences (see ▶ Fig. 12.7 and ▶ Fig. 12.10c). Proteinaceous contents or intracystic hemorrhage produce high-amplitude internal echoes at ultrasound, increased signal intensity on T1 W images, and heterogeneous signal intensity on T2 W images. The cysts have smooth margins on CT scans, and attenuation values in the cysts depend on protein content (see ▶ Fig. 12.7, ▶ Fig. 12.10c, ▶ Fig. 12.15, and ▶ Fig. 12.21a).

▶ **Clinical features.** Cysts of the uterus, vulva, and vagina usually do not produce clinical symptoms.

▶ **Differential diagnosis.** Bartholin's cysts may become superinfected (bartholinitis) and may undergo secondary abscess formation or even malignant transformation resulting in Bartholin's gland carcinoma (p. 455).

▶ **Brief definition.** Most simple cystic lesions of the ovary are functional cysts (developing from an unruptured graafian follicle) smaller than 3 cm in diameter. Lesions must measure more than 3 to 4 cm to qualify as "ovarian cysts." They may have thin internal septa and may show intracystic hemorrhage. Corpus luteum cysts develop from the remnants of a ruptured graafian follicle. They may reach several centimeters in size and often show a thickened, irregular wall.[15,31,32] The terms "polycystic ovary syndrome" or "Stein–Leventhal syndrome" refer to a disease in which a hormonal disorder leads to a firm, thickened ovarian capsule on both sides that prevents follicular rupture. A peripheral string-of-beads row of multiple, equal-sized follicles, usually found in an enlarged ovary with a dense central stroma, is pathognomonic for polycystic ovary syndrome.[15]

▶ **Imaging signs.** Simple functional and benign ovarian cysts have contents of fluid attenuation, have a smooth and thin cyst wall, and display posterior acoustic enhancement on ultrasound. They do not show wall thickening, internal septa, or solid components. The cyst contents may show higher echogenicity, increased signal intensity, or increased attenuation due to proteinaceous

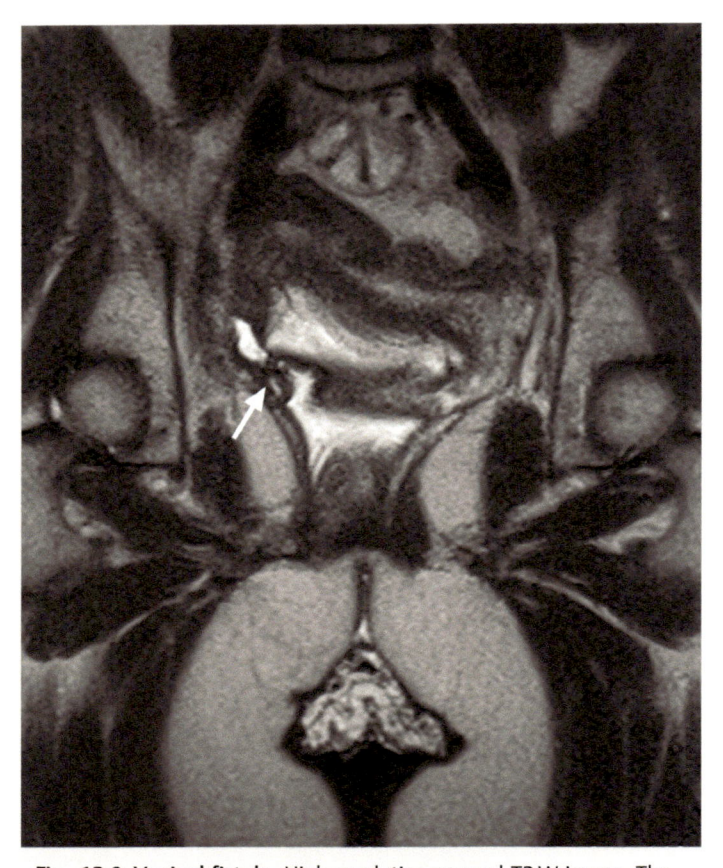

Fig. 12.9 Vaginal fistula. High-resolution coronal T2 W image. The fluid-filled bladder is seen cranial to the vaginal stump, which is distended with ultrasound gel. The fluid-filled bean-shaped structure on the right side is a collection resulting from a posthysterectomy vesicovaginal fistula (arrow). The surrounding soft tissue does not show an associated inflammatory reaction.

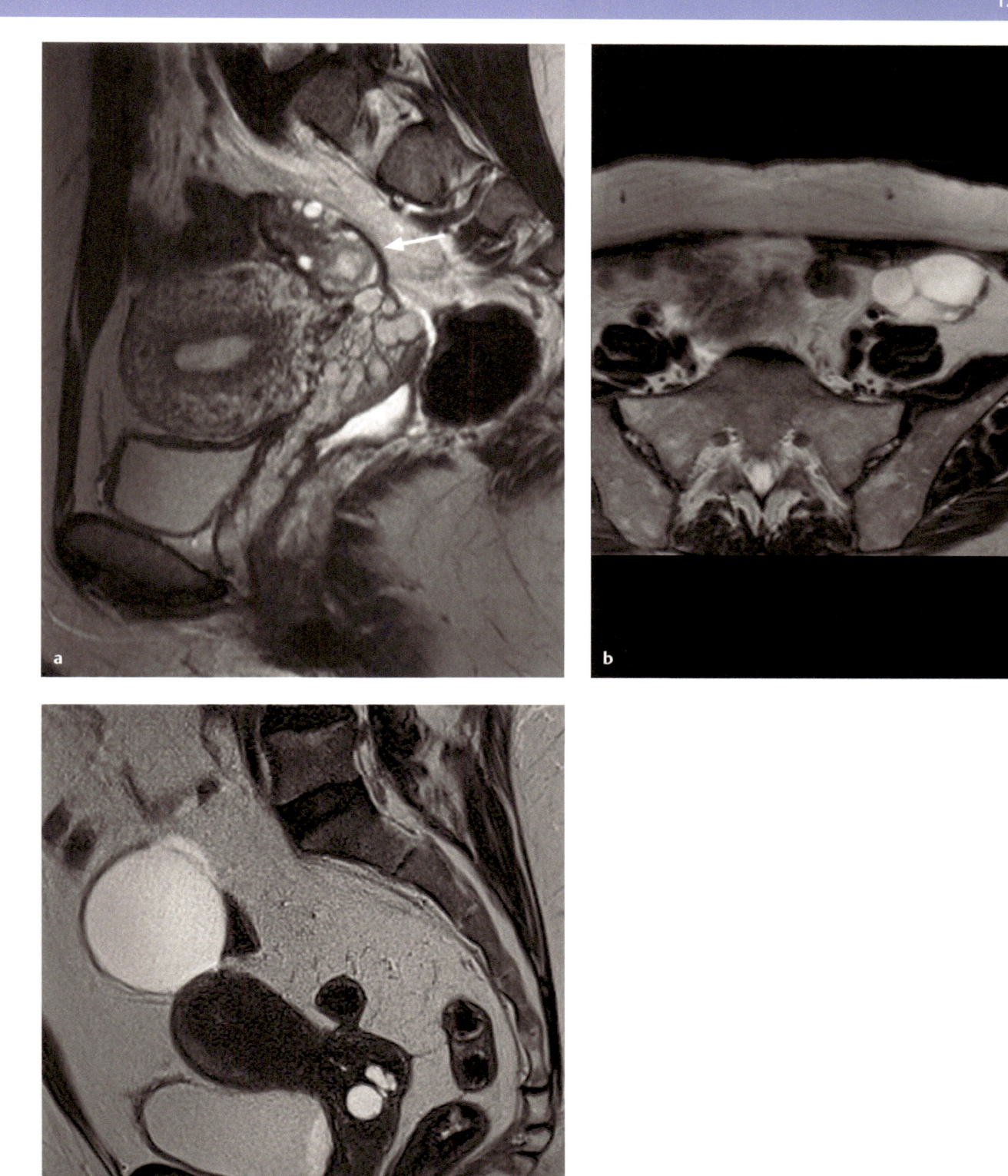

Fig. 12.10 Benign cystic lesions of the ovary. MRI appearance. **(a)** High-resolution sagittal T2W image. The thick-walled cystic lesion with a slightly irregular appearance in the lower part of the ovary is a corpus luteum cyst (arrow). Several follicles at various stages of maturity are also visible in the cortex. **(b)** High-resolution axial T2W image shows multiple simple cysts in the left ovary anterior to the psoas muscle. **(c)** High-resolution sagittal T2W image. A large, simple ovarian cyst abuts the uterine fundus. Several simple nabothian follicles are visible within the cervix.

material or intracystic hemorrhage. A corpus luteum cyst usually has a thick, irregular wall, is often hemorrhagic, and shows intense contrast enhancement, which can make it difficult to distinguish from a malignant process[15,33] (▶ Fig. 12.10).

> **Caution**
> If a hemorrhagic ovarian cyst is suspected, a sonographic follow-up should be scheduled 6 weeks after the initial examination (an acyclic schedule, therefore subject to a different hormone status). Alternatively, MRI should be performed for further differentiation.[33]

▶ **Clinical features.** Functional and benign ovarian cysts are usually asymptomatic and have a strong tendency to regress over time. On reaching a certain size, however, they may cause dull, diffuse lower abdominal pain by exerting pressure on adjacent organs. They may also cause bladder and bowel dysfunction and back pain. Sudden, excruciating pain with possible nausea and vomiting may signify a ruptured cyst or twisted pedicle.[17]

▶ **Differential diagnosis**[34]
- Cystadenoma.
- Endometrioma (hyperintense in unenhanced T1 W sequences, hypointense in T2 W sequences).
- Cystadenocarcinoma (check for malignancy criteria).

▶ **Pitfalls.** Follicles at different stages of maturity, sometimes coexisting with functional or benign ovarian cysts, are a common finding in women of reproductive age. This normal pattern should not be erroneously described as a "polycystic ovary" (▶ Fig. 12.11).

Ovarian and Tubal Torsion

▶ **Brief definition.** Twisting of the ovary on its vascular pedicle may result from abrupt body movements in a patient with a large ovarian cyst or tumor. Isolated torsion of the fallopian tube is extremely rare (1:1.5 million). Risk factors are a long mesosalpinx, hydrosalpinx, acute pelvic inflammatory disease, hypermotility of the fallopian tube, or trauma. The incidence is highest in women of reproductive age, but children may also be affected. Adnexal torsion more commonly occurs on the right side. This could relate to a hypermobile ileocecal pole on the right side, or the fact that the left half of the pelvic cavity is mostly occupied by the sigmoid colon, leaving little room for tubo-ovarian torsion to occur.[23,28,35,36]

▶ **Imaging signs**
- *Ovarian torsion*: The ovary may show edematous swelling and wall thickening. The fallopian tube may also be thickened, and follicles may be arranged in a ringlike pattern at the periphery of the twisted ovary. Ascites is often detectable. Ovarian torsion is confirmed by an absence of flow signals on Doppler ultrasound (▶ Fig. 12.12) or absence of enhancement on sectional imaging after IV administration of contrast medium. Frequently the uterus is tilted toward the side of the torsion.[15,18,37]
- *Tubal torsion*: The fallopian tube is dilated and its wall may be thickened. The ipsilateral ovary may appear normal. It is common to find ascites and a perifocal inflammatory reaction.[38]

▶ **Clinical features.** The classic clinical presentation of acute torsion is severe unilateral pain of sudden onset, muscular guarding, possible nausea and vomiting, and possible laboratory signs of inflammation. Patients with gradual torsion present with lower abdominal pain, possible guarding, fever, nausea, and vomiting. Torsion of the pedicle initially leads to hemorrhagic infarction (due to venous stasis). Additional involvement of the arteries may lead to ovarian necrosis with hemorrhage and shock, sometimes accompanied by paralytic ileus. The pain resulting from tubal torsion may radiate to the groin or thigh.[15,17,28,39]

▶ **Differential diagnosis**[28]
- Ruptured ovarian cyst.
- Tubo-ovarian abscess.
- Hydrosalpinx.
- Acute abdomen from a different cause.

Polyps

▶ **Brief definition.** Polyps of the uterine corpus or cervix are common incidental findings. They may be sessile or they may protrude into the lumen attached to the mucosa by a pedicle. They may be hypertrophic, atrophic, or functional. The risk of endometrial cancer is increased 9-fold in patients with endometrial or cervical polyps.[31]

▶ **Imaging signs.** Polyps appear sonographically as hyperechoic masses. On MRI they are iso- to hypointense to endometrium in

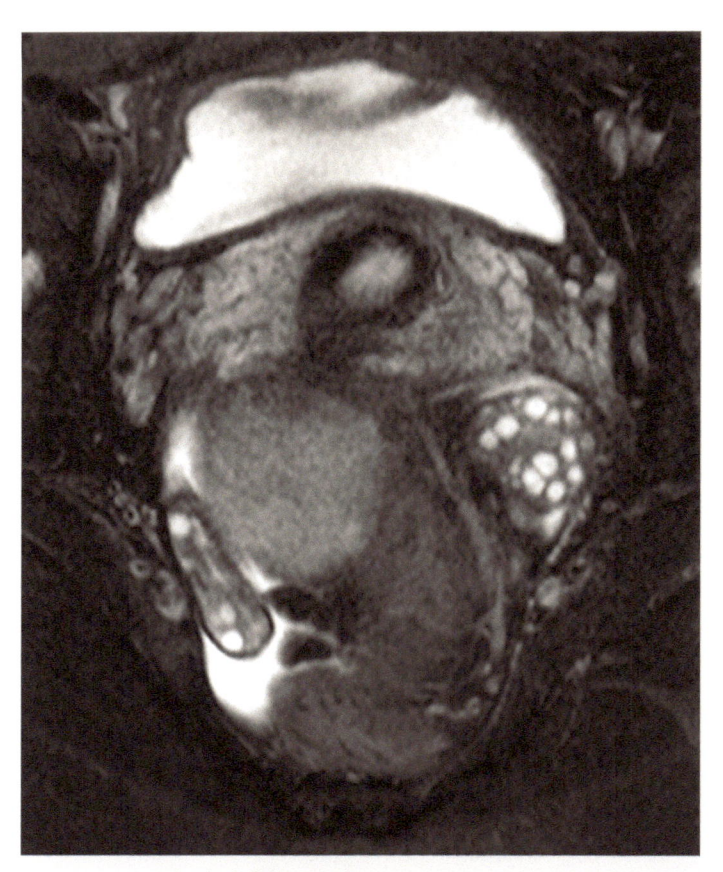

Fig. 12.11 Multiple follicles. Both ovaries contain multiple follicles of varying size and maturity in a young woman not taking hormonal contraceptives. Physiologic amounts of free fluid are visible in the lesser pelvis.

unenhanced T2 W sequences. After IV administration of contrast medium, small polyps show higher signal intensity (due to greater enhancement) than large polyps.[40]

▶ **Clinical features.** Patients may complain of hypermenorrhea (increased bleeding due to decreased uterine contractility), menorrhagia (bleeding for more than 6 days), or metrorrhagia (acyclic bleeding), depending on the size of the endometrial polyp. Polyps may also cause postmenopausal bleeding. The torsion of a pedunculated polyp may cause cramping, laborlike pains. Cervical polyps are usually asymptomatic.[31]

▶ **Differential diagnosis**
- Leiomyomas.
- Endometrial hyperplasia.
- Endometrial carcinoma.
- Cervical carcinoma.

Leiomyomas

▶ **Brief definition.** Leiomyomas (fibroids) are benign, estrogen-sensitive neoplasms derived from smooth muscle cells. More than 90% are located in the uterus. Approximately 25 to 35% of women of reproductive age have leiomyomas. New leiomyomas cease to form after menopause, and existing fibroids tend to regress. Leiomyomas have a pseudocapsule and smooth margins, and are classified by their location as submucosal (growth directed toward the lumen), intramural, or subserosal (growth directed outward). Pedunculated leiomyomas also occur. Besides the uterine cavity, fibroids may also occur at cervical, vaginal, and intraligamentous sites.[40]

▶ **Imaging signs.** The diagnosis is usually based on pelvic examination and ultrasound, which depicts leiomyomas as rounded, heterogeneous masses with smooth margins. High-resolution pelvic MRI is useful for evaluating leiomyomas that are large or have increased in number, for planning treatment (especially embolization, ultrasound thermoablation, and MRI-guided ablation with focused ultrasound), and for the exclusion of a malignant process (▶ Fig. 12.13, ▶ Fig. 12.14). The MRI signal characteristics of leiomyomas vary with their composition:[40]

- *Leiomyomas without degenerative changes*: These are rounded, sharply circumscribed, fibrocyte-rich tumors that are slightly hypointense to myometrium in T1 W sequences and very hypointense in T2 W sequences. The signal pattern is usually inhomogeneous after IV administration of contrast medium, and a pseudocapsule can often be identified (see ▶ Fig. 12.13).[10]
- *Leiomyomas with degenerative changes*: These tumors tend to show heterogeneous signal intensity even in unenhanced sequences due to internal calcifications or the presence of hyaline, fatty, myxomatous, or liquid components (see ▶ Fig. 12.13).

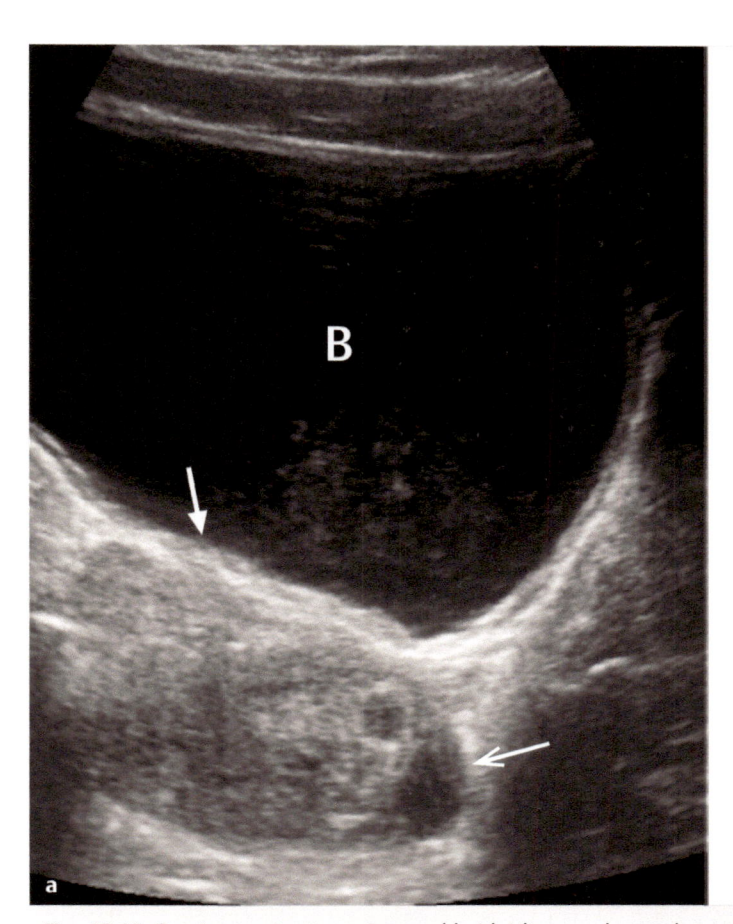

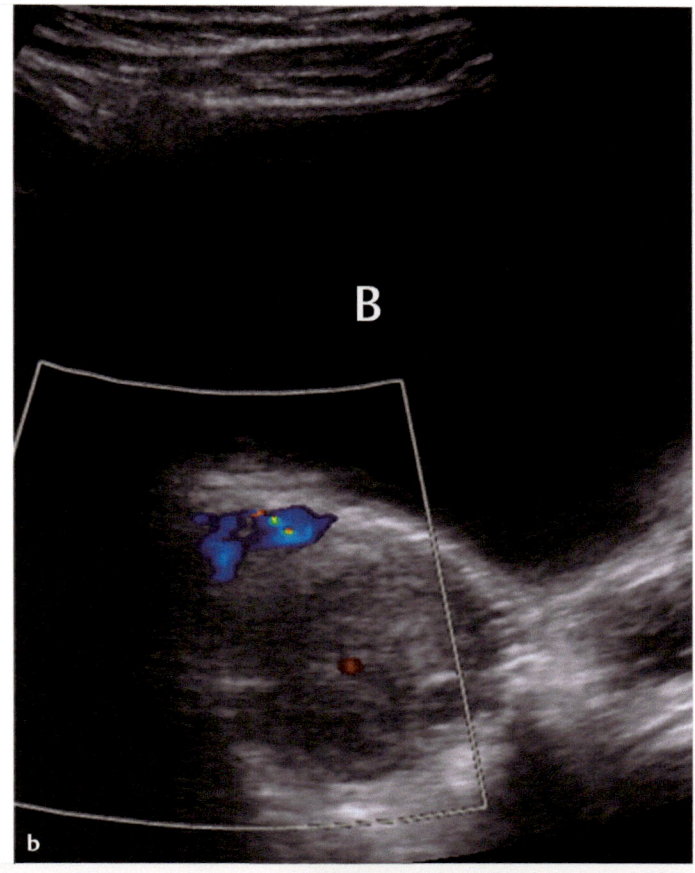

Fig. 12.12 **Ovarian torsion** in an 8-year-old girl. Ultrasound scan shows an enlarged ovary ([a], arrow) bordered by free fluid ([a], open arrow). Normal Doppler signals are almost completely absent in the twisted pedicle (b). T2 W images show enlargement of the affected right ovary ([c], [d], arrows). The follicles are arranged in a ring pattern at the periphery of the ovary. The left ovary appears normal ([c], [d], open arrows). In the contrast-enhanced T1 W GRE images, the affected ovary is markedly enlarged (e) and shows less enhancement than the left ovary (f). (a) Ultrasound. (b) Color Doppler ultrasound.

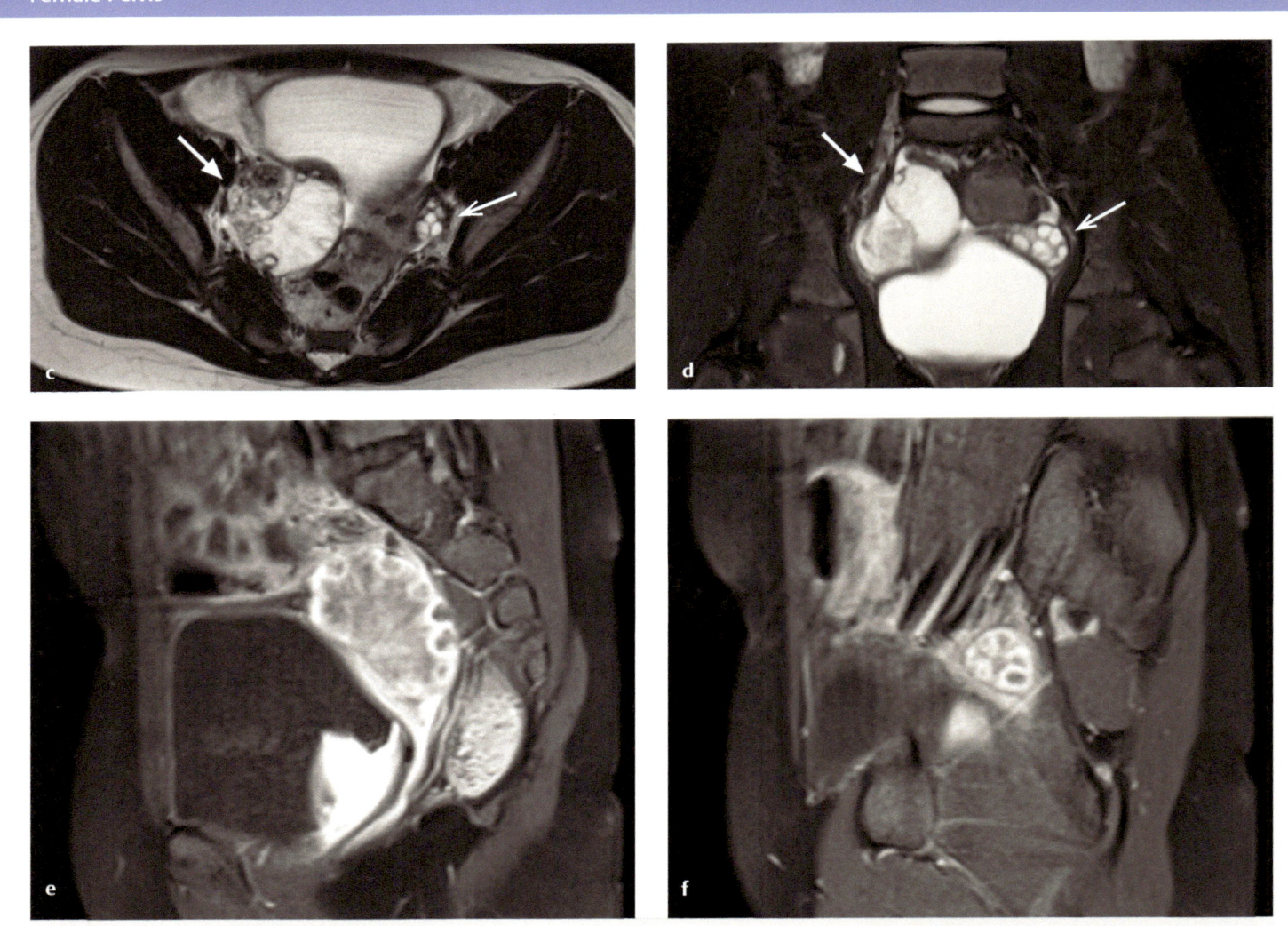

Fig. 12.12 (continued) (**c**) Axial T2 W image without fat suppression. (**d**) Coronal T2 W image with fat suppression. (**e**) Sagittal T1 W GRE image after IV administration of contrast medium. Right ovary. (**f**) Sagittal T1 W GRE image after IV administration of contrast medium. Left ovary.

When leiomyomas are detected incidentally in a CT examination, they show early arterial enhancement and are usually hypodense on delayed scans. Attenuation tends to be homogeneous in small leiomyomas and heterogeneous in large ones. Internal calcifications are frequently present and are demonstrated better by CT than by MRI. Hyperdense inclusions on CT may signify intratumoral hemorrhage, while hypodense areas are suggestive of necrosis or infection.

▶ **Clinical features.** Leiomyomas of the uterine corpus are usually asymptomatic. Some 25 to 50% of women with fibroids have no symptoms. Depending on their size and location, leiomyomas may present clinically with hypermenorrhea (increased bleeding due to decreased uterine contractility), menorrhagia (bleeding for more than 6 days), metrorrhagia (acyclic bleeding), or even cramping pains. Primarily nongynecologic symptoms may also occur,[40] such as:
- Pollakiuria.
- Bladder dysfunction.
- Urgency or stress incontinence (especially with anterior wall leiomyomas or vaginal fibromyomas).
- Dyspareunia (especially with vaginal leiomyomas).
- Defecation complaints (especially with posterior wall leiomyomas).
- Hydronephrosis (due to ureteral compression by a leiomyoma).

▶ **Differential diagnosis**
- Polyps (from subserosal leiomyomas).
- Adenomyosis (from intramural leiomyomas).
- Uterine sarcoma (mainly requires differentiation from intramural or fast-growing leiomyomas).
- Leiomyosarcoma of the cervix or vagina.
- Ovarian fibroma (mainly requires differentiation from a serous or pedunculated leiomyoma).
- Ovarian carcinoma (mainly requires differentiation from a serous or pedunculated leiomyoma).

Endometriosis

▶ **Brief definition.** After leiomyomas, endometriosis is the second most common gynecologic disease in women of reproductive age. The average prevalence is approximately 10 to 15%.[41] The disease is characterized by the presence of endometrial tissue outside the uterine cavity. The ovaries are most commonly affected (endometrioma, chocolate cyst). Other sites of involvement are:[41,42,43,44]
- Fallopian tubes.
- Sacrouterine ligaments.
- Torus uterinus (upper portion of the posterior lip of the cervix).
- Vagina (especially the upper portion of the posterior vaginal wall, the rectovaginal pouch, or the posterior part of the vaginal fornix).

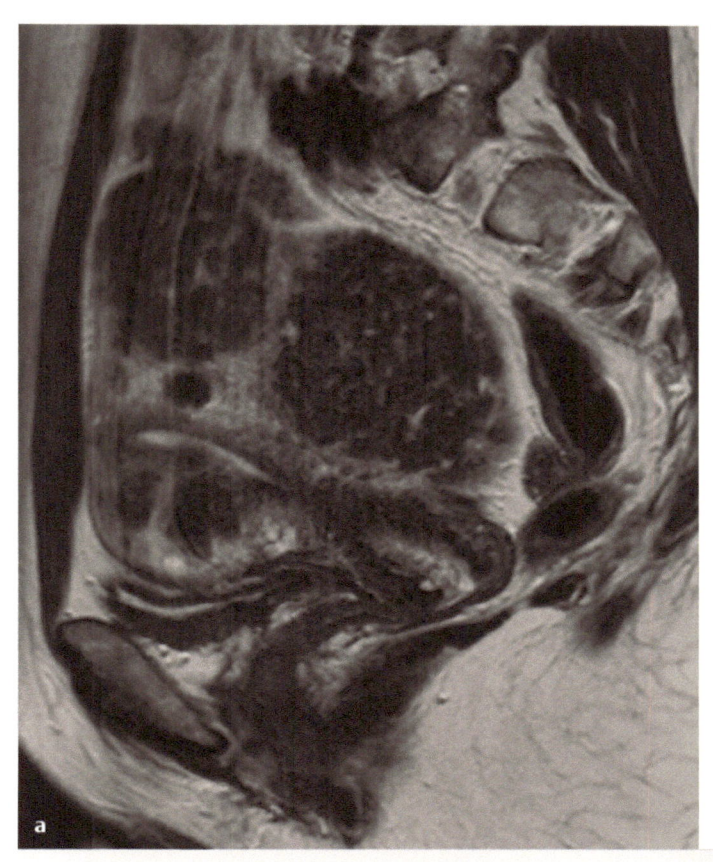

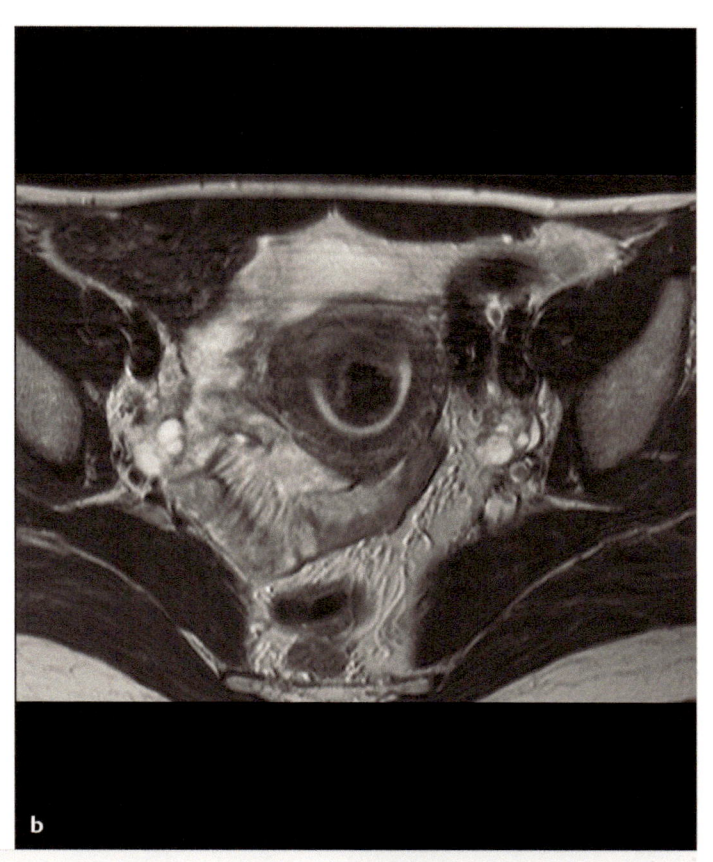

Fig. 12.13 Localization of leiomyomas. (a) Sagittal T2 W image displays three small, hypointense intramural leiomyomas and two large subserosal leiomyomas with degenerative changes in the posterior wall of the uterine corpus. The anteflexed uterus abuts the bladder roof. (b) Axial T2 W image in a different patient shows a submucosal leiomyoma protruding into the uterine cavity. Both ovaries, which contain follicles and functional cysts, are visible on the pelvic wall.

- Bladder wall.
- Detrusor muscle.
- Urethra.
- Rectum.
- Bowel.
- Pelvic wall.
- Peritoneum.
- Abdominal wall.

Because these tissue implants are estrogen-sensitive like the endometrium itself, they are also subject to hormonal stimulation. The risk of malignant transformation is approximately 2.5%.[45]

▶ **Imaging signs.** The pelvic examination (palpation, speculum examination) and ultrasound are usually sufficient to establish a noninvasive diagnosis of ovarian endometriosis. But if the endometrium has an atypical sonographic appearance, if there is suspicion of extraovarian or deep infiltrating endometriosis, or if the patient has unexplained dysmenorrhea, MRI is recommended.[41,43,44] The sonographic and MRI findings are as follow.

- *Endometrioma (chocolate cyst)*: Endometrioma has a heterogeneous ultrasound appearance with low central echogenicity and hyperechoic mural foci. No intraluminal Doppler signals are recorded.[44,46] On MRI, endometrioma has high signal intensity in the unenhanced T1 W sequence. The T2 W sequence usually shows decreased signal intensity due to an increased iron content from recurrent intralesional hemorrhages with a possible fluid level or "shading" caused by blood breakdown products at different stages (▶ Fig. 12.15).[33,47]
- *Deep infiltrating endometriosis*: Nodules of extraovarian endometriosis are visible on MRI when they measure approximately 7 mm or larger. The foci of endometriosis are hypointense in unenhanced T1 W sequences and in T2 W sequences (▶ Fig. 12.16, ▶ Fig. 12.17). Hyperintense spots may be visible in T1 W images.[42,48] Foci of endometriosis in the abdominal wall appear hyperintense in unenhanced fat-saturated T1 W sequences.

Note

Whenever endometriosis is suspected, the MRI sequences should be angled relative to the long axis of the uterine corpus to permit better evaluation of the sacrouterine ligament, torus uterinus (posterior cervix or isthmus, at the insertion of the sacrouterine ligaments), and vaginal fornix. The slice thickness should be no more than 3 to 4 mm so that small nodules can be detected.[44]

CT is not indicated in the diagnostic work-up of endometriosis.[33] Laparoscopy is an invasive procedure that can be both diagnostic and therapeutic.

▶ **Clinical features.** Symptomatic patients usually present with chronic lower abdominal pain. Symptoms depend on the site of involvement by endometriosis and may include hypermenorrhea

Female Pelvis

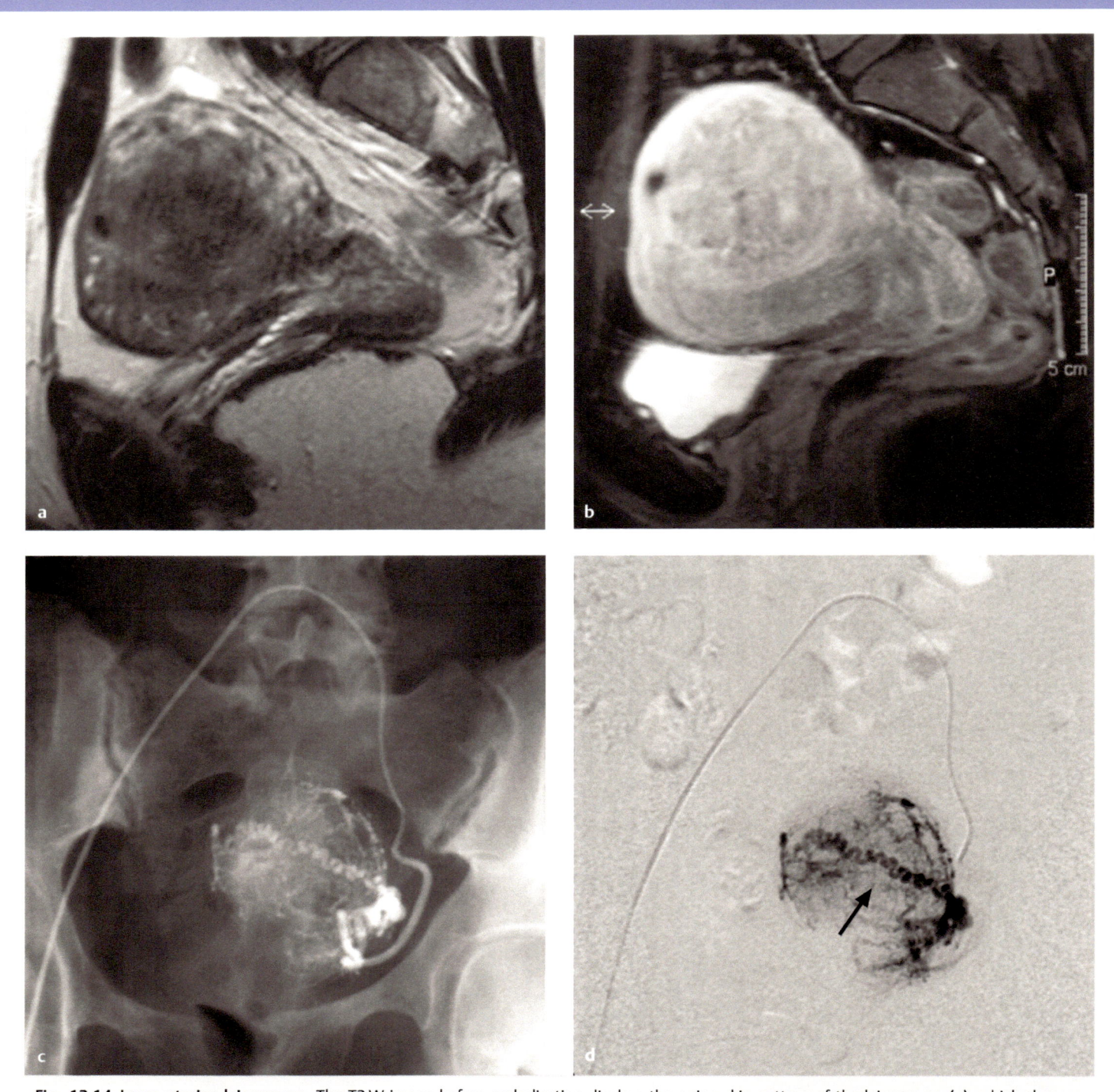

Fig. 12.14 Large uterine leiomyoma. The T2 W image before embolization displays the onion-skin pattern of the leiomyoma (a), which shows homogeneous enhancement after administration of contrast medium (b). First the left and then the right uterine artery are catheterized with a Roberts catheter introduced via the right femoral artery and are embolized with particles 500 to 900 µm in diameter (c, d). The corkscrew-shaped vessels, visible prior to embolization ([d], arrow), are occluded after embolization (e, f). In the T2 W image after embolization (g), the leiomyoma is less hyperintense than in the preembolization image. The postcontrast T1 W image (h) shows complete absence of enhancement in the leiomyoma (M) while the myometrium and cervix continue to show normal enhancement. (a) Preembolization T2 W image. (b) Preembolization T1 W image after administration of contrast medium. (c) Catheter position. (d) Corkscrew vessels before embolization (arrow). ▶

or dysmenorrhea, dyspareunia, painful defecation during menses, or even bladder dysfunction. Endometriosis may cause acyclic complaints and may be a cause of infertility.[41,44,49] ▶ Table 12.2 lists the most frequent sites of involvement by deep infiltrating endometriosis and the resulting symptoms.

▶ **Differential diagnosis.** The following entities need to be differentiated from endometrioma:[44,50]

- *Mature teratoma or dermoid cyst* (usually have a heterogeneous appearance due to cystic and solid components, internal calcifications, hairs, etc.).
- *Functional or hemorrhagic cysts* (hemorrhagic cysts shrink or resolve within a short time).
- *Ovarian fibroma* (ultrasound shows hypoechoic mass with small vessels; MRI shows unenhanced low T1 W and T2 W signal intensity).

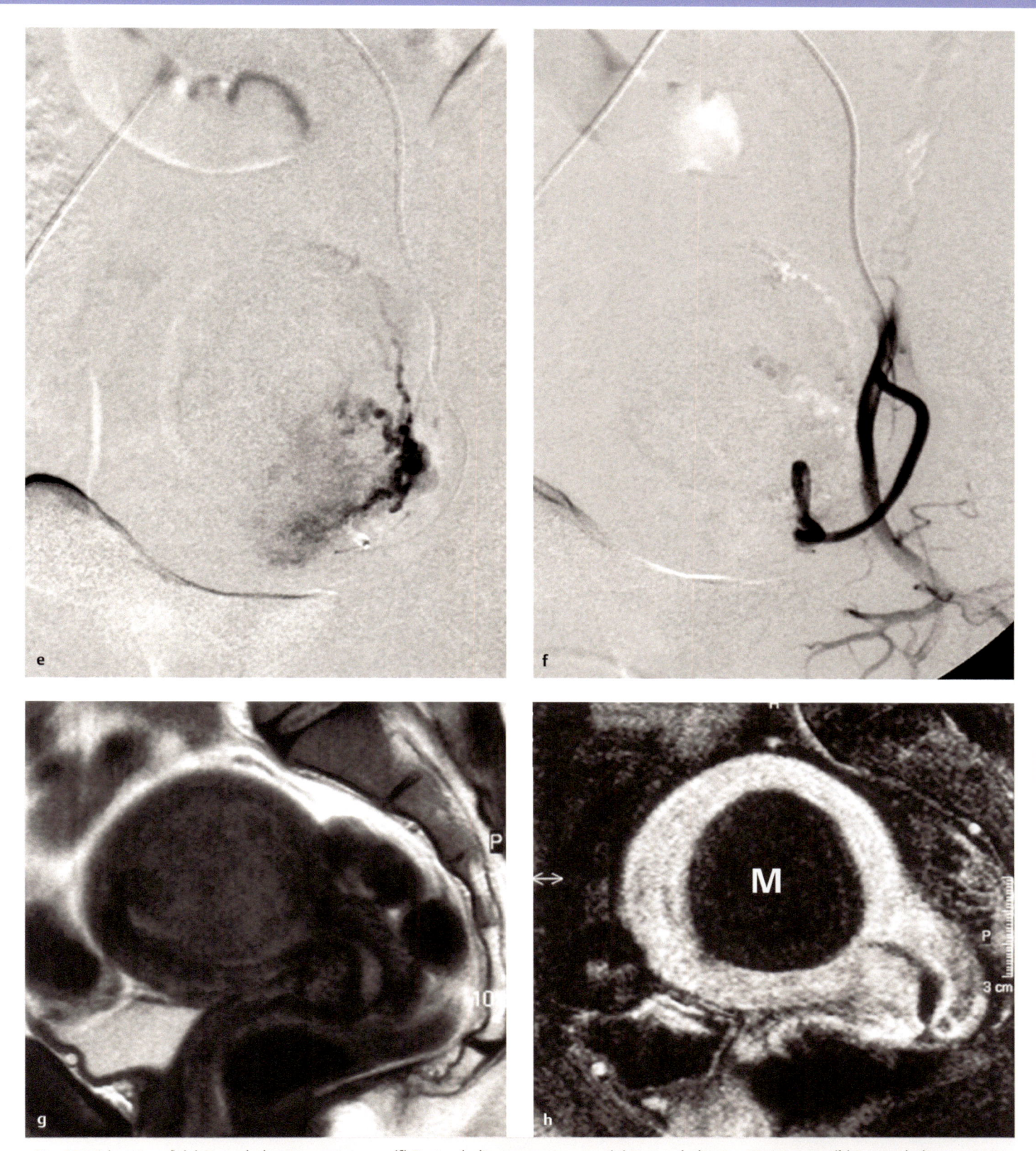

Fig. 12.14 (*continued*) (**e**) Preembolization angiogram. (**f**) Postembolization angiogram. (**g**) Postembolization T2 W image. (**h**) Postembolization T1 W image after injection of contrast medium.

- Tubo-ovarian abscess.
- Ovarian carcinoma (wall thickening, rich vascular supply, positive malignancy criteria).

▶ **Key points.** The MRI protocol for the detection of deep infiltrating endometriosis should include the following sequences:[44]

- High-resolution T2 W TSE sequence with a 3- to 4-mm slice thickness in sagittal and axial oblique or coronal oblique orientation relative to the uterine corpus.
- Unenhanced T1 W (T)SE sequence with and without fat saturation.
- Contrast-enhanced T1 W sequence with fat saturation (in the plane that best demonstrates the pathology).

Female Pelvis

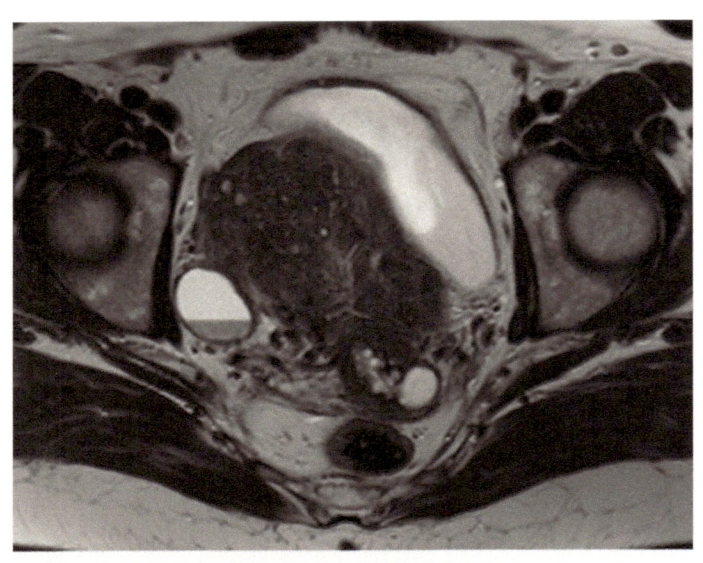

Fig. 12.15 Endometriotic cyst and uterine adenomyosis. High-resolution axial T2W image shows a cystic lesion with a fluid level in the right ovary due to varying proportions of blood breakdown products (confirmed as an endometriotic cyst). The uterine corpus shows diffuse wall thickening and small hyperintense spots caused by the implantation of endometrial cells in uterine adenomyosis. Simple cysts are visible in the cervix.

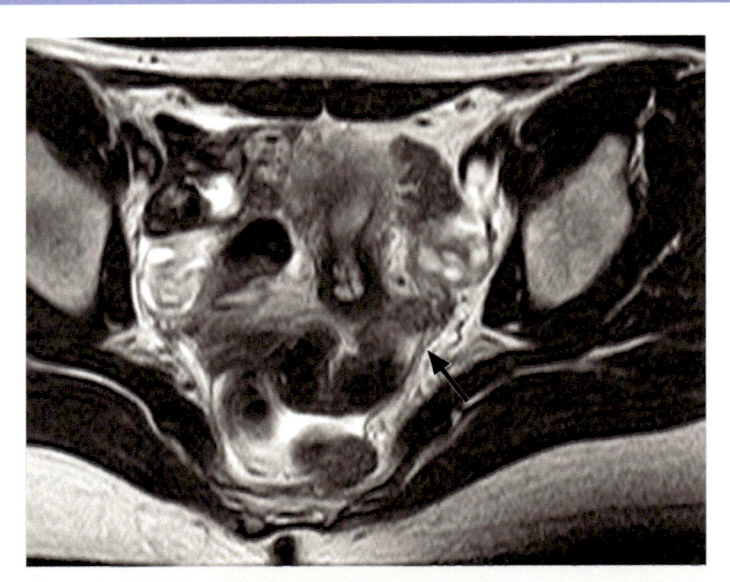

Fig. 12.16 Deep infiltrating endometriosis. High-resolution axial T2W image demonstrates a hypointense nodular mass at the 3 o'clock to 4 o'clock position in the left posterolateral quadrant of the cervix (arrow). The mass represents a focus of endometriosis at the junction of the torus uterinus and sacrouterine ligament. Physiologic amounts of free fluid are noted in the lesser pelvis.

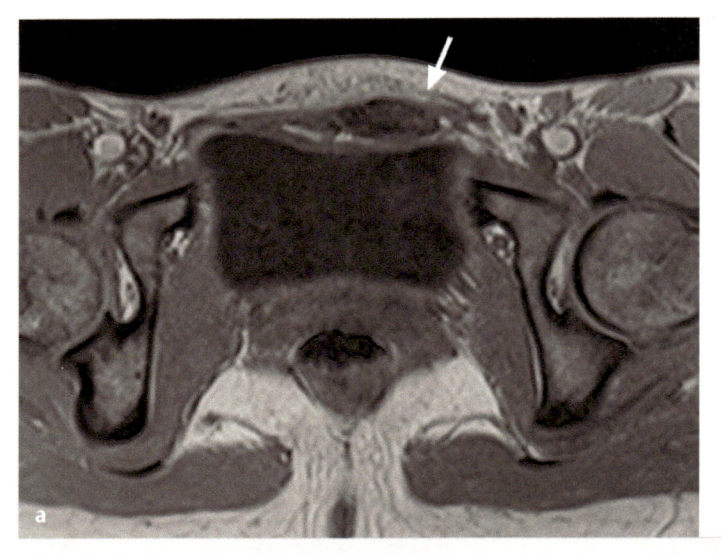

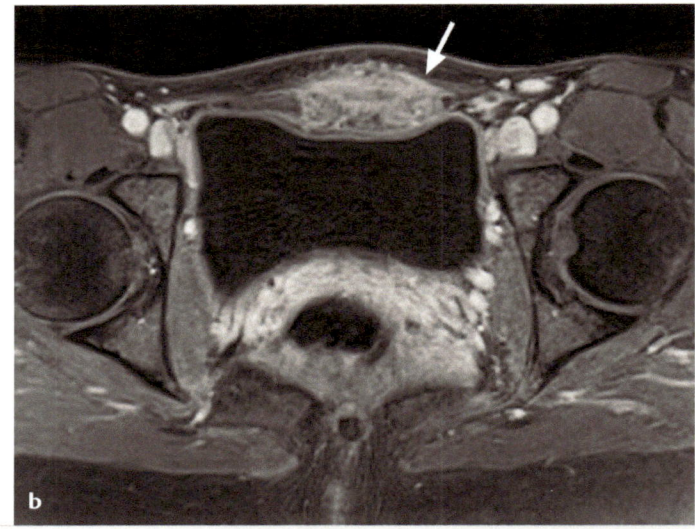

Fig. 12.17 Deep infiltrating endometriosis in the abdominal wall. (a) Unenhanced axial T1W image shows unilateral circumscribed thickening of the left rectus abdominis muscle (arrow). **(b)** T1W after administration of contrast medium. The focus of endometriosis in the abdominal wall shows intense enhancement (arrow).

Subtype: Adenomyosis

▶ **Brief definition.** Adenomyosis is a subtype of subperitoneal endometriosis that is located in the myometrium or junctional zone of the uterus. A focus of endometriosis located within the myometrium is called an adenomyoma. Uterine adenomyosis is characterized by the presence of ectopic endometrial tissue distributed diffusely in the uterine wall.

▶ **Imaging signs**
- *Adenomyoma*: Adenomyoma tends to have an oval shape and be somewhat less sharply delineated from surrounding myometrium than an intramural leiomyoma (▶ Fig. 12.18). They have the same MRI signal characteristics as leiomyomas.
- *Uterine adenomyosis*: Adenomyosis has ill-defined sonographic margins and shows heterogeneous echogenicity that may include cystic elements. MRI typically shows thickening of the junctional zone to more than 12 mm (▶ Fig. 12.19, ▶ Fig. 12.20; ≤ 5 mm is normal), and a discrepancy is usually noted between the anterior and posterior uterine walls (see ▶ Fig. 12.20).[18]

▶ **Clinical features.** Patients may complain of heavy or painful menstrual bleeding and may have bleeding between periods.

12.4 Diseases

▶ **Differential diagnosis**
- Leiomyoma.
- Uterine sarcoma.

12.4.3 Malignant Lesions

Endometrial Carcinoma

▶ **Brief definition.** With an incidence of approximately 25:100,000 women, endometrial carcinoma is the fourth most common malignant tumor in women and the most common gynecologic malignancy (as of June, 2016).[51] Risk factors are overstimulation by estrogens, metabolic syndrome, diabetes mellitus, polycystic ovarian syndrome, nulliparity, breast cancer, and use of tamoxifen. Peri- and postmenopausal women are predominantly affected. The peak age of incidence is approximately 75 to 80 years. Adenocarcinoma is the main type of endometrial cancer, accounting for 80 to 90% of cases. The depth of myometrial invasion correlates strongly with the risk of lymph node metastasis.[52]

▶ **Imaging signs.** Ultrasound can detect endometrial thickening or a tumor mass; the diagnosis is confirmed histologically by fractional curettage. Pretherapeutic contrast-enhanced MRI of the pelvis has a sensitivity of 91% in determining the depth of myometrial invasion.[53] MRI is also helpful in the pretherapeutic evaluation of retroperitoneal lymph nodes, as lymphatic drainage may be discontinuous and initial lymph node metastasis may occur to para-aortic nodes.[9] In current international guidelines, however, pretherapeutic MRI is recommended only as a guide for planning radiotherapy in patients deemed inoperable due to comorbid conditions.

Table 12.2 Common sites of involvement by endometriosis and resulting symptoms

Sites of involvement	Symptoms
Uterus, cul-de-sac	Dysmenorrhea
Uterosacral ligament, torus uterinus	Dyspareunia
Vagina, cul-de-sac, rectum	Painful defecation during menstruation
Small intestine	Acyclic pains
Bladder	Bladder symptoms

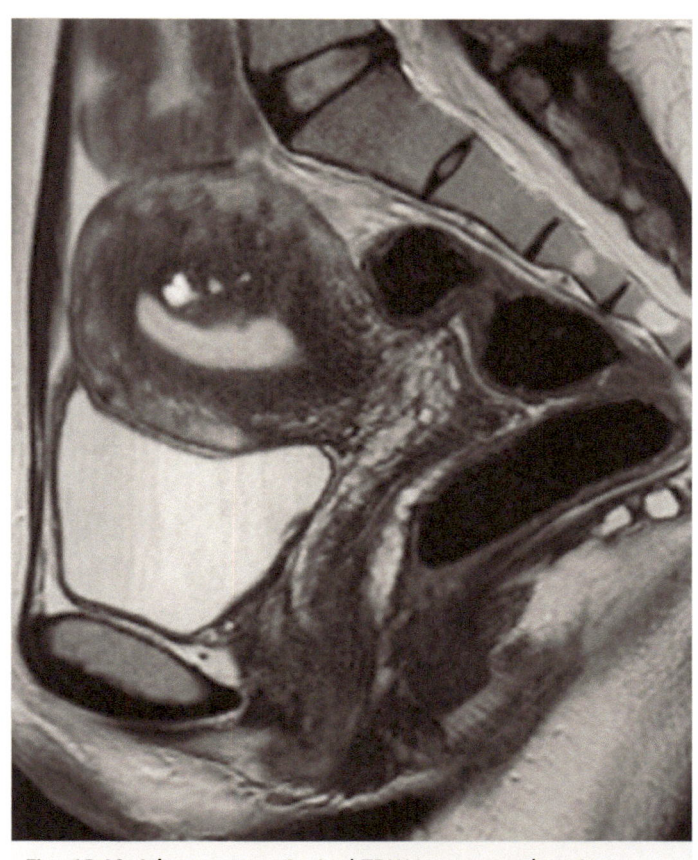

Fig. 12.18 **Adenomyoma.** Sagittal T2W image reveals a circumscribed, fibroidlike mass in the posterior uterine wall protruding into the uterine cavity. The mass contains focal hyperintensities and is poorly delineated from surrounding myometrium, consistent with an adenomyoma.

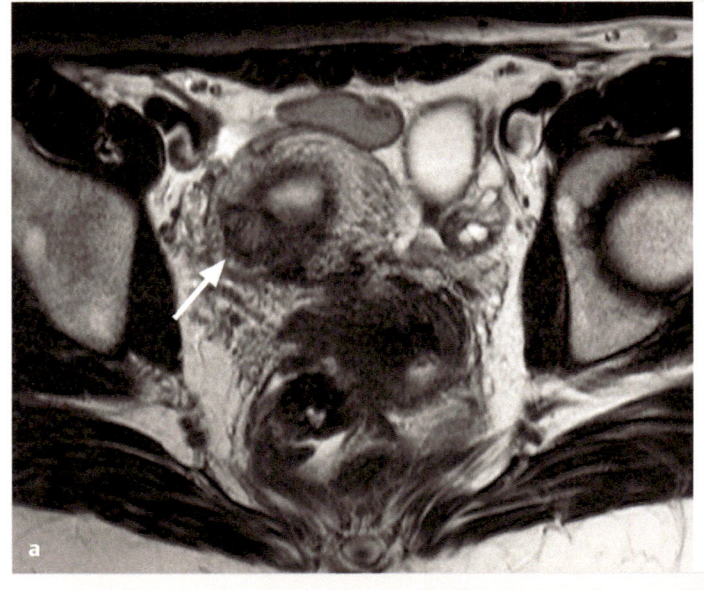

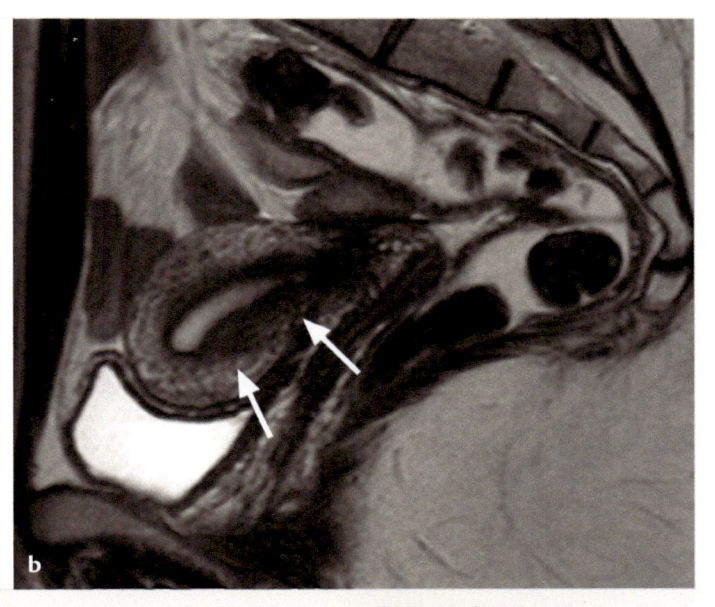

Fig. 12.19 **Focal adenomyosis.** Circumscribed thickening of the junctional zone (arrows). **(a)** Axial T2W image. **(b)** Sagittal T2W image.

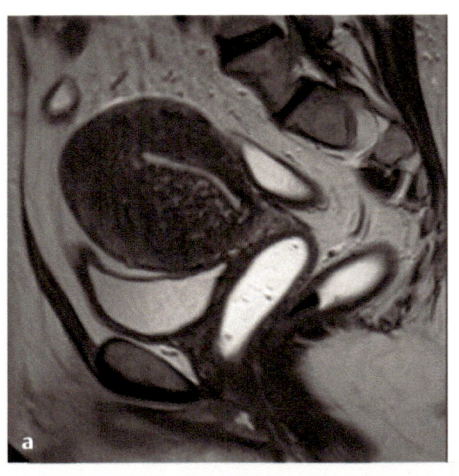

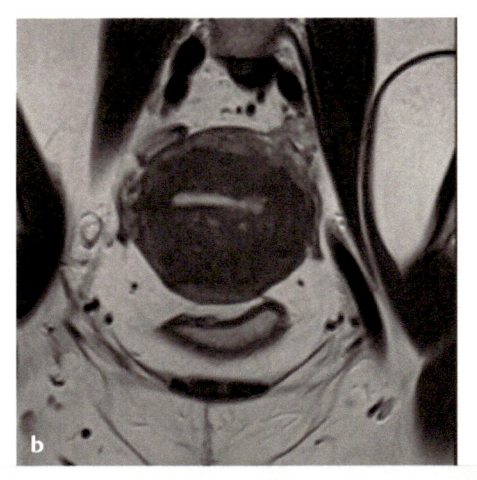

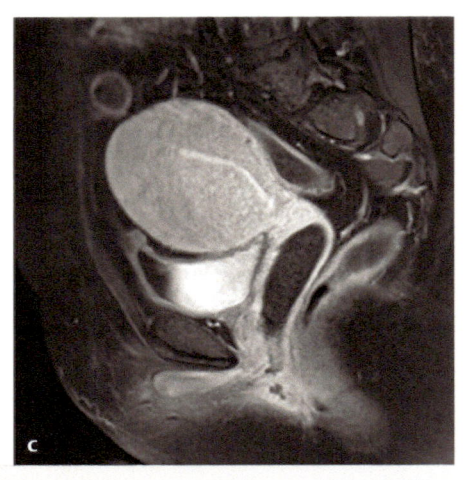

Fig. 12.20 Diffuse adenomyosis. Thickening of the junctional zone is noted throughout the uterus and is most pronounced in the anterior wall. The T2 W images display the typical hyperintense glands **(a, b)**. The uterus shows homogeneous enhancement after administration of contrast medium **(c)**. **(a)** T2 W image sagittal to the uterus. **(b)** T2 W image paracoronal to the uterus. **(c)** Fat-suppressed T1 W image after injection of contrast medium.

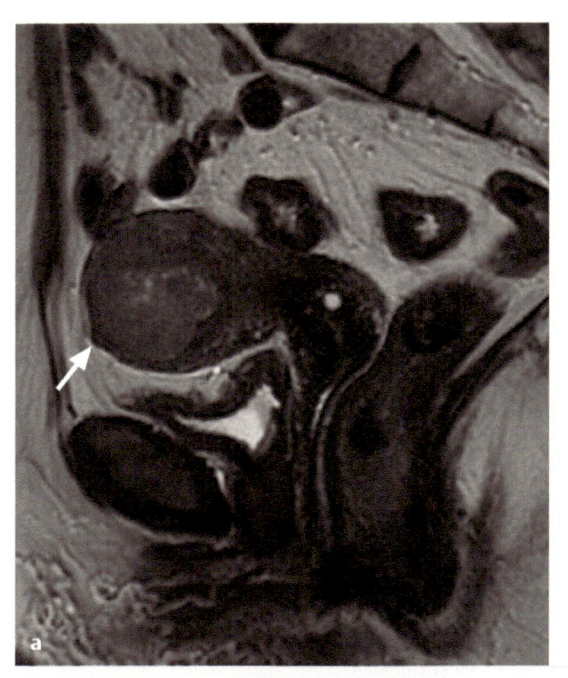

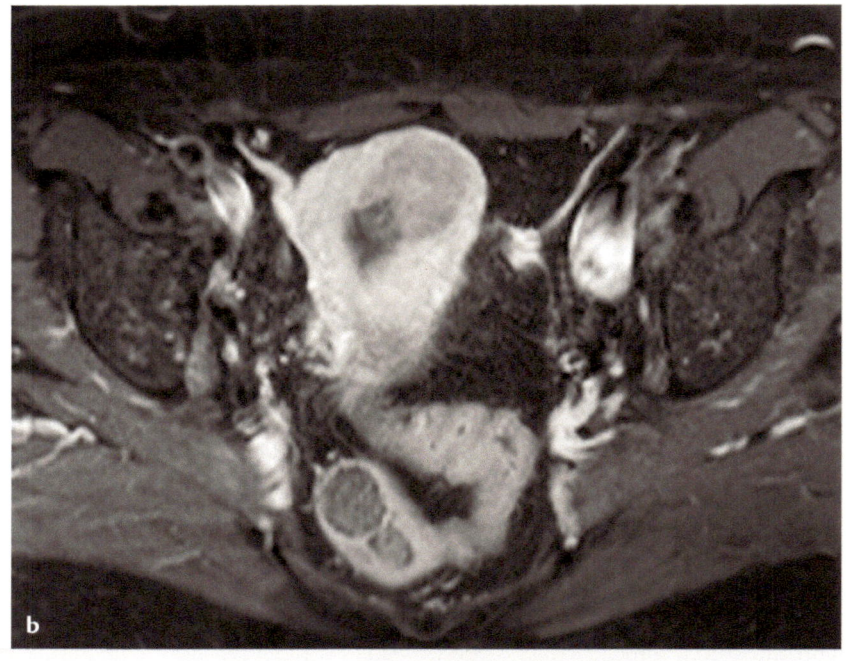

Fig. 12.21 Stage pT1b pN0 endometrial carcinoma. (a) High-resolution sagittal T2 W image shows a moderately hyperintense tumor growing from the endometrium into the myometrium of the anterior uterine wall and showing greater than 50% myometrial invasion (arrow). Tumor does not extend to the serosa. **(b)** Axial fat-saturated T1 W image after administration of contrast medium. The hypointense tumor is demarcated relative to the myometrium. The image confirms absence of serosal involvement.

The endometrium always appears hyperintense in the unenhanced T2 W sequence, regardless of hormonal status. The junctional zone is hypointense, and the outer layer of the myometrium shows intermediate signal intensity.[54] In most cases endometrial carcinoma is moderately hyperintense in the T2 W sequence, although small tumors may be isointense to endometrium in the T2 W sequence, making detection difficult without administration of contrast medium. A contrast-enhanced T1 W sequence with fat saturation is helpful in these cases for detection of the lesion and its delineation from surrounding endometrium and myometrium, owing to the hypointense appearance of the tumor in this sequence (conspicuity is best approximately 2 minutes after injection of contrast medium; ▶ Fig. 12.21).[9] Diffusion-weighted imaging (DWI) can also aid detection, as the tumor shows greater loss of signal intensity in the ADC map than surrounding myometrium.[14] A key criterion for recognizing incipient invasion of the bladder or rectal mucosa is obliteration of the fat plane between the organs (best appreciated in the unenhanced T1 W sequence) and thickening of the organ walls in the T2 W sequence or contrast-enhanced T1 W sequence.[9] Staging is based on the current 2010 version of the UICC staging criteria (▶ Fig. 12.22).[55,56]

CT imaging is not indicated for local staging but is used for radiotherapy planning or screening for distant metastasis (especially to lung, liver, and retroperitoneal lymph nodes). If contrast-enhanced CT is available from a study done for a different indication, venous-phase images will portray endometrial carcinoma as a hypodense mass within the uterine cavity. The depth of myometrial invasion is difficult to assess due to the low

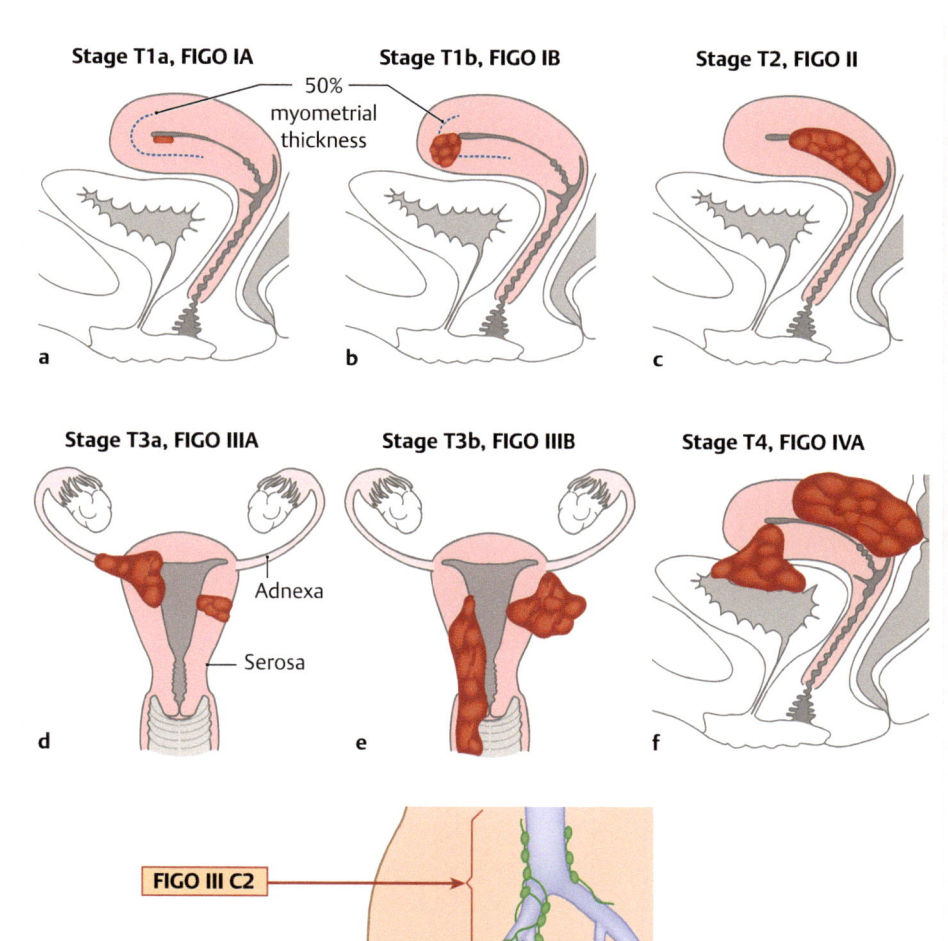

Fig. 12.22 Staging of primary endometrial carcinoma.[55,56] (a) Tumor is confined to the endometrium or shows less than 50% myometrial invasion. (b) Tumor is confined to the uterine corpus and shows at least 50% myometrial invasion. (c) Tumor extends through the uterine isthmus to involve the cervix. (d) Tumor invades the serosa or adnexa. (e) Vaginal or parametrial involvement. (f) Invasion of surrounding structures such as bladder or bowel. (g) The FIGO system for lymph node staging distinguishes between stage IIIc1 disease (positive pelvic lymph nodes) and stage IIIc2 disease (positive para-aortic lymph nodes with or without pelvic nodes). Involvement of inguinal and other intra-abdominal lymph nodes is classified as distant metastasis (FIGO IVb M1).

soft tissue contrast of CT, and sensitivity is only about 58 to 61%. Invasion should be suspected if the cervix appears heterogeneous and thickened. Tumor spread beyond the serosa (adnexa, parametria) appears as indistinct, increased periuterine reticular markings. Obliteration of the fat plane suggests bladder or rectal invasion, and this is confirmed by the presence of solid intraluminal densities.[57] PET-CT has a role in the detection of distant metastases and recurrence.[9]

▶ **Clinical features.** The clinical hallmark of endometrial carcinoma is postmenopausal bleeding. Atypical intermenstrual bleeding may occur in perimenopausal women.

▶ **Differential diagnosis**
- Leiomyoma.
- Endometrial hyperplasia.
- Carcinosarcoma.
- Uterine sarcoma.

▶ **Key points.** The following sequences should be included in the MRI protocol for the pretherapeutic staging of endometrial carcinoma (compare with ESUR guidelines):[9]

- High-resolution sagittal, axial oblique (parallel to short axis of uterine corpus), and coronal oblique (parallel to long axis of uterine corpus) T2 W sequences.
- Unenhanced T1 W sequence coronal to the body axis (for evaluating retroperitoneal lymph nodes).
- Contrast-enhanced sagittal and axial oblique T1 W sequence with fat saturation (optimal enhancement between 90 and 150 seconds after injection of contrast medium).

Cervical Carcinoma

▶ **Brief definition.** The incidence of cervical carcinoma according to the WHO is 13 per 100,000 women in the United States and 67 per 100,000 women in Europe).[51] There are large differences in incidence between countries worldwide. Infection with the human papillomavirus is causative in almost all cases, especially infection with the high-risk types 16 and 18. Histologically, approximately 80% of cervical cancers are squamous cell carcinomas and 20% are adenocarcinomas. The average age at diagnosis is 52 years. The decision between primary surgical treatment or primary chemoradiotherapy or brachytherapy depends mainly on tumor size and the presence of parametrial invasion.[8] With increasing spread of cervical carcinoma along the parametria to the pelvic wall or lower third of the vagina, the likelihood of positive para-aortic or inguinal lymph nodes increases. Metastases to liver, lung, or bone may be detectable in advanced tumor stages.

▶ **Imaging signs.** According to the International Federation of Gynecology and Obstetrics (FIGO), the clinical staging of cervical carcinoma is based on a pelvic examination that includes bimanual palpation and may include cystorectoscopy, depending on stage. Ultrasound is often inadequate for the evaluation of local disease but is useful for the exclusion of urinary tract obstruction and hepatic metastases. At FIGO stage Ib2 or higher, MRI is recommended in the Society for Gynecology and Obstetrics guidelines for the pretherapeutic evaluation of locoregional tumor spread; MRI also has a role in radiotherapy planning and post-treatment follow-up.[8,58]

The cervical mucosa is hyperintense in the unenhanced T2W sequence, and the cervical stroma is hypointense.[54] Cervical carcinoma is hypointense to surrounding stromal tissue in the unenhanced T2W sequence (▶ Fig. 12.23). In rare cases the tumor is isointense to surrounding tissue in the T2W sequence or is too small in diameter for MRI detection, as it may represent residual tumor tissue following curettage. These cases can be evaluated by DWI or contrast-enhanced T1W imaging with fat saturation for tumor detection.[8] The tumor shows loss of signal intensity in the ADC map. In the fat-saturated T1W sequence after administration of contrast medium, the tumor is hypointense to surrounding tissue or myometrium in the early phase (optimal contrast approximately 15–30 seconds after injection of contrast medium), whereas the tumor is hyperintense to myometrium in the late phase.[59,60] A dynamic contrast study is advantageous, therefore.

> **Caution** ⚠
>
> It is essential to angle the axial slices parallel to the short axis of the cervix, especially for the evaluation of parametrial invasion. That is the only orientation in which the T2W sequence displays a ring or "doughnut" pattern formed by the hypointense stromal ring and hyperintense lumen, and any disruption in that pattern is easily detected.

Staging is based on the current 2010 version of the UICC criteria (▶ Fig. 12.24).[55,56] CT is used for primary imaging only if MRI is contraindicated; its main role is in radiotherapy planning and the detection of distant metastases (lung, liver, bone) or peripheral lymph node metastases.[58,61] If contrast-enhanced CT is available, cervical carcinoma will usually appear as an eccentric thickening of the cervical tissue to more than 3.5 cm.[57] Ill-defined thickening or convexity of the cervical margins (see ▶ Fig. 12.23c) is an indicator of parametrial invasion.[60] Invasion of the bladder wall or rectum is manifested by irregular wall thickening or a solid mass protruding into the lumen; it is also indicated by obliteration of the fat plane.[57] PET-CT has a role in locally advanced cervical carcinoma, in the detection of recurrence, and especially the detection of lymph node metastases that have a normal initial imaging appearance.[62]

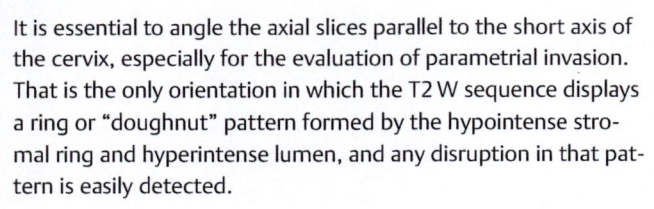

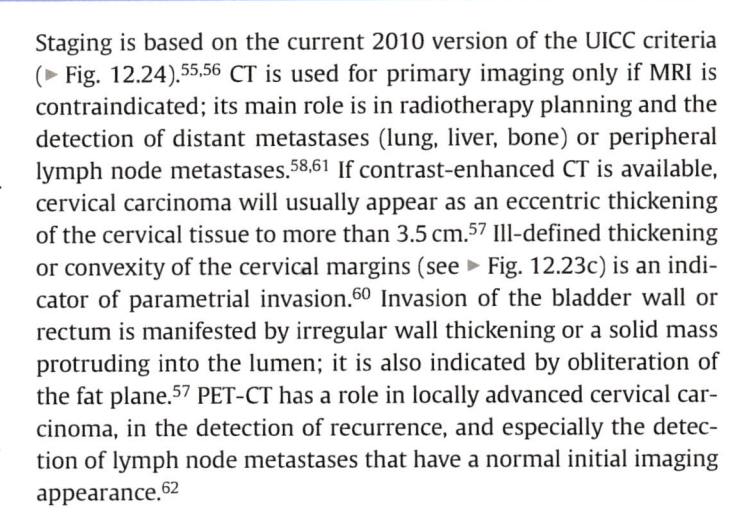

▶ **Clinical features.** Cervical carcinoma is frequently asymptomatic in its early stage. With advanced cervical cancer, bleeding may occur after sexual intercourse, strenuous athletic activity such as bicycling or horseback riding, or straining at stool.

▶ **Differential diagnosis**[18]
- Endometrial carcinoma.
- Lymphoma.
- Sarcoma.
- Metastasis.
- Complicated cervicitis.
- Cervical polyp, cervical leiomyoma.

▶ **Key points.** While IV administration of contrast medium may be unnecessary for primary lesion detection, since most tumors are clearly visualized in the unenhanced T2W sequence, the use of IV contrast medium is essential in the follow-up of brachytherapy, chemoradiation, or surgery so that recurrent tumor can be differentiated from scar tissue.[8] The following sequences should be used for the pretherapeutic staging of cervical carcinoma (see ESUR guidelines)[8]:
- High-resolution sagittal and axial oblique T2W sequence (parallel to the short axis of the cervix).

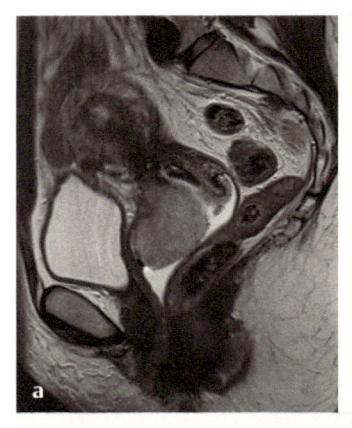

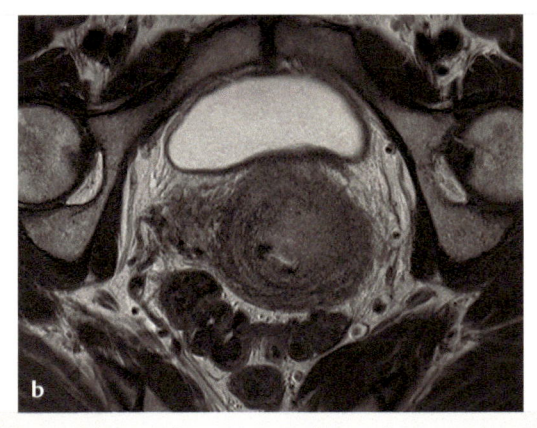

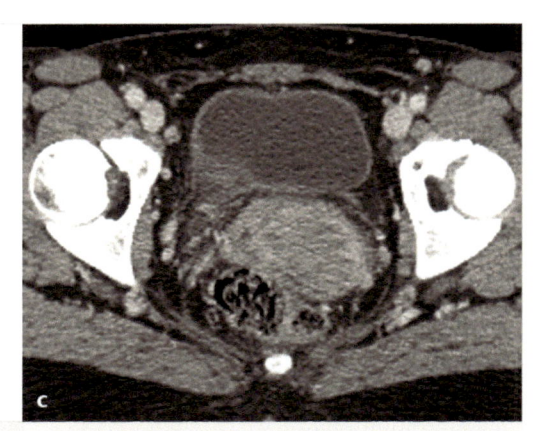

Fig. 12.23 Stage T2b cervical carcinoma. (a) Sagittal T2W image shows a hyperintense tumor with its main bulk on the anterior lip of the cervix. The tumor has infiltrated the anterior vaginal wall but has not yet penetrated the vaginal wall to reach the bladder. **(b)** Angled axial T2W image. The hypointense stromal ring of the cervix is interrupted between the 12 o'clock and 4 o'clock positions. There is general thickening of the paracervical tissue. Invasion of the left parametrium has probably occurred but is not very pronounced in this case. **(c)** Contrast-enhanced CT in the same patient shows increased cervical tissue density with no further morphological details. The extent and slightly ill-defined margins suggest that parametrial invasion has occurred.

12.4 Diseases

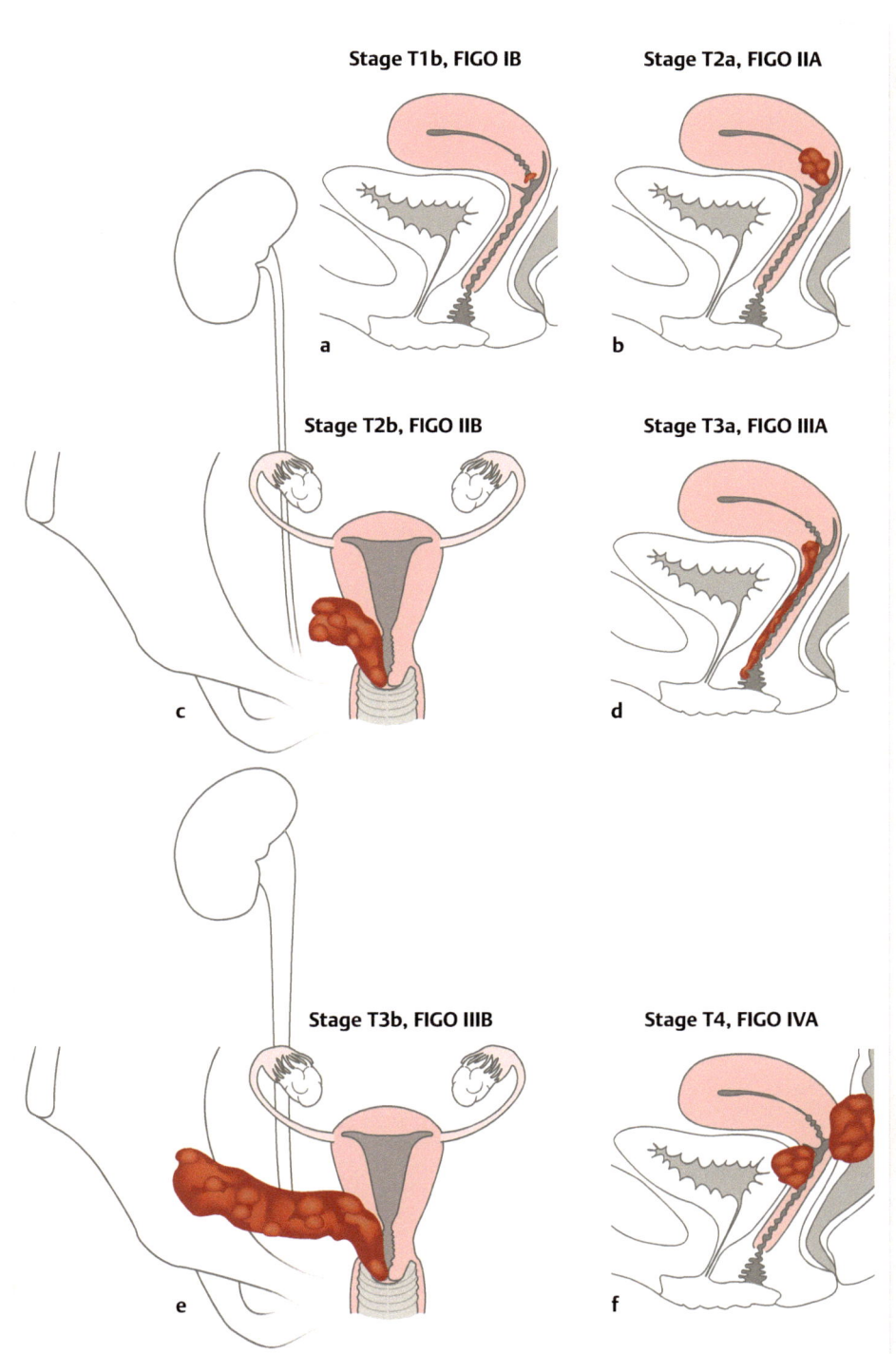

Fig. 12.24 Staging of primary cervical carcinoma.[55,56] (a) The carcinoma is confined to the cervix; it is ≤ 4 cm in greatest dimension (stage T1b1) or > 4 cm in greatest dimension (T1b2). (b) The carcinoma invades the isthmus, uterine corpus, or upper two-thirds of the vagina; it is ≤ 4 cm in greatest dimension (stage T2a1) or > 4 cm in greatest dimension (T2a2). (c) The carcinoma invades the parametrium but not to the pelvic wall. (d) The carcinoma involves the lower third of the vagina. (e) The carcinoma extends to the pelvic sidewall and/or causes hydronephrosis or a nonfunctioning kidney. (f) The carcinoma extends beyond the lesser pelvis and invades the posterior bladder wall or anterior rectal wall.

- Unenhanced axial T1 W sequence relative to the body axis (from the symphysis to the left renal vein), mainly for the detection of lymphadenopathy or bone metastasis.
- DWI with a *b*-value between 500 and 1000 (mainly for the detection of residual tumor tissue or small suspicious lymph nodes).
- Sagittal and axial oblique T1 W enhancement dynamics with fat saturation sagittal oblique and axial oblique (most helpful for distinguishing small tumors or suspected recurrence from scar tissue).

Note
A fat-saturated T2 W sequence does not contribute to the diagnosis of cervical carcinoma or the detection of parametrial invasion.[8]

Vaginal Carcinoma

▶ **Brief definition.** Approximately 90% of primary vaginal cancers are squamous cell carcinomas. Vaginal carcinoma has a low incidence of approximately 0.7 new cases per 100,000 population per year and comprises approximately 2% of all female pelvic tumors.[63] Most vaginal malignancies invade the vagina secondarily from surrounding pelvic organs or metastasize from more distant sites. A major risk factor for the development of primary vaginal carcinoma is human papillomavirus infection, especially with the high-risk type 16.

Note

If a vaginal tumor invades the cervix, it is considered to be primary cervical carcinoma. If it infiltrates the vulva, the tumor is staged like a primary vulvar carcinoma. But if a vaginal tumor is detected 5 years after successful treatment for cervical carcinoma, it is staged like a primary vaginal carcinoma.[57]

▶ **Imaging signs.** MRI is helpful in determining whether a lesion is primary vaginal carcinoma or a tumor that has invaded the vagina from a different site of origin. In most cases the tumor is found on the vaginal fornix or posterior vaginal wall and protrudes into the lumen.[63] Contrast-enhanced CT may be indicated for the detection of distant metastasis (especially to lung, liver, and bone) but has no role in the evaluation of local disease. The vaginal mucosa is hyperintense in the unenhanced T2 W sequence; the submucosa and muscularis are hypointense, and the adventitia is hyperintense. Vaginal carcinoma is (moderately) hyperintense in the unenhanced T2 W sequence (▶ Fig. 12.25). A perifocal inflammatory response is not uncommon and increases the apparent tumor size. Circumscribed enhancement of the bladder or rectal wall is suspicious for invasion. The invasion of muscle tissue is best appreciated in the T2 W sequence.[64]

Note

Vaginal distention with 20 to 40 mL of (sterile) ultrasound gel is recommended for the MR imaging of vaginal carcinoma, as it enables positive identification of the primary tumor site.

The staging of vaginal carcinoma is based on the 2010 version of the UICC criteria (▶ Fig. 12.26).[56]

▶ **Clinical features.** Affected women are usually asymptomatic in the early stages. Advanced tumors may be associated with diffuse lower abdominal pain, difficulty urinating or passing stool, or a bloody discharge.

▶ **Differential diagnosis**[64]
- Lymphoma.
- Metastasis from another genital tumor.
- Melanoma.
- Sarcoma.

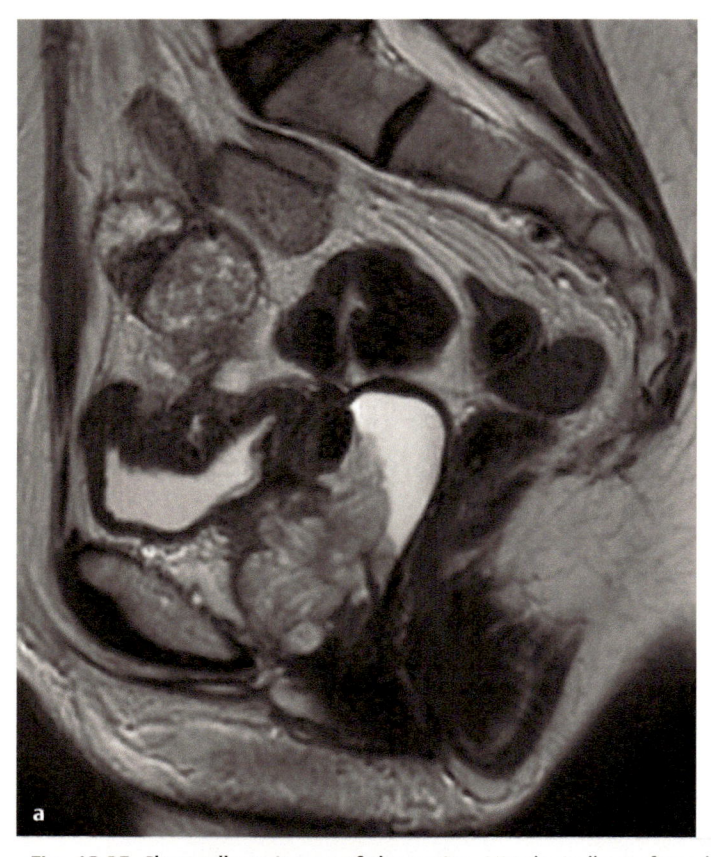

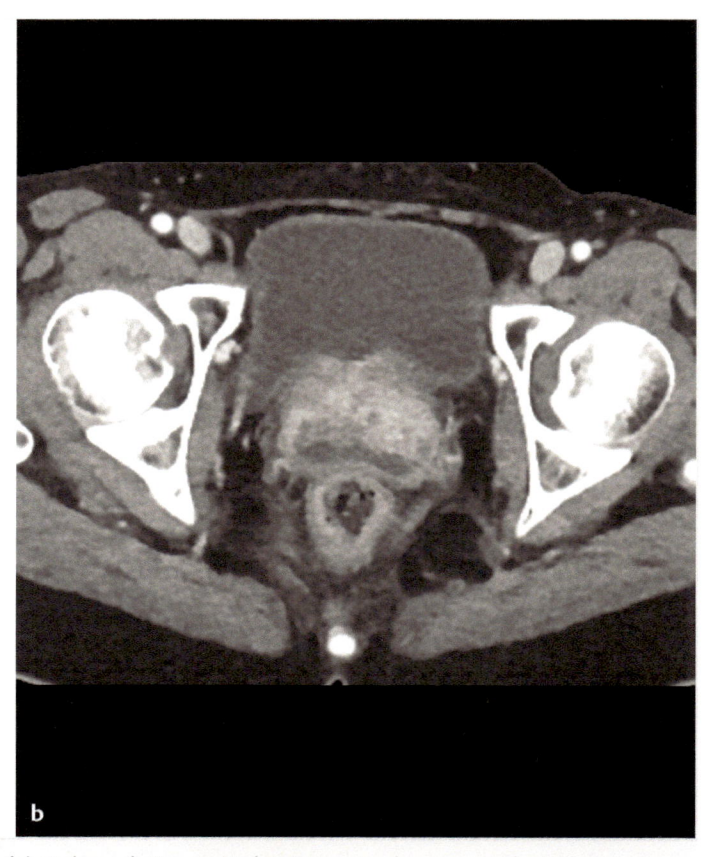

Fig. 12.25 **Clear-cell carcinoma of the vagina.** Histologically confirmed. (a) High-resolution sagittal T2 W image shows a streaky hyperintense tumor on the anterior vaginal wall that encases the urethra and extends to the bladder floor. Vaginal distention helps to confirm that the posterior vaginal wall is clear. (b) Axial CT scan in the venous phase shows that tumor has penetrated the anterior vaginal wall. The posterior vaginal wall and rectum are not involved.

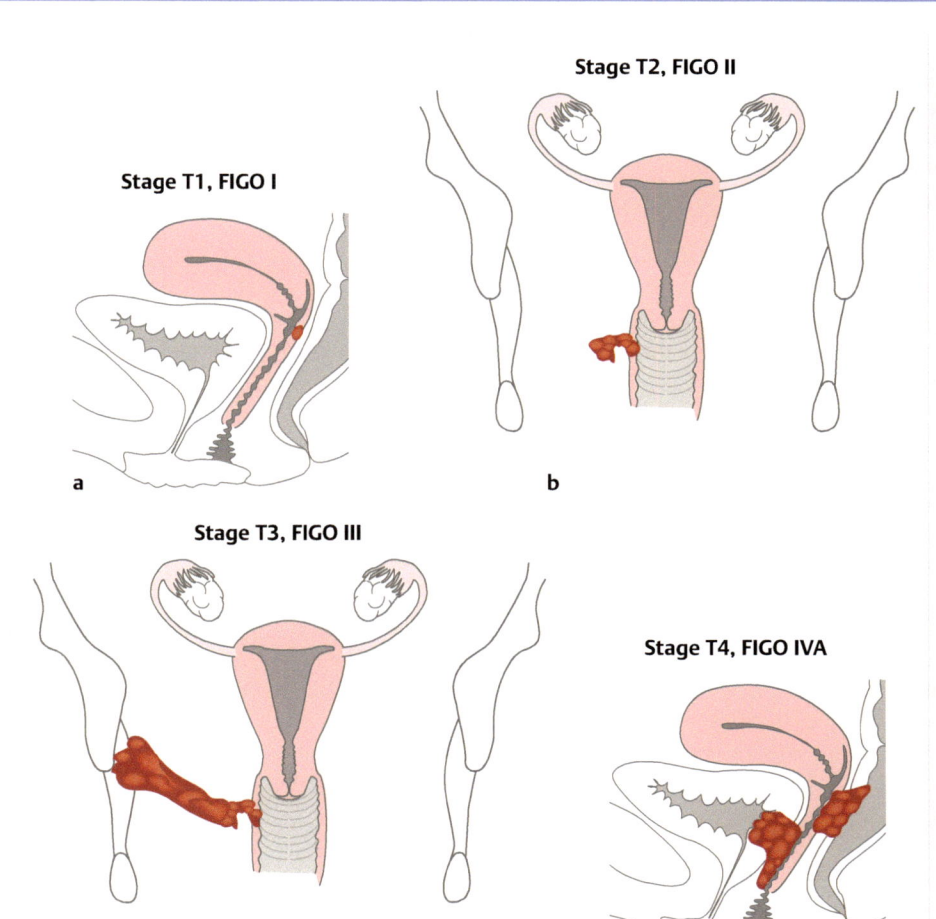

Fig. 12.26 Staging of primary vaginal carcinoma.[56] (a) The carcinoma arises from the posterior vaginal wall, less commonly from the anterior wall, and is confined to the vagina. (b) The carcinoma invades paravaginal tissues. (c) The carcinoma extends to the pelvic sidewall. (d) The carcinoma invades the bladder or rectal mucosa or shows direct extension beyond the lesser pelvis.

▶ **Key points.** The MRI protocol for the pretherapeutic staging of vaginal carcinoma should include the following sequences:[64,65]
- High-resolution sagittal and axial oblique T2 W TSE sequences (parallel to the short axis of the vagina).
- Unenhanced axial T1 W sequence relative to the body axis.
- Contrast-enhanced sagittal and axial oblique T1 W sequences with fat saturation.

Vulvar Carcinoma

▶ **Brief definition.** Approximately 2.4:100 000 women will develop vulvar carcinoma per year in the United States.[106] In approximately 40 to 60% of cases the cancer is linked to infection with human papillomavirus (especially the high-risk types 16, 18, 33, and 39). Other risk factors include infection with herpes simplex virus type 2, lichen sclerosis, and squamous cell hyperplasia.[5,63] The most common sites of primary tumor occurrence are the labia majora and minora (approximately 80% of cases). Less common sites are the clitoris (approximately 10% of cases) and the posterior commissure (approximately 10% of cases). Approximately 90% of the lesions are squamous cell cancers. Vulvar carcinoma spreads contiguously to surrounding structures (urethra, vagina, and anus). Lymph node metastasis occurs chiefly to inguinal or femoral lymph nodes and very rarely to pelvic nodes.[63] Distant metastases are a very late occurrence and consist mainly of cutaneous manifestations on the lower abdomen or trunk. Other potential sites are the liver, lung, pleura, kidneys, myocardium, brain, spinal column, and spleen.[5]

▶ **Imaging signs.** The diagnosis is suggested by visible and palpable findings and is confirmed by biopsy. Small local tumors usually do not require sectional imaging. Moreover, superficial tumors with an invasion depth less than 3 mm are associated with less than a 10% risk of lymph node metastasis.[5] If invasion of the urethra, vagina, or anus is suspected, however, MRI can add important information on local extent and lymph node status and is recommended for lesions at FIGO stage II or higher in the guidelines of the Society for Gynecology and Obstetrics.[66]

> **Caution**
>
> Vulvar carcinoma is multifocal in approximately 10 to 15% of cases, so it is important to look for a second carcinoma of the cervix or vagina or possible perianal involvement.[67]

Tumors with a mass effect are already detectable as hyperintense lesions in the unenhanced T2 W sequence. Local invasion, especially of the urethra, is manifested by obliteration of the fat plane (best appreciated in the high-resolution unenhanced T2 W sequence or the T1 W sequence without fat saturation).[64,65] Positive detection, then, requires an axial plane oriented parallel to the distal urethra. The tumor is hypointense to surrounding tissue after IV administration of contrast medium, which is particularly effective in revealing smaller tumors or plaquelike lesions (▶ Fig. 12.27).

Female Pelvis

> **Note**
>
> The FIGO staging of vulvar carcinoma differs from the TNM system in both the advanced T stage and the N stage (▶ Fig. 12.28 and ▶ Table 12.3).[56] Thus, a detailed description of the findings is essential for appropriate treatment planning. If necessary, the corresponding FIGO stage can also be indicated.

Staging is based on the current 2010 version of the UICC criteria (see ▶ Fig. 12.28).[56] The staging of lymph node metastases is based on number and size (N1a/b, N2a/b/c, N3 versus FIGO IIIA–C and IVa; see Table 12.3). Contrast-enhanced CT of the abdomen can detect lymph node metastases and/or distant metastases and can help direct treatment planning in patients with advanced disease.

▶ **Clinical features.** Patients often have somewhat nonspecific symptoms such as burning, itching, soreness, or dyspareunia.

▶ **Differential diagnosis**
- Vulvar intraepithelial neoplasia (VIN 3).
- Sarcoma.
- Melanoma.

▶ **Key points.** The MRI protocol for the pretherapeutic staging of vulvar carcinoma should include the following sequences[65]:
- High-resolution sagittal and axial oblique T2 W sequence (parallel to the short axis of the distal urethra), supplemented if necessary by a coronal oblique T2 W sequence (parallel to the long axis of the urethra).

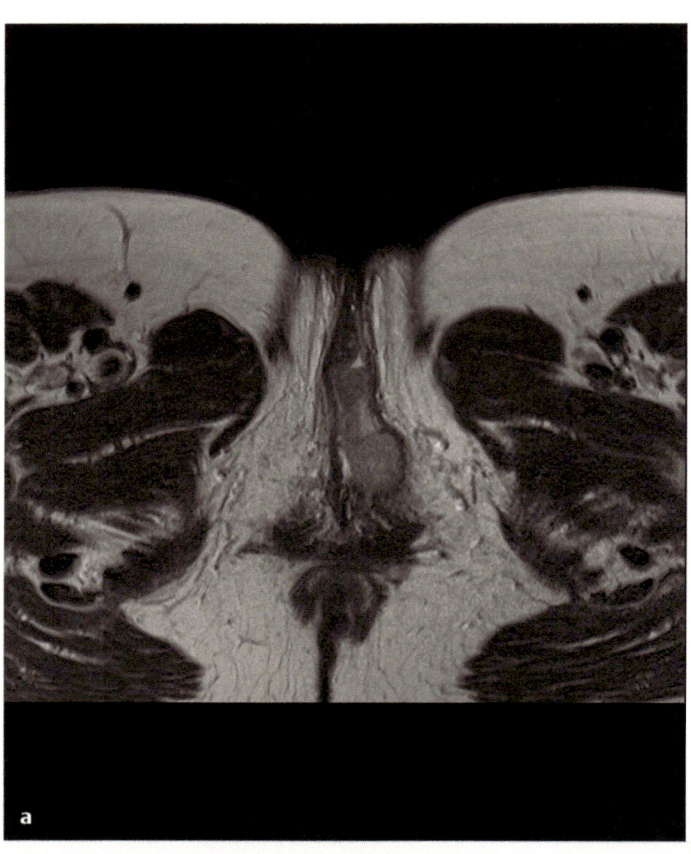

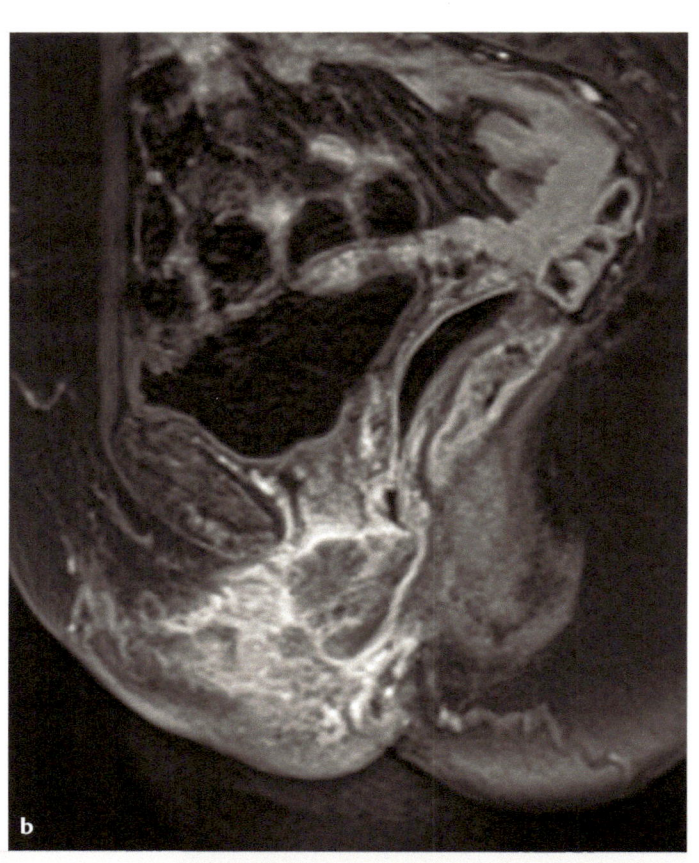

Fig. 12.27 **Stage T2 vulvar carcinoma.** (a) Axial high-resolution T2 W image shows a moderately hyperintense mass arising from the left labium and showing subclitoral-to-perineal extension. (b) Contrast-enhanced fat-saturated T1 W image. The tumor is hypointense to surrounding tissue and has invaded the distal urethra and vagina, with extension to the anus.

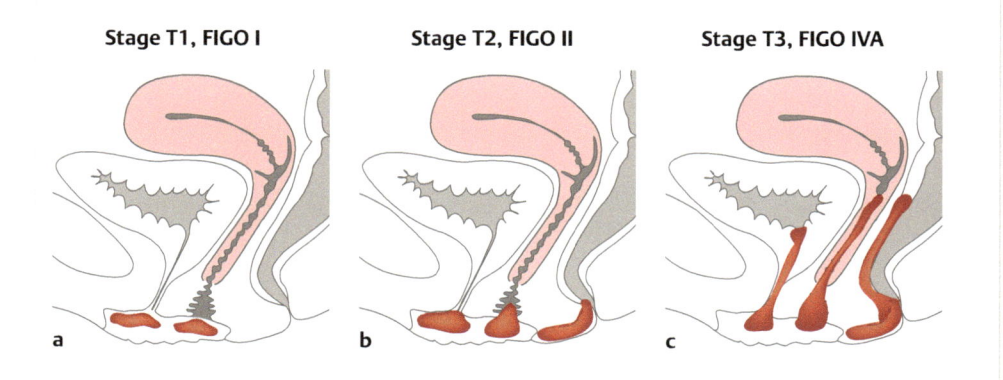

Fig. 12.28 **Staging of primary vulvar carcinoma.**[55,56,68] (a) The carcinoma is confined to the vulva (labia, clitoris) or perineum; it is ≤ 2 cm in greatest dimension (stage T1a) or > 2 cm (T1b). (b) The carcinoma invades the lower third of the urethra and/or the lower third of the vagina and/or the anus. (c) Advanced invasion with involvement of the upper two-thirds of the urethra and/or vagina, invasion of the bladder or rectal wall, and fixation to the pelvic wall is classified as T3, which corresponds to FIGO stage IVa.

Table 12.3 Current N staging system for primary vulvar carcinoma[56]

TNM	FIGO	Regional lymph node involvement
N1a	IIIA	One or 2 lymph node metastases, each > 5 mm
N1b	IIIA	One lymph node metastasis ≥ 5 mm
N2a	IIIB	Three or more lymph node metastases, each < 5 mm
N2b	IIIB	Two or more lymph node metastases ≥ 5 mm
N2c	IIIC	Lymph node metastasis with extracapsular spread
N3	IVA	Fixed or ulcerated lymph node metastasis

- Unenhanced axial T1 W sequence relative to the body axis.
- Contrast-enhanced sagittal, axial oblique, and coronal oblique T1 W sequences with fat saturation.

Bartholin Gland Carcinoma

▶ **Brief definition.** Bartholin gland carcinoma accounts for 1 to 7% of all vulvar carcinomas. The main histological types are squamous cell carcinoma, adenocarcinoma, and adenoid cystic carcinoma.[69] In 33 to 47% of cases, ipsilateral lymph node metastasis is already present at the time of diagnosis. Contralateral lymph nodes are involved in 5 to 14% of cases.[70]

▶ **Imaging signs.** MRI is helpful for defining extent and evaluating lymph node status. Images will usually show a wall-thickened Bartholin's cyst with liquid or necrotic contents that is contiguous with a perineal or vaginal tissue mass. The tumor may be predominantly solid with some cystic components. It appears moderately hyperintense to isointense in the unenhanced T2 W sequence and may enhance intensely in the postcontrast T1 W sequence.[70]

▶ **Clinical features.** Clinical examination reveals unilateral labial swelling, possibly associated with signs of inflammation, pain, itching, or bleeding. The tumor is often misinterpreted initially as bartholinitis or an abscess.

▶ **Differential diagnosis**[71]
- Bartholinitis.
- Bartholin's gland abscess.
- Vulvar carcinoma.

Recurrent Tumors

▶ **Brief definition**
- *Recurrence of endometrial carcinoma*: Endometrial carcinoma that has been treated by primary surgery will most commonly recur within the first 2 years. Metastases appear as solid soft tissue masses, usually located in the vagina and parametria or affecting the lymph nodes. Recurrent endometrial carcinoma after primary radiotherapy is often located in the uterus or ovaries.[31]
- *Recurrence of cervical carcinoma*: Approximately 10 to 42% of cervical cancers recur after primary surgery, 60 to 70% within the first 2 years. They often present as a solid mass on the vaginal stump but may also be manifested in the vagina, parametria, pelvic wall, or bone.[31,57,72]
- *Recurrence of vulvar or vaginal carcinoma*: Approximately 80% of recurrent vulvar or vaginal carcinomas after primary surgery occur during the first 2 years, and most recurrences are local. The risk of recurrent vulvar carcinoma increases if lymph node metastases were detected initially.[5,73]

Note
Recurrent tumor requires differentiation from fibrous scar tissue. This can be particularly difficult during the first 6 months after surgery, when the fibrous tissue will frequently show enhancement after IV administration of contrast medium.[60]

▶ **Imaging signs.** If there is clinical suspicion of postoperative tumor recurrence in the lesser pelvis, contrast-enhanced MRI is useful for localizing the recurrence and defining its extent. Both scar tissue and recurrent tumor tissue are moderately hyperintense in the unenhanced T2 W sequence. Differentiation is aided by the contrast-enhanced fat-saturated T1 W sequence: scar tissue is hypointense in that sequence due to lack of uptake of contrast medium, while inflammatory or neoplastic tissue concentrates more contrast medium and is therefore hyperintense.[60] PET-CT should be used in patients with a suspected small residual tumor and for detection of occult metastasis.[72]

▶ **Clinical features.** Recurrent tumors are frequently asymptomatic and are detected during follow-up. Vaginal bleeding and lower abdominal complaints may occur, depending on the size and location of the recurrence.

▶ **Key points.** MR images are oriented relative to the vaginal stump in patients who have had a hysterectomy for primary endometrial, cervical, or vaginal carcinoma. Image orientation relative to the primary tumor, as in the initial work-up, is prescribed only after chemoradiotherapy. Vaginal opacification with (sterile) ultrasound gel is important because it distends the vaginal walls and facilitates the detection of recurrent tumor tissue on the vaginal stump.

▶ **Pitfalls.** In young women selected for irradiation of the pelvis, the ovaries are often transposed out of the proposed radiotherapy field to preserve ovarian function. Usually they are fixed to the lower paracolic gutter or anterior to the psoas muscle. In that position they may be mistaken for an ovarian mass, lymph node metastasis, recurrence, or peritoneal mass if the surgical history is unknown.[74,75,76]

Sarcomas of the Pelvic Organs

Uterine Sarcoma

▶ **Brief definition.** Approximately 2 to 3% of all genital malignancies are uterine sarcomas. They are divided into three histological subtypes:[56]
- *Leiomyosarcoma* (usually arising in the myometrium).
- *Endometrial stromal sarcoma.*
- *Adenosarcoma* (usually arising in the endometrium).

Female Pelvis

▶ **Imaging signs.** The standard initial imaging study is transvaginal sonography. MRI can add significant information on tumor extent. Contrast-enhanced CT can provide an overview of local invasion, distant metastases, ascites, and peritoneal seeding.[77] PET-CT has yielded very promising results on sarcoma staging, grading, and response to treatment.[78] Generally speaking, the differentiation between leiomyoma and leiomyosarcoma is difficult to accomplish with MRI. Suggestive signs are rapid growth, a large heterogeneous mass, and central necrotic components.[18] Adenosarcoma often appears as a large, cystic mass with multiple internal septa and heterogeneous solid components within the uterine cavity. The solid components are usually hypointense in the unenhanced T2W sequence and show intense enhancement after administration of contrast medium (▶ Fig. 12.29).[68] Staging is based on the current 2010 version of the UICC criteria (Table 12.4).[56]

▶ **Clinical features.** Uterine sarcoma is frequently asymptomatic. It may occasionally cause (postmenopausal) bleeding or lower abdominal pain.

▶ **Differential diagnosis**
- Leiomyoma.
- Endometrial carcinoma.

▶ **Key points.** Leiomyosarcoma and endometrial stromal sarcoma at the T1 stage are classified according to tumor size, while adenosarcoma is classified according to the depth of myometrial invasion (see ▶ Table 12.4). The staging of carcinosarcoma is similar to that of endometrial cancer, and the same imaging protocol is followed; thus in this case as well, the MRI sequences should be oriented relative to the uterine corpus.

Vaginal Sarcoma

▶ **Brief definition.** Approximately 2% of malignant vaginal tumors are sarcomas. Rhabdomyosarcoma is the most common soft tissue tumor in girls up to 5 years of age, while leiomyosarcoma does not occur until adulthood.[79] Distant metastasis is common and occurs mainly by the hematogenous route.

▶ **Imaging signs.** Nodular thickening of the vaginal wall may be palpable on physical examination. Tumor detection relies on ultrasonography. Contrast-enhanced MRI is used to evaluate surrounding structures and confirm distant metastases. CT has no role in local tumor diagnosis due to its poor morphological discrimination, but it can be used to screen for distant metastasis.[77] PET-CT has yielded promising results for grading, staging, and follow-up.[78] MRI signs are as follows:

- *Rhabdomyosarcoma*: This tumor often shows a heterogeneous signal pattern after administration of contrast medium. It is usually hypointense in the unenhanced T1W sequence and hyperintense in the T2W sequence. Some tumors have a pseudocapsule, which is hypointense in T1W and T2W sequences.[80]
- *Leiomyosarcoma*: This tumor often appears as a mixed cystic–solid mass with irregular, infiltrating margins. It tends to be

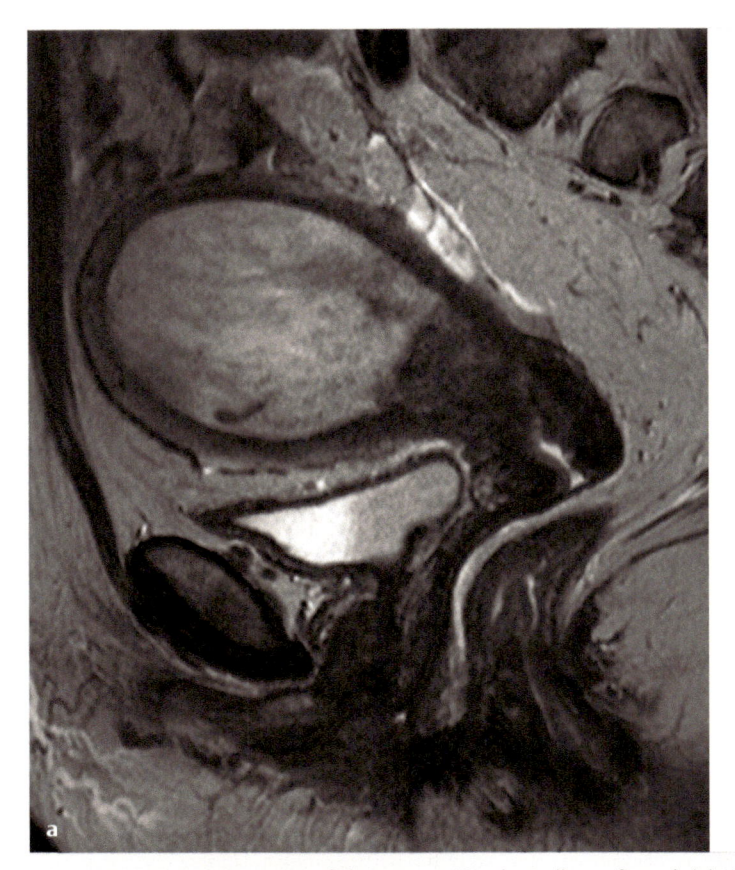

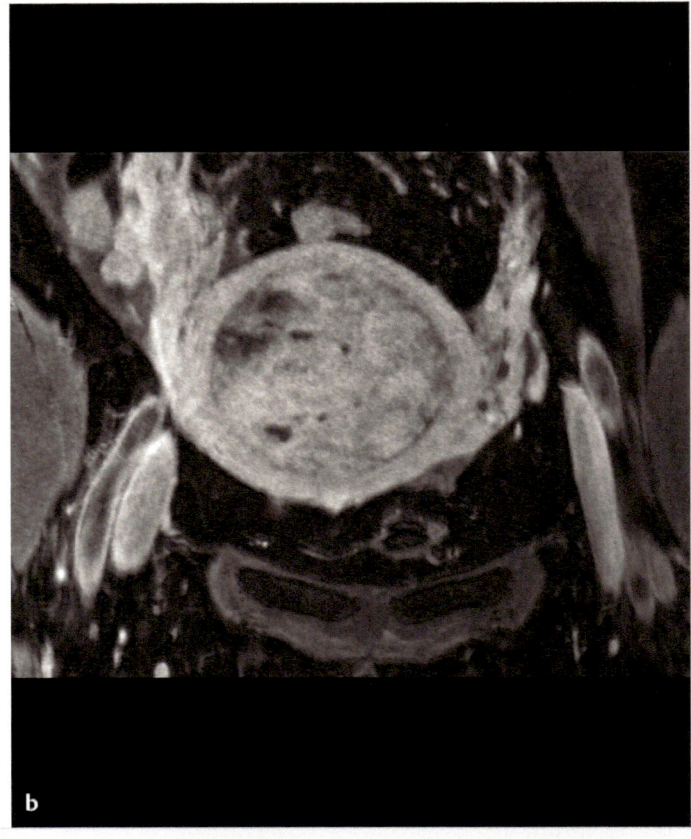

Fig. 12.29 Carcinosarcoma of the uterus. Histologically confirmed. **(a)** High-resolution sagittal T2W image. The uterine corpus is distended by a hyperintense, inhomogeneous mass. The myometrium is thinned, the serosa is intact. Decreased signal intensity is noted in the isthmic portion of the mass. The cervix appears normal. **(b)** Axial oblique postcontrast T1W image with fat saturation. The tumor shows intense enhancement with an overall heterogeneous appearance and smooth margins.

hyperintense on T2 W images but hypointense on T1 W images. It shows a high affinity for gadolinium-based contrast medium.[81]

▶ **Clinical features.** Patients may complain of diffuse lower abdominal pain or specific pain in the vagina, bladder, or rectum. Luminal obstruction of the vagina may lead to hematocolpos or hematometra.

Table 12.4 Current staging system for uterine sarcoma[56]

Tumor stage	Tumor extent
T1	Tumor confined to the uterus
• T1a versus T1b	Leiomyosarcoma and endometrial stromal sarcoma: tumor ≤ 5 cm in greatest dimension versus > 5 cm
• T1a versus T1b versus T1c	Adenosarcoma: tumor confined to the endometrium or endocervix versus < 50% myometrial involvement versus ≥ 50% myometrial involvement
Tumor extends beyond the uterus, within the lesser pelvis	
T2a	Involves adnexa
T2b	Involves other pelvic tissues (except the bladder and rectum)
T4	Invades the bladder or rectum
Tumor extends beyond the lesser pelvis	
T3a	Infiltrates abdominal tissues at one site
T3b	Infiltrates abdominal tissues at more than one site
N1	Regional lymph node metastasis
M1	Distant metastasis

▶ **Differential diagnosis**
- Vaginal carcinoma.
- Melanoma.
- Metastasis.

Pelvic Lymphoma

▶ **Brief definition.** Involvement of the uterus and cervix by non-Hodgkin's lymphoma is very rare (fewer than 1% of non-Hodgkin's lymphomas). Primary vulvovaginal lymphoma is also rare, accounting for just 1% of all extranodal lymphomas. Women at any age from 20 to 80 years may be affected.[79]

▶ **Imaging signs.** Ultrasound is suitable for local tumor detection but may be unable to define the full extent of lymphomatous involvement, so sectional imaging is helpful. In cases where spread of the disease beyond the lesser pelvis is already suspected clinically, contrast-enhanced whole-body CT is indicated for treatment planning and follow-up.[82] Contrast-enhanced MRI of the pelvis is the modality of choice for the evaluation of local findings.
- *Uterine lymphoma*: This lesion usually appears on MRI as a homogeneous mass of high T2 W signal intensity that is poorly delineated from surrounding tissue and shows intense enhancement.[83]
- *Vulvovaginal lymphoma*: Typically this tumor is homogeneously hypointense in the unenhanced T1 W sequence, is moderately hyperintense in the T2 W sequence (▶ Fig. 12.30), and shows homogeneous enhancement. It has infiltrating margins and may present a lobulated appearance.[79]

▶ **Clinical features.** Patients may be asymptomatic or may complain of irregular vaginal bleeding or nonspecific lower abdominal complaints. Depending on the size and location of the tumor, patients may experience postcoital bleeding or voiding difficulties (especially with primary cervicouterine lymphoma), a

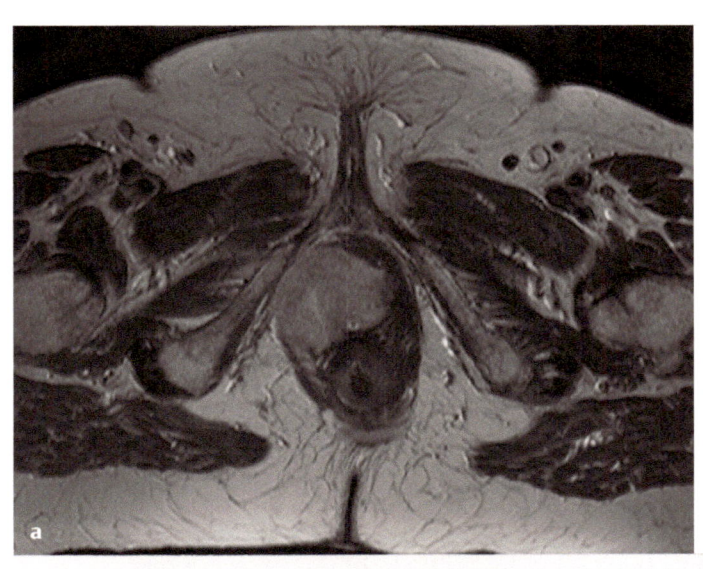

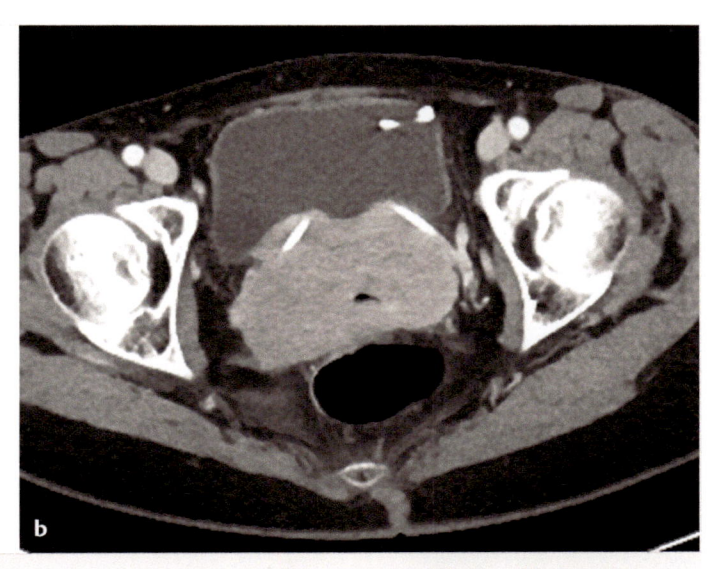

Fig. 12.30 Vulvovaginal lymphoma. (a) High-resolution axial T2 W image. The lymphoma, located in the perineal region, is moderately hyperintense and has smooth margins but presents a somewhat polygonal shape. Histologically, the tumor is a B-cell lymphoma. (b) Axial CT scan in the venous phase shows intense, homogeneous enhancement of the lymphoma, which has infiltrated the bladder wall and both ostia. Bilateral indwelling ureteral stents are noted to be present. The lymphoma also extends to the anterior rectal wall. It was identified histologically as diffuse large cell B-cell lymphoma.

nonspecific pressure sensation on the pelvic floor, or persistent discharge (especially with vulvovaginal lymphoma).[68]

▶ **Differential diagnosis.** The diagnostic possibilities depend upon location and extent:
- Leiomyoma with degenerative changes.
- Endometrial carcinoma.
- Cervical carcinoma.
- Vaginal carcinoma
- Vulvar carcinoma.
- Metastasis.

Ovarian Tumors

▶ **Brief definition.** Ovarian carcinoma is the sixth most common malignancy in women, with an incidence of 12 cases per 100,000 women per year in the United States, and is the leading cause of gynecologic cancer deaths.[84] Risk factors are a *BRCA-1* or *BRCA2* mutations and hereditary nonpolyposis colorectal cancer (HNPCC). Ovarian cancer is often asymptomatic, causing a delay in diagnosis until the tumor has reached an advanced stage.[85] Ovarian tumors show considerable variation in their biological origin and behavior. Approximately two-thirds are of epithelial origin, approximately one-fourth are germ-cell tumors, and just 10% are sex cord-stromal tumors (▶ Table 12.5).[31] Secondary tumors of the ovary may be metastatic to a primary tumor of the gastrointestinal tract (e.g., Krukenberg's tumor, gastric signet-ring carcinoma), pancreas, or breast. Ovarian tumors may also be secondary to melanoma or lymphoma. Sarcoma may also involve the ovary.[13,15,18,31] A special type of epithelial tumor is pseudomyxoma peritonei, caused by intraperitoneal seeding from a primary mucinous tumor of the ovary, pancreas, or appendix due to spontaneous rupture, biopsy, or surgery.[31,33] Meigs's syndrome denotes a triad of findings consisting of a benign ovarian tumor (usually fibroma), ascites, and pleural effusion.

▶ **Imaging signs.** Current gynecologic guidelines describe transvaginal ultrasound as the most important imaging modality for ovarian cancer owing to its high availability. It is unsuitable for staging, however, as it provides limited visualization of the pelvis as a whole.[13,85] Current guidelines recommend CT, MRI, and PET-CT for more detailed investigations and to narrow the differential diagnosis.[85] MRI provides better characterization of the lesion owing to its high soft-tissue contrast and can detect malignancies with an accuracy of 93%.[86] It also supplies information on surrounding structures and locoregional manifestations but, like ultrasound, is inadequate for the complete pretherapeutic staging of suspected cancer.

Note

Contrast-enhanced multidetector CT is the imaging modality of choice for staging an ovarian tumor because it supplies all relevant information for treatment planning.[13]

Besides the evaluation of existing hepatic, lymphogenous, or pulmonary metastasis, multidetector CT can detect peritoneal nodules ≥ 5 mm in size with a sensitivity of 100% and accuracy of 80%.[87] PET-CT is particularly rewarding in the detection of lymph node metastases, peritoneal deposits, therapeutic follow-up, and the investigation of equivocal lesions or recurrence in patients with clinical suspicion of recurrent disease.[85,88,89]

Note

The use of MRI for the further differentiation of a sonographically indeterminate ovarian mass can aid therapeutic decision making by reducing the rate of false-positive malignancies: while a benign tumor is treatable by local excision, a malignant process, if operable, will require major oncologic surgery (including complete preliminary staging).[47,90]

Staging is based on the current 2010 version of the UICC criteria (▶ Fig. 12.31).[56] Metastases on the liver capsule (peritoneal nodules) correspond to a T3–FIGO III tumor, whereas metastases in the hepatic parenchyma correspond to M1–FIGO IV. Stage T1c is based partly on the presence of malignant cells in ascites, and stage T2c is based entirely on that criterion. Stage T3a includes microscopic peritoneal deposits that are not definable by sectional imaging. Pleural effusion requires positive cytology in order to be classified as M1 or FIGO IV.[56]

The ovaries in women of reproductive age normally measure approximately 3 cm in diameter. The ovarian cortex is more hypointense than the medulla in the unenhanced T2W sequence. The cortex contains hyperintense mature and immature follicles, which range from 0.5 to 4 cm in size.[15,33] The corpus luteum may be demonstrable as a more complex structure in the ovary. It may contain hemorrhagic foci and shows prominent enhancement.[47]

Note

Postmenopausal ovaries are atrophic and have a greater proportion of fibrous stroma, which is hypointense in T1W and T2W sequences and shows little or no enhancement. Fatty components or even isolated small cysts may also be detectable.[15,47]

Table 12.5 WHO classification of ovarian tumors[18,31,65,85]

Epithelial tumors	Germ cell tumors	Sex cord-stromal tumors
• Serous tumor • Mucinous tumor • Endometrioid carcinoma • Clear cell tumor • Transitional cell tumor (Brenner's tumor) • Squamous cell carcinoma • Mixed epithelial tumor • Undifferentiated carcinoma	• Mature teratoma (dermoid; with possible malignant degeneration) • Immature teratoma • Dysgerminoma • Endodermal sinus tumor (yolk sac carcinoma) • Carcinoid • Embryonal carcinoma • Choriocarcinoma (malignant trophoblastic tumor)	• Granulosa cell tumor • (Malignant) thecoma • Fibroma • Sertoli–Leydig cell tumor (androblastoma) • Sclerosing stromal tumor

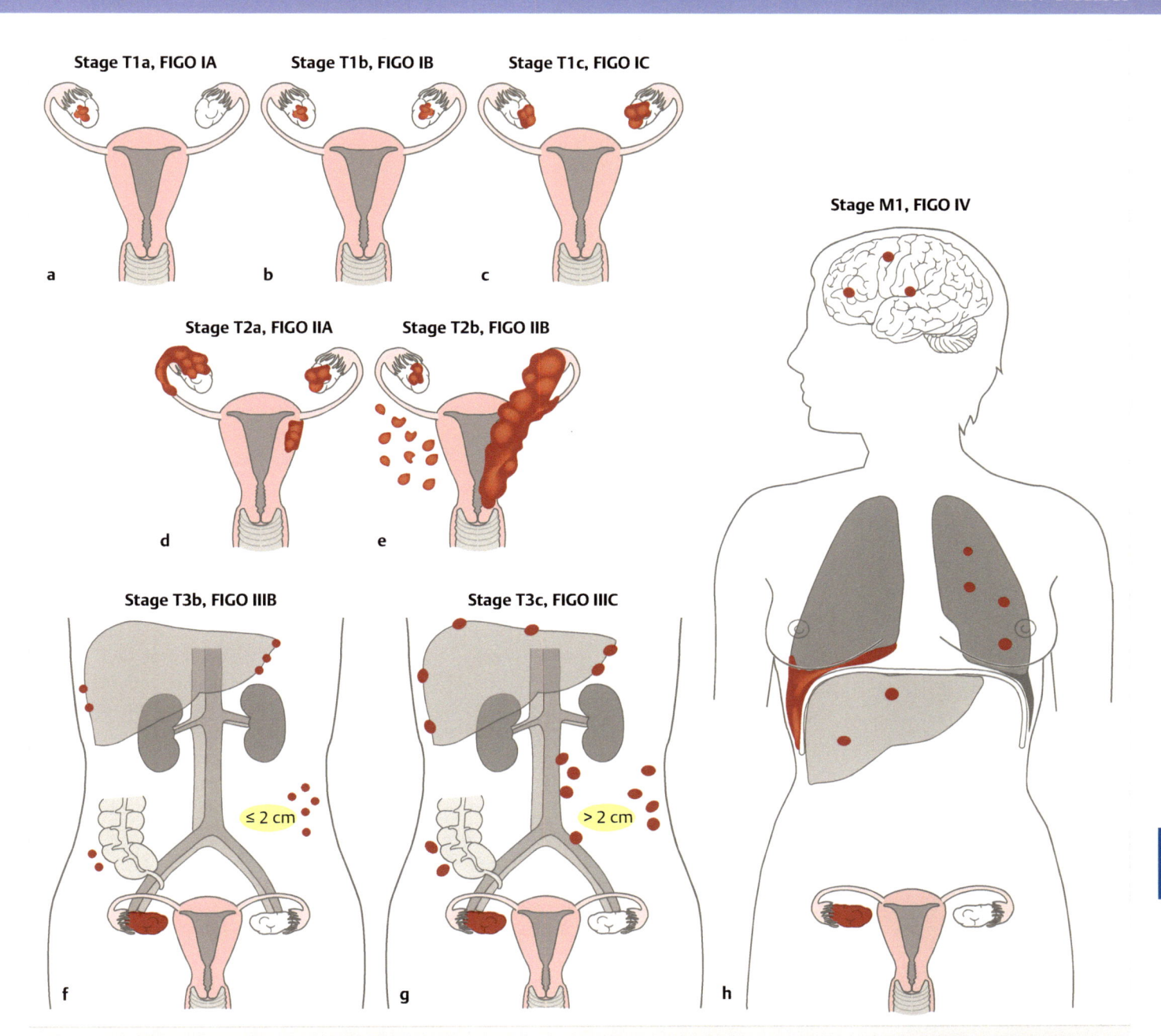

Fig. 12.31 Staging of primary ovarian carcinoma.[56] Grossly visible disease. **(a)** Tumor is limited to one ovary, the capsule is intact, there is no visible tumor on the surface. **(b)** Tumor involves both ovaries, the capsule is intact, there is no tumor on the surface. **(c)** Tumor involves one or both ovaries with capsular rupture or tumor on the surface. **(d)** Tumor involves one or both ovaries with extension and/or implant on the uterus and/or fallopian tubes. **(e)** Tumor involves one or both ovaries with extension to other pelvic intraparietal tissues. **(f)** Tumor involves one or both ovaries with macroscopic, extrapelvic peritoneal metastasis ≤ 2 cm in greatest dimension. **(g)** Tumor involves one or both ovaries with macroscopic, extrapelvic peritoneal metastasis >2 cm in greatest dimension. **(h)** Distant metastases to liver, lung, pleura, and brain.

Ovarian tumors may be predominantly cystic, may contain solid components, or may display mixed features (see ▶ Table 12.6). It may be difficult to definitely characterize the lesion by imaging because of the similar morphologies of different subtypes, but there are several suggestive morphological criteria that can narrow the differential diagnosis for a given tumor. For example, the detection of papillary growth within a cystic ovarian mass is a strong predictor of malignancy.[33] Some morphological signs of malignancy, especially nodular or papillary growth or the presence of intralesional necrosis, may be appreciated only after IV administration of contrast medium.[33] The following are recognized as criteria for malignancy:

- Cystic ovarian mass greater than 4 cm in diameter.
- Cyst wall thickness greater than 3 mm.
- Nodular changes in the cyst wall.
- Papillary growth.
- Solid or predominantly solid tumor components.
- Necrotic foci in solid tumor components.
- Concomitant detection of ascites, contiguous invasion, and lymphadenopathy.

Female Pelvis

Table 12.6 Differential diagnosis of ovarian tumors based on their morphological composition and benign/malignant classification[33,50]

Benign or malignant	Predominantly cystic	Predominantly solid	Mixed cystic-solid	Fatty components
Benign	• Serous cystadenoma • Mucinous cystadenoma	• Fibroma • Thecoma • Sclerosing stromal tumor		
Usually benign		• Brenner tumor	• Mature teratoma (dermoid)	• Mature teratoma (dermoid)
Low-grade malignancy	• Borderline tumors	• Sertoli–Leydig cell tumor		
Malignant	• Serous cystadenocarcinoma	• Granulosa cell tumor • Dysgerminoma	• Mucinous cystadenocarcinoma • Endometrioid carcinoma • Immature teratoma • Clear cell carcinoma	• Immature teratoma

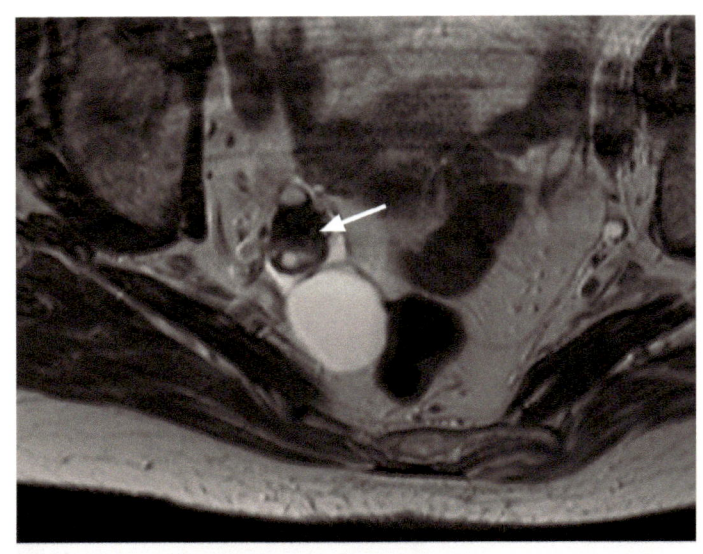

Fig. 12.32 **Cystadenofibroma.** Axial T2 W image displays the right ovary with follicles, a thin-walled ovarian cyst, and a hypointense solid central component in the ovary with no criteria of malignancy. The lesion was confirmed histologically as cystadenofibroma (arrow).

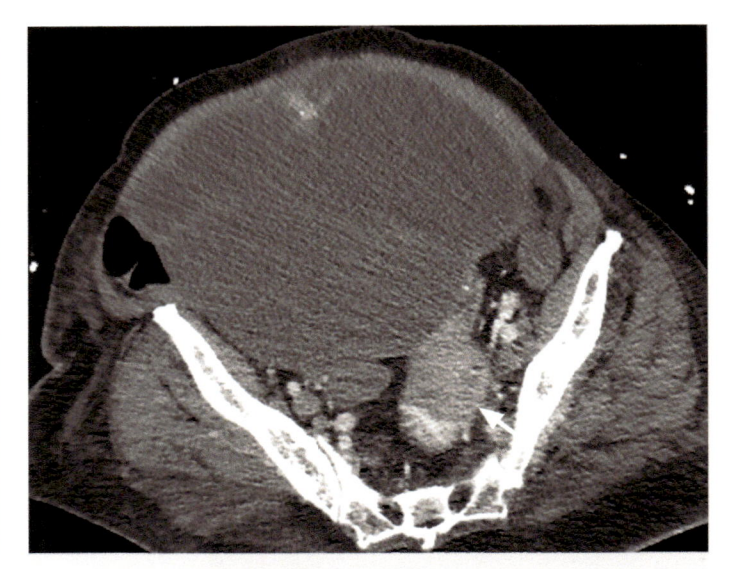

Fig. 12.33 **Cystadenofibroma.** Axial venous CT scan in a different patient shows a giant cystic mass of the right ovary that occupies most of the lesser pelvis. The anterior portion of the mass includes a small solid structure with stippled internal calcifications. Other than its size, the mass shows no apparent criteria of malignancy, although soft-tissue contrast is poorer than in MRI. The mass was identified histologically as cystadenofibroma. A regressive cystic teratoma, also confirmed histologically, is noted in the left ovary as an incidental finding.

▶ **Clinical features.** Ovarian tumors may be asymptomatic for a long time and may be detected incidentally in routine examinations. Depending on the growth tendency of a lesion and whether it is benign or malignant, patients may present with increased abdominal circumference (due to tumor size or ascites) or with nonspecific symptoms such as lower abdominal pain, a bloated feeling, or back pain.[31]

▶ **Differential diagnosis**
- Tubo-ovarian abscess.
- Meigs's syndrome.
- Actinomycosis.
- Tuberculosis.

The various ovarian tumor entities are reviewed in ▶ Table 12.6. Illustrative images are shown in ▶ Fig. 12.32, ▶ Fig. 12.33, ▶ Fig. 12.34, ▶ Fig. 12.35, ▶ Fig. 12.36, and ▶ Fig. 12.37.

▶ **Key points.** The following series of MRI sequences should be performed for the local evaluation of an ovarian tumor, particularly from the standpoint of determining whether the tumor is benign or malignant (see ESUR guidelines).[13,47]
- Basic sequences:
  - High-resolution sagittal T2 W TSE sequence (to detect an ovarian lesion that is lateral, anterior, or posterior to the uterus).
  - High-resolution T2 W and unenhanced T1 W sequences, coronal if the lesion is lateral to the uterus, or axial if the lesion is anterior or posterior to the uterus, using a 4- to 5-mm slice thickness across the ovarian lesion.
- Special sequences for further differentiation:
  - Unenhanced T1 W sequence with fat saturation (STIR not recommended, as it is not specific for fat).
  - T1 W sequence after administration of contrast medium, with fat saturation, in at least two planes.
  - If necessary, DWI with a b-value between 800 and 1000s/mm^2.

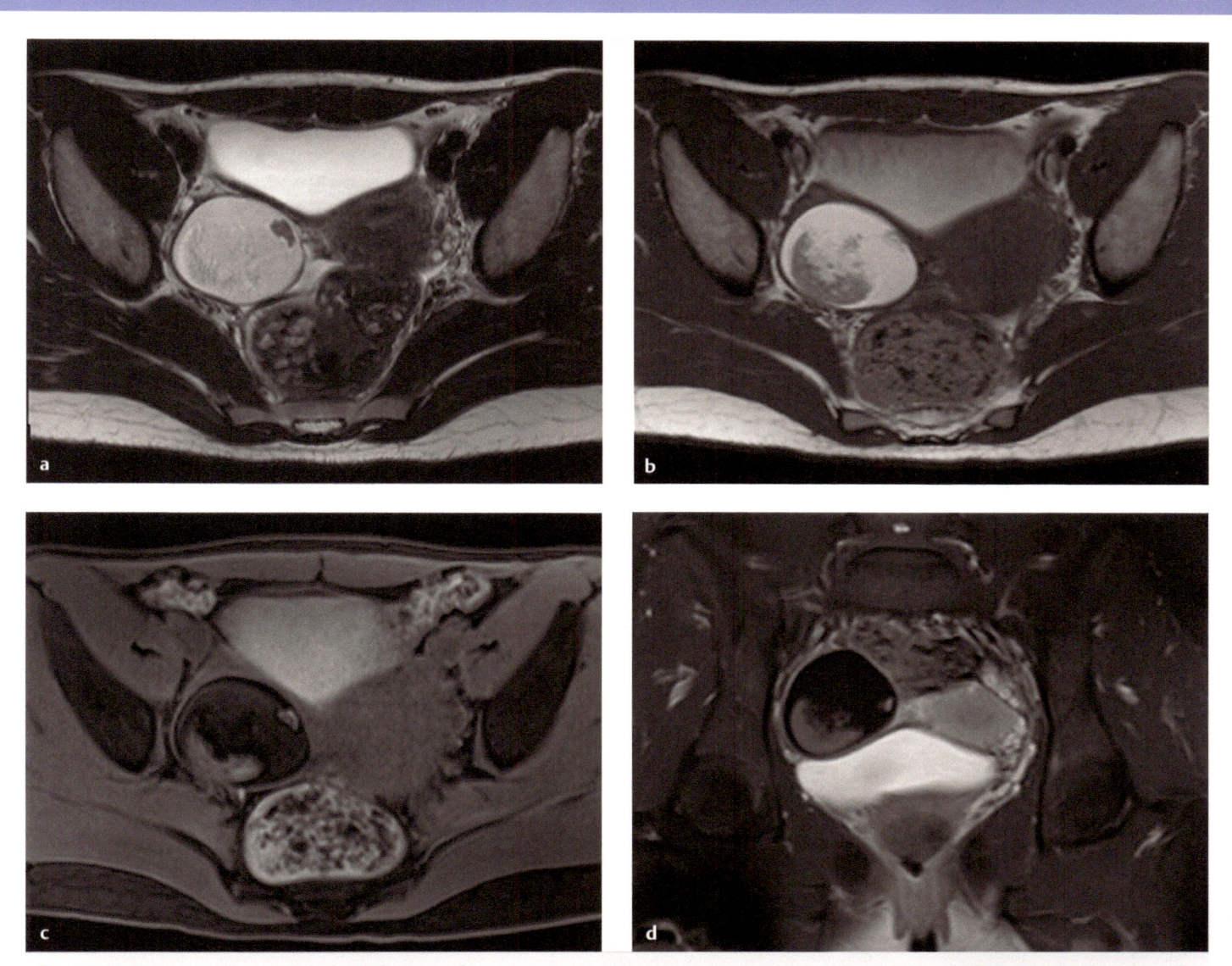

Fig. 12.34 Mature teratoma. Typical MRI features of a mature teratoma in a young woman. **(a)** High-resolution axial T2 W image shows a well-circumscribed cystic lesion of the right ovary with an internal, sharp-edged hypointense structure and a somewhat patchy posterior hypointensity. The uterine corpus is displaced toward the left pelvic wall. The left ovary with follicles is visible between the left pelvic wall and corpus. Coprostasis is noted within the rectum. Physiologic amounts of free fluid are present. **(b)** Axial unenhanced T1 W image. The lumen appears hyperintense, also with a patchy posterior hypointensity. **(c)** Axial unenhanced fat-saturated T1 W image. The lumen is homogeneously hypointense except for the posterior patchy areas. This is suggestive of fatty contents. **(d)** Coronal T1 W image after IV administration of contrast medium. Only the solid components within the cyst show enhancement.

▶ Fig. 12.38 presents an algorithm for the differential diagnosis of ovarian tumors based on their signal characteristics in the basic and special MRI sequences.

Note

When CT is used for the imaging evaluation of an ovarian tumor, the examination should be preceded by oral administration of water or contrast medium and, if necessary, rectal administration of contrast medium for better delineation of bowel loops. Reconstruction of the portal venous phase in three planes with a 3- to 5-mm slice thickness is essential because papillary growth and solid components in particular may not yet show enhancement in the arterial phase.[13]

Fallopian Tube Carcinoma

▶ **Brief definition.** Fallopian tube carcinoma has a very low incidence of 3.6 per 1 million women per year and comprises approximately 0.5% of all gynecologic malignancies. Given its close histological resemblance to papillary serous ovarian carcinoma, the actual number of primary fallopian tube cancers is probably underestimated.[91,92,93] Women in the sixth to seventh decades are most commonly affected, and association with a *BRCA1* or *BRCA2* gene mutation has been described.[94] Fallopian tube carcinoma directly infiltrates surrounding structures (transluminal spread to the ovary and uterus, transmural spread to the bladder, rectum, and pelvic wall). Lymphogenous metastasis may occur anywhere in the abdomen (inguinal, iliac, para-aortic to infrarenal levels) due to the extensive lymphatic network that drains nearby organs and ligaments. Hematogenous metastasis is usually detected only at an advanced stage, the most common sites being the liver, pleura, vagina, lung, and brain.

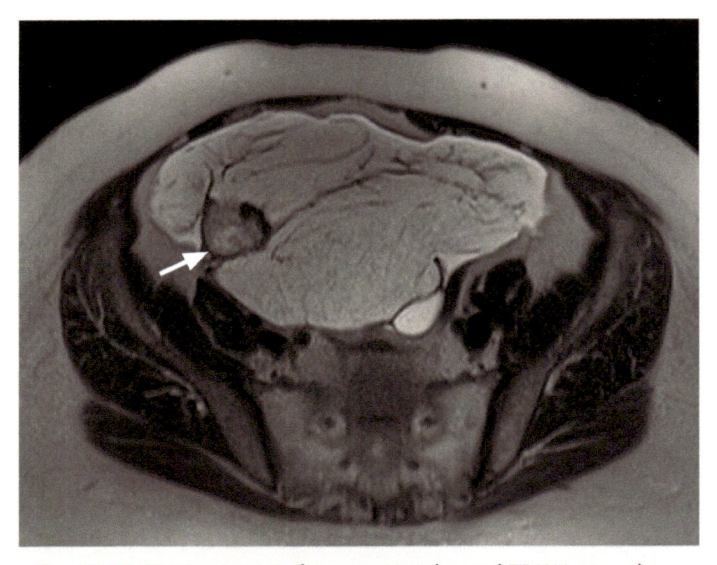

Fig. 12.35 **Mucinous cystadenoma.** Unenhanced T2W image shows a polygonal cystic mass permeated by multiple thin septa and streaks. It was identified histologically as mucinous cystadenoma of the left ovary with no evidence of malignancy. A predominantly solid, hypointense structure is noted incidentally in the right ovary, identified histologically as a dermoid (arrow).

▶ **Imaging signs.** CT is the imaging modality of choice for the preoperative staging of primary fallopian tube carcinoma. MRI aids in the primary local differentiation of cystic adnexal lesions. DWI is helpful in the detection of small deposits, and the combination of DWI and administration of contrast medium will increase the accuracy of detection.[95,96] It is common to find a dilated, fluid-filled fallopian tube with a papillary growth or solid nodule on the tubal wall. Increased fluid production by the tumor may distend the tube into a sausage shape.[97] The cystic components have fluid-equivalent density and signal intensity on CT and MRI but may appear more heterogeneous depending on their composition (blood, debris). Papillary and nodular components show increased enhancement on CT and MRI, but enhance less than the myometrium.[98] It is common to find ascites, which has a high positive predictive value for peritoneal metastases.[99] The staging system for primary fallopian tube carcinoma is like that for ovarian carcinoma (see ▶ Fig. 12.31).[31,56] 18F-FDG PET-CT has yielded promising results in the detection of recurrence and screening for metastasis.[100,101]

▶ **Clinical features.** Fallopian tube carcinoma is frequently asymptomatic. Some patients experience lower abdominal pain, which may be dull or colicky, as well as vaginal bleeding, discharge, or a palpable mass in the lower abdomen. Serum levels of CA-125 are elevated in approximately 92% of patients with primary fallopian tube carcinoma.[102,103]

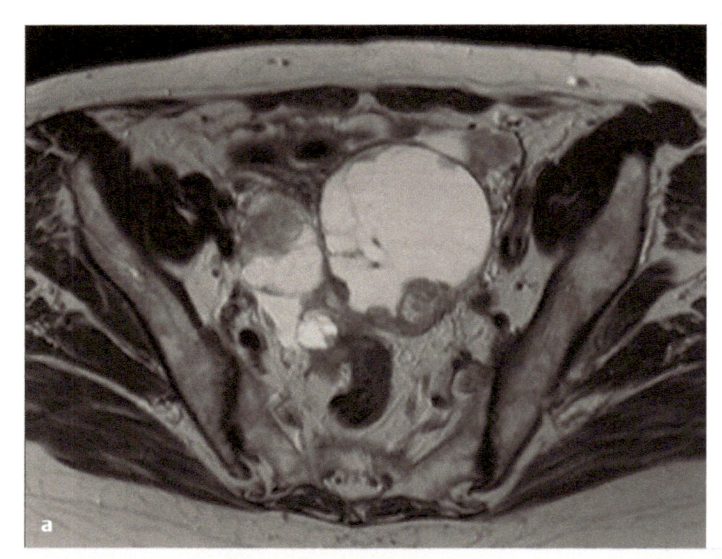

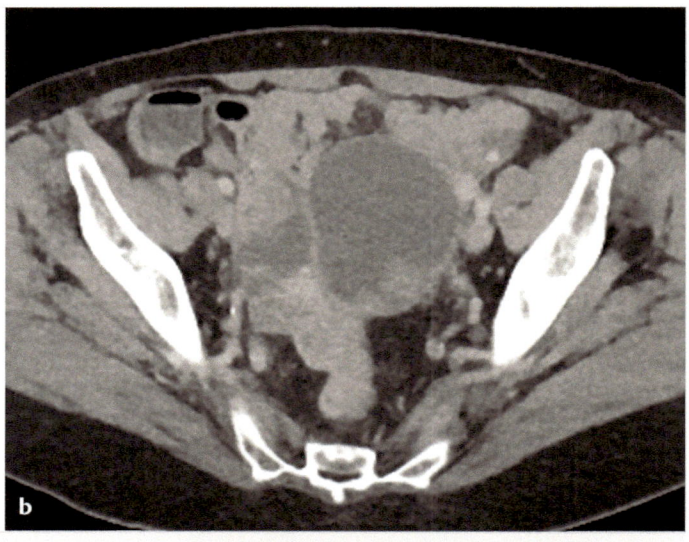

Fig. 12.36 **Serous papillary adenocarcinoma of both ovaries.** Histologically confirmed. (a) High-resolution axial T2W image demonstrates cystic and solid components, septa, and nodular growth. The ovaries are clearly differentiated from each other. (b) Corresponding axial CT scan in the venous phase. The cystic and solid components are visualized, but the relatively poor soft-tissue contrast limits further differentiation and delineation from adjacent intestinal structures.

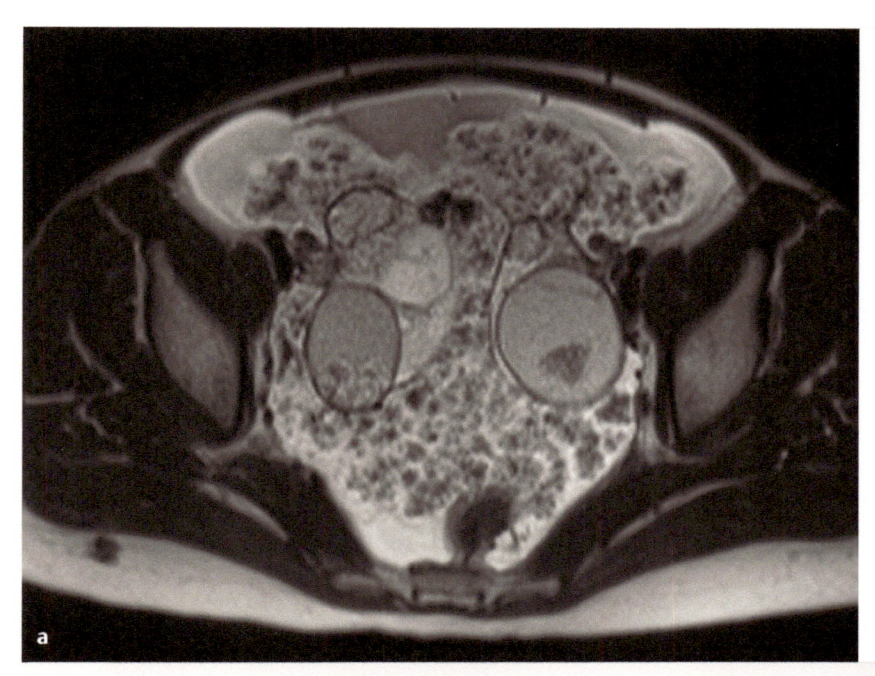

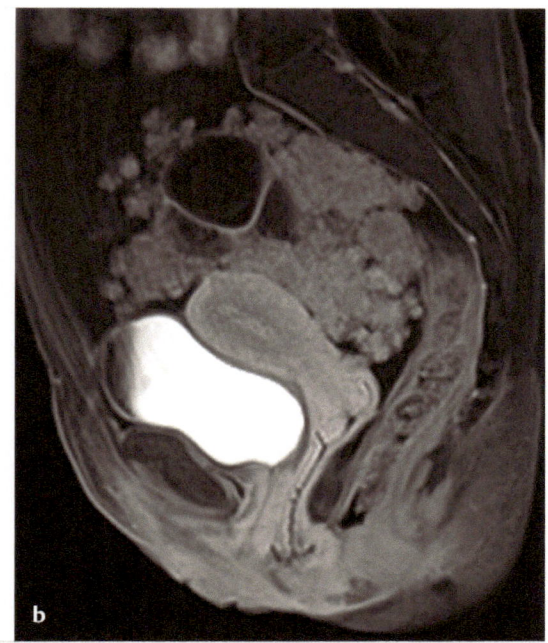

Fig. 12.37 Bilateral serous borderline tumors. Histologically confirmed. **(a)** Axial T2 W image shows multiple cystic lesions in both ovaries with prominent septa, papillary growth, and ascites. **(b)** Sagittal contrast-enhanced T1 W image. The papillary structures show intense enhancement. The cyst wall is thickened and also shows prominent enhancement. Ascites has spread throughout the abdominal cavity. The outlines of the uterus, cervix, bladder, urethra, and rectum are clearly defined. The cul-de-sac is distended by ascites.

▶ **Differential diagnosis**[104]
- Papillary serous ovarian carcinoma.
- Serous epithelial ovarian carcinoma (arising directly in the ovary).
- Hydrosalpinx, hematosalpinx, or pyosalpinx in a setting of inflammation (distinguished by an absence of solid mural changes; the only changes are in the fluid composition, due mainly to blood or debris).
- Tubo-ovarian abscess.
- Ectopic pregnancy.

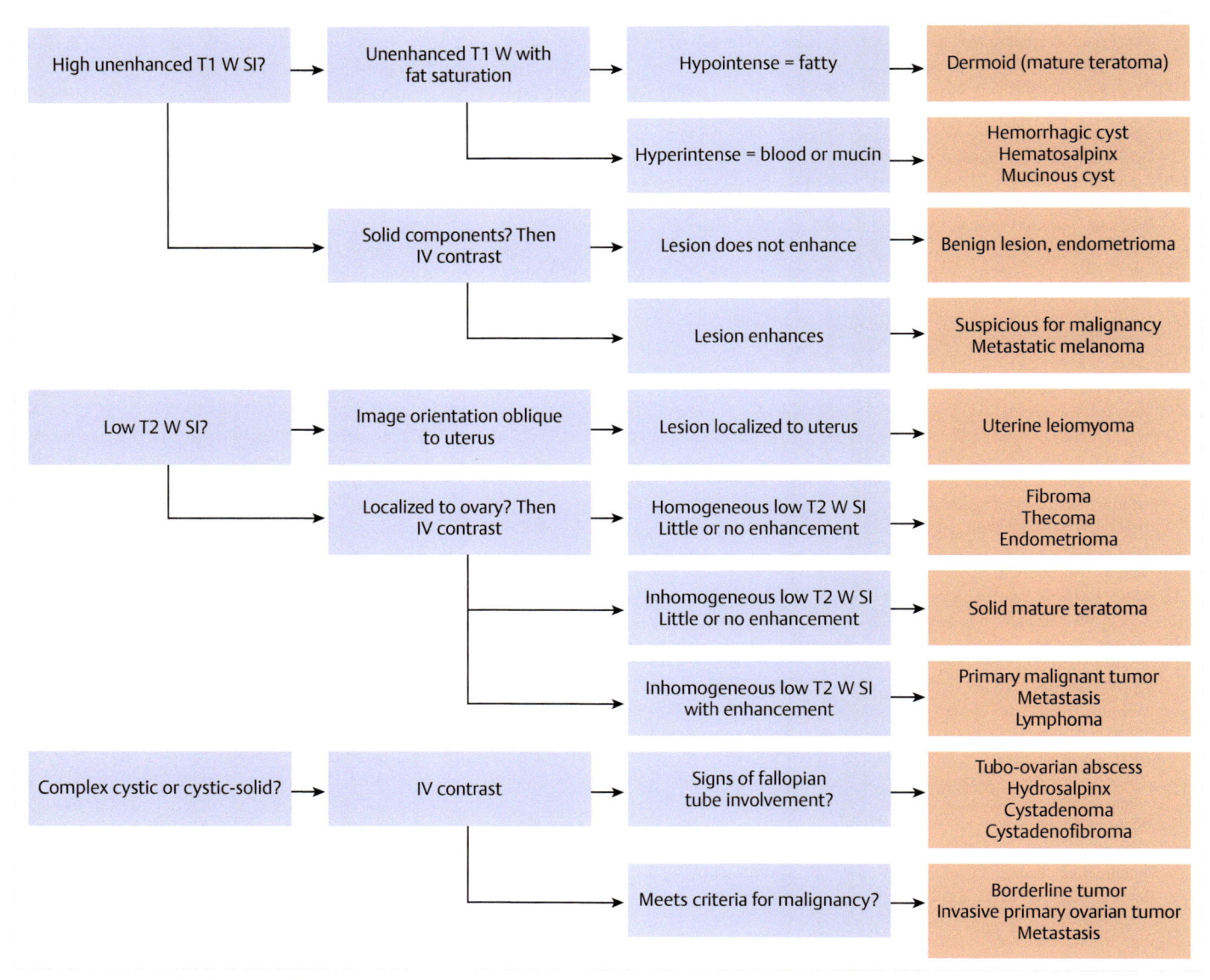

Fig. 12.38 Algorithm for the imaging evaluation and differential diagnosis of ovarian tumors.[68]

Bibliography

[1] Lippert H, Deller T. Lehrbuch Anatomie. München: Urban & Fischer; 2003
[2] Pfisterer J, Ludwig M, Vollersen E. Funktionelle Anatomie der weiblichen Genitalorgane. In: Diedrich K, Holzgreve W, Jonat W, Schneider K-T, Schultze-Mosgau A, Weiss J, eds. Gynäkologie und Geburtshilfe. Berlin: Springer; 2007:3–18
[3] Pfleiderer A, Kaufmann M. Anatomie, Topographie und Funktion der weiblichen Genitalorgane. In: Breckwoldt M, Kaufmann M, Pfleiderer A, eds. Gynäkologie und Geburtshilfe. Stuttgart: Thieme; 2011:14–25
[4] Kommoss F. Anatomie und Embryologie. In: Kreienberg R, Bois A, Pfisterer J, Schindelmann S, Schmalfeldt B, eds. Management des Ovarialkarzinoms Interdisziplinäres Vorgehen. Heidelberg: Springer; 2009:17–22
[5] Costa S. Vulva. In: Kaufmann M, Costa S, Scharl A, eds. Die Gynäkologie. Berlin: Springer; 2013:416–428
[6] De Gaetano AM, Calcagni ML, Rufini V, et al. Imaging of gynecologic malignancies with FDG PET-CT: case examples, physiologic activity, and pitfalls. Abdom Imaging. 2009; 34(6):696–711
[7] Harry VN. Novel imaging techniques as response biomarkers in cervical cancer. Gynecol Oncol. 2010; 116(2):253–261
[8] Balleyguier C, Sala E, Da Cunha T, et al. Staging of uterine cervical cancer with MRI: guidelines of the European Society of Urogenital Radiology. Eur Radiol. 2011; 21(5):1102–1110
[9] Kinkel K, Forstner R, Danza FM, et al. European Society of Urogenital Imaging. Staging of endometrial cancer with MRI: guidelines of the European Society of Urogenital Imaging. Eur Radiol. 2009; 19(7):1565–1574
[10] Kirchhoff SMR. Vagina, Uterus, Adnexe. In: Scheffel H, Alkadhi H, Boss A, Merkle E, eds. Praxisbuch MRT Abdomen und Becken. Berlin: Springer; 2012:181–194
[11] Thomassin-Naggara I, Darai E, Bazot M. Gynecological pelvic infection: what is the role of imaging? Diagn Interv Imaging. 2012; 93(6):491–499
[12] Beddy P, Moyle P, Kataoka M, et al. Evaluation of depth of myometrial invasion and overall staging in endometrial cancer: comparison of diffusion-weighted and dynamic contrast-enhanced MR imaging. Radiology. 2012; 262(2):530–537
[13] Forstner R, Sala E, Kinkel K, Spencer JA, European Society of Urogenital Radiology. ESUR guidelines: ovarian cancer staging and follow-up. Eur Radiol. 2010; 20(12):2773–2780
[14] Shen SH, Chiou YY, Wang JH, et al. Diffusion-weighted single-shot echoplanar imaging with parallel technique in assessment of endometrial cancer. AJR Am J Roentgenol. 2008; 190(2):481–488
[15] Scheidler J. Bildgebende Diagnostik der inneren weiblichen Genitalorgane - Adnexe. In: Adams S, Nicolas V, Freyschmidt J, eds. Urogenitaltrakt, Retroperitoneum, Mamma. Berlin: Springer; 2004:221–240
[16] Horton KM, Sheth S, Corl F, Fishman EK. Multidetector row CT: principles and clinical applications. Crit Rev Computed Tomogr. 2002; 43(2):143–181

[17] Finas D, Altgassen C. Notfälle. In: Diedrich K, Holzgreve W, Jonat W, Schneider K-T, Schultze-Mosgau A, Weiss J, eds. Gynäkologie und Geburtshilfe. Berlin: Springer; 2007:594–598

[18] Roth CG. Fundamentals of body MRI. Philadelphia: Elsevier Saunders; 2012:261–368

[19] Gätje R. Chronisches Unterbauchschmerzsyndrom. In: Kaufmann M, Costa S, Scharl A, eds. Die Gynäkologie. Berlin: Springer; 2013:345–351

[20] Ludwig M, Bonatz G, Küpker W, et al. Sexuelle Differenzierung und Entwicklung. In: Diedrich K, Holzgreve W, Jonat W, Schneider K-T, Schultze-Mosgau A, Weiss J, eds. Gynäkologie und Geburtshilfe. Berlin: Springer; 2007:37–58

[21] Alt C, Gebauer G. Uterus. In: Hallscheidt P, Haferkamp A, eds. Urogenitale Bildgebung. Berlin: Springer; 2011:232–301

[22] Brucker S, Oppelt P, Ludwig K, et al. Vaginale und uterine Fehlbildungen. Teil 2. Geburtshilfe Frauenheilkd. 2005; 65:R221–R244

[23] Rezvani M, Shaaban AM. Fallopian tube disease in the nonpregnant patient. Radiographics. 2011; 31(2):527–548

[24] Imaoka I, Wada A, Matsuo M, Yoshida M, Kitagaki H, Sugimura K. MR imaging of disorders associated with female infertility: use in diagnosis, treatment, and management. Radiographics. 2003; 23(6):1401–1421

[25] Yitta S, Hecht EM, Slywotzky CM, Bennett GL. Added value of multiplanar reformation in the multidetector CT evaluation of the female pelvis: a pictorial review. Radiographics. 2009; 29(7):1987–2003

[26] Ha HK, Lim GY, Cha ES, et al. MR imaging of tubo-ovarian abscess. Acta Radiol. 1995; 36(5):510–514

[27] Kim SH, Kim SH, Yang DM, Kim KA. Unusual causes of tubo-ovarian abscess: CT and MR imaging findings. Radiographics. 2004; 24(6):1575–1589

[28] Forstner R, Schneider A. Acute and chronic pelvic pain disorders. In: Hamm B, Forstner R, eds. MRI and CT of the Female Pelvis. Berlin: Springer; 2007:355–378

[29] Weisner D. Entzündungen der weiblichen Genitalorgane und der Brust. In: Diedrich K, Holzgreve W, Jonat W, Schneider K-T, Schultze-Mosgau A, Weiss J, eds. Gynäkologie und Geburtshilfe. Berlin: Springer; 2007:188–209

[30] Uhl B. Benigne Veränderungen. In: Uhl B, ed. Gynäkologie und Geburtshilfe compact: alles für Station, Praxis und Facharztprüfung. Stuttgart: Thieme; 2010: 407–490

[31] Jonat W, Bauerschlag D, Schem C, et al. Gut- und bösartige gynäkologische Tumoren. In: Diedrich K, Holzgreve W, Jonat W, Schneider K-T, Schultze-Mosgau A, Weiss J, eds. Gynäkologie und Geburtshilfe. Berlin: Springer; 2007:211–298

[32] Mitchell DG, Gefter WB, Spritzer CE, et al. Polycystic ovaries: MR imaging. Radiology. 1986; 160(2):425–429

[33] Radeleff B. Ovarien. In: Hallscheidt P, Haferkamp A, eds. Urogenitale Bildgebung. Berlin: Springer; 2011:303–346

[34] Mettler L, Schmutzler A. 2007

[35] Gross M, Blumstein SL, Chow LC. Isolated fallopian tube torsion: a rare twist on a common theme. AJR Am J Roentgenol. 2005; 185(6):1590–1592

[36] Nichols DH, Julian PJ. Torsion of the adnexa. Clin Obstet Gynecol. 1985; 28(2):375–380

[37] Lubarsky M, Kalb B, Sharma P, Keim SM, Martin DR. MR imaging for acute nontraumatic abdominopelvic pain: rationale and practical considerations. Radiographics. 2013; 33(2):313–337

[38] Pedrosa I, Zeikus EA, Levine D, Rofsky NM. MR imaging of acute right lower quadrant pain in pregnant and nonpregnant patients. Radiographics. 2007; 27(3):721–743, discussion 743–753

[39] Distler W, Riehn A. Gynäkologische Notfälle. In: Distler W, Riehn A, eds. Notfälle in Gynäkologie und Geburtshilfe. 3rd ed. Heidelberg: Springer; 2006:43–62

[40] Kröncke T. Benign uterine lesions. In: Hamm B, Forstner R, eds. MRI and CT of the Female Pelvis. Berlin: Springer; 2007:61–100

[41] Schindler A. Epidemiologie, Pathogenese und Diagnostik der Endometriose. J Fertil Reprod. 2007; 17:22–27

[42] Bazot M, Darai E, Hourani R, et al. Deep pelvic endometriosis: MR imaging for diagnosis and prediction of extension of disease. Radiology. 2004; 232(2):379–389

[43] Del Frate C, Girometti R, Pittino M, Del Frate G, Bazzocchi M, Zuiani C. Deep retroperitoneal pelvic endometriosis: MR imaging appearance with laparoscopic correlation. Radiographics. 2006; 26(6):1705–1718

[44] Kinkel K, Frei KA, Balleyguier C, Chapron C. Diagnosis of endometriosis with imaging: a review. Eur Radiol. 2006; 16(2):285–298

[45] Van Gorp T, Amant F, Neven P, Vergote I, Moerman P. Endometriosis and the development of malignant tumours of the pelvis. A review of literature. Best Pract Res Clin Obstet Gynaecol. 2004; 18(2):349–371

[46] Patel MD, Feldstein VA, Chen DC, Lipson SD, Filly RA. Endometriomas: diagnostic performance of US. Radiology. 1999; 210(3):739–745

[47] Spencer JA, Forstner R, Cunha TM, Kinkel K, ESUR Female Imaging Sub-Committee. ESUR guidelines for MR imaging of the sonographically indeterminate adnexal mass: an algorithmic approach. Eur Radiol. 2010; 20(1):25–35

[48] Bazot M, Gasner A, Ballester M, Daraï E. Value of thin-section oblique axial T2-weighted magnetic resonance images to assess uterosacral ligament endometriosis. Hum Reprod. 2011; 26(2):346–353

[49] Fauconnier A, Chapron C, Dubuisson JB, Vieira M, Dousset B, Bréart G. Relation between pain symptoms and the anatomic location of deep infiltrating endometriosis. Fertil Steril. 2002; 78(4):719–726

[50] Forstner R, Kinkel K. Adnexal masses: characterization of benign ovarian lesions. In: Hamm B, Forstner R, eds. MRI and CT of the Female Pelvis. Berlin: Springer; 2007:197–232

[51] Globocan, Estimated Cancer Incidence, Mortality and Prevalence Worldwide. Available at: http://globocan.iarc.fr/Pages/fact_sheets_cancer.aspx. Accessed January 03, 2018

[52] Boronow RC, Morrow CP, Creasman WT, et al. Surgical staging in endometrial cancer: clinical-pathologic findings of a prospective study. Obstet Gynecol. 1984; 63(6):825–832

[53] Kinkel K, Kaji Y, Yu KK, et al. Radiologic staging in patients with endometrial cancer: a meta-analysis. Radiology. 1999; 212(3):711–718

[54] Sala E, Hricak H. Female pelvis. In: Reiser MF HH, Semmler W, ed. Magnetic resonance romography. Berlin: Springer; 2008:964–997

[55] Pecorelli S. Revised FIGO staging for carcinoma of the vulva, cervix, and endometrium. Int J Gynaecol Obstet. 2009; 105(2):103–104

[56] Wittekind C, Meyer H-J. International Union against Cancer. TNM: Klassifikation maligner Tumoren. Weinheim: Wiley-Blackwell; 2010

[57] Brant W. Pelvis. In: Webb W, Brant W, Major N, eds. Fundamentals of Body CT. Philadelphia: Saunders: 2006:355–376

[58] Leitlinienprogramm Onkologie: S3-Leitlinie Diagnostik, Therapie und Nachsorge der Patientin mit Zervixkarzinom. Kurzversion 1.0, 2014, AWMF 032/033OL

[59] Naganawa S, Sato C, Kumada H, Ishigaki T, Miura S, Takizawa O. Apparent diffusion coefficient in cervical cancer of the uterus: comparison with the normal uterine cervix. Eur Radiol. 2005; 15(1):71–78

[60] Zaspel U, Hamm B. Cervical cancer. In: Hamm B, Forstner R, eds. MRI and CT of the Female Pelvis. Berlin: Springer; 2007:121–180

[61] Brocker KA, Alt CD, Eichbaum M, Sohn C, Kauczor HU, Hallscheidt P. Imaging of female pelvic malignancies regarding MRI, CT, and PET/CT : part 1. Strahlenther Onkol. 2011; 187(10):611–618

[62] Pandharipande PV, Choy G, del Carmen MG, Gazelle GS, Russell AH, Lee SI. MRI and PET/CT for triaging stage IB clinically operable cervical cancer to appropriate therapy: decision analysis to assess patient outcomes. AJR Am J Roentgenol. 2009; 192(3):802–814

[63] Thill MBM, Bohlmann MK, Dittmann C, et al. Diagnostik und operative Therapie des Vulva- und Vaginalkarzinomes. Der Onkologe. 2009; 15(1):28–39

[64] Zaspel U, Hamm B. Vagina. In: Hamm B, Forstner R, eds. MRI and CT of the Female Pelvis. Berlin: Springer; 2007:275–292

[65] Alt CD, Brocker KA, Eichbaum M, et al. Imaging of female pelvic malignancies regarding MRI, CT, and PET/CT: Part 2. Strahlenther Onkol. 2011; 187(11): 705–714

[66] Deutsche Krebsgesellschaft e. V. (DKG), Deutsche Gesellschaft für Gynäkologie und Geburtshilfe e. V. (DGGG), Arbeitsgemeinschaft fur Gynäkologische Onkologie (AGO). Diagnostik und Therapie des Vulvakarzinoms und seiner Vorstufen. AWMF-Register-Nr. 015/059; 2008.

[67] Rheinthaller A, Leodolter S. Vulvakarzinom. In: Gnant M, Schlag P, eds. Chirurgische Onkologie: Strategien und Standards für die Praxis. Wien: Springer; 2008: 441–447

[68] Nucci MR, Oliva E. Gynecologic Pathology. Edinburgh: Churchill Livingstone; 2009

[69] Lee SI, Oliva E, Hahn PF, Russell AH. Malignant tumors of the female pelvic floor: imaging features that determine therapy: pictorial review. AJR Am J Roentgenol. 2011; 196(3) Suppl:S15–S23, S24–S27

[70] Kraemer B, Guengoer E, Solomayer EF, Wallwiener D, Hornung R. Stage I carcinoma of the Bartholin's gland managed with the detection of inguinal and pelvic sentinel lymph node. Gynecol Oncol. 2009; 114(2):373–374

[71] Pinn M, Austin L, Schomas D, et al. Case report from Mayo Clinic: locally advanced Bartholin gland carcinoma. Radiol Oncol. 2007; 41(2):72–79

[72] Sala E, Rockall AG, Freeman SJ, Mitchell DG, Reinhold C. The added role of MR imaging in treatment stratification of patients with gynecologic malignancies: what the radiologist needs to know. Radiology. 2013; 266(3):717–740

[73] Costa S. Vagina. In: Kaufmann M, Costa S, Scharl A, eds. Die Gynäkologie. Berlin: Springer; 2013:429–436

[74] Bashist B, Friedman WN, Killackey MA. Surgical transposition of the ovary: radiologic appearance. Radiology. 1989; 173(3):857–860

[75] Goldberg RE, Sturgeon JF. Surgically transposed ovary presenting as an intraperitoneal mass on computed tomography. Can Assoc Radiol J. 1995; 46(3):229–230

[76] Saksouk FA, Johnson SC. Recognition of the ovaries and ovarian origin of pelvic masses with CT. Radiographics. 2004; 24 Suppl 1:S133–S146

[77] Kortmann B, Reimer T, Gerber B, Klautke G, Fietkau R. Concurrent radiochemotherapy of locally recurrent or advanced sarcomas of the uterus. Strahlenther Onkol. 2006; 182(6):318–324

[78] Benz MR, Tchekmedyian N, Eilber FC, Federman N, Czernin J, Tap WD. Utilization of positron emission tomography in the management of patients with sarcoma. Curr Opin Oncol. 2009; 21(4):345–351

[79] Griffin N, Grant LA, Sala E. Magnetic resonance imaging of vaginal and vulval pathology. Eur Radiol. 2008; 18(6):1269–1280

[80] Elsayes KM, Narra VR, Dillman JR, et al. Vaginal masses: magnetic resonance imaging features with pathologic correlation. Acta Radiol. 2007; 48(8):921–933

[81] Yang DM, Kim HC, Jin W, Lee JM, Lim SJ, Lim JW. Leiomyosarcoma of the vagina: MR findings. Clin Imaging. 2009; 33(6):482–484

[82] Tateishi U, Terauchi T, Inoue T, Tobinai K. Nodal status of malignant lymphoma in pelvic and retroperitoneal lymphatic pathways: PET/CT. Abdom Imaging. 2010; 35(2):232–240

[83] Kim YS, Koh BH, Cho OK, Rhim HC. MR imaging of primary uterine lymphoma. Abdom Imaging. 1997; 22(4):441–444

[84] Cancer Stat Facts: Vulvar Cancer. Available at: http://seer.cancer.gov/statfacts/html/vulva.html. Accessed February 2,2017

[85] Leitlinienprogramm Onkologie der AWMF, Deutschen Krebsgesellschaft e. V. und Deutschen Krebshilfe e. V. S3-Leitlinie "Diagnostik, Therapie und Nachsorge maligner Ovarialtumoren". AWMF-Register-Nr. 032/035OL; 2013, and http://www.esmo.org/Guidelines/Gynaecological-Cancers/Newly-Diagnosed-and-Relapsed-Epithelial-Ovarian-Carcinoma, accessed January 03, 2018

[86] Hricak H, Chen M, Coakley FV, et al. Complex adnexal masses: detection and characterization with MR imaging—multivariate analysis. Radiology. 2000; 214(1):39–46

[87] Buy JN, Ghossain MA, Sciot C, et al. Epithelial tumors of the ovary: CT findings and correlation with US. Radiology. 1991; 178(3):811–818

[88] De Iaco P, Musto A, Orazi L, et al. FDG-PET/CT in advanced ovarian cancer staging: value and pitfalls in detecting lesions in different abdominal and pelvic quadrants compared with laparoscopy. Eur J Radiol. 2011; 80(2):e98–e103

[89] Saif MW, Tzannou I, Makrilia N, Syrigos K. Role and cost effectiveness of PET/CT in management of patients with cancer. Yale J Biol Med. 2010; 83(2):53–65

[90] Sohaib SA, Mills TD, Sahdev A, et al. The role of magnetic resonance imaging and ultrasound in patients with adnexal masses. Clin Radiol. 2005; 60(3): 340–348

[91] Kurman RJ, Shih IeM. The origin and pathogenesis of epithelial ovarian cancer: a proposed unifying theory. Am J Surg Pathol. 2010; 34(3):433–443

[92] Piek JM, van Diest PJ, Zweemer RP, et al. Dysplastic changes in prophylactically removed Fallopian tubes of women predisposed to developing ovarian cancer. J Pathol. 2001; 195(4):451–456

[93] Schneider C, Wight E, Perucchini D, Haller U, Fink D. Primary carcinoma of the fallopian tube. A report of 19 cases with literature review. Eur J Gynaecol Oncol. 2000; 21(6):578–582

[94] Koo YJ, Im KS, Kwon YS, et al. Primary fallopian tube carcinoma: a clinicopathological analysis of a rare entity. Int J Clin Oncol. 2011; 16(1):45–49

[95] Kyriazi S, Collins DJ, Morgan VA, Giles SL, deSouza NM. Diffusion-weighted imaging of peritoneal disease for noninvasive staging of advanced ovarian cancer. Radiographics. 2010; 30(5):1269–1285

[96] Low RN, Sebrechts CP, Barone RM, Muller W. Diffusion-weighted MRI of peritoneal tumors: comparison with conventional MRI and surgical and histopathologic findings-a feasibility study. AJR Am J Roentgenol. 2009; 193(2): 461–470

[97] Schünke M, Schulte E, Schumacher U. Prometheus. LernAtlas der Anatomie: Innere Organe. 2nd ed. Stuttgart: Thieme; 2009. Illustrated by M. Voll/K. Wesker

[98] Kawakami S, Togashi K, Kimura I, et al. Primary malignant tumor of the fallopian tube: appearance at CT and MR imaging. Radiology. 1993; 186(2):503–508

[99] Coakley FV, Choi PH, Gougoutas CA, et al. Peritoneal metastases: detection with spiral CT in patients with ovarian cancer. Radiology. 2002; 223(2):495–499

[100] Karlan BY, Hoh C, Tse N, Futoran R, Hawkins R, Glaspy J. Whole-body positron emission tomography with (fluorine-18)-2-deoxyglucose can detect metastatic carcinoma of the fallopian tube. Gynecol Oncol. 1993; 49(3):383–388

[101] Makhija S, Howden N, Edwards R, Kelley J, Townsend DW, Meltzer CC. Positron emission tomography/computed tomography imaging for the detection of recurrent ovarian and fallopian tube carcinoma: a retrospective review. Gynecol Oncol. 2002; 85(1):53–58

[102] Gadducci A, Landoni F, Sartori E, et al. Analysis of treatment failures and survival of patients with fallopian tube carcinoma: a cooperation task force (CTF) study. Gynecol Oncol. 2001; 81(2):150–159

[103] Puls LE, Davey DD, DePriest PD, et al. Immunohistochemical staining for CA-125 in fallopian tube carcinomas. Gynecol Oncol. 1993; 48(3):360–363

[104] Kaufmann M, Pfleiderer A. Tumoren und Veränderungen der weiblichen Geschlechtsorgane. In: Breckwoldt M, Kaufmann M, Pfleiderer A, eds. Gynäkologie und Geburtshilfe. Stuttgart: Thieme; 2011:161–237

[105] Schünke M, Schulte E, Schumacher U. Prometheus. LernAtlas der Anatomie: Allgemeine Anatomie und Bewegungssystem. 3rd ed. Stuttgart: Thieme; 2011. Illustrated by M. Voll/K. Wesker

[106] Shaaban AM, Rezvani M. Imaging of primary fallopian tube carcinoma. Abdom Imaging. 2013; 38(3):608–618

13 Male Pelvis

Tobias Franiel

13.1 Testis and Epididymis

13.1.1 Imaging

Ultrasonography, including color duplex sonography and power Doppler, is still the primary modality for imaging diseases of the testis and epididymis. MRI is a valuable adjunct that can add significant information owing to its excellent soft tissue contrast; it is used mainly to resolve discrepancies between clinical and sonographic findings. MRI is particularly helpful in the investigation of sonographically indeterminate lesions.

13.1.2 Anatomy

The normal testis in an adult is oval in shape with a long-axis diameter of 3 to 5 cm and a short-axis diameter of 2 to 4 cm (▶ Fig. 13.1). It is normal for the two testes to differ slightly in size. The testis consists of approximately 250 to 400 lobules, which are compartmentalized by a radial pattern of septa. These septa extend into the testis from the outer fibrous capsule, the tunica albuginea, and coalesce to form the mediastinum testis, which also transmits branches of the testicular artery and vein. The testicular lobules are composed of multiple tortuous seminiferous tubules, which converge centrally to form the rete testis. The rete is drained by approximately 10 to 15 excretory ducts, the efferent ductules, which transport sperm from the rete testis to the epididymis.

The elongated epididymis consists mostly of the tightly coiled epididymal duct and is approximately 6 to 7 cm long. It is located on the posterolateral side of the testis and is divisible into a head, body, and tail. The head is located at the upper pole of the testis, the tail at its lower pole. The tail gives rise to the vas deferens (ductus deferens), which enters the abdomen in the spermatic

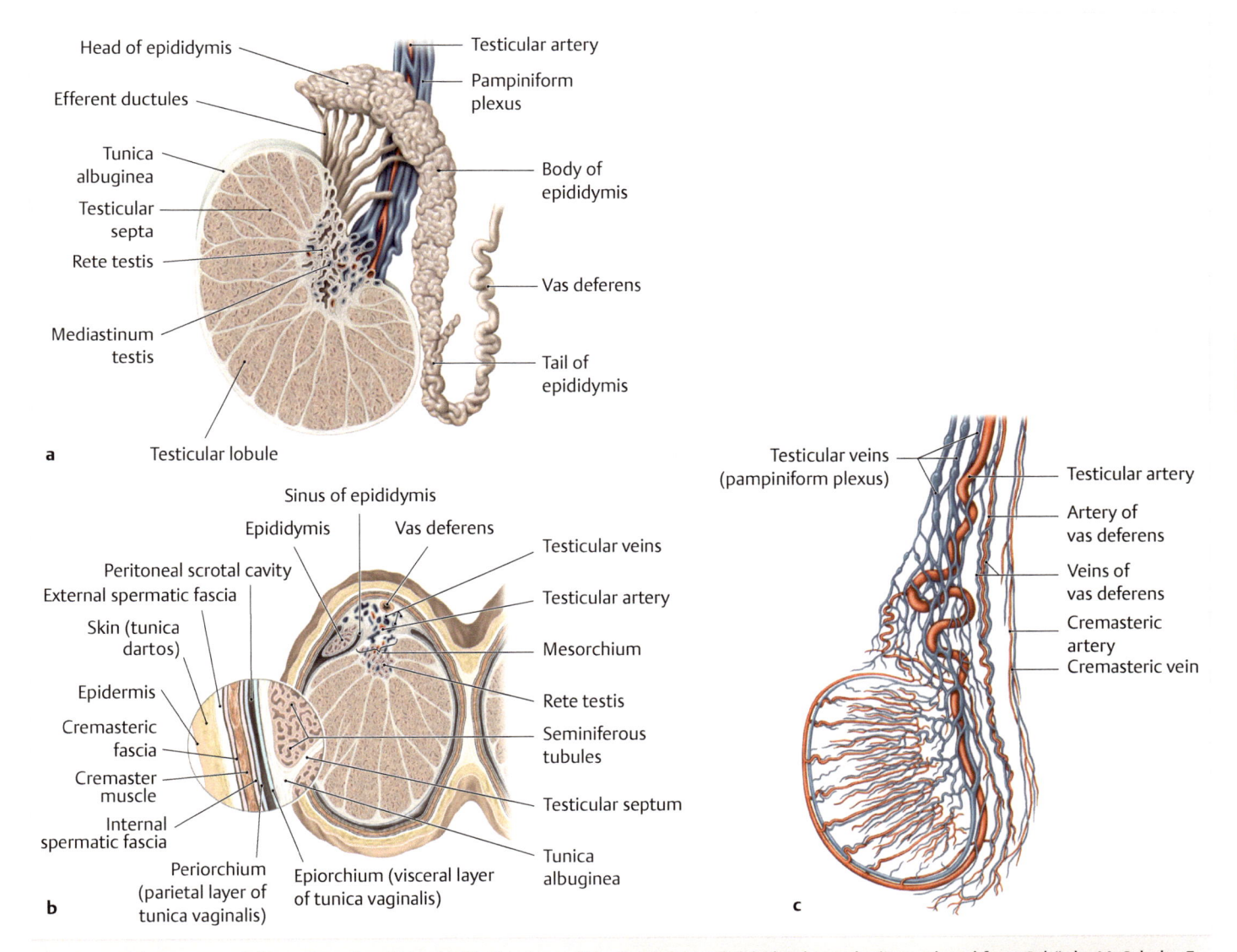

Fig. 13.1 (a) Structure of the testis and epididymis. (b) Structure of the testicular wall. (c) Blood vessels. (Reproduced from Schünke M, Schulte E, Schumacher U. Prometheus. LernAtlas der Anatomie: Innere Organe. Illustrated by M. Voll/K. Wesker. 2nd ed. Stuttgart: Thieme; 2009 and 2011.)

Male Pelvis

cord and runs from there to the prostate. The spermatic cord also transmits the testicular artery and vein, the pampiniform plexus, and the nerves and lymphatics of the testis.

The tunica vaginalis, composed of a parietal and a visceral layer, is the part of the peritoneum that preceded the descent of the testis from the abdomen into the scrotum. It forms a pouch that envelops almost all of the testis except where it connects to the epididymis. The communication between the pouch and peritoneal cavity is obliterated after birth. A small amount of fluid is normally present between the two layers of the tunica vaginalis, creating a mobile interface. The tunica vaginalis is continuous externally with the cremaster muscle, which is covered by scrotal skin. The testes are separated from each other by a fibromuscular septum derived from the subcutaneous tissue of the scrotal skin.

The testis receives its blood supply from the testicular artery. Both the right and left arteries arise from the aorta just below the renal arteries. The testicular vein collects blood from the pampiniform plexus; it opens directly into the inferior vena cava on the right side and into the left renal vein on the left side.

▶ **Sonographic landmarks.** The testis has a homogeneous, intermediate echogenicity that is interrupted only by the eccentrically placed, hyperechoic mediastinum testis (▶ Fig. 13.2). The tunica albuginea that encloses the testis appears as a thin, hyperechoic line upon the testis. The scrotal cavity, with its thin echo-free fluid rim, is most clearly visible at the head of the epididymis. The head of the epididymis, like the epididymis as a whole, is isoechoic or slightly hypoechoic and has a slightly coarser echo texture than the testis. Differentiation of the testis and epididymis is most easily accomplished in longitudinal scans.

▶ **MRI landmarks.** The testes are hyperintense on T2 W images and has homogeneous intermediate signal intensity on T1 W images (▶ Fig. 13.3). The tunica albuginea is most clearly depicted on T2 W images as a thin, hypointense band surrounding the testis. The eccentrically placed mediastinum testis is also hypointense on T1 W and T2 W images (▶ Fig. 13.4). The epididymis is slightly more heterogeneous than the testis, appearing hypo- to isointense on T1 W images and hypointense on T2 W images. The

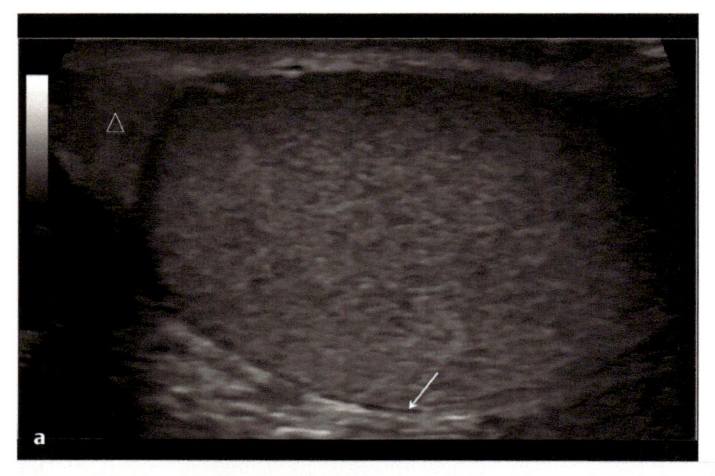

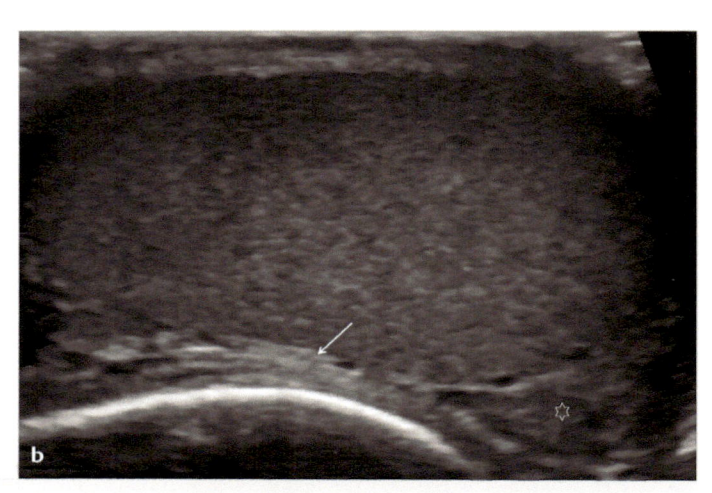

Fig. 13.2 Normal ultrasound appearance of the testis. (a) Normal testis of moderate echogenicity, viewed in longitudinal scan. Note the hyperechoic tunica albuginea bordered by a small amount of hypoechoic fluid between the parietal and visceral layers of the tunica vaginalis (arrow). The wedge-shaped feature at upper left is the head of the epididymis (triangle), which is less echogenic than the testis and shows a slightly coarser texture. (b) This scan displays the tail of the epididymis (star) and the hyperechoic mediastinum testis (arrow), which occupies an eccentric, posterolateral position.

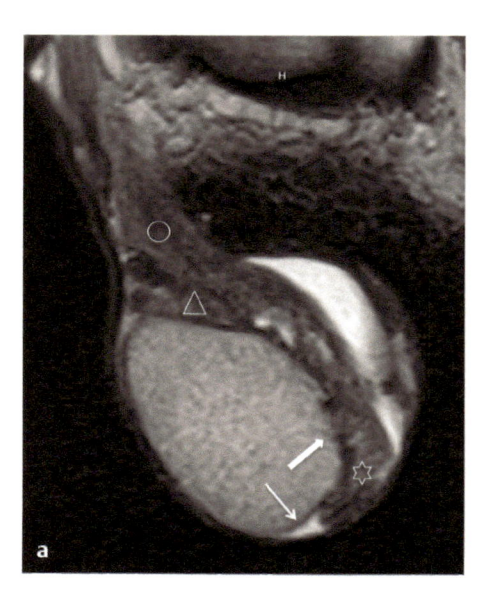

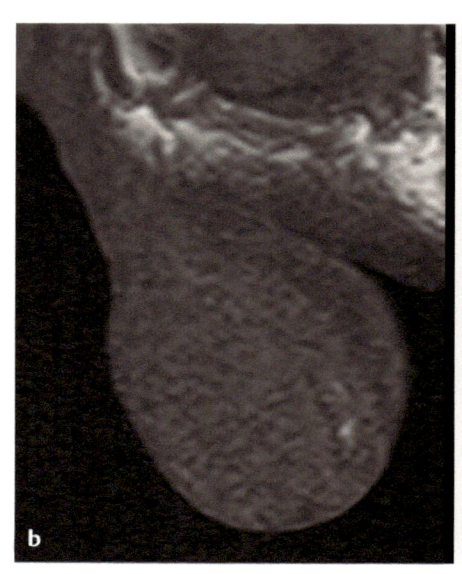

Fig. 13.3 Normal MRI appearance of the testis. Parasagittal images. (a) T2 W image. The testicular parenchyma appears hyperintense. The tunica albuginea enclosing the testis appears as a linear hypointensity (thin arrow). The mediastinum testis with the rete testis (thick arrow) forms a hypointense connection between the testis and epididymis. The head of the epididymis (star), tail of the epididymis (triangle), and spermatic cord (circle) are clearly visualized. (b) T1 W image. The testis and epididymis are poorly differentiated from each other on T1 W images, as both appear hypointense.

13.1 Testis and Epididymis

epididymis enhances more than the testis after IV administration of contrast medium.

13.1.3 Congenital Disorders: Cryptorchidism (Undescended Testis)

▶ **Brief definition.** Normally the testis descends through the inguinal canal and into the scrotum during the 36th week of gestation. Cryptorchidism is a condition in which the testis remains undescended or maldescended, causing it to be absent from the scrotum. An incompletely descended testis is usually within the inguinal canal and will complete its descent during the first year of life. An undescended testis may also be located within the abdomen or at ectopic sites outside the normal track of descent.

▶ **Imaging signs.** The undescended testis appears small and hypoechoic on ultrasound (▶ Fig. 13.5). If the testis is not found during ultrasound scanning, it should be located by MRI or, alternatively, by laparoscopy. On MRI the undescended testis is hypointense in the T1 W sequence and hyperintense in the T2 W sequence. If the testis is atrophic, it will show decreased signal intensity on T2 W images. An undescended testis often shows little or no enhancement after IV administration of contrast medium.

▶ **Clinical features.** Failure of a testicle to descend during the first year of life may result in infertility because the intra-abdominal body temperature is higher than the scrotal temperature. This temperature differential also increases the risk of developing testicular cancer.

▶ **Pitfalls.** The undescended testis may be misinterpreted as a lymph node.

▶ **Key points.** Cryptorchidism refers to a maldescended or undescended testis. The testis is often located in the inguinal canal, where it is easily identified with ultrasound. An intra-abdominal testis is detectable by laparoscopy or MRI. Cryptorchidism is associated with an increased risk of testicular cancer.

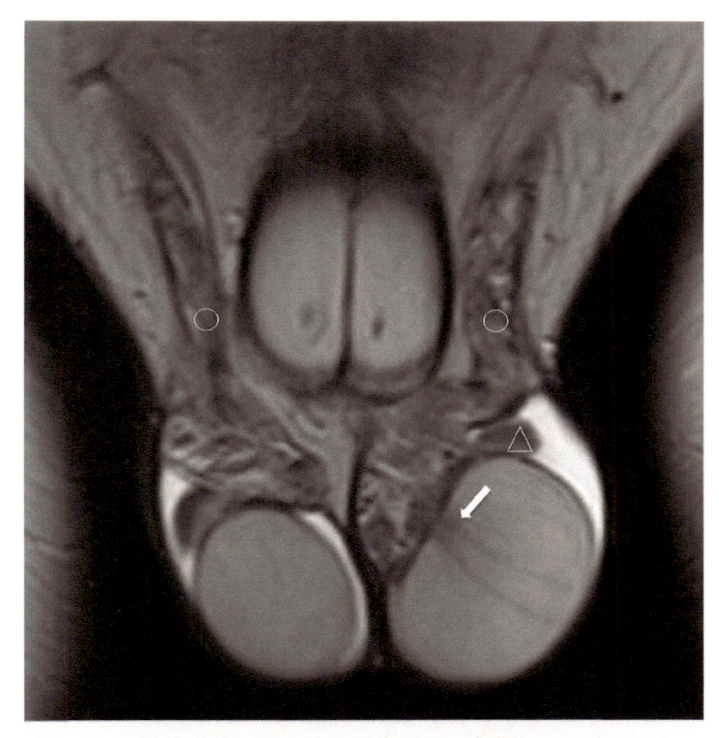

Fig. 13.4 Normal MRI appearance of the testis. The septa permeating the testis and the mediastinum testis (arrow) appear hypointense in this paracoronal T2 W image. The head of the epididymis (triangle) and the spermatic cords (circles) in the inguinal canal are also clearly displayed. The medial oval structures are the corpora cavernosa of the penis.

13.1.4 Vascular Diseases

Varicocele

▶ **Brief definition.** A varicocele is formed by dilated, tortuous veins in the pampiniform plexus. Idiopathic varicocele results from incompetent venous valves and is a frequent cause of infertility. A secondary varicocele is caused by hampered venous return in the testicular vein due to a rise of retroperitoneal pressure (e.g., retroperitoneal mass or hydronephrosis) or inferior vena cava thrombosis.

▶ **Imaging signs.** Ultrasound scans should be performed in both the standing and supine positions and should include a Valsalva maneuver. The probe can be moved down along the spermatic

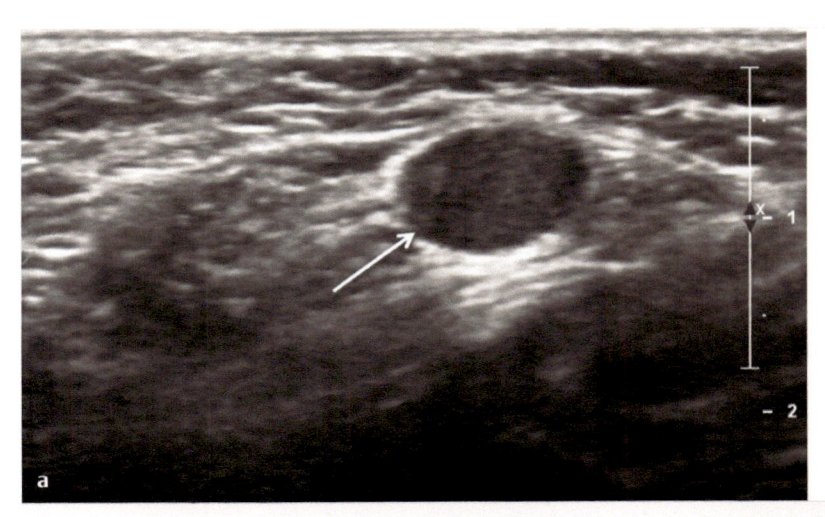

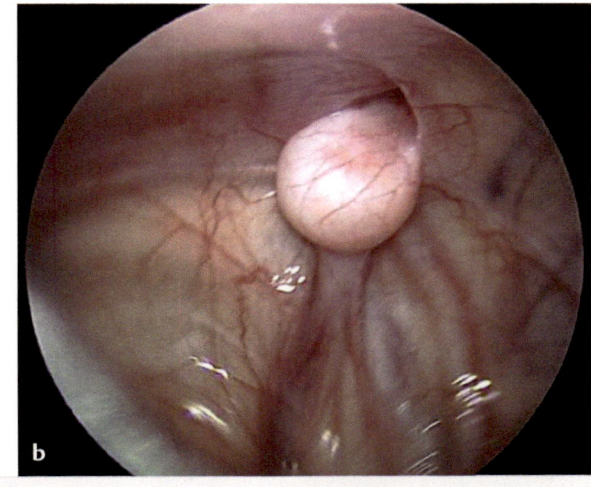

Fig. 13.5 Cryptorchidism (undescended testis). (a) Ultrasound B-mode image reveals the small, hypoechoic undescended testis (arrow) in the inguinal canal at the level of the internal (superficial) inguinal ring. (b) Corresponding laparoscopic view.

cord to the pampiniform plexus. Scans at that level will demonstrate multiple dilated, tortuous veins more than 2 to 3 mm in diameter in the spermatic cord and around the epididymis. Blood flow in the affected area is very slow and can be detected by color duplex sonography at sensitive settings. Idiopathic varicoceles tend to drain when the patient is positioned supine, whereas secondary varicoceles persist; MRI does not have a role in making this determination. The internal spermatic vein is classified into different anatomical types based on the presence of collateral vessels to renal capsular vessels, lumbar veins, or the inferior vena cava. The collaterals are visualized during interventional therapy by injecting contrast material into the left renal vein or by selective catheterization. The presence of collaterals will determine the risk of reflux of sclerosant and the risk of recurrence after interventional sclerotherapy.

▶ **Clinical features.** Most varicoceles are asymptomatic and are often detected incidentally in a morphologically normal scrotum. They are more common on the left side because the testicular vein drains at a 90° angle into the left renal vein. Symptomatic patients may complain of tension or position-dependent pain that is exacerbated by standing or walking. These cases can be treated by interventional sclerotherapy with access through the (right) common femoral vein and selective catheterization of the left testicular vein.

▶ **Pitfalls.** The varicocele may be missed if the examination is performed only in the supine position and/or without a Valsalva maneuver.

▶ **Differential diagnosis.** The clinical differential diagnosis includes hydroceles, spermatoceles, hernias, and testicular tumors. These conditions are easily differentiated from one another by imaging.

▶ **Key points.** Varicoceles are caused by dilated, tortuous veins in the pampiniform plexus. They are diagnosed by B-mode ultrasound imaging and color duplex scanning in both the standing and supine positions, aided by a Valsalva maneuver. The diagnosis of a secondary varicocele requires the exclusion of a retroperitoneal mass (e.g., renal tumor).

Testicular Torsion

▶ **Brief definition.** Supravaginal testicular torsion, which is more common in newborns, is distinguished etiologically from intravaginal torsion of the spermatic cord, which is much more common in adolescents and adults. A predisposing factor for intravaginal torsion is the "bell clapper" deformity, in which the tunica vaginalis completely surrounds the testis, allowing the spermatic cord to become twisted on its longitudinal axis. The degree of spermatic cord torsion dictates the severity of decreased arterial blood flow. Interruption of venous drainage leads to hemorrhagic infarction of the testicular parenchyma.

▶ **Imaging signs.** Both sides should be imaged sonographically and the affected testis compared with the nonpainful side. In the acute stage of testicular torsion (the first 6 hours), the testis is enlarged and has a heterogeneous, hypoechoic appearance. The epididymis is also enlarged and is heterogeneously hypoechoic. A thin hydrocele may additionally be present. In cases where the torsion is undiagnosed, the subacute stage (the next 5 days) is marked by increasing enlargement of the testis and epididymis, which exhibit a more heterogeneous echo pattern. Unless the torsion is reduced, the testis will become atrophic and show decreasing echogenicity. Absence of flow signal in the affected testis on color duplex sonography or power Doppler confirms the diagnosis of testicular torsion (▶ Fig. 13.6). Milder degrees of torsion (less than 360°) may initially compromise only venous flow in the affected testis while arterial blood flow is still detectable, although it is often diminished relative to the opposite side.

▶ **Clinical features.** Testicular torsion presents with acute pain of sudden onset in the affected testis or scrotum.

▶ **Pitfalls.** Detectable blood flow in the affected testis does not exclude testicular torsion, especially if it is decreased relative to the opposite side.

Note

In doubtful cases where testicular torsion is suspected but blood flow is present, the testis should be surgically exposed.

▶ **Differential diagnosis.** After acute epididymitis or epididymo-orchitis, testicular torsion is the second most common cause of acute testicular or scrotal pain. Absence of flow signal in the affected testis confirms testicular torsion, while increased blood flow is suggestive of epididymo-orchitis. Another differential diagnosis is torsion of the testicular or epididymal appendix.

▶ **Key points.** Testicular torsion is marked by acute onset of severe pain in the testis or scrotum. The cause is torsion of the spermatic cord about its long axis, compromising arterial blood flow to the testis. The testis may be devoid of flow signal by color duplex and power Doppler ultrasonography, or milder degrees of torsion may cause diminished flow relative to the opposite side.

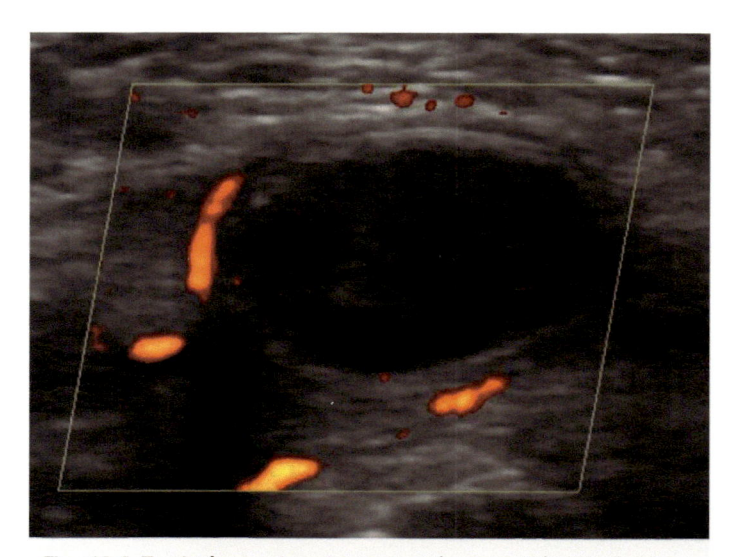

Fig. 13.6 Testicular torsion. Power Doppler image shows a hypoechoic testis that is devoid of flow signals and occupies an abnormally high position. The absence of detectable blood flow confirms testicular torsion. The hypoechoic testicular parenchyma indicates an older process.

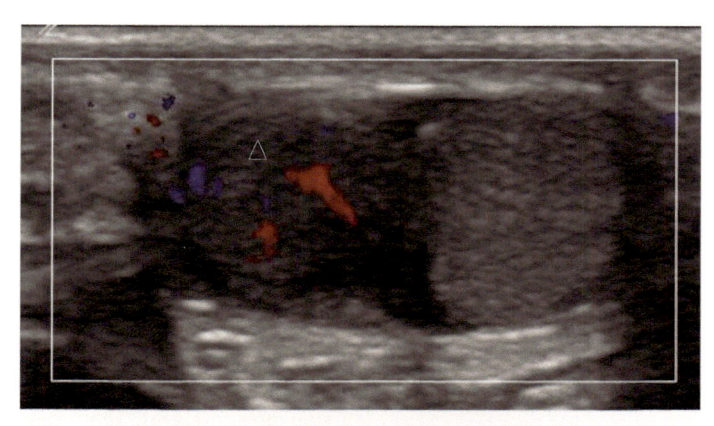

Fig. 13.7 Epididymitis. Longitudinal ultrasound scan of the testis shows an enlarged epididymal head (triangle) with increased color flow signals.

13.1.5 Inflammatory Diseases: Epididymitis and Epididymo-orchitis

▶ **Brief definition.** Inflammations of the epididymis and testis are the most frequent cause of acute testicular and scrotal pain. Acute epididymitis very often results from an ascending bacterial infection of the lower urinary tract. It usually affects the head of the epididymis, although the entire epididymis may be involved. Isolated orchitis may occur in a setting of mumps.

▶ **Imaging signs.** Sonographically, the affected portions of the epididymis are enlarged and hypoechoic to normal surrounding tissue. Color duplex and power Doppler ultrasonography show increased blood flow (▶ Fig. 13.7). If the testis is also affected (acute epididymo-orchitis), it appears enlarged and shows increased blood flow by color duplex and power Doppler ultrasonography. Its echo pattern in the B-mode image is heterogeneously hypoechoic. In more severe cases of epididymo-orchitis, the inflammatory process may give rise to a testicular abscess. Ultrasound in this case will show a heterogeneous fluid collection with a hypervascular rim within the enlarged testis. On MRI, the affected epididymis is enlarged and shows a heterogeneous, predominantly hyperintense signal pattern on T2W images. Cases complicated by intrascrotal hemorrhage show variable T1W and T2W signal characteristics depending on the age of the hemorrhage. Inflamed areas enhance intensely after administration of gadolinium contrast. In the case of orchitis, affected areas show homogeneous to heterogeneous hyperintensity on T2W images.

▶ **Clinical features.** Epididymitis and epididymo-orchitis present clinically with increasing pain that is exacerbated by pressure and movement. Physical lifting of the testis relieves pain due to epididymitis (positive Prehn's sign). Fever and voiding problems may also be present.

▶ **Differential diagnosis.** Differentiation is required mainly from testicular torsion. In contrast to epididymitis, increased blood flow is not seen on color duplex sonography. A testicular tumor may cause diagnostic confusion, especially in patients with chronic inflammatory testicular changes.

▶ **Key points.** Inflammatory changes in the testis and epididymis account for the majority of acute, painful scrotal diseases. On ultrasound the affected areas are enlarged and heterogeneously hypoechoic. Color duplex and power Doppler ultrasonography show increased blood flow.

13.1.6 Traumatic Disorders: Testicular Trauma

▶ **Brief definition.** The testis is susceptible to injury by blunt or penetrating trauma. Testicular rupture constitutes a urological emergency, in which ultrasound plays a key diagnostic role.

▶ **Imaging signs.** The ruptured testis has indistinct margins and an irregular contour. Sonographically, the testicular parenchyma shows heterogeneous echogenicity as a result of intratesticular hemorrhage and infarction. Extratesticular blood collections (epididymal hemorrhage, hematocele) may hinder the examination. Switching to color duplex and/or power Doppler mode during the examination is very helpful in distinguishing between vascularized testicular parenchyma and nonvascularized hematoma. MRI is excellent for evaluating the integrity of the tunica albuginea on T2W images. Additionally, the injured testis appears hypointense to the uninjured side on T2W images and shows less enhancement on T1W images after administration of gadolinium contrast medium. The appearance of intratesticular hematomas depends on the age of the collection. Acute hematomas show decreased signal intensity on T1W images and increased signal intensity on T2W images. Chronic hematomas, on the other hand, are hyperintense in both T1W and T2W sequences.

▶ **Clinical features.** The testis is painful and the scrotal skin shows livid discoloration. Extensive hematomas are most often found in association with blunt trauma.

▶ **Pitfalls.** A common error is to omit daily ultrasound follow-ups of hematomas that have not been surgically evacuated.

▶ **Key points.** The testis may be injured as a result of acute or blunt trauma. The initial imaging study of choice is ultrasonography. The affected testis shows a heterogeneous echo pattern due to intratesticular hemorrhage and infarction. Extratesticular hematomas are a common associated finding. MRI is best for assessing the integrity of the tunica albuginea.

13.1.7 Benign Intrascrotal Masses

Hydrocele

▶ **Brief definition.** Hydrocele is a collection of excessive fluid (small amounts are normal) between the parietal and visceral layers of the tunica vaginalis and is the most common cause of testicular swelling. Congenital hydrocele results from persistent patency of the vaginal process; this type will resolve as the process obliterates during the first year of life. Acquired hydroceles may result from prior trauma, epididymitis or epididymo-orchitis, inguinal hernia, or a testicular tumor. Acquired hydroceles may also be idiopathic.

▶ **Imaging signs.** Idiopathic hydrocele is composed of serous fluid that appears echo-free on ultrasound (▶ Fig. 13.8). This differs from traumatic hematocele and pyocele in a setting of acute

Male Pelvis

epididymitis or epididymo-orchitis, which are hypoechoic and contain echogenic septa and protein precipitates that create internal echoes. On MRI, hydroceles are diagnosed in association with other testicular diseases and show typical fluid signal characteristics (hypointense in T1 W sequences, hyperintense in T2 W sequences). MRI is not used for the initial diagnosis of hydroceles. Testicular and epididymal appendices are most clearly visualized when a hydrocele is present. They are embryonic remnants that are normally only a few millimeters long and may be found at the upper pole of the testis or epididymis.

▶ **Clinical features.** Hydroceles are painless and may gradually increase in size. The enlargement may be perceived as a sensation of pressure or heaviness.

▶ **Pitfalls.** A hydrocele with internal septa may be mistaken for a spermatocele in the B-mode image.

▶ **Differential diagnosis.** Pyoceles and hematoceles have internal echoes and sometimes contain septa. Color duplex and power Doppler scans show the presence of flow signals in spermatoceles.

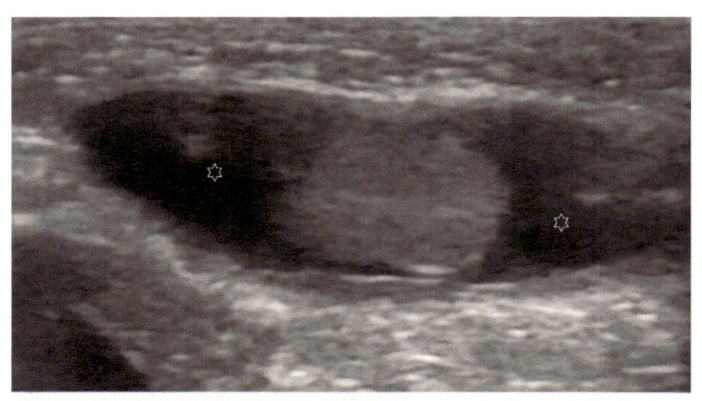

Fig. 13.8 **Testicular hydrocele.** With a hydrocele (stars), the normal testis is surrounded by an abnormally increased volume of serous fluid.

▶ **Key points.** Hydrocele is a painless fluid collection between the two layers of the tunica vaginalis. The imaging modality of choice is ultrasound, which shows an echo-free fluid collection devoid of flow signals. Acquired hydroceles contain internal echoes caused by precipitated proteins and are often septated.

Spermatocele

▶ **Brief definition.** Spermatoceles are located within the head of the epididymis. They may result from prior trauma or epididymitis. Spermatocele is composed of protein-rich fluid with cellular breakdown products.

▶ **Imaging signs.** A spermatocele appears sonographically as a well-circumscribed, echo-free to hypoechoic mass with internal echoes and posterior acoustic enhancement (▶ Fig. 13.9). On MRI it displays typical cystlike fluid characteristics (hypointense in T1 W sequences, hyperintense in T2 W sequences; ▶ Fig. 13.10).

▶ **Clinical features.** Spermatoceles do not cause complaints. They are often noted as incidental findings. Spermatoceles may be associated with a dull aching sensation.

▶ **Differential diagnosis**
- *Simple epididymal cyst*: This lesion is less common than spermatocele and may occur anywhere in the epididymis. It is echo-free on ultrasound and shows posterior acoustic enhancement. On MRI it presents smooth margins and is hypointense in T1 W sequences and hyperintense in T2 W sequences (▶ Fig. 13.11).
- *Testicular and tunica cysts*: A testicular cyst is located within the testis close to the mediastinum, while a tunica cyst is located in the tunica albuginea (▶ Fig. 13.12).

▶ **Key points.** A spermatocele is composed of protein-rich fluid and is located in the epididymal head. It presents smooth margins. Sonographically it is echo-free to hypoechoic with internal echoes and shows posterior acoustic enhancement. The differential

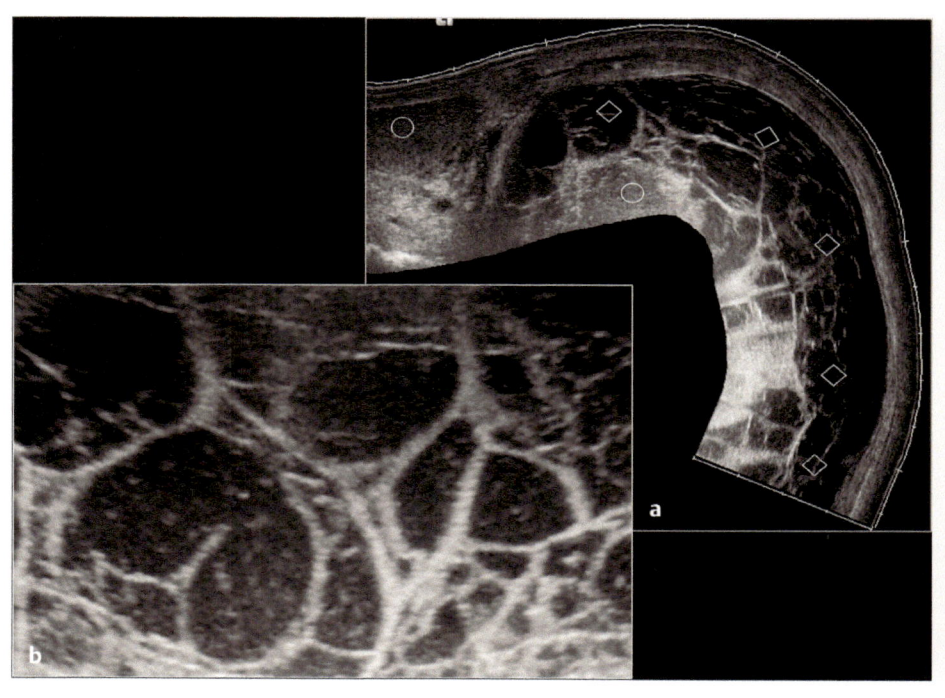

Fig. 13.9 **Large spermatocele.** (a) Composite longitudinal ultrasound scans of a spermatocele (diamonds) permeating the entire epididymis. The scans include sections of normal testis (circles) on the ipsilateral and contralateral sides. (b) Magnified view displays the hypoechoic cystic structures with internal echoes.

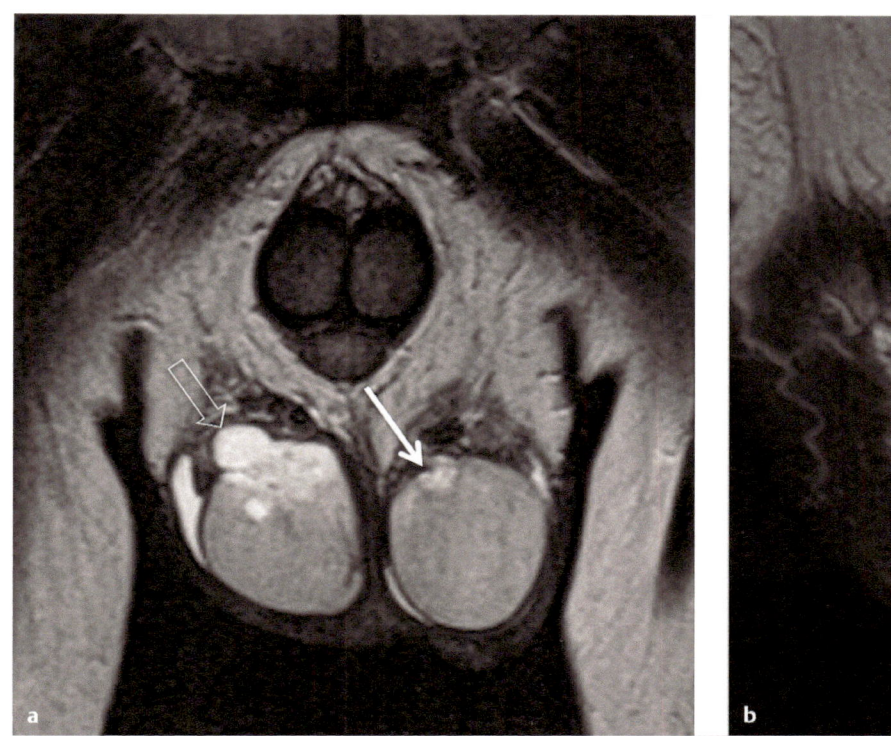

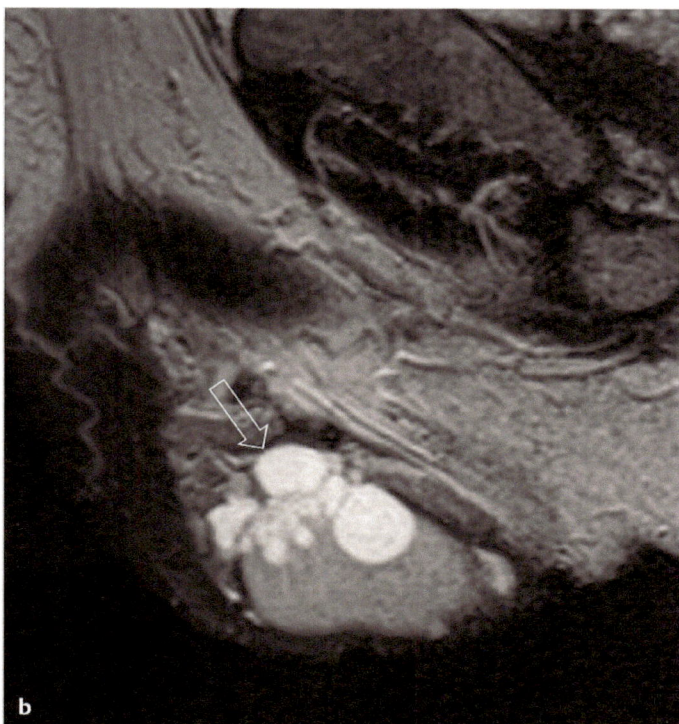

Fig. 13.10 Spermatocele in the head of the epididymis. T2W images of a spermatocele in the right epididymal head ([a], [b], open arrows). A smaller spermatocele in the left epididymal head ([a], arrow) is also shown. (a) Coronal T2W image. (b) Sagittal T2W image.

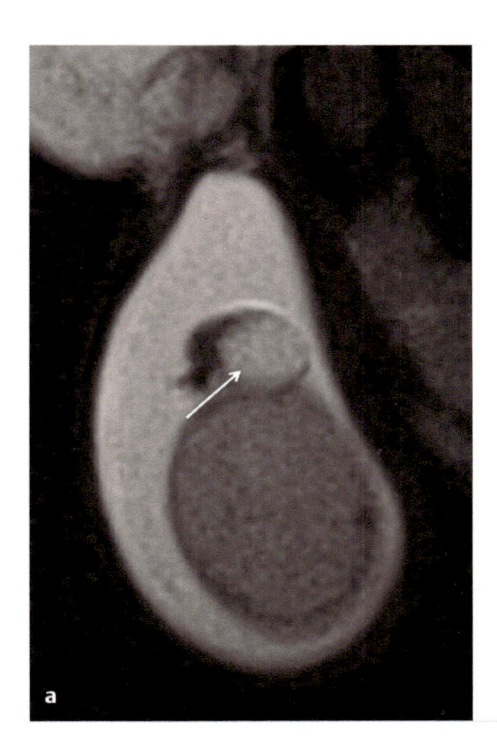

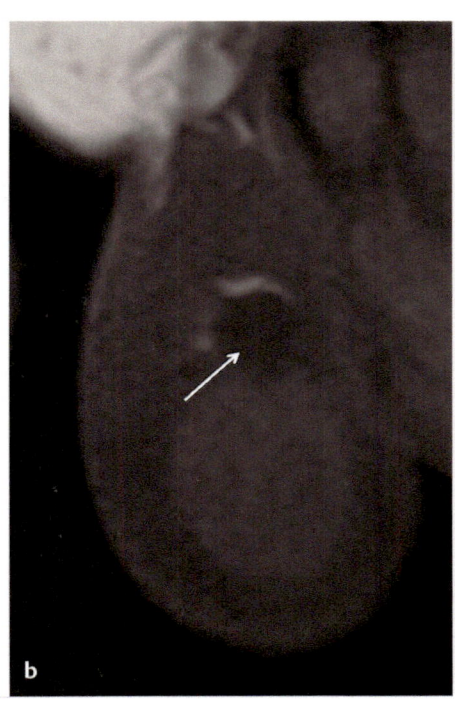

Fig. 13.11 Simple epididymal cyst. Typical appearance of a simple cyst in the epididymal head ([a], [b], arrows). The well-circumscribed cyst is hyperintense in the T2W image (a) and hypointense in the T1W image (b). A hydrocele is also present. (a) T2W image. (b) T1W image.

diagnosis includes simple epididymal cysts as well as testicular and tunica cysts.

Testicular Microlithiasis

▶ **Brief definition.** Testicular microlithiasis is defined as the presence of multiple microcalcifications in a normal or undescended testis. The microcalcifications are 1 to 2 mm in size and are located in the seminiferous tubules of the testicular lobules. The pathogenesis of testicular microlithiasis is not fully understood, but it is currently believed that the calcifications result from cellular necrosis. Testicular microcalcifications are a predisposing factor for the development of testicular cancer. Consequently, these patients should be scheduled for regular ultrasound follow-ups and laboratory tests for tumor markers.

▶ **Imaging signs.** Ultrasound shows multiple 1- to 2-mm hyperechoic lesions distributed diffusely in the testicular parenchyma

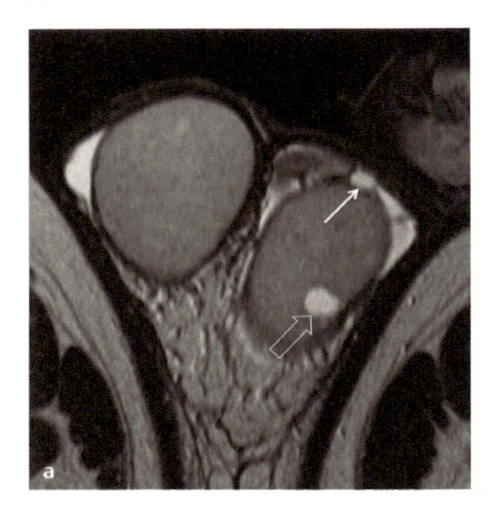

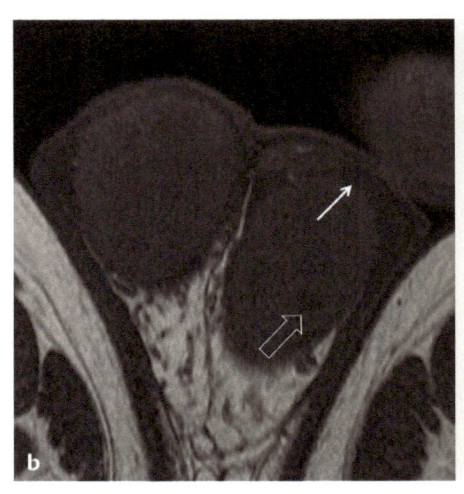

Fig. 13.12 Testicular cyst and tunica cyst. The testicular cyst ([a], [b], open arrows) and tunica cyst ([a], [b], arrows) show typical high signal intensity in the T2W image (a) and low signal intensity in the T1W image (b). (a) Axial T2W image. (b) Axial T1W image.

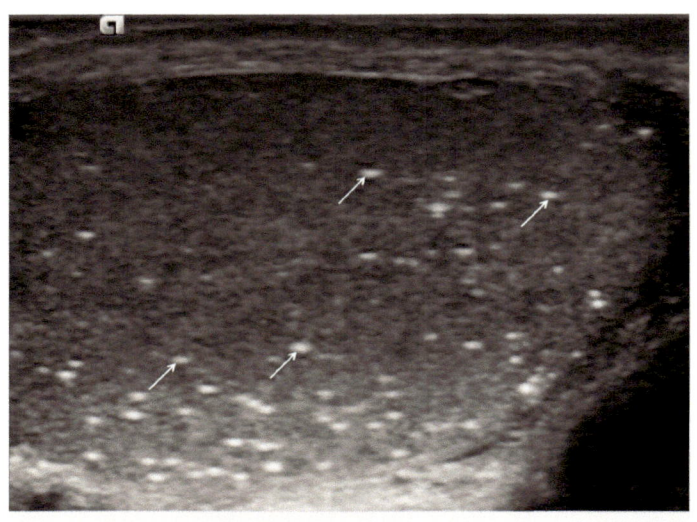

Fig. 13.13 Testicular microlithiasis. The diffusely distributed microcalcifications in testicular microlithiasis appear sonographically as small hyperechoic foci (arrows) in the testicular parenchyma, which shows normal echogenicity.

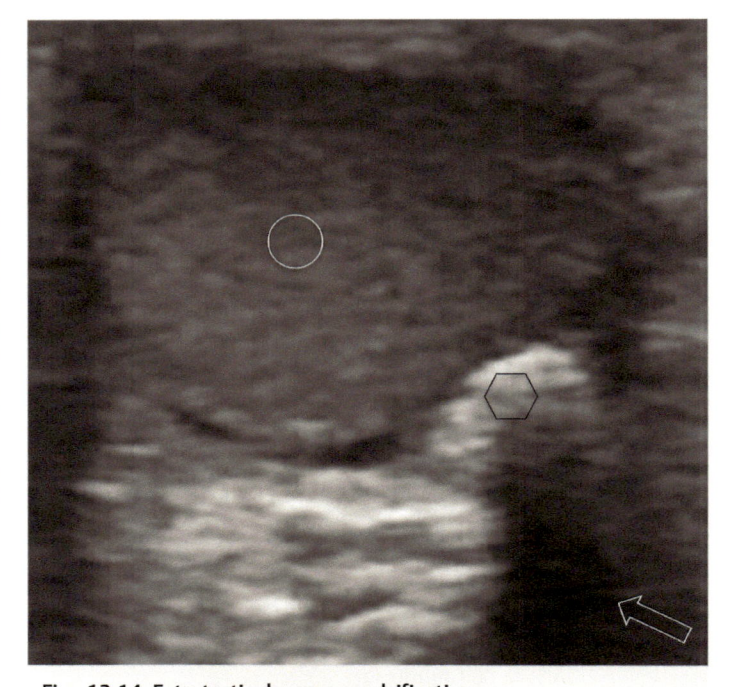

Fig. 13.14 Extratesticular macrocalcification. A macrocalcification (hexagon) is found outside the testis (circle) following trauma with an associated hematoma. An acoustic shadow (arrow) is present posterior to the macrocalcification.

(▶ Fig. 13.13). MRI aids in the detection or exclusion of suspicious focal lesions revealed by ultrasound.

▶ **Clinical features.** Testicular microlithiasis is an incidental finding and does not cause complaints.

▶ **Pitfalls.** A common error is failure to maintain follow-up in patients with microlithiasis.

▶ **Differential diagnosis.** Differentiation is mainly required from microcalcifications associated with testicular tumors or previous trauma (▶ Fig. 13.14).

▶ **Key points.** Ultrasound in patients with testicular microlithiasis shows multiple, diffusely distributed echogenic lesions 1 to 2 mm in size (microcalcifications).

> **Note**
>
> Microlithiasis has a strong association with testicular tumors and these patients should be scheduled for regular ultrasound follow-ups.

13.1.8 Malignant Neoplasms

Testicular Tumors

▶ **Brief definition.** Testicular tumors are subdivided into three main groups:
- Germ cell tumors (ca. 90% of all testicular tumors).
- Sex cord-stromal tumors (ca. 5% of all testicular tumors).
- Lymphomas and metastases.

They are the most common tumors in males 20 to 40 years of age. Three different classifications are currently used for the description of testicular tumors and their metastasis:
- TNM classification (▶ Table 13.1).
- Lugano classification for staging and response assessment (▶ Table 13.2).
- Classification of the International Germ Cell Cancer Collaborative Group (IGCCCG) for defining prognostic groups.

Table 13.1 TNM classification of testicular cancer

Designation	Description
Primary tumor	
Tx	Primary tumor cannot be assessed
T0	No evidence of a primary tumor (e.g., if only scar is found in the testis, same as burned-out tumor)
Tis	Intratubular germ cell neoplasia (carcinoma in situ)
T1	Tumor limited to the testis and epididymis
T2	Tumor limited to the testis and epididymis, with involvement of lymphatics or blood vessels of the tunica vaginalis
T3	Tumor invades the spermatic cord
T4	Tumor invades the scrotum
Regional lymph nodes	
Nx	Regional lymph nodes cannot be assessed
N0	No regional lymph node metastasis
N1	Metastasis with a lymph node mass ≤ 2 cm in greatest dimension and ≤ 5 nodes positive
N2	Metastasis with a lymph node mass > 2 cm but ≤ 5 cm in greatest dimension; or > 5 nodes positive, none > 5 cm
N3	Metastasis with a lymph node mass > 5 cm in greatest dimension
Distant metastasis	
M0	No distant metastasis
M1	Distant metastasis
Serum tumor markers	
Sx	Marker studies not available
S0	Marker study levels within normal limits
S1	LDH < 1.5 times normal *and* β-HCG < 5,000 mIU/mL *and* AFP < 1,000 ng/mL
S2	LDH 1.5–10 times normal *or* β-HCG 5,000–50,000 mIU/mL *or* AFP 1,000–10,000 ng/mL
S3	LDH > 10 times normal *or* β-HCG > 50,000 mIU/mL *or* AFP > 10,000 ng/mL

Abbreviations: AFP, alpha-fetoprotein; hCG, human chorionic gonadotropin; LDH, lactate dehydrogenase.

▶ **Clinical features.** Testicular tumors present clinically as a firm, painless testicular mass that slowly enlarges over time and may be accompanied by a hydrocele. Bleeding into the tumor or tunica is associated with acute pain. Hormone-secreting tumors may lead to gynecomastia, premature virilization, and decreased libido.

▶ **Pitfalls.** The presence of a hydrocele may direct attention away from a possible coexisting tumor.

▶ **Differential diagnosis.** Testicular tumors require differentiation from focal orchitis. The testis in patients with focal orchitis contains solitary or multiple hypoechoic areas. The chronic form in particular is difficult to distinguish from a testicular tumor.

Table 13.2 Lugano classification of testicular cancer. Stages based on CT or MRI are indicated by the prefix "c" (for "clinical"). Stages based on postoperative histology are indicated by the prefix "p" (for "pathology")

Stage	Description
I	No evidence of metastases
IIA	Retroperitoneal lymph node metastases < 2 cm
IIB	Retroperitoneal lymph node metastases 2–5 cm
IIC	Retroperitoneal lymph node metastases > 5 cm
III	Supradiaphragmatic lymph node metastases and/or hematogenous metastases

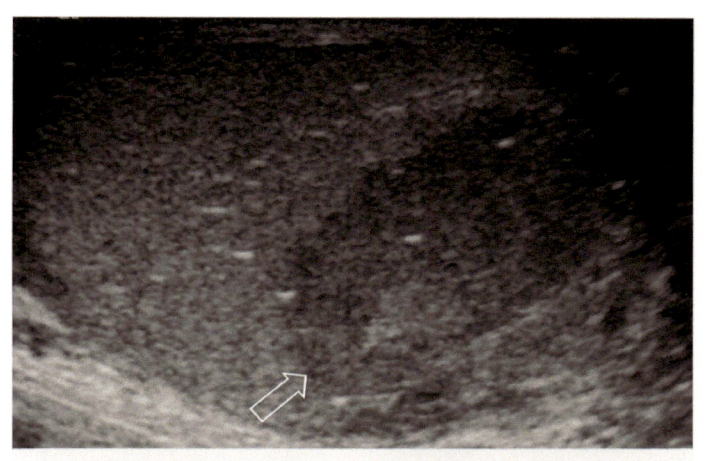

Fig. 13.15 **Seminoma.** Ultrasound depicts a homogeneously hypoechoic mass (arrow) in the testis with testicular microlithiasis, which is a predisposing factor for testicular cancer.

Infarction in the setting of epididymo-orchitis with associated hemorrhage may likewise appear as a heterogeneous hypoechoic area. The radiological differential diagnosis also includes abscesses and granulomas. Most testicular tumors measuring 1.5 cm or more in diameter will show increased blood flow by Doppler ultrasound. While this method cannot provide a more specific tumor diagnosis, it can clearly differentiate a vascularized testicular tumor from an avascular hematoma. This is particularly important in patients with a known trauma history.

Germ Cell Tumors

Seminoma

▶ **Brief definition.** Seminoma is the most common cell type (40% of testicular tumors), with a peak incidence between 30 and 50 years of age. Seminomas are round to oval-shaped tumors and may have smooth or ill-defined margins.

▶ **Imaging signs.** When imaged with ultrasound, seminomas are homogeneously hypoechoic to surrounding testicular tissue (▶ Fig. 13.15). They may contain cysts. Color duplex and power Doppler sonography show a heterogeneous flow signal within the tumor. On MRI, these tumors typically show homogeneous low signal intensity on T2W images and are isointense on T1W images. Heterogeneous areas within the seminoma are due to regressive changes (e.g., necrosis). Seminomas show inhomogeneous enhancement after administration of gadolinium contrast medium. Neither ultrasound nor MRI can supply an accurate histological classification or positively distinguish seminomas from nonseminomatous tumors and sex cord-stromal tumors.

▶ **Key points.** Seminomas present clinically as a painless mass that is sometimes accompanied by a hydrocele. They are homogeneously hypoechoic on ultrasound scans but may contain cystic components. On MRI they are isointense in T1 W sequences and hypointense in T2 W sequences. Cysts, when present, produce a heterogeneous appearance.

Nonseminomatous Tumors

▶ **Brief definition.** Nonseminomatous tumors comprise approximately 50% of all testicular tumors. They include teratoma, embryonal cell carcinoma, yolk sac tumor, and choriocarcinoma:
- *Teratoma*: Teratomas occur predominantly in children and in young adults of 25 to 30 years of age. They can be classified as mature, immature, or teratomas with malignant transformation.
- *Embryonal cell carcinoma*: These tumors are most common in patients between 25 and 35 years of age. Generally they are more aggressive and tend to invade the tunica albuginea and metastasize outside the testis.
- *Choriocarcinoma*: Choriocarcinoma is the rarest germ cell tumor and occurs in patients 20 to 40 years of age. It is very aggressive and often metastasizes by both the lymphogenous and hematogenous routes. Choriocarcinoma can metastasize even in the absence of a detectable solid intratesticular tumor. It is common in these cases to find a "burned-out" tumor in the testis, presumably because rapid, aggressive tumor growth has outstripped the blood supply.

▶ **Imaging signs.** Nonseminomatous tumors have a more heterogeneous sonographic appearance than seminomas due to the presence of echo-free cysts, echogenic calcifications with acoustic shadows, and hypoechoic hemorrhagic areas with internal echoes (▶ Fig. 13.16). In the case of teratoma, the calcifications are often found within areas of cartilage, bone and/or fibrous tissue. Embryonal cell carcinoma, like choriocarcinoma, generally has ill-defined lobulated margins. As a rule, however, the different entities cannot be positively distinguished from one another by B-mode ultrasound, color duplex, or power Doppler due to a broad overlap of findings. Nonseminomatous tumors have a

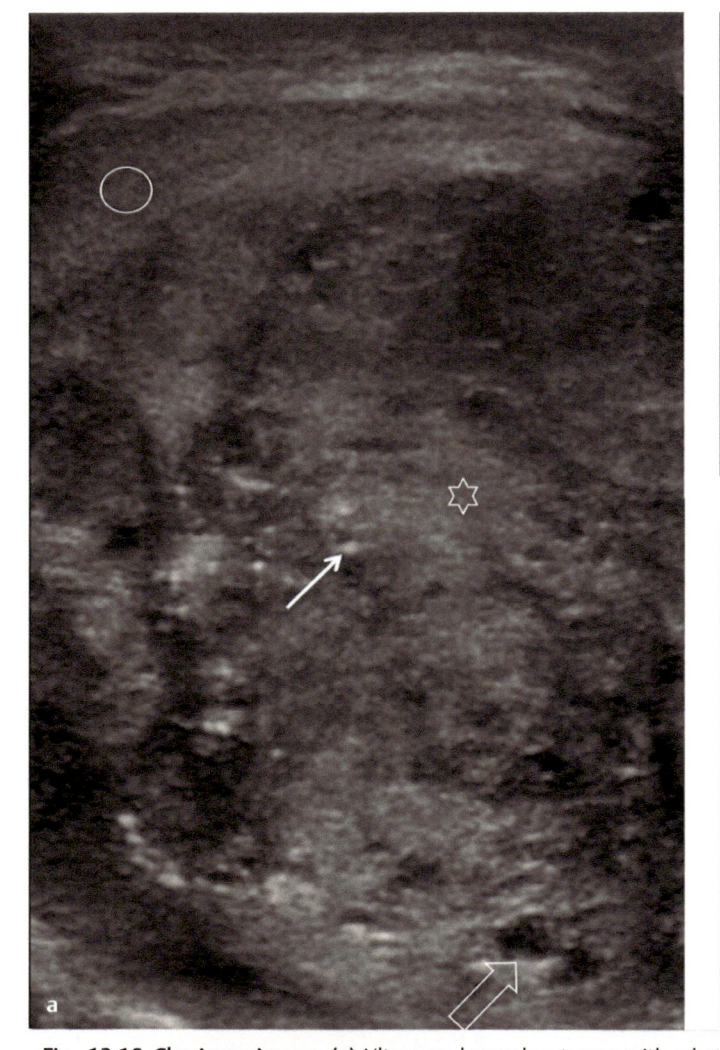

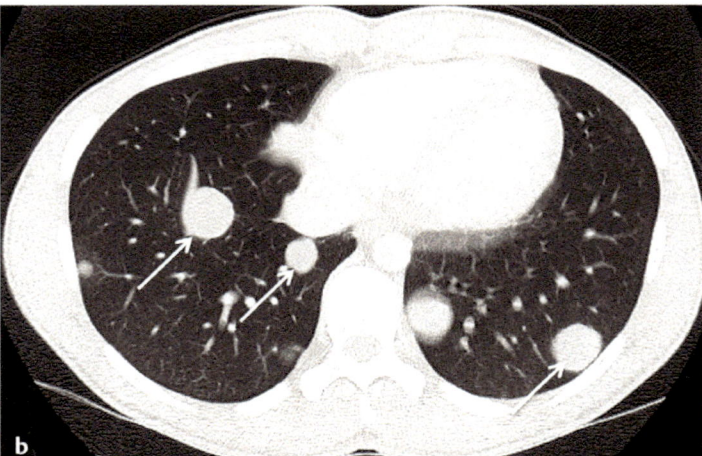

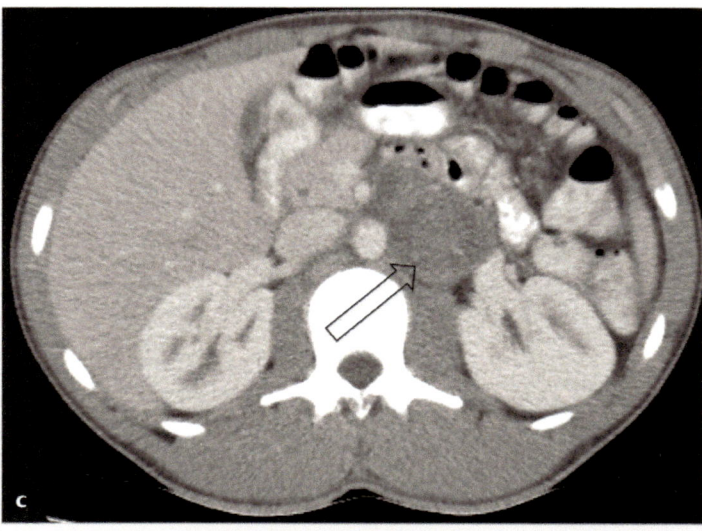

Fig. 13.16 Choriocarcinoma. (a) Ultrasound reveals a tumor with a heterogeneous echo pattern due to coexisting calcifications (arrow), solid components (star), and hypoechoic hemorrhagic areas (open arrow). Normal testicular parenchyma is visible at the upper left (circle). (b) Pulmonary metastases (arrows) on axial CT. (c) Para-aortic lymph node metastasis (arrow).

heterogeneous color-duplex and power-Doppler appearance with areas of increased and/or reduced blood flow within the testis. A burned-out tumor appears sonographically as an echogenic scar or hyperechoic calcification with an acoustic shadow in the testicular parenchyma. On MRI, the tumors are often heterogeneous due to hemorrhage, necrosis, and calcifications with an isointense signal on T1 W images and a hypointense signal on T2 W images. After administration of gadolinium contrast medium, the tumors show a heterogeneous pattern with areas of increased and/or decreased blood flow, similar to their ultrasound appearance.

▶ **Key points.** Nonseminomatous tumors, like all testicular tumors, present as a painless mass that may be accompanied by a hydrocele. At ultrasound they show a heterogeneously hypoechoic pattern due to a combination of echo-free cysts, hypoechoic hemorrhage with internal echoes, and hyperechoic calcifications. This pattern is more common with nonseminomatous tumors than with seminomas. Color duplex and power Doppler ultrasound show areas of increased and decreased blood flow. On MRI, nonseminomatous tumors are isointense on T1 W images and hypointense on T2 W images with heterogeneous components due to hemorrhage, necrosis, and calcifications.

Sex Cord-Stromal Tumors

▶ **Brief definition.** These tumors arise from the testicular stroma and are mostly benign. They may consist of stromal cells of one type, or they may contain a mixture of cell types showing different grades of differentiation. The most common sex cord-stromal tumor is the Leydig cell tumor. Its age distribution is bimodal with peaks occurring at 3 to 6 years and 20 to 40 years. Other sex cord-stromal tumors are Sertoli cell tumors and granulosa cell tumors.

▶ **Imaging signs.** Small tumors are hypoechoic at ultrasound, while larger tumors are often heterogeneous due to necrosis and intralesional hemorrhage. On MRI, small tumors are isointense to normal testis in the T1 W sequence and hypointense in the T2 W sequence.

Lymphoma and Metastases

▶ **Brief definition**
- *Lymphoma*: Lymphoma (generally non-Hodgkin's lymphoma) may occur as a primary intratesticular tumor or may be a manifestation of systemic disease.
- *Metastases*: Tumors that commonly metastasize to the testis are, in descending order of frequency, lung cancer, prostate cancer, renal carcinoma, tumors of the gastrointestinal tract, and malignant melanoma.

▶ **Imaging signs.** Sonographically, intratesticular lymphoma is hypoechoic and well vascularized. It may appear as a well-circumscribed tumor or may diffusely infiltrate the normal testicular parenchyma. It is extremely rare to find areas of necrosis, intralesional hemorrhage, or calcifications. Lymphomas are generally isointense or hypointense to normal testis on T1 W images and hypointense on T2 W images. Metastases have a similar appearance but may also appear slightly hyperintense in T1 W images depending on the identity of the primary tumor (e.g., metastases from melanoma).

Epididymal Tumors

Epididymal tumors are extremely rare. The most common is adenomatoid tumor, which is most likely to occur in the body of the epididymis. Adenomatoid tumor is usually no larger than 5 to 20 mm and has smooth margins and a solid hyperechoic appearance.

13.2 Penis

13.2.1 Imaging

Ultrasound is the modality of first choice in the initial urological evaluation of the penis. MRI, with its excellent soft tissue contrast, is used for the further investigation of sonographically indeterminate lesions.

13.2.2 Anatomy

The penis consists of three cylindrical, cavernous masses of erectile tissue: the paired dorsolateral corpora cavernosa and the single ventral corpus spongiosum (▶ Fig. 13.17). The proximal portions of the corpora cavernosa form the penile crura, which attach to the inferior pubic rami. The center of each corpus cavernosum is traversed by a cavernosal artery. The corpora cavernosa are separated from each other by a fibrous septum. The corpus

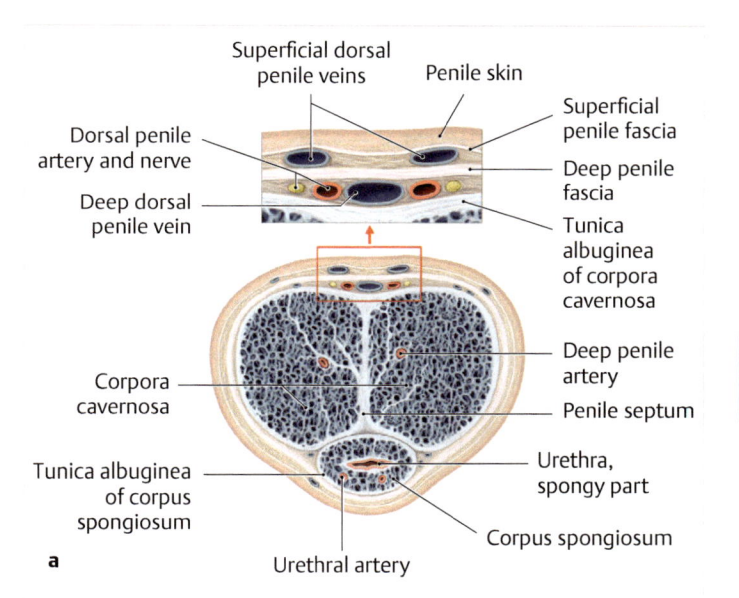

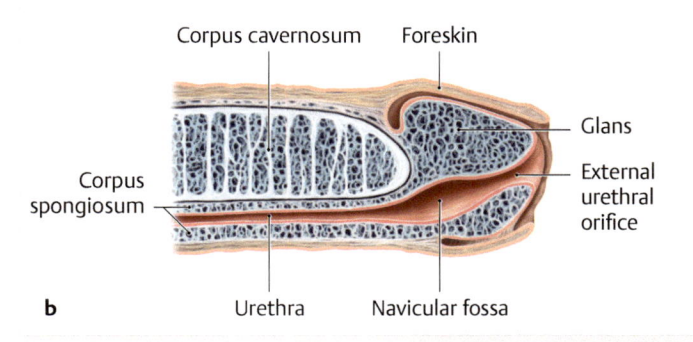

Fig. 13.17 Anatomy of the penis. (a) Cross section. (b) Longitudinal section through the distal penis. (Reproduced from Schünke M, Schulte E, Schumacher U. Prometheus. LernAtlas der Anatomie: Allgemeine Anatomie und Bewegungssystem. Illustrated by M. Voll/ K. Wesker. 3rd ed. Stuttgart: Thieme; 2011.)

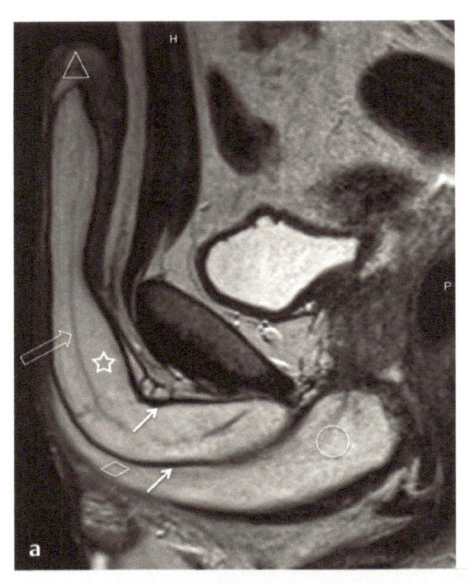

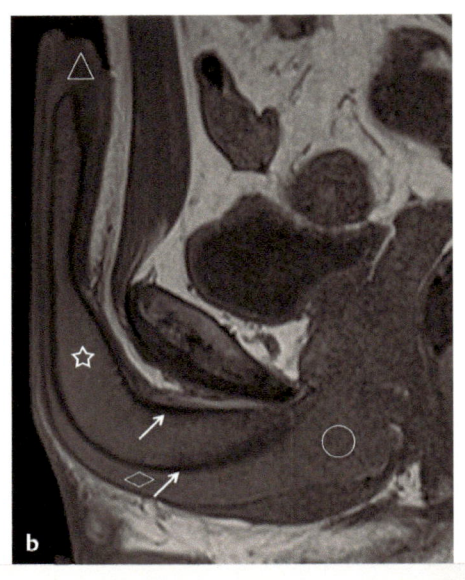

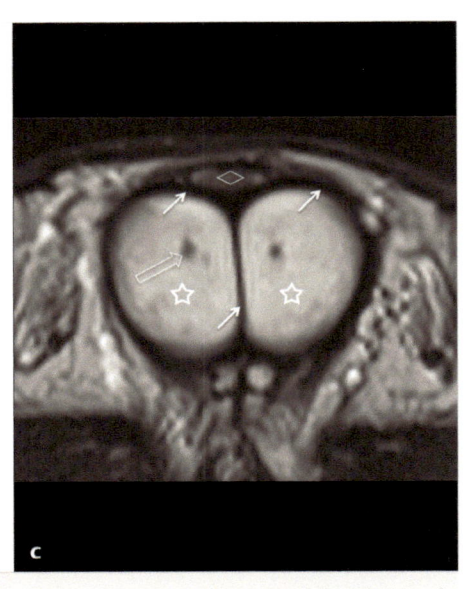

Fig. 13.18 Normal MRI appearance of the penis. Note the corpus spongiosum (diamonds) with the penile bulb (circles), glans penis (triangles), and corpora cavernosa (stars). The tunica albuginea and Buck's fascia are indistinguishable on MRI, both appearing as a hypointense line (arrows) in T1 W and T2 W images. The cavernous artery appears as a hypointense line at the center of the corpora cavernosa in the sagittal T2 W image (open arrow [a]) and as a hypointense point in the axial image (open arrow [c]). The subcutaneous connective tissue, devoid of fat, and the penile skin are also well defined. (a) Sagittal T2 W image. (b) Sagittal T1 W image. (c) Axial T2 W image.

spongiosum forms the penile bulb posteriorly at the level of the urogenital diaphragm, and it forms the glans penis anteriorly. The spongy part of the urethra runs through the corpus spongiosum. Each corporal body is surrounded by an approximately 1-mm-thick layer of connective tissue, the tunica albuginea. External to the tunica albuginea is a thicker fibrous layer called the Buck's fascia. It encloses all three corporal bodies and separates the corpora cavernosa from the corpus spongiosum. The penis is enclosed externally by lean subcutaneous connective tissue and the penile skin. The deep and superficial dorsal veins are located in the subcutaneous tissue on the dorsal midline.

▶ **MRI landmarks.** The signal characteristics of the dorsal corpora cavernosa vary with blood flow; generally they show intermediate signal intensity on T1 W images and high signal intensity on T2 W images (▶ Fig. 13.18). The cavernosal artery at the center of each corpus cavernosum appears as a hypointense tubular structure on T2 W images. The corpus spongiosum is traversed by the spongy part of the urethra, which is sometimes visible on T2 W images as a hypointensity within the hyperintense corpus spongiosum. The tunica albuginea that envelops each of the corporal bodies and the outer Buck's fascia that encloses all three corpora cannot be resolved as separate structures with the MRI scanners in current clinical use. Thus they appear as a hypointense line on both T2 W and T1 W images. The penis is bounded externally by lean subcutaneous connective tissue and the penile skin. These structures appear hyperintense to the underlying Buck's fascia and tunica albuginea on T2 W images. The superficial and deep dorsal penile veins are rarely visualized by MRI.

13.2.3 Vascular Disorders

Priapism

▶ **Brief definition.** Priapism is the term applied to a prolonged, often painful erection. Approximately 90% of cases are caused by decreased venous outflow from the corpora cavernosa (low-flow priapism) and approximately 10% by increased arterial inflow due to a traumatic arteriolacunar fistula (high-flow priapism).

> **Caution**
>
> Untreated low-flow priapism leads to infarction with subsequent fibrosis and is a urological emergency.

▶ **Imaging signs.** MRI can determine the extent of infarction in patients with low-flow priapism. Dynamic T1 W images after administration of contrast medium show absence of enhancement. With high-flow priapism, on the other hand, dynamic postcontrast T1 W images will show earlier enhancement of the affected corpus cavernosum relative to the contralateral, unaffected corpus cavernosum. Often a fistula can be detected on these images, in which case T2 W images will show a heterogeneous signal with flow voids. A fistula is also detectable by B-mode and color duplex sonography. Selective arteriography can define the fistula and also provide access for superselective embolization (▶ Fig. 13.19).

▶ **Clinical features.** Low-flow priapism is generally more painful than high-flow priapism. Low-flow priapism is associated with a violaceous discoloration and penile edema, whereas the penis in high-flow priapism is warm and well perfused. Pulsations are often palpable at the site of the arteriolacunar fistula in high-flow priapism. Clinical examination and determination of blood oxygen level in the corpora cavernosa are often sufficient to differentiate the low-flow and high-flow forms.

▶ **Differential diagnosis.** The clinical differential diagnosis mainly consists of penile edema and penile hematoma with associated penile swelling due to trauma. The corporal bodies in these cases have a normal imaging appearance.

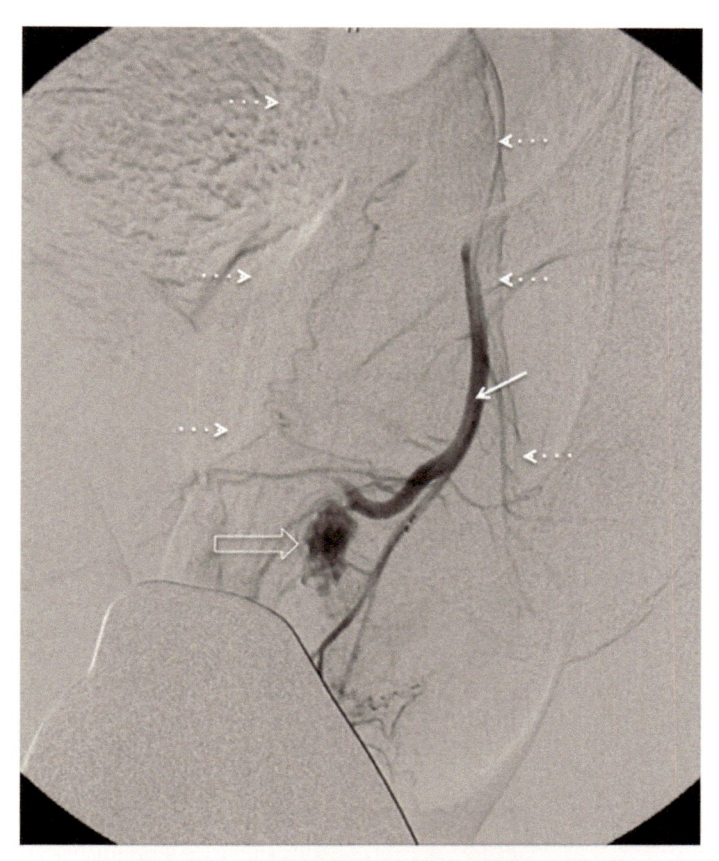

Fig. 13.19 Posttraumatic high-flow priapism. The patient developed a sustained erection (dotted arrows) approximately one week after a traumatic injury to the proximal portions of the corpora cavernosa. Selective angiography of the distal branches of the left internal pudendal artery (arrow) opacifies the arteriovenous fistula (open arrow) at the level of the penile crura. The fistula was occluded by superselective embolization with a mixture of Gelaspon and contrast medium.

▶ **Key points.** Low-flow priapism is caused by decreased venous outflow from the corpora cavernosa. High-flow priapism is caused by an arteriocavernous fistula, often due to trauma. The two forms are often distinguishable by clinical examination and blood gas analysis. In the case of high-flow priapism, MRI helps to determine the extent of infarction. An arteriocavernous fistula causing high-flow priapism can be identified by dynamic contrast-enhanced T1 W imaging, ultrasound imaging with color duplex sonography, and selective arteriography; the last procedure also establishes access for superselective embolization.

Cavernosal Thrombosis

▶ **Brief definition.** Thrombosis of the corpus cavernosum is usually segmental, affecting only one corpus. It may result from low-flow priapism, trauma, or a hypercoagulable state.

▶ **Imaging signs.** The affected corpus cavernosum is distended and filled with clotted blood (▶ Fig. 13.20). It may compress the normal, contralateral corpus. MR signal intensities vary with the age of the blood. Thrombosis in the subacute stage has intermediate to high signal intensity on T1 W and T2 W images. The signal intensities diminish over time, and an organized thrombus has low signal intensity on both T1 W and T2 W images.

▶ **Clinical features.** Partial cavernosal thrombosis presents clinically as partial priapism.

▶ **Differential diagnosis.** Fibrosis of the corporal bodies does not cause a mass effect and, unlike fresh thrombosis, is hypointense to the corpus spongiosum on both T1 W and T2 W images. A penile fracture is distinguished by a discontinuity in the tunica albuginea. It is also common to find associated soft tissue edema.

▶ **Key points.** Thrombosis of the corpus cavernosum is usually segmental. MR signal intensities vary with the age of the blood. The thrombosis is T1 hyperintense and T2 hypointense at the time of the examination.

13.2.4 Inflammatory Disorders: Peyronie's Disease

▶ **Brief definition.** Peyronie's disease, known also as induratio penis plastica, is a localized inflammation of the tunica albuginea that is characterized in the acute stage by pain and focal thickening of the affected tunica albuginea, forming a fibrous plaque. The chronic stage is characterized by less pain and increased localized fibrosis of the tunica albuginea.

▶ **Imaging signs.** The affected area may undergo partial or complete calcification, which is visible with CT or ultrasound. MRI can additionally detect nonpalpable plaques, which appear hypointense on both T1 W and T2 W images. Inflammatory activity can be assessed after IV administration of contrast medium, as the affected area will show marked enhancement in the acute stage (▶ Fig. 13.21).

▶ **Clinical features.** The affected portion of the tunica albuginea may be painful and causes penile deviation. The inflamed or fibrotic area is palpable.

▶ **Differential diagnosis.** Scar tissue after a penile fracture also shows low signal intensity on T1 W and T2 W images but does not enhance after administration of contrast medium.

▶ **Key points.** Peyronie's disease is a localized inflammation of the tunica albuginea associated with focal thickening of the affected tunica. The affected area is hypointense on T1 W and T2 W images and enhances in the acute stage. Most urologists do not resect the plaques in the initial stage; surgery is postponed until the active inflammatory stage has subsided.

13.2.5 Traumatic Disorders: Penile Fracture

▶ **Brief definition.** Penile fracture is defined as a tear in the tunica albuginea, usually caused by blunt trauma to the erect penis (e.g., during intercourse).

▶ **Imaging signs.** The integrity of the tunica albuginea is most accurately assessed with MRI. A tear in the tunica albuginea most commonly occurs in the distal two-thirds of the penis, appearing

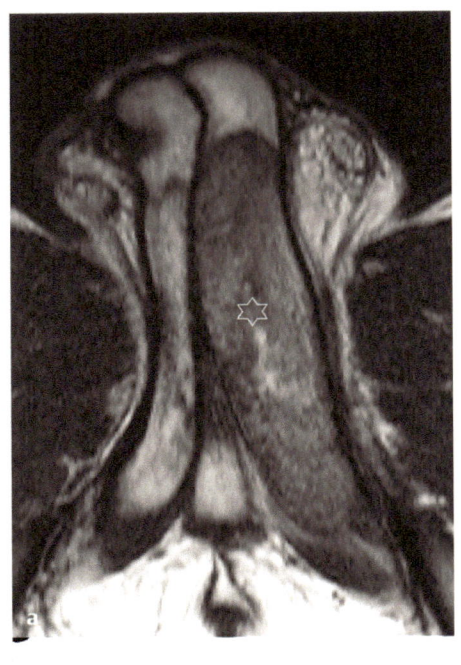

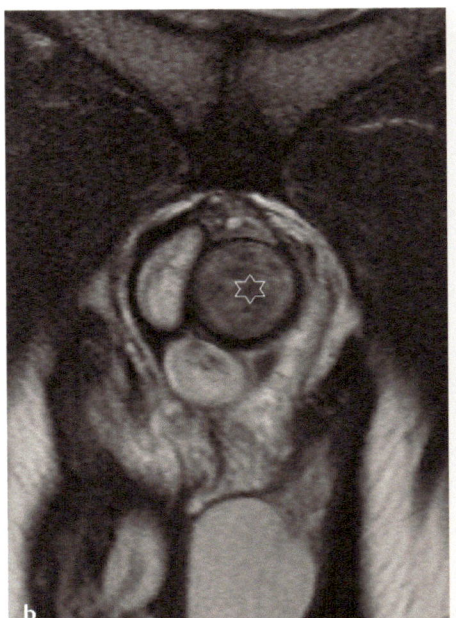

Fig. 13.20 **Organized thrombosis of the left corpus cavernosum.** The left corpus cavernosum ([a]–[d], stars) is enlarged and has displaced the right corpus cavernosum toward the opposite side. The affected portion of the left corpus cavernosum shows heterogeneous low signal intensity on T2 W images (a, b). The corresponding low signal intensities in the T1 W image (c) support the suspicion of organized thrombosis. The affected portion does not enhance after administration of gadolinium contrast medium, unlike the normal portion ([d], arrow), due to the absence of blood flow. (a) Axial T2 W image. (b) Coronal T2 W image. (c) T1 W image before administration of contrast medium. (d) T1 W image after administration of contrast medium.

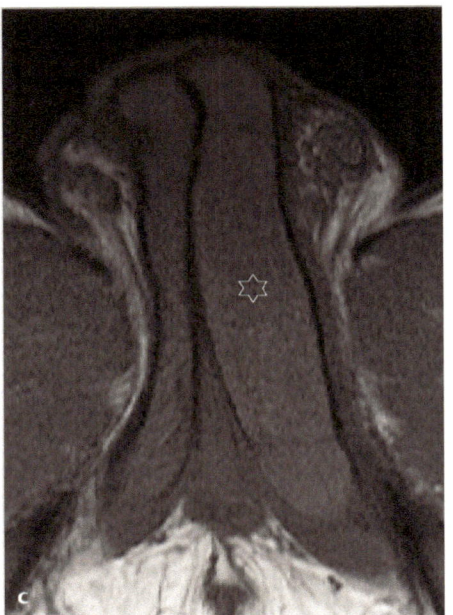

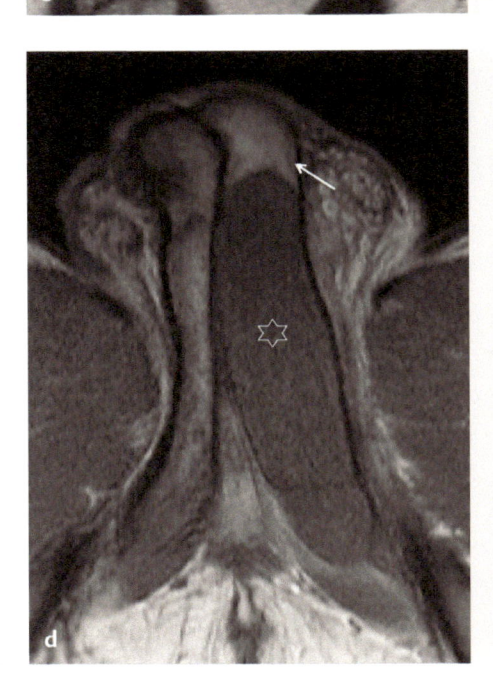

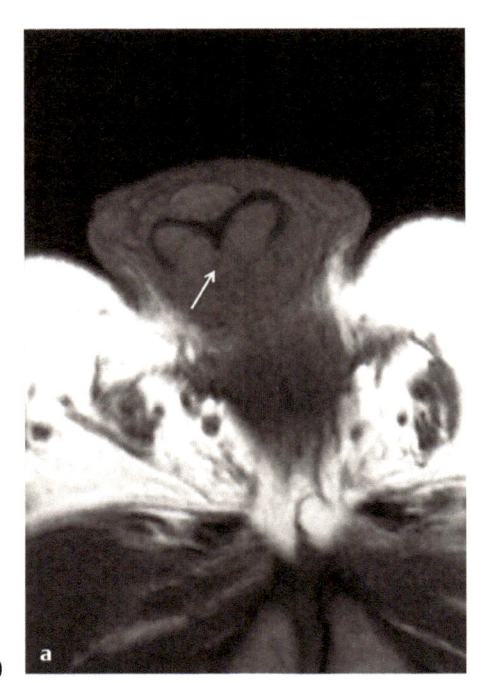

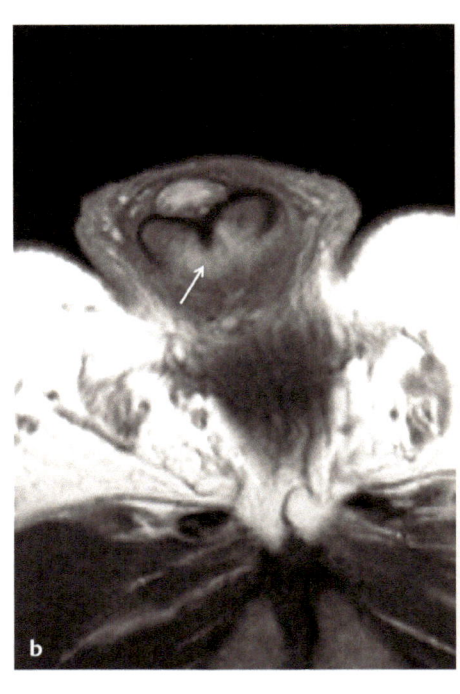

Fig. 13.21 **Peyronie's disease in the acute stage.** (a) The tunica albuginea of the corpora cavernosa is obscured posteriorly by inflammatory plaque (arrow). (b) Postcontrast image shows marked enhancement at that site, indicating active inflammation (arrow).

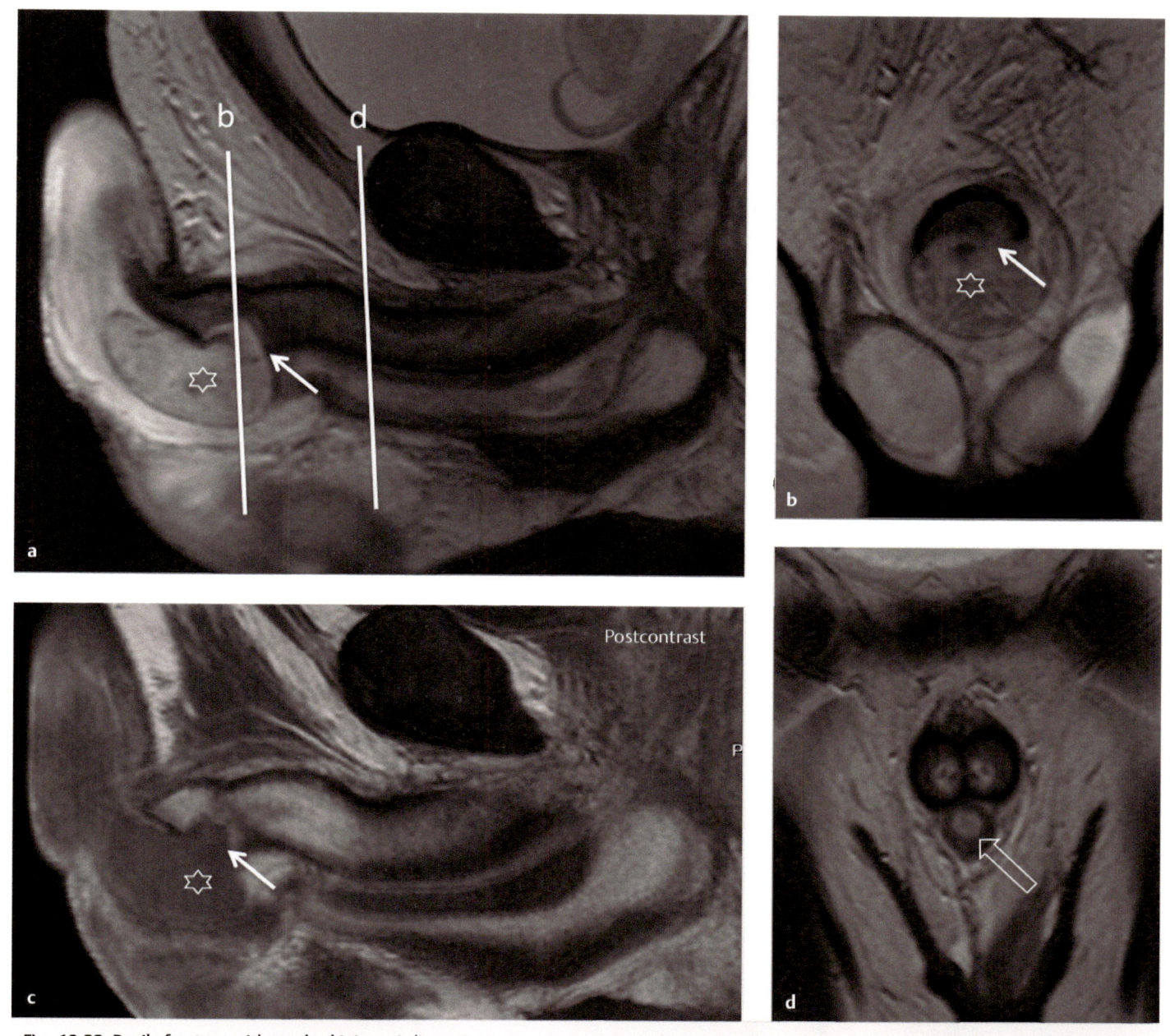

Fig. 13.22 **Penile fracture with urethral injury.** A discontinuity is present at a typical site in the tunica albuginea (arrows) at the junction of the middle and distal thirds of the penis. The penile fracture is associated with a hematoma (stars) and urethral fracture. The ureter proximal to the fracture site is dilated and filled with blood ([d] open arrow). (a) Sagittal unenhanced MR image (T2W). (b) Sagittal MR image in the plane labeled "b" in panel (a). (c) Sagittal MR image after administration of contrast medium (T1W). (d) Paracoronal MR image in the plane labeled "d" in panel (a).

on both T1 W and T2 W images as a discontinuity in the hypointense tunica albuginea (▶ Fig. 13.22). The contrast is generally depicted more clearly on T2 W images, although an accompanying hematoma can mask a tear. In these cases the absence of hematoma enhancement after administration of contrast medium will suggest the correct diagnosis.

▶ **Clinical features.** A penile fracture usually causes an audible snap at the time of injury, accompanied by sudden onset of pain and immediate loss of erection. Associated hematoma is often present and is generally confined to the penis but may spread to the scrotum, perineum, and thigh.

Caution

Fracture of the penis is a surgical emergency. Untreated cases lead to deformity and erectile dysfunction. Associated injury to the urethra may lead to hematuria and dysuria.

▶ **Pitfalls.** Concomitant urethral injury may be missed, so the corpus spongiosum should be carefully evaluated at imaging.

▶ **Key points.** A traumatic fracture of the tunica albuginea is associated with a snapping sound and pain of sudden onset. MRI

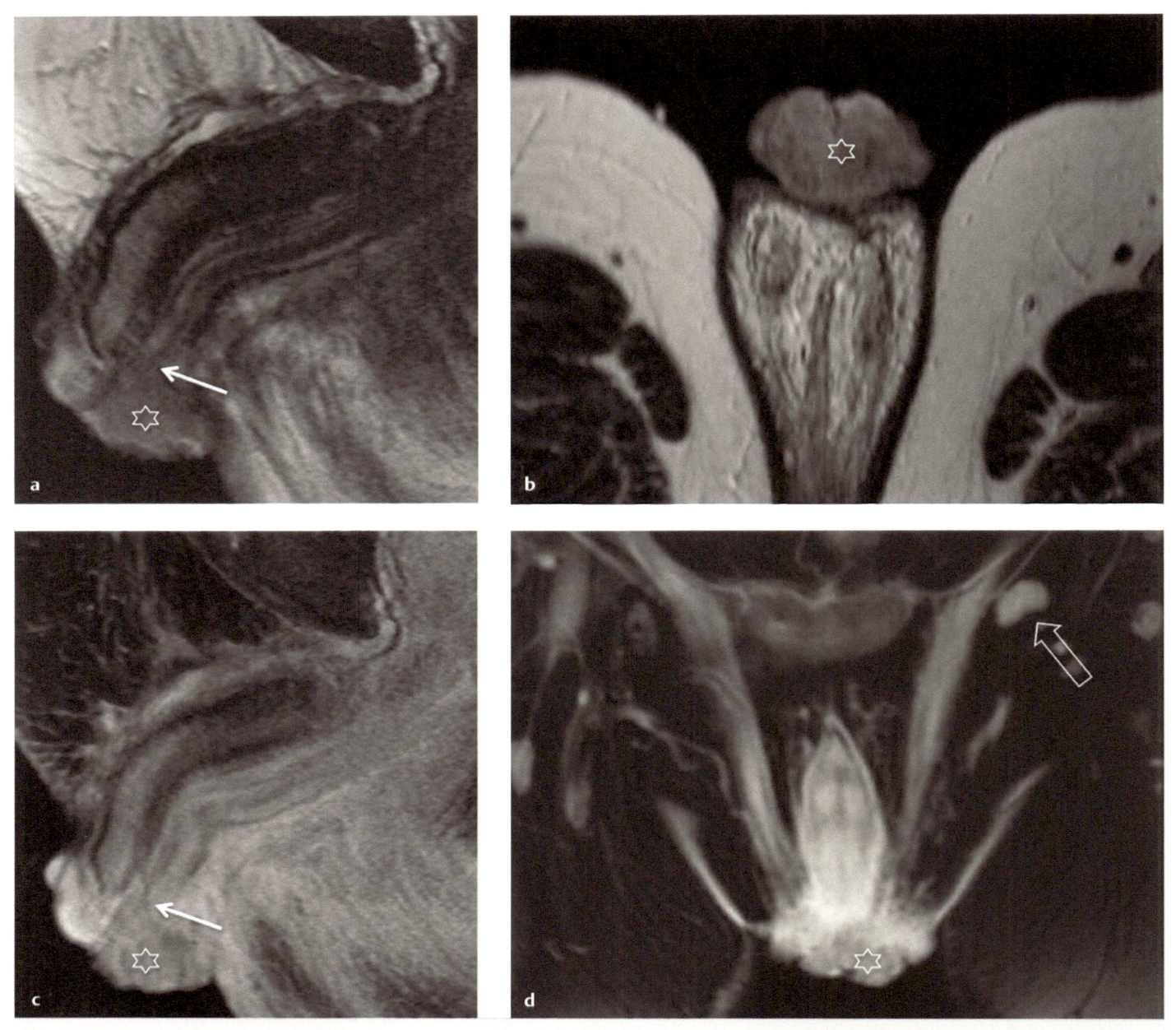

Fig. 13.23 **Carcinoma of the glans penis.** The penile carcinoma (stars) is slightly hypointense to the corporal bodies in the T2 W images (**a, b**). The carcinoma shows less enhancement than the corporal bodies after administration of contrast medium (**c, d**). Invasion of the corpus spongiosum is a poor prognostic sign (arrows). The inguinal lymph nodes exhibit normal size and shape on both sides (open arrow), indicating that inguinal lymph node metastasis has not occurred. (**a**) Sagittal T2 W image. (**b**) Axial T2 W image. (**c**) Sagittal T1 W image after administration of contrast medium. (**d**) Coronal T1 W image after administration of contrast medium.

can clearly demonstrate the discontinuity in the hypointense tunica albuginea on both T1 W and T2 W images. MRI can also define the extent of associated hematoma and urethral injury.

13.2.6 Penile Carcinoma

▶ **Brief definition.** Most penile cancers are squamous cell carcinomas. Penile carcinoma is a very rare tumor, accounting for less than 1% of all male cancers. It has a peak incidence between 60 and 70 years of age. An association with human papillomavirus types 16 and 18 has been described.

▶ **Imaging signs.** Imaging is necessary for the staging of penile carcinoma; MRI is superior to CT for evaluating the primary lesion. On MRI, squamous cell carcinoma of the penis is hypointense to the corporal bodies on T1 W and T2 W images (▶ Fig. 13.23); it shows less enhancement than the corpora on postcontrast images.

▶ **Clinical features.** Squamous cell carcinoma of the penis often presents initially as a painless, focal epithelial thickening on the glans penis; there may be an associated ulcer. The treatment of choice is penectomy. The prognosis is good in the absence of corporal invasion or lymph node metastasis.

▶ **Pitfalls.** A common error is failure to evaluate the inguinal lymph nodes for metastatic involvement on MRI.

▶ **Differential diagnosis.** The clinical differential diagnosis includes soft or hard chancre and condylomata acuminata. If

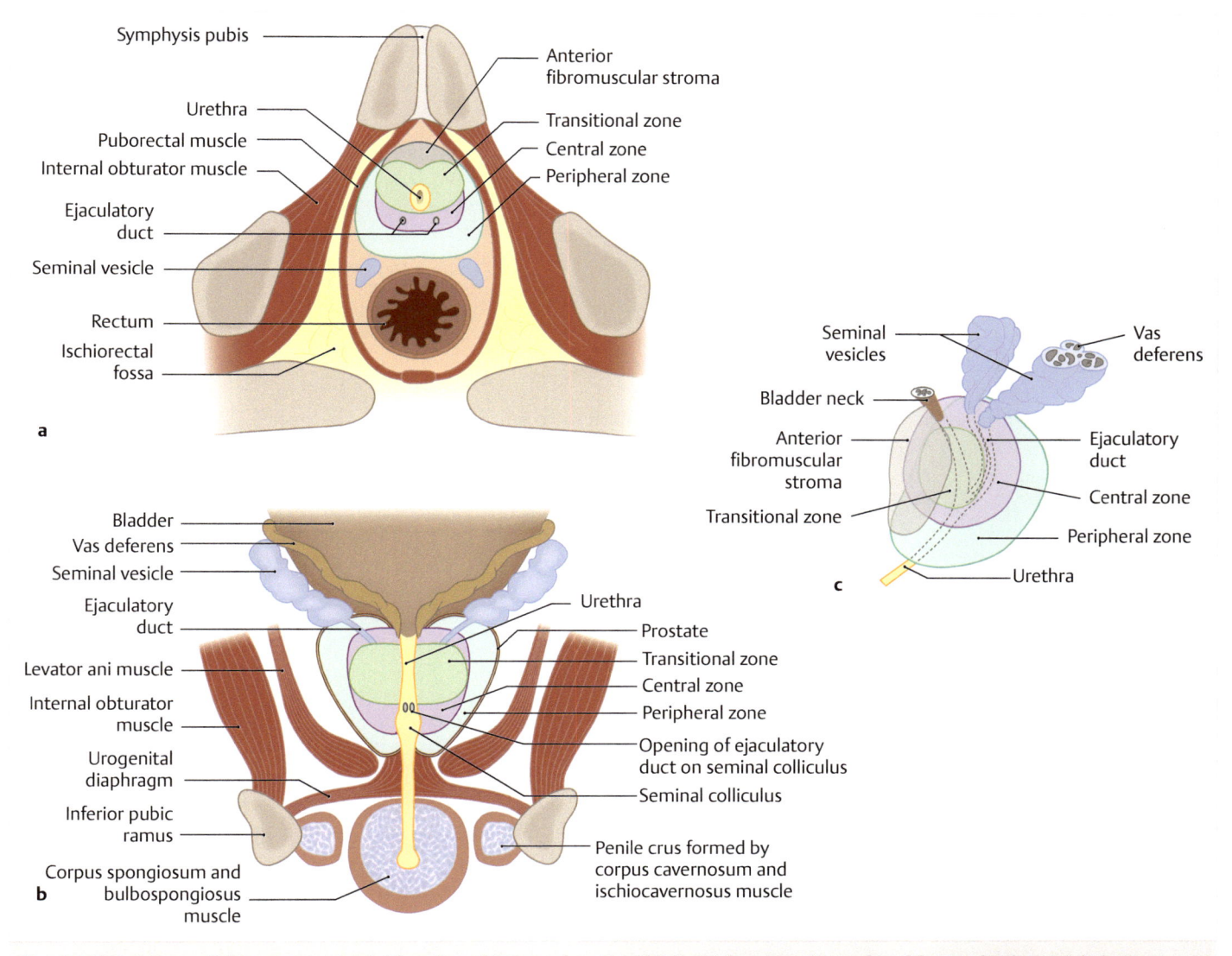

Fig. 13.24 Anatomy of the prostate. (a) Axial section. (b) Coronal section. (c) Sagittal section. (Reproduced from Schünke M, Schulte E, Schumacher U. Prometheus. LernAtlas der Anatomie: Innere Organe. Illustrated by M. Voll/K. Wesker. 2nd ed. Stuttgart: Thieme; 2009.)

penis carcinoma has invaded the urethra or prostate (stage T3) or other adjacent structures (stage T4), the radiological differential diagnosis should include carcinoma of the anterior urethra. Both penile and urethral carcinoma are hypointense to the corporal bodies on T1 W and T2 W images. Very rare penile malignancies are sarcomas and metastases to the penis.

▶ Key points. Most penile carcinomas are squamous cell carcinomas and are manifested on the glans penis. MRI is necessary for staging. Squamous cell carcinoma of the penis is hypointense to the corporal bodies on T1 W and T2 W images. The tumor enhances less than the corpora after administration of contrast medium.

13.3 Prostate and Seminal Vesicles

13.3.1 Imaging

The prostate is usually examined initially with transrectal ultrasound. MRI provides more detailed images that can define the zonal anatomy of the prostate and detect prostatic abnormalities. MRI is the modality of choice for imaging prostate cancer owing to its excellent soft tissue contrast and the increased sensitivity afforded by spectroscopic and perfusion imaging.

13.3.2 Anatomy

The healthy prostate is a walnut-sized gland that encircles the urethra between the bladder and urogenital diaphragm and is bounded externally by a thin, compressed tissue layer (▶ Fig. 13.24). Cephalad to the base of the prostate and lateral to the vas deferens are the paired, elongated seminal vesicles, which resemble clusters of grapes. The excretory duct of each seminal vesicle joins with the ipsilateral vas deferens to form the ejaculatory duct, which opens into the urethra on the seminal colliculus. Neurovascular bundles surround the prostate chiefly on the posterolateral side. The nerves and vessels that penetrate the prostate are sites of predilection for the extracapsular extension of prostate cancer. The prostate consists of four zones:
- Peripheral zone.
- Transitional zone.
- Central zone.
- Very small, proximal periurethral zone.

The peripheral zone of the prostate is separated from the central gland (i.e., the central and transitional zones) by a narrow fibromuscular band. The peripheral zone accounts for approximately 70% of the prostate volume in young men, the central zone 25%, and the transitional zone 5%. With aging, the prostate not only enlarges but also shows a change in relative zonal volumes as the transitional zone and, to a lesser degree, the periurethral zone become predominant as a result of benign prostatic hyperplasia (p. 486). Each zone consists of stromal and epithelial components, the latter being greater in the peripheral zone than in the central gland. Approximately 70% of prostatic adenocarcinomas arise in the peripheral zone, 25% in the transitional zone, and 10% in the central zone.

▶ **MRI landmarks.** The zonal anatomy of the prostate is clearly depicted in T2 W images (▶ Fig. 13.25, ▶ Fig. 13.26). The peripheral zone generally shows high signal intensities due to its large glandular component while the central gland show lower, heterogeneous signal intensities due to a larger stromal component. The grapelike seminal vesicles are located cephalad to the base of the prostate and appear hyperintense on T2 W images. Medial to each seminal vesicle is the vas deferens. The urethra appears as a triangular midline structure in the posterior third of the central gland. The seminal colliculus with the opening of the ejaculatory duct is best displayed on coronal images. The neurovascular bundles are located along the posterolateral aspect of the left and right sides of the gland and appear hyperintense with tubular structures on T2 W images. Anterior to the prostate is a caplike layer of fibromuscular tissue that is separated from the symphysis by fat. Posterior to the prostate is the rectum, which is distended when an endorectal coil is used. Lateral to the prostate are the muscular structures of levator ani and obturator internus. The prostate appears homogeneously hypointense on T1 W images (▶ Fig. 13.27).

13.3.3 Prostatitis

▶ **Brief definition.** Prostatitis syndrome is subdivided into several clinical forms:
- Acute bacterial prostatitis.
- Chronic bacterial prostatitis.
- Chronic prostatitis or chronic pelvic pain syndrome without detectable bacteria.
- Asymptomatic inflammatory prostatitis in which inflammatory cells can be detected by prostatic biopsy or in fluid expressed from the gland.

The most common form is chronic abacterial prostatitis. Less common are acute and chronic bacterial prostatitis, which are usually caused by gram-negative organisms. Complications of acute bacterial prostatitis include prostatic abscess, cystitis, ascending pyelonephritis, and epididymitis.

▶ **Imaging signs.** MRI is not indicated in patients with clinical symptoms of prostatitis. It does have a role in differentiating chronic forms of prostatitis from prostate cancer: both appear hypointense on T2 W images, but prostatitis is more likely to show a triangular configuration with a streaky appearance (▶ Fig. 13.28). Chronic prostatitis cannot be positively differentiated from prostate cancer, however. Prostatitis is hypointense on T1 W images. Even modern MR techniques of proton magnetic resonance spectroscopy (MRS), diffusion-weighted imaging

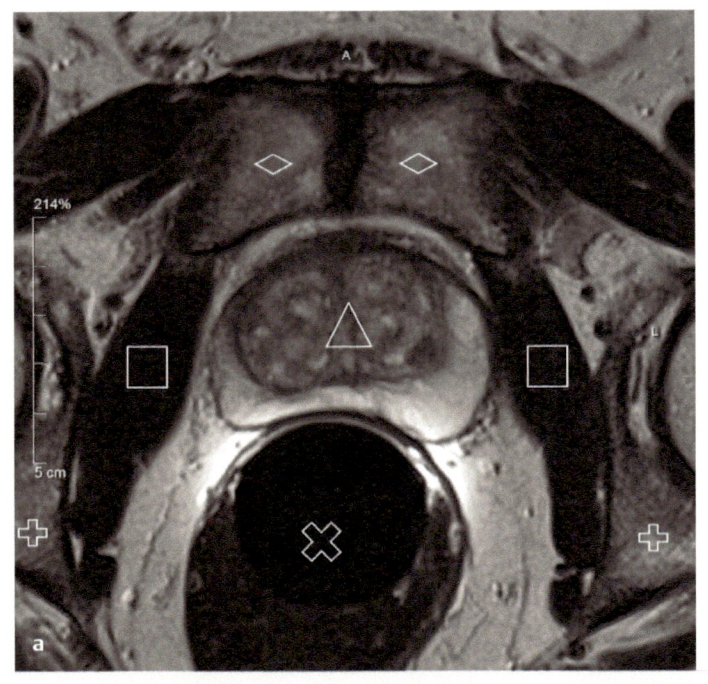

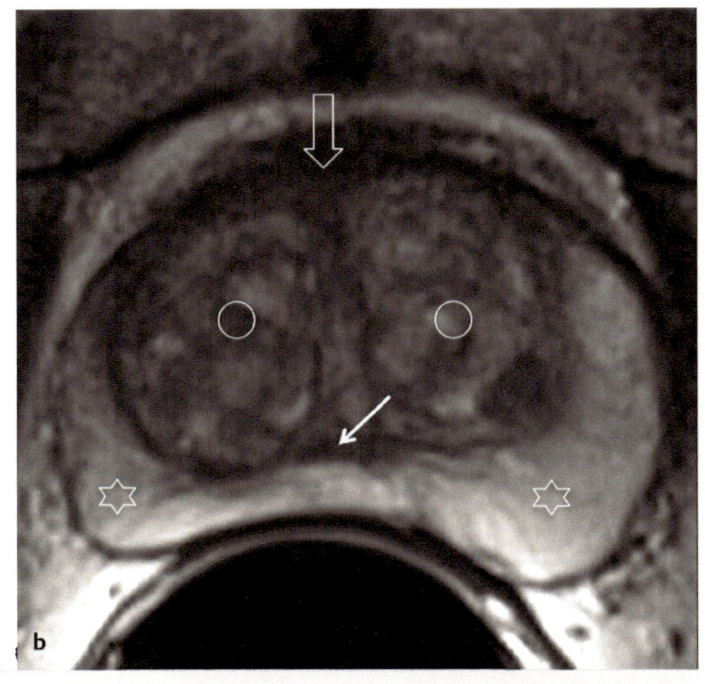

Fig. 13.25 **Normal MRI appearance of the prostate.** Axial T2 W images in a 53-year-old man. (a) T2 W survey image of the lesser pelvis: prostate (triangle), endorectal coil inside the rectum (cross) with fecal residues, obturator internus muscle (squares), symphysis (diamonds), and acetabulum (plus signs). (b) Magnified view clearly demonstrates the hyperintense peripheral zone (stars), the large, heterogeneous transitional zone (circles), the urethra (arrow), and anterior fibromuscular connective tissue (open arrow).

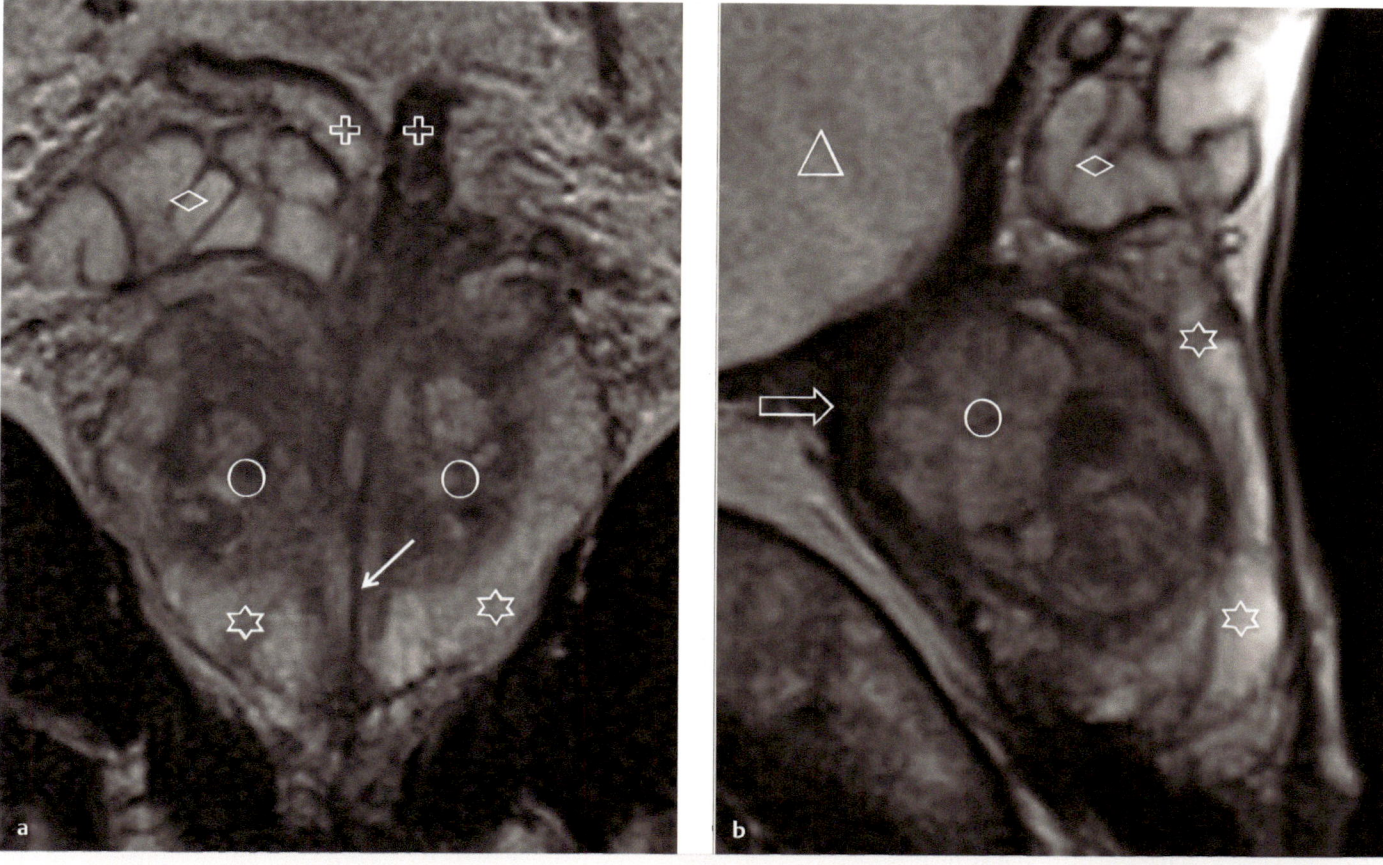

Fig. 13.26 Normal MRI appearance of the prostate. Coronal and sagittal T2W images. Both images display the hyperintense peripheral zone (stars), the enlarged, heterogeneous transitional zone (circles), and the hyperintense seminal vesicles with their grapelike configuration (diamonds). The vas deferens (plus signs) and urethra (arrow) are displayed in the coronal image (**a**), and the anterior fibromuscular tissue (open arrow) and bladder (triangle) are visible in the sagittal image (**b**). (**a**) Coronal T2W image. (**b**) Sagittal T2W image.

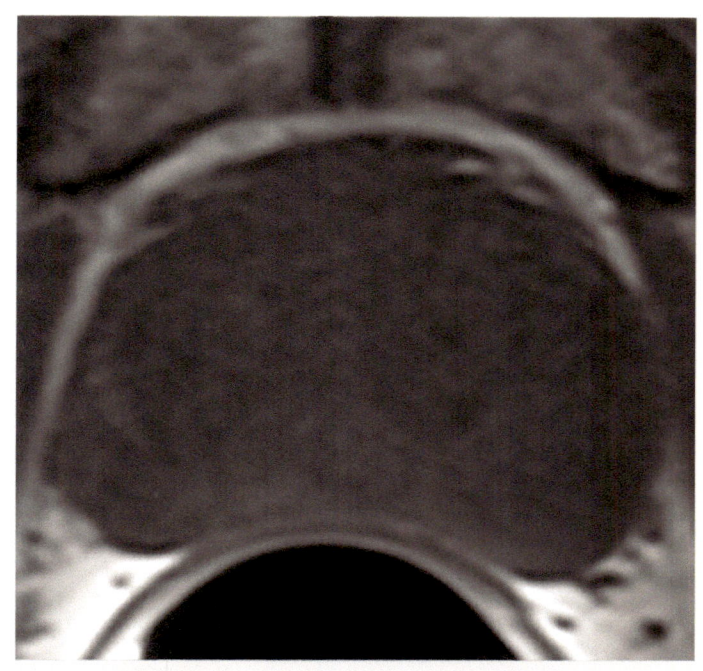

Fig. 13.27 Normal MRI appearance of the prostate. Axial T1W image. The prostate appears homogeneously hypointense. Its zonal anatomy is not defined.

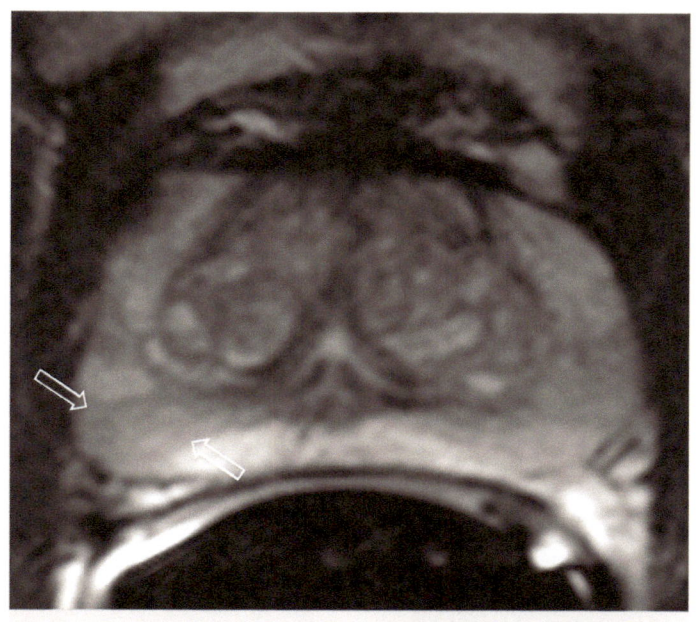

Fig. 13.28 Chronic prostatitis. An area of chronic prostatitis (arrows) is visible in the peripheral zone on the right side. The streaky hypointense pattern in the T2W image is a typical finding.

Male Pelvis

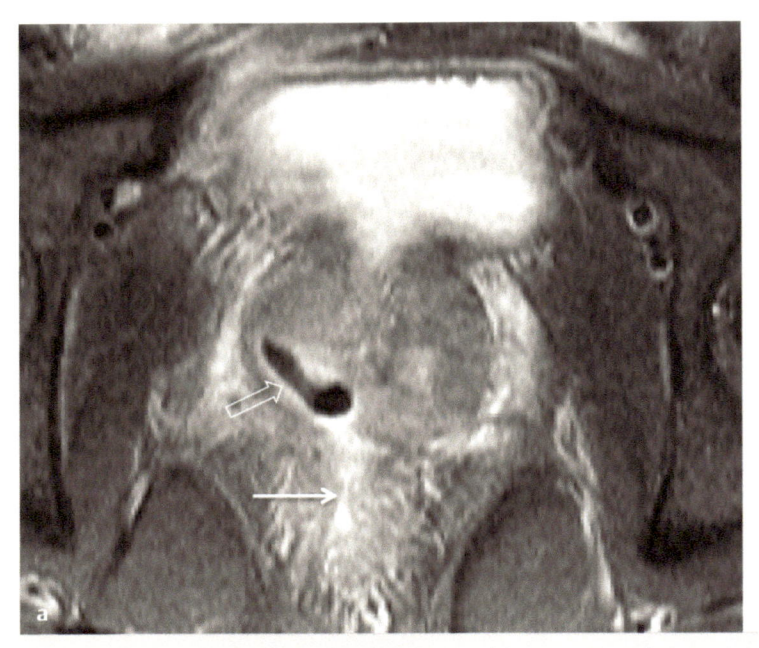

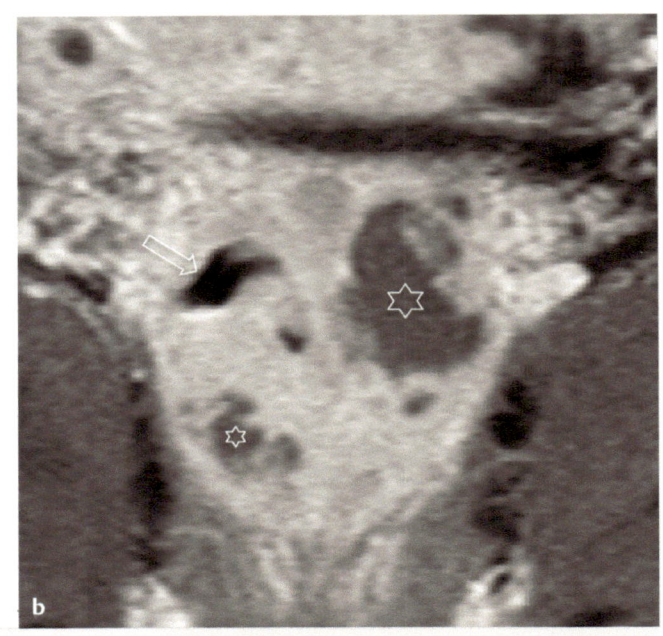

Fig. 13.29 Prostatitis with abscess formation. (a) T2 W image shows extensive prostatitis with abscess formation. Note the fistulous tract to the rectum (arrow) and air inclusions (open arrow). (b) T1 W image after administration of contrast medium clearly defines the areas of inflammatory liquefaction (stars) within the prostate.

(DWI), and dynamic contrast-enhanced MRI are unable to establish a definitive diagnosis of chronic prostatitis. The central liquefaction in a prostatic abscess is hyperintense on T2 W images and hypointense on T1 W images (▶ Fig. 13.29). The surrounding inflammatory wall shows increased enhancement after administration of contrast medium.

▶ **Clinical features.** Acute bacterial prostatitis and prostatic abscess are typically associated with fever, painful urination, and perineal and back pain. The symptoms of chronic bacterial and abacterial prostatitis are nonspecific. They are often associated with recurrent urinary tract infections.

▶ **Pitfalls.** Be aware that imaging studies are limited in their ability to differentiate prostatitis from other conditions.

▶ **Differential diagnosis.** The most important differential diagnosis is prostate cancer. Low-grade cancers in particular may have imaging features that are indistinguishable from chronic prostatitis. High-grade prostate cancers tend to show more homogeneous hypointensity on T2 W images than chronic prostatitis. Hematoma is another differential diagnosis on T2 W images. Hematoma appears hyperintense on T1 W images, in contrast to prostatitis. Fibrosis (e.g., after radiotherapy) is hypointense on T2 W and T1 W images.

▶ **Key points.** Acute or chronic prostatitis may be bacterial or abacterial. Imaging cannot positively differentiate chronic prostatitis from prostate cancer. Both conditions are hypointense on T2 W images, but chronic prostatitis is more likely to appear wedge-shaped with a streaky signal pattern. Even modern MRI techniques of proton MRS, DWI, and dynamic contrast-enhanced MRI cannot provide a definitive diagnosis. Acute prostatitis has a typical clinical presentation that includes fever, painful urination, and perineal and back pain; generally, therefore, imaging is unnecessary in the diagnosis of prostatitis. Nevertheless, the nonspecific features of chronic prostatitis should always be considered in the differential diagnosis of prostate cancer.

13.3.4 Benign Prostatic Hyperplasia

▶ **Brief definition.** Benign prostatic hyperplasia (BPH) is a benign disorder that occurs predominantly in older men. It is caused by a progressive hyperplasia of the stromal and epithelial components of the transitional zone.

▶ **Imaging signs.** BPH appears sonographically as heterogeneous tissue with hypoechoic and hyperechoic areas in the central gland. On MRI, the enlarged transitional zone is clearly depicted in T2 W images (▶ Fig. 13.30). It consists of multiple nodules with a heterogeneous appearance due to the combined presence of stroma-rich (hypointense) and gland-rich (hyperintense) areas. The typical nodule in BPH is bordered by a hypointense rim on T2 W images. The enlarged transitional zone is hypointense on T1 W images, like the peripheral zone.

▶ **Clinical features.** Increasing enlargement of the prostate leads to obstructive symptoms such as incomplete bladder emptying and storage symptoms such as pollakiuria and nocturia. The urinary obstruction leads to increasing trabeculation and diverticulum formation in the bladder. A serious complication is acute urinary retention, which may be drug-induced or may result from local or general anesthesia.

▶ **Pitfalls.** Inexperienced practitioners in particular may misinterpret the enlarged transitional zone as prostate cancer.

▶ **Differential diagnosis.** Stroma-rich hypointense areas in the enlarged transitional zone are difficult to distinguish from prostate cancer. As in prostate cancer, nodules that form in BPH may show early, intense enhancement on dynamic contrast-enhanced

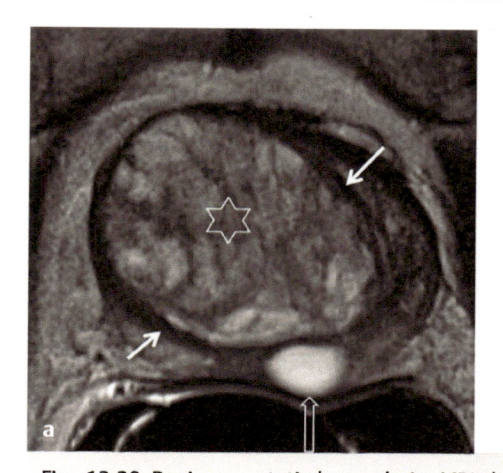

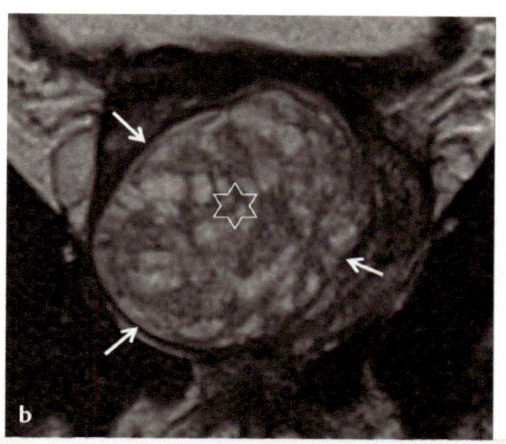

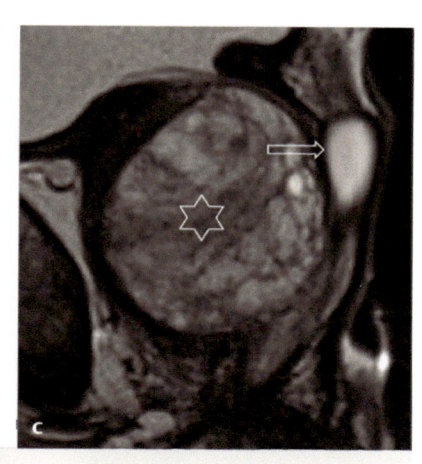

Fig. 13.30 Benign prostatic hyperplasia. MRI shows a large, heterogeneous nodule (a–c, stars) in the setting of BPH with a typical hypointense peripheral rim (a, b, arrows). A prostatic utricle cyst (a, c, open arrows) is noted incidentally at a typical site. **(a)** Axial T2 W image. **(b)** Coronal T2 W image. **(c)** Sagittal T2 W image.

MRI, restricted diffusion on DWI, and elevated choline levels and relatively low creatine levels on proton MRS.

▶ **Key points.** Benign prostatic hyperplasia is a benign disorder of the prostate. It is caused by progressive hyperplasia of the stromal and epithelial components of the transitional zone with increasing age, which leads to voiding and storage symptoms. On MRI, the enlarged transitional zone is best demonstrated in T2 W images. It consists of multiple nodules, which typically appear heterogeneous with a hypointense rim. A diagnostic challenge is to differentiate the stroma-rich hypointense areas of BPH from hypointense prostate cancer in the transitional zone.

13.3.5 Prostate Cancer

▶ **Brief definition.** Prostate cancer is the most common malignant tumor in males and the second leading cause of cancer deaths. The risk of developing prostate cancer increases with aging. Histopathologically, the most common type of prostate cancer is adenocarcinoma. It is usually multifocal and rarely unifocal. Approximately 70% of prostatic adenocarcinomas arise in the peripheral zone and approximately 30% in the central gland. The malignancy of adenocarcinoma is often graded with the Gleason score, which describes the deviation from normal glandular architecture. Since the tumors are often heterogeneous, a two-part Gleason score is used, the first number denoting the tumor grade that comprises most of the tumor:
- Low-grade prostate cancer: Gleason score 3 + 3.
- Intermediate-grade prostate cancer: Gleason score 3 + 4.
- High-grade prostate cancer: Gleason score at least 4 + 3.

The staging of prostate cancer follows the TNM classification (▶ Table 13.3). Initial lymphogenous metastasis occurs to the lymph nodes of the obturator fossa and along the iliac vessels. Sites of predilection for hematogenous metastasis are the bones. Less common sites are parenchymal organs such as the lung and liver.

▶ **Imaging signs.** Prostate cancer is hypointense on T1 W images, like normal prostatic tissue. On T2 W images, prostate cancer typically appears as a focal lesion of decreased signal intensity (▶ Fig. 13.31, ▶ Fig. 13.32, ▶ Fig. 13.33). This finding is not specific, however, and so T2 W and T1 W sequences are increasingly supplemented by DWI, proton MRS, and dynamic contrast-enhanced MRI (▶ Fig. 13.34). Proton MRS can provide a noninvasive analysis of the chemical composition of tissue based on the chemical shift of hydrogen-containing molecules. Choline-containing molecules and citrate are important in the diagnosis of prostatic disease. Choline levels are typically elevated in prostate cancer, while citrate levels are decreased. This contrasts with the low choline and high citrate levels found in normal prostatic tissue. On DWI, prostate cancer is typically characterized by a decreased ADC value relative to normal tissue. Dynamic contrast-enhanced MRI measures the change of R1 relaxivity in tissue over time after the administration of gadolinium contrast medium. When the time–signal intensity curves are analyzed, prostate cancer is characterized by an earlier and steeper upslope than normal surrounding prostatic tissue and by more rapid washout as a result of tumor angiogenesis and the resulting increase in tissue permeability. The varied and complex information supplied by time–signal intensity curves can be condensed to just a few parameters by using pharmacokinetic models that describe the histology and physiology of tissue microcirculation in terms of mathematical formulas. Prostate cancer typically shows increased transfer constants relative to normal prostatic tissue based on the pharmacokinetic models in current clinical use.

▶ **Clinical features.** The symptoms of prostate cancer depend on the stage of the disease. Patients with early disease confined to the prostate are asymptomatic. Advanced stages present with

Table 13.3 TNM classification of prostate cancer

Designation	Description
T1	Tumor confined within the prostate and detectable only by biopsy
T2	Tumor confined within the prostate
T3	Tumor extends through the prostatic capsule
• T3a	Unilateral or bilateral extracapsular extension
• T3b	Tumor invades the seminal vesicle(s)
T4	Tumor fixed or invades adjacent structures other than seminal vesicles (e.g., bladder, levator muscles, pelvic wall)

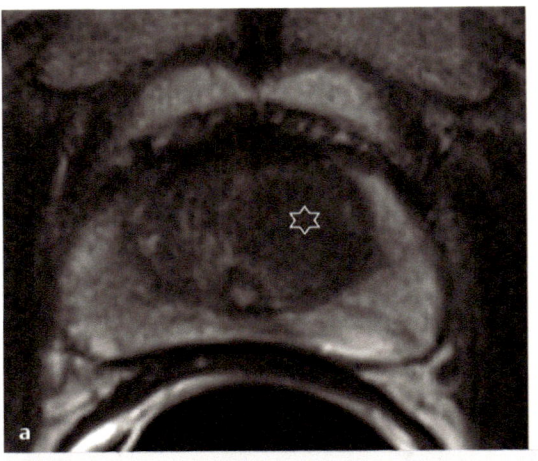

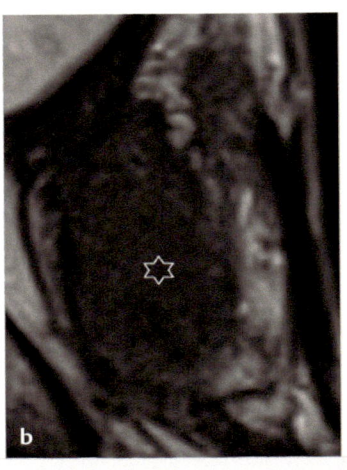

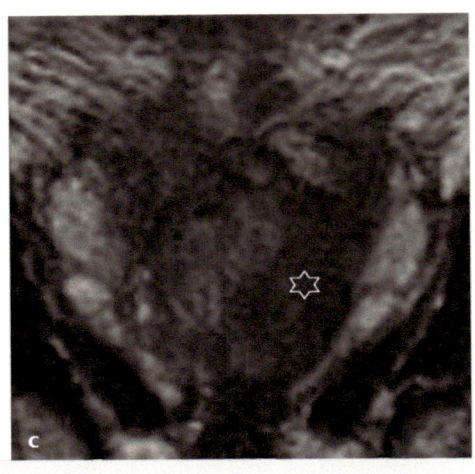

Fig. 13.31 **Prostate cancer** in a 69-year-old man with a serum PSA of 16.0 ng/mL. A large prostatic carcinoma (Gleason score 3 + 4) in the left transitional zone has a typical homogeneously hypointense appearance on T2W images ([a]–[c], stars). **(a)** Axial T2W image. **(b)** Sagittal T2W image. **(c)** Coronal T2W image.

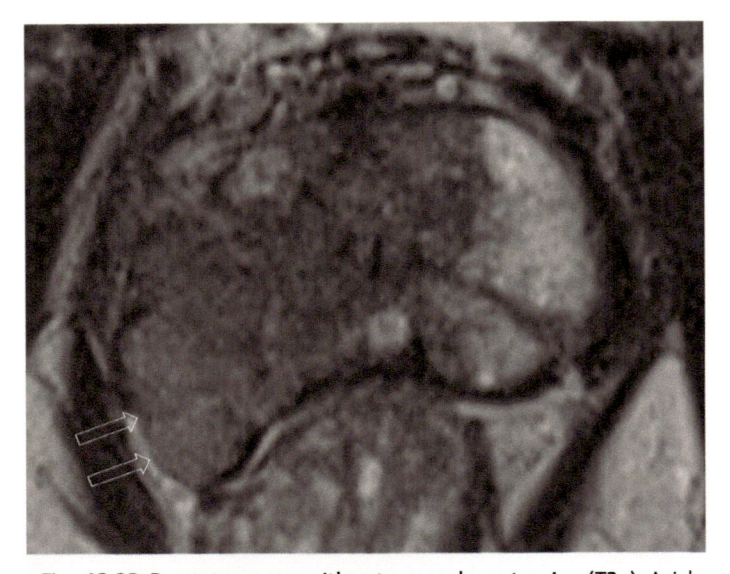

Fig. 13.32 **Prostate cancer with extracapsular extension (T3a).** Axial T2W image of the prostate in a 74-year-old man with a serum PSA of 20.8 ng/mL and biopsy-proven prostate cancer with a Gleason score of 4 + 5. MRI shows extracapsular extension (arrows) toward the right side with obliteration of the rectoprostatic angle.

obstructive complaints and hematuria. Serum levels of prostate-specific antigen (PSA) are of major importance in early diagnosis. The reference ranges for normal PSA levels vary with age, and the following upper limits are widely accepted:
- Men 50 years of age or older: 2.5 ng/mL.
- Men 60 years of age or older: 3.5 ng/mL.
- Men over 60 years of age: 4.0 ng/mL.

The diagnostic accuracy of the PSA level can be improved by determining the molecular fractions of the total PSA value. A ratio of unbound to total PSA less than 15% is suspicious for prostate cancer, while higher values are more consistent with BPH. Determining the age-adjusted rate of change in PSA levels also improves the specificity of the PSA value. The diagnostic work-up of patients with initial suspicion of prostate cancer should include a systematic ultrasound-guided transrectal biopsy. Patients with at least one negative core-needle biopsy will benefit from MRI, however. It has been shown that MRI and subsequent MRI-assisted biopsy in these patients can detect more prostate cancers with fewer biopsies.

▶ **Pitfalls.** The following mistakes are common:
- MRI is withheld from patients with at least one negative ultrasound-guided biopsy and continued suspicion of prostate cancer. Tumors located at an apical, far lateral, or anterior site in the gland may escape detection by systematic ultrasound-guided transrectal core-needle biopsy.
- MRI of the prostate is withheld in patients with discrepant clinical findings on prostate cancer risk. Besides the accurate visualization of prostate cancer, MRI can also detect extracapsular extension.
- MRI of the prostate is performed too soon after prior ultrasound-guided biopsy. Postbiopsy hemorrhage can degrade the findings on proton MRS and DWI, making the tests difficult to interpret. For this reason, MRI should be scheduled at least 6 weeks after biopsy.

▶ **Differential diagnosis**
- *Chronic prostatitis*: Chronic prostatitis cannot be positively distinguished from prostate cancer even with multiparametric MRI, so it should always be considered in the differential diagnosis. The clinical course or directed, image-guided biopsy can establish the diagnosis.
- *Benign prostatic hyperplasia*: The nodules that form in BPH also require differentiation from prostate cancer. Multiparametric MRI cannot positively distinguish hyperplastic nodules from cancer. However, the detection of a hypointense rim on T2W images of the nodules can confirm a diagnosis of BPH. Thus, the latest MRI techniques should always be interpreted in conjunction with the T2W image findings. It is still challenging to differentiate a stroma-rich, rimless nodule in BPH from prostate cancer.
- *Hypointense fibrosis*: Hypointense fibrosis on T2W and T1W images of the prostate can be differentiated from prostate cancer by dynamic contrast-enhanced MRI and proton MRS. An area of fibrosis does not have an increased transfer constant on pharmacokinetic maps compared with prostate cancer, and fibrosis does not show a choline-to-citrate ratio that is suspicious for cancer.

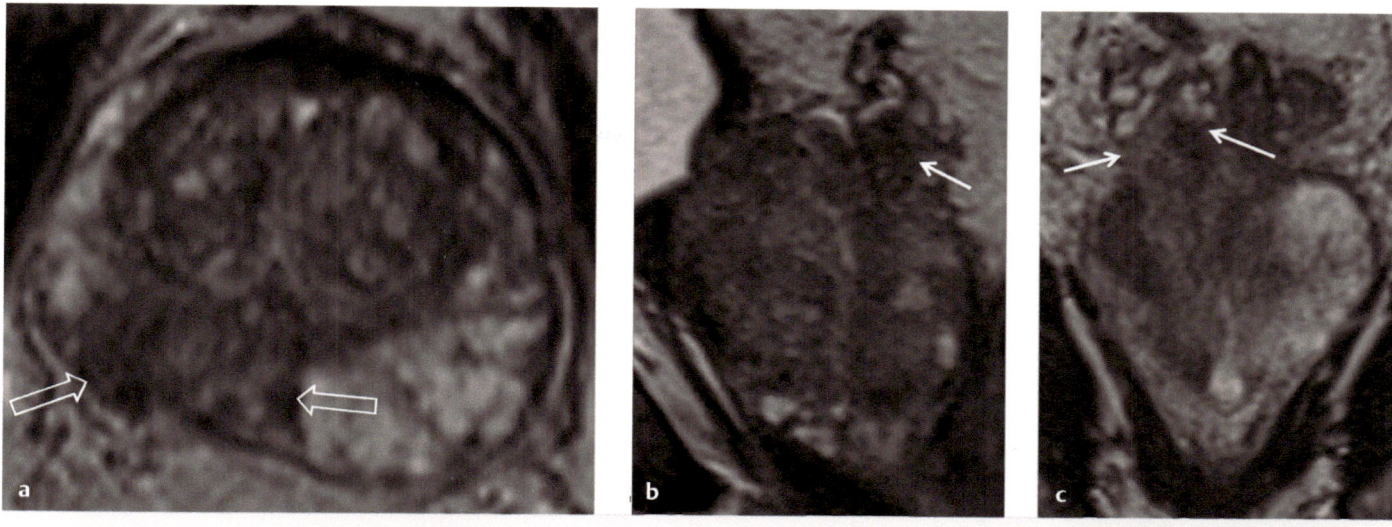

Fig. 13.33 Prostate cancer with invasion of the right seminal vesicle (T3b). T2 W images of the prostate in a 69-year-old man with a serum PSA of 16.2 ng/mL and biopsy-proven prostate cancer with a Gleason score of 4 + 5. The axial image demonstrates the prostate cancer ([a], open arrows) in the right peripheral zone. Invasion of the right seminal vesicle is clearly apparent in the sagittal and coronal images ([b], [c], arrows). (a) Axial T2 W image. (b) Sagittal T2 W image. (c) Coronal T2 W image.

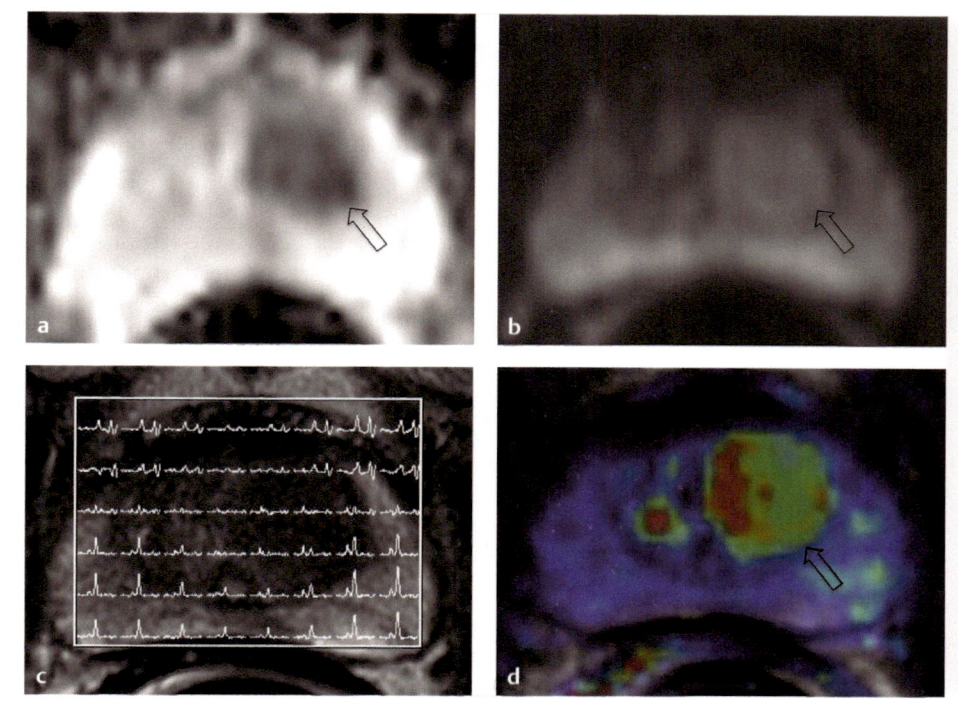

Fig. 13.34 Prostate cancer. The same patient as in ▶ Fig. 13.31. Multiparametric MRI. (a) ADC map. The prostate cancer (arrow) is characterized by restricted diffusion relative to normal surrounding tissue. (b) Corresponding b-800 image. The prostate cancer (arrow) is hyperintense. (c) MRS. This area shows decreased citrate and elevated choline levels relative to normal tissue. (d) The transfer constant K_{trans} calculated from signal intensities on dynamic contrast-enhanced MRI shows elevated values in prostate cancer (arrow) compared with normal tissue.

- Postbiopsy *hemorrhage*: Hemorrhage after needle biopsy may appear as a focal T2 W hypointensity that resembles prostate cancer. But an older hemorrhage is hyperintense on T1 W images and this will suggest the correct diagnosis.

▶ **Key points.** Prostate cancer is the most common malignant tumor in males. The aggressiveness of the tumor is assessed with the Gleason grade or Gleason score. Staging is based on the TNM classification. In this system a T1 tumor is detectable only by biopsy, a T2 tumor is confined to the prostate, a T3 tumor shows extracapsular extension, and a T4 tumor has invaded adjacent structures. Prostate cancer typically appears as a focal hypointensity on T2 W images. The specificity of this feature is increased by the modern techniques of proton MRS, DWI, and dynamic contrast-enhanced MRI. Chronic prostatitis is the main condition that requires imaging differentiation from prostate cancer.

Bibliography

▶ **Testis and Epididymis**

[1] Andipa E, Liberopoulos K, Asvestis C. Magnetic resonance imaging and ultrasound evaluation of penile and testicular masses. World J Urol. 2004; 22(5):382–391
[2] Cramer BM, Schlegel EA, Thueroff JW. MR imaging in the differential diagnosis of scrotal and testicular disease. Radiographics. 1991; 11(1):9–21

[3] Dogra VS, Gottlieb RH, Oka M, Rubens DJ. Sonography of the scrotum. Radiology. 2003; 227(1):18–36

[4] Hamm B. Differential diagnosis of scrotal masses by ultrasound. Eur Radiol. 1997; 7(5):668–679

[5] Hamm B, Asbach P, Beyersdorff D, Hein P, Zaspel U, eds. Urogenitales System. Stuttgart: Thieme; 2007

[6] Hautmann R. Urologie. 4th ed. Heidelberg: Springer; 2010

[7] Kubik-Huch RA, Hailemariam S, Hamm B. CT and MRI of the male genital tract: radiologic-pathologic correlation. Eur Radiol. 1999; 9(1):16–28

[8] Leonhardt WC, Gooding GA. Sonography of intrascrotal adenomatoid tumor. Urology. 1992; 39(1):90–92

[9] Müller-Leisse C, Bohndorf K, Stargardt A, et al. Gadolinium-enhanced T1-weighted versus T2-weighted imaging of scrotal disorders: is there an indication for MR imaging? J Magn Reson Imaging. 1994; 4(3):389–395

[10] Tsili AC, Tsampoulas C, Giannakopoulos X, et al. MRI in the histologic characterization of testicular neoplasms. AJR Am J Roentgenol. 2007; 189(6):W331–W337

▶ Penis

[11] Andresen R, Wegner HE, Miller K, Banzer D. Imaging modalities in Peyronie's disease. An intrapersonal comparison of ultrasound sonography, X-ray in mammography technique, computerized tomography, and nuclear magnetic resonance in 20 patients. Eur Urol. 1998; 34(2):128–134, discussion 135

[12] Kalash SS, Young JD, Jr. Fracture of penis: controversy of surgical versus conservative treatment. Urology. 1984; 24(1):21–24

[13] Kirkham A. MRI of the penis. Br J Radiol. 2012; 85(Spec No 1):S86–S93

[14] Kirkham AP, Illing RO, Minhas S, Minhas S, Allen C. MR imaging of nonmalignant penile lesions. Radiographics. 2008; 28(3):837–853

[15] McCance DJ, Kalache A, Ashdown K, et al. Human papillomavirus types 16 and 18 in carcinomas of the penis from Brazil. Int J Cancer. 1986; 37(1):55–59

[16] Pretorius ES, Siegelman ES, Ramchandani P, Banner MP. MR imaging of the penis. Radiographics. 2001; 21(Spec No):S283–S298, discussion S298–S299

[17] Uder M, Gohl D, Takahashi M, et al. MRI of penile fracture: diagnosis and therapeutic follow-up. Eur Radiol. 2002; 12(1):113–120

[18] Vapnek JM, Hricak H, Carroll PR. Recent advances in imaging studies for staging of penile and urethral carcinoma. Urol Clin North Am. 1992; 19(2):257–266

▶ Prostate and Seminal Vesicles

[19] Choi YJ, Kim JK, Kim N, Kim KW, Choi EK, Cho KS. Functional MR imaging of prostate cancer. Radiographics. 2007; 27(1):63–75, discussion 75–77

[20] Engelbrecht MR, Huisman HJ, Laheij RJ, et al. Discrimination of prostate cancer from normal peripheral zone and central gland tissue by using dynamic contrast-enhanced MR imaging. Radiology. 2003; 229(1):248–254

[21] Franiel T. Multiparametrische Magnetresonanztomografie der Prostata-Technik und klinische Anwendungen [Multiparametric magnetic resonance imaging of the prostate—technique and clinical applications]. RoFo. 2011; 183:607–617

[22] Franiel T, Stephan C, Erbersdobler A, et al. Areas suspicious for prostate cancer: MR-guided biopsy in patients with at least one transrectal US-guided biopsy with a negative finding–multiparametric MR imaging for detection and biopsy planning. Radiology. 2011; 259(1):162–172

[23] Leitlinienprogramm Onkologie der AWMF, Deutsche Krebsgesellschaft e. V. und Deutsche Krebshilfe e. V. Interdisziplinäre Leitlinie der Qualität S3 zur Früherkennung, Diagnose und Therapie der verschiedenen Stadien des Prostatakarzinoms. Version 2.0. AWMF-Register-Nr. 043–022OL; 2011

[24] McNeal JE. The zonal anatomy of the prostate. Prostate. 1981; 2(1):35–49

[25] McNeal JE, Redwine EA, Freiha FS, Stamey TA. Zonal distribution of prostatic adenocarcinoma. Correlation with histologic pattern and direction of spread. Am J Surg Pathol. 1988; 12(12):897–906

[26] Moseley ME, Butts K, Yenari MA, Marks M, de Crespigny A. Clinical aspects of DWI. NMR Biomed. 1995; 8(7–8):387–396

[27] Mountford CE, Doran S, Lean CL, Russell P. Proton MRS can determine the pathology of human cancers with a high level of accuracy. Chem Rev. 2004; 104(8):3677–3704

[28] Nelson AW, Harvey RC, Parker RA, Kastner C, Doble A, Gnanapragasam VJ. Repeat prostate biopsy strategies after initial negative biopsy: meta-regression comparing cancer detection of transperineal, transrectal saturation and MRI guided biopsy. PLoS One. 2013; 8(2):e57480

[29] Qayyum A, Coakley FV, Lu Y, et al. Organ-confined prostate cancer: effect of prior transrectal biopsy on endorectal MRI and MR spectroscopic imaging. AJR Am J Roentgenol. 2004; 183(4):1079–1083

[30] Schiebler ML, Tomaszewski JE, Bezzi M, et al. Prostatic carcinoma and benign prostatic hyperplasia: correlation of high-resolution MR and histopathologic findings. Radiology. 1989; 172(1):131–137

[31] Schünke M, Schulte E, Schumacher U. Prometheus. LernAtlas der Anatomie: Innere Organe. 2nd ed. Stuttgart: Thieme; 2009. Illustrated by M. Voll/K. Wesker

[32] Schünke M, Schulte E, Schumacher U. Prometheus. LernAtlas der Anatomie: Allgemeine Anatomie und Bewegungssystem. 3rd ed. Stuttgart: Thieme; 2011. Illustrated by M. Voll/K. Wesker

[33] Siegel R, Naishadham D, Jemal A. Cancer statistics, 2012. CA Cancer J Clin. 2012; 62(1):10–29

[34] Swanson MG, Vigneron DB, Tabatabai ZL, et al. Proton HR-MAS spectroscopy and quantitative pathologic analysis of MRI/3D-MRSI-targeted postsurgical prostate tissues. Magn Reson Med. 2003; 50(5):944–954

[35] White S, Hricak H, Forstner R, et al. Prostate cancer: effect of postbiopsy hemorrhage on interpretation of MR images. Radiology. 1995; 195(2):385–390

Index

Note: Page numbers set bold or *italic* indicate headings or figures, respectively.

A

abscess
- cholangiogenic 268
- hepatic 215, *219*
-- amebic 219
-- multiple abscesses *219*
-- with cholangitis 289
- lung 141
- lymph node 364
- prevertebral 387
- prostatic 487
- renal 416
- splenic 358, *359*
- tubo-ovarian 438
-- tubercular 438
absorption atelectasis 133, *133*
accessory renal arteries 394, *395*
accessory spleen 354, *354*
achalasia 323, *325*
acinar cell carcinoma 310, *312*
acute aortic syndrome 82
acute interstitial pneumonia 155, *156*
adenocarcinoma
- colorectal 217, 348
- esophageal 327
- gallbladder 275
- lung 148
- ovarian 461
- pancreatic 300, *303*, 310
-- classification 302
-- staging 302
- small bowel 342
-- classification 343
adenoma 203
- adrenal 384
- Conn 379
- hepatocellular 202, *205*
adenomyoma 448, *448*
adenomyomatosis 256, 270, *273*, 276
adenomyosis 447, *447*, 448
- diffuse *449*
- focal *448*
adenosarcoma 458
adhesive atelectasis 133
adrenal glands
- adenoma 384
- anatomy 371
- carcinoma 373
- cysts 383
- functional diseases 377
- hematoma *374*, 388
- imaging 371
-- adults 371
-- children 371
-- computed tomography (CT) 373
-- magnetic resonance imaging (MRI) 375
-- positron emission tomography-computed tomography (PET-CT) 374
-- ultrasound 371
- incidentaloma *372*, 375
- lung cancer staging 376–377
- metastases 385
- myelolipoma 383, *385*
adrenal vein sampling 375
adrenocortical carcinoma 373, **388**, *389*
- classification 389
adrenocortical insufficiency 382
adrenogenital syndrome 382
adult respiratory distress syndrome (ARDS) 171, *172*
- diagnostic criteria 171
adventitia 71
alpha-antitrypsin deficiency 130
alveolar microlithiasis 169, *170*
alveolar proteinosis 169, *171*
alveoli 126
amebic abscess 219
amyloidosis 45, *45*, *168*, 168
aneurysm
- aortic 78, *81*
-- abdominal 80, 84
-- ascending 81
-- causes 79
-- classification *81–82*
-- diameter related to complication rates 84
-- mycotic 81
-- thoracoabdominal 83
- pulmonary artery 111, *113*
-- classification 113
-- iatrogenic *114*
- splenic artery 361, *362*
angina pectoris
- stable 37
- unstable 37
angiofollicular hyperplasia 21
angiomyelolipoma 193
angiomyolipoma 193, *195–196*, 401, *403–405*
angiosarcoma *57*, 57
- hepatic 198
- inferior vena cava 97
annular pancreas 294, *295*
anthracosis 162
aorta 71
- abdominal 71
-- aneurysm 80
- acute aortic syndrome 82
- anatomy 71, *71*
- ascending *3*, *31*, 71
-- aneurysm 81
- coarctation 75, *75*, *76*
-- infantile *76*
- congenital anomalies *72*, *78*
-- variants in the origins of supra-aortic vessels 73, *73*, *73*, *74*
- coral reef 93, *94*
- descending *3*, *31*, 71
- development *72*, 72
- intramural hematoma 86, *87*
- penetrating ulcer *88*, 88
aortic aneurysms 78, *81*
- abdominal 80
-- follow-up 84
-- causes 79
-- Crawford classification 82
-- diameter related to complication rates 84
-- Estrera classification 81
-- metastases 385
-- mycotic 81
-- thoracoabdominal 83
aortic arch 71
- classification 72
- double 76, *77*
- right *77*, *78*
aortic dissection 84, *86*
- classification 85
aortic fistulas 97
aortic insufficiency *62*, 62
aortic nipple 81, *84*
aortic root 71
aortic rupture 89, *90*
- spontaneous 90
- traumatic *89*, 90
aortic stenosis 60, *60*, *61*
- congenital abdominal 78
- coral reef aorta 93, *94*
- grading 60
aortic vascular rings 76, *77*
aortitis 94
- causes 94, *94*
aortocaval fistula 98
aortoenteric fistula 97, *98*
aortoiliac stenoses, classification 93, *93*
aortopulmonary fistula 97–98
aortopulmonary window 2
aplasia
- pericardial 68
- pulmonary 134
appendicitis 345, *345*
arcuate uterus 436, *436*
arrhythmogenic right ventricular cardiomyopathy *44*, 45
arterial hypovascular hepatic lesions 190–191
arteriovenous malformations 117, 118–119
- Rendu-Osler-Weber disease 192
asbestosis 161, *163*
- mesothelioma 176, *176*
- pulmonary fibrosis 163
aspergilloma 143, *144*
aspergillosis 143
- allergic bronchopulmonary 143–144, *145*
- invasive 144
-- angioinvasive 143, *145*
aspiration events *165*, 165, *166*
asplenia 354
atelectasis 132, *134*
- absorption 133, *133*
- adhesive 133
- compression 133, *133*
- contraction 133
atherosclerosis 33
atresia
- biliary 249, *252*, 294
- esophageal 326, *328*
-- classification 327, *328*
atrial septum
- lipomatous hypertrophy 52, *54*
- myxoma *52*
atrium
- left 31
-- lipoma *53*
-- myxoma *52*
-- right *2*, 31

-- lipoma *53*
-- thrombus *56*
atypical pneumonia 138
autoimmune pancreatitis 300
azygos continuation 103
azygos vein *3*, 101

B

B-cell lymphoma 20, *23*
Bartholin gland carcinoma 456
Bartholin's cysts 439
benign mesenchymal tumors in children 195
benign prostatic hyperplasia **488**, *488*, 490
β-thalassemia 319
bicornuate uterus *436*, 436, *437*
bifid ureter 393, *424*
bile ducts 239, *240*
- benign tumors 270
- common 239, *241*
-- carcinoma 278, *279*, 289
- dilatation 244
-- cystic 248
- intraductal papillary mucinous neoplasm 272, *274*
- obstruction 261
-- intrahepatic 244, *284*
- postoperative changes
-- cholecystectomy 283, *284*
-- endoscopic retrograde cholangiopancreatography 285, *286*
-- percutaneous transhepatic cholangiodrainage 285, *287–288*
- variants 246, *249–251*
bile plug syndrome 249
biliary atresia 246, 249, *252*
biliary capillaries 239
biliary cystadenocarcinoma 277, *277*
biliary fluid 239
- flow in liver 240
biliary hamartomas of interlobular ducts 244
biliary obstruction 244, 261, 284
biliary pancreatitis 260
biliary stricture 282, 285
biliary tract, *see* bile ducts
- anatomy 239
-- variants 244
- developmental anomalies 244
-- classification 245, *248*
- imaging 242
- pathophysiology 240
- trauma 281
biliary-cutaneous fistula 285
biliary-vascular fistula 288
biloma 282, 285
bladder masses 420, *426*
- carcinoma 425, *427*
Bochdalek hernia 26, *27*
Bochdalek triangle 26
brachiocephalic trunk 3
brachiocephalic veins *3*, 101
broad ligament *431*, 433
bronchi *2–3*, *123*
- *See also* lung
- bifurcation angle 122

491

Index

- mucocele 129
- tracheal bronchus 127
bronchial arteries 122, 124
- hypertrophy 124
bronchial tree 126
bronchiectasis 128
- cystic fibrosis 129, 160
bronchiolitis 128, 130
- constrictive 130, 131
bronchiolitis-associated interstitial lung disease 154, 154
bronchitis 130
bronchogenic cysts 16, 16, 136
bronchopneumonia 138–139, 140
BuddChiari syndrome 187, 187
Burkitt's lymphoma 201, 366

C

calcification
- alveolar 170
- coronary arteries 37
-- Agatston score 37
- extratesticular macrocalcification 476
- gallbladder 263
- pericardial 68–69
- renal cyst 398
- silicosis 161
- splenic cyst 358
carcinoids 12, 12, 343
- See also neuroendocrine tumors
- mediastinal 12
- small intestine 344
- thymic 12
carcinoma, see adenocarcinoma
- acinar cell 310, 312
- adrenocortical 373, 388, 389
-- classification 389
- Bartholin gland 456
- bladder 425, 427
- bronchogenic, see lung cancer
- cervical 449, 451
-- recurrence 456
-- staging 452
- cholangiocellular 269, 277
- colorectal 348
-- classification 349
-- staging 349
- common bile duct 278, 279, 289
- cystic duct 278
- embryonic cell 14, 463
- endometrial 448, 450
-- recurrence 456
-- staging 451
- esophageal 327, 330
-- classification 330
-- staging 30
- fallopian tube 464
- fibrolamellar 206, 206, 207
- gallbladder 275, 276
-- staging 276
- gastric 334, 334
- hepatic duct bifurcation 278
- hepatocellular 206, 208–211, 375
- lung, see lung cancer
- ovarian 447, 461
-- staging 458
- pancreatic 280, 300, 303
-- classification 302

-- staging 302
- penile 482, 484
- prostate 483, 489
-- classification 489
- renal cell 405
-- classification 410
-- clear cell 406, 408
-- papillary 406, 409
- small intestine 342
- testicular 476
- thymic 10, 11
- thyroid 9
- urothelial 420, 425, 427
- vaginal 453, 453
-- recurrence 456
-- staging 454
- vulvar 454, 455
-- recurrence 456
-- staging 455, 456
carcinomatosis, pericardial 69
cardiac cycle 39
cardiac function assessment
- global 38
- regional 38
cardiac tumors 48
- benign primary tumors 51
-- children 55
- malignant primary tumors 57
- malignant secondary tumors 59
-- contiguous spread 59
-- metastases 59, 59
-- transvascular invasion 59, 59
- sites of occurrence 51
cardinal ligament 433
cardinal veins 102
cardiomyopathies 41
- arrhythmogenic right ventricular 44, 45
- dilated 43, 44
- hypertrophic 29, 33, 46, 49–50
- noncompaction 48
- restrictive 45
- Takotsubo 46, 48
cardiothoracic ratio 35
Caroli's disease 250
Caroli's syndrome 244, 250, 254
carotid artery
- common 3
- variants in origin 73–74
Castleman's disease 21, 23, 368, 368
cavernosal thrombosis 480, 481
cavernous hemangioma 193
celiac trunk 178, 180, 292, 293
- biliary-vascular fistula 288
cervical carcinoma 449, 451
- recurrence 456
- staging 452
cervical rib syndrome 100, 100
chemotherapy-induced cholangitis 288
chemotherapy-induced cholecystitis 288, 290
chloroma 215, 218
chocolate cyst 444
cholangiocarcinoma 277
- growth patterns 278
- staging 279
cholangiocellular carcinoma 269, 277
cholangiogenic abscesses 268
cholangitis
- ascending 266, 268

- chemotherapy-induced 288
- following long-term drainage 289
- primary sclerosing 267, 267, 269
- secondary sclerosing 267, 269
cholecystectomy, cystic duct leak 235, 283, 285
cholecystitis 260
- chemotherapy-induced 288, 290
- chronic 262, 264, 276
cholecystolithiasis 245, 255, 257, 260
choledochal cysts 249
- classification 248
- type I 253
choledocholithiasis 258–260, 281
cholelithiasis 253
- See also gallstones
- silent 254
cholestasis 240, 243
- nonobstructive 241
- obstructive 241
cholesterolosis 270, 273
choriocarcinoma 463, 478
chorionic epithelioma 14
chronic lymphocytic leukemia 365
chronic obstructive pulmonary disease (COPD) 130
ChurgStrauss syndrome 166, 167
cirrhosis, liver 222, 225–226, 269
- alcoholic 355–356
- portal venous collaterals 227
coarctation of the aorta 75, 75, 76
- infantile 76
colitis
- pseudomembranous 346, 346
- ulcerative 346, 347
-- clinical features 347
-- imaging signs 347
-- versus Crohn's disease 342
collateral pathways
- hepatic cirrhosis 227
- Leriche syndrome 91, 91
- portal hypertension 225
colon 320, 324
- diseases 344
- diverticula 348
- transverse 323
colonic carcinoma 349, 350
- colorectal, sigmoid colon 349
colorectal carcinoma 348
- classification 349
- staging 349
community-acquired pneumonia 139
compression atelectasis 133, 133
congenital adrenal hyperplasia 382
congenital diaphragmatic hernia 136, 137, 137
congenital hepatic fibrosis 244
congenital lobar emphysema 136, 136
Conn adenoma 379
connective tissue diseases 167
- manifestations 167
constrictive bronchiolitis 130, 131
constrictive pericarditis 66, 68–69
coral reef aorta 93, 94
coronary arteries 31, 38
- calcification 37
-- Agatston score 37
- plaques 38
coronary heart disease 33
coronary occlusion 36

coronary stenosis 35
costoclavicular syndrome 100, 101
CREST syndrome 167
Crohn's disease 339, 341–342
- versus ulcerative colitis 342
cryptogenic organizing pneumonia 154, 155
cryptorchidism 470, 470
Cullen's sign 297, 297
Cushing's syndrome 377
cutaneous T-cell lymphoma 366
cystadenocarcinoma, biliary 277, 277
cystadenofibroma 459
cystadenoma
- mucinous 461
- serous 306, 307
cystic adenomatoid malformation of the lung 135, 136
cystic artery 240, 241
cystic duct
- carcinoma 278
- leak 235, 283, 285
cystic fibrosis 159, 160, 311
- bronchiectasis 129, 160
- pseudohypertrophy of the pancreas 315
- with pancreatic lipomatosis 314
cystic hygroma 18
cysts
- adrenal 383
- bronchogenic 16, 16, 136
- chocolate 444
- choledochal 249
-- classification 248
-- type I 253
- dermoid 13, 446
- endometriotic 447
- epidermoid 13
- epididymal 473, 474
- esophageal duplication 18, 18
- hepatic 184, 194, 197
-- multilocular 198
- ovarian 440, 462
- pancreatic 305, 312
-- differential diagnosis 310
- pericardial 17, 17
- renal 394, 396–399
-- See also polycystic kidney disease
-- Bosniak classification 395
-- cystic renal degeneration 398
-- with solid components 399–400
- splenic 357, 358
-- calcified 358
-- hemorrhagic 328
- testicular 473, 475
- thymic 11, 12
- tunica 473, 475
- unilocular 305
- urachal 426
-- infected 429
- uterine 439
- vaginal 439
- vulvar 439

D

delayed enhancement 39, 41
dermatomyositis 167
dermoid cysts 13, 446

Index

desquamative interstitial pneumonia 154, *155*
diaphragm *26*
– hernias 26
– – congenital 136, *137*, 137
– – rupture *234*
diffuse large B-cell lymphoma 367
dilated cardiomyopathy 43, *44*
diverticula
– duodenal 329, *331*
– esophageal 324, *325*
– gastric 329, *331*
– Kommerell 73, *74*
– Meckel's *335*, 335
– pericardial *17*, 17
– Zenker's 324
diverticulitis *348*, 348
diverticulosis *348*, 348
double aortic arch 76, *77*
double crush syndrome 101
Dressler's syndrome 66
drowning, near 165, *165*
ductal adenocarcinoma, pancreatic 300, *303*
– classification 302
– staging 302
duodenal diverticulum 329, *331*
duodenum 319
– blood supply 293
– ulcer 330
duplex kidney 418, *422*, *424*
duplex ureter 393, *425*

E

Echinococcus granulosus (dog tapeworm) 220, 220, *221–222*
Echinococcus multilocularis (fox tapeworm) 220, *222–223*
ectopic thyroid tissue 10
edge-on effect 3
embryonic cell carcinoma 14, 476
emphysema 130, *132*
– congenital lobar *136*, 136
empyema
– gallbladder 259, *263*, 267
– pleural *176*, 176
endometrial carcinoma 448, *450*
– recurrence 456
– staging *451*
endometrioma 444
endometriosis 444
– deep infiltrating 444, *447*
– sites of involvement 449
endometriotic cyst *447*
endometritis 437
endometrium 431
endoscopic retrograde cholangiopancreatography (ERCP) 259
– complication 267
– postoperative changes 285, *286*
epidermoid cysts 13
epididymal cysts 473, *474*
epididymal tumors 479
epididymis
– anatomy *468*
– imaging 468
epididymitis *472*, 472
epididymo-orchitis 472
epiploic appendagitis *346*, 346

esophageal carcinoma 327, *330*
– classification 330
– staging 330
esophageal duplication cysts *18*, 18
esophagus 3, 319
– achalasia 323, *325*
– anatomy 319, *321*
– atresia 326, *328*
– – classification 327, *328*
– carcinoma, *see* esophageal carcinoma
– constrictions 319
– diverticula 324, *325*
– – epiphrenic 325
– – parabronchial 325, *326*
– – pulsion 324
– – traction 324
– – Zenker's 324
– varices 325, *326–327*
extragonadal germ cell tumors 12, *14*
– markers 14
extramedullary hematopoiesis *26*, 26
extratesticular macrocalcification 476
extrinsic allergic alveolitis 163, *164*

F

fallopian tubes *431–432*
– carcinoma 464
– torsion 441
fatty liver, *see* hepatic steatosis
female pelvis
– anatomy *431–432*, *434*
– – benign tumors and pseudotumors 439
– – blood supply *432*, 433
– – genitalia 431
– – lymphatic drainage 433
– – pelvic floor 433
– congenital anomalies 436
– differential diagnosis 435
– imaging 433
– – computed tomography (CT) 435
– – magnetic resonance imaging (MRI) 434, 435, *435*
– – transabdominal ultrasound 434
– inflammatory changes 437
– malignant lesions 448
– suspensory apparatus 433
fibroadenoma *54*
fibroelastoma 53, *54–55*
fibrolamellar carcinoma 206, *206*, *207*
fibroma 55–56, 447
fibromuscular dysplasia 414, *421*
fibropolycystic liver disease 246
fibrosarcoma, cardiac 57
fibrosclerosis, multifocal 5
fibrosis, *see* cystic fibrosis
– asbestosis 163
– congenital hepatic 244
– idiopathic pulmonary 151, *152*
– mediastinal 8
– retroperitoneal 416, 418
fire-related pulmonary trauma 164
fistula
– aortic 97
– biliary-cutaneous 285
– biliary-vascular 288
– tracheoesophageal 326
– vaginal *439*, 439

focal fatty infiltration of the liver 221, *224*
focal fatty sparing in the liver 221, *224*
focal nodular hyperplasia *202*, 202, *204*
foreign body aspiration 165, *166*
Franz's tumor 311

G

gallbladder 239
– benign tumors 270
– – hyperplasia of the gallbladder wall 270
– blood vessels 240, *241*
– – variants *242*
– empyema 259, *263*, 267
– hydrops 259, *262*
– imaging 242
– – computed tomography (CT) 243
– – conventional radiography 242
– – magnetic resonance cholangiopancreatography 243
– – magnetic resonance imaging (MRI) 243
– – ultrasonography 242, *245*
– innervation 240
– lymphatics 240
– malignant tumors 275
– – carcinoma 275, 276, *276*
– – metastases 270, 276
– pathophysiology 240
– polyps 256, 270, *271–272*, 276
– porcelain 262, *264*
– – Mirizzi's syndrome *266*
– sludge 256, *257*
– trauma 281, *282*
– tumor 256
– variants 245, *249*
gallstones 253, *255–258*, *264*, 270
– *See also* cholecystolithiasis
ganglioneuroblastoma 386–387
ganglioneuroma 386–387
Gartner's duct cysts 439
gastric artery 180
gastric carcinoma *334*, 334
gastric diverticulum 329, *331*
gastric juice aspiration 165
gastric lymphoma 333, *334*
gastrinoma 304
gastrinoma triangle 304
gastroduodenal artery 180
gastrointestinal stromal tumors (GIST) *333*, 333
– classification 333
gastrointestinal tract
– anatomy 319
– imaging 322
– – computed tomography (CT) 323
– – contrast media 323
– – magnetic resonance imaging (MRI) 323
– – radiography 322
– imaging landmarks 320
– wall layers 319, *322*
germ cell tumors, extragonadal 12, *14*
– markers 14
– mixed 14
Gerota's fascia 392, *393*
giant cell arteritis 95
goiter 8, *9*

– multinodular *9*
Goodpasture's syndrome 168, *169*
Grey-Turner sign *297*, 297

H

hairy cell leukemia 366
hamartoma 150, *152*
– biliary, of interlobular ducts 244
– mesenchymal 195, 197, *200*
heart
– anatomy 29
– – cardiac borders 29, *30*
– – cardiac chambers 29, *31*
– – slice orientations *32*
– cardiomyopathies 41
– coronary heart disease 33
– thrombi *56*, 56
– tumors 48
– – benign primary tumors 51
– – malignant primary tumors 57
– – malignant secondary tumors 59
– – sites of occurrence 51
heart failure 31
– imaging signs 32, *35–36*
hemangioendothelioma, infantile 195, 197, *198–199*
hemangioma
– capillary 194
– cardiac 55
– cavernous 193
– giant 194
– hepatic 182, 190, *192*
– splenic 359, *360*
hemangiosarcoma, hepatic 200
hematoma
– adrenal *374*, 388
– intramural 86, *87*
– newborn 387
hematosalpinx 437
hemiazygos continuation 103
hemiazygos vein 3, 101
hemochromatosis 44, 225, *228*, 314, 316
– secondary, *see* hemosiderosis
hemoperitoneum 234
hemorrhage
– gastrointestinal 339, *340–341*
– intrapulmonary 168
– splenic cyst 359
hemosiderosis 44, *228*, 228, *229*, 316
hepatic abscess, *see* liver
hepatic artery 240, *241*
– common 180
– pseudoaneurysm following biliary drain removal 287
hepatic cyst 184, 194, 197
– multilocular 198
hepatic hemangioma 182,
– adult 190
– capillary 194
– cavernous 193
– giant 194
– pediatric 190
hepatic steatosis 230
hepatitis, neonatal
hepatoblastoma 2
– staging 213, 2
hepatocellular c
211, 375

Index

hernia
- Bochdalek 26, 27
- congenital diaphragmatic 136, 137, 137
- hiatal 327, 328–329
- Larrey 26
- Morgagni 26, 27

hiatal hernia 327, 328–329
histiocytosis X 158
Hodgkin's lymphoma 19, 22, 365, 368
- staging 366
horseshoe kidney 394, 394, 395
hydatid disease
- dog tapeworm 220, 220, 221–222
- fox tapeworm 220, 222–223
- imaging features 220

hydrocele 472, 473
hydronephrosis 423
- radiological grades 391
hydrosalpinx 437–438, 438
hymenal atresia 436
hyperaldosteronism 378, 379
hypercortisolism 377
hypertrophic cardiomyopathy 29, 33, 46, 49–50
hypertrophic pyloric stenosis 329, 331

I

ileocolic intussusception reduction 337
ileum 320, 323
- diseases 335
iliac veins 101, 432
- thrombosis 106
immunocytoma 367
incidentaloma 372, 375
- management algorithm 379
infant respiratory distress syndrome (IRDS) 173
- stages 173, 174
infantile hemangioendothelioma 195, 197, 198–199

- reduction 337
iron storage diseases 225
ischemic cascade 36
Islet cell tumor 304

J

jaundice, obstructive 240, 244, 260–261, 283–284
jejunum 320, 323
- diseases 335
jugular vein 101

K

kidney
- abscess 416
- agenesis 393
- anatomy 392
-- blood supply 396
-- congenital variants 393
-- positional variants 393
-- cysts 394, 396–399
-- See also polycystic kidney disease
-- Bosniak classification 395
-- cystic renal degeneration 401
-- with solid components 399–400
-- duplex 418, 422, 424
- horseshoe 394, 394, 395
- imaging 391
-- computed tomography (CT) 391
-- corticomedullary phase 392
-- diffusion-weighted imaging (DWI) 392
-- magnetic resonance imaging (MRI) 392
-- parenchymal phase 392
-- radiography 391
-- ultrasound 391
-- urographic phase 392
-- venous phase 392
-- voiding cystourethrography 391
- inflammatory changes 409
- medullary sponge 400
- pediatric tumors 406
-- nephroblastoma 406, 411
-- neuroblastoma 408, 412
- solid masses 400
-- angiomyolipoma 401, 403–405
-- lymphoma 402, 406–407
-- oncocytoma 400, 402–403
-- renal cell carcinoma 405
- transplantation 416
-- postoperative period 416
-- preoperative evaluation 416
- vascular changes 413

Klatskin tumor 278, 280
Kommerell diverticulum 73, 74

- without degenerative changes 442
leiomyosarcoma
- cardiac 57
- uterine 458
- vaginal 460

Leriche syndrome 91
- acute 91, 92
- chronic 91, 92

leukemia
- chronic lymphocytic 365
- hairy cell 366

lipoma 15, 16
- cardiac 52, 53
- hepatic 193
- pancreatic 310, 313–314
- retroperitoneal 418

lipomatosis mediastinalis 15, 16
lipomatous hypertrophy of the atrial septum 52, 54
liposarcoma 15, 15
- cardiac 57
- retroperitoneal 418

liver
- abscess 215, 219
-- amebic 219
-- with cholangitis 289
- anatomy 178, 179
-- variants 178
- arterial hypovascular lesions 190–191
- bile flow 240
- blood flow 240
- cirrhosis 222, 225–226, 269
-- alcoholic 355–356
-- portal venous collaterals 227
- differential diagnosis of focal lesions 189–192
- imaging 178
-- chemical shift technique 181, 183
-- computed tomography (CT) 179, 181
-- contrast-enhanced imaging techniques 181, 182, 184–185
-- diffusion-weighted imaging 181, 184
-- extracellular contrast agents 181
-- landmarks 178
-- magnetic resonance imaging (MRI) 180
-- ultrasonography 178
-- unenhanced imaging techniques 181
- inflammatory changes 215
- mesenchymal tumors
-- benign 190, 195
-- malignant 198
- metastases 184–185, 213, 214–215
- parasitic lesions 219
- parenchymal pseudolesions 221
- primary hepatocellular lesions 202
-- benign 202
-- malignant 206
- trauma 232, 282
-- contusion 234
-- injury scale 233
-- laceration 233–234
- vascular diseases 182

lung
- abscess 141
- anatomy 121, 122

-- interlobar fissures 121, 121
-- pulmonary segments 121, 123
- congenital malformations 134
-- cystic adenomatoid malformation 135, 136
-- vascular anomalies 135
- infections 138
- neoplasms 146
- parenchyma 126
- trauma 164
- vessels 122

lung cancer 59, 148, 148, 149
- central cell carcinoma 150
- classification 148, 151
- mediastinal cell carcinoma 150
- squamous cell carcinoma 149
- staging 151, 376–377

lupus erythematosus 167
lymph nodes
- abscess 364
- anatomy 362
- chest 19, 20
- differential diagnosis of enlargement 364
- imaging 362
-- computed tomography (CT) 363, 364
-- magnetic resonance imaging (MRI) 363
-- positron emission tomography-computed tomography (PET-CT) 364, 364
-- radiography 363
-- ultrasound 363, 363
- metastases 363, 364, 366
-- retroperitoneal 418

lymphadenitis, tuberculous 365
lymphadenopathy, reactive 364
lymphangioleiomyomatosis 159, 159
lymphangioma 18, 18, 136
- splenic 359
lymphoid interstitial pneumonia 156
lymphoma 19
- Burkitt's 201, 367
- cardiac 58, 58
- cutaneous T-cell 366
- diffuse large B-cell 367
- gastric 333, 334
- hepatic 199, 201
- Hodgkin's 19, 22, 365, 368
-- staging 366
- malignant 364
- MALT 366
-- pulmonary 366
-- vocal cord 367
- mantle cell 367
- marginal zone 366
- non-Hodgkin's 20, 365, 367
-- B-cell 23, 367
-- staging 366
- pelvic 460
- renal 402, 406–407
- splenic 356–357, 358
- testicular 477
- uterine 461
- vulvovaginal 457, 461

M

malacoplakia 417

Index

malignant lymphoma 364
- *See also* lymphoma
MALT lymphoma 366
- pulmonary 366
- vocal cord 367
mantle cell lymphoma 367
marginal zone lymphoma 366
May-Thurner syndrome 105, *106*
MayerRokitanskyKüsterHauser syndrome 437
Meckel's diverticulum *335*, 335
media 71
mediastinitis 8
- acute 3
- chronic 5
mediastinum
- anatomy 1
-- CT landmarks 1, *3*
-- divisions 1, *2*
-- radiographic landmarks 1, *2*
- masses 7
-- anterior mediastinum 8
-- cystic 16
-- middle mediastinum 19
-- posterior mediastinum 23
- radiographic evaluation 1
-- edge-on effect *3*
-- silhouette sign 1, *5–6*
- traumatic injury 27
medullary cystic kidney disease 400
medullary sponge kidney 400
melanoma 364
mesenteric artery
- inferior 180
- superior 180, 292, *293*
-- pseudoaneurysm in chronic pancreatitis *298*
mesenteric ischemia 337
mesenteric vein
- inferior 180, *293*
- superior 180, *293*
mesonephros 393
mesothelioma *176*, 176
mesothelioma, pericardial 67
metanephros 393
metastases
- adrenal 385
- cardiac *59*, 59
- gallbladder 270, 276
- hepatic 184–185, *213*, *214*
-- hypervascular 213, *215–216*
-- hypovascular 213, *216–217*
-- lymph node 363, 364, 366
-- retroperitoneal 418
-- pancreas 304, 305, 306
-- pheochromocytoma 382
-- phrenic nerve *4*
-- splenic 360, *360*, *361*
-- testicular 477
microlithiasis, alveolar 169, *170*
Mirizzi's syndrome 265, *266*
mitral insufficiency *63*, 63, *64*
mitral stenosis 62
- grading 63
Morgagni hernia 26, *27*
mucinous cystadenoma 461
mucinous cystic neoplasm 308, *311*
mucocele 129
multifocal fibrosclerosis 5
multiple myeloma 368, *369*

myelolipoma, adrenal 383, *385*
myocardial hypertrophy 29, *33*, 46, *49*
myocardial infarction *33*, *41–42*
myocardial perfusion
- assessment 39, *39*
- defect *40*
myocarditis 41, *43*
myolipoma 193
myometrium 431
myxoma 51, *52*

N

near-drowning 165, *165*
nephroblastoma 406, *411*
- classification 411
neurinoma 23, *24*
neuroblastoma 6, 24, *25*, 386, 408, 412
- staging 386, 388, 412
neuroendocrine tumors, *see* carcinoids
- classification 343
- pancreas 303
- thymus 12
neurofibroma 23, *24*
neurogenic tumors 23
non-Hodgkin's lymphoma 20, 365, 367
- B-cell 23, 367
- staging 366
nonalcoholic steatohepatitis (NASH) 230, *231*
noncompaction cardiomyopathy 48
nosocomial pneumonia 139
nutcracker syndrome 104

O

obstructive jaundice 240, *244*, *261*, *283–284*
Ogilvie's syndrome 350, *351*
oncocytoma 400, *403*
- multiple 402
oophoritis 437
Ormond's disease 416, *418*, *421–422*
osteosarcoma, cardiac 57
ovarian artery *432*, 433
ovarian carcinoma 447, *461*, 461
- staging 458
ovarian cysts 440, *462*
ovarian torsion 441, *442*
ovarian tumors 461
- *See also* ovarian carcinoma
- borderline 462
- classification 462
- differential diagnosis 463
-- algorithm *464*
ovarian vein 432
ovaries 431, *432*, *432*
- follicles, multiple 441

P

pancreas 304
- anatomy 292
-- blood supply 292, *293*
-- body 292
-- head 292
-- position 292
-- tail 292
-- variants 294
-- annular 294, *295*

- carcinoma 280, 300, *303*
-- classification 302
-- staging 302
- congenital anomalies 294
- cystic lesions 305, 312
-- classification 306
-- differential diagnosis 310
-- macrocystic 308, *311*
-- microcystic 306, *307*
-- with solid components 310
- development 292, *294*
- hypervascular masses 304
- imaging landmarks 292
- lipoma 310, *313–314*
- metastases 304, 305, 306
- neuroendocrine tumors 303
- nonneoplastic diseases 292
- pseudohypertrophy in cystic fibrosis 315
- tumor types 301
pancreas divisum *294*, 294
- incomplete 295
pancreatic arteries 293
pancreatic veins 293
pancreaticoduodenal arteries 293
pancreaticoduodenal veins 293
pancreatitis
- acute 294, *296*
-- paraduodenal 296, *296*
- autoimmune 300
- biliary 260
- chronic 281, 297, *298–299*
-- infected necrotic area 299
papillary fibroelastoma 53, *54–55*
paraduodenal pancreatitis 296, *296*
paraganglioma *25*, 25
parametria 433
parasitic infections, hepatic 219
patent ductus arteriosus 73
peanut aspiration 165, *166*
pectoralis minor syndrome *100*, 101
pelvic inflammatory disease 437
penile carcinoma *482*, *484*
penis
- anatomy *479*, 479
- fracture *482*, *483*
- imaging *479*, *480*
- inflammatory disorders 481
- vascular disorders 479
percutaneous transhepatic cholangio-drainage (PTCD) 243, 267
- postoperative changes 285, *287–288*
pericardial aplasia 68
pericardial cysts *17*, 17
pericardial diverticula *17*, 17
pericarditis 66, *67–68*
- constrictive 66, *68–69*
- infectious 66
pericardium 64, *65–66*
- anatomy 64, *65*
- diseases 66
- masses 67
perimetrium 431
Peyronie's disease 481, *482*
pheochromocytoma 371, *380*, 380
- cystic 384
- management algorithm *381*
- metastatic 382
phrenic nerve 1
- mediastinal metastasis *4*

pleura 121, 173
- mesothelioma *176*, 176
pleural effusion 174, *175*
pleural empyema *176*, 176
pleural plaques 162, *163*
pleuroparenchymal fibroelastosis 156
pneumatosis intestinalis 337, *338*
pneumobilia 245
- postoperative 285, *286*
pneumoconioses 160, 162
- collagenous 162
- noncollagenous 163
Pneumocystis pneumonia 139, *140*
pneumomediastinum 27, *28*
pneumonia 138
- aspiration 165
- community-acquired 139
- cryptogenic organizing 154, *155*
- interstitial 138–139
-- acute 150, 155
-- chronic fibrosing 151
-- desquamatve 154, *155*
-- idiopathic 150–151, 152, *152*, 154
-- lymphoid 156
-- nonspecific *153*, 153
-- smoking-related 154
-- subacute 150
-- usual 151
- nosocomial 139
pneumothorax 27, 173, *174*
polycystic kidney disease 198, *402*
- adult 399
- autosomal dominant (ADPKD) 244, *247*, 399
- autosomal recessive (ARPKD) 398
- infantile 398
- intermediate 399
- juvenile 399
- neonatal 399
polymyositis 167
polyps
- gallbladder 256, 270, *271–272*, 276
- uterine 441
polysplenia 354
porcelain gallbladder 262, *264*
- Mirizzi's syndrome 266
portal hypertension, collateral pathways 225
portal vein thrombosis 182, *185–186*
portal venous system 180
prevertebral abscess 387
priapism 479, *480*
primary hemochromatosis, *see* hemochromatosis
primary hepatocellular lesions 202
- benign 202
- malignant 206
primary hyperaldosteronism 378
primary seminomas 13
pronephros 393
prostate
- anatomy 484, *485–487*
- benign prostatic hyperplasia 488, 488, 490
- imaging 483
prostate cancer 488, *489–491*
-- classification 489
prostatitis 485, *487*
- abscess formation 487
- chronic 490

495

Index

proteinosis, alveolar 169, *171*
pseudoaneurysm following biliary drain removal 287
pseudocysts, pancreas *221*, 305
pseudomembranous colitis *346*, 346
pulmonary agenesis 134, *135*
pulmonary aplasia 134
pulmonary arteries *2–3*, 122
- agenesis 109, *111*
- aneurysm 111, *113*
-- classification 113
-- iatrogenic 114
- sling 110, *111*
pulmonary embolism 113, *114–115*
- septic emboli 140, *141*
pulmonary hypertension 116, *117*
- classification 116
pulmonary infarction 170, *171*
pulmonary nodules 146
- follow-up recommendations 147
- solid 146
- subsolid 147
pulmonary sequestration 137, *138*
pulmonary trauma 164
pulmonary trunk 31
pulmonary veins 124, *125*
pulmonary vessels 109
- *See also* pulmonary arteries; pulmonary veins
- anatomy 109
- aneurysm classification 113
- anomalous pulmonary venous return 111, *112*
- arteriovenous malformations 117, *118–119*
- congenital anomalies 109, 110
- development 109
pyelonephritis 409, *414–415*
- xanthogranulomatous 412, *418–419*
pyloric stenosis 329, *331*
pyosalpinx 437

R

radiofrequency ablation 208
rectal carcinoma 349, *350*
- *See also* colorectal carcinoma
rectum diseases 344
recurrent laryngeal nerve 1, *4*
- compression 7
renal agenesis 393
renal artery *180*, 396
- accessory 394, *395*
- atherosclerotic stenosis 413, *421*
renal cell carcinoma 405
- classification 410
- clear cell 406, *408*
- papillary 406, *409*
renal cysts 394, *396–399*
- *See also* polycystic kidney disease
- Bosniak classification 395
- with solid components 399–400
renal vein 432
Rendu-Osler-Weber disease 187
- arteriovenous malformations 188
- phenotypes 188
respiratory bronchiolitis-associated interstitial lung disease *154*, 154
respiratory distress syndrome 171
- adult (ARDS) 171, *172*
- infant (IRDS) 173
-- stages 173, *174*
restrictive cardiomyopathies 45
retroperitoneal fibrosis 416, 418
retroperitoneal masses 416
rhabdomyoma 55
rhabdomyosarcoma 15, 59, 425, 460
rheumatoid arthritis 167–168
right aortic arch 77, *78*
right ventricular outflow tract 31
round ligament 431–432, *433*

S

sacrouterine ligaments 431
Salmonella aortitis 94
salpingitis 437
- tubercular 438
sarcoidosis 19, *21*, 46, *47*, 156, *157–158*, *255*, 368
- staging 20, 157
sarcomas 15
- cardiac 57
- uterine *457*, 458
-- staging 459
-- vaginal 459
scalenus syndrome *100*, 101
schwannoma 23
scimitar syndrome 111, *112*
scleroderma 167
seminomas 13, 476, *478*
septate uterus *436*, 436
serous cystadenoma 306, *307*
sex cord-stromal tumors 477
Sharp's syndrome 167
siderosis 162
sigmoid volvulus 344
silent cholelithiasis 254
silhouette sign 1, *6*
silicosis 161, *161*, *162*
SIRT (selective internal radiation therapy) 208
Sjögren's syndrome 167
small intestine 319, *320*, 323
- adenocarcinoma 342
-- classification 343
- carcinoid tumor 344
- carcinoma 342
- hemorrhage 340–341
- intussusception 337
- obstruction 324, 335, *336*
- tumor characteristics 343
smoke inhalation 164
smoking-related idiopathic interstitial pneumonia 154
solid pseudopapillary tumor 310, *311*
spermatocele 473, *473*, *474*
spleen
- abscess 358, *359*
- anatomy 352
- angiosarcoma 360
- anomalies and variants 354
-- accessory spleen *354*, 354
- cyst 357, *358*
-- calcified 358
-- hemorrhagic 359
- diseases 355
- hamartoma 360
- hemangioma 359, *360*
- imaging 352
-- computed tomography (CT) 352–353, 353
-- magnetic resonance imaging (MRI) 354
-- ultrasound 353, *353*
- lymphangioma 359
- lymphoma 356–357, 358
- metastases 360, *360*, *361*
- rupture 361, 361
splenic artery 180
- aneurysm 361, *362*
splenic infarction 356, *357*
splenic vein *180*, 293
splenomegaly 355
- differential diagnosis 355
splenosis 354
spring water cysts 17
sternocostal triangle 26
stomach 319, *322*
- anatomy 320–321
- carcinoma *334*, 334
- gastric diverticulum 329, *331*
- lymphoma 333, *334*
- ulcer 330
subclavian artery 3
- aberrant 73, *75*
subclavian steal syndrome *99*, 99
subclavian vein 101
subseptate uterus *436*, 436
superior vena cava (SVC) *2–3*, 31, 101
- congenital anomalies 103
- obstruction 7, *8*
- persistent left 102, *104*
superior vena cava syndrome 105, *107*
supra-aortic branch vessels 1, *3*
SwyerJamesMacLeod syndrome *146*, 146

T

T-cell lymphoma 20
TACE (transarterial chemoembolization) 208, *210*
- response evaluation 208, 211
Takayasu's arteritis 95, *96*
Takotsubo cardiomyopathy 46, *48*
tapeworm infection
- dog tapeworm 220, *220*, *220*, *221–222*
- fox tapeworm 220, *222–223*
tension pneumothorax 173, *174*
teratomas 446
- mediastinal 13, *13*
- ovarian 460
- testicular 476
testicular cysts 473, *475*
testicular microlithiasis 474, *475*
testicular torsion *471*, 471
testicular tumors 475
- germ cell tumors 476
- nonseminomatous tumors 476
- testicular cancer classification 477
testis
- anatomy *468*, 468
- congenital disorders 470
- imaging 468, *469–470*
- trauma 472
- undescended *470*, 470
- vascular disorders 470
thoracic artery, internal 3

thoracic duct 1
thoracic inlet syndrome 100
thoracic outlet syndrome 100, *101*
thoracic vein, internal 3
thrombi, cardiac *56*, 56
thrombosis
- cavernosal 480, *481*
- iliac veins 106
- portal vein 182, *185–186*
- vena cava 105, *108*
thymoma *5*, 10, *11*
thymus 10, *10*
- carcinoids 12
- carcinoma 10, *11*
- cysts *11*, 12
- hyperplasia 10
- neuroendocrine tumors 12
thyroid gland
- carcinoma 9
- ectopic thyroid tissue 10
- enlargement 9
- goiter 8, *9*
torsion
- fallopian tubes 441
- ovaries 441, *442*
- testicular *471*, 471
toxic gas inhalation 164
trachea 121
- displacement 8, *9*
- narrowing of 7
tracheal bronchus *127*, 127
tracheal stenosis 128
tracheobronchial system 127
tracheoesophageal fistula 326
tracheomalacia 9, *9*
tracheopathia osteochondroplastica *128*, 128
trauma
- aortic rupture *89*, 90
- diaphragm 234
- gallbladder 281, *282*
- liver 232, *233–234*, 282
-- injury scale 233
- mediastinal 27
- penis 482, *483*
- pulmonary 164
-- inhalation trauma *164*, 164
- testicular 472
tricuspid insufficiency *64*, 64
tricuspid stenosis 64
tuberculosis 141
- genital tract 438
- healed 143
- miliary 142, *143*
- postprimary *142*, 142
- primary 141, *142*
tuberculous lymphadenitis 365
tuberous sclerosis, pulmonary involvement 159
tubo-ovarian abscess 438
- tubercular 438
tubo-ovarian complex 438
tunica cysts 473, *475*

U

ulcer
- aortic, penetrating *88*, 88
- gastrointestinal 330
-- perforated 332

ulcerative colitis 346, *347*
- clinical features 347
- imaging signs 347
- versus Crohn's disease 342
undescended testis *470*, 470
unilocular cysts, pancreas 305
urachal cysts 426
- infected *429*
ureter
- bifid 393, *424*
- duplex 393, *425*
- female *431*
ureteral stones 426
ureterocele *423*
urinary tract 416
- congenital variants 418
- retroperitoneal masses 416
urolithiasis *428*
urothelial carcinoma *420*, 425, *427*
uterine cysts 439
uterine lymphoma 461
uterine polyps 441
uterine sarcoma *457*, 458
- staging 459

uterovaginal agenesis 437
uterus *431–432*
- adenomyosis *447*
- congenital anomalies *436*, 436, *437*
- positional variants 431
uterus didelphys *436*, 436

V

vagina 431, *431–432*
- cysts 439
- uterovaginal agenesis 437
vaginal carcinoma *453*, 453
- recurrence 456
- staging *454*
vaginal fistula *438*, 439
vaginal sarcoma 459
vagus nerve 1, *4*
varices, esophageal 325, *326–327*
varicocele 470
vascular tumors, malignant 96
vasculitides 165
vasculitis 95
- classification 95

vena cava, *see* inferior vena cava (IVC); superior vena cava (SVC)
- thrombosis 105, *108*
- tumor thrombi 107, *109–110*
-- causes 109
venous system *102*
- congenital anomalies 102
- development *103*
ventricles 33
- hypertrophy 29, *33*
-- *See also* hypertrophic cardiomyopathy
-- concentric *35*
- left *31, 33, 35*
-- segmentation *34*
-- thrombus *54*
- right *31, 33*
vertebral artery, variant in origin *74*
vesicoureteral reflux grading *413*, *413*
virilization 381
vitelline veins 102
voiding cystourethrography 391
volvulus 344
- sigmoid *344*

vulvar carcinoma 454, *455*
- recurrence 456
- staging *455*, 456
vulvar cysts 439
vulvovaginal lymphoma *457*, 461

W

Waldenström disease 367
Wegener's granulomatosis 165, *166*
Wilm's tumor 387
Wunderlich's syndrome 401, *403*

X

xanthogranulomatous pyelonephritis 412, *418–419*

Z

Zenker's diverticulum 324
Zollinger-Ellison syndrome *332*, 332